BSAVA Manual of Reptiles
third edition

T0178804

Editors:

Simon J. Girling
BVMS(Hons) DZooMed DipECZM(Zoo Health Management) CBiol FRSB EurProBiol FRCVS
The Royal Zoological Society of Scotland,
134 Corstorphine Road, Edinburgh EH12 6TS, UK

Paul Raiti
DVM DipABVP(Reptile & Amphibian Practice)
Beverlie Animal Hospital,
17 West Grand Street, Mount Vernon, NY 10552, USA

Published by:

British Small Animal Veterinary Association
Woodrow House, 1 Telford Way,
Waterwells Business Park, Quedgeley,
Gloucester GL2 2AB

A Company Limited by Guarantee in England
Registered Company No. 2837793
Registered as a Charity

3807PUBS18

Titles in the BSAVA Manuals series

For further information on these and all BSAVA publications, please visit our website: **www.bsava.com/shop**

Contents

Contributors

Mads F. Bertelsen
DVM DVSc DipACZM DipECZM(Zoo Health Management)
Copenhagen Zoo,
Roskildevej 38, DK-2000 Frederiksberg, Denmark

Sarah J.L. Brown
MA VetMB CertZooMed GPCert(ExAP) MRCVS
Holly House Veterinary Hospital,
468 Street Lane, Moortown, Leeds LS17 6HA, UK

Donal M. Boyer
Curator of Herpetology, Bronx Zoo,
Wildlife Conservation Society,
2300 Southern Boulevard, Bronx, NY 10460, USA

Ian Calvert†
BSc BVSc CertZooMed CBiol MIBiol MRCVS
Strathmore Veterinary Clinic,
6 London Road, Andover, Hampshire SP10 2PH, UK

John Chitty
BVetMed CertZooMed CBiol MRSB MRCVS
Anton Vets,
Unit 11 Anton Mill Road, Andover SP10 2NJ, UK

John E. Cooper
DTVM FRCPath FRSB CBiol FRCVS
Durrell Institute of Conservation and Ecology (DICE),
The University of Kent, CT2 7NZ, UK

Stephen J. Divers
BSc(Hons) BVetMed DZooMed DipECZM(Herpetology, Zoo Health Management) DipACZM FRCVS
College of Veterinary Medicine,
University of Georgia, 2200 College Station Road,
Athens GA 30602, USA

Kevin Eatwell
BVSc(Hons) DZooMed DipECZM(Herpetology, Small Mammals) MRCVS
Royal (Dick) School, Hospital for Small Animals,
Easter Bush Vet Centre, Roslin EH25 9RG, UK

Mary A. Fraser
BVMS PhD CertVD CBiol FRSB FRSPH PGCHE FHEA MAcadMEd FRCVS
Vets Now Ltd.,
Penguin House, Castle Riggs,
Dunfermline KY11 8SG, UK

Simon J. Girling
BVMS(Hons) DZooMed DipECZM(Zoo Health Management) CBiol FRSB EurProBiol FRCVS
The Royal Zoological Society of Scotland,
134 Corstorphine Road, Edinburgh EH12 6TS, UK

Darryl Heard
BSc BVMS PhD DipACZM
College of Veterinary Medicine,
University of Florida, Gainesville FL 32608, USA

Joanna Hedley
BVM&S DZooMed(Reptilian) DipECZM(Herpetology) MRCVS
Beaumont Sainsbury Animal Hospital,
Royal Veterinary College, Royal College Street,
London NW1 0TU, UK

Ben Hynes
MA VetMB CertVC(Veterinary Cardiology) MRCVS
Abbey Veterinary Centre,
St Arvans Chambers, Abergavenny NP7 5PR, UK

Jay D. Johnson
DVM
Arizona Exotic Animal Hospital,
744 North Center St, Mesa AZ 85201, USA

Sid (Zdenek) Knotek
DVM PhD DipECZM(Herpetology)
Avian and Exotic Animal Clinic,
Faculty of Veterinary Medicine,
University of Veterinary and Pharmaceutical Sciences,
Palackeho trida 1946/1, CZ 612 42 Brno,
Czech Republic

Ross A. Machin
DVM GPCert(ExAP) PgC(EAS) MRCVS
Reptiland,
Hawley Road, Hinckley LE10 0PR, UK

Rachel E. Marschang
PD DrMedVet DipECZM(Herpetology) FTA Mikrobiologie ZB Reptilien
Laboklin GmbH & Co. KG,
Steubenstrasse 4, 97688 Bad Kissingen, Germany

Adam D. Naylor
BVetMed MScWAH CertAVP(ZM) DipACZM MRCVS
The Royal Zoological Society of Scotland,
134 Corstorphine Road, Edinburgh EH12 6TS, UK

Terry Norton
DVM DipACZM
Georgia Sea Turtle Center/Jekyll Island Authority,
214 Stable Rd, Jekyll Island GA 31527, USA

Michael Pees
ProfDrMedVet DipECZM(Avian, Herpetology)
Clinic for Birds and Reptiles,
University of Leipzig An den Tierkliniken 17,
04103 Leipzig, Germany

Sarah Pellett
BA VetMB BSc CertAVP DZooMed(Reptilian) MRCVS
Animates Veterinary Clinic,
2 The Green, Thurlby PE10 0EB, UK

Aidan Raftery
MVB CertZooMed CBiol MRSB MRCVS
Avian and Exotic Animal Clinic,
221 Upper Chorlton Road,
Manchester M16 0DE, UK

Paul Raiti
DVM DipABVP(Reptile & Amphibian Practice)
Beverlie Animal Hospital,
17 West Grand Street, Mount Vernon,
NY 10552, USA

Louise J. Rayment-Dyble
BVetMed CertZooMed MRCVS
All Creatures Healthcare Ltd,
Brackenwood, Sandy Lane, Horsford,
Norwich NR10 3FB, UK

Drury R. Reavill
DVM DipABVP(Avian, Reptile & Amphibian Practice) DipACVP
Zoo/Exotic Pathology Service,
6020 Rutland Drive,
Carmichael CA 95608, USA

Matthew Rendle
RVN
Association of Zoo and Exotic Veterinary Nurses
(AZEVN), PO Box 10637,
Market Harborough LE16 0HG, UK

Estelle Rousselet
DVM PhD
College of Veterinary Medicine,
University of Florida,
Gainesville FL 32608, USA

T. Franciscus Scheelings
BVSc MVSc MANZCVSc(Med Aust Wildl) DipECZM(Herpetology)
School of Biological Sciences,
Monash University, Wellington Rd,
Clayton 3800, Australia

Nicole Stacy
DVM DrMedVet DipACVP(Clinical)
College of Veterinary Medicine,
University of Florida, Gainesville FL 32608, USA

Molly Varga
BVetMed CertZooMed DZooMed(Mammalian) MRCVS
Rutland House Veterinary Referrals,
St Helens WA9 4HU, UK

Jim Wellehan
DVM MS PhD DipACZM DipACVM(Virology, Bacteriology/Mycology)
College of Veterinary Medicine,
University of Florida, Gainesville FL 32608, USA

David Williams
MA MEd VetMD PhD DECAWBM CertVOphthal CertWEL FHEA FRCVS
Department of Veterinary Medicine,
University of Cambridge, Madingley Road,
Cambridge CB3 0ES, UK

Kevin Wright[†]
DVM DipABVP(Reptile & Amphibian Practice)
Arizona Exotic Animal Hospital,
744 North Centre St, Mesa AZ 85201, USA

Foreword

It is truly astonishing how our knowledge of reptiles has expanded since I first started treating them in the early 90s. I have since moved on to pastures new and treat reptiles infrequently nowadays and so this new manual provides a welcome and extremely detailed reference for those cases I do still see. The range of species seen has also increased enormously and each comes with its own very specific husbandry and nutritional requirements – deficiencies in which are often the underlying cause of problems. All aspects of clinical care from diagnosis to surgery, aftercare and therapeutics are covered with reference to individual species where appropriate.

There is extensive use of colour illustrations and photographs which prove invaluable in identifying pathology and demonstrating surgical techniques together with liberal use of bullet points and tables that make this a really useful manual in a practice setting where time is pressing and getting information in a concise and practical manner is paramount.

The authors and editors are to be commended on this major update to a manual that was already the 'go-to' manual for reptile vets. This new manual provides a wealth of information and practical advice which will benefit both the general practitioner seeing a small number of reptiles or a more specialist practitioner dealing with these species on a daily basis. This manual has the breadth of topics and the detail required to provide a really useful resource within any practice and is a valuable addition to the extensive range of BSAVA Manuals.

Philip Lhermette BSc(Hons) CBiol FRSB BVetMed FRCVS
BSAVA President 2018–2019

Preface

This third edition of the *BSAVA Manual of Reptiles* is another milestone in the commitment of the BSAVA to exotic species medicine and builds on the previous edition with some considerable changes and updates. Reptile medicine and surgery is now being accepted as a mainstream discipline within the veterinary world, reflected in the growing number of textbooks covering the discipline and also the appearance of postgraduate qualifications which have appeared in Europe and the USA.

This new manual retains the same structure as previously and is divided into three main parts:

Part one focuses on husbandry aspects including captive maintenance and nutrition and sees the addition of a new chapter on reptile anatomy and physiology. We have elected also to keep the chapter on breeding and neonatal care, and despite the sad loss of our colleague Dr Kevin Wright, this chapter has been updated by Dr Paul Raiti and we keep Dr Wright's name on the chapter in memoriam.

Part two contains all of the details necessary to carry out successful clinical examination, anaesthesia, surgery (including endoscopy), treatment (including emergency and critical care), non-invasive imaging, laboratory testing, clinical and post-mortem examination as well as humane euthanasia. Extensive use is made of new images in chapters covering surgery, endoscopy and diagnostic imaging in particular.

Part three addresses disease by organ system and, as before, chapters covering parasitology and infectious disease provide a different perspective which helps to unify the text and introduce emerging diseases.

Additionally, there is a new chapter on marine turtle rehabilitation as well as updates on the handling of venomous species and also a chapter dedicated to crocodilians.

As previously, the common names for reptiles have been used throughout, however, for the purists, an appendix for common and scientific names has been included. The appendix on differential diagnosis by clinical signs has been updated as has the reptile formulary. Finally, we have also kept and updated the appendices on legislation and conversion units for certain clinical pathology parameters.

This manual has been long in the making and we would like to thank all the contributors as well as the excellent editorial staff at BSAVA for their perseverance and determination to get this important text to print. We owe you all a debt of gratitude.

Simon J. Girling
Paul Raiti
November 2018

Chapter 1

Anatomy and physiology

T. Franciscus Scheelings

Biologically speaking, reptiles were an evolutionary masterstroke. The development of a reproductive modality not dependent on water and an integumentary system that was resistant to desiccation, able to withstand ultraviolet irradiation and survive the daily mechanical trauma of a terrestrial lifestyle was a pivotal moment in the history of Earth's biodiversity. These adaptations allowed reptiles (amniotes) to fill ecological niches that were previously inaccessible to the anamniotic species (fish and amphibians) and led to an explosion in diversification of life on Earth. Reptiles first emerged during the late Devonian period and by the late Triassic period were the dominant terrestrial vertebrates. For the next 160 million years reptiles ruled the air, land and sea, and many of the attributes that made them so successful persist in modern reptiles.

There are over 9000 species of extant reptiles, each of which has evolved in response to the unique environmental pressures of its native habitat. Reptiles are found on every continent except Antarctica. Therefore, the assortment of form and function seen in the Reptilia is immense, and to adequately encapsulate it in a single text is difficult. However, there are a number of anatomical and physiological features that are common throughout the taxon, and a sound understanding of these basic principles is essential for the successful management of pathological conditions in herpetofauna.

Thermoregulation

All reptiles are *poikilothermic* (sometimes referred to as *ectothermic*) animals; that is, they derive their preferred body temperature by moving between areas of hot and cold, a process known as thermoregulation (Figures 1.1 and 1.2). This behaviour allows them to maintain a fairly constant body temperature in order for normal physiological processes, such as immune surveillance and cardiovascular function, to occur. Terrestrial reptiles are considered *stenothermal* because they are able to accurately control their body temperature within a very narrow range. Arboreal or aquatic reptiles are *eurythermal* because they allow their body temperature to vary widely according to external temperatures. Some species, such as marine iguanas, also rely on social interactions to aid in thermoregulation, and it has been shown that some species of marine turtles display a certain degree of *homeothermy*.

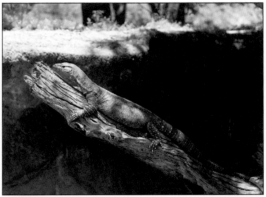

1.1 Reptiles such as this lace monitor are ectothermic animals and regulate their body temperature by moving between areas of hot and cold.

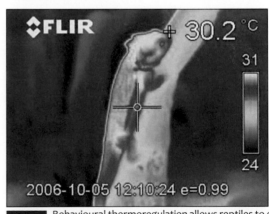

1.2 Behavioural thermoregulation allows reptiles to elevate their body temperature above ambient temperature.

Each species of reptile has its own characteristic 'Preferred Optimal Temperature Zone' (POTZ) (Figure 1.3) and it is essential that they be provided with the means to achieve this temperature when designing an enclosure. This fact also has important ramifications for the clinician as all sick reptiles should be maintained as close to their POTZ as possible to facilitate healing and optimal metabolism of drugs.

The reliance on behavioural traits for thermoregulation has both costs and benefits. Poikilothermy avoids the expense associated with maintaining a high basal metabolic rate, and animals can endure prolonged periods of food and water deprivation. However, behavioural thermoregulation also has significant costs as animals need

Species	Geographical range	Lifestyle	Habitat	POTZ	UV light required
Chelonians					
Common long-necked turtle (*Chelodina longicollis*)	Eastern Australia	Semiaquatic, diurnal	Temperate	26–28°C	Yes
Macquarie River turtle (*Emydura macquarii*)	Eastern Australia	Semiaquatic, diurnal	Temperate	26–28°C	Yes
Red-eared slider (*Trachemys scripta elegans*)	Southern and central USA	Semiaquatic, diurnal	Temperate	20–24°C	Yes
Box turtles (*Terrapene* spp.)	North America and Mexico	Terrestrial, diurnal	Temperate to semi-desert	25–32°C	Yes
Leopard tortoise (*Stigmochelys pardalis*)	Sub-Saharan Africa	Terrestrial, diurnal	Savannah to semi-desert	25–35°C	Yes
African spurred tortoise (*Centrochelys sulcata*)	Sub-Saharan Africa	Terrestrial, diurnal	Savannah to semi-desert	25–35°C	Yes
Lizards					
Knob-tailed geckos (*Nephrurus* spp.)	Central Australia	Terrestrial, nocturnal	Semi-desert to desert	29–32°C	Unknown
Leopard gecko (*Eublepharis macularius*)	India and Pakistan	Terrestrial, crepuscular	Semi-desert	25–30°C	Possibly low levels
Day geckos (*Phelsuma* spp.)	Islands of the Indian Ocean	Arboreal, diurnal	Tropical	30–32°C	Yes
Green iguana (*Iguana iguana*)	Central and South America	Arboreal, diurnal	Tropical	29–32°C	Yes
Panther chameleon (*Furcifer pardalis*)	Madagascar	Arboreal, diurnal	Tropical	27–29°C	Yes
Jackson's chameleon (*Trioceros jacksonii*)	East Africa	Arboreal, diurnal	Semi-tropical to montane	24–29°C	Yes
Bearded dragons (*Pogona* spp.)	Widespread distribution over Australia	Semi-arboreal, diurnal	Temperate to desert	25–35°C	Yes
Blue-tongue lizards and shingleback lizards (*Tiliqua* spp.)	Widespread distribution over Australia	Terrestrial, diurnal	Temperate to tropical	32–36°C	Yes
Savannah monitor (*Varanus exanthematicus*)	Sub-Saharan Africa	Terrestrial, diurnal	Semi-desert	26–38°C	Yes
Spiny-tailed monitors (*Varanus* spp.)	Central to north-western Australia	Terrestrial, diurnal	Desert to dry tropical	35–50°C	Yes
Water monitors (*Varanus* spp.)	Northern Australia	Semiaquatic, diurnal	Tropical to dry tropical	35–40°C	Yes
Lace monitor (*Varanus varius*)	Eastern Australia	Semi-arboreal, diurnal	Temperate to tropical	35–45°C	Yes
Snakes					
Garter snake (*Thamnophis sirtalis*)	North America	Terrestrial, semiaquatic, diurnal	Temperate	21–28°C	Unknown
Corn snake (*Pantherophis guttatus*)	North America	Terrestrial, diurnal	Semi-arid	25–30°C	Unknown
Boa constrictor (*Boa constrictor*)	Central and South America	Terrestrial, semi-arboreal, semiaquatic, nocturnal	Tropical	28–30°C	Unknown
Burmese python (*Python bivittatus*)	South East Asia	Terrestrial, nocturnal	Tropical	28–30°C	Unknown
Coastal carpet python (*Morelia spilota mcdowelli*)	Eastern Australia	Arboreal, nocturnal	Tropical	30–35°C	Unknown
Green tree python (*Morelia viridis*)	North-eastern Australia, Papua New Guinea	Arboreal, nocturnal	Tropical	28–32°C	Unknown

1.3 Preferred optimal temperature zone (POTZ) for some commonly kept reptile species.

to expend energy for locomotion when moving between sun and shade, and they are also at increased risk of predation while basking. Additionally, poikilotherms are more vulnerable to temperature fluctuations and they are unable to maintain high metabolic activity for as long as endotherms.

The body temperature of reptiles may be raised by the conduction of heat from the substratum, air or water, or by absorption of infrared radiation. Conversely, the core temperature of reptiles may be lowered by the loss of heat through conductance, convection or by loss of body fluids. Thermoreception is thought to be mediated by a combination of specialized peripheral nerve endings and the pineal gland. In response to environmental temperature, cardiac output may increase or decrease along with

a corresponding fluctuation in blood flow to limbs, resulting in cooling or heating of the animal. Many species of reptiles have adapted skin appendages to trap and conserve thermal energy or are able to vary the surface area available for thermoregulation by altering their posture or position relative to the sun (Figure 1.4). Some reptiles are also able to vary absorption of radiant heat by altering their colour. This is achieved via melanophores within the skin and is controlled by hormonal pathways.

Temperate species of reptiles undergo periods of brumation during winter where their body temperatures gradually decrease below their POTZ in response to lowering environmental temperatures. During this time their metabolic rate decreases dramatically and, as such, their requirements for oxygen are much lower. Brumating

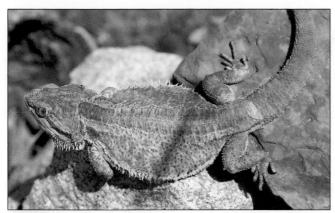

1.4 Some species of reptiles can enhance their ability to absorb thermal radiation by altering their posture or body position relative to the sun. This inland bearded dragon is increasing its surface area by flattening out.

reptiles rely on metabolism of fat stores for energy and therefore animals that are in poor body condition prior to brumation may not survive the winter. Brumation can be an important trigger for reproduction in many temperate species. Tropical species of reptiles do not generally brumate, and maintaining them at temperatures below their POTZ for prolonged periods of time may have deleterious effects on their health. Additionally, reptiles should not be subjected to temperatures greatly above their POTZ, as this may result in decreased immune function and clinical signs of heat stress similar to those seen in mammals.

Integument

In order to survive the terrestrial environment, the skin of reptiles needed to undergo dramatic alteration from that of their amphibious predecessors. It was imperative that the integument combat the loss of fluids from deeper tissues to the dehydrating environment, protect against a novel army of invading pathogens and withstand daily mechanical trauma. The advent of such a protective barrier was a pivotal moment in Earth's history.

Anatomy

The scales of reptiles represent a folding of the epidermis and, for the most part, cover the entirety of the reptile integument. The greatest folding is seen in snakes, where adjacent scales overlap and are joined by a flexible hinge region (Jacobson, 2007). They are exquisitely arranged in precise patterns with regional specificity and usually form the basis for species identification. Reptilian scales can vary greatly in size and shape and some have undergone modification to form horns, crests, spines, rattles and dewlaps.

The integument of reptiles consists of two layers: the outer epidermis and the underlying dermis. The epidermis is covered by either alpha- or beta-keratin. In chelonians and crocodilians, alpha- and beta-keratins in epidermal scales alternate horizontally, while in squamates the keratins in the outer portion of scales alternate vertically (Jackson, 2007). In most chelonians the shell is covered by beta-keratin except for soft-shelled chelonians, in which alpha-keratin covers the carapace and plastron. The epidermis is comprised of multiple distinct layers. From superficial to deep, these are (Maas, 2013):

- **Oberhautchen:** the outermost portion of the beta-layer, characterized by serrations, surface ornaments and pits
- **Beta stratum:** inelastic tough stratified epithelial layer, composed primarily of beta-keratin (the hinge area between scales is lacking this layer)
- **Mesostratum:** transitional cells between the alpha- and beta-layers
- **Alpha stratum:** soft flexible epithelial layer composed primarily of alpha-keratin
- **Lacunar stratum:** innermost layer of the outer portion of the skin, tightly adhered to newly forming Oberhautchen
- **Inner generation layer:** the newly developing Oberhautchen and alpha- and beta-layers
- **Stratum germinativum:** deepest basal layer of progenitor columnar epithelium.

The dermis is highly vascular and contains sensory tissue, chromatophores (pigment cells) and osteoderms in some species. It is the complex arrangement (both vertically and horizontally) of pigment cells within the dermis that gives each reptile its unique coloration. Four basic chromatophores have been identified in reptiles and include: melanophores containing melanin; erythrophores and xanthophores containing pteridines and carotenoids; and iridophores containing reflecting platelets of guanine, adenine, hypoxanthine and uric acid (Jackson, 2007).

Osteoderms are mineralized bones entrenched within the dermis and are characteristic of the skin of crocodilians, chelonians and some squamates (Figure 1.5). Osteoderm development is asynchronous; they first form along the cervical vertebrae where they then extend down towards the tail and outwards to the lateral extremities of the body. Undoubtedly, the most extreme example of osteoderm development is the chelonian shell. In essence, the shell is composed of a series of osseous elements united into dorsal (carapace) and ventral (plastron) components. The plastron is fused to portions of the pectoral girdle, including the coracoid and epicoracoid bones, and the carapace encompasses the ribs and vertebrae (Figure 1.6). The shell is covered by thick epidermal scales known

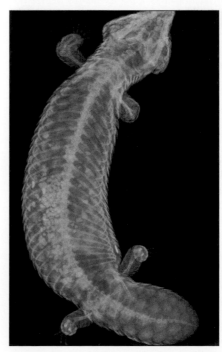

1.5 Osteoderms are a prominent feature of reptilian skin. Note the presence of large calcified scales in this radiograph of a shingleback lizard.

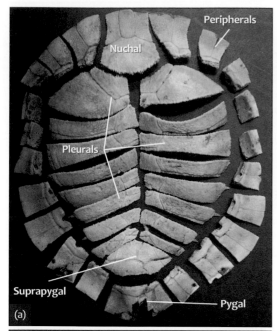

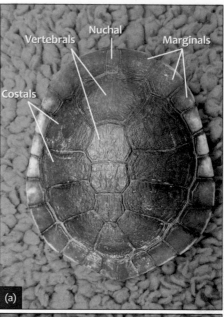

1.7 (a) Dorsal and (b) ventral views of the scutes of the chelonian shell.

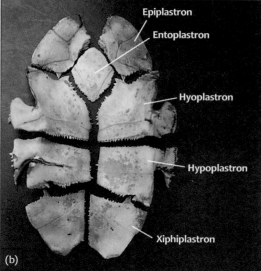

1.6 (a) Dorsal and (b) ventral views of the osteoderms of the shell of a semiaquatic chelonian; the common long-necked turtle.

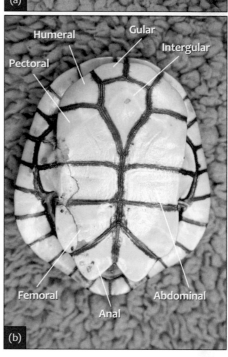

as scutes. Scutes do not precisely overlap the bones of the shell and they show regional differentiation (Figure 1.7).

The skin of reptiles contains relatively few glands. In many lizards, the males develop prominent femoral pores associated with sexual maturity (Figure 1.8). These glands are located along the ventral surface of the hindlimbs (or just caudal to the vent in some species, such as leopard geckos) and their function is to secrete pheromones and a thick waxy substance that aids in adhering the male to the female. Snakes possess paired anal scent glands in the base of the cloaca that may be used as a deterrent against predators and for marking territory. Other secretory glands in reptiles that are used for defence against predation include the Rathke's gland of chelonians, located between the dorsal corners of the bridge/carapace junction, caudal to the foreleg, and cranial to the hindleg (Figure 1.9). In some species, this gland emits a foul-smelling liquid when the animal has been disturbed.

Labial pits (Figure 1.10) are utilized by boas, pythons and vipers to sense infrared radiation to aid the apprehension of prey. In pythons and boas they are located along the edges of the labial scales and cover almost the entire

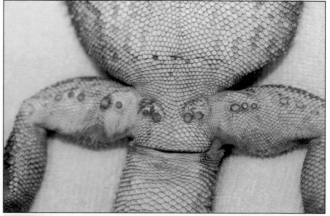

1.8 Femoral pores are prominent in some male lizards when they reach sexual maturity as is the case with this inland bearded dragon.

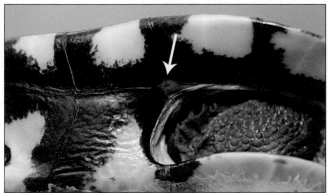

1.9 In this common long-necked turtle, the Rathke's gland is arrowed and is used by some chelonians as a deterrent against predation.

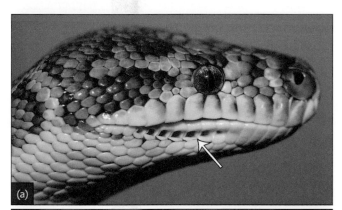

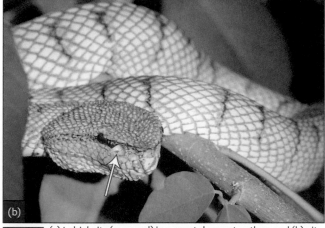

1.10 (a) Labial pits (arrowed) in a coastal carpet python and (b) pit organ (arrowed) in a Wagler's pit viper.

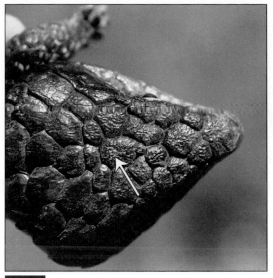

1.11 Shingleback lizard parietal eye (arrowed).

upper or lower lip. In vipers they are found bilaterally, midway between the nostril and the eye and are focused in a forward direction.

The parietal eye (Figure 1.11) is a structure unique to lizards and is most well developed in the tuatara. It is located on the dorsal head, and consists of a rudimentary lens and retina. Its function is to relay environmental cues to the pineal gland, thus stimulating hormone production and influencing thermoregulation.

Physiology

In most reptiles, colour is influenced by sex, social status and environment. Although most animals exhibit a changeless or slowly changeable colour pattern (morphological colour change), some species of reptiles possess the ability to rapidly change colour in response to environmental stimuli such as background colour, light intensity or

changing social context. This colour alteration is known as physiological colour change and is achieved by repositioning of the pigment granules within the cytoplasm of chromatophores by microscopic intracellular microorganelles. This process is affected by the nervous and endocrine systems and, depending on the species, reptiles may use one or a combination of both systems. Physiological colour change is especially important in species such as the chameleon, where physical appearance of individuals is a major component of communication (Figure 1.12).

Morphological colour change, such as the ontogenetic colour adjustment that occurs in the green tree python, usually reflects a shift in lifestage requirements and an adaptation to a new ecological niche. It results from altered pigment cell number and/or amount of pigment within cells. The dramatic change in colour from juvenile to adult green tree python occurs primarily as the diet of young animals alters from small ground-dwelling heliothermic reptiles and invertebrates found on the forest fringes to the adult diet of mammals and birds located within dense rainforest (Wilson *et al.*, 2007). The colour of

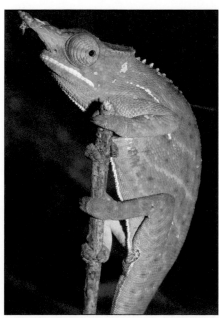

1.12 Chameleons are able to change colour rapidly and spectacularly. The primary function of their colour change is communication.

adult and juvenile green tree pythons appears to help them avoid avian predators in the habitats that the snakes prefer (Wilson *et al.*, 2007). It is suspected that similar selective pressures have resulted in the ontogenetic colour change of emerald tree boas, and this is an astonishing example of convergent evolution.

The integument of many desert-dwelling reptiles has also evolved the ability to harvest free-standing water or rain. The skin of these animals has developed hygroscopic properties that allow direct uptake of water from dew, wet foliage, standing water and damp sand. This process is achieved by the presence of minute interscalar capillary channels about 5–50 μm wide that support a pressure head of about 10 cm of water. As water is drawn into these conduits it is directed towards the labial scales where it is mixed with saliva and imbibed.

Perhaps the most spectacular and identifiable physiological property of reptilian skin is ecdysis (Figure 1.13). All reptiles periodically renew the outer layer of skin in a process colloquially known as 'shedding'. There is some variation between species:

- **Lizards:** shed in large patches over a period of days (discontinuous)
- **Snakes:** shed entire skin at once, usually as a complete skin (discontinuous)
- **Chelonians:** scutes shed intermittently over weeks (continuous).

The process of ecdysis can be divided into resting phases (consisting of three subdivisions) and five stages of renewal. In summary:

- **Resting stage:** outer epidermis is complete, no cellular differentiation or proliferation
- **Renewal stage:** stratum germinativum undergoes hypertrophy and cellular migration. Cells begin to differentiate and mature into new alpha-, beta- and Oberhautchen layers. Animals may appear to have a blue tinge and in snakes and geckos the spectacle may become cloudy
- **Cleavage:** lymphatic fluids enzymatically cleave the outer skin from the new skin underneath. The newly formed outer layers then undergo a brief period of drying and maturation as the keratin stiffens.

Ecdysis appears to be under the influence of the pituitary–thyroid axis. Factors that influence the rate of shedding in reptiles include:

- Age: young growing animals shed more frequently
- Frequency and volume of food consumed
- Temperature

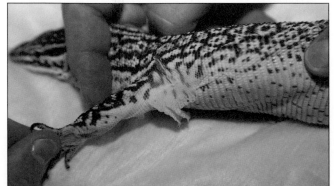

1.13 Some lizards, such as this spiny-tailed monitor, shed in patches and the entire skin is shed over a period of weeks.

- Humidity
- Season, e.g. photoperiod
- Ectoparasitism
- General health.

Skeletal system

The adaptations of the reptilian skeletal system reflect the need for ambulation in a dry environment and for feeding on a more diverse range of food items. The head is usually carried off the ground, on a well developed neck. Aquatic reptiles also show further specialization for swimming and feeding in water. The reptilian skull is made up of a series of dermal bones with a varying number of fossae in the temporal region, which provide space for the temporal muscles. The number and position of the temporal openings are an important means by which reptiles (and in fact many vertebrates) are classified:

- **Chelonians:** no temporal fossa – anapsida (Figure 1.14)
- **Lizards and snakes:** two temporal fossae – diapsida (Figure 1.15).

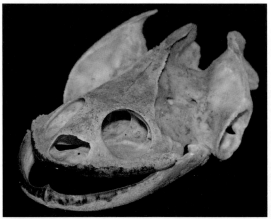

1.14 The skulls of chelonians are classified as anapsid (no temporal fossa).

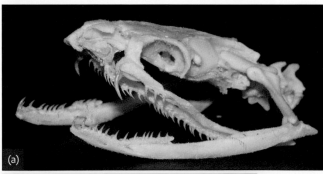

(a)

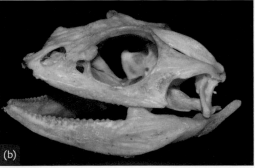

(b)

1.15 The skulls of squamates such as (a) the eastern tiger snake and (b) the inland bearded dragon are diapsid (two temporal fossae).

Chelonians lack teeth but instead have a specialized keratin mouth part known as a rhamphotheca, which covers both the maxilla and mandible. Almost all other reptiles possess teeth in one form or another. The teeth of lizards are generally pleurodont (attached to the sides of the mandible without sockets), but in Agamidae, Chamaeleonidae and Sphenodontidae they are acrodont (attached to the biting edges of the jaws without sockets) (Figure 1.15). Pleurodont teeth (Figure 1.16) are regularly shed and replaced throughout life. Acrodont teeth are not replaced except in young specimens.

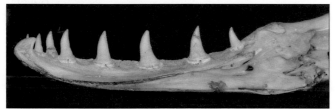

1.16 Varanids have pleurodont dentition. The teeth are attached to the medial aspect of the jaw.

The dental arrangement of snakes is more complex and varies between species. In general, snake teeth are described as being ankylosed to the rim of a low socket in a type of modified thecodont dentition. Viperid snakes have a moveable maxilla and tubular front fangs; elapids have a fixed tubular front fang; the Atractaspididae have a tubular moveable front fang; and the fourth group, the Colubridae, have enlarged posterior fangs that may be grooved or ungrooved but are never tubular (Jackson, 2003).

All colubroid snakes possess teeth on the maxillary, palatine, pterygoid and dentary bones and in all venomous species the fang is a modified maxillary tooth (Jackson, 2003). The teeth of all snakes are routinely shed and replaced throughout life. In elapids, viperids and atractaspidids the fang is positioned at the rostral end of the maxilla, and in viperids and atractaspidids the maxilla is reduced and there are no teeth other than the fangs (Jackson, 2003). In order to accommodate the elongated fangs of viperids and atractaspidids, the maxilla can rotate so that the fangs point caudally when the mouth is closed and are erect when the mouth is opened (Jackson, 2003).

The spinal column of reptiles shows regional differentiation. The divisions of the spine are cervical, trunk, sacral and caudal vertebrae. The first two cervical vertebrae are modified to form the atlas and axis and all vertebrae articulate with each other by a system of interlocking processes. There are no intervertebral discs between the spaces of successive vertebrae in reptiles. Ribs are attached to every trunk vertebra in all species of reptiles (Figure 1.17). Fracture planes have evolved in the caudal vertebrae of some lizards, allowing them to lose a portion of the tail. This process, known as autotomy, is a defensive measure used to avoid predation. Not all species can regenerate the tail once it has been lost but in those that can the tail is usually morphologically different to the original tail and bone is replaced with cartilage.

The limbs of reptiles show marked variation depending on individual ecology. Terrestrial reptiles may have adaptations for digging, arboreal reptiles may have elongated toes equipped with sharp claws, and aquatic chelonians often have webbed feet or flippers to aid in swimming (Figure 1.18). In some species, such as legless lizards and snakes, limbs have been lost altogether. In members of the Boidae and Pythonidae, a vestigial pelvic girdle exists in the form of femoral spurs, which are used by the male to stimulate the female during copulation (Figure 1.19).

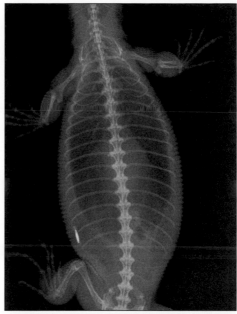

1.17 Ribs are attached to every trunk vertebra in all species of reptiles.

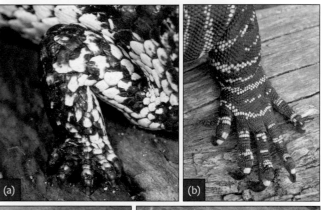

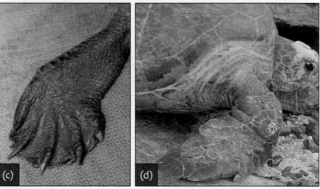

1.18 The limbs of reptiles show variation depending on ecology: (a) terrestrial – shingleback lizard; (b) arboreal – lace monitor; (c) semiaquatic – Macquarie river turtle; (d) marine – green sea turtle.

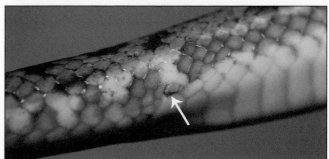

1.19 In members of the Boidae and Pythonidae, a vestigial pelvic girdle exists in the form of femoral spurs. Cranial is to the right of the picture.

Cardiovascular system

Owing to its relatively simple gross morphological appearance, the reptilian heart is often erroneously referred to as a primitive precursor to the modern avian or mammalian heart. The historical view that evolution forms a linear progression from a simple to a complex body design is outdated and does not take into consideration the intricate branching nature of an organism's natural history.

Anatomy

The cardiovascular anatomy of reptiles varies with taxon, and even between species. Morphological and physiological adaptations of reptilian hearts reflect the varied demands of individual life traits. Generally speaking, though, there are two major designs. The first is found in squamates and chelonians, and the second is found in crocodilians. This chapter will not detail the anatomy or physiology of crocodilian hearts (see Chapter 26).

The location of the heart varies between species but it typically sits roughly along the axial midline (Wyneken, 2009).

- **Chelonians:** the heart lies deep to the margins of the humeral and pectoral scutes. It is usually caudal to the acromium processes and cranial to the distal procoracoid process–procoracoid cartilage junction (Figure 1.20).
- **Lizards:** the heart may be located within the gular region (some geckos) or more commonly within the pectoral girdle (Figure 1.21). In varanids, Gila monsters and tegus the heart lies more caudally within the coelom (Figure 1.22).
- **Snakes:** in most species the heart is found at 22–33% of the snout–vent length (Figures 1.23 and 1.24). In aquatic species the heart may be more caudal at 25–45% snout–vent length. For organ location for surgery in snakes, the reader is strongly advised to refer to the excellent descriptions in McCracken (1999).

The non-crocodilian heart has four distinct chambers (Figures 1.25 to 1.27):

- A dorsal sinus venosus
- Two cranially situated atria
- A single caudal ventricle, which is further divided into three subchambers.

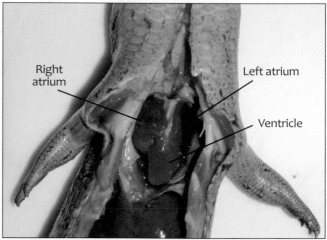

1.21 As shown in this eastern blue-tongue lizard, the heart of lizards is commonly located within the pectoral girdle.

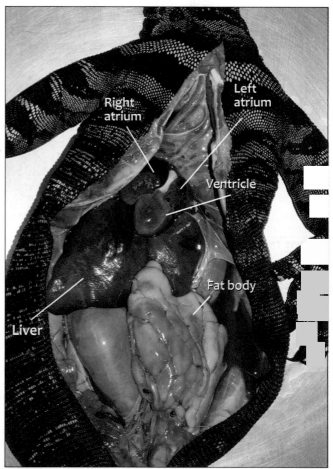

1.22 In some lizards, such as varanids, the heart lies caudally within the coelom as demonstrated in this lace monitor.

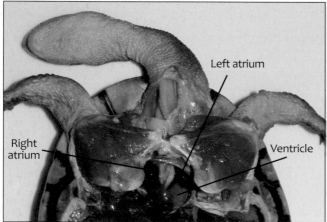

1.20 The chelonian heart, as shown in this common long-necked turtle, lies deep to the margins of the humeral and pectoral scutes.

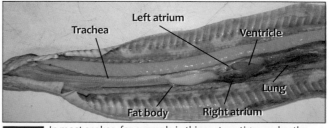

1.23 In most snakes, for example in this eastern tiger snake, the heart is found at 22–33% of the snout–vent length.

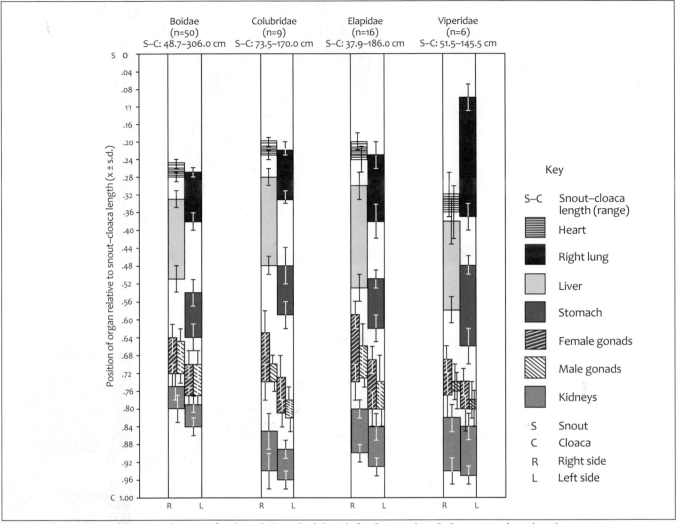

1.24 The positions of the internal organs of snakes relative to body length; family mean data. S–C = snout to cloaca length.
(Courtesy of Helen McCracken)

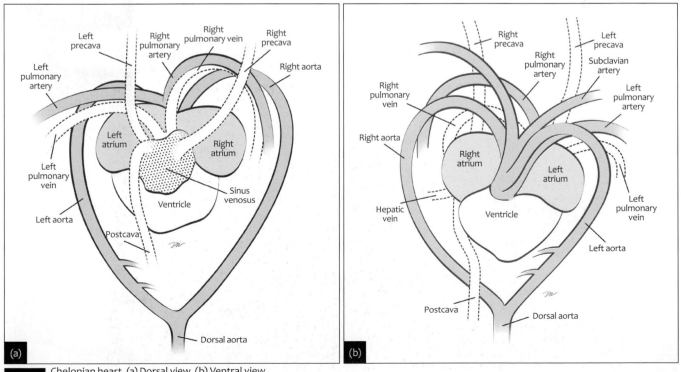

1.25 Chelonian heart. (a) Dorsal view. (b) Ventral view.
(Courtesy of Jeanette Wyneken and reproduced from Mader (2006) with permission from Elsevier)

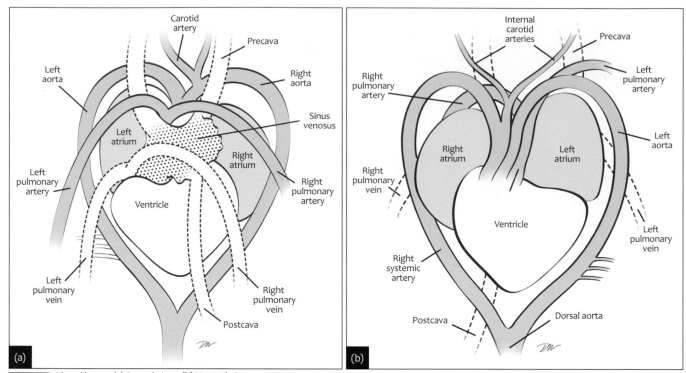

1.26 Lizard heart. (a) Dorsal view. (b) Ventral view.
(Courtesy of Jeanette Wyneken and reproduced from Mader (2006) with permission from Elsevier)

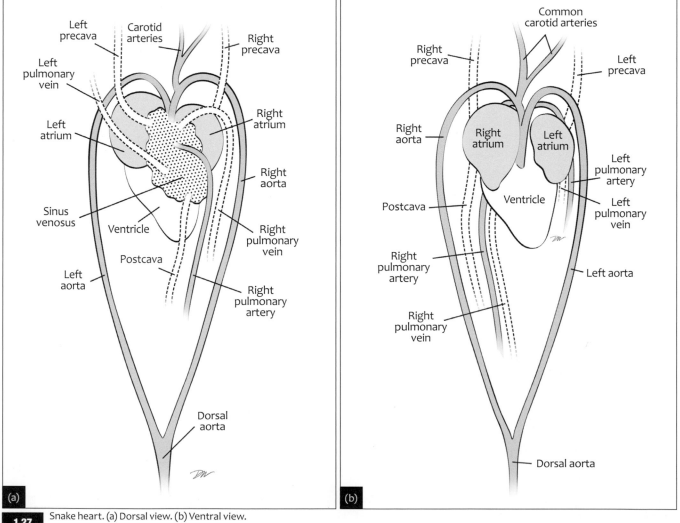

1.27 Snake heart. (a) Dorsal view. (b) Ventral view.
(Courtesy of Jeanette Wyneken and reproduced from Mader (2006) with permission from Elsevier)

Sinus venosus

The sinus venosus is the first chamber to receive systemic blood in all reptiles. It is a thin sac-like structure that is located dorsal to the atria. In chelonians and tuataras it is undivided and in squamates it is partially divided by an incomplete septum. The sinus venosus is supplied by venous blood from the left precava, the right precava, the left hepatic vein and the postcava. It empties into the right atrium via a sino-atrial aperture.

Atria

The atria are separate from each other and the left atrium is typically smaller.

- The left atrium receives oxygenated blood from the pulmonary vein, which in some species is guarded from backflow by a valve.
- The right atrium receives deoxygenated blood from the sinus venosus and in some species is much larger than the left atrium (e.g. snakes).

The atria communicate with the single ventricle by atrioventricular funnels.

Ventricle

The single non-crocodilian ventricle is internally divided by a muscular septum into three subchambers:

- Cavum arteriosum is located dorsally and receives blood from the left atrium
- Cavum venosum is also located dorsally and receives blood from the right atrium
- Cavum pulmonale is the most ventral subchamber and receives blood from the cavum venosum.

The ventricular septum that separates the subchambers is poorly developed in chelonians but is well developed in varanids and pythons, leading to functional separation of the pulmonary and systemic circulation. The ventricle is separated from the atria by sino-atrial valves that are either bell-shaped or bicuspid.

Great vessels

The great vessels are the major conduits of blood from the ventricle. These include the left aorta, the right aorta and the pulmonary trunk (see Figures 1.25 to 1.27). They have thick muscular walls and in aged animals their cartilaginous bases may become calcified. The pulmonary trunk emerges from the cavum pulmonale to supply blood to the lungs. In species with two lungs the pulmonary trunk is branched. The aortas emerge from the cavum venosum to supply blood to the rest of the body.

The left aorta initially arches to the left and then traverses caudally. It supplies blood to the abdominal viscera. The right aorta arches right before it also heads in a caudal direction. It supplies blood to the head, stomach, pancreas, spleen and intestines. Blood flow from the ventricle to the aortas is controlled by a semilunar valve. Both aortas unite caudal to the heart to form the dorsal aorta.

Renal portal system

The renal portal system is found in all species of reptiles. Its significance, along with its function, is discussed in detail later in this chapter.

Haemopoiesis

The blood of reptiles consists of both cellular and acellular components. Reptilian haematology and biochemistry are heavily influenced by a number of factors including age, sex, reproductive status, nutrition, season and environmental conditions. Therefore, it requires careful assessment of these factors when interpreting results. Haemopoiesis in reptiles occurs in bone marrow, liver and spleen.

Haemopoietic marrow is found in a range of bones including the dermal bones of chelonian shells, the long bones of lizards, and the vertebral bodies and ribs of snakes. The bone marrow is the primary site for erythropoiesis, granulopoiesis and thrombopoiesis (Campbell and Ellis, 2007).

The spleen functions as an organ of leucopoiesis in reptiles. In early life it is primarily involved in granulopoiesis but during later development it becomes predominately involved with lymphopoiesis (Campbell and Ellis, 2007). The spleen of reptiles is relatively small. It may be a separate organ or combined with the pancreas as a spleno-pancreas (snakes).

The thymus, located within the cervical region in close proximity to the carotid arteries, is predominately involved in lymphocyte maturation. Lymphoid precursors from the yolk sac or bone marrow infiltrate the thymus during embryonic development where they undergo further differentiation into T lymphocytes. T cells that originate in the thymus then spread to the spleen, liver and other tissues containing lymphoid aggregates (Campbell and Ellis, 2007). The origin of B lymphocytes in reptiles is unknown.

Physiology

The heart rate of reptiles is much slower than in endotherms of a comparable size. This is in part due to the low metabolic rate of poikilothermic animals. The heart rate of reptiles is further influenced by a number of other factors, including environmental temperature, blood oxygen saturation, respiratory rate, stress, sensory stimulation and feeding. Cardiac function of reptiles is maximal when they are maintained within their POTZ.

The vagus nerve innervates the reptile heart. Vagal parasympathetic (cholinergic) nerve fibres provide inhibitory control, and the sympathetic nervous system exerts mild adrenergic excitatory control.

Due to the three-chambered arrangement of the non-crocodilian heart, the flow of blood through this structure is complex. Under conditions of normal respiration a series of muscular contractions and pressure differentials act to create a functionally dual circulatory system. This is summarized in Figure 1.28.

Atrial diastole

- Blood drains from the sinus venosus into the right atrium via the sino-atrial aperture.
- The left atrium receives blood from the pulmonary vein, which is guarded from backflow with a flap or valve.

Atrial systole

- Blood is pushed from both atria simultaneously into the single ventricle. The right atrium supplies deoxygenated blood to the cavum venosum, whereas oxygenated blood flows into the cavum arteriosum from the left atrium.

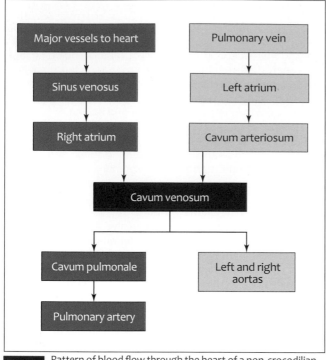

1.28 Pattern of blood flow through the heart of a non-crocodilian reptile.

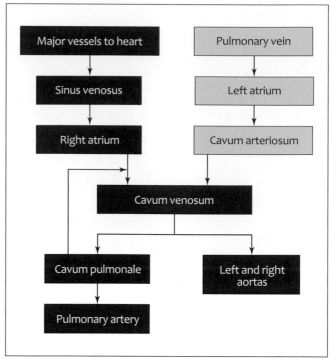

1.29 Pattern of blood flow through the heart of a non-crocodilian reptile with a right-to-left shunt.

Ventricular diastole

- Blood moves from the cavum venosum into the cavum pulmonale.

Ventricular systole

- Blood exits the cavum pulmonale into the pulmonary artery and then to the lungs. It is also pushed from the cavum arteriosum into the cavum venosum where it enters the aortic trunk, and from there it flows to the head and the rest of the body.
- Separation of blood occurs via movement of muscular ridges and minute differences in contraction times for the different regions of the ventricle.
- A small amount of blood may enter the left aorta from the cavum pulmonale during ventricular systole.

Such a blood flow system results in a left-to-right shunt due to pressure differentials. Under normal respiration approximately 60% of the cardiac output is directed towards the pulmonary circulation, and the remaining 40% enters the systemic circulation. In aquatic reptiles, diving and breath holding results in a dramatic increase in pulmonary pressure and a subsequent right-to-left shunt as blood bypasses the pulmonary system (Figure 1.29). Regulation of shunting in reptiles is by the autonomic nervous system. During periods of anoxia, reptiles are able to rely on anaerobic glycolysis to fuel metabolism. They are able to do this far more efficiently than endothermic animals and some species of reptiles may tolerate low oxygen levels for up to 30 hours.

The cardiovascular system is a critical component of thermoregulation in reptiles. When animals bask the temperature of the skin rapidly increases resulting in vasodilation and pooling of peripheral blood. The resulting decrease in systemic pressure supports a right-to-left cardiac shunt, which allows continued perfusion of the brain and other vital organs via the right aortic arch. As the warm cutaneous blood returns to the central circulation the core body temperature of the reptile is increased. Conversely, when reptiles are cold, peripheral vasoconstriction and central vasodilation result in core venous pooling of blood and decreased cutaneous heat loss.

Respiratory system

The respiratory system of reptiles is anatomically and functionally distinct from all other vertebrates. Significant differences also occur between orders, and even between species of the same order. In general, reptiles lack a bronchial tree leading to terminal alveolar sacs. Air exchange surfaces are formed by small crypts in the lung parenchyma known as ediculae and faveolae (Figure 1.30). Additionally, all non-crocodilian reptiles lack a true diaphragm.

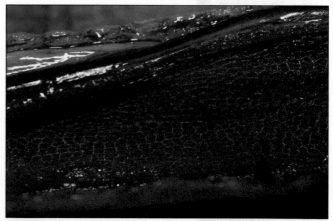

1.30 The air exchange surfaces of reptiles are known as ediculae and faveolae and they have a honeycomb-like appearance as seen in this Stimson's python.

Anatomy

Chelonians

In chelonians, paired nares open into a keratinized vestibule separated by a septum into left and right sides, and lined with olfactory epithelium. The vestibule then gives rise to a single dorsal passage that opens into the pharynx. The glottis is caudal to the fleshy tongue (Figure 1.31a) and the trachea is short with complete cartilaginous rings. It bifurcates in the cervical region (Figure 1.32) and the paired bronchi then enter the lungs in the dorsocranial coelomic cavity.

The lungs of chelonians are paired sac-like organs located in the dorsal coelomic space (Figure 1.33). The lungs are of equal size and extend to the cranial poles of the kidneys (Figure 1.34). Depending on species, the lungs may be subdivided into 3 to 11 subchambers. Although chelonians do not possess a true diaphragm, the cranial coelomic cavity is separated from the caudal coelomic cavity by a non-muscular pseudodiaphragm known as the septum horizontale. This separation is not seen in marine turtles.

While the added protection the shell provides chelonians is self-evident, its development did not come without considerable anatomical rearrangement and subsequent physiological sacrifices. Unlike that of any other tetrapod, the morphology of chelonians is unique in that both the pelvic and pectoral girdles are located within the bony shell. This is equivalent to other species having their hips and shoulder blades inside their ribcage (Landberg *et al.*, 2003). Coupled with the fixed volume of the shell space, these anatomical anomalies exert significant constraints on lung ventilation. The amalgamation of ribs and dermal bones means that chelonians cannot rely on intercostal muscles to expand the chest and draw air into the lungs under negative pressure like mammals or other reptiles. Consequently, chelonians must rely on well developed sheet-like abdominal muscles to drive ventilation (Landberg *et al.*, 2003). Therefore, both inspiration and expiration are active processes in chelonians.

Two abdominal muscles, the transverse abdominis and the oblique abdominis, appear to be the primary muscles involved in chelonian respiration (Landberg *et al.*, 2009). The oblique abdominis is a thin muscle that spans the

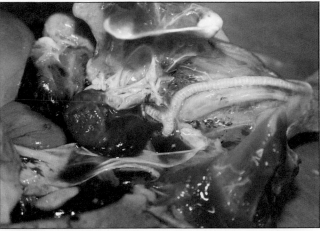

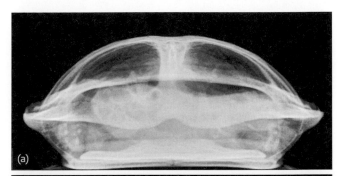

1.32 The trachea of chelonians is short and usually bifurcates in the cervical region. Cranial is to the right of the picture.

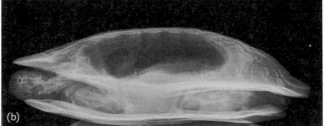

(a)

(b)

1.33 The lungs of chelonians are located in the dorsal coelomic space as indicated by these (a) craniocaudal and (b) lateral whole-body radiographs. Cranial is to the left of the picture.

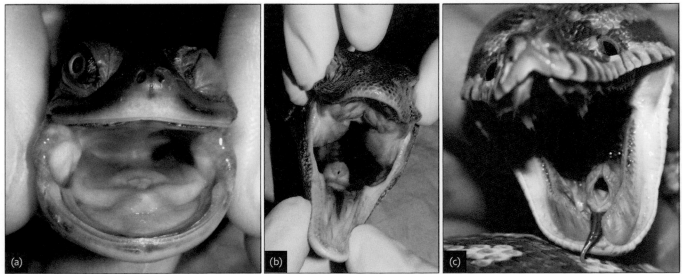

(a) (b) (c)

1.31 (a) The chelonian glottis is located at the base of the fleshy tongue. (b) The position of the lizard glottis varies depending on species and can be situated rostrally, as in this monitor, or more caudally. (c) The snake glottis is located rostrally near the base of the tongue.

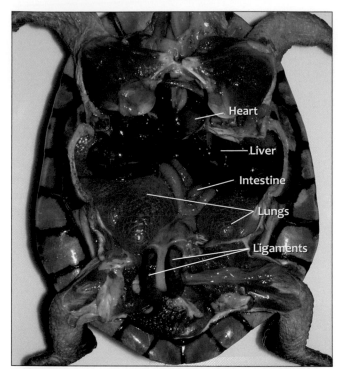

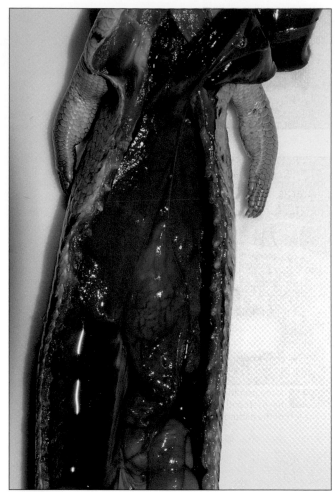

1.34 The lungs of chelonians are of equal size and extend to the cranial poles of the kidneys, as exposed in this common long-necked turtle. Note: the kidneys are obscured by the lungs.

inguinal limb pockets cranial to each hindlimb between the carapace and plastron. Contraction of this muscle expands the coelomic cavity, resulting in reduced intra-pulmonary pressure, and subsequently inhalation. The transverse abdominis originates on the inside of the cara-pace and cups the cranial half of each lung. As it contracts it raises intrapulmonary pressure resulting in exhalation (Landberg *et al.*, 2009). This reliance on abdominal muscu-lature for respiration has implications for some chelonians during locomotion. The skeletal muscles responsible for limb movement are located within the coelomic cavity and their activity results in functional changes in coelomic volume. Ventilation is not affected by ambulation in terres-trial turtles, but it has variable effects on aquatic species. In semiaquatic chelonians the mechanical consequences of locomotion are offset by smaller tidal movements during limb movement. The most extreme effects are seen in marine turtles, in which breathing ceases entirely during terrestrial locomotion (Landberg *et al.*, 2009).

Some aquatic chelonians are capable of supplemental cloacal, pharyngeal or cutaneous respiration.

Lizards

The upper respiratory tract of lizards is similar to that of chelonians. Some species possess paired salt glands that discharge into the nares. The nasal septum of lizards is continuous and so paired choanae open into the pharynx. The location of the glottis is variable and is largely influ-enced by the feeding strategy of the lizard. In carnivorous species it is rostrally placed, but in other species it is found more caudally at the base of the tongue (see Figure 1.31b). The tracheal rings are incomplete and bifurcate in the coelomic cavity near the base of the heart. An excep-tion to this is Old World chameleons, in which some species possess an accessory lung located in the ventral cervical region. The function of this structure is unknown.

The lungs of lizards are of comparable size and occupy the cranial portion of the coelomic cavity (Figure 1.35).

1.35 The lungs of lizards are of comparable size and occupy the cranial portion of the coelomic cavity. The liver has been retracted in this picture of an eastern blue-tongue lizard, to expose the lungs. Cranial is to the top of the picture.

They differ in structure depending on species. Members of the families Iguanidae, Agamidae and Chamaeleonidae have transitional lungs and members of the families Varanidae and Helodermatidae have multichambered lungs (Jacobson, 2007). The caudal segment of the lung is analogous to the avian air sac and is not involved in gas exchange. In some species, such as varanids, a mem-brane separates the heart and lungs from the rest of the coelomic cavity, but it has no respiratory function.

Similarly to chelonians, both inspiration and expiration are active processes in lizards. Respiration is achieved by contraction of intercostal muscles. Some species utilize smooth muscle within the lungs to aid in inspiration.

Snakes

The glottis of snakes is situated rostrally within the oral cavity and is highly mobile to permit respiration during food consumption (see Figure 1.31c). The trachea is C-shaped with incomplete tracheal rings and enters the lung near the base of the heart. Some species possess a 'tracheal lung' that is essentially a cranial extension of the functional lung tissue into the dorsal trachea. In some species this can be inflated for defensive purposes.

Most snakes have a single lung, with the left side being vestigial or absent altogether (Figure 1.36). The left lung is typically only found in more primitive species such as boids (Figure 1.37). The lung is elongate and gradually

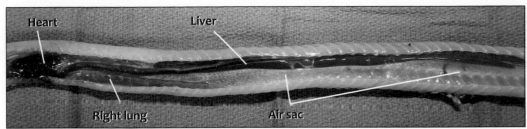

1.36 Most snakes have a single lung with the left side being vestigial or absent altogether, as seen in this lowland copperhead. The functional lung transitions into a non-respiratory air sac caudally. Cranial is to the left of the picture.

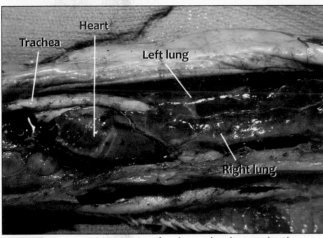

1.37 More primitive species of snakes such as boas and pythons have left and right lungs as seen in this olive python. Cranial is to the left of the picture.

transitions into a non-respiratory air sac at its caudal end (see Figure 1.36). The air sac extends to the gall bladder in terrestrial species and as far distally as the cloaca in aquatic species. In boids and colubrids the respiratory portion of the lung lies between the heart and the cranial pole of the liver, and in viperids and elapids it is situated cranial to the heart (Jacobson, 2007). In most species the lungs are single chambered, except for the families Anomalepididae, Typhlopidae and Acrochordidae, which have multichambered lungs (Jacobson, 2007).

In snakes, respiration is both an active and a passive process. Expiration is achieved by contraction of dorso-lateral (muscularis transversus dorsalis and muscularis costalis internus superior) and ventrolateral (muscularis transversus abdominus and muscularis obliquus abdominus internus) muscles (active) and relaxation of the inspiratory muscles as well as the natural recoil of the lungs (passive). Inspiration occurs by relaxation of the expiratory muscles (passive) and elevation of the ribs caused by contraction of the muscularis levator costarum and retractor costarum (active) (Wood and Lenfant, 1976).

Physiology

As mentioned earlier, reptiles are able to withstand long periods of anaerobic metabolism. Unique buffering systems within the circulatory system enable reptiles to tolerate high levels of lactic acid and hydrogen ions that would be fatal to endothermic animals. This is of clinical importance to veterinary surgeons (veterinarians) as these compensatory mechanisms mean that reptiles are able to conceal respiratory disease until it is severe and advanced.

Respiration in reptiles is controlled by hypoxia and hypercapnia as well as environmental temperature. An increase in ventilation is observed during periods of low O_2

and high CO_2. In most reptiles, hypercapnia causes an increase in tidal volume, and hypoxia causes an increase in respiratory rate (Schumacher, 2011). An exception to this phenomenon is seen in chelonians, in which hypercapnia results in an increase in respiratory rate and hypoxia results in a decrease in respiratory rate. The stimulus to breathe in reptiles is driven by low oxygen concentration in the blood. The higher demand for oxygen that accompanies an increase in body temperature, or during diving in aquatic species, is met by increasing tidal volume and not respiratory rate. A decrease in both respiratory rate and tidal volume is observed in reptiles exposed to conditions of high oxygen tension, such as supplementation with hospital oxygen (Schumacher, 2011).

Gastrointestinal system

Although the alimentary tract of reptiles is simple in comparison to other vertebrates, there is marked variation in morphology between species. This diversity is a function of the immense range of food items that are consumed by reptiles. As is the case with mammals, carnivorous reptiles tend to have a short digestive system, while herbivorous reptiles tend to have a longer intestinal tract with a large sacculated caecum. Omnivorous reptiles have a combination of both. In all species, the alimentary system terminates at the cloaca, which is a combined excretory–reproductive organ.

Anatomy
Oral cavity

Great variety exists in the shape and complexity of reptile tongues. The chelonian tongue is thick and fleshy and contains numerous taste buds and salivary glands. It has limited mobility but aids in swallowing food and water.

For most lizards the tongue is thick and mobile, and it is important for catching and manipulating food as well as swallowing. The most extreme example of this is seen in chameleons, in which the large prehensile tongue is covered in sticky saliva and shoots out from a sheath connected to the hyoid apparatus to capture prey many body lengths away (Figure 1.38).

Snakes (and varanid lizards) have a thin forked mobile tongue that plays no role in prehension of food (Figure 1.39). Snake tongues are aglandular and are heavily keratinized. The primary function of the snake tongue is chemosensory. While exploring their environment snakes will constantly flick the tongue in and out. Chemical scents are collected on the surface of the tongue and are processed by the vomeronasal (Jacobson's) organ in the roof of the mouth as the tongue is retracted into the oral cavity.

The fangs of venomous snakes are supplied by the venom gland (Figure 1.40), which when present in colubrids is known as Duvernoy's gland. Both venom and

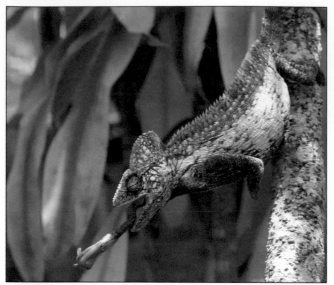

1.38 Chameleons, as demonstrated by this Oustalet's chameleon, have a large prehensile tongue that they use to capture prey many body lengths away.

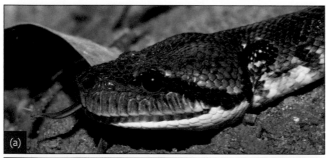

(a)

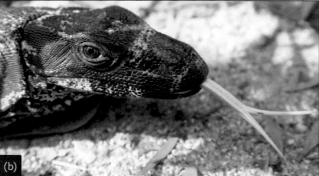

(b)

1.39 (a) Snakes (e.g. the Madagascar ground boa) and (b) varanid lizards (e.g. the lace monitor) have a thin forked mobile tongue that plays no role in prehension of food.

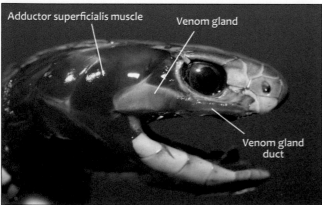

Adductor superficialis muscle — Venom gland

Venom gland duct

1.40 The fangs of venomous snakes, such as this lowland copperhead, are supplied by the venom gland.

Duvernoy's glands are innervated by the maxillary branch of the trigeminal nerve with contributions from the facial nerve. Blood supply comes from branches of the internal carotid artery (Jackson, 2003). In all species the venom gland is sheathed in fibrous connective tissue to which muscles adhere; however, the shape of the gland differs greatly among the three families. Viperids have a triangular gland with a large lumen that stores much of the venom; conversely the elapid venom gland is ovoid with a narrow lumen and much of the venom storage occurs within the cells lining the gland (Jackson, 2003). The atractaspidid venom gland is cylindrical with a central lumen and in some species it extends beyond the head. Considerable anatomical variation exists between the species that possess Duvernoy's glands but generally it is located behind the eye, is composed mostly of serous cells and empties at the base of the posterior fang via a short duct (Jackson, 2003).

In comparison to venomous snakes, the venom system of helodermatids (Gila monster and beaded lizard) is relatively simple and has evolved primarily as a defensive weapon, playing only a minor role in prey capture and immobilization (Bogert and Del Campo, 1956; Strimple *et al.*, 1997) (Figure 1.41). The venom is produced by a pair of lobular glands on the rostral portion of the lower jaw from which three to four ducts supply a specialized fold of mucous membrane (the dental sac) that lies between the lip and the lower jaw (Bogert and Del Campo, 1956; Strimple *et al.*, 1997). This dental sac acts as a venom reservoir and it is from here that venom is drawn up by capillary action to supply the row of grooved teeth that lies along the length of the mandible (Bogert and Del Campo, 1956; Strimple *et al.*, 1997). The teeth of helodermatids are regionally differentiated, are pleurodont and are regularly shed and replaced. The largest and most heavily grooved teeth, and therefore the best adapted for introducing venom into a wound, are centrally located on the lower jaw.

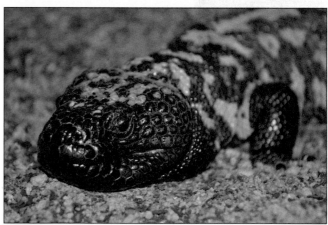

1.41 The Gila monster is a lizard that has evolved a venomous bite to aid in defence.
(Courtesy of Damian Goodall)

Oesophagus

The oesophagus primarily acts as a conduit for transfer of food from the oral cavity to the stomach. Occasionally the oesophagus may play a role in food storage and may also aid in digestion both mechanically and enzymatically. The length of the oesophagus varies significantly. It is longest in snakes and much shorter in the other orders. An exception to this is the pleurodiran (side-necked) turtles of Australia, which have a proportionally very long oesophagus.

There is variation in anatomy and function of the oesophagus between reptile groups, based on differences in diet. The oesophagus of marine turtles is lined with a series of heavily keratinized papillae that protect the turtle from potentially harmful food items. In snakes, the oesophagus is thin-walled and highly distensible to accommodate large prey items. In boid snakes, gut-associated lymphoid tissue (GALT) is arranged into oesophageal tonsils.

Stomach

In all reptiles, the oesophagus empties into the stomach, which stores and digests food. The stomach of chelonians has a greater and lesser curvature, lizards have oval stomachs and snakes posses an elongate stomach that appears as an extension of the oesophagus. The stomach is separated from the oesophagus by a sphincter and it can be divided into two sections, the corpus (fundus) and the pars pylorica. The mucosa of reptilian stomachs is arranged in longitudinal folds of varying degrees. In lizards and chelonians there is relatively little folding, whereas in snakes prominent folds allow for marked gastric expansion for digestion of whole prey (Figure 1.42).

Digestion in reptiles occurs using a combination of mechanical and enzymatic processes. Similarly to that of mammals, the mucosa of reptilian stomachs secretes a variety of enzymes, including hydrochloric acid and pepsin. Strong muscular contractions and the ingestion of gastroliths in some species also aid in the breakdown of food. The rate of digestion depends on a number of factors, including temperature and meal type and size, as well as general health. The venom of snakes may aid the digestive process in some species.

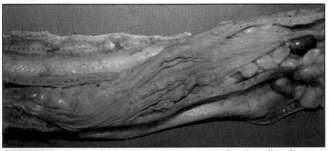

1.42 Prominent folds in the gastric mucosa of snakes allow for marked expansion of the stomach for digestion of large prey items. Cranial is to the left of the picture.

Intestine

From the stomach, ingesta is moved into the intestines, where the process of digestion continues. In the proximal small intestine, continued mixing of enzymes, chyme and bile results in further processing of food for absorption in the small intestine. The pH of the intestine is generally alkaline or slightly acidic. Depending on species, the small intestine may be long and convoluted (herbivores) or short and straight (carnivores). Carnivorous reptiles also tend to have extensive longitudinal and transverse intestinal folds to increase the surface area available and maximize absorption.

Following the small intestine is the colon. In herbivorous reptiles the colon is greater in length and volume compared to carnivorous reptiles and it may be sacculated or divided into numerous partitions or compartments. Herbivorous reptiles also possess a large caecum, which is typically rudimentary in most carnivores. The caecum is located in the right caudal coelomic cavity and acts as a site for hindgut fermentation in some reptiles. Oxyurid nematodes are also commonly encountered in the caecum and colon of reptiles, and they are thought to aid in the mechanical breakdown of intestinal contents (Figure 1.43).

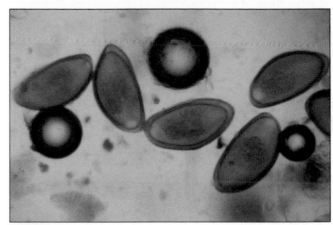

1.43 Oxyurid nematodes are common in the caecum and colon of reptiles, and they are thought to aid in the mechanical breakdown of intestinal contents.

Cloaca

The cloaca represents the terminal portion of the gastrointestinal, urinary and reproductive systems. It can be divided into three distinct compartments:

- **Urodeum:** dorsocranial and contains openings to the ureters, the oviducts/vas deferens and the bladder (when present)
- **Coprodeum:** lies between the urodeum and proctodeum and receives faeces from the distal colon
- **Proctodeum:** most caudal portion of the cloaca and receives outflow from the other two compartments, where it can be deposited into the outside world.

Liver and gall bladder

The liver of reptiles is similar in function to that of other vertebrates. In chelonians and lizards the liver is bilobed and closely attached to the stomach by the hepatoduodenal ligament. In snakes the liver is flattened and elongate, and it attaches to the dorsal surface of the lung and stretches caudally towards the air sac. The gall bladder of chelonians and lizards is nestled within the right liver lobe but in snakes it lies caudal to the liver and is associated with the pancreas and spleen (Figure 1.44).

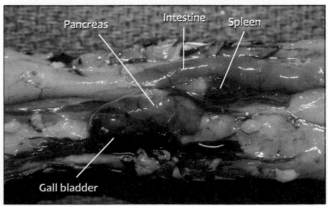

1.44 In snakes, the gall bladder lies caudal to the liver and is associated with the pancreas and spleen. Cranial is to the left of the picture.

The liver of reptiles is important for lipid, glycogen and protein metabolism. It acts as a fat and energy storage organ and is involved in the production of clotting factors and vitamin D metabolism. The appearance and function of the liver is affected by various physiological processes such as lipid mobilization during hibernation, or vitellogenesis in female reptiles.

Pancreas

In chelonians and lizards, the pancreas is located in the mesenteric border of the duodenum in close association with the spleen. In snakes, it is caudal to the pylorus. The pancreas of reptiles has both exocrine and endocrine functions and, in contrast to mammals, there is no clear demarcation between the two pancreatic segments.

The exocrine secretions of the pancreas include digestive enzymes and alkalinizing agents to neutralize the acidic pH of the intestinal contents. In general, reptiles produce amylase, lipase and protease (including chitinase in insectivorous species), but the proportion of each enzyme that is produced is dependent on the diet of the reptile.

The endocrine portion of the reptilian pancreas is poorly understood. Histologically the pancreas contains islets of Langerhans and it is presumed that these produce insulin and glucagon in a similar manner to mammals.

Physiology
Feeding strategies

Reptiles employ a range of methods to detect, apprehend and ingest food items. Like mammals, reptiles can be divided into herbivores, omnivores and carnivores. The feeding strategy of reptiles is heavily influenced by environment, presence or absence of sympatric species or competitors, and the productivity of their habitat. This complex interplay of factors means that myriad behavioural and physiological adaptations have evolved in reptiles designed entirely around acquisition of food.

Herbivorous reptiles rely on microbial fermentation to convert indigestible cellulose to volatile fatty acids. All herbivorous reptiles are hindgut fermenters and utilize an enlarged caecum or sacculated colon as the fermentation vat.

In general, carnivorous and omnivorous reptiles employ one of two strategies to hunt prey: sit-and-wait (ambush predators) or active foraging. Each methodology has costs and benefits. Active foraging is energetically expensive and therefore requires a higher caloric intake. It also increases the likelihood of exposure to other predators. Conversely, ambush hunters are harder for predators to detect and their caloric requirements are lower, but they may have to go for long periods without food, which can further impact other physiological processes such as reproduction.

Reptiles have evolved a range of sensory organs to aid in the detection of food. Visual acuity is sharp in chelonians and lizards and is the primary route by which they locate nutrients. Chemosensory detection of food is also common in chelonians and squamates, and the Jacobson's organ is an important component in this method, especially in snakes and varanids. Infrared sensory organs have evolved in a number of snake species to detect minute changes in environmental temperatures.

Once a reptile has detected a potential prey item, a number of tactics may be utilized in order to subdue the animal. Some reptiles simply crush smaller prey items with powerful jaws (Figure 1.45), while others, such as pythons and boas, quickly suffocate the animal by tightly coiling around it. Perhaps the most sophisticated method of prey

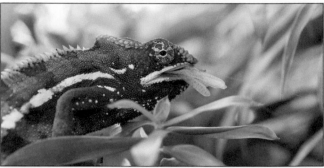

1.45 Some reptiles kill their prey by crushing it with powerful jaws, which is the technique demonstrated here by the panther chameleon.

acquisition to have evolved in reptiles was the venom-delivery system of venomous snakes (Figure 1.46). The components of snake venom are designed to disable normal physiological pathways on a number of levels. Broadly speaking they are able to influence neuromuscular function and haemodynamics, as well as cause lysis of muscle, fat and blood cells.

The most important factor that influences the function of the gastrointestinal system of reptiles is body temperature. Digestion of food items is not possible below 7°C and only occurs very slowly between 10 and 15°C. Digestion is optimal within an animal's preferred optimal temperature range (Jacobson, 2007).

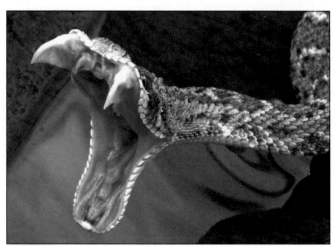

1.46 Venomous snakes, such as this western diamondback rattlesnake, incapacitate prey items by delivering venom through a bite.

Gastrointestinal microflora

The gastrointestinal microflora of reptiles is composed of aerobic and anaerobic Gram-positive and Gram-negative bacteria, yeast and protozoa. Few studies exist detailing the composition of the intestinal microcosm of reptiles and, like in mammals, it is probable that the array of microbes that resides within a reptilian host is influenced by factors such as environment and diet. Genera that have been identified as potential commensal organisms include *Escherichia*, *Proteus*, *Aeromonas*, *Pseudomonas*, *Yersinia*, *Salmonella*, *Candida* and *Cryptosporidium*. Many of these organisms have been implicated in cases of reptile-associated zoonoses and therefore care should be taken when handling any reptile.

The acquisition of intestinal microbial flora by reptiles can occur at any time during a number of early life stages. Some species of bacteria (such as *Salmonella*) are capable of transovarian passage and can infect the young while they are still *in utero*. The surface of eggs may become contaminated as they pass through the cloaca and are deposited into the soil. Coprophagia and ingestion of soil may also play an important role in gut colonization.

Urinary system

The evolution of reptiles and their terrestrial existence required modifications to the urinary system for improved conservation of water and greater control of homeostasis. Although there are species-specific differences, the basic components of the urinary system are relatively well conserved among reptile species. In general, it consists of paired kidneys and ureters, and a urinary bladder in some individuals (Figure 1.47).

Taxon	Bladder
Chelonians	Present in all
Snakes	Absent in all
Lizards	
Agamidae	Present in most, some vestigial
Anguidae	Present
Chamaeleonidae	Present
Gekkonidae	Present
Helodermatidae	Present
Iguanidae	Present in most, some vestigial
Lacertidae	Present
Pygopodidae	Absent
Scincidae	Present
Teiidae	Absent
Varanidae	Absent
Xantusiidae	Present

1.47 Presence of a urinary bladder in reptile taxa.

Anatomy
Kidneys

All reptiles have lobulated paired kidneys that are approximately equal in size. The location of the kidneys varies among the different orders and suborders.

- **Chelonians:** the kidneys are short and broad and located near the pelvic canal, adhered to the dorsocaudal carapace (Figure 1.48).
- **Lizards:** in most lizards the kidneys are located deep within the pelvic canal and in some species extend into the tail base (Figure 1.49). An exception to this is varanid lizards, in which the kidneys are found in the caudal coelom (Figure 1.50).
- **Snakes:** the kidneys are located in the caudal coelomic cavity with the right kidney situated cranially to the left kidney (Figure 1.51).

As in other vertebrates, the functional unit of the kidney is the nephron. Compared with mammalian kidneys, reptilian kidneys are sparsely populated by nephrons. Renal corpuscles consisting of a Bowman's capsule and a glomerulus are found in almost all reptiles, with the exception of a few lizard and snake species. The glomeruli of reptiles are poorly vascularized in comparison with birds and mammals. There is no loop of Henle.

The kidney of snakes and lizards shows microscopic sexual dimorphism. The males have an enlarged portion, known as the sexual segment, located within the distal tubule before the collecting tubule. During the breeding season this segment enlarges and secretes a mucoid substance that becomes incorporated into the seminal fluid. The purpose of this secretion is unknown but it has been hypothesized to aid in formation of seminal plugs in females to prevent rival males from copulating.

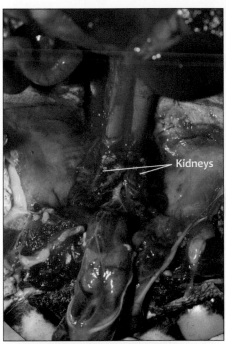

1.48 In chelonians, the kidneys are located near the pelvic canal, adhered to the dorsocaudal carapace. Cranial is to the top of the picture.

Kidneys

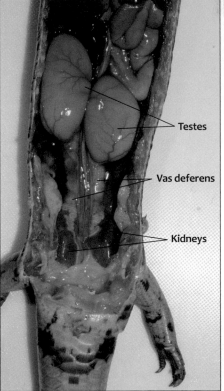

1.49 Eastern blue-tongue lizard: in most lizards the kidneys are located deep within the pelvic canal and in some species extend into the tail base. Cranial is to the top of the picture.

Testes

Vas deferens

Kidneys

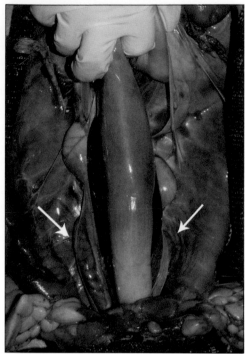

1.50 The kidneys of varanids (arrowed) are found in the caudal coelom as seen in the lace monitor.

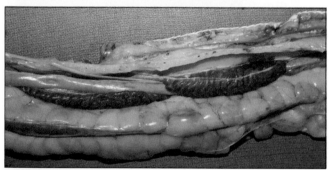

1.51 The kidneys of snakes are located in the caudal coelomic cavity with the right kidney situated cranially to the left kidney.

All reptiles have a renal portal system. Arterial blood to the kidneys is supplied by a variable number of vessels that arise directly from the aorta. In all species, venous blood from the tail and the hindlimbs can be diverted from the caudal vein into paired renal portal veins and then into the kidneys. The blood that enters the kidneys is then used to perfuse the renal tubules and does not pass through the glomeruli. From there, blood leaves the kidneys and re-enters the general circulation via the efferent renal portal veins (Holz, 2006). For a schematic representation of the renal vasculature of reptilian species, see Figures 1.52 to 1.54.

Urinary bladder

- **Chelonians:** present in all species (Figure 1.55). In terrestrial tortoises the bladder is a major site for water storage. It is supplied by the ureters, which enter the neck in a similar manner to those in mammals. It empties into the cloaca via a short urethra.
- **Lizards:** presence is variable (Figure 1.56). The bladder is never connected directly to the ureters and empties into the urodeum via the urethra.
- **Snakes:** absent in all species. The ureters empty directly into the urodeum. A small volume of urine can be stored in the distal colon or in the distal ureters.

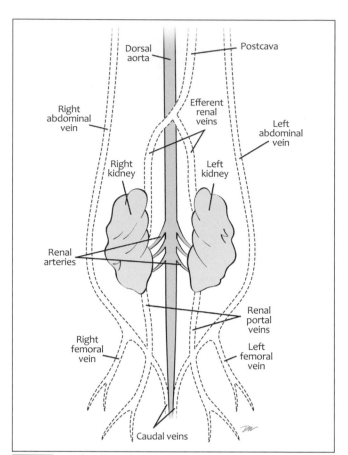

1.52 Renal and vascular anatomy of the generic chelonian.
(Courtesy of Jeanette Wyneken and reproduced from Mader (2006) with permission from Elsevier)

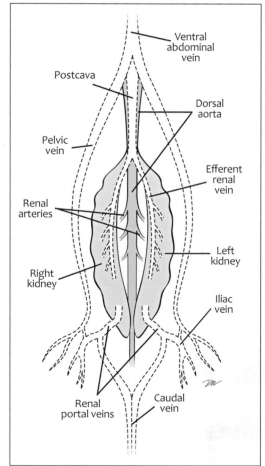

1.53 Renal and vascular anatomy of the generic lizard.
(Courtesy of Jeanette Wyneken and reproduced from Mader (2006) with permission from Elsevier)

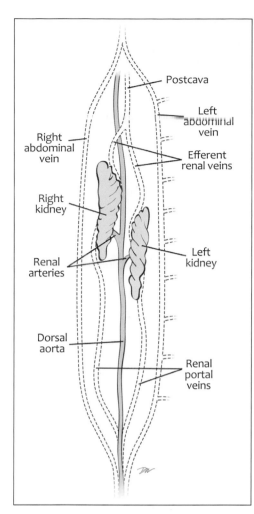

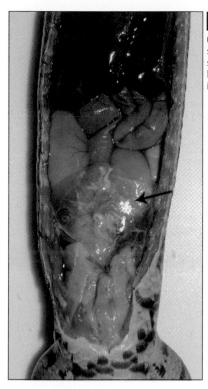

1.54 Renal and vascular anatomy of the generic snake. (Courtesy of Jeanette Wyneken and reproduced from Mader (2006) with permission from Elsevier)

1.56 A urinary bladder (arrowed) is only present in some species of lizards, such as this eastern blue-tongue lizard. Cranial is to the top of the picture.

Physiology

The byproduct of protein metabolism is nitrogenous waste. Reptiles are able to excrete nitrogen in the form of ammonia, urea or uric acid, but the proportions of these products vary with ecology. Ammonia is metabolically inexpensive but it is highly soluble and highly toxic. Therefore, its production only occurs in marine and aquatic freshwater chelonians where access to water is not restricted. In some species ammonia may comprise up to 25% of the total nitrogenous waste. Urea is less soluble than ammonia but more soluble than uric acid. It has an intermediate metabolic cost. As it must be excreted in solution, its production is also limited to semiaquatic species that have regular access to water. Uric acid is the least soluble product of nitrogen metabolism and thus its production is not limited by low water availability. However, its creation carries a high metabolic cost. It is primarily utilized by terrestrial species, including tortoises, lizards and snakes, where accessibility of water may be variable. Uric acid binds to proteins and either sodium (herbivores) or potassium (carnivores) and is passed into the urodeum. It is then retropulsed back into the rectum so that reabsorption of bound protein can occur and is excreted from the body via the cloaca (Holz, 2006).

Reptiles lack a loop of Henle and thus are unable to concentrate urine above blood osmolarity. During times of water deprivation reptiles conserve fluid by decreasing glomerular filtration. This is achieved by constriction of the afferent arterioles, mediated by arginine vasotocin released by the posterior pituitary gland. As blood flow through the glomeruli decreases, the renal tubule cells become at risk of developing ischaemic necrosis. This risk is mitigated by venous blood from the caudal body being shunted through the kidneys via a series of valves, maintaining perfusion to the tubules (renal portal system). The physiological methods by which this process is controlled in reptiles are not well understood. Some species of reptiles can further concentrate urine by use of well developed nasal salt glands. These glands enable excretion of excessive electrolytes without increasing water loss via the kidneys.

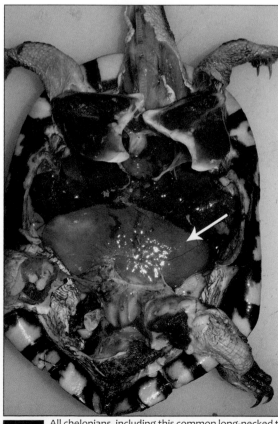

1.55 All chelonians, including this common long-necked turtle, possess a urinary bladder (arrowed).

Reproductive system

Reptiles were the first vertebrate species to evolve a reproductive system that did not rely on water. This conferred on them an enormous teleological advantage and led to their eventual global radiation and subsequent diversification. Reptilian reproduction shows further specialization from lower vertebrates in that fertilization is internal and, in all modern species except for the tuatara, specific organs for copulation, derived from the cloacal wall, have evolved in the male.

Anatomy

Male reproductive anatomy

The testes of male reptiles are paired and are located within the dorsomedial coelomic cavity. They vary in size depending on season and are largest during spermatogenesis. Semen travels from the testes into the ductus deferens, which empties into the cloaca. Variation exists in morphology of the copulatory organ but, in all species, it is not associated with the urinary system.

- **Chelonians:** have a single median phallus that originates in the cranioventral cloaca. It comprises a midline groove that lies between two longitudinal ridges that curl together during erection to form the seminal groove. Semen travels through the seminal groove (Figure 1.57).

- **Snakes and lizards:** have paired hemipenes (Figure 1.58) that are inverted caudally into the base of the tail. They are held in place by a retractor muscle and only one hemipenis is everted into the female's cloaca during copulation. Semen travels from the Wolffian ducts to the base of the hemipenis and is delivered to the female by the sulcus spermaticus on the outside of the hemipenis. In some species of lizards (varanids), the hemipenes are characterized by the presence of ossified hemibacula (Figure 1.59).

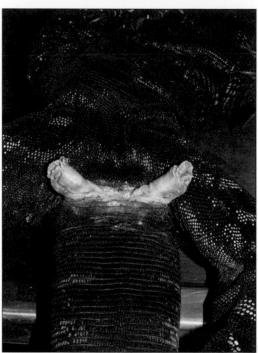

1.58 Snakes and lizards (e.g. lace monitor pictured) have paired hemipenes located within the tail base that evert for copulation.

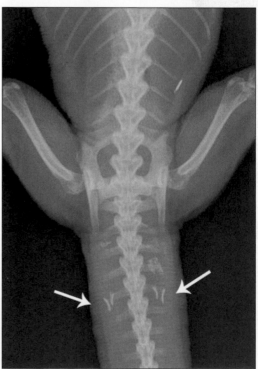

1.59 In some species of lizard, such as varanids (e.g. lace monitor pictured), the hemipenes are characterized by the presence of ossified hemibacula (arrowed).

1.57 Common long-necked turtle: the reproductive tract of the male chelonian in relationship to other organs. L = ligament; LL = left liver lobe; LU = lung; RL = right liver lobe; T = testis.

Female reproductive anatomy

The female reproductive tract consists of paired ovaries similarly located to the testes (Figure 1.60). The gross appearance of the ovaries varies with the stages of oogenesis. An inactive follicle appears as a small sphere and during maturation enlarges to form a sac-like structure filled with vitellogenic material. In snakes the ovaries occupy the caudal half of the coelomic cavity and the right ovary is cranial to the left ovary.

The paired oviducts lie immediately caudal to the ovaries and are suspended by the mesovarium (Figure 1.61). In species that lay eggs, the shell membranes are deposited in the isthmus and calcification occurs in the oviducts. Some species can store eggs in the oviducts until laying conditions are ideal, and some can also store semen in the oviducts for indefinite periods.

Physiology

Sexual maturation in reptiles is determined by size and body condition. Therefore, in wild animals, the advent of reproductive capacity is dependent entirely on environmental conditions. Similarly, in captive animals, the onset of sexual maturity is heavily influenced by husbandry circumstances. Age is an inaccurate indicator for the reproductive capabilities of any reptile. A number of reproductive modalities have evolved in reptiles, including oviparity (egg laying), viviparity (live bearing) and parthenogenesis (asexual reproduction).

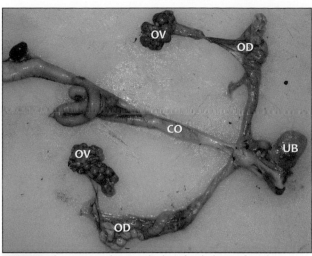

1.61 The common long-necked turtle, chelonian female reproductive system dissected from the body. CO = colon; OD = oviduct; OV = ovary; UB = urinary bladder. Cranial is to the left of picture.

Reproductive cycle

In many species, reproduction is intimately linked with season to take advantage of favourable environmental conditions and food availability. This is especially evident in temperate species, in which brumation is an important component of their life history. Tropical species are less inclined to have such demarcated reproductive periods, as their environment tends to be more stable. This phenomenon is commonly observed in a range of northern Australian reptiles, in which breeding may occur year-round. For animals that do have distinct reproductive cyclical activity, the cues to initiate follicular development and sperm production are an increase in day length, warmer ambient temperature, barometric pressure differentials and alternations in relative humidity.

Hormonal regulation of reproduction in reptiles is likely to be similar to that in mammals. Pituitary gonadotropins similar to follicle-stimulating hormone (FSH) and luteinizing hormone (LH) have been identified in chelonians, and a single FSH-like compound has been found in squamates. These pituitary hormones stimulate gonadal activity resulting in oestrogen secretion from the ovaries, and testosterone secretion from the testes. In female reptiles an increase in oestrogen levels results in hepatic conversion of stored lipid to vitellogenin. During this time the liver enlarges dramatically and may become yellow in appearance. Vitellogenin is then sequestered by the developing ovaries. A range of ovulation patterns have been described in female reptiles and include:

- **Polyautochronic:** simultaneous ovulation of many ova from both ovaries
- **Monoautochronic:** a single ovum is ovulated simultaneously from each ovary
- **Monoallochronic:** one ovum is ovulated from either ovary and alternates between ovaries for each single-egg clutch.

In some female reptiles, stimulation from males is required in order for ovulation to occur. Important stimuli include observation of ritualistic combat between rival males, detection of pheromones, or the act of copulation. If these cues are not provided then ovulation may be incomplete and serious reproductive disease can ensue. Fertilization is internal in all reptiles and occurs near the cranial end of the oviduct.

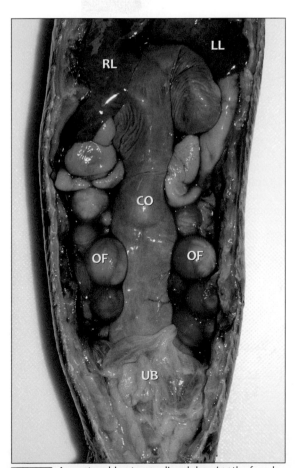

1.60 An eastern blue-tongue lizard showing the female reproductive tract which consists of paired ovaries similarly located to the testes. CO = colon; LL = left liver lobe; OF = ovarian follicle; RL = right liver lobe; UB = urinary bladder.

Oviparity: Oviparous reptiles lay eggs at varying species-specific stages of embryonic development at or beyond the blastula stage. The ovum becomes an egg when albumen and a shell are added in the oviduct. The degree of calcification of reptilian eggs varies between species, ranging from soft and rubbery (snakes, most lizards and some chelonians) to hard or papery (some chelonians, crocodilians and geckos) (Figure 1.62). Once the female is content that conditions are right, the eggs are then deposited into a nest. The incubation chamber may simply consist of a shallow hole dug into soft soil or may be more complex, such as seen in the lace monitor, in which females utilize termite mounds to incubate eggs. Incubation periods for eggs are highly variable and may be as short as a few weeks to as long as 18 to 24 months.

An advantage of oviparity is that multiple clutches may be produced in a single year, thus maximizing reproductive potential. Disadvantages to oviparity are that incubation is almost entirely dependent on environmental conditions and deposited eggs are at an increased risk of predation.

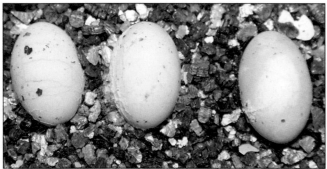

1.62 The eggs of reptiles show varying degrees of calcification. Chelonian eggs such as these are typically more rubbery.

Viviparity: More than 140 species of reptile have independently evolved to be viviparous. However, viviparity has never evolved in chelonians or crocodilians and is restricted solely to squamates (Rafferty *et al.*, 2013). In viviparous reptiles nutrients are provided to the developing young through lecithotrophy (yolk) or matrotrophy (placentation). Viviparity is advantageous in that females have greater control over embryonic development through behavioural thermoregulation. For this reason it is commonly seen in temperate reptiles. However, viviparity also has costs. The developing embryos appropriate nutrients that could otherwise be utilized by the mother. In addition, they occupy a substantial proportion of the coelomic volume and inhibit normal gastrointestinal function. As a result, only one clutch is usually possible per year and postpartum females are typically in poor body condition.

Parthenogenesis: Parthenogenesis is uncommon in reptiles but has been described in a number of lizard and snake species. Species that employ this method of reproduction can alternate between sexual and asexual reproduction. Species in which parthenogenesis has been described include the blind snake, the yellow-spotted monitor and the Komodo dragon.

Temperature-dependent sex determination: The sex ratios within a clutch of some species of reptiles (both oviparous and viviparous) may be influenced by temperature. This phenomenon has been observed in chelonians, crocodilians and lizards and the exact temperatures at which each sex is produced are dependent on the species.

Nervous system

The reptilian nervous system is relatively simple in comparison to that of mammals. It can be broadly divided into the central nervous system (CNS) and the peripheral nervous system (PNS). The CNS consists of the linearly organized brain and the spinal cord. The PNS includes all of the sensory and motor neurons outside of the CNS.

Brain

The brain of reptiles is housed in a tubular braincase. Reptiles have both subdural and epidural spaces within the braincase. The brain can be divided into various segments that can be distinguished both by gross morphology and microscopically (Figure 1.63). From cranial to caudal these are the prosencephalon (forebrain), cerebrum (telencephalon), diencephalon, mesencephalon (midbrain) and rhombencephalon (hindbrain). The pineal complex arises just caudal to the cerebrum and regulates pigmentation and biological rhythms. It is most well developed in the tuatara and poorly developed in snakes and crocodilians.

The brain and spinal cord are bathed in clear cerebrospinal fluid (CSF) that also fills the ventricles and the central canal of the spinal cord. It is produced by the tela choroidea in the midbrain and is resorbed in the distal end of the central spinal canal in the terminal ventricle.

Two meninges cover the brain and spinal cord, the pia-arachnoid and the dura mater. CSF is found between the two layers and not in the subarachnoid space. Reptiles have a poorly studied blood–brain barrier.

There are 12 cranial nerves (CN) that emerge from the brain:

- **CN I (olfactory):** olfaction (sensory), carries information from the nose and Jacobson's organ
- **CN II (optic):** vision (sensory), carries information from the retina to the thalamus
- **CN III (oculomotor):** controls movement of the eye (motor)
- **CN IV (trochlear):** controls movement of the eye (motor)
- **CN V (trigeminal):** sensory from skin around eye, labial pits and controls muscles of mastication (motor)
- **CN VI (abducens):** controls movement of the eye (motor)
- **CN VII (facial):** sensory from skin around the side of the face, controls muscles associated with maxilla and neck (motor)

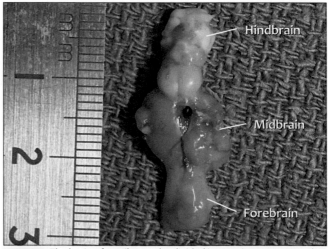

1.63 The brain of reptiles can be divided into various segments that can be distinguished both by gross morphology and microscopically.

- **CN VIII (statoacoustic):** hearing and balance (sensory)
- **CN IX (glossopharyngeal):** taste (sensory), controls muscle of the tongue (motor)
- **CN X (vagus):** sensory and motor to heart, glottis and viscera
- **CN XI (spinal accessory):** controls trapezius and sternomastoid muscles (motor)
- **CN XII (hypoglossal):** controls hyoid muscles and tongue (motor).

Spinal cord

The spinal cord of reptiles extends from the foramen magnum down the entire length of the vertebrae to the tip of the tail. There is no cauda equina. The spinal cord of reptiles possesses regional locomotor control centres that are autonomous of the brain. Histologically the spinal cord is similar in structure to that of mammals. Paired spinal nerves arise from each vertebra via intervertebral foramina. Each spinal nerve has a dorsal (sensory) and ventral (motor) root. The number of spinal nerves is dependent on the number of vertebrae, so snakes have far more spinal nerves than any other species.

The autonomic nervous system of reptiles shows homology with that of higher vertebrates. The sympathetic neurotransmitter is primarily noradrenaline (norepinephrine). Stimulation of the sympathetic nervous system results in activation of the flight-or-fight response and a subsequent increase in heart rate, metabolism and vasodilation. Parasympathetic stimulation is cholinergic and restores the body to its resting state.

Peripheral nervous system

Similarly to mammals, reptiles possess peripheral nerves that are responsible for transmitting sensory information (sight, smell, hearing, temperature, etc.) back to the brain. These sensory nerves are complemented by motor neurons, which innervate skeletal muscles and allow reptiles to act in response to environmental stimulation. The mechanism of action of these neuronal pathways is considered to be the same as in mammals; that is, by electrical signals and neurotransmitters that diffuse across synapses.

References and further reading

Alibardi L (2003) Adaptation to the land: the skin of reptiles in comparison to that of amphibians and endotherm amniotes. *Journal of Experimental Zoology* **298B**, 12–41

Bennet T (2011) The chelonian respiratory system. *Veterinary Clinics of North America: Exotic Animal Practice* **14**, 225–239

Bogert CM and Del Campo RM (1956) The Gila monster and its allies: the relationships, habits and behavior of the lizards of the family Helodermatidae. *Bulletin of the American Museum of Natural History* **109**, 1–238

Campbell TW and Ellis CK (2007) Hematology of reptiles. In: *Avian and Exotic Animal Hematology and Cytology, 3rd edn*, ed. TW Campbell and CK Ellis, pp. 51–82. Blackwell Publishing, Oxford

Cowles RB and Bogert CM (1944) A preliminary study of the thermal requirements of desert reptiles. *Bulletin of the American Museum of Natural History* **83**, 261–296

Funk RS (2002) Lizard reproductive medicine and surgery. *Veterinary Clinics of North America: Exotic Animal Practice* **5**, 579–613

Holz P (2006) Renal anatomy and physiology. In: *Reptile Medicine and Surgery, 2nd edn*, ed. DR Mader, pp. 135–144. Elsevier, St. Louis

Huey RB and Slatkin M (1976) Costs and benefits of lizard thermoregulation. *Quarterly Review of Biology* **51**, 363–384

Innis CJ and Boyer TH (2002) Chelonian reproductive disorders. *Veterinary Clinics of North America: Exotic Animal Practice* **5**, 555–578

Jackson K (2003) The evolution of venom-delivery systems in snakes. *Zoological Journal of the Linnean Society* **137**, 337–354

Jacobson ER (2007) Overview of reptile biology, anatomy and histology. In: *Infectious Diseases and Pathology of Reptiles*, ed. ER Jacobson, pp. 1–30. CRC Press, Boca Raton

Jenson B, Nielson JM, Axelsson M et al. (2010) How the python separates pulmonary and systemic blood pressures and blood flows. *Journal of Experimental Biology* **213**, 1611–1617

Landberg T, Mailhot JD and Brainerd EL (2003) Lung ventilation during treadmill locomotion in a terrestrial turtle, *Terrapene Carolina*. *Journal of Experimental Biology* **206**, 3391–3404

Landberg T, Mailhot JD and Brainerd EL (2009) Lung ventilation during treadmill locomotion in a semi-aquatic turtle, *Trachemys scripta*. *Journal of Experimental Zoology* **311A**, 551–562

Landmann L (1986) Epidermis and dermis. In: *Biology of the Integument Volume 2, Vertebrates*, ed. J Bereiter-Hahn, AG Matoltsy and S Richards, pp. 150–187. Springer-Verlag, Berlin

Maas AK (2013) Vesicular, ulcerative, and necrotic dermatitis of reptiles. *Veterinary Clinics of North America: Exotic Animal Practice* **16**, 737–755

Mader DR (ed.) (2006) *Reptile Medicine and Surgery, 2nd edn*. Saunders Elsevier, St Louis

McCracken HE (1999) Organ location in snakes for diagnostic and surgical evaluation. In: *Zoo and Wild Animal Medicine Current Therapy, 4th edn*, ed. ME Fowler and RE Miller, pp. 243–248. W.B. Saunders Company, Philadelphia

Mitchell M (2009) Reptile cardiology. *Veterinary Clinics of North America: Exotic Animal Practice* **12**, 65–79

Mitchell M and Diaz-Figueroa O (2005) Clinical reptile gastroenterology. *Veterinary Clinics of North America: Exotic Animal Practice* **8**, 277–298

Rafferty AR, Evans RG, Scheelings TF and Reina RD (2013) Limited oxygen availability *in utero* may constrain the evolution of live birth in reptiles. *American Naturalist* **181**, 245–253

Rivera S (2008) Health assessment of the reptilian reproductive tract. *Journal of Exotic Pet Medicine* **17**, 259–266

Schumacher J (2011) Respiratory medicine of reptiles. *Veterinary Clinics of North America: Exotic Animal Practice* **14**, 207–224

Seebacher F and Franklin CE (2005) Physiological mechanisms of thermoregulation in reptiles: a review. *Journal of Comparative Physiology B* **175**, 533–541

Stahl SJ (2002) Chelonian reproductive disorders. *Veterinary Clinics of North America: Exotic Animal Practice* **5**, 615–636

Strimple PD, Tomassoni AJ, Otten EJ and Bahner D (1997) Report on envenomation by a Gila monster (*Heloderma suspectum*) with a discussion of venom apparatus, clinical findings and treatment. *Wilderness and Environmental Medicine* **8**, 111–116

Vickaryous MK and Sire JY (2009) The integumentary skeleton of tetrapods: origin, evolution, and development. *Journal of Anatomy* **214**, 441–464

Wilson D, Heinsohn R and Endler JA (2007) The adaptive significance of ontogenetic colour change in a tropical python. *Biological Letters* **3**, 40–43

Wood SC and Lenfant CJ (1976) Respiration: mechanics, control and gas exchange. In: *Biology of the Reptilia, Volume 5*, ed. C Gans. Academic Press, San Diego

Wyneken J (2007) Reptilian neurology: anatomy and function. *Veterinary Clinics of North America: Exotic Animal Practice* **10**, 837–853

Wyneken J (2009) Normal reptile heart morphology and function. *Veterinary Clinics of North America: Exotic Animal Practice* **12**, 51–63

Young JZ (1989) Life on land: the reptiles. In: *The Life of Vertebrates, 3rd edn*, ed. JZ Young, pp. 276–291. Oxford University Press, Oxford

Chapter 2

Reptile pet trade and welfare

Louise Rayment-Dyble

Keeping reptiles as pets is a relatively recent idea, as historically reptiles have been surrounded by fear, myth and legend. Some people are less than enthusiastic, but with new knowledge and less fear, reptiles are becoming more mainstream as pets and in fact are now hugely popular with many people. In a modern society, where busy lives make time for pets less available, they are seen as easier to manage and are also increasingly available. For example, where a few years ago specialist reptile breeders found it difficult to obtain import permission for the first bearded dragons to be brought in from Australia, they are now bred in vast numbers and have exceeded iguanas to be the most popular lizard pet. They are even for sale in less specialist locations, such as large pet superstores, which have also expanded their range of accessories for reptiles to take up a large section of the shop floor (Figures 2.1 and 2.2).

There are many opposed to the keeping of exotic pets in general, who have concerns about their welfare and risk of zoonotic disease, but in the author's opinion they can make good and safe pets as long as the best husbandry practices are used. As veterinary surgeons (veterinarians), treating them in practice can be both interesting and rewarding and our experience can add to the rapidly expanding field of knowledge of reptile medicine, which further improves their welfare. They are not 'cuddly' pets, nor are they cheap – the general rule is that you should spend more on the vivarium and husbandry set-up than

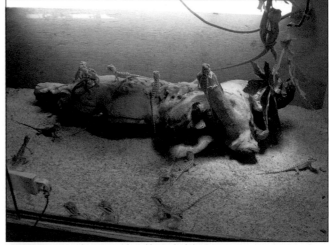

2.2 Juvenile captive-bred bearded dragons.
(With permission from the Grooms at Reptile Crazy, Norwich)

the pet itself. It is important that owners are educated and do not take on a pet reptile for the wrong reasons. It is our responsibility as veterinary surgeons to give the best and correct advice, care, education and recommendations to ensure the welfare of our reptile patients.

As clinicians we are increasingly presented with reptile clinical challenges and opportunities to learn and progress. From a business point of view it also makes sense to consider these cases seriously and carry out a professional assessment. Our first challenge, therefore, is to identify what species we have been presented with.

The class Reptilia

The class Reptilia (Figure 2.3) includes over 9000 species. There is a great variety, including huge strict carnivores like crocodiles, tiny insectivorous lizards such as the anoles, true vegetarians such as green iguanas, and even some that eat other reptiles, e.g. snake-eating kingsnakes.

Reptiles are distributed throughout almost all climates and ecosystems on the planet. They are colloquially known as 'cold-blooded', but the more correct term 'ectothermic' better describes their physiology. Reptiles use their behaviour to regulate their core body temperature and have the ability to hibernate or aestivate in extremes of cold or heat, respectively. Their anatomy is well adapted to suit their lifestyle and in this respect they are fascinatingly varied.

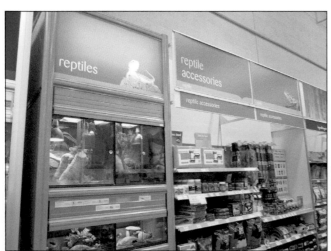

2.1 Reptile section in Pets at Home.
(With permission from Pets at Home; © Louise Rayment-Dyble)

Order	Suborder	Family	Examples
Chelonia	Pleurodira (side-necked chelonians)	Chelidae	Side-necked turtles
		Pelomedusidae	Side-necked turtles
	Cryptodira (hidden-necked chelonians)	Carettochelyidae	Fly River turtle
		Cheloniidae	Green turtle, hawksbill turtle, loggerhead turtle
		Chelydridae	Snapping turtles
		Dermatemydidae	Central American river turtles
		Dermochelyidae	Leatherback turtle
		Emydidae	Freshwater terrapins and turtles
		Kinosternidae	Mud and musk turtles
		Platysternidae	Big-headed turtle
		Testudinidae	Tortoises
		Trionychidae	Soft-shelled turtles
Squamata	Amphisbaenia	Amphisbaenidae	Worm lizard
		Bipedidae	Two-legged worm lizard
		Rhineuridae	Florida worm lizard
		Trogonophidae	Old World amphisbaenids
	Lacertilia	Agamidae	Agamas, bearded dragons, frilled lizard, water dragons
		Anguidae	Slow worms
		Chamaeleonidae	Chameleons
		Cordylidae	Plated lizards
		Dibamidae	Blind lizards
		Eublepharidae	Geckos
		Gekkonidae	Geckos
		Gymnophthalmidae	Tegus
		Helodermatidae	Gila monster
		Iguanidae	Anoles, iguanas, chuckwallas
		Lacertidae	Sand lizards, wall lizards
		Scincidae	Skinks
		Teiidae	Ameivas, tegus, whiptails
		Varanidae	Monitor lizards
		Xantusiidae	Night lizards
		Xenosauridae	Knob-scaled lizards
	Serpentes	Acrochordidae	Elephant trunk snakes
		Aniliidae	Pipe snakes
		Anomalepididae	Blind snakes
		Atractaspididae	Mole vipers
		Boidae	Common boa, pythons
		Bolyeriidae	Round Island boa
		Colubridae	Hognose snakes, kingsnakes, milk snake, ratsnakes
		Elapidae	Cobras, coral snake, sea snakes
		Leptotyphlopidae	Blind snakes
		Loxocemidae	Mexican burrowing python
		Typhlopidae	Blind worm snake
		Uropeltidae	Shield-tailed snake
		Viperidae	Rattlesnakes, vipers
		Xenopeltidae	Sunbeam snake
Crocodilia		Alligatoridae	Alligators
		Crocodylidae	Crocodiles
		Gavialidae	Gavials
Rhynchocephalia		Sphenodontidae	Tuatara

2.3 Taxonomy of reptiles.

Husbandry is therefore hugely important. Get it wrong and you can cause a lot of issues; get it right and you can equally prevent or resolve many issues. They require keeping at their Preferred Optimal Temperature Zone (POTZ), outside of which they cannot function or metabolize normally, so it is important to identify the species and the POTZ. We also need to know from what climate the species originates (Figure 2.4): is it an arboreal species (i.e. does it climb or live on the ground or in a burrow)? Does it live in a rainforest or a desert? What does it eat?

As clinicians, we cannot therefore apply one set of rules or put all reptiles into one category or we would be doing the vast majority a disservice. However, one should not be put off tackling a reptile case presented in practice. General principles of veterinary medicine and surgery can be applied; with these, along with some knowledge of commonly kept species, an ability and curiosity to find other sources of information, and a large amount of common sense, we are well prepared to deal with the growing number of reptile patients. Husbandry and welfare play a huge part in the medical treatment of these animals, perhaps more so than any other group of species we are faced with.

The first question is to establish the species and sex and it is a good idea to have your nurse or receptionist ask this of the owner. It can be useful to use more detailed questionnaires, which can be completed while owners are waiting for their consultation, to aid information gathering and save time. With this in mind, though, it does happen that owners do not know what species or sex their pet is – the pet may have been rescued or the owner may not have been given the right information from the vendor, so it is worth double-checking. (Figure 2.5 shows some common species to aid with identification; in rare cases, there are always online search engines with an image tag.) Sexing

individuals can also be a challenge and there is no shame in saying you cannot accurately sex an individual reptile – some species such as *Uromastyx* spp. and some monitors are notoriously difficult, especially when young, immature and kept alone, and some animals do not show clear sexual differentiation (see Chapter 1).

Reptiles are a long way from domestication; however, there is a large trade in colour morph forms of certain species – i.e. they have been bred to have a genetic mutation which gives their skin a particular colour or pattern. The most common species bred in this way are corn snakes and royal or ball pythons: there are over 100 colour morphs of corn snakes listed and the number of these is growing. Some herpetologists and hobbyists use colloquial abbreviations or jargon in referring to their reptiles, which can be confusing. Figure 2.6 shows some of the terms used, but is by no means exhaustive. There are a number of websites with good photographs to aid identification. Some of these rarer colours are highly prized and can change hands for considerable sums of money.

Handouts and care sheets for various commonly kept species can be found online – the author recommends Lifelearn and Lafeber among others (see References and further reading). Booklets on bearded dragons, leopard geckos, corn snakes, red-eared sliders, etc., are also available from The Herpetocultural Library.

The reptile trade

As we have established, the UK trade in pet reptiles is increasing. On the one hand the number of captive-bred reptiles has vastly increased and many species could perhaps now be supplied virtually exclusively from captive breeding; on the other hand there is still an increase in the number of reptiles being imported as 'wild-caught'. It is extremely difficult to gain comprehensive and accurate figures on the number of reptiles sold into the UK. It is even more difficult to obtain figures on the illegal trade, where smuggled reptiles are often crammed into small containers, in poor conditions, and many die in transit or shortly after. There are individuals sold as 'captive-bred' that may have been taken from the wild as hatchlings. A Royal Society for the Prevention of Cruelty to Animals (RSPCA) report showed that in 2005 1.6 million reptiles were imported under CITES (Convention on International Trade of Endangered Species of Wild Flora and Fauna) regulations, and in 2009 between 5.9 and 9.8 million individuals were imported: a five-fold increase. As only 8% of the known worldwide species are listed under CITES, the trade could be significantly greater. There is a theory that the 2005 ban on wild bird importation could have meant that trappers and hobbyists have moved over to reptiles as they are more easily traded internationally (Figure 2.7).

Captive breeding is extremely specialized, as reptiles require complex habitats to mimic their natural surroundings and stimulate the behaviours that lead to successful reproduction (Figure 2.8). There are still problems associated with just captive maintenance of some species, let alone trying to breed, incubate and rear healthy offspring. With time and progress, knowledge is rapidly expanding and many more species are being bred successfully. There are commercial farms, for example those in South America, which rear green iguanas for the pet trade in the USA and beyond. Along with this comes a growing amount of legislation to try and stop the illegal trade and reduce pressure on wild stocks.

2.4 Chameleons in mesh vivarium.
(With permission from the Grooms at Reptile Crazy, Norwich; © Louise Rayment-Dyble)

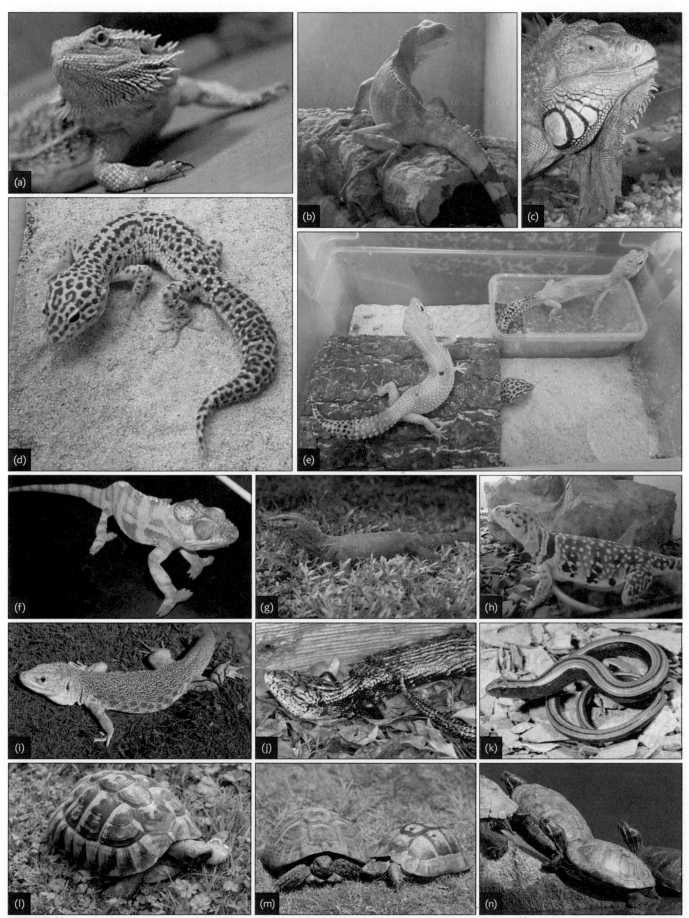

2.5 (a) Bearded dragon; (b) water dragon; (c) green iguana; (d) leopard gecko; (e) 'high yellow' leopard gecko; (f) panther chameleon; (g) Bengal monitor lizard; (h) collared lizard; (i) eyed lizard; (j) blue-tongued skink; (k) slow worm (UK non-venomous); (l) Greek spur-thighed tortoise; (m) Hermann's tortoise; (n) red-eared terrapin (UK non-venomous). (continues) ▶

(a, b, d–f, h, o, x–z, © Louise Rayment-Dyble; c, g, i–n, p–w, ai–ci, © Joe Blossom; b, d, e, h, z, with permission from the Grooms at Reptile Crazy, Norwich)

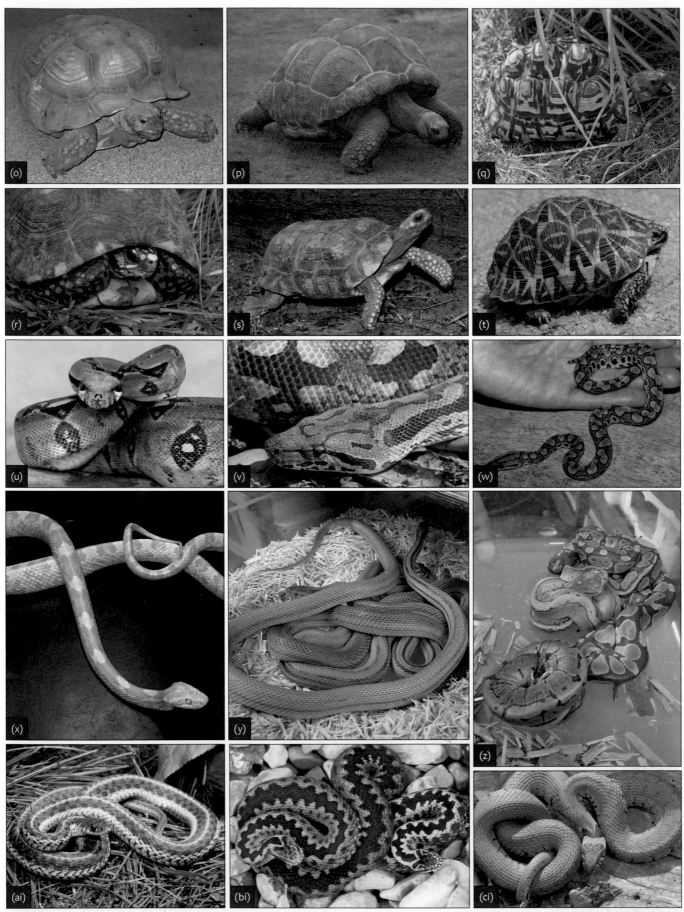

2.5 (continued) (o) sulcata tortoise; (p) Aldabra tortoise; (q) leopard tortoise; (r) red-footed tortoise; (s) yellow-footed tortoise; (t) Indian star tortoise; (u) boa constrictor; (v) Dumeril's boa; (w) rainbow boa; (x) corn snake: yellow colour morph; (y) corn snake: pinstripe colour morph; (z) royal python colour morphs; (ai) garter snake; (bi) adders (UK venomous); (ci) grass snake (UK non-venomous).
(a, b, d–f, h, o, x–z, © Louise Rayment-Dyble; c, g, i–n, p–w, ai–ci, © Joe Blossom; b, d, e, h, z, with permission from the Grooms at Reptile Crazy, Norwich)

Term	Description
BCI	Boa constrictor snake of the subspecies *imperator*
BCC	As above but subspecies *constrictor*
RI	Respiratory infection
Anery	Anerythristic – lacking red pigment; tend to look grey
Amel	Amelanistic – no black pigment
Pins	Pinstriped longitudinally
Bee stripe	Striped perpendicularly to body length
Stripe	Striped longitudinally, i.e. along body length
Axanthic	Lacking yellow pigment
Pastels	A paler or dilute version of the original or normal colour
Microscaled	Bred with a reduced number of scales

2.6 Glossary of colloquial terms used by herpetologists.

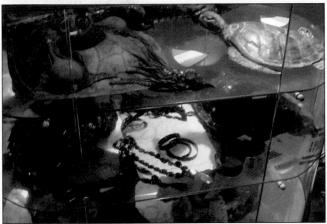

2.7 Illegally imported reptile goods seized by customs.
(© Louise Rayment-Dyble)

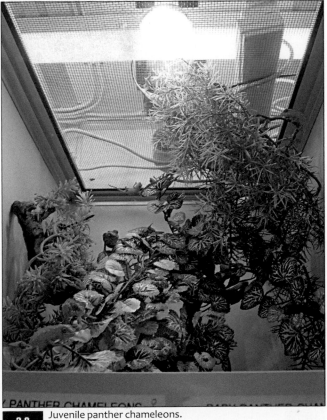

2.8 Juvenile panther chameleons.
(With permission from the Grooms at Reptile Crazy, Norwich; © Louise Rayment-Dyble)

Legal considerations

The UK Government's Department of the Environment, Food and Rural Affairs (DEFRA) website states that there are no animal health import requirements for individual pet reptiles. They can be brought into the UK as long as they are accompanied by their owner and a letter from a veterinary surgeon or the owner stating that the animals are fit and healthy to complete the journey. Up to five pet invertebrates, pet reptiles and pet amphibians, accompanied by their owner, can be brought into the UK without the need to undergo veterinary checks on entry, and, therefore, they do not need to be imported via a Border Inspection Post (BIP). However, DEFRA recommends that you should contact the airline to ensure that it is prepared to carry the animal(s). Commercial consignments, unaccompanied pets and consignments of more than five pets from outside the EU (except Norway, Switzerland and Liechtenstein) coming into the UK must be imported through a BIP and must meet the commercial import conditions.

CITES

The Convention on International Trade of Endangered Species of Wild Flora and Fauna lists species that are prohibited from being taken from the wild and thus require permits to be imported and sold. Interestingly, the CITES definition of 'captive-bred' actually refers to F2-generation individuals, whose parents were bred in captivity. First-generation offspring from a wild-caught pair brought into captivity cannot be defined or sold as 'captive-bred' under CITES regulations. This raises the possibility that many pets labelled as 'captive-bred' may not be. Policing these regulations is difficult and once species are banned from trade it can put pressure on other similar species to replace them. For example, the ban on Mediterranean tortoise (*Testudo*) species means that there is increased trade in other terrestrial tortoises that are perhaps more challenging to maintain. Additionally, customs officers have to be capable of identifying species to ensure they match their labelled containers.

Micro-chipping has recently become the 'gold standard' for identifying individuals as the chips are universally easy to read and difficult to tamper with. The British Veterinary Zoological Society's (BVZS) guidelines for sites for placement of microchip transponders are shown in Figure 2.9. Normal-sized chips can be implanted into tortoises of 10 cm straight carapace length and above. Mini-microchips are also available, which can be implanted into smaller tortoises of 6.5 cm and above and other small individual reptiles. The skin should be cleansed thoroughly with an iodine-based solution before and after implantation (a toothbrush is useful), and it is recommended that tissue glue is placed over the needle entry site.

Dangerous Wild Animals Act

The Dangerous Wild Animals Act 1976 (UK) was reviewed in 2007 and has applications to reptile species. A licence granted by the local authority is required to keep all the venomous species of snakes and lizards, e.g. Gila monster, and all species of the order Crocodilia. The requirements include a protocol for dealing with escapes, and aspects of health and safety (see Appendix 5).

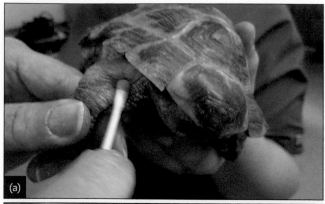

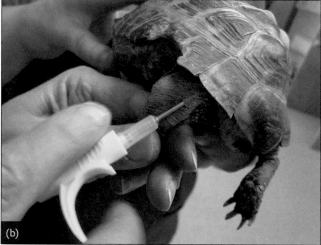

2.9 (a) Preparation of the skin for microchip implantation in a tortoise. (b) Placing of the microchip implant.
(© Louise Rayment-Dyble)

Zoonotic infections

One much discussed issue in relation to reptiles is that of zoonotic disease, most specifically salmonellosis. It is safest to assume that most, if not all, reptiles have the ability to carry and shed *Salmonella* spp. in their faeces and thus pose a risk to people; with a higher risk for certain groups of people, such as the elderly, small children and those with impaired immune systems due to disease or medication. Infection can be avoided by prevention of handling by these groups and supervision of others. Practice of good hygiene using disinfection, hand washing with hot soapy water and care with where in the house the reptile is allowed to roam (e.g. bathrooms and kitchen surfaces are best avoided) will also help avoid contamination and infection.

This should not be a reason *not* to keep a reptile as a pet, unless personal health issues make it inadvisable; in fact, for some older children with allergies a reptile can be a more suitable pet than a furred mammal. (There is a client advice leaflet available from the Health Protection Agency at www.hpa.org.uk.)

Other examples of potentially zoonotic infectious agents that reptiles can carry are *Cryptosporidium* (but there are so far no known reports of transmission), *Pseudomonas*, *Escherichia coli*, *Mycobacterium*, tick-borne rickettsiae (e.g. Q fever) and pentastomid parasites. There may also be other infections not yet identified and zoonotic risks should always be considered when handling any species.

Setting up your practice for treating reptile patients

Why do I want to treat reptiles in my practice?

This is a reasonable question to ask; most of us feel we were not taught very much about them at undergraduate level, although this is improving. Most veterinary surgeons who treat exotics in practice have not had very much formal training, but have expanded knowledge from their own experience as hobbyists and enthusiasts. Therefore, if we do not come from that background we can feel out of our depth and intimidated by the reptile patients – not just clinically, but they can be a bit scary to the uninitiated! From a clinical point of view, reptiles present a new and interesting variety and challenge, and successful cases can be extremely rewarding. The human–animal bond is just as strong with reptile pets (Figure 2.10). Many owners develop close relationships with their pet reptile and as such, demand the same level of clinical expertise and service they receive with their other species of pets. We are now more often presented with reptile patients and requests for treatment and advice, so as a profession it is almost expected of us: part of a growing trend and challenge to the profession, similar to that faced by our farm colleagues treating dogs and cats in the 1950s. The type of client varies enormously and although there are more experienced specialist veterinary surgeons around, some clients cannot afford this or just need simple first-opinion advice. From a purely business point of view it also makes sense. As of 2016, reptiles alone account for almost 10% of the author's practice turnover and we now offer health plans to reptile owners to try and encourage a more prophylactic approach to their management and health. There is a school of thought that says clients may be impressed with the versatility of a veterinary surgeon who can treat a wider range of species – so much so that they are more likely to bring their more traditional companion pets to a practice that offers appointments for the more exotic (Figures 2.11 and 2.12). Further specialization in herpetological medicine is possible within the European College of Zoological Medicine, the American Board of Veterinary Practitioners and the American College of Zoological Medicine.

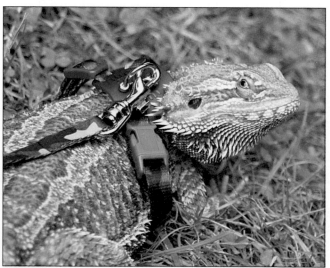

2.10 A pet bearded dragon in a harness.
(© Louise Rayment-Dyble)

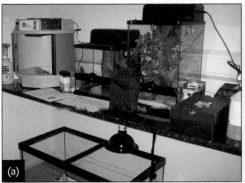 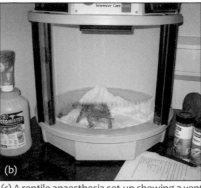 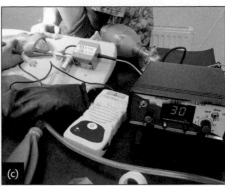

2.11 (a) A reptile ward. (b) A reptile hospital cage. (c) A reptile anaesthesia set-up showing a ventilator and Doppler monitor.
(© Louise Rayment-Dyble)

Basics (starting to see reptiles – you may already have most of these in your surgery)

- Scales – able to weigh a variety of sizes down to a few grams
- Aquarium
- Water containers, crocks that cannot be overturned
- Towels, cloth bags and pillow cases – for restraint
- Plastic trays and boxes for soaking
- Digital thermometer
- Gauntlets
- Latex gloves
- Povidone iodine compounds that are safe for topical application in reptiles
- Cotton buds and cotton wool
- Fenbendazole, ivermectin, metronidazole
- Vitamin and mineral supplements
- Injectable calcium gluconate and oxytocin
- Antibiotics such as enrofloxacin and marbofloxacin
- Anti-inflammatories – meloxicam and carprofen
- Tissue glue
- Microchips – normal size and mini-chips for small tortoises and lizards
- Hospital cage/intensive care unit/basic vivarium that can give heat and ideally ultraviolet (UV) light – can use lamp on a stand
- Oral fluids such as glucose, electrolytes, concentrated food supplements and probiotics
- Butterfly cannulae for fluids
- Crystalloid fluids, such as normal saline and Hartmann's

Mid-level (starting to see reptiles regularly)

- Microscope, slides and coverslips – for faecal examination
- Stains for cytology
- Doppler – for monitoring heart rate and confirming death in euthanasia or dead-on-arrival cases (e.g. 'my tortoise didn't wake up from hibernation')
- A range of vivaria for differently sized reptiles and several lamps including UV, red bulbs, ceramic heaters and heat mats
- Water sprays/humidifiers/sphagnum moss
- Thermometers and hygrometers for vivaria (and to retail to clients)
- Feeding support – nutritional formulae for debilitated and recovering reptiles
- Metal ball-tipped straight gavage tubes/oral specula
- Red rubber feeding tubes and small feeding tubes – for placing pharyngostomy tubes
- Propofol, ketamine, oxfendazole, ceftazidime, medical grade disinfectants safe for use topically and in nebulizers, etc., isoflurane or sevoflurane
- Small uncuffed endotracheal tubes – dog catheters and cannulae can be cut down for tiny patients and attached to a 3.5 mm endotracheal tube connector
- Small circuits such as Ayre's T-pieces
- Nebulizer
- Radiography – small, fine detail, e.g. mammography film or digital

Advanced (wanting to progress with reptiles and second opinions)

- Small animal ventilator
- Bag valve mask/manual resuscitator for ventilation in recovery
- Hobby tool/drill and oscillating saw for tortoise surgery and postmortem
- Snake sexing probes
- Snake hooks and tubes
- Feeding tongs
- Hoof or dental repair adhesives
- Adhesive plastic drapes
- Hooks and eyes and surgical wire for tortoise shell repairs
- Expoxy adhesive glue
- An in-house blood machine that can measure small volumes and test uric acid and ionized calcium
- A rigid endoscope with air insufflation pump
- An ultrasound scanner with a small-footprint high frequency probe
- Anaesthesia monitors, electrocardiography machine, apnoea alert, pulse oximeter and/or capnograph
- Digital thermometer probe
- Vascular clips
- Radiosurgical unit
- Haemostatic aids, e.g. cellulose matrix

2.12 Equipment list for treating reptiles.

How do I attract reptile owners to my practice?

Once you feel confident about seeing reptiles, it is time to get the word out and let people know. Clubs and societies are useful points of contact and giving lectures can be a good way of informing people. Tortoise worming events or 'parties' can be a good way of bringing clients into the practice and educating them. Social media is a hugely powerful tool in marketing, and developing a relationship with local suppliers, breeders and reptile shops is useful as they will refer and recommend clients (Figure 2.13).

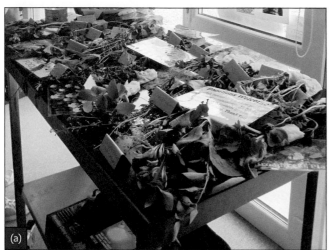

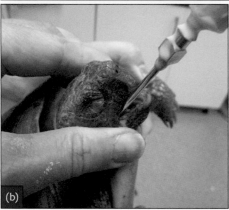

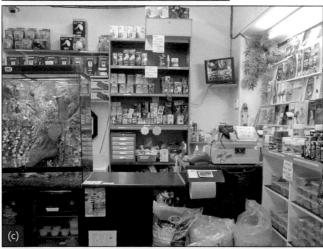

2.13 (a) Example weeds on display on a tortoise open day in practice. (b) A tortoise being wormed. (c) The reptile shop 'Reptile Crazy'.
(© Louise Rayment-Dyble; c, with permission from the Grooms at Reptile Crazy, Norwich)

Welfare

Along with the increase in numbers and despite better husbandry there are more welfare cases presented by the RSPCA and other sources. Behaviour can be used as a way of assessing welfare and stress.

Perhaps the most widely recognized yardstick for animal welfare is the discussion of the 'Five Freedoms', which can also be applied to captive reptiles (Figure 2.14).

Freedom	Comments
Freedom from thirst, hunger and malnutrition	Feed the correct diet and present in recognizable form. For example, royal pythons may not recognize white rodents as prey as they do not resemble their normal coloured rodent prey. Water may not be accepted in a dish, e.g. some chameleons require water to be sprayed on to vivarium vegetation or furniture. Feed a vegetarian diet to herbivores – iguanas and tortoises fed animal protein can develop gout and renal failure. Avoid obesity – common in large pythons, boas and monitor lizards – encourage exercise and limit food intake. Provide the correct mineral balance including UVB light, calcium and vitamin D3 to avoid nutritional secondary hyperparathyroidism, also called metabolic bone disease
Freedom from thermal and physical discomfort	All reptiles must be kept at their POTZ in order to function, metabolize, digest, etc. Provide the correct level of humidity to avoid dysecdysis (problems with skin shedding), especially common in desert species that use the microclimate of a burrow to aid shedding, e.g. bearded dragons and leopard geckos
Freedom from fear and distress	Use behaviour assessment to establish if the animals are stressed due to their environment. Do not mix species, avoid overcrowding and allow plenty of access to facilities, e.g. basking area large enough for all to use. Minimize handling, provide hides for security and privacy from view and other reptiles
Freedom from pain and disease	Practice good hygiene and prophylactic care to avoid parasitism. Ensure correct temperature and thermal gradient – if too cold, snakes may coil around heat sources or towards heat mats and incur thermal burns
Freedom to express normal patterns of behaviour	Allow sufficient space, substrate, vivarium furniture and habitat for normal behaviour. However 'natural' it may be, feeding of live vertebrate prey is illegal

2.14 The 'Five Freedoms'. POTZ = preferred optimal temperature zone.

Sources of information for owners and veterinary surgeons

There is a growing number of continuing professional development courses and conferences that can be attended both in the UK and abroad, including the British Small Animal Veterinary Association (BSAVA) Congress, the North American Veterinary Conference and European meetings. Membership of societies, such as the BVZS, the BSAVA and the Association of Reptilian and Amphibian Veterinarians, can provide more specialist knowledge and their meetings give the opportunity to meet with other colleagues, as personal communication is always a good way to learn. There is a large number of excellent textbooks published on the subject of reptile husbandry and medicine, and the internet is also there for reference, although some information can be anecdotal and needs to be viewed with this in mind.

References and further reading

Alderton D (1986) *A Petkeeper's Guide to Reptiles and Amphibians*. Salamander, London

Carpenter JW (2013) *Exotic Animal Formulary*. Elsevier, Missouri

Divers SJ (2013) Get endoscopy savvy. *BSAVA Companion* (March edn), 4–7

Ebenhack A (2012) *Healthcare and Rehabilitation of Turtles and Tortoises*. Living Art Publishing, Oklahoma, USA

Fowler ME (1986) *Zoo and Wild Animal Medicine, 2nd edn*. WB Saunders, Philadelphia

Fowler ME (1993) *Zoo and Wild Animal Medicine: Current Therapy 3*. WB Saunders, Philadelphia

Fowler ME (1999) *Zoo and Wild Animal Medicine: Current Therapy 4*. WB Saunders, Philadelphia

Frye FL (1995) *Reptile Clinician's Handbook*. Krieger, Florida

Frye FL and Williams DL (1995) *Self-Assessment Colour Review of Reptiles and Amphibians*. Manson, London

Girling SJ and Raiti P (2004) *BSAVA Manual of Reptiles, 2nd edn*. BSAVA Publications, Gloucester

Jessop M (2009) Identification of tortoises. *In Practice* **31**, 46–57

Johnson-Delaney C (1996) *Exotic Companion Medicine Handbook for Veterinarians*. Wingers Publishing, Lake Worth, Florida

Krautwald-Junghanns ME, Pees M, Reese S and Tully T (2011) *Diagnostic Imaging of Exotic Pets, Birds, Small Mammals and Reptiles*. Schültersche Verlagsgesellschaft, Hanover, Germany (English Translation)

Mader D (1996) *Reptile Medicine and Surgery*. WB Saunders, Philadelphia

Mader D (2006) *Reptile Medicine and Surgery, 2nd edn*. Saunders Elsevier, St Louis

Meredith A and Johnson-Delaney C (2010) *BSAVA Manual of Exotic Pets, 5th edn*. BSAVA Publications, Gloucester

RSPCA (2010) Welfare indicator: the number of imported wild-taken reptiles and birds as a proportion of the total trade into the UK and the EU. In: *The Welfare State: Five Years Measuring Welfare in the UK, 2005–2009*, pp. 109–112. Available at: www.rspca.org.uk/utilities/aboutus/reports/animalwelfareindicators

Seal J (1999) The reptile house. In: *The Snakebite Survivors' Club*, pp. 4–5. Macmillan, London

Smith L (2013) Tortoise parties. *BSAVA Companion* (February edn), 18–21

Thompson L (2013) Basic care of reptiles: husbandry requirements and fluid therapy. *Animal Health Advisor* **2(9)**, 16–18

Warwick C, Arena P, Lindley S, Jessop M and Steedman C (2013) Assessing reptile welfare using behavioural criteria. *In Practice* **35**, 123–131

Webster AJF (1994) *Animal Welfare: A Cool Eye Towards Eden*. Blackwell Science, Oxford

Useful websites

www.britishcheloniagroup.org.uk

www.tortoiseclub.org

www.thetortoisetable.org.uk – for lists and pictures of edible plants for tortoises

www.politicalanimal.org.uk – reference for RSPCA and import data

www.lafebervet.com – resource for CPD, techniques and client handouts

www.lifelearn.co.uk – client handouts

www.tortoisetrust.org

www.uvguide.co.uk

www.vetronic.co.uk – for ventilators

www.meadowsanimalhealthcare.co.uk – for feeding tubes and nebulizers

Chapter 3

Captive maintenance

Molly Varga

Since this chapter was originally written over a decade ago, the number and variety of reptiles being kept as pets has increased exponentially. Likewise, there is an increased requirement for these animals to be provided with good healthcare. There are many positive improvements to reptile keeping in the UK, including the improved accessibility of suitable equipment and feed stuffs, and the provision of medical insurance for reptiles. However, despite the increased interest in reptiles as pets (both from the owner and the veterinary side) many conditions seen are still directly related to deficiencies in basic husbandry. This raises two areas of concern: firstly, many of these problems are inherently preventable; and secondly, the information available is often contradictory or, occasionally, unreliable.

Until definitive research is done, the advice given should be based on a critical review of the information currently available. It is perfectly possible to provide a good captive environment for many species of reptiles, allowing freedom from disease and encouraging normal behaviour.

The aim of this chapter is to provide a practical guide for advising on the captive maintenance of reptiles in general, with specific information on commonly held species, concentrating on the physiological and ethological concepts behind the recommendations. The aim is to achieve an improvement in overall welfare by improving standards of husbandry and evaluating the success of this using the 'Five Freedoms' used to define animal welfare in captivity (see also Chapter 2):

- Freedom from malnutrition
- Freedom from thermal and physical discomfort
- Freedom from injury and disease
- Freedom to express most normal patterns of behaviour
- Freedom from fear and stress.

Figure 3.1 defines some commonly used, and frequently misinterpreted, terms.

Terms	Definitions
Endotherm	An animal whose thermal energy is a byproduct of its own metabolism. This includes mammals, birds and some reptiles. For example, female pythons regulate their body temperature during egg brooding cycles using shivering thermogenesis
Ectotherm	An animal that regulates its body temperature by using energy derived from external sources. This term accurately describes the thermogenic behaviour of most reptiles
Homeotherm	An animal whose body temperature is relatively consistent (±2°C). Some reptiles can regulate their body temperature within a narrower range than this, especially during periods of activity (Ackerman, 1998)
Poikilotherm	An animal whose body temperature is variable. This is *not* the same as an ectotherm; indeed, many mammals, particularly those that undergo hibernation, could correctly be termed poikilothermic
Preferred Optimum Temperature Zone (POTZ)	The range of temperatures within which a specific ectotherm functions optimally *overall*. It is the thermal environment within which a reptile will engage in normal activities. It is important to note that all physiological functions have a temperature at which they function optimally but, within a species, not all functions are optimized at the same temperature. The term POTZ is somewhat misleading, since it implies a conscious choice. Activity temperature range (ATR) may be a better term as it is less anthropomorphic (DeNardo, 2002)
Selected body temperature (T_s)	The temperature selected by an individual when placed in an artificial thermal gradient. This will vary over time, as the temperature selected will mirror the optimal temperature for the physiological function perceived as most important at that time. It is synonymous with preferred body temperature (T_p). This is sometimes expressed as a *range* of temperatures, which reflects the middle 50–67% of the body temperatures measured during an animal's circadian temperature fluctuation (De Nardo, 2002)
Minimum and maximum critical temperatures	The upper and lower thermal tolerance limits where the righting reflex is lost in 50% of animals
Heliothermy	Deriving most thermal energy from the sun's radiation (all diurnal reptiles)
Thigmothermy	Deriving most thermal energy by conduction from items in the environment (many nocturnal or crepuscular reptiles)

3.1 Definitions of some commonly used terms.

BSAVA Manual of Reptiles, third edition. Edited by Simon J. Girling and Paul Raiti. ©BSAVA 2019

Housing

Environmental design

The aim of environmental design is to provide a habitat that:

- Encourages natural behaviour
- Allows the maintenance of animals in good health
- Minimizes the stresses associated with captivity and the diseases related to these pressures.

An understanding of a species' behaviour in the wild and an appreciation that there are different ways to achieve these aims are important. The two extremes of animal display are clinical and naturalistic habitats (see below). Many people use a combination of these in order to provide an environment that suits their particular needs. With larger specimens it may not be possible to provide a suitable naturalistic environment due to space constraints, particularly in private homes. Each set-up should be judged on its own merits.

Clinical habitats

The clinical environment is one with minimal cage furniture and a basic substrate, aimed towards easiest access for observation and cleaning, such as a plastic or glass vivarium with a hide box and newspaper as substrate (Figures 3.2 and 3.3). This type of set-up uses disposable substrate and furniture, and frequent cleaning is required. It is perhaps most suitable for in-clinic use, pet shops and breeding facilities. Ideally, this should be a short-term solution for most small specimens, as some of the factors that provide psychological benefits to the inhabitant may be compromised. For example, deep sand is required for burrowing species such as the sand boa.

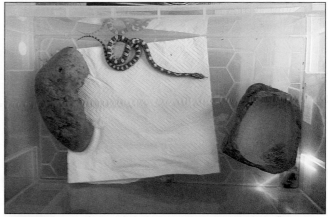

3.3 Corn snake in a clinical environment: note the lack of vivarium furniture and substrate. Everything within the environment is disposable or amenable to easy cleaning and disinfection.

The primary disadvantage of these systems is that they necessitate frequent handling of occupants, which may cause significant stress in the more timid species (e.g. royal python). However, clinical settings are commonly used for larger specimens, such as giant snakes (>2 m), due to the effective use of available space.

Naturalistic habitats

The naturalistic display is one with extensive naturally derived cage furniture and substrate that provides a reasonably detailed 'caricature' of the native environment (Figures 3.4 and 3.5). This type of environment is more suitable for private owners or collection displays.

The 'landscaping' of the vivarium needs to take into account how the animal behaves in the wild. For example, green iguanas are arboreal and therefore require a degree

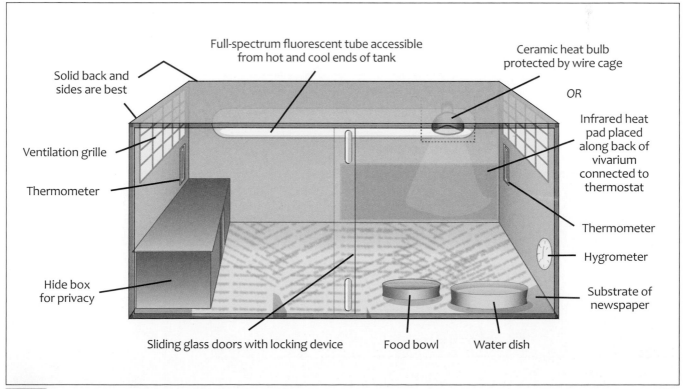

Solid back and sides are best

Full-spectrum fluorescent tube accessible from hot and cool ends of tank

Ceramic heat bulb protected by wire cage

OR

Ventilation grille

Thermometer

Infrared heat pad placed along back of vivarium connected to thermostat

Thermometer

Hygrometer

Hide box for privacy

Sliding glass doors with locking device

Food bowl

Water dish

Substrate of newspaper

3.2 Clinical environment: plastic or glass vivarium with a hide box and newspaper as substrate.

of vertical as well as horizontal freedom within their enclosures. In this instance, the floor area required is less than that needed by a comparably sized terrestrial lizard, such as a Savannah monitor, but the vertical rise of the tank needs to be significantly greater. In order for the animal to make use of the vertical rise, provision must be made to allow climbing, e.g. by including shelves or tree branches in the overall design.

The more naturally derived tank 'furniture' that is used, the greater is the potential for pathogen build-up if close attention is not paid to hygiene. For example, snake mite *Ophionyssus natricis* infestation can escalate when natural wood fomites are not changed or adequately treated. In parallel with recent trends in fish keeping, the trend with naturalistic environments is to encourage a 'pseudo-ecosystem' with exploitation of natural biological processes, such as denitrifying bacteria for waste management.

Even with the simplest naturalistic vivaria, full cleaning does not need to be as frequent as is necessary for clinical tanks because they are managed as a 'deep litter' system (De Vosjoli, 1999). Spot cleaning of waste matter should be carried out when necessary; organic waste should be removed as rapidly as possible, scooping out only the soiled substrate. Complete changing of substrate can be

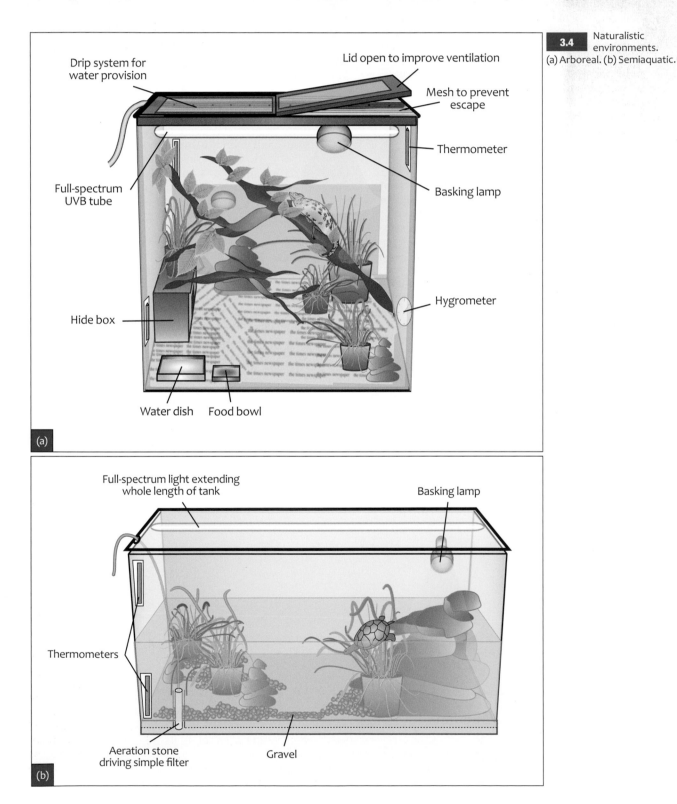

3.4 Naturalistic environments. (a) Arboreal. (b) Semiaquatic.

(a)
- Drip system for water provision
- Lid open to improve ventilation
- Mesh to prevent escape
- Thermometer
- Full-spectrum UVB tube
- Basking lamp
- Hide box
- Hygrometer
- Water dish
- Food bowl

(b)
- Full-spectrum light extending whole length of tank
- Basking lamp
- Thermometers
- Aeration stone driving simple filter
- Gravel

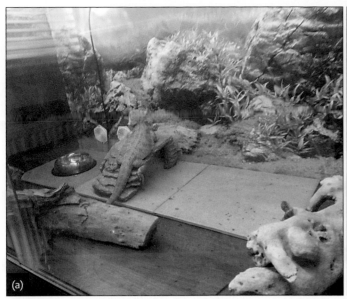 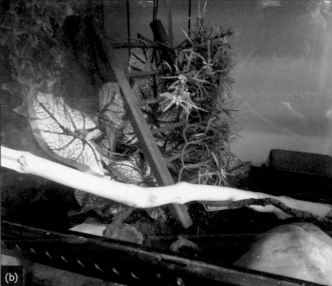

3.5 (a) Bearded dragon in a semi-naturalistic environment. This type of environment attempts to provide a more natural living space for the animal while retaining much of the ability to be easily cleaned and disinfected; note the lack of substrate and minimal amount of furniture. (b) Chameleon in a naturalistic vivarium. This type of enclosure attempts to closely mimic the environment an animal would inhabit in the wild; again, note the amount of internal furniture and substrate present. While this makes for a more complex and interesting environment and is suitable for a healthy individual, it is more difficult to keep clean and it is practically impossible to disinfect most of the elements.

undertaken considerably less frequently, depending on the vivarium size and number of occupants (the smaller the enclosure size or the greater the number of occupants, the more frequently a complete clean-out should be done).

Aside from the appearance, the primary advantage of this type of set-up is the provision of psychological and potentially stress-reducing benefits, such as natural cover, infrequent handling of cage inhabitants and a range of microclimates.

Building materials

A great variety of materials can potentially be used successfully to build reptile enclosures. The ideal building material should be:

- Strong enough to enclose the specimen in question
- Durable enough to last for the expected life of the vivarium
- Non-toxic
- Easy to clean
- Non-porous
- Preferably cheap and easy to obtain.

Most vivaria are a combination of more than one type of structural material. Examples include:

- Glass/safety glass
- Perspex (tends to scratch easily with routine cleaning)
- Fibreglass
- Sealed or melamine-covered wood (untreated wood is not a suitable material as it is very porous, will rot when in contact with wet organic waste, and can also harbour bacteria, fungi and parasitic mites)
- Plastic-covered wire mesh (mesh must be small enough not to entrap the limbs of the tank occupant).

It is worth noting that any glue or other fixatives should also conform to the general criteria of being non-toxic and easy to clean.

Many reptiles will not see glass or Perspex walls as a barrier and will repeatedly knock or rub their snouts on them, causing potentially severe rostral abrasions. This is a particular concern in Asian water dragons. A tape strip placed outside the tank at reptile nose level allows the animal to appreciate that a barrier exists and can help correct this problem.

A secure system of closing and locking the vivarium is a sensible precaution, particularly when dealing with snakes, and becomes imperative when dealing with dangerous or venomous specimens.

Size

Vivarium size will depend on the size, activity levels and number of specimens to be housed within. At the minimum, the size of the enclosure should be large enough to permit a temperature gradient to be set up and maintained. Using a clinical-type set-up will allow more efficient use of space and, therefore, a somewhat smaller vivarium for a similar sized animal than a naturalistic habitat. It is worth remembering that there needs to be sufficient floor space available for the inhabitants to move around, thermoregulate, feed and defecate. As a guide, at least 30–40% of the floor space should be available for these activities. Smaller faster specimens such as green anoles require more space relative to their body size than do larger more torpid animals such as adult boa constrictors.

Some recommendations for minimum tank size are given in Figure 3.6. As a general rule, the largest area possible should be provided for each animal; large enough at least that the desire to escape is diminished or that when startled the animal can get outside its flight zone without colliding with the wall of the enclosure. This facilitates the provision of a variety of microhabitats with different temperatures and humidities. Animals kept in confined spaces have little opportunity to exercise and may become obese. Other welfare implications of enclosures that are too small include the inability to express normal behaviours and stress caused by inability to move away from perceived threats.

Group	Lifestyle	Dimensions
Chelonians	Terrestrial	Area: 5 x animal's length squared
	Semiaquatic	Longest side: 5 x animal's length Shortest side: 3 x animal's length Height: high enough to prevent escape; allow half animal's length in water depth
Lizards	Terrestrial	Longest side: 3 x animal's length Shortest side: 2 x animal's length Height: high enough to prevent escape
	Arboreal	Longest side: 3 x animal's length Shortest side: 2 x animal's length Height: 2–3 x animal's length
	Burrowing	Longest side: 3 x animal's length Shortest side: 2 x animal's length Height: ½ body length above substrate; allow at least 30 cm of substrate
Snakes	Terrestrial	Longest side: ¾ of body length Shortest side: ⅓ of body length Height: ½ body length
	Arboreal	Longest side: ¾ of body length Shortest side: ⅓ of body length Height: allow for body length
	Burrowing	Longest side: ¾ of body length Shortest side: ⅓ of body length Height: ½ body length above substrate; allow at least 30 cm of substrate

3.6 Recommendations for vivarium size for various types of reptile. (Data from Barnard (1996))

Substrate

The substrate is the material used to cover the floor of the vivarium; different things are required from it depending on species behaviour. For example, substrate is less critical for arboreal species, such as the emerald tree boa, as so little time is spent in contact with the floor. In contrast, terrestrial species such as the inland bearded dragon are much more sensitive to improper substrate selection. Burrowing species, such as skinks, should be provided with a floor covering that allows them to display their normal behaviour. Substrates need to be:

- Non-toxic
- Non-irritant
- Easy to clean
- Easy to obtain
- Preferably cheap.

Properties of a variety of substrate materials are compared in Figure 3.7. As the properties of each substrate vary, consideration should be given to using more than one type, particularly in naturalistic vivaria. The author advocates the use of several substrates, often placed in shallow removable containers. This allows for the provision of varying humidities and the creation of humidity gradients/microhabitats, while making cleaning achievable.

Substrate	Easy to clean?	Easy to replace?	Cheap?	Aesthetic?	Disease risk	Comments
Newspaper	Yes	Yes	Yes	No	Low	Lead in ink can cause irritation and make animals dirty
Sand	Relatively frequent scooping; less frequent full changes	Yes	Yes	Yes	Risk of gut impaction if ingested with food	
Astroturf®	Yes	Yes	Relatively	Yes	Low	Not suitable for burrowing species
Calcisand	Yes (see sand)	Yes	Slightly more expensive	Yes, but often highly coloured	Can discolour skin; calcium uptake unknown	Should not be used as a substitute for a proper diet as it has been associated with gut impaction in leopard geckos
Corn cobs	Yes, but particles larger so organic waste less easy to scoop thoroughly	Yes	Relatively	Relatively	Can harbour chiggers and mites; risk of inappropriate ingestion	Not recommended
Wood chip	Yes, but larger particles make thorough scooping more difficult	Yes	Yes	Yes	Organic so can harbour chiggers and mites; risk of inappropriate ingestion	Chippings from aromatic woods such as cedar should not be used as the oils may cause dermal and/or respiratory irritation
Wood shavings	Yes	Yes	Yes	Yes	As for wood chip; also retains humidity, with increased risk of mould build-up	Not recommended
Bark	Yes; NB: particle size	Yes	Yes	Relatively	As for wood chip; also retains humidity, with increased risk of mould build-up	
Peat moss	Harder to see organic waste and remove it thoroughly	Yes	Yes	Yes	Deep litter system allows microbe build-up	Need to pay attention to proper cleaning
Aquarium gravel	Yes	Yes	Moderately	Moderately	Can cause mechanical irritation to skin; risk of inappropriate ingestion	Not a very common natural habitat; easy to disinfect

3.7 A comparison of available substrates. (continues) ▶

Substrate	Easy to clean?	Easy to replace?	Cheap?	Aesthetic?	Disease risk	Comments
Cat litter	Yes	Yes	Yes	No	Clay litter can be dusty, causing respiratory inflammation; wood-based litter has problems as for wood shavings; risk of inappropriate ingestion	Not recommended
Earth	Yes, but can be difficult to see organic waste and remove it properly	Yes	Yes	No	Can import bacteria, fungal spores and ecto/endoparasites	Not recommended

3.7 (continued) A comparison of available substrates.

Temperature

All reptiles are, to a greater or lesser extent, ectothermic. Environmental temperature is one of the most important factors governing reptile biology because the rate of all physiological processes depends upon it, although the details are still poorly understood. Temperature is closely related to humidity and ventilation and altering one of these parameters will affect both of the others. Figure 3.8 gives the thermal requirements of some commonly kept species.

Temperature gradient

Each animal should have access to a suitable range of temperatures within the tank so that behavioural thermoregulation is possible. This necessitates providing a temperature gradient such that one end of the tank is at or below the lower end of the Preferred Optimal Temperature Zone (POTZ) and the other end is at or above the higher end of the POTZ. (It should be noted that the POTZ varies between day and night and, in some species, seasonally.) The gradient should be across useable areas of the tank and should be measured by placing thermometers on the tank walls at levels where the animal is likely to bask. Heat mats placed on 33–50% of the back wall of the tank are commonly used to elevate the ambient temperature above room temperature and provide the basic gradient (see Figure 3.2). Unlike mats available for dog and cat use, these heat pads provide radiant heat and are not pressure-sensitive. For tanks with a vertical rise, the temperature gradient should be in both the horizontal and vertical planes. An additional focal heat source is placed at one end of the tank and this also contributes to the temperature gradient. This could be a radiant bulb or an additional underfloor heat mat.

Heat sources

How the heat is applied is very important and should reflect the way that the animal thermoregulates in the wild:

- Species such as inland bearded dragons and collared lizards that bask in the sun should be provided with a radiant heat source such as a ceramic or incandescent bulb
- For nocturnal or crepuscular species, such as leopard geckos, which gain heat from conduction, electric heat mats or lights shining on to (and thereby warming) cage furniture are more suitable.

Where a light source is used to provide the hot end of the temperature gradient, thought should be given to alternative provision to maintain a gradient at night because reptiles should not be constantly exposed to light. Ceramic bulbs, heating tape or heating pads are useful in this instance (Figure 3.9). It should be noted that the POTZ varies diurnally and, while a temperature gradient is still required to allow thermoregulation overnight, the temperatures attained will need to be lowered to reflect normal nocturnal cooling.

Species	Geographical range	Lifestyle	Habitat	Preferred Optimal Temperature Zone (POTZ)	Relative humidity (RH)	UVB light required?	Comments
Spur-thighed tortoise, Hermann's tortoise	Mediterranean to Asia Minor	Terrestrial	Temperate	20–28°C	30–50%	Yes	Will thrive in lower temperatures outside in the summer
African spurred tortoise	Sub-Saharan Africa	Terrestrial	Semi-arid to desert	25–35°C	40–75%	Yes	
Leopard tortoise	Sub-Saharan Africa	Terrestrial	Savannah to semi-arid to desert	25–35°C	40–75%	Yes	
Bell's hingeback tortoise	West Africa	Terrestrial	Savannah to rainforest	24–28°C	50–80%	Yes	
Red-eared terrapin	Southern and central USA	Semiaquatic	Temperate	20–24°C	60–90%	Yes	
Red-footed tortoise	Panama to northern Argentina	Terrestrial	Grasslands, savannah, forest edges	21–27°C	50–60%	Yes	

3.8 Environmental requirements of some commonly kept species. (continues)

Species	Geographical range	Lifestyle	Habitat	Preferred Optimal Temperature Zone (POTZ)	Relative humidity (RH)	UVB light required?	Comments
Yellow-footed tortoise	Northern South America	Terrestrial	Rainforest	25–27°C	75–80%	Yes	
Green iguana	Latin America	Arboreal, terrestrial	Rainforest	25–35°C	75–100%	Yes	
Asian water dragon	China and South East Asia	Arboreal, semiaquatic	Rainforest	24–30°C	80–90%	Yes	
Bell's dab lizard	Northern Africa	Terrestrial, burrowing	Desert	32–38°C	20–50%	Yes	Dry heat required
Inland bearded dragon	Eastern Australia	Terrestrial	Desert	25–35°C with basking area of 38–42°C	30–40%	Yes	Requires increased RH or humid microhabitats during shedding
Leopard gecko	India and Pakistan	Terrestrial, crepuscular	Semi-arid	25–30°C	30–40%	Controversial; probably do but possibly less than other species	May be more sensitive to UV light. Requires humid microhabitats
Veiled chameleon	Yemen	Arboreal	Semi-arid	21–38°C	75–80%	Yes	Requires a drip system or misting for water provision
Savannah monitor	Western Africa	Terrestrial	Savannah to semi-arid	26–38°C	20–50%	Yes	Eats whole prey so less reliant on UV light
Garter snake	North America	Terrestrial, semiaquatic	Temperate	21–28°C	50–80%	Not determined	It is probable that most species of snake would benefit from some UV exposure but this remains undetermined
Kingsnake	North America	Terrestrial	Semi-arid scrubland	25–30°C	30–70%	Not determined	
Corn snake	North America	Terrestrial	Semi-arid scrubland	25–30°C	30–70%	Acierno *et al.* (2008) demonstrated that corn snakes increase calcidiol levels when exposed to UVB	Upper range of humidity useful when shedding
Common boa	South America	Terrestrial, semi-arboreal and semiaquatic	Rainforest	28–30°C	50–80%	Not determined	Upper range of humidity useful when shedding
Emerald tree boa	South America	Arboreal	Rainforest	25–35°C	60–80%	Not determined	
Sand boa	Southern Europe to Central Africa, Asia and the Middle East	Burrowing	Desert	25–30°C	20–30%	Not determined	
Royal python	West and Central Africa	Terrestrial	Scrubland	25–30°C	50–80%	Not determined	Upper range of humidity useful when shedding
Burmese python	Burma, southern China, Indochina	Terrestrial, semi-arboreal	Rainforest	25–30°C	50–80%	Not determined	Upper range of humidity useful when shedding

3.8 (continued) Environmental requirements of some commonly kept species.

Type of heat source	Advantages	Disadvantages
Heat pads	Good range of sizes and wattages, therefore versatile. Best used external to the tank, either underneath or behind one of the vertical walls	Often do not provide high enough basking temperatures for heliotherms. Hazardous heat build-up can occur when using with large specimens, where heat is not absorbed as fast as it is produced (thermal blocking). Specimens that are weak and unwell may not be able to move off the heat source
Ceramic lamps	Provide high levels of heat; a range of strengths are available; suitable for basking specimens	Must always be used with a thermostat, and can cause severe burns to both cage inhabitants and owners if direct contact occurs. Bulbs used within a vivarium MUST have a non-conductive protective guard surrounding them to prevent the reptile coming into direct contact
Incandescent bulbs	These are useful for providing visual hot spots (some species appear to favour these); temperatures achieved depend on the wattage of the bulb	May not provide a warm enough basking spot for some species. Must be used with a protective guard and a dimming switch. They should not be left on overnight and are therefore not suitable as the sole source of heat
Heating tape	Can precisely control where the heat is supplied	Does not provide a warm enough ambient temperature for many species and should not be relied upon as the only heat source. Should be viewed as a tool to give thermal heterogeneity in a vivarium heated in another fashion
Hot rocks		The heat produced is at best unpredictable and often excessive, leading to thermal burns. These are not recommended

3.9 A comparison of the available types of heat source.

In all cases, tank inhabitants should be protected from direct contact with intense heat sources to prevent thermal burns. Bulbs should be protected with wire cages or placed out of the animal's reach. Heat pads should not be placed under more than 33–50% of the floor area, allowing escape from the heat source if needed. As many heating pads, especially older models, generate enough heat to break vivarium glass, the pad should be positioned a few millimetres away from the tank wall and on the outside. This has the added benefit of removing the possibility of contamination by urine and faeces. Underfloor heating is not suitable for species such as sand boas that use burrowing as a cooling strategy. Anecdotally, it is also less suitable for tortoises as it appears to cause maldigestion. Perhaps the best way of avoiding thermal burns is to ensure that the ambient background temperature is high enough, meaning that the tank inhabitants are not stimulated to seek close approximation to the focal heat sources.

De Vosjoli (1999) and Arena and Warwick (1995) suggest that the size of the heat source relative to the size of the reptile is important. Both groups found that when large specimens are attempting to elevate their whole-body temperature using small but intense heat sources, problems such as thermal burns are more likely to occur.

All devices used to heat vivaria should be controlled using a preset thermostat to prevent overheating or over-cooling. There are three types of thermostat easily available to hobbyists:

- **On/off thermostats:** the heat source is 'on' until the set temperature is reached, and then 'off' until the temperature falls enough to trigger a restart. This means the temperature inside the vivarium varies between the set upper temperature and the lower temperature at which the 'restart' is triggered; therefore, the temperature inside the vivarium is not constant. This is the simplest and cheapest option
- **Pulse proportional thermostats:** these are a more expensive option, suitable for use with non-light-emitting heat sources (e.g. ceramic lamps). They allow much finer control of the temperature range within the vivarium by altering the flow of electricity to the heat source in response to the vivarium temperature. They are not suitable for use with light-emitting bulbs because the variation in electrical flow would cause the bulb to flicker
- **Dimming thermostats:** these are suitable for use with light bulbs (of some types) as well as with heaters. They also alter the flow of electricity in response to changing temperatures, but this is achieved by reducing the current, meaning that there is no flicker. This type of thermostat gives very specific control of temperature within a specified range.

Care should be taken to avoid contact of any electrical equipment with water, urine and faeces; additionally, smoke detectors and fire-fighting equipment should be in place. It is important to remember that even though thermostats can be set to deliver specific temperatures, this is not always what is achieved in reality and true temperatures attained should still be measured using a separate thermometer placed at an appropriate level within the tank. Thermostat probes should be placed so that they will measure temperature at a sensible point within the vivarium (in an area the animal is able to use, not where the animal cannot access) and not one that will give a false idea of the temperature being attained.

Relative humidity

The relative humidity (RH) requirements of commonly held species are listed in Figure 3.8. Many common disease problems are caused by low humidity, e.g. chronic renal failure in green iguanas and shedding problems in snakes. Bacterial and fungal dermatitis in snakes and lizards can be caused by excessive humidity. Inappropriate humidity may arise through lack of measurement. Hygrometers are readily available and should be used to measure RH.

Ventilation should not be compromised in order to maintain correct humidity. It is far easier to maintain a 'wet' tank where there is little or no air movement, but this type of atmosphere will allow rapid build-up of airborne bacteria, viruses, fungal spores and chemicals.

Humidity can be increased by spraying/misting; inclusion of waterfalls/water features/commercial humidifiers; strategic placement of water bowls (e.g. in the focal hot spot or over a heat pad); increasing the surface area of water provided; and the use of substrates that tend to retain humidity, such as sphagnum moss and peat. Many semi-arid species such as leopard geckos can be kept at room humidity (20–50% typically) and benefit from substrates such as sand that tend to favour dryness. Even for arid-adapted species, humid microhabitats are often essential. These can be contrived within hide areas by using damp substrate or daily misting. Providing different substrates within the same vivarium can aid in the provision of a heterogeneous humidity environment, meaning that the inhabitant can regulate its humidity more closely.

Ventilation

Ventilation requires complete air changes to be achieved within a vivarium rather than simply circulating air in a closed system. It is measured as the number of air changes in the vivarium per unit time. Ventilation allows for dissemination of suspended particles, airborne bacteria, viruses and fungal spores, and reduces any odour associated with the enclosure.

It is harder to maintain adequate temperature and humidity within an enclosure when ventilation is good. This is because increasing air movement has a cooling effect and will also move suspended water particles, making it necessary to replace the lost heat and moisture continuously. Temperature and humidity should be closely monitored.

The type of enclosure will direct the sort of ventilation required. For example, vertically oriented arboreal vivaria can become stagnant near the bottom, so that ventilation needs to be provided in the vertical plane as well as the horizontal.

In small vivaria increasing ventilation can be as simple as adjusting the size of the vent holes in the top. For larger more complex habitats an active system is required. This could comprise a clean air inlet, a 'dirty' air exhaust and a method of moving air. Fans can be placed that simply increase air circulation within the vivarium and thereby increase diffusion through vents. For larger vivaria, fans that actively draw in clean air, with passive outflow through ventilation holes or active exhaust by extractor fans, can be very effective.

Light

Both quality (wavelength and intensity) and quantity (periodicity) of light provision for captive reptiles are vitally important. Light initiates its effects on the body by hitting photoreceptors in the skin and central nervous system (in the retina and pineal gland; see Chapter 21) and triggering photochemical reactions. Light affects mineral metabolism, reproduction and behaviour.

Light is made up of infrared (3000 nm–1 mm), visible (380–780 nm) and ultraviolet A, B and C band (100–380 nm) wavelengths. In general terms the infrared band is responsible for imparting thermal energy to bodies, allowing warming. Visible light initiates reproductive behaviour in many species, and the ultraviolet A band also affects behaviour, whereas UVB (290–320 nm) affects vitamin D production and calcium metabolism.

Most lizards and chelonians benefit from full-spectrum lighting (UVA, UVB, visible and infrared wavelengths emitted from a single fluorescent bulb) when kept in captivity. Many snakes have been successfully kept without access to the full spectrum of light (diamond pythons appear to be an exception to this rule).

Species that are found in areas of intense sun radiation in the wild (e.g. inland bearded dragons and arboreal chameleons) have melanin in the skin and also in the coelom, which limits the penetration of UV radiation. Care should be taken when choosing lighting for species typically found in shaded areas, such as boa constrictors, as their innate protection from radiation damage may not be as good.

UVB and vitamin D3

Some species, e.g. green iguanas, require UVB in order to synthesize previtamin D3 in the skin and to maintain blood levels of the active vitamin. Research has questioned the effectiveness of vitamin D uptake from the gut in this species (Allen and Oftedal, 1994). Other species such as Savannah monitors have been kept successfully using a dietary vitamin D3 supplement. Species living in areas of high UV intensity are more reliant on dermal synthesis of vitamin D3, and little is stored, whereas those from more shaded areas and nocturnal species absorb oral forms of vitamin D3 that are stored in the liver (Calvert, 2002). In addition, those species that ingest whole prey, such as snakes, are less reliant on skin formation of vitamin D3.

Light sources

Until the synthesis of vitamin D and the qualities of light required to achieve this are better understood, it is difficult to make definite recommendations regarding UV provision. It has been suggested that high-output bulbs (e.g. ZooMed ReptiSun 5.0) are ideal for UV-reliant species such as the green iguana, whereas lower-rated bulbs (e.g. ZooMed ReptiSun 2.5) may be more suitable for species exposed to less sunlight in the wild (e.g. leopard geckos) (N. Gentz, personal communication). It is also worth noting that endogenous vitamin D3 synthesis is temperature dependent and so providing useful light in the absence of appropriate temperature will not have as great a benefit. It is strongly recommended that reptiles should

not be required to choose between light and heat; therefore, the UV provision and the radiant heat source should ideally be placed close together so that heat and light emanate from the same position.

The use of UVB-only bulbs or 'black lights' is discouraged, as intense sources can cause retinal damage to the owner and potentially to the animal. Full-spectrum bulbs appear to be much safer and also emit some UVA radiation, which exerts behavioural effects. Very few bulbs available on the market at this time have been tested objectively with regard to the intensity of the various wavelengths emitted.

There is significant reduction of UV intensity as distance from the light source increases (the inverse square rule states that the intensity of light is reduced with the square of the distance from the source). Ultraviolet radiation does not penetrate glass or Perspex®, so UV sources should always be placed within the vivarium. In practical terms this means that basking areas should be within 30 cm of full-spectrum bulbs. Often the best position is to place the full-spectrum bulb along the back wall of the vivarium, so the focal basking hot spot is within the suggested 30 cm distance. For arboreal tanks it may be sensible to consider using two fluorescent bulbs placed perpendicularly, so that most of the available space has adequate UV intensity. Semiaquatic species such as the red-eared terrapin also require ultraviolet light; however, UV radiation does not penetrate far beneath the water surface and so the bulb should be positioned such that surface basking areas are within a suitable distance. It is worth considering that research has shown reptiles behaviourally control the amounts of UV light to which they are exposed, in a similar manner to thermoregulation. This implies that it is beneficial to provide a UV gradient as well as refuges where vivarium inhabitants can avoid UV light if necessary. Too much UV light is as bad as too little and can be implicated in both dermal and ocular lesions.

Types of UV bulb

There are two main types of UV-emitting bulb available commercially in the UK: UV-emitting fluorescent bulbs and ballasted UV lamps (of which there are two types) (Figure 3.10).

Fluorescent bulbs emit low to mid-range amounts of UV light, with virtually no heat. This type of lamp is the most frequently encountered in hobbyist vivaria and the limitations associated with its use must be understood. The amount of UV emitted attenuates with time and bulbs will need to be changed every 6 months. Fluorescent tube bulbs also require specific electrical attachments for use, in which endplates and an external ballasting unit are included. Fluorescent bulbs are now also available in a compact form that fits into normal light bulb fittings. In order to assess the amount of UV being emitted, the use of a UV meter is recommended. This can assist with assessment of the

Characteristic	UV-emitting fluorescent tubes	Internally ballasted UV lamps	Externally ballasted UV lamps
UV wavelengths emitted	UVA and some UVB	UVA, UVB and UVC	UVA, UVB and UVC
Lifespan	6–9 months	Up to 18 months	Up to 18 months
Heat emitted	No	Yes	No
Dimming/control capability	Yes	No	No
Cost	Relatively cheap	Relatively expensive	Relatively expensive

3.10 A comparison of the pros and cons of the available types of UV-emitting bulbs.

tube's placement within the vivarium as well as in deciding when the tube needs to be changed. There are two types of fluorescent tubes available in the UK, those that are made specifically to produce UVB output (actually give out UVA and some UVB) and those that supposedly simulate daylight (give out UVA but very little UVB). The former type is more suitable for most vivaria. Studies using UV meters suggest that the output from these lamps is similar to the amount of UV measured in shaded areas, so more intense sources may be more suitable for those species that live in high-intensity UV areas. Ballast units of suitable wattage should be used in combination with these bulbs to ensure correct functioning; however, some studies show that the type of ballast unit used can affect the UV output of the bulb.

Internally ballasted high-intensity discharge lamps (mercury vapour and metal halide UV lamps) emit UV light over a broad spectrum (including UVA, UVB and UVC) as well as producing heat. Ballasting refers to an electrical device built into the lamp that limits or controls the amount of current passing through the lamp, making explosion and failure less of a risk. Due to the way these lamps are constructed, dimming is not a possibility, making them less flexible for use in a domestic vivarium because the heat produced is significant and cannot be adjusted. These lamps can be fitted using a standard light bulb fitting.

Externally ballasted mercury vapour UV lamps are the newest addition to the commercial market in the UK. In common with the internally ballasted bulbs, these lamps emit UV light over a broad spectrum. The advantage of these bulbs is that the ballasting device (the part of the unit that produces heat in the process of controlling the current throughput) is located outside of the light-producing portion. This means that they are much more suitable for use in domestic vivaria because the bulb portion does not produce much heat. These lamps also cannot be dimmed.

UV meters

While manufacturers of UV bulbs make certain claims regarding their output and longevity, these are not always accurate. Independent trials have found that the quality and quantity of UV output can vary widely between bulbs and from what is claimed by the manufacturers. Veterinary surgeons (veterinarians) are encouraged to use a good quality UV meter (e.g. the Solarmeter 6.5 UV Index Meter, Solartech Inc.) to measure the UV output of the bulbs being used for their patients (both in the home vivaria and in hospital) to ensure that this is adequate. Owners should also be encouraged to measure the UV output of their bulbs.

Adverse effects of UV light

Some skin cells may be damaged or killed in response to incorrect UV provision. Death of skin cells results in a condition similar to 'sunburn' in humans, and this may well cause pain and distress to the individual. Damage to the surviving skin cells affects the DNA and RNA, and may predispose to certain types of dermatological neoplasia as well as suppressing the immune system. Toxic syndromes, hyperkeratosis, anorexia and death have also been reported.

Ocular damage secondary to excessive UV exposure has been widely reported in mammals; however, there are only anecdotal reports in reptiles. Conditions reported include photokeratoconjunctivitis and cataracts. Photokeratoconjunctivitis is a rapid response to excessive UV exposure, while cataractous change tends to be a more chronic response.

Clearly the provision of UV light should not be taken lightly and any UV source should be treated with respect. It is important to remember that any human reptile keeper who is in direct contact with inappropriate UV light provision may also suffer physical damage in the same way as the reptile inhabitants.

In ALL cases, reptiles should be provided with refuge areas that allow them to remove themselves from UV light if they feel it is necessary. Exposure to UVB light in excess of that required for vitamin D production is not beneficial.

Periodicity

The length of time for which there is light within the tank is also important. A good rule is to be guided by the geographical origin of the species. Animals that originate from equatorial regions require a 12 hour light/12 hour dark regime, whereas animals from further north or south will benefit from varying the light period from 9 to 14 hours on a seasonal basis. Light sources should never be left on all the time, as 24-hour light exposure is a significant source of stress (Arena and Warwick, 1995).

Furniture

There may be little or no cage furniture other than food pots and hide areas but with the naturalistic type of tank a lot more is required. Any organic material that is brought into the tank can be a potential source of disease, so it is suggested that this be properly disinfected initially, either by baking in an oven or by scalding with boiling water. Wood and other porous items may harbour organisms such as mites and perpetuate an existing disease problem. Any cage furniture should be cleaned and disinfected or changed regularly. In common with construction materials and substrate, furniture should be non-toxic, of a suitable size and should not cause physical damage to inhabitants.

Increased variety within the environment can be created using different items such as logs, branches, rocks, living plants and hide boxes. However, all these items take up space so, unless the animal can utilize the areas above or underneath them, an increase in floor space should be allowed for. An interesting environment is more likely to provide scope for an animal to exhibit normal behaviour. It has been suggested that moving environmental landmarks around slightly may provide added interest; however, totally changing the environment may prove stressful (Chiszar et al., 1995).

In addition to the psychological benefits that vivarium furniture may provide, physical requirements should also be met. For example, adding rocks or rough branches to a snake vivarium can aid in shedding when other environmental considerations such as humidity are already suitable.

Hide areas

Hide areas, in general one hide box per animal plus one, should be used to provide a place where the animal can avoid observation and also small localized areas of increased humidity, lower temperature and shade. Hide areas are an easy way to increase the thermal heterogeneity of the tank. They should be large enough for the specimen in question to fit inside but small enough to give a sense of security. Provision of an 'escape' area can help in cases of intraspecific aggression where multiple individuals are housed together. Many snakes, such as the royal python, prefer to ingest prey in the privacy of a dark hide area and will become anorexic if one is not provided.

Water

All reptiles should be provided with a source of water regardless of whether they are likely to drink. It should be noted that many species will bathe in water as a cooling mechanism, some semiaquatic species require it for swimming, and it is very useful for providing a focus of humidity. The simplest source is a flat shallow water bowl with a relatively large surface area – preferably one that is hard to tip over, with a ramp or some other provision to allow escape if a reptile falls in by mistake. Size should be matched to the size of the proposed inhabitant. For semiaquatic species that often bask at the water surface, the ultraviolet light and focal hot spot should be placed to accommodate this requirement. Water temperature should be approximately 5°C lower than air temperature.

Water can also be provided in other ways, such as drip systems, misting sprays and waterfalls. Looking at how the animal obtains water in the wild will dictate what should be provided in captivity. Many reptiles (including veiled chameleons and green iguanas) only take water from droplets on leaves; thus, spraying the cage foliage several times a day or setting up a constant drip system so that the leaves are constantly wet is far more effective than providing a water bowl.

Water quality

In vivaria where there is a permanent water feature the water quality should be monitored. This can be done using a proprietary test kit or by any aquatic shop. Minimum parameters to check are ammonia, nitrate and nitrite. These factors are directly related to build-up of organic waste within the system. High levels may be toxic directly, may indicate a general hygiene problem or be related to overstocking.

Water changes should be done regularly, at least 30% every 2 weeks, and water should either be dechlorinated using commercial tablets or allowed to stand for 24 hours prior to use. Changing the water basically dilutes contaminants.

Filtration reduces suspended particulate matter and chemical contaminants. The water area and volume will tend to dictate the type of filtration used. Small volumes with low stocking densities will not need anything other than regular water changes. Under-gravel filters (where an aquarium pump draws water through a 5–7 cm layer of gravel sitting on top of a filter plate on the bottom of the tank) are easy to set up and have a wide application. The filtration is both mechanical and biological, since denitrifying bacteria can colonize the gravel. The amount of faeces produced by species such as red-eared terrapins may overpower simple filtration systems. Feeding in a separate tank may help, or more powerful pump filtration systems may be indicated.

Cleaning

One of the most important aspects of reptile maintenance is good hygiene. It has been suggested that it is necessary to balance the regularity of cleaning with degree of 'shyness' of the animal but cleanliness should not be compromised. It is important to emphasize the importance of cleaning and thoroughly removing organic debris, and to differentiate this from disinfection. Organic waste must be completely removed before disinfection is undertaken because it can 'inactivate' disinfectants, and also the physical presence of organic matter can prevent pathogenic organisms from coming into contact with the disinfectant.

The degree of cleaning required will depend on the type of set-up. Organic waste products should be removed as soon as possible after being voided. Clinical habitats will require a full change of substrate each time this happens, but with particulate substrate used in more natural habitats a thorough scooping is enough. Regardless of set-up, each vivarium should be cleaned thoroughly on a weekly basis and disinfected monthly. Figure 3.11 lists some common disinfectants.

Waste matter from reptile vivaria should be disposed of carefully as it is a potential source of *Salmonella* and other infectious organisms. Latex or rubber gloves should be

Chemical	Examples of trade products	Spectrum of activity	Comments
Phenol/cresol	Lysol	Effective against a wide range of microorganisms. Will kill acid-fast organisms but have less activity against fungi, and none against spores	*Toxic.* Not for use where may contact animal, as may cause skin irritation. Adsorbs on to porous material and is hard to rinse off
Formaldehyde	Formula H	Wide range of effectiveness. May inactivate most viruses	*Toxic* but suitable for use in empty vivaria. Risks to human user
Quaternary ammonium compounds	Ark-Klens, Cetrimide, F10 (in combination with biguanidine)	Broad antibacterial efficacy (except *Pseudomonas*), but very poor against fungi and spores. Inactivated by organic debris	Addition of biguanidine improves effectiveness against fungi, spores and viruses. Safe, but ingestion/inhalation can cause respiratory paralysis. Not suitable for animal contact
Chlorhexidine	Hibitane, Savlon	Broad spectrum of activity, even in the face of organic debris. Very poor activity against mycobacteria, spores and non-enveloped viruses. Not effective against *Pseudomonas* spp.	Safe. Suitable for animal contact. NB: reports of toxicosis occurring when used as a bath for topical treatment – signs included neuropathies and emesis
Hypochlorites	Bleach, Milton's solution	Broad spectrum but not active against fungal or bacterial spores or Coccidia	Relatively safe. Effectiveness reduced by organic debris. Less stable in dilute solution and in presence of UV light. Fumes are irritant to mucous membranes
Iodophors	Tamodine, Betadine, Pevidine	Good activity against Gram-positive and Gram-negative bacteria, fungi and viruses. Little activity against acid-fast bacteria and spores	Safe. May cause discoloration. Can be relatively expensive. Reduced activity in presence of organic debris
Dodecyl-di-(aminoethyl) glycine	Amprotect	Good spectrum of activity	Safe

3.11 Disinfectants for reptile housing.

worn during cleaning and disinfection. Equipment and tanks should not be cleaned in any area that is used for food preparation, nor is it desirable to use bathing facilities. If the bathroom must be used, it should be thoroughly cleaned and disinfected before its next use.

Social structure

Where more than one individual is to be housed in the same vivarium, thought should be given to the social structure of the groups created. Reference should be made to how the particular species behaves in the wild. For example, corn snakes are solitary except during the breeding season, so keeping them housed in groups is a potential stressor. In contrast, inland bearded dragons may be kept in groups of one male with two or more females if the vivarium is large enough (Raftery, 2002). Specimens should be matched for size to reduce bullying, and adequate space is required to avoid competition for food and basking sites.

In general it is hard to recommend that different species of reptile be kept in the same vivarium, as husbandry requirements vary so greatly (see Figure 3.8). Care should be taken to avoid introducing disease problems such as inclusion body disease (IBD) when pythons are kept in the same environment as boas. IBD can be spread when boas and pythons are kept in the same airspace (not necessarily the same vivarium). Spread is thought to be by aerosol formation, fomites or mechanical vectors such as mites. The boa is a clinically silent carrier and the python is very susceptible to disease. IBD has also been recorded in other species of snake, e.g. the Eastern kingsnake and the palm viper.

Generally, species from different geographical origins should not be kept in the same vivarium, as differing disease susceptibility is unknown. Exposing a naïve animal to a disease that is endemic in another part of the world is likely to result in disaster, as inborn resistance will not be present. It is obviously not advisable to keep potential predators and prey together.

Special considerations

Record keeping

Record keeping provides the owner and veterinary surgeon with a lot of information, particularly where subtle changes are occurring over long periods of time. A diary should be kept of when the reptile feeds, when it sheds, and when faeces and urates are passed, and whether those are normal in colour and consistency. Regular weighing on accurate scales should be encouraged and graphs kept of the results. Cleaning and disinfection days should also be noted. Frequency of exhibiting normal behaviours and change in behaviours should be recorded and noted; however, the amount of time spent observing the animals must be taken into account.

Preventive medicine

All reptile owners should have a preventive medicine programme tailored to suit the needs of their particular collection. As a minimum, routine yearly physical examinations; faecal sample evaluations for nematodes, trematodes, cestodes and protozoan infections (these are particularly important when the reptile is being fed on live

food); and blood smears to check for haemoparasites (of significance in imported specimens) are recommended. Treatment of any parasite burden should be undertaken as necessary. Many veterinary surgeons advocate taking routine baseline biochemistry and haematology samples as well as radiographs to allow the establishment of normal databases. This would be ideal if money is not an area of concern, because it permits subclinical problems to be diagnosed early. There are currently no vaccines available for reptiles.

Quarantine procedures

Quarantine periods are utilized in order to prevent the introduction of pathogens into a collection by the addition of a new individual. A quarantine period should always be advised when introducing a new specimen into an existing collection. Simply put, quarantine allows the owner and veterinary surgeon to make certain that the new individual is healthy prior to introduction. The incoming animal should be kept in optimum conditions but in an airspace separate from other animals. In this instance, a simple clinical tank is most appropriate because it allows good visualization and monitoring of the newcomer, as well as easy and effective cleaning. Separate utensils and cage furniture should be used, and feeding or cleaning should be undertaken after the rest of the collection has been dealt with. In larger collections and zoos, the owner or caretaker should not contact the main collection after touching the new specimen until they have showered and changed clothes and shoes, to avoid transmission of disease on fomites.

- Quarantine should last from a minimum of 1–2 months up to 9–12 months (Divers, 1996), depending on the situation.
- During the period of quarantine each new acquisition should be monitored closely to check it is exhibiting normal behaviour and also eating.
- Each specimen should be examined by a veterinary surgeon.
- Faecal samples should be checked for parasitic ova and pathogenic protozoa; three successive negative samples are required to pronounce the animal free of the parasites.
- A blood smear to check for haemoparasites is also advisable.
- It may also be sensible in certain situations to consider testing for other infectious diseases (e.g. mycoplasmosis, herpesvirus infection, inclusion body disease). Decisions regarding testing should be made with knowledge of the specimen's origin and also the disease status of its proposed destination.

Even with all the above precautions, no single animal can be guaranteed free of disease; quarantine simply improves the statistical likelihood that an animal is healthy. Obviously, moving to new premises (for example when an animal is put into quarantine, or when introduced into a new collection/group) can cause stress, meaning that previously subclinical diseases may become clinical. If this happens when the animal is put into quarantine it is advantageous because it allows disease to be identified and addressed prior to introduction; however, the stress of introduction may be the point at which disease is revealed.

Testing for the presence of *Salmonella* is controversial since it can be a normal commensal in many species and unlikely to cause disease in other reptiles. It is questionable whether *Salmonella* should be treated even if found, owing to the risks of inducing resistant forms and the improbability of actually clearing the infection reliably. If an animal is tested for *Salmonella* and found to be negative, all this really means is that the organism was not being shed at the time of sampling, not that it is not present. All reptiles should be suspected of harbouring the organism and handled accordingly. Measures for preventing the spread of salmonellosis to humans are given in Chapters 2 and 6.

Aggression

Aggression is frequently encountered in captive reptiles and is often a cause for presenting the animal to a veterinary surgeon (Figure 3.12). Posturing, dewlap extension, head bobbing, biting, striking and tail whipping are examples of aggressive behaviour. It should be noted that aggression may be a part of normal species behaviour, e.g. in adult male green iguanas, and is one reason why it is not recommended to keep these animals in groups. Interspecific aggression should be taken into account when considering housing different species in the same environment, either in the same vivarium or within the same visual field, because appreciation of a potentially aggressive animal will cause significant stress to individuals of less dominant species.

When directed against human handlers, aggression may relate to previous negative stimuli during handling. Regular handling when young may reduce the fight/flight response as an individual matures, making it less likely that an aggressive response will be elicited during human–reptile interaction. Human-directed aggression may pose a significant health and safety risk to reptile keepers, particularly if the specimen in question is large. Other potential causes of aggression are:

- Seasonal hormonal changes related to breeding
- Natural timidity
- Defensive responses in the face of perceived attack
- A poorly organized and restrictive environment
- Pain.

Female owners of male green iguanas may find their animals become increasingly aggressive to them during their menstrual period. Therefore, a thorough evaluation of both environment and animal should be undertaken before any decision is made regarding the management of aggressive behaviour.

Iguanas are known to exhibit intraspecific aggressive behaviour. This is seen particularly in adult males during the breeding season. It has been shown that castration of males before the onset of sexual maturity may help reduce the incidence of aggressive behaviours directed against other pets and human handlers (Bradley, 2002; Lock and Bennett, 2015); however, the development of secondary sexual characteristics such as the dewlap and crest will be affected. Castration at a later stage is less likely to be as successful, although some have found it effective, the greatest effect being seen during the subsequent breeding season. Other suggestions are: reducing the number of daylight hours that aggressive iguanas are allowed; eliminating contact with conspecifics, both males and females; and slightly reducing environmental temperature. It is important to stress to owners that aggressive behaviour can be normal in iguanas, and that environmental measures designed to modify this behaviour should not be extreme enough to compromise the animal's welfare or cause it stress.

References and further reading

Acierno MJ, Mitchell MA, Zachariah TT *et al.* (2008) Effects of ultraviolet radiation on plasma 25-hydroxyvitamin D3 concentrations in corn snakes (*Elaphe guttata*). *American Journal of Veterinary Research* **69(2)**, 294–297

Ackerman L (1998) *Biology, Husbandry and Health Care of Reptiles, Volume 2. The Husbandry of Reptiles*. TFH Publications Inc., Neptune, NJ

Allen ME and Oftedal OT (1994) The nutrition of carnivorous reptiles. In: *Captive Management and Conservation of Amphibians and Reptiles*, ed. JB Murphy *et al.*, pp. 71–82. Society for the Study of Reptiles and Amphibians, Ithaca, NY

Association of Reptilian and Amphibian Veterinarians (2003) *Salmonella Bacteria and Reptiles: Client Education Handout*. ARAV Special Publications. Available at: www.ARAV.org

Barnard SM (1996) *Reptile Keeper's Handbook*. Krieger, Malabar, FL

Bradley T (2002) Reptile behaviour basics for the veterinary clinician. *Proceedings of the Association of Reptilian and Amphibian Veterinarians Annual Conference*, pp. 165–169

Calvert I (2002) Light – putting the sun in a box. In: *Proceedings of the British Veterinary Zoological Society, Spring Meeting*, pp. 22–27

Chiszar D, Tomlinson WT, Smith HM, Murphy JB and Radcliffe CW (1995) Behavioural consequences of husbandry manipulations: indicators of arousal, quiescence a nd environmental awareness. In: *Health and Welfare of Captive Reptiles*, ed. C Warwick *et al.*, pp. 186–204. Chapman and Hall, London

DeNardo DF (2002) Reptile thermal biology: a veterinary perspective. *Proceedings of the Association of Reptilian and Amphibian Veterinarians Annual Conference*, pp. 157–161

De Vosjoli P (1999) Designing environments for captive amphibians and reptiles. *Veterinary Clinics of North America Exotic Animal* **2**, 43–68

Divers SJ (1996) Basic reptile husbandry, history taking and clinical examination. *In Practice* **18**, 51–65

Divers SJ and Mader DR (2005) *Reptile Medicine and Surgery, 2nd edn*. WB Saunders, Philadelphia

Hernandez-Divers SJ (2001) Clinical aspects of reptile behaviour. *Veterinary Clinics of North America Exotic Animal* **4**, 599–612

Lock B and Bennett A (2015) Changes in plasma testosterone and aggressive behaviour in male green iguanas (*Iguana iguana*) following orchidectomy. *Journal of Herpetological Medicine and Surgery* **25(3–4)**, 107–115

Mitchell MA and Shane SM (2001) Salmonella in reptiles. *Seminars in Avian and Exotic Pet Medicine* **10**, 25–35

Raftery AP (2002) *Pet Owner's Guide to the Bearded Dragon*. Ringpress Books, Dorking

Warwick C (1995) Psychological and behavioural principles and problems. In: *Health and Welfare of Captive Reptiles*, ed. C Warwick *et al.*, pp. 205–238. Chapman and Hall, London

Warwick C, Frye FL and Murphy JB (2013) Miscellaneous factors affecting health and welfare. In: *Health and Welfare of Captive Reptiles*, ed. C Warwick *et al.*, pp. 263–283. Springer Science and Business Media, Dordrecht

Warwick C and Steedman C (1995) Naturalistic *versus* clinical environments in husbandry and research. In: *Health and Welfare of Captive Reptiles*, ed. C Warwick *et al.*, pp. 113–130. Chapman and Hall, London

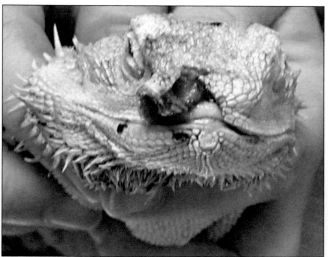

3.12 This inland bearded dragon was injured by a cagemate during feeding time.
(Courtesy of Paul Raiti)

Chapter 4

Nutrition

Matthew Rendle

Veterinary herpetologists have been slow to recognize that nutrition is key in maintaining healthy and reproductively successful animals; this is in no small way owing to a lack of information that is science based rather than extrapolation from personal experience of similar species.

Reptiles will often survive being fed an inappropriate or inadequate diet, sometimes for several years, but many of the medical problems seen in these pet reptiles are to a large extent caused by poor nutrition. However, making an assessment of the diet being fed can be very challenging in some species, who in the wild would show different dietary requirements at different life stages, and this is complicated further as there are often also seasonal alterations in the food eaten in the wild. Replication of these variations is optimal but problematic as nutritional information on even the most commonly kept species in the wild is hard to find, let alone replicate.

Commercially produced diets are available for some species, but it will be some time before we see whether manufacturers' claims of their nutritional content and suitability are established.

It is well established that a more sophisticated approach to nutrition is crucial both to preserving appropriate habitat and to successful captive breeding of many endangered reptiles (Oftedal and Allen, 1996).

Species	Temperature (°C)	Food passage time
Chelonians		
Galapagos tortoise	NR	7–20 days
Lizards		
European wall lizard	NR	33–40 hours
Italian wall lizard	NR	33–40 hours
European green lizard	NR	32–45 hours
Green iguana	27.5	6–8 days
Whiptail lizard	NR	20–23 hours
Snakes		
Burmese python	NR	38 days
Yellow-bellied racer	NR	4 days
Eastern kingsnake	23	3 days
Eastern ribbon snake	21–26	4–5 days
Eurasian water snake	25	6–7 days
Speckled rattlesnake	NR	5–6 days
Tortuga Island rattlesnake	NR	9 days

4.1 Time required for food to pass through the gut in a variety of reptiles (normal gut transit time). NR = not recorded (field data).

Special features of reptile nutrition

Many of the approaches used in the development of suitable diets for other pet species can be applied to reptiles, but there are important additional factors that are not usually encountered in mammals.

Digestion

Gut transit time

Normal gut transit time varies enormously between reptile species (Figure 4.1).

Temperature effects

Environmental temperature can profoundly affect digestive processes in reptiles. An iguana kept at 28°C may eat, but it will not digest its food properly (Lichtenbelt, 1992). Low temperatures also have adverse effects on assimilation in monitor lizards (Buffenstein and Lou, 1982). In the Burmese python, digestive efficiency is not affected by temperature but the rate of digestion is (Wang et al., 2003). Fluctuating temperature can pose particular problems when a reptile like the Hermann's tortoise is kept outdoors at latitudes more northerly than its native habitat. Suboptimal temperatures can lead to maldigestion and bloat or constipation. These can be life-threatening conditions in chelonians as pressure inside the shell tends to compress the lungs and occlude major blood vessels (see Figure 4.8).

Energy requirements

In mammals and birds energy requirements are based on measurements of the basal metabolic rate (BMR). This is defined as energy expenditure when fasted in the dark, resting, and at an environmental temperature identical to the animal's internal body temperature.

Similar measurements have been made for reptiles and amphibians but, because these animals are ectotherms, their body temperature varies with environmental temperature. The reptilian equivalent of BMR is termed the standard metabolic rate (SMR). Because SMR varies with environmental temperature, it should always be quoted for a specific temperature. In the wild the actual daily energy expenditure, field metabolic rate (FMR), is usually 1.25 to 2 times SMR, depending on the reptile's activity level.

The SMRs of reptiles (Figure 4.2) are much lower than the BMRs of birds and mammals of equivalent size: a resting 100 g lizard at 37°C has a metabolic rate that is only about 15% of that of a same-sized mammal resting at the same environmental temperature. In the wild, a lizard may spend 30–70% of the day at a much lower body temperature, further reducing its energy requirements. FMR studies on iguanas have shown that a 100 g lizard has a daily energy requirement that is only 5.5% of that of a similar-sized rodent in the same environment (8.9 kJ/day *versus* 162 kJ/day) (Nagy, 1982). Consequently, reptiles do not need to feed nearly as frequently as mammals. A study of wild green iguanas found that they spent on average only 9 minutes a day feeding, over an observation period of 15 days (Rand *et al.*, 1990).

Captive reptiles usually expend less energy obtaining food than do their wild counterparts, and therefore have even lower energy requirements. Reptile owners often severely overestimate their pets' daily dietary needs; obesity (Figure 4.3) and fatty liver syndrome (see Chapter 17) are commonly encountered, and preventable, causes of morbidity and mortality.

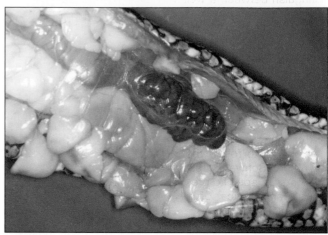

4.3 Coelomic cavity of a pet snake that had been grossly overfed by its owner. Note the large quantities of adipose tissue around the kidneys.

Species	Temperature (°C)	SMR, BMR or FMR (kJ/kg per day)	Allometric equation (kJ/day; M = mass in kg)	Reference
Rodents	37	757.23 (FMR)	757.23 $M^{0.67}$	Nagy (1982)
General placental mammal	37	293.07 (BMR)	293.07 $M^{0.75}$	Kleiber (1961)
General reptile SMR	30	21.69	21.69 $M^{0.80}$	Andrews and Pough (1985)
	30	33.68	33.68 $M^{0.77}$	Bennett and Dawson (1976)
Chelonians				
Desert tortoise	Variable	35.9[a]		Nagy and Medica (1986)
	31	19.9	19.9 $M^{0.75}$ [b]	Barboza (1995)
	30	12.5	12.5 $M^{0.75}$ [c]	
Painted turtle	30	5.28	5.28 $M^{0.33}$	Kepenis and McManus (1974)
Lizards				
General lizard	37	51.37	51.37 $M^{0.82}$	Bennett and Dawson (1976)
Bell's dab lizard	35 $Q_{10} = 2.4$ [d]	87.24	87.24 $M^{0.80}$	Zari (1996)
Eastern fence lizard	35	29.8		John-Alder and Joos (1991)
		54[a]		Angilletta (2001)
Green iguana	Variable	56.27[a]	56.27 $M^{0.80}$	Nagy (1982)
	30	36.78	36.78 $M^{0.734}$	Maxwell *et al.* (2003)
Inland bearded dragon	37	52.85	52.85 $M^{0.80}$	Brand *et al.* (1991)
Namib sanddiver[e]	Variable	167.76[a]		Nagy (1982)
Monitor lizards[e]	35	95.04	95.04 $M^{0.86}$	Thompson and Withers (1994)
		91.6	91.6 $M^{0.84}$	Secor and Phillips (1997)
Snakes				
Boid snakes	20	7.48	7.48 $M^{1.09}$	Galvao *et al.* (1965)
Colubrid snakes	20 $Q_{10} = 2.4$	18.36	18.37 $M^{0.98}$	Galvao *et al.* (1965)

4.2 Some representative SMRs for various reptiles compared with the FMR of a rodent (compiled from a range of species) and the BMR of a general placental mammal. Note the variation between different reptile groups. [a] FMR, data from free-living animals. [b] Maintenance energy requirement measured in tortoises acclimated to outdoor metabolism cages. [c] SMR measured in laboratory. [d] Q_{10} over the 20–30°C range was determined from some groups. [e] These lizards have an active foraging lifestyle and hence higher SMR. BMR = basal metabolic rate; FMR = field metabolic rate; M = mass in kg; SMR = standard metabolic rate. NB: Q_{10} temperature coefficient is a measure of the rate of change of a biological or chemical system as a consequence of increasing the temperature by 10 °C.

Conversely, a well fed reptile can easily survive a one-third loss in bodyweight. Based on SMR values, a 700 kg crocodile would have a large enough calorie store to survive a 2-year fast (Coulson, 1984). It can be difficult to distinguish between a well fed reptile that is undergoing a 'normal fast' and one that is anorexic because of an underlying medical problem.

Chemoreception

Lizards and snakes possess a vomeronasal system which, at least in some species, seems to take precedence over olfaction in triggering feeding responses. When a rattlesnake strikes at a mouse it learns a chemosensory signature of that individual prey item in a split second, and it then prefers to follow the trail of that mouse rather than any others (Schwenk, 1995). Exposure of snakes while still in the egg to specific prey odours can also condition their subsequent choice of prey (Burghardt, 1992; Weldon et al., 1994).

Assessment of growth and body condition

In theoretical terms it is possible to calculate a reasonable estimate of the daily energy requirements of a particular reptile, but applying this information in practice may be difficult. The precise energy content of the actual diet fed may not be known, and there will also always be individual differences in metabolic and digestive efficiency. It is therefore important to record regularly other measures of nutritional status, such as amounts and types of food eaten, weight, snout–vent length (SVL), faecal and urate output, faecal transit time, body condition score, and general feeding behaviour. Such data can help to identify 'changes' at a stage early enough to take corrective measures, and are invaluable in determining whether a reptile is truly anorexic.

Condition scoring

On a basic level it is useful to keep records of gross body condition based on a simple scoring system: 1 = emaciated; 2 = underfed; 3 = normal; 4 = well fed; 5 = obese. In lizards this can be based on the appearance of the tail base (Figure 4.4) or on palpation of the fat bodies. Photographs of the relevant reptile body part(s) alongside a ruler can provide an excellent record that may pick up more subtle changes, in addition to the more obvious visual signs of body condition (Figure 4.5). This sort of assessment is frequently performed by biologists; more detailed information can be found in Bradshaw and Death (1991).

Growth curves

For some species 'normal' growth curves have been determined (Figure 4.6) and can be useful in identifying gross dietary deficiency or excess. Many of these, however, do not distinguish between the sexes, which may grow at different rates and have different energy requirements at different times of the year. Often they also do not quote the temperature at which the animals were kept. The growth of a wild reptile follows a mathematically defined curve (Andrews, 1982), where weight (W) is related to SVL (L) by species-specific coefficients:

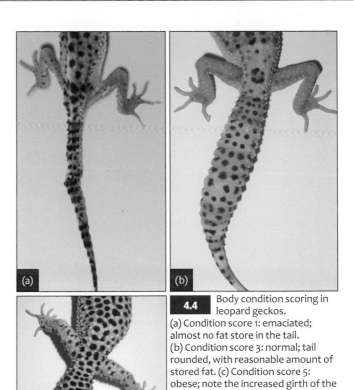

4.4 Body condition scoring in leopard geckos. (a) Condition score 1: emaciated; almost no fat store in the tail. (b) Condition score 3: normal; tail rounded, with reasonable amount of stored fat. (c) Condition score 5: obese; note the increased girth of the legs as well as the tail.

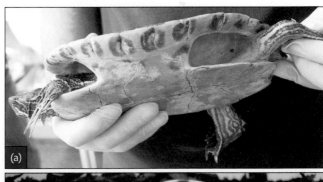
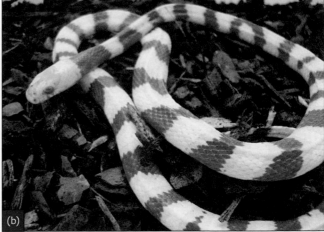

4.5 (a) A malnourished slider and (b) a malnourished snake.

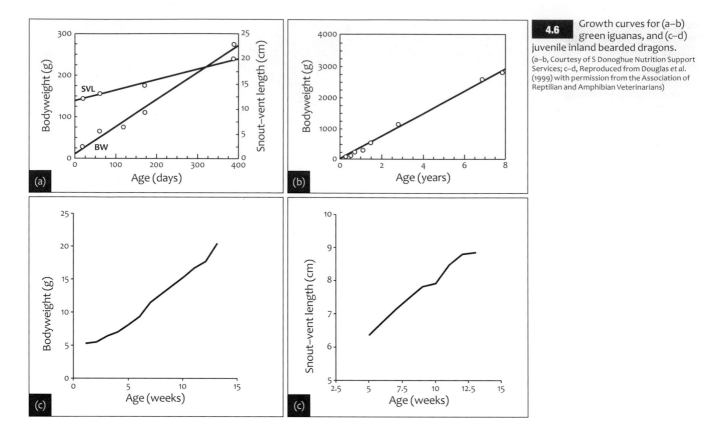

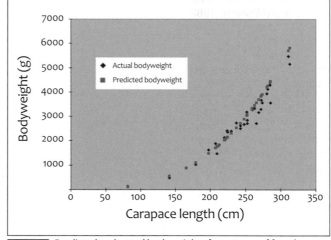

4.6 Growth curves for (a–b) green iguanas, and (c–d) juvenile inland bearded dragons. (a–b, Courtesy of S Donoghue Nutrition Support Services; c–d, Reproduced from Douglas *et al.* (1999) with permission from the Association of Reptilian and Amphibian Veterinarians)

$$W = c \times L^d$$

The coefficients c and d have been determined for a limited number of species; Andrews (1982) contains a useful appendix with growth and size data on a wide range of species.

Chelonians

Jackson's ratio is used to assess body condition in Hermann's and spur-thighed tortoises (Figure 4.7; see also Chapter 6):

$$W = 0.191 \times L^3$$

where W = bodyweight (g) and L is carapace length (cm). It should be noted that the coefficients are species specific. If this equation were used for marginated tortoises, a normal animal would seem to be overweight; a Horsfield's tortoise would seem to be underweight. Equations for these two species have sadly not been formulated yet.

Green iguanas

Donoghue *et al.* (1998) found that in healthy green iguanas bodyweight could be related to SVL by the equation:

$$W = (61 \times SVL) - 859$$

where W is bodyweight (g) and SVL is measured in cm. An even more accurate prediction of adult bodyweight can be obtained using the equation:

$$W = (31.8 \times SVL) + (73 \times TC) + (25.6 \times AG) - (29 \times TBC) - 848$$

where W = bodyweight (g), SVL is measured in cm, TC = right thigh circumference (cm), AG = mid-abdominal girth (cm) and TBC = tail base circumference (cm).

4.7 Predicted and actual bodyweights for a group of female spur-thighed tortoises just prior to hibernation. Data collected at British Chelonia Group tortoise weigh-in.

Water

Although not strictly speaking a nutrient, water is an extremely important part of a reptile's diet. Providing sufficient daily water should be a simple matter, but dehydration, hyperuricaemia and subsequent kidney failure or bladder stone formation (Figure 4.8) are common causes of sickness in captive reptiles. Dehydration is particularly hazardous in herbivores because plants contain large concentrations of potassium ions; accumulation of extracellular potassium ions when kidney tubules are damaged can lead to cardiac problems.

Reptiles have evolved to have accessory excretory glands to deal with excess potassium, such as the nasal and periocular glands.

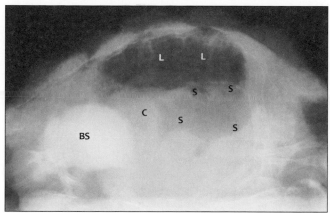

4.8 Respiratory distress in this juvenile Hermann's tortoise was caused by severe constipation and gas production. In this case, failure to provide a suitable source of water appears to have led to the formation of a bladder stone and subsequent intestinal blockage. BS = bladder stone; C = colon; L = compressed lungs; S = stomach outline.

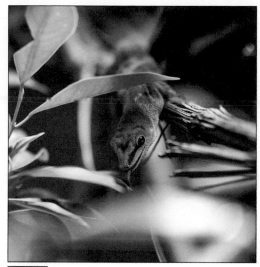

4.9 Green Madagascar gecko drinking.

Requirements

Water turnover rates in the wild (field water budgets) have been determined for a range of lizards and tortoises and indicate a general relationship between water turnover and bodyweight, which can be described by the equation:

$$R = 20.6\ W^{0.84}$$

where R = water turnover or loss (ml/day) and W = bodyweight (kg) (Minnich, 1982). This provides a starting benchmark for average water intake in reptiles of about 20–30 ml/kg per day.

Some desert species are known to exist almost entirely on water metabolized from food, for example dab lizards (Munsey, 1972); some species will also obtain water by transpulmonic absorption from being in burrows that contain high levels of condensation owing to changes in temperature. In some circumstances, requirements may be higher than predicted by the equation, especially if a tropical forest reptile is kept in low humidity and has recently shed its skin. For several days after ecdysis the water permeability of reptilian skin increases dramatically because of the loss of surface lipids. When the calcium intake of birds is increased, water consumption increases up to fourfold; thus, mineral supplementation of reptile diets might increase fluid requirements.

Some herpetology books advocate withdrawing water from anorexic reptiles for several days in the hope that the dehydrated animal will be more willing to eat food to try to satiate its thirst. However, this strategy is very dangerous for those reptiles that excrete waste mainly as uric acid. This is a low-solubility product and crystallizes out of solution easily, causing irreversible damage to kidney tubules when the glomerular filtration rate is severely reduced. Cachexic reptiles should always be suitably hydrated prior to oral alimentation, if necessary by tube feeding water or other fluids or, in more serious cases, by intravenous, intracoelomic or intraosseous fluids (see Chapter 11).

Presentation

In the wild, reptiles such as chameleons, green iguanas, desert lizards and arboreal snakes usually get water by licking droplets of condensation off leaves or from their food (Figure 4.9). These reptiles may ignore dishes containing static water and it is therefore important to spray vegetation or use a drip system, ultrasonic humidifier or misting system to present the water in an appropriate form (see also Chapter 3).

Quality

Some tropical rainforest snakes that would normally drink soft acidic water appear to be reluctant to drink water taken straight from a domestic water supply, possibly because chemicals or dissolved minerals (in hard water areas) alter the taste. Water pH affects mineral content; heavy metals like lead, aluminium, copper and zinc tend to form non-toxic precipitates in alkaline solutions but even low levels can be toxic in acidic solutions (Tucker, 1993). Water intake can often be improved by offering spring water or leaving tap water to stand for several days to allow dissolved gases to be released.

Hygiene

In a heated vivarium, water can soon become contaminated with bacteria, especially if an animal defecates in the water; therefore, regular changes are essential. Some reptiles such as iguanas and blood pythons seem to prefer to defecate in water.

When providing water in static pools it is useful to use a three-bowl system: one in use, one soaking in disinfectant and one bowl drying overnight for use the next day.

When large volumes of water are being sprayed regularly into a vivarium to maintain humidity, problems can arise with *Aeromonas* spp. infections or waterborne parasites. This is best avoided by providing moss-covered drainage in the base of the vivarium. Sphagnum moss has a low surface pH and will help to reduce bacterial growth and retain ammonia in the less toxic ionized form if placed on top of a drainage tray (Barnett *et al.*, 2001).

Reptile trophic groups

For convenience, it is useful to consider reptile diets under the feeding categories of herbivores, omnivores and carnivores. Some reptiles are highly specialized feeders (e.g. the Bengal monitor feeds largely on dung beetles (Auffenberg, 1994)), while others are opportunists with less specific tastes. Some species show changes in dietary preference as they grow. The Gray's monitor even changes its dentition, jaw bones and masseter muscles to cope with its adult diet of specific fruits and molluscs (Auffenberg, 1988). Others are adapted to exploit different food sources and different quantities of food at different times of the year. Generalizations are therefore difficult to make and can be misleading. It is important to always reflect on the wild feeding patterns of the species for which you are trying to provide a balanced and complete captive diet. There is often marked seasonal variation in the available food items. This can be clearly seen in species of European vipers such as the Hungarian meadow viper whose venom becomes more potent during the seasons when it eats rodents and less potent during the seasons when it eats insects. Wherever possible, the formulation of a particular reptile diet should start with reference to field observations, even if the diet cannot be easily replicated in a captive situation. Field studies may at least indicate why problems are being encountered and suggest possible solutions.

None of the diets presented in this chapter should be regarded as definitive; modifications will no doubt need to be made as data from more controlled studies become available.

Herbivore diets

A rough guide to feeding commonly encountered herbivorous reptiles is given in Figure 4.10. Some chelonians and lizards will be almost entirely herbivorous throughout their lives (Figure 4.11), with distinctive dietary requirements.

Herbivorous lizards

The only reptilian herbivore that has been researched in any detail is the green iguana, but much of the information is probably relevant to other reptile herbivores.

A complete chemical (proximate) analysis of a diet used successfully by Philadelphia Zoo for herbivorous reptiles is shown in Figure 4.12 to illustrate current ideas on target levels for various minor dietary components.

Some of the research data have been used to formulate an appropriate iguana diet. This basic 'salad' can probably be used as a basis for other herbivore diets (see Figure 4.10). An extensive discussion on the evolution of iguana diets and practical aspects of iguana feeding can be found in Kaplan (2002). Even an ideal diet will be unbalanced if the reptile selectively eats some components and leaves others, so it is important to present food in a way that prevents this and also to identify components that are not eaten.

Feeding herbivorous reptiles

Average dietary composition (percentage dry matter)

Protein	Carbohydrate	Fat	Crude fibre
13–35%	55–75% (includes fibre)	<10%	15–40%

General principles
Feed herbivores diets that:

- Are HIGH in slowly digested carbohydrate (e.g. cellulose), calcium (juveniles need higher concentrations than adults) and vitamin A
- Have APPROPRIATE amounts of plant-based proteins and are of appropriate energy density. Feed at appropriate frequency
- Are LOW in quickly fermented sugars (e.g. low fruit content), fat, thiocyanates (goitrogens), phosphorus, oxalates and phytates.

Chelonians
Testudo species

- These do best on a mixture of leafy weeds and grasses, e.g. dandelion, clover, plantain, land cress, watercress, coriander, pea leaves and pods, timothy grass, alfalfa. Shop-bought salads often have a high water content compared with home-grown greens and thus have a lower nutritional value on a dry weight basis.
- Fruit should only be a very small part of the diet.
- Based on faecal analysis in the natural habitat, consumption of animal protein is very rare.

Spur-thighed tortoise: wild diet = 30% *Plantago* (plantain), 26% Compositae (daisy family), 10% Rubiaceae (bedstraw family).

Hermann's tortoise: wild diet = 25% Rubiaceae, 22% Leguminosae (pea flower family), 10% Compositae, 8% Ranunculaceae (buttercup family). Seed mixes are available; grow these on limed soil to maximize calcium content.

Horsfield's tortoise: despite difference in habitat, has wild diet similar to Hermann's tortoise, but with high calcium to phosphorus ratio (3.5:1).

Leopard tortoise
This should be given a diet similar to the Mediterranean tortoises but with a higher proportion of grasses; add about 20% of good quality chopped timothy hay or dried alfalfa.

Lizards
Green iguana
A suitable 'iguana salad' consists of:

- 32% carotenoid-containing high-calorie vegetable, e.g. winter squash, red pepper, sweet potato, parsnip. These are low in oxalates and a good source of vitamins A and C. Microwaving the squash improves palatability and digestibility
- 24% green beans and peas, e.g. runner bean, French bean, mangetout, peas in pods. These are a good protein and fibre source, although they contain oxalates and phytates which will reduce available calcium
- 16% alfalfa hay. This is a good protein, fibre and calcium source. (It is very difficult to produce a diet with a high enough protein and low oxalate/phytate content unless alfalfa is used)
- 15% green leafy vegetable, ideally home-grown on calcium-enriched soil, e.g. dandelion, watercress, land cress, spring greens, coriander, Chinese cabbage, kale, broccoli, plantain, mulberry leaves, nasturtium leaves. These are a source of water (iguanas often will not drink from bowls). Use them to increase activity level and stimulate foraging behaviour by distributing them around the vivarium. Try to select greens high in calcium and low in oxalates (see Figure 4.15). Brassicas are nutritious but should be fed in moderation because of their goitrogenic thiocyanate content. Most iguanas also relish flowers: dandelion, nasturtium, pansy, viola, rose and carnation are suitable

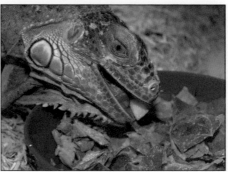
Green iguana

4.10 A rough guide to feeding herbivorous reptiles. (continues) ▶

Feeding herbivorous reptiles

- 4% fruit, e.g. blueberry, cranberry, raspberry, fig, papaya, melon, strawberry, grape, apple, peach, apricot, dates, banana (in skin), tomato. These enhance palatability and provide antioxidants and trace minerals. Feed sparingly, however, as they contain quickly fermenting sugars, which can upset cellulose-digesting bacteria. Figs usually have a high calcium content.

Everything except leafy greens should be served finely chopped and mixed to reduce selective feeding. The mixture can be made up and frozen but should then be used within a month. Thiaminases reduce thiamine in defrosted vegetables; a small amount of vitamin B1 can be added (pure vitamin or brewer's yeast – latter contains high phosphate) if frozen vegetables are used.

Despite attempting to reduce oxalates and use calcium-rich vegetables, it is likely that this diet will still be calcium deficient. Supplement with calcium: 3 g per 100 g wet weight of vegetable mix for juveniles and reproductively active females, or 1 g per 100 g for adults (>2 years). Over-supplementing with calcium can reduce the uptake of other trace minerals and high levels are toxic.

Rhinoceros iguana
Feed 95% green iguana diet (as above) plus 5% animal matter. In the wild they eat a very small amount of insect and vertebrate prey, usually opportunistically.

Prehensile-tailed skink
These lizards are almost totally herbivorous. Feed as green iguanas. In the wild the bulk of the diet is made up of leaves of the creeper *Epipremnum pinnatum* and leaves and fruit of the epiphytic vine *Scindapsus*. Several zoos grow *E. aureum* as a food plant. A colony at

Philadelphia Zoo is fed on a mixture of cos (romaine) lettuce, endives, bananas, apples and hard-boiled egg, at a ratio of 510:340:136:3:1 wet weight, to which is added a comprehensive vitamin and mineral supplement.

These lizards frequently eat their own faeces; this coprophagy may be important for the conservation of cellulose-digesting bacteria.

Spiny-tailed lizards
Feed on:

- Dandelion, nasturtium, pumpkin, pansy and other edible flowers; dandelion greens, watercress, peas, green beans, lentils, sweetcorn, winter squash, carrots, sweet potatoes, kale, spring and turnip greens; alfalfa pellets; and occasional pieces of fruit, e.g. chopped fig
- Some keepers leave a bowl of red and green lentils, yellow and green split peas, millet, sesame seeds, wheat, bee pollen granules and organic cereal grains in the vivarium, although these can cause impaction. A better alternative is to grind this into a coarse powder
- An occasional insect. Field studies showed that insects are eaten occasionally and make up about 1% of the diet.

These lizards maintain high diurnal body temperatures (38–41°C) in the wild, which may be necessary to digest food properly. They tend to eat little and often and are probably adapted to eat a high proportion of dry fruit (seeds). Such diets can be high in oxalates and phytates, and may lower calcium availability. Access to high levels of UVB is therefore crucial.

In the wild, spiny-tailed lizards obtain all their water from food and dew.

4.10 (continued) A rough guide to feeding herbivorous reptiles.

Chelonians
Tortoises
African spurred tortoise, Aldabran tortoise, chaco tortoise, desert tortoise, Egyptian tortoise, gopher tortoise, Hermann's tortoise, Horsfield's tortoise, Indian star tortoise, leopard tortoise, marginated tortoise, pancake tortoise, radiated tortoise, spur-thighed tortoise
Terrapins
Indian roofed terrapin
Turtles
Flatback, green, hawksbill, Kemp's, leatherback, loggerhead and olive ridley turtles. Most of these marine turtles are omnivorous as juveniles but become primarily herbivorous as adults
Lizards
Iguanids (almost all species), prehensile-tailed skink, spiny-tailed lizards

4.11 Reptiles considered to be, almost exclusively, herbivorous.

Nutrient type	Nutrient	Dry matter percentage
Protein/fat/fibre	Crude protein	21%
	Fat	6%
	Crude fibre	13%
Amino acids	Arginine	1.05%
	Cystine	0.54%
	Isoleucine	1.06%
	Lysine	1%
	Methionine	0.4%
	Threonine	0.86%
	Tryptophan	0.2% ▶

Nutrient type	Nutrient	Dry matter percentage
Amino acids *continued*	Tyrosine	0.66%
	Valine	1.2%
Minerals	Calcium	1.0%
	Copper	8 mg/kg
	Iodine	0.3 mg/kg
	Iron	113 mg/kg
	Magnesium	0.2%
	Manganese	40 mg/kg
	Phosphorus	0.7%
	Potassium	2.1%
	Selenium	0.2 mg/kg
	Sodium	0.2%
	Zinc	47 mg/kg
Vitamins	Carotene	69 mg/kg
	Choline	1345 mg/kg
	Vitamin A	3300 IU/kg
	Biotin	0.87 mg/kg
	Folacin (folic acid)	6 mg/kg
	Niacin	61 mg/kg
	Pantothenate	58 mg/kg
	Riboflavin	14 mg/kg
	Thiamine	9 mg/kg
	Vitamin B12	0.029 mg/kg
	Vitamin C	1330 mg/kg
	Vitamin D3	1400 IU/kg
	Vitamin E	21 IU/kg

4.12 Proximate analysis (based on dry matter) of salad diet used by Philadelphia Zoo for herbivorous reptiles. (Data adapted from Bentley *et al.*, 1997)

Fibre

All herbivorous lizards have enlarged proximal colons, with varyingly developed transverse septa (Figure 4.13) that form lunar or semicircular valves in most species (Iverson, 1980). This anatomical development appears to be associated with the development of hindgut fermentation and is believed to slow the movement of fibre (Iverson, 1982). This allows time for cellulose to be digested by bacterial and protozoan symbionts. Large numbers of nematodes (Oxyuridae and Atractidae with direct life cycles) are found in many iguana colons, which has prompted the suggestion that these helminths may also be symbionts that play a role in the mechanical mixing and breakdown of vegetation or even in the regulation of bacterial and protozoan intestinal fauna (Iverson, 1982).

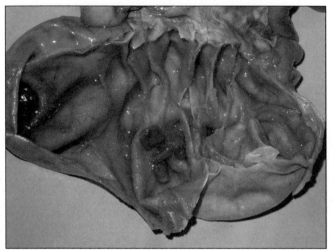

4.13 Iguana colon showing ileocolic valve and transverse septa. Wood chips and other foreign bodies often get trapped in these folds, which can lead to impaction.

The production and absorption of volatile fatty acids from fibre digestion has been documented in several species of iguana (McBee and McBee, 1982) and tortoise (Barboza, 1995). These herbivores are able to derive 23–64% of their digestible energy from fibre, which is the reason why they are able to achieve digestive efficiencies of 35–40% (at least equivalent to mammalian herbivores).

In herbivorous mammals, such as cattle, fibre-digesting microorganisms convert toxic waste produced by the host, such as ammonia and urea, into peptides. This provides extra protein for the cow and reduces the workload on the kidneys. However, peptide production depends critically on the quantity and quality of fibre supplied to the microbes (Webster, 1996). Very little is known about this interplay in the gut fermentation biochemistry of reptiles but it is highly likely that ensuring a similar balance is also important in these herbivores (Foley et al., 1992).

Feeding insufficient dietary fibre or excessive quickly fermented carbohydrates can lead to rapid and detrimental changes in the intestinal bacterial flora in mammalian herbivores, and similar problems are encountered in reptiles; however, energy and dry matter intake in juvenile green iguanas declines when 'neutral detergent fibre' exceeds 24% of dry matter (DM) in diets containing 29% protein (Baer et al., 1997).

Protein

Iguanids studied in the wild show complex foraging strategies, with the diet consisting of 21–70 different plants, depending on species and season. Leaves and berries selected have a significantly higher protein content (20–25% DM) than the average in the environment (Wouter and van Marken Lichtenbelt, 1993). Protein intake also varies with season. Young leaves that develop at the end of the dry season are consumed preferentially and contain high levels of protein.

A study of yearling green iguanas found that increasing the plant protein in the diet produced an increase in growth rate until levels exceeded 30% DM, when no further increase was observed (Donoghue et al., 1998). Whether this level of protein is good for long-term health is not known, but it helps to put an upper limit on the protein requirement.

Although current wisdom suggests that animal protein should not be fed to true herbivores, in the wild herbivorous reptiles are very occasionally observed eating animal protein, often in the form of carrion or mammalian faeces. This may be a response to seasonal dietary impoverishment or just opportunistic. As our knowledge of digestion in herbivorous reptiles is extremely rudimentary and because captive reptiles cannot regulate their own diets, it is probably sensible to only provide plant protein sources, even though field observations may document occasional ingestion of animal proteins.

It is, however, quite difficult to produce diets containing these levels of plant protein using shop-bought vegetables; as the diet must also have high fibre levels, high calcium levels, low oxalate and goitrogen levels, and a suitable energy density, many herbivorous reptiles simply fed on shop-bought 'greens' are likely to be receiving very deficient diets.

Excessive purine production as a result of high protein intake has been suggested as a cause of hyperuricaemia and kidney failure in herbivorous reptiles. Although plausible, there are very few controlled scientific studies that have addressed this issue (e.g. Christian and Torregrosa, 1986) and this is unlikely to be a problem in home-produced plant-based diets. The effect of proteins on kidney function in a wide range of animals has recently been reviewed by Singer (2003). It is likely that herbivorous reptiles would very occasionally feed on animal protein, normally in the form of carrion, but it is not advisable to suggest this to owners with emaciated reptiles as a method for weight gain as it will inevitably result in large amounts of inappropriate animal protein being regularly fed.

Some literature suggests that there is a developmental shift in the food requirements of herbivorous reptiles, with juveniles having a higher protein requirement which can only be supplied by the ingestion of animal-based food. Consequently, owners may be wrongly advised to practise supplementary feeding with insects or with cat and dog food. Although supplying extra protein for growth sounds logical, studies with wild iguanas have shown that juveniles achieve this end by a different strategy. They select plant material higher in digestible protein and digest the food 1.3 times more rapidly than adults. Shorter transit times are achieved by maintaining higher body temperatures (Troyer, 1984).

Calcium and phosphorus

The importance of feeding diets with calcium:phosphorus ratios >2:1 is often stressed because of the frequent occurrence of metabolic bone disease in reptiles (see Chapter 22). Details of the composition of a wide range of cultivated vegetables and fruit can be accessed easily via the Internet (Figure 4.14). Although these lists are widely quoted, the tables contain average values that can vary widely

Information source	Description
Dr Duke's Phytochemical and Ethnobotanical Databases: https://phytochem.nal.usda.gov	Contains links to a range of plant databases containing data compiled mainly by the United States Department of Agriculture (USDA). Data on most food plants can be accessed. NB: figures are *averages*, and composition varies with soil, fertilizer and watering
USDA Food Composition Databases: http://ndb.nal.usda.gov	Provides access to the USDA National Nutrient Database for Standard Reference, containing detailed analysis of the average composition of a huge range of foods
Guinea Lynx Oxalic Acid Chart: http://www.guinealynx.info/diet_oxalic.html	Short list of common plants containing oxalic acid

4.14 Internet sources of useful nutritional information. NB: web addresses may change but sites should then be located using search engines.

depending on the location and soil type on which the plant is grown and the season. One approach to this problem is to grow food plants (e.g. dandelions) in soil that has been treated with lime to maximize calcium uptake. Alternatively, mineral supplements can be added to the diet.

Phytotoxins

Many plants produce toxic chemicals to deter browsing by herbivores; levels tend to be highest in older leaves. Several phytotoxins have important adverse nutritional effects. It is almost impossible to produce varied diets that contain none of these compounds, but careful selection of foods can reduce their levels.

Oxalates and phytates: These are important as they chelate calcium and inhibit its uptake from the intestine. Addition of high-oxalate plant material to the diet is a common way in which owners unwittingly cause considerable reduction in the effective calcium content of the food ration. Parsley, spinach, spring (or collard) greens and cos (romaine) lettuce are commonly used vegetables that have relatively high oxalate contents (Figure 4.15). Phytates found in cereals and legumes reduce the uptake of phosphorus, calcium and iron.

Goitrogens: Hypothyroidism can be a problem if the diet contains large amounts of thiocyanate-containing brassicas (broccoli, kale, cabbage, Brussels sprouts, bok-choi) or soya-based products such as tofu. Hypothyroidism is more commonly encountered in large herbivores; e.g.

Oxalate content	Food source
Very high oxalate (>1.00 g/100 g)	Cassava, chives, parsley, purslane
High oxalate (0.51–1.00 g/100 g)	Beet leaves, spinach
Medium oxalate (0.26–0.50 g/100 g)	Brussels sprouts, carrots, dandelions, French beans, spring (collard) greens, cos (romaine) lettuce, radish, watercress
Low oxalate (0.10–0.25 g/100 g)	Asparagus, aubergine, broccoli, cabbage, cauliflower, celery, chicory, endive, sweet potato, turnip
Very low oxalate (<0.10 g/100g)	Coriander, cucumber, kale, okra, onion, parsnip, pea, pepper (capsicum), potato, squash, sweetcorn, tomato, turnip greens

4.15 Oxalate content of some commonly fed plants.

cabbage leaves are often used as a cheap, easily available source of food for giant tortoises. Fed in moderation, however, brassicas are a nutritious food source and some varieties, such as spring greens, usually have reasonably high calcium levels.

Herbivorous chelonians

Many chelonians are almost completely herbivorous but different groups appear to vary with respect to their preferred fibre intake. The Mediterranean tortoises are essentially browsers of herbaceous plants and consume a wide range of these in the wild. They seem to do best when allowed to roam in well planted gardens. It is now possible to buy seed mixes that enable owners to grow collections of wild flowers that appear to be relished by and safe for tortoises, and these are a good way of providing dietary variety that is pesticide-free. However, no research has been done on the energy content and chemicals these plants contain. If using such mixes it is probably sensible to grow them in containers using soil from different locations to which extra lime has been added to maximize trace mineral content in the diet.

The leopard and African spurred tortoises of the African savannah are thought to require a higher fibre diet than Mediterranean tortoises, based on a higher intake of grasses and hays. Some keepers recommend that 70–75% of the diet should be grass based, but studies on the leopard tortoise in the wild indicate that some populations may eat a higher percentage of herbaceous plants (Kabigumila, 2000). The same study also usefully determined the average growth rate of these tortoises in the wild (7 mm/month as juveniles and subadults; 5.7 mm/month in adult females and 3.2 mm/month in adult males; measured as increase in carapace length); this provides a useful reference point for assessing the effect of diet on growth in captive specimens.

Giant Aldabran and Galapagos tortoises should also do best on high-fibre diets, considering the available food in their island habitats; however, adapting captive tortoises to new diets can be difficult (Wright *et al.*, 1997). Surprisingly, Horsfield's tortoise, which lives on the Russian Steppe, eats very little grass; like the Mediterranean tortoises, in the wild it eats mainly herbaceous plants. However, the Horsfield's tortoise is unusual because extreme conditions in its native habitat limit its activity to just 3 months of the year. Even during its active season it spends 90% of the time inactive, and usually only feeds for about 15 minutes each day (Lagarde *et al.*, 2002, 2003). It has been estimated that even in a good year this tortoise will spend less than 20 hours in feeding activity! Obesity is therefore likely to be a problem with this tortoise in captivity. Growth rates in the wild have been documented by Lagarde *et al.* (2001).

Omnivore diets

Reptiles that normally live in food-rich environments tend to be selective feeders, whereas those from impoverished environments, such as deserts, are often omnivores. Active foragers are often specialists, whereas more sedentary animals have more varied tastes (Pianka, 1986). It is possible to predict a lizard's trophic group from intestinal length (Figure 4.16).

Many lizards and a few chelonians are omnivorous. Some are omnivores from birth, while others change their dietary intake at different life stages. Several species of

Trophic group	Whole intestine	Small intestine	Large intestine
Herbivores	293	195	97
Omnivores	184	129	55
Insectivores	131	87	34

4.16 Length of the intestine as a percentage of body length in different trophic groups of lizards.
(Data from Skoczylas, 1978)

turtle are carnivorous as juveniles but predominantly herbivorous as adults (Ernst and Barbour, 1989; Bjorndal and Bolton, 1990), such as the Giant Asian pond turtle. The inland bearded dragon is primarily insectivorous as a juvenile but changes to a diet that includes about 20–50% plant material as an adult (Greer, 1989; Macmillan *et al.*, 1989). Day geckos eat both insects and fruit as adults. A rough guide to feeding omnivorous reptiles is provided in Figure 4.17.

Feeding omnivorous reptiles

Average dietary composition (percentage dry matter)

Protein	Carbohydrate	Fat
15–40%	20–75%	5–40%

General principles
Information on the dietary requirements of omnivores is often confusing. This reflects both ignorance and the variety of dietary strategies that span the continuum between herbivory and carnivory. Dietary requirements may vary for different life stages and sexes, and in different seasons. In addition, variation in the dietary preferences of individuals within the same species undoubtedly exists. Offering a varied, well balanced diet is, in theory, the best strategy, but this does not always guarantee that the reptile will eat appropriately. Omnivores therefore need careful monitoring to avoid dietary imbalances and excess.

Chelonians
Hingeback tortoises
Feed:

- 80% vegetable matter: 'iguana salad' (see Figure 4.10) without alfalfa but with mushrooms. Alfalfa is not required as a protein source and would probably provide too much fibre; add calcium carbonate as part of a vitamin supplement. Fungi form an important component of the wild diet
- 20% slugs, snails, millipedes, woodlice, earthworms, waxworms, spiders.

Expected dry matter intake at 30°C is 5 g/kg.

Box turtles

- In the wild, box turtles are opportunistic omnivores. Wild diet = earthworms, snails, grubs, dung beetles, caterpillars, grasshoppers, cicadas, grasses, fallen fruit, berries, mushrooms, flowers, herbaceous plants.
- They tend to feed in the morning and are attracted to yellow and orange foods. They can be finicky feeders and it may take several weeks to implement dietary changes.
- Vitamin A deficiency is common; ensure diet contains a good proportion of beta-carotene containing plants.
- Take care with cage substrate, as this may be eaten.

Eastern box turtle: Feed:

- 50–70% animal matter: millipedes, woodlice, snails, beetles, slugs, earthworms, waxworms, spiders, 'pinkie' mice, crickets, caterpillars
- 30–50% vegetable matter: 70–80% as 'iguana salad' (see Figure 4.10) without alfalfa but with mushrooms
- 20–30% fruit and flowers, e.g. berries, melon, peach, pear, apple, plum, fig, tomato and edible flowers.

Ornate box turtle: This is more carnivorous than the Eastern box turtle. Feed:

- 90% animal matter
- 10% green leafy vegetable matter.

Malayan box turtle: More aquatic than other box turtles; it is assumed to be omnivorous but in the wild it seems to eat mainly vegetation. Requirements for animal matter still to be determined. Suggest feed green leafy diet plus aquatic plants (e.g. duckweed, *Elodea*, water hyacinth) plus 10–20% animal matter.

Red-eared terrapin
Feed:

- 60–70% animal matter: *Zophobas*, crickets, waxworm larvae,

earthworms, *Tubifex*, water snails, raw (whole) small fish, trout or low-fat dog-food pellets. Avoid the use of raw or cooked meats, especially for juveniles, as these contain very little calcium. NB: *Tubifex* and water snails may harbour parasites
- 20–30% green leafy vegetables or aquatic plants.

Several commercially produced foods are available (see text). Wild diet = snails, slugs, insects, crayfish, other aquatic invertebrates, tadpoles, small fish, carrion, algae and aquatic plants. Younger terrapins are more carnivorous than adults and become more herbivorous as they mature. Aquatic plants such as duckweed, water lettuce and water hyacinth, plus other aquatic and bog plants, form a substantial portion of the adult diet.

Feed adults 2–3 times a week and no more than can be consumed in 30–40 minutes. Ideally, feed in a separate tank to avoid water contamination.

Painted turtle and musk turtle
Both these have similar dietary requirements to the red-eared terrapin. To ensure that aquatic reptiles get vitamin supplements, a chopped mixture of animal food, greens and vitamin supplement powder can be mixed with gelatin solution, allowed to set and then cut into cubes for feeding. These can be frozen for later use.

Lizards
Asian water dragon
Asian water dragons are mainly carnivorous but adults eat a small amount of vegetable matter. Feed:

- 80–95% animal matter: varied insect diet (feed high-fat insects, e.g. waxworms, sparingly), earthworms, spiders, millipedes, woodlice, snails, small fish, very occasional 'pinkie' mouse
- 10–15% vegetable matter: very finely chopped 'iguana salad' (see Figure 4.10).

These lizards can store large quantities of fat and are easily overfed; feed adults every 3 days and monitor weight.

Inland bearded dragon
Feed:

- 60% varied insect diet
- 40% finely chopped 'iguana salad' (see Figure 4.10).

Feed juveniles (<6 months) 5-times a week and adults 3-times a week. Studies in the wild suggest that the adult diet is 20–50% vegetable matter. As obesity is a common problem it is probably best to feed a relatively high proportion of vegetable matter unless gravid.

Blue-tongued skink
Feed:

- 50% vegetables: peas/beans in pods, root vegetables, chopped green leaves and stalks
- 25% whole, minced or chopped rodents. Dog food (of low-fat type) can be substituted and giant mealworms fed occasionally. Also, occasionally feed a few live crickets to stimulate exercise
- 25% soft fruit.

Two or three meals a week should be adequate. These lizards are prone to obesity, so weight should be monitored carefully by the owner.

Pink-tongued skink
This is a specialist mollusc feeder. Feed:

- 80% snails and slugs
- 20% chopped greens and vegetables.

Shingleback skink
This has a very varied wild diet. Feed fruit, green leafy vegetables, a wide range of invertebrates and an occasional 'pinkie' mouse.

4.17 A rough guide to feeding omnivorous reptiles. (continues) ▶

Feeding omnivorous reptiles

Plated lizards

Feed:

- 50% insects and small rodents
- 50% 'iguana salad' (see Figure 4.10), small amounts of fruit occasionally.

Tegus

These lizards are the New World equivalent of monitors, but their diet has a substantial vegetarian component. Feed:

- 50% rodents, small insects (e.g. crickets, mealworms), low-fat dog food
- 50% fruit.

A commercial tegu diet has been produced. Juvenile tegus generally require more protein than adults. Take care when feeding as these animals bite.

Veiled chameleon

Feed:

- 85–95% insects and other invertebrates (as for other chameleons)
- 5–15% vegetable matter: chopped green leafy herbaceous plant matter, e.g. the mix fed to Mediterranean tortoises or 'iguana salad' (see Figure 4.10).

Lives in mountainous desert regions where daytime temperatures reach 38°C. Insects are scarce and young chameleons grow slowly. Metabolic bone disease (see Chapter 22) commonly occurs if growth is too rapid and diet is calcium deficient. High UVB and calcium supplementation are essential. Adults survive by consuming some plant matter as well as animal matter; high body temperatures may be necessary for digesting plant matter. The chameleon obtains water by licking dew.

4.17   (continued) A rough guide to feeding omnivorous reptiles.

Investigations

Food intake has been investigated extensively to explain omnivory as a dietary strategy in birds and mammals (Krebs, 1978) but very little research has been done on reptiles.

Omnivorous tortoises

A study by Hailey *et al.* (1998) on the omnivorous Speke's hingeback tortoise, which feeds on fungi, leaves and invertebrates, provides useful insights and illustrates how omnivorous diets can be investigated (Figure 4.18). This African tortoise has a much shorter large intestine and gut retention time than herbivorous tortoises, and a poor ability to process coarse vegetation (Hailey, 1997). Most animals forage for diets that maximize energy intake. On this basis, the Speke's hingeback tortoise should prefer to eat fungi, as these provide most energy (69 kJ/kg/day, compared with 42 and 31 kJ/kg/day for leaves and millipedes, respectively). However, it chooses to eat a mixture even when fungi are present in excess. Total consumption was limited by dry mass intake (5 g/kg/day at 30°C), rather than energy or wet mass. This is similar to the consumption reported for the desert tortoise (4.6 g/kg/day (Nagy and Medica, 1986)).

Omnivory may arise because the most energy-rich food is in short supply, contains dose-dependent toxins or is deficient in specific nutrients, or because other foods enhance the digestion of the optimal food (Bowen *et al.*, 1995). In the Speke's hingeback tortoise, eating a mixture reduced digestive efficiency related to energy intake (measured as the apparent digestive coefficient for energy intake) from 74% to 64%. Further analysis found that nutrient deficiency provided the best explanation for the diet. The gross protein contents of fungi, leaves and invertebrates were similar, but fungi contain limited amounts of essential amino acids (Crisan and Sands, 1978). Mineral content differed quite considerably: calcium was low in leaves and even lower in fungi, but quite high in millipedes. Calcium is known to be deficient in herbivorous diets for tortoises and this is probably the reason why tortoises ingest bones or soil (Marlow and Tollestrup, 1982; Esque and Peters, 1994). High potassium:sodium dietary ratios may also be an important constraint in animals that eat vegetation, especially when this is in their growth phase (Belovsky, 1978; Nagy and Medica, 1986); this has been suggested as the reason why leopard tortoises seek out and eat soils high in sodium (Hailey and Coulson, 1996). In addition to their calcium content, millipedes also have a higher sodium:potassium ratio than fungi and leaves and may therefore help to provide additional sodium. The results indicate that African millipedes are eaten to provide scarce minerals and possibly amino acids, but can probably be replaced by appropriate mineral supplementation or other calcium-rich invertebrates.

Measurements of digestibility are extremely useful when trying to provide a suitable diet for reptiles, since they may highlight crucial dietary elements that need to be replicated or modified, and are part of the database that commercial food manufacturers should provide to support the efficacy of their diets.

Based on phylogeny it is likely that the *Kinyxis* genus of hingeback tortoises arose from herbivorous ancestors and has adapted to a habitat where vegetation is seasonal and deficient in calcium by becoming omnivorous. The yellow-footed and red-footed tortoises occupy a similar ecological niche in South America and consume large quantities of fruit in addition to fungi and animal protein (Moskovits and Bjorndal, 1990). Environments with high humidity and easy access to water seem to be important requirements of omnivorous tortoises, which may be related to the higher dietary protein levels and the need to flush more uric acid out through the kidneys.

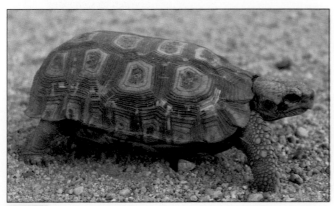

4.18   Hingeback tortoise.

Omnivorous lizards

Inland bearded dragons seem to be primary insectivores that can digest and utilize vegetable matter annually when prey becomes scarce owing to the hot and harsh environment. They may therefore represent the opposite end of the omnivorous spectrum. Figure 4.19 proposes a diet of watercress and crickets. Studies comparing commercial food for inland bearded dragons with two other diets containing different proportions of crickets and watercress were carried out by Mobray and Smith (1999). While the diets could all supply reasonable amounts of energy, the apparent digestibility of nitrogen was poor, especially when there was a high proportion of watercress. These results suggest that protein type and availability may be important factors in designing appropriate diets for these lizards. Witz and Lawrence (1993) reported an apparent digestive coefficient of 83% for domestic crickets in a six-lined racerunner lizard, so some species may be more efficient at digesting chitin. It is important to consider species variation in a food item's bioavailability, especially if the prey item is not eaten in the wild.

In some situations limited protein intake may be beneficial in captive lizards. Limited nitrogen consumption inhibits the development of prehibernatory ovarian follicles in the desert tortoise (Henen and Oftedal, 1999), whereas egg production is stimulated when these tortoises have protein reserves (Henen, 2002). If this situation is true for other reptiles, as in birds (Drent and Daan, 1980), then regulating protein intake might be a useful way of either stopping or stimulating the production of ovarian follicles (Figure 4.20). Owners of omnivorous reptiles often struggle to feed vegetable matter as they tend to anthropomorphise the positive reaction and increased activity they get at the time they feed insects and other animal based proteins to their pets; most omnivorous reptiles are hardwired to seek out animal protein as it represents high levels of energy compared with vegetable matter. This anthropomorphic tendency can lead to obesity and metabolic bone disorder.

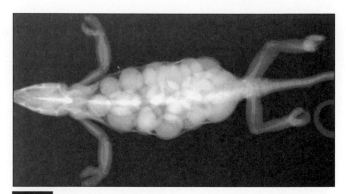

4.20 Chameleon with retained eggs.

Carnivore diets

Reptilian carnivores can be divided into those that feed largely on vertebrates and those that feed primarily on invertebrates. Feeding frequency needs to be related to the age of the animal and metabolic requirements. There are also quite marked differences in feeding frequency in different snake genera (Figure 4.21). A rough guide to feeding carnivorous reptiles is provided in Figure 4.22.

Variety of snake	Feeding interval
Pythons	*Python:* 40 days (longer for giant species)
Boas	*Lichanura:* 30 days *Boa:* 35 days
Pit vipers	*Crotalus:* 38 days
Colubrids	*Pituophis:* 14 days *Lampropeltis:* 12 days *Masticophis:* 10 days *Coluber:* 8 days

4.21 Average feeding intervals observed in adult wild snakes. (Data from Secor and Diamond, 2000)

What quantity of watercress and crickets should be fed to a juvenile male 100 g inland bearded dragon?

- Diet should be ~80% invertebrates and ~20% vegetable matter on an 'as fed' basis.
- Energy content of 80 g crickets = 392.8 kJ (calculated from Figure 4.26). Energy content of 20 g watercress = 9.2 kJ (see Figure 4.14), but watercress can vary widely in water content; dandelions seem to have a more consistent water content. Energy content of mixture = 402 kJ.
- If digestibility of diet is assumed to be 80%, the metabolizable energy content (ME) = 321.6 kJ/100 g = 3.22 kJ/g.
- SMR of bearded dragons is 0.109 ml O_2/h/g (Brand *et al.*, 1991) at 37°C = 261.6 ml O_2/day per 100 g. For an omnivore, the energy equivalent of 1 ml O_2 = 20.43 J, so SMR = 5.34 kJ/day.
- Assume needs of 1.5 SMR in captivity = 8.01 kJ/day. Thus, 8.01/3.22 = 2.49 g of mix should be fed per day per 100 g bodyweight = 1.99 g of crickets and 0.5 g of watercress per day.

Owners commonly feed 4–5 times this amount, which may explain why fatty livers are common in this species. In some situations it is helpful to get owners to feed every other, or every third, day as a way of reducing the calorific intake.

If this were an adult lizard it would be better to increase the ratio of crickets to greens to 50:50. (Assuming ~70% digestibility, the energy content of a mix of 100 g crickets plus 100 g watercress is theoretically 1.9 kJ/g, and for a similar dandelion mix is 2.4 kJ/g.)

Notes
- When feeding calculated diets it is essential to check the animal's weight on a regular basis. Weight loss indicates that calculated levels are inadequate and might also indicate that vivarium temperature is too high. Weight gain could indicate the reverse.
- Inland bearded dragons are fairly sedentary, so exercise levels are likely to be low and energy requirements are probably about 1.25 SMR for adults, although calorific requirements can rise to 2 x SMR in a female producing eggs.
- It is important to recognize that although this sort of diet can provide adequate energy levels it may be deficient in other components. The digestibility of plant protein, for example, may be much lower than that of animal protein.
- Very little research has been done on captive diets for inland bearded dragons, so the optimal components for the plant-based portion of the diet are unknown. A multicomponent leafy greens salad as used for green iguanas (see Figure 4.10) may provide a more balanced diet with a higher overall digestibility.
- The invertebrate component should be varied, using cockroaches, mealworms, earthworms, spiders, isopods and others (de Vosjoli and Mailloux, 1993) to ensure an adequate supply of essential amino acids.
- Most diets will be calcium deficient and can be improved by the addition of calcium carbonate or other calcium salts, but this often reduces palatability and it is difficult to ensure known intake.

4.19 Feeding inland bearded dragons.

Feeding carnivorous reptiles

Average dietary composition (percentage dry matter)

Protein	Carbohydrate	Fat
25–60%	<10%	30–60%

General principles

These are generally the easiest reptiles to feed. Try to vary the food of insectivorous lizards and ensure that fat-rich food (e.g. waxworms) does not form the major part of the diet.

Chelonians

Mata mata

In the wild feeds almost entirely on fish, but can be trained to eat mice.

Snapping turtles

Feed mice, chicks and fish. Juveniles also eat insects and other aquatic invertebrates. There is some evidence that adults also eat small amounts of aquatic plants.

Lizards

Insectivorous lizards

These include skinks, whiptails, lacertids, zonures and most chameleons. The veiled chameleon also eats small quantities of vegetation (see Figure 4.17).

- General diet for insectivorous lizards: flies, cockroaches, crickets, grasshoppers, locusts, silkworms, snails, spiders, millipedes, woodlice, mealworms, giant mealworms (*Zophobas* sp.), waxworms, Mediterranean flour moths (*Anagasta kuehniella*), hawkmoth caterpillars (e.g. *Manduca sexta*), stick insects, praying mantids. Most species lose appetite if fed the same insects continually. Variety can be enhanced by using different foods to 'gut load' crickets.
- Some species will also take small earthworms.
- Some of the larger species will take beetles.

Try to feed a much wider range of invertebrates than those commonly sold by pet shops. Some insect species can be obtained as eggs from specialist companies and reared for food; fruit flies and house flies are also relatively easy to culture, as are snails. Others can be obtained by sweep netting countryside vegetation during the summer months (ensure the area has not been treated with herbicides or insecticides). Calcium-rich invertebrates, such as snails, spiders, millipedes and woodlice, are usually easy to obtain. Millipedes and woodlice can be easily cultured in bins of leaves and vegetable waste, to which calcium carbonate can be added. The pill millipede *Glomeris marginata* is a particularly good source of calcium.

- Feed ground-dwelling lizards in a separate bare-floored vivarium, as ingestion of vivarium substrates and subsequent gut impaction is a common occurrence.
- Feed chameleons by placing prey in small plastic open-topped containers.
- Avoid feeding prey with hard exoskeletons that are larger than the distance between the lizard's eyes.

Geckos

Most species are insectivores (see above). Do not feed insects that are too large, as they may attack the lizard. Remove any uneaten crickets and fruit from the enclosure after a few hours. Calcium supplementation is essential; add to food or leave a small dish of a ground calcium source in the vivarium.

Tokay gecko: These also eat small rodents and lizards.

Day geckos: Feed:

- 90% insects
- 10% soft fruits (e.g. papaya, banana, peach, mango, melon) or baby food fruit purée. Nectar foods formulated for lorikeets can also be fed instead of fruit.

Anoles, basilisks and desert spiny lizards

These are primarily insectivores but many species (especially the larger ones) will also eat small amounts of fruit and greens.

Collared lizards

These are mainly insectivorous but in the wild also prey on small lizards.

Monitor lizards

These large lizards are mainly opportunistic carnivores and scavengers (although one species, Gray's monitor, is a frugivore).

Savannah monitor:

- Normally fed on various life stages of mice, day-old chicks and the occasional egg. There is some debate as to whether this is an appropriate diet, as it differs markedly from the wild diet (see below).
- Often ignore small insects. Feed large species, e.g. locust, black field cricket, Argentinean wood cockroach.
- Juvenile African land snails and Roman snails are useful additions.
- Will also eat fish.

Wild diet = beetle larvae, beetles, millipedes and centipedes early in the wet season, replaced by orthopterans (grasshoppers) later in the year; also mantids, hymenopterans, lepidopterans, scorpions, snails, crustaceans, amphibians, and eggs of agamids and of their own kind. During the height of the wet season, ingested food may be 10% of bodyweight.

In some locations these lizards undergo long seasonal fasts from December to late May, living off accumulated body fat. Obesity is a common problem and periods of fasting may be helpful.

Spiny-tailed monitor: This very small monitor feeds mainly on invertebrates (particularly orthopterans and beetles) and other lizards (geckos, agamids and skinks). Feed an insect-based diet with the occasional small mouse. They are known to be cannibalistic in captivity but can usually be kept in small groups of similar-sized animals.

Slow worm

Slow worms should be fed soft-bodied invertebrates, especially slugs and earthworms.

Snakes

Garter snakes and Eurasian water snakes

These live in wetland habitats and feed largely on fish and amphibians. They will usually adapt to feeding on thawed frozen fish or fish strips, or freshly killed small fish, e.g. goldfish, guppies, swordtails. Thiamine deficiency can occur if fed on improperly defrosted fish. Commercial diets can be used and appear to provide appropriate nutrition.

Green snakes

The comments on feeding invertebrate-eating lizards probably also apply to these snakes. Unlike mammal-eating snakes, it is likely that these diurnally active snakes also require UVB light or a vitamin D source.

Rough green snake: Feed crickets and other insects, woodlice, millipedes, earthworms.

Smooth green snake: Feed insects and spiders.

Oriental green snake: Feeds largely on earthworms.

Snail-eating snakes

These snakes have specially adapted jaws that enable them to extract snails from their shells. They will usually accept *Helix* garden snails.

Hognose snakes

These eat frogs and especially toads. The western and dusky subspecies can usually be converted to rodents.

Ratsnakes, gopher snakes, bullsnakes, pine snakes, racers and whipsnakes

Feed: mice, small rats, birds (usually nestlings).

Indigo snake, kingsnakes and milk snakes

These feed mainly on lizards and other snakes in the wild, but can usually be converted to mice and birds if this is done soon after hatching. In some areas indigo snakes also consume small turtles.

Pythons and boas

Feed: mice, rats, rabbits and piglets (depending on the size of the snake). Calorific requirements are about 2.5 times less than those of the commonly kept colubrids (see Figure 4.2).

Egg-eating snakes

Feed raw hens' eggs. Will need biotin supplement to counteract anti-vitamin avidin in unfertilized eggs.

4.22 A rough guide to feeding carnivorous reptiles.

Diets comprising vertebrates

Most, though not all, snakes prey on other vertebrates. In the wild, a common pattern is for juveniles to feed on lizards, amphibians or invertebrate prey and then to switch to mammals and/or birds after reaching a larger size (Rodríguez-Robles and de Jesús-Escobar, 1999; Rodríguez-Robles, 2002).

Feeding live vertebrate prey is unethical, and can lead to severe bite injuries to the snake. Most snakes will eat dead prey, provided it is thoroughly defrosted, warm and dry. If food is rejected, freshly killed prey can sometimes stimulate a feeding response, as can exposing the brain tissue or viscera of a defrosted rodent. Olfactory manipulation can be used, for example, in bird-eating species (such as green tree pythons). Applying feathers or yolk from a day-old chick to a rodent will improve acceptability, or rubbing rodents on dampened pieces of sloughed lizard skin for juveniles that prefer to eat lizards (such as kingsnakes). An alternative strategy is to put cotton wool soaked in mouse flavouring close to hatching eggs. Various scenting strategies have been discussed by Burghardt (1992) and Weldon et al. (1994).

The time at which food is offered can also be important, as some species are primary nocturnal or diurnal feeders.

Rodents

In captivity many snakes will usually eat various life stages of mice or rats, and a proximate analysis of these is detailed in Figure 4.23. Using SMRs and data from proximate analysis, it is possible to construct spreadsheets that predict feeding requirements (Figure 4.24), but these should always be correlated with data from the particular animal as there is bound to be variation in both the energy density of food items and individual digestive efficiency. There are quite marked differences in the energy requirements of colubrids compared with pythons and boids (Galvao et al., 1965), and quantities fed need to reflect these differences.

Royal pythons are commonly regarded as difficult feeders, although this is often because owners have previously kept more active colubrids that feed more frequently. Like other pythons, the royal is a sit-and-wait predator but tends to be a nocturnal feeder. It spends long periods in underground burrows, and inappropriate husbandry can lead to non-feeding. In the wild it preys on rodents related to gerbils and jerboas; prey acceptance can be improved by using olfactory manipulation, such as scenting a mouse with some used bedding from a gerbil cage or some feathers from a bird. Offering various types of rodents will often tempt a reluctant reptile to feed; species such as the Natal multimammate mouse (*Mastomys natalensis*) are readily available frozen from pet stores and are highly palatable in some species such as blood pythons. In the wild some snake species have refused to change their preferred diet even in the face of a population crash and when a plentiful supply of other suitable mammalian prey was available (Diller and Johnson, 1988).

Birds

Green tree pythons and South American tree boas are reputed to eat a high proportion of birds in the wild, and the feeding of feathered prey has been advocated to prevent constipation. However, a study has shown that in the wild the main diet of the emerald tree boa is arboreal rodents, although birds are occasionally taken (Stafford and Henderson, 1996). Constipation is more likely to be caused by dehydration (these snakes drink rainwater from their coils and ignore water in bowls) and inactivity (Figure 4.25). Defecation can often be stimulated by allowing the snake to swim in shallow lukewarm water.

Fish

The availability of appropriately sized and good-quality fish has improved recently, and they can be purchased from most good angling shops. Whole fish are similar in nutrient

Food item	Mass (g)	Length (cm)	Water (%)	Protein (% DM)	Fat (% DM)	Ash (% DM)	Vitamin A (IU/kg DM)	Vitamin E (IU/kg DM)
Mouse								
'Pinkie'	1.7	3	82	64.2	15.2	9.7	35,533	39.1
'Fuzzie'	3.8	3.7	70.8	41.8	46.7	8.4	16,933	40.7
'Crawler'	6.5	4.7	69	46.6	46.6	8.5	16,667	47.9
Medium	14.8	7	69.7	58.6	19.9	17	59,033	40.4
a'Normal'	25.5		65.8	51.8	26	15.3		
Large	36.2	8.2	62.9	45	32.1	13.6	287,033	55.2
Rat								
'Pinkie'	10	5.2	79.2	57.9	23.7	12.2	21,333	470.4
Small	54.1	12.6	70	56.1	27.5	14.8	45,633	143.1
Large	256.9	19.9	65.2	51.3	35.1	8.8	335,300	152.3
Others								
Chick	b30		77.6	64.7	13.9	8.9	35,600	51,300
Smelt	b12		84	67.6	18.2	9.1		
Frog	c12		77.5	71.18	10.23	13.43	25,109	82.22

4.23 Proximate analysis of vertebrate prey commonly used to feed snakes and lizards. DM = dry matter. a 'Normal' = averaged from medium and large data.

(Data from Douglas et al., 1994, except for b Allen and Oftedal, 1994 and c Schairer et al., 1998)

Feeding requirements of colubrid snakes									
	C	D	E	F	G	H	I	J	K
Calculation		C^0.98	D x 18.37	E x 7	F x 1.4[a]	F/6.09[b]	G/6.09	G/3.77	I x 1.5
	Weight (kg)	Scaled weight	Standard metabolic rate (SMR) (kJ/day) at 20°C	Energy requirement (kJ/wk) at 20°C	Energy requirement (kJ/wk) at 25°C (Q10 for snakes for 20–30°C = 2.4)	Estimated minimum requirement for maintenance (g fresh mouse or rat per wk) at 20°C	Minimum requirement (g mouse per wk) at 25°C	Lafeber – Emeraid Carnivore required (ml/wk) at 25°C (4 kJ/ml), minimum for anorexic snake[c] (frequency of feeding will be dictated by the species)	Food requirement to allow for growth (g mouse per wk); SMR x 1.5 at 25°C
	0.1	0.1	1.92	13.47	18.86	2.21	3.10	5.00	4.64
	0.15	0.16	2.86	20.03	28.04	3.29	4.60	7.44	6.91
	0.175	0.18	3.33	23.3	32.62	3.83	5.36	8.65	8.03
	0.25	0.26	4.72	33.05	46.27	5.43	7.60	12.27	11.40
	0.3	0.31	5.65	39.52	55.33	6.49	9.09	14.68	13.63
	0.35	0.36	6.57	45.96	64.34	7.55	10.57	17.07	15.85
	0.4	0.41	7.48	52.39	73.35	8.6	12.04	19.46	18.07
	0.45	0.46	8.4	58.8	82.32	9.65	13.52	21.84	20.28
	0.5	0.51	9.31	65.19	91.27	10.7	14.99	24.21	22.48
	0.55	0.56	10.23	71.58	100.21	11.75	16.46	26.58	24.68
	0.6	0.61	11.14	77.95	109.13	12.8	17.92	28.95	26.88
	0.65	0.66	12.04	84.31	118.03	13.84	19.38	31.31	29.07
	0.7	0.71	12.95	90.66	126.92	14.89	20.84	33.67	31.26
	0.75	0.75	13.86	97	135.80	15.93	22.30	36.02	33.45
	0.8	0.8	14.76	103.33	144.66	16.97	23.75	38.37	35.63
	0.85	0.85	15.67	109.66	153.52	18.01	25.21	40.72	37.81
	0.9	0.9	16.57	115.98	162.37	19.04	26.66	43.07	39.99
	0.95	0.95	17.47	122.29	171.21	20.08	28.11	45.41	42.17
	1	1	18.37	128.59	180.03	21.11	29.56	47.75	44.34
	1.5	1.49	27.33	191.33	267.86	31.42	43.98	71.05	65.98
	2	1.97	36.23	253.64	355.10	41.65	58.31	94.19	87.46

4.24 This spreadsheet can be used to estimate how much to feed a growing male corn snake, or the quantity of an enteral preparation to feed an anorexic colubrid snake. Such tables should always be used in conjunction with regular weighing of the animal, and modified as necessary. Spreadsheet analysis helps to produce a scientifically based estimate which provides at least a rational starting point for evaluating a snake's diet. A similar sheet can be produced for pythons and boids by substituting 'C^1.09' in the calculation in column D and 'D x 7.48' in column E. Column G refers to a 'normal' mouse (see Figure 4.23) and will need to be modified based on the type of rodent fed. By substituting values for 'pinkies', a similar chart can be produced as a guide to feeding juveniles. *Note that the values are temperature dependent.* The average Q_{10} for snakes is 2.4 (Andrews and Pough, 1985); this value can be used as a multiplier to estimate standard metabolic rate (SMR) at a different temperature. [a] Original determination of snake SMR done at 20°C; as preferred temperature zone for colubrids is ~25°C, an adjustment has to be made for the increased temperature. Q_{10} values for snakes for 20–30°C is 2.4; as this is a figure based on a logarithmic scale, the value for a 5°C increase is ~1.4. [b] This figure is calculated from normal mouse data in Figure 4.23. [c] Before starting the feeding plan dehydration and/or hypovolemia must be corrected. Emeraid is an excellent semi-elemental diet for short-term use but it is not a balanced diet. ^ = Excel symbol for 'to the power of'. NB: Q_{10} temperature coefficient is a measure of the rate of change of a biological or chemical system as a consequence of increasing the temperature by 10 °C.

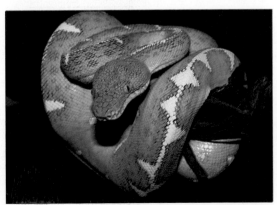

4.25 Tree boas and pythons perch with coils that trap rainwater from which they drink.

composition to small mammals, but fat content can vary widely with species and season. Many species have high levels of the fat-soluble vitamins A, D and E. However, the polyunsaturated fatty acids in fish undergo rapid oxidation after death, which quickly depletes the vitamin E content (Allen and Baer, 1989). Nutrient quality can also decline rapidly, secondary to bacterial spoilage, if the fish is not stored at low temperatures soon after being caught. The flash freezing of fish in small batches can maintain the nutritional content. Steatitis and fat necrosis secondary to vitamin E deficiency has been recorded in alligators fed poor-quality fish (Larsen *et al.*, 1983). Thiaminases can also degrade thiamine when fish are defrosted, which can lead to deficiencies; this tends to be a problem of saltwater fish which are used as reptile food as they are cheap and readily available (see Chapter 22).

Special requirements

Obligate mammalian carnivores such as cats are known to have specific nutritional requirements. Extrapolating from these, it would be expected that carnivorous reptiles that feed on vertebrate prey are likely to require diets that have elevated levels of arginine, methionine, cystine and taurine, vitamin A, niacin, and linoleic and arachidonic acids. However, experiments with green anoles and red-eared terrapins indicated that neither has the expected elevated requirement for arginine (Coulson and Hernandez, 1970). Similarly, adding taurine to the alligator diet described by Brisbin et al. (1990) did not improve the growth of hatchling and juvenile alligators (Kercheval and Little, 1990). Another study showed that bullsnakes can synthesize adequate amounts of niacin (Bartkiewicz et al., 1982). Staton (1990) found that alligator growth was improved by adding arachidonic acid to the diet, but the requirement for linoleic acid was more equivocal. Based on these limited studies, it seems prudent to exercise care with extrapolations from mammalian carnivores until more information is available.

In practice, nutritional problems with reptiles that feed on whole vertebrate prey are relatively uncommon, provided the food is fed uneviscerated and unfasted and has not been frozen for excessively long periods. The visceral organs are a source of trace minerals (e.g. copper, zinc, iodine, calcium, phosphorus, magnesium) and fat-soluble vitamins (A, D, E), and the ingesta are a source of vitamins B12, C and K. However, diet can considerably affect trace mineral composition of rodents, and some may be deficient in copper and manganese (Dierenfeld and Barker, 1995).

Spontaneous skin rupture secondary to vitamin C deficiency has been documented in snakes (Frye, 1991) as a result of being fed fasted mice.

Diets comprising invertebrates

A few reptiles, e.g. thread snakes and blind snakes, are specialist insectivores that feed mainly on ants and termites. Others, like the more commonly encountered green snakes, are usually more generalist feeders; insects form a large proportion of the diet of the North American rough and smooth green snakes, while mainly earthworms are eaten by the Asian species. Among lizards, a few species, e.g. North American horned lizards, are primarily ant feeders. However, most carnivorous lizards are generalist invertebrate consumers, although, like the snakes, some are active foragers and others are sit-and-wait predators. The more sedentary predators are likely to have lower SMRs than active ones and feed less frequently.

Some montane chameleons seem to be the reptile equivalent of sloths, in that they feed less frequently and maintain bodyweight on smaller quantities of food than more active lizards like the lacertids, although SMRs have not yet been measured in this group. When satiated, chameleons are fairly sedentary but they become quite active and restless when hungry. Like a number of other lizards, some chameleons seem deliberately to reduce their metabolism during certain months of the year, even when given access to a hot basking spot within the vivarium (Davidson, 1997). In the wild this is probably a mechanism for dealing with seasonal food paucity, driven by endogenous hormonal factors that persist even in captivity. Inland bearded dragons show similar behaviour. This is related to a period of aestivation that they undergo in the wild during the hottest part of the year when food is scarce. Similar fasts occur in other reptiles (see Chapter 22).

Nutrients

Analysis of a wide range of insects indicates that they are potentially a good source of protein, potassium and magnesium, a variable source of sodium and iron, and usually a poor source of calcium and vitamin A (Studier and Sevick, 1992). Given the opportunity, many insectivores will supplement their diets with other invertebrates. Spiders, millipedes, isopods (woodlice) and gastropods are excellent sources of calcium. Earthworms are a variable source of calcium and are eaten by many species (Reichle et al., 1969). A study of the Trinidad gecko showed that it ate invertebrates from at least 16 different orders, with females selecting a higher proportion of gastropods, reflecting higher calcium demands (Miranda and Andrade, 2003). In several species studied in the wild there is ecological partitioning of habitat and food resources between different age groups. Juvenile lacertid lizards feed mainly on orthopterans (e.g. grasshoppers) and spiders, whereas adults concentrate on beetles and isopods (Angelici et al., 1997).

Studies on chickens and rats have suggested that arginine and methionine may be limiting amino acids in diets based on Mormon crickets (Anabrus simplex) and mealworms (Tenebrio molitor) (Finke et al., 1989). Tryptophan levels are also low in both insects, and cysteine levels are low in crickets. The addition of methionine to fly larvae meal improved the growth of rats fed on this diet (Onifade et al., 2001).

In the wild some lizards appear to select insect prey based on species rather than size; this probably reflects a need to ensure adequate amino acid intake (Magnussen and Da Silva, 1993). Seasonal changes in the abundance of particular insects and dietary selection will also increase variation in the diet (Allen et al., 1993). Some lizards appear to have colour preferences for prey. For example, feeding crickets on alfalfa or Spirulina powder turns them green and seems to make them more acceptable to some chameleons.

In contrast, captive lizards are often fed on a very restricted range of insects and it is then important to improve amino acid and mineral content prior to feeding. Analysis of the commonly fed house cricket Acheta domestica shows that both adults and newly hatched 'pinhead' crickets contain levels of magnesium, manganese, iron, copper and zinc that would be adequate to meet the dietary requirements of mammals, and are also good sources of protein. However, they are a poor source of calcium and vitamin A, in common with other insects, although 'pinheads' contain considerably higher levels of calcium than adults (Barker, 1997). More recent studies indicate that silk moth larvae and stick insects fed on mulberry leaves accumulate high levels of calcium, vitamin E and fibre (Dierenfeld, 2001). If this were reproducible, irrespective of the plant's location, these insects would have considerable potential as food for captive insectivores. Proximate analysis of commonly fed invertebrates is shown in Figure 4.26. Some of the commonly fed insects, e.g. waxworms, are high in fat and should not be fed in excess.

Owners should feed the widest range of insects possible; in the summer collecting insects from local fields by taking sweepings using an entomology net can be a useful source of a variety of insects, but it is of paramount importance to get permission to take the sweepings from the landowners and also to make sure no pesticides are being used in the area. These swept insects should be fed without delay to prevent the inevitable loss of their nutritional value.

Species	Water	Protein (% of DM)	Fat (% of DM)	Carbohydrate (% of DM)	Total ash (% of DM)	Ca (mg/kg DM)	Mg (mg/kg DM)	Cu (mg/kg DM)	Fe (mg/kg DM)	Mn (mg/kg DM)	Zn (mg/kg DM)	Vitamin A (IU/kg DM)	Vitamin E (IU/kg DM)	Carotenoids identified
Mealworm Tenebrio molitor	62.9 ± 3.6	51.8 ± 5.3	31.1 ± 3.9	12.8	4.3 ± 3.7	0.1 ± 0.1	0.3 ± 0.02	17.7 ± 4.7	39.7 ± 19.2	6.8 ± 4.2	131 ± 7	811 ± 324	30 ± 3	None
Super mealworm Zophobas morio	57.0 ± 1.4	42.9 ± 1.4	40.8 ± 2.3	12.8	3.5 ± 0.6	0.12 ± 0.2	0.2 ± 0.02	13.9 ± 3.1	50.3 ± 6.5	1.5 ± 0.6	88 ± 4	972 ± 570	32 ± 6	NA
Waxworm Galleria mellonella	61.9 ± 2.1	41.1 ± 2.8	51.4 ± 5.4	4.2	3.3 ± 1.0	0.06 ± 0.01	0.1 ± 0.01	3.1 ± 1.3	77.3 ± 13.1	3.3 ± 0.8	79 ± 6	150 ± 160	509 ± 23	Lutein, zeaxanthin
House cricket Acheta domestica	73.2 ± 1.9	64.1 ± 2.2	22.8 ± 1.5	6	5.1 ± 1.4	0.21 ± 0.03	0.1 ± 0.01	8.5 ± 1.0	112.3 ± 58.1	30 ± 5	186 ± 16	811 ± 849	81 ± 41	Beta-carotene
Pinhead cricket	62.9 ± 11.2	55.1 ± 3.4	9.8 ± 1.4	23.9	11.2 ± 8.2	2.1 ± 2.7	0.2 ± 0.06	10.4 ± 1.1	224 ± 91	56 ± 22	157 ± 20	628 ± 600	80 ± 46	
Locust Melanopus[a]	71	58	30	12		NA	NA	NA	NA	NA	NA			
Grasshopper (wild)		NA	NA		NA	NA	NA	NA	NA	NA	NA	1034 ± 1327	NA	Beta-carotene, lutein, canthaxanthin
American cockroach	66.7	10.16												
Silkworm larvae Bombyx mori[a]		54	43	3	0.5	0.5								
Fruit fly Drosophila melanogaster	67.2 ± 4.3	56.3 ± 0.8	16.7 ± 2.1		5.3 ± 0.8	0.2 ± 0.02	0.1 ± 0.03	7.3 ± 3.6	473 ± 41	16.1 ± 2.7	158 ± 82	0	16 ± 7	
Dung beetle	53.3 ± 1.4	62.6 ± 3.4	12.3 ± 1.7		3.1 ± 0.8	0.1 ± 0.01	0.1 ± 0.01	20.7 ± 5.3	238 ± 51	61.1 ± 25.4	128 ± 8	192 ± 171	57 ± 35	Phytofluene, carotenes
Earthworm Lumbricus terrestris (commercial)	75.8 ± 4.8	50.4 ± 9.4	10.6 ± 1.7		24.9 ± 11.4	1.2 ± 0.03	0.2 ± 0.03	8.1 ± 1.7	5802 ± 2324	113 ± 51	231 ± 56	328 ± 171	229 ± 8	None
Earthworm (wild-caught)	74.5 ± 2.0	32.2 ± 6.6	2.6 ± 1.0		45.7 ± 6.6	1.0 ± 0.3	0.3 ± 0.03	32.9 ± 18	11087 ± 2938	199 ± 45	271 ± 89	2400 ± 279	70 ± 12	
Snail												317 ± 569	NA	Beta-carotene, lutein, zeaxanthin

4.26 Proximate analysis of commonly fed invertebrate prey, mean ± SD. DM = dry matter; NA = data not available. (Data from Dierenfeld and Barker, 1995; [a] Additional values from Donoghue, 1995)

Commercial diets

Commercially produced formulated diets could, in theory, provide a way of ensuring that reptiles get a correctly balanced diet; several diets are available. Many commercial diets claim to be nutritionally complete but, in the absence of scientifically tested and agreed recommended daily allowances, such claims are questionable.

Formulated diets have been used successfully to raise green iguanas commercially in Costa Rica and as part of a conservation plan for captive Galapagos land iguanas (Oftedal and Allen, 1996). Juvenile inland bearded dragons fed a formulated diet achieved higher bodyweights compared with those fed on a cricket and vegetable diet; however, the formulated diet contained 46.9% protein *versus* 22% in the latter (Douglas *et al.*, 1999).

In contrast, one study that measured growth rates in green iguanas on three commercial diets compared with a greens and salad diet, found that dry matter intake and growth were reduced in the animals fed commercial diets (Donoghue, 1994). This may in part relate to palatability problems and animals having difficulty recognizing the material as food. The latter is a particular problem in the context of diets for carnivorous species, where visual and olfactory cues are essential triggers for feeding responses. One solution currently being tested is to expose developing eggs to specific odours that are incorporated into the commercial diet so that neonates more easily recognize the diet as food. Point light sources played over the food will often illicit a chase-and-eat response in insectivorous lizards. Some species of snake seem to take 'mouse sausage' made from minced rodents, and one product is designed to help prevent thiamine deficiency in garter snakes. Acceptance is usually best in all carnivores when the diet is fed from birth.

Quality control is an issue with commercial products, since two studies have found that the actual dietary content did not always correspond to what was declared on the label (Hurty *et al.*, 2001). Ideally, all nutritional products sold for reptiles should be independently regulated so that owners can be assured of both the quality of the product and of the scientific research on which the formulation is based.

Dietary supplementation

Daily requirements

Although supplementation of the diets of captive herbivorous and insectivorous reptiles is likely to be necessary, very little research has been done to establish specific daily nutrient needs. Optimal supplementation levels are likely to vary with gross diet, age, body size, sex, activity level, physiological state, health status, concurrent drug therapy and other factors. Allen and Oftedal (1994) have proposed a set of minimum nutrient levels for carnivorous reptiles (Figure 4.27) based on recommended dietary amounts (RDAs) for other carnivores, and Philadelphia Zoo has published a proximate analysis of the diet formulated by its nutritionists for reptile herbivores, which is based on extrapolation from RDAs of other herbivores. At the moment these are estimates which will no doubt be refined in the light of further research.

Nutrient	Minimum dietary level
Crude protein	30–50%
Ether extract	10–15%
Linoleic acid 3	1.0%
Arginine	1.00%
Isoleucine	0.50%
Lysine	0.8%
Methionine + cystine	0.75%
Threonine	0.70%
Tryptophan	0.15%
Calcium	0.8–1.0%
Copper	5–8 ppm
Iodine	0.3–0.6 ppm
Iron	60–80 ppm
Magnesium	0.04%
Manganese	5 ppm
Phosphorus	0.5–0.9%
Potassium	0.4–0.6%
Selenium	0.1–0.3 ppm
Sodium	0.2%
Zinc	50 ppm
Vitamin A	5000–10,000 IU/kg
Biotin	70–100 ppb
Choline	1250–2400 ppm
Folate	200–800 ppb
Niacin	10–40 ppm
Pantothenate	10 ppm
Riboflavin	2–4 ppm
Thiamine	1–5 ppm
Vitamin B12	20 ppb
Vitamin B6	1–4 ppm
Vitamin C	Reptiles are thought to be able to synthesize sufficient quantities of vitamin C from intestinal microflora but during periods of chronic illness dosages of 10–20 mg/kg/feed may be beneficial
Vitamin D	500–1000 IU/kg
Vitamin E	100 IU/kg

4.27 Suggested minimum nutrient levels in diets of captive carnivorous reptiles. Amounts are on a dry matter basis. ppb = parts per billion; ppm = parts per million. (Data from Allen and Oftedal, 1994)

Calcium

Calcium deficiency is a common problem in both herbivores and insectivores. Precise calcium requirements have not been determined for most reptiles, and extrapolations are usually made from studies on birds and domestic mammals. These advise 1.8–3 mg of calcium per kilocalorie of metabolizable energy, or about 1% of the dry matter (Arnaud and Sanchez, 1990). A study (van der Wardt *et al.*, 1999) of Drakensberg crag lizards found that calcium balance was maintained in this species when calcium uptake was 1.4–5.6% of dry matter intake, which is slightly higher than the levels used for poultry. In contrast, Allen (1989a,b) found that growth and calcium retention could be met by calcium at 0.85% of dry matter intake in leopard geckos, similar to that recommended for growing kittens. This subject is discussed in more detail in Chapter 22.

There are two main methods of supplementation of calcium. One method is dusting: all food items are placed in a bag and high-calcium powder added. The items are coated and hopefully some powder will remain on the food items until ingestion. This, in practical terms, is not always that reliable as the powder often falls off. The second, and in the author's opinion the more suitable, method is to feed naturally high-calcium plants for herbivores, and for insectivores the feeder insects should be provided with an appropriate high calcium diet (and water) at all times. The second method does require a level of protein intake that mimics the wild diet. Species such as green iguanas and bearded dragons would, in the wild, have what appears to be a low-protein diet that most owners would consider impoverished. However this low-protein diet allows a growth rate that the volume of ingested calcium can support. Both these methods must be used in conjunction with the provision of light in the UVB spectrum (see Chapter 22).

Vitamin D3 is very unstable and although it is often present in reptile supplements, it is at an inappropriately low level and is denatured very quickly by heat and light. If supplementation with oral D3 is administered at the same time as naturalistic levels of UV light this is likely to result in ectopic calcification, which can be hard to diagnose and impossible to remobilize.

Complex supplements

While many of these supplements are likely to help correct deficiencies in captive diets, in the absence of scientific data documenting tissue nutrient levels and long-term feeding effects in controls and animals fed a particular supplement, it is difficult to give any firm recommendations. Product manufacturers should be able to supply documented evidence to provide assurance of quality control, efficacy, tolerance and safety (Bauer, 2001).

Many vitamins are relatively labile chemicals and contact with moisture and trace minerals will catalyse oxidation, leading to reduced activity. Tamper-proof expiry dates ought therefore to be an important feature of these products. Independent assessment of both the quality and efficacy of products for reptiles is rare, and so it is important to obtain products from trusted sources. Commercial reptile foods and supplements have been found to differ in content from the label (Donoghue and Dzanis, 1995). Equally importantly, the product should not contain toxic substances such as heavy metals, pesticide residues, hormones, nitrosamines, mycotoxins or toxic levels of nutrients.

Several multivitamin–multimineral products aimed specifically at reptiles are available and appear to reduce the number of issues in most species. However, this is reliant on owners using the supplement at the recommended level, and ideally they should be bought in small quantities so, once opened, they are used within a month, and during this time stored appropriately, i.e. in a fridge or at least in a dark area out of direct sunlight.

Probiotics

Probiotics fall into a similar category to vitamin and mineral supplements. Anecdotally and clinically, these appear to be beneficial in some situations, particularly when dietary upsets are present or during the administration of antibiotics. Probiotics appear to be beneficial in herbivorous

and omnivorous reptiles, but are considered of limited use in carnivorous reptiles that consume whole vertebrae prey, such as mammals and birds. However, their efficacy in humans, where controlled studies have been conducted, is disputed (Atlas, 1999). So far no efficacy studies have been conducted in any veterinary species.

Until appropriate studies have been carried out it is probably best to keep an open but critical mind, which is probably equally true for many areas of reptile nutrition.

References and further reading

Abate A (1997) Nutrition. Part IV: vitamins, minerals and other nutrients from supplementation. *Chameleon Information Network Bulletin* **25**, 9–25

Allen ME (1989a) Nutritional Aspects of Insectivory. PhD dissertation, Michigan State University

Allen ME (1989b) Dietary induction and prevention of osteodystrophy in an insectivorous reptile *Eublepharis macularius*: characterisation by radiography and histopathology. *Third International Colloquium on the Pathology of Reptiles and Amphibians*, pp. 83–84

Allen ME (1997) From blackbirds to thrushes … to the gut-loaded cricket: a new approach to zoo animal nutrition. *British Journal of Nutrition* **78**, S135–S143

Allen ME and Baer DJ (1989) Fat soluble vitamin concentrations in fish commonly fed to zoo animals. *Proceedings of the American Association of Zoo Veterinarians*, p. 104

Allen ME and Oftedal OT (1994) The nutrition of carnivorous reptiles. In: *Captive Management and Conservation of Amphibians and Reptiles*, ed. JB Murphy et al., pp. 71–83. Society for the Study of Amphibians and Reptiles, Ithaca, NY

Allen ME, Oftedal OT and Ullrey DE (1993) Effect of dietary calcium concentrations on mineral composition of fox geckos (*Hemidactylus garnoti*) and Cuban tree frogs (*Osteophilus septentrionalis*). *Journal of Zoo and Wildlife Medicine* **24**, 118–128

Andrews RA and Pough FH (1985) Metabolism of squamate reptiles: allometric and ecological relationships. *Physiological Zoology* **58**, 214–231

Andrews RM (1976) Growth rate in island and mainland anoline lizards. *Copeia*, 477–482

Andrews RM (1982) Patterns of growth in reptiles. In: *Biology of the Reptilia, Volume 13*, ed. C Gans and FH Pough, pp. 273–319. Academic Press, London and New York

Andrews RM (1984) Energetics of sit-and-wait and widely-foraging lizard predators. In: *Vertebrate Ecology and Systematics – A Tribute to Henry S. Fitch*, ed. RA Siegel et al., pp. 137–145. University of Kansas, Lawrence, KS

Angelici FM, Luiselli L and Rugiero L (1997) Food habits of the green lizard, *Lacerta bilineata*, in central Italy and a reliability test of faecal pellet analysis. *Italian Journal of Zoology* **64**, 267–272

Angilletta MJ (2001) Variation in metabolic rate between populations of a geographically widespread lizard. *Physiological and Biochemical Zoology* **74**, 11–21

Arnaud CD and Sanchez SD (1990) Calcium and phosphorus. In: *Present Knowledge in Nutrition, 6th edn*, ed. ML Brown, pp. 212–223. Nutrition Foundation, Washington DC

Atlas RM (1999) Probiotics: snake oil for the new millennium? *Environmental Microbiology* **1**, 377

Auffenberg W (1988) *Gray's Monitor*. University of Florida Press, Gainesville, FL

Auffenberg W (1994) *The Bengal Monitor*. University of Florida Press, Gainesville, FL

Avery RA (1970) Utilization of caudal fat by hibernating common lizards, *Lacerta vivipara*. *Comparative Biochemistry and Physiology* **37**, 119–121

Baer DJ, Oftedal OT and Rumpler WV (1997) Dietary fibre influences nutrient utilization, growth and dry matter intake of green iguanas (*Iguana iguana*). *Journal of Nutrition* **127**, 1501–1507

Barboza PS (1995) Digesta passage and functional anatomy of the digestive tract in the desert tortoise (*Xerobates agassizii*). *Journal of Comparative Physiology B* **165**, 193–202

Barker D (1997) Preliminary observations on nutrient composition differences between adult and pinhead crickets (*Acheta domestica*). *Bulletin of the Association of Reptilian and Amphibian Veterinarians* **7(1)**, 10–13

Barnett SL, Cover JF and Wright KM (2001) Amphibian husbandry and housing. In: *Amphibian Medicine and Surgery*, ed. K Wright and B Whitaker, pp. 35–61. Krieger, Malabar, FL

Bartkiewicz SE, Ullrey DE and Trapp AL (1982) A preliminary study of niacin needs of the bull snake (*Pituophis melanoleucus sayi*). *Journal of Zoo Animal Medicine* **13**, 55–62

Bauer JE (2001) Evaluation of nutraceuticals, dietary supplements, and functional food ingredients for companion animals. *Journal of the American Veterinary Medical Association* **218**, 1755–1760

Belovsky GE (1978) Diet optimization in a generalist herbivore: the moose. *Theoretical Population Biology* **14**, 105–134

Bennett AF and Dawson WR (1976) Metabolism. In: *Biology of the Reptilia, Volume 5*, ed. C Gans and WR Dawson, pp. 127–223. Academic Press, New York

Bentley A, Toddes B and Wright K (1997) Evolution of diets for herbivorous and omnivorous reptiles at Philadelphia Zoo: from mystery towards science. *Proceedings of the Nutrition Advisory Group*, pp. 65–74

Bentley PJ and Schmidt-Nielsen K (1966) Cutaneous water loss in reptiles. *Science* **151**, 1547–1549

Bjorndal KA and Bolton AB (1990) Digestive processing in a herbivorous freshwater turtle: consequences of small intestine fermentation. *Physiological Zoology* **63**, 1232–1247

Bowen SH, Lutz EV and Ahlgren MO (1995) Dietary protein and energy as determinants of food quality: trophic strategies compared. *Ecology* **76**, 899–907

Boyer TH and Boyer DM (1993) Breeding season anorexia in snakes. *Bulletin of the Association of Reptilian and Amphibian Veterinarians* **3(1)**, 6

Bradshaw SD and Death G (1991) Variation in condition indexes due to climatic and seasonal factors in an Australian desert lizard, *Amphibolurus nuchalis*. *Australian Journal of Zoology* **39**, 373–385

Brand MD, Couture P, Else PL, Withers KW and Hulbert AJ (1991) Evolution of energy metabolism. *Journal of Biochemistry* **275**, 81–86

Brisbin LI, McCreedy CD, Zippler HS and Staton MA (1990) Extended maintenance of American alligators on a dry formulated ration. In: *Crocodiles: Proceedings of the 10th Working Meeting of the Crocodile Specialist Group of the Species Survival Commission of the IUCN*, pp. 16–31. IUCN – World Conservation Union, Gland, Switzerland

Bronikowski AM (2000) Experimental evidence for the adaptive evolution of growth rate in the garter snake *Thamnophis elegans*. *International Journal of Organic Evolution* **54**, 1760–1767

Buffenstein R and Lou G (1982) Temperature effects on bioenergetics of growth, assimilation efficiency and thyroid activity in juvenile varanid lizards. *Journal of Thermal Biology* **7**, 197–200

Burghardt GM (1992) Prior exposure to prey cues influences chemical prey preference and prey choice in neonatal garter snakes. *Animal Behaviour* **44**, 787–789

Christian K and Torregrosa D (1986) Effect of diet on nitrogenous wastes of the iguana *Cyclura nubila*. *Comparative Biochemistry and Physiology A* **85**, 761–764

Coulson RA (1984) Metabolic rate and habit in reptiles. *Symposia of the Zoological Society of London* **52**, 155–176

Coulson RA and Hernandez T (1970) Nitrogen metabolism and excretion in the living reptile. In: *Comparative Biochemistry of Nitrogen Metabolism, Volume 2: The Vertebrates*, ed. JW Campbell, pp. 639–710. Academic Press, New York

Crisan EV and Sands A (1978) Nutritional value. In: *The Biology and Cultivation of Edible Mushrooms*, ed. ST Chang and WA Hayes, pp. 137–168. Academic Press, New York

Davidson LJ (1997) *Chameleons, Their Care and Breeding*. Hancock House, Surrey, British Columbia

de Vosjoli P and Mailloux R (1993) *The General Care and Maintenance of Bearded Dragons*. Advanced Vivarium Systems, Lakeside, CA

Dierenfield ES (2001) Some preliminary observations on herbivorous insect composition: nutrient advantages from a green leaf diet? *Proceedings of the Comparative Nutrition Society*, p. 99

Dierenfield ES and Barker D (1995) Nutrient composition of whole prey commonly fed to reptiles and amphibians. *Proceedings of the Association of Reptilian and Amphibian Veterinarians Annual Conference*, pp. 3–15

Diller LV and Johnson DR (1988) Food habits, consumption rates, and predation rates of western rattlesnakes and gopher snakes in southwestern Idaho. *Herpetologica* **44**, 228–233

Donoghue S (1994) Growth of juvenile green iguanas (*Iguana iguana*) fed four diets. *Journal of Nutrition* **124**, 2626S–2629S

Donoghue S (1995) Clinical nutrition of reptiles and amphibians. *Proceedings of the Association of Reptilian and Amphibian Veterinarians Annual Conference*, pp. 16–37

Donoghue S and Dzanis DA (1995) Evaluating commercial diets. *Proceedings of the Association of Reptilian and Amphibian Veterinarians Annual Conference*, pp. 74–82

Donoghue S, Vidal J and Kronfeld D (1998) Growth and morphometrics of green iguanas (*Iguana iguana*) fed four levels of dietary protein. *Journal of Nutrition* **128**, 2587S–2589S

Douglas KE, Saker KE, Smith SA, Robertson JL and Holladay SD (1999) A preliminary feeding study in bearded dragon lizards *Pogona vitticeps*. *Bulletin of the Association of Reptilian and Amphibian Veterinarians* **9(3)**, 42–46

Douglas TC, Pennino M and Dierenfeld ES (1994) Vitamins E and A and proximate composition of whole mice and rats used as feed. *Comparative Biochemistry and Physiology A* **107**, 419–424

Drent RH and Daan S (1980) The prudent parent: energetic adjustments in avian breeding. *Ardea* **68**, 225–252

Ernst CH and Barbour RW (1989) *Turtles of the World*. Smithsonian Institute Press, Washington DC

Esque TC and Peters EL (1994) Ingestion of bones, stones and soil by desert tortoises. In: *Biology of North American Tortoises*, ed. RB Bury and DJ Germano, pp. 105–111. Fish and Wildlife Research, US Department of the Interior, Washington DC

Finke MD, DeFoliart GR and Benevenga NJ (1989) Use of a four-parameter logistic model to evaluate the quality of protein from three insect species when fed to rats. *Journal of Nutrition* **119**, 864–871

Foley WJ, Boulskila A, Shkolnik A and Choshniak I (1992) Microbial digestion in the herbivorous lizard *Uromastyx aegyptius* (Agamidae). *Journal of Zoology* **226**, 337–398

Frye, FL (1991) *Biomedical and Surgical Aspects of Captive Reptile Husbandry, 2nd edn*. Krieger, Melbourne, FL

Galvao PE, Tarasantchi J and Guertzenstein P (1965) Heat production of tropical snakes in relation to body weight and body surface. *American Journal of Physiology* **209**, 501–506

Greer AE (1989) *Biology and Evolution of Australian Lizards*. Surrey Beatty & Sons, Chipping Norton, NSW

Hailey A (1997) Digestive efficiency and gut morphology of omnivorous and herbivorous African tortoises. *Canadian Journal of Zoology* **75**, 787–794

Hailey A, Chidavaenz RL and Loveridge JP (1998) Diet mixing in the omnivorous tortoise *Kinixys speckii*. *Functional Ecology* **12**, 373–385

Hailey A and Coulson IM (1996) Differential scaling of home-range area to total daily movement distance in two African tortoises. *Canadian Journal of Zoology* **74**, 97–102

Henen BT (2002) Tortoise reproductive nutrition. *Integrative and Comparative Biology* **42**, 43–50

Henen BT and Oftedal OT (1999) The importance of dietary nitrogen to the reproductive output of female desert tortoises (*Gopherus agassizii*). *Proceedings of the Second Comparative Nutrition Society Symposium*, pp. 83–88

Hurty CA, Diaz DE, Campbell JL and Lewbart GA (2001) Chemical analysis of six commercial adult iguana (*Iguana iguana*) diets. *Journal of Herpetological Medicine and Surgery* **11**, 23–26

Iverson JB (1980) Colic modification in the iguanine lizards. *Journal of Morphology* **163**, 79–93

Iverson JB (1982) Adaptations to herbivory in iguanine lizards. In: *Iguanas of the World: Their Behavior, Ecology, and Conservation*, ed. GM Burghardt and AS Rand, pp. 60–76. Noyes Publications, Park Ridge, NJ

John-Alder HB and Joos B (1991) Interactive effects of thyroxine and experimental location on running endurance, tissue masses, and enzyme activities in captive versus field-active lizards (*Sceloporus undulatus*). *General and Comparative Endocrinology* **81**, 120–132

Kabigumila J (2000) Growth and carapacial colour variation in the leopard tortoise *Geochelone pardalis* in northern Tanzania. *African Journal of Ecology* **38**, 217–227

Kaplan M (2002) *Iguana Care: Feeding and Socialization*, pp. 23–47. Available at: www.anapsid.org/iguana/icfs

Kepenis V and McManus JJ (1974) Bioenergetics of young painted terrapin *Chrysemys picta*. *Comparative Biochemistry and Physiology A* **48**, 309–317

Kercheval DR and Little P (1990) Comparative growth rates of young alligators utilizing rations of plant and/or animal origins. In: *Crocodiles: Proceedings of the 10th Working Meeting of the Crocodile Specialist Group of the Species Survival Commission of the IUCN*, pp. 286–312. IUCN – World Conservation Union, Gland, Switzerland

Kleiber M (1961) *The Fire of Life: An Introduction to Animal Energetics*. John Wiley, New York

Krebs JR (1978) Optimal foraging: decision rules for predators. In: *Behavioural Ecology: An Evolutionary Approach*, ed. JR Krebs and NB Davies, pp. 23–63. Blackwell, Oxford

Lagarde F, Bonnet X, Corbin J et al. (2003) Foraging behaviour and diet of an ectothermic herbivore: *Testudo horsfieldi*. *Ecography* **26**, 236–241

Lagarde F, Bonnet X, Henen BT et al. (2001) Sexual size dimorphism in steppe tortoises (*Testudo horsfieldi*): growth, maturity, and individual variation. *Canadian Journal of Zoology* **79**, 1433–1441

Lagarde F, Bonnet X, Nagy K et al. (2002) A short spring before a long jump: the ecological challenge to the steppe tortoise (*Testudo horsfieldi*). *Canadian Journal of Zoology* **80**, 493–502

Larsen REC, Buergelt PT, Cardeilhac PT and Jacobson ER (1983) Steatitis and fat necrosis in alligators. *Journal of the American Veterinary Medical Association* **183**, 1202–1204

Lichtenbelt WDV (1992) Digestion in an ectothermic herbivore, the green iguana (*Iguana iguana*): effect of food composition and body temperature. *Physiological Zoology* **65**, 649–673

McBee RH and McBee VH (1982) The hindgut fermentation in the green iguana (*Iguana iguana*). In: *Iguanas of the World: Their Behavior, Ecology, and Conservation*, ed. GM Burghardt and AS Rand, pp. 73–87. Noyes Publications, Park Ridge, NJ

Macmillan RE, Augee ML and Ellis BA (1989) Thermal ecology and diet of some xerophilous lizards from western New South Wales. *Journal of Arid Environments* **16**, 193–201

Madsen T and Shine R (2000) Energy versus risk: costs of reproduction in free-ranging pythons in tropical Australia. *Australian Journal of Ecology* **25**, 670–677

Magnussen WE and Da Silva EV (1993) Relative effects of size, season and species on the diets of some Amazonian savannah lizards. *Journal of Herpetology* **27**, 380–383

Marlow RW and Tollestrup K (1982) Mining and exploitation of natural mineral deposits by the desert tortoise *Gopherus agassizii*. *Animal Behaviour* **30**, 475–478

Maxwell L, Jacobson ER and McNab BK (2003) Intraspecific allometry of metabolic rate in green iguanas (*Iguana iguana*). *Comparative Biochemistry and Physiology A* **136**, 301–310

Menon J, Shah RV and Hiradhar PK (1981) Effect of thyroidectomy on carbohydrate metabolism during tail regeneration in the gekkonid lizard *Hemidactylus flaviviridis*. *Indian Journal of Experimental Biology* **19**, 1018–1026

Minnich JE (1982) The use of water. In: *Biology of the Reptilia, Volume 12*, ed. C Gans and FH Pough, pp. 323–395. Academic Press, London and New York

Miranda JP and Andrade GV (2003) Seasonality in diet, perch use and reproduction of the gecko *Gonatodes humeralis* from Eastern Brazilian Amazon. *Journal of Herpetology* **07**, 133–138

Mobray RM and Smith TMG (1999) *Investigating the Digestibility of a New Formulated Diet in Comparison to a Conventional Diet for Bearded Dragons (Pogona vitticeps)*. BVSc dissertation, University of Bristol

Moskovits DK and Bjorndal K (1990) Diet and food preferences of the tortoises *Geochelonia carbonaria* and *Geochelone denticulata* in northwestern Brazil. *Herpetologica* **46**, 207–218

Munsey LD (1972) Water loss in five species of lizards. *Comparative Biochemistry and Physiology A* **43**, 781–794

Nagy KA (1982) Energy requirements of free-living iguanid lizards. In: *Iguanas of the World*, ed. GM Burghardt and AS Rand, pp. 49–59. Noyes Publications, Park Ridge, NJ

Nagy KA and Medica PA (1986) Physiological ecology of desert tortoises in southern Nevada. *Herpetologica* **42**, 73–92

National Research Council (1995) *Nutrition Requirements of Laboratory Animals, revised 4th edn*. National Academy Press, Washington DC

Oftedal OT and Allen ME (1996) Nutrition as a major facet of reptile conservation. *Zoo Biology* **15**, 491–497

Onifade AA, Oduguwa OO, Fanimo AO *et al*. (2001) Effects of supplemental methionine and lysine on the nutritional value of housefly larvae meal (*Musca domestica*) fed to rats. *Bioresource Technology* **78**, 191–194

Pianka ER (1986) *Ecology and Natural History of Desert Lizards: Analyses of the Ecological Niche and Community Structure*. Princeton University Press, Princeton, NJ

Rand AS, Dugan BA, Monteza H and Vianda D (1990) The diet of a generalized folivore: *Iguana iguana* in Panama. *Journal of Herpetology* **24**, 211–214

Reichle DE, Shanks MH and Crossley DA (1969) Calcium, potassium and sodium content of forest floor arthropods. *Annals of the Entomological Society of America* **62**, 57–66

Rodríguez-Robles JA (2002) Feeding ecology of North American gopher snakes (*Pituophis catenifer*, Colubridae). *Biological Journal of the Linnean Society* **77**, 165–179

Rodríguez-Robles JA, Bell CJ and Greene HW (1999) Gape size and evolution of diet in snakes: feeding ecology of erycine boas. *Journal of Zoology* **248**, 49–58

Rodríguez-Robles JA and de Jesús-Escobar JM (1999) Molecular systematics of New World lampropeltinine snakes (Colubridae): implications for biogeography and evolution of food habits. *Biological Journal of the Linnean Society* **68**, 355–385

Schairer ML, Dierenfeld ES and Fitzpatrick MP (1998) Nutrient composition of whole green frogs *Rana clamitans* and southern toads *Bufo terrestris*. *Bulletin of the Association of Reptilian and Amphibian Veterinarians* **8(3)**, 17–21

Schwenk K (1995) Of tongues and noses: chemoreception in lizards and snakes. *Trends in Ecology and Evolution* **10**, 7–12

Secor SM and Diamond J (2000) Evolution of regulatory responses to feeding in snakes. *Physiological and Biochemical Zoology* **73(2)**, 123–141

Secor SM and Phillips JA (1997) Specific dynamic action of a large carnivorous lizard *Varanus albigularis*. *Comparative Biochemistry and Physiology A* **117**, 515–522

Singer MA (2003) Dietary protein-induced changes in excretory function: a general animal design feature. *Comparative Biochemistry and Physiology B* **136**, 785–801

Skoczylas R (1978) Physiology of the digestive tract. In: *Biology of the Reptilia, Volume 8*, ed. C Glans, pp. 589–717. Academic Press, London and New York

Stafford PJ and Henderson RW (1996) *Kaleidoscopic Tree Boas: The Genus Corallus of Tropical America*. Krieger, Malabar, Fl

Staton MA (1990) Essential fatty acid nutrition of the American alligator (*Alligator mississippiensis*). *Journal of Nutrition* **120**, 674–685

Studier EH and Sevick SH (1992) Live mass, water content, nitrogen and mineral levels in some insects from South-Central Michigan. *Comparative Biochemistry and Physiology A* **103**, 579–595

Thompson GG and Withers PC (1994) Standard metabolic rate of two small Australian varanid lizards (*Varanus caudolineatus* and *V. acanthurus*). *Herpetologica* **50**, 494–502

Troyer K (1984) Diet selection and digestion in *Iguana iguana*: the importance of age and nutrient requirements. *Oeologia* **69**, 1566–1574

Tucker CS (1993) Water analysis. In: *Fish Medicine*, ed. MK Stoskopf, pp. 166–197. WB Saunders, Philadelphia

van der Wardt ST, Kik MJ, Klaver PS, Janse M and Beynen AC (1999) Calcium balance in Drakensberg Crag lizards (*Pseudocordylus melanotus melanotus*; Cordylidae). *Journal of Zoo and Wildlife Medicine* **30**, 541–544

Wang T, Zaar M, Arvedsen S, Vedel-Smith C and Overgaard J (2003) Effects of temperature on the metabolic response to feeding in *Python morulus*. *Comparative Biochemistry and Physiology A* **133**, 519–527

Webster J (1996) Digestion and metabolism. In: *Understanding the Dairy Cow, 2nd edn*, pp. 40–61. Blackwell Scientific, Oxford

Weese JS (2002) Microbiologic evaluation of commercial probiotics. *Journal of the American Veterinary Medical Association* **220**, 794–797

Weissman C, Kemper M and Hyman AI (1989) Variation in the resting metabolic rate of mechanically ventilated critically ill patients. *Anaesthetics and Analgesics* **68**, 457–461

Weldon PJ, Demeter BJ, Walsh T and Kliester JSE (1994) Chemoreception in the feeding behaviour of reptiles: considerations for maintenance and management. In: *Captive Management and Conservation of Amphibians and Reptiles*, ed. JB Murphy, K Adler and JT Collins, pp. 61–70. Society for the Study of Amphibians and Reptiles, Ithaca, NY

Witz BW and Lawrence JM (1993) Nutrient absorption efficiencies of the lizard *Cnemidophorus sexlineatus* (Sauria: Teiidae). *Comparative Biochemistry and Physiology A* **105**, 151–155

Wood SC, Hicks JW and Dupre RK (1987) Hypoxic reptiles: blood gases, body temperature and control of breathing. *American Zoologist* **27**, 21–29

Wouter D and van Marken Lichtenbelt W (1993) Optimal foraging of a herbivorous lizard, green iguana, in a seasonal environment. *Ecologia* **95**, 246–256

Wright KM, Toddes B and Donoghue S (1997) To form the more perfect stool: feeding trials on the Galapagos (*Geochelone nigra*) and Aldabra (*Geochelone gigantea*) tortoise population at the Philadelphia Zoo. *Proceedings of the American Association of Zoo Veterinarians*, pp. 11–15

Zari TA (1996) Effects of body mass and temperature on standard metabolic rate of the herbivorous desert lizard *Uromastyx philbyi*. *Journal of Arid Environments* **33**, 457–461

Chapter 5

Breeding and neonatal care

Kevin Wright[†] and Paul Raiti

Many people keep reptiles as pets without any intention of breeding them, while others enjoy propagating them and selling or trading the offspring.

Proper husbandry and a nutritionally complete diet are essential for reproduction to be a consistent and predictable event for most reptiles (Figure 5.1). Detailed record-keeping is an important tool for breeding reptiles and should include data on age, ancestry or pedigree, food consumption, defecation, weight, sheds, medical problems and reproductive output, so that successful practices are documented and any problems may be analysed. Parameters of the physical environment, such as photoperiod, temperature, relative humidity and significant shifts in barometric pressure should also be noted so that important influences on reproduction can be recognized.

A reptile must be in good physical condition and free of clinical and subclinical diseases in order to have sufficient energy stores to support reproduction. This is especially true for females as their nutritional status and body condition determine the investment they are able to make in offspring. Females that are underweight, have received suboptimal diets or are small in size for their age produce fewer and smaller eggs or young than do robust females.

Problems of the reproductive system, such as egg binding and prolapse, are described in Chapter 20.

Reproduction in reptiles

- The majority of reptiles are oviparous and produce shelled eggs that incubate in the environment before hatching (Figure 5.2a).
- A number of reptiles are viviparous; their embryos are retained in the oviduct (shell gland) until they are fully developed and are born live (Figure 5.2b). The method of viviparous development varies as some groups have offspring that develop depending entirely on yolk, a state formerly referred to as ovoviparity, while others have a chorioallantoic placenta that nurtures the offspring ('true' viviparity).

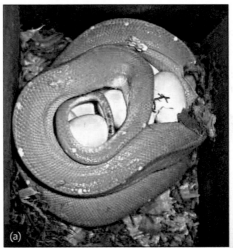

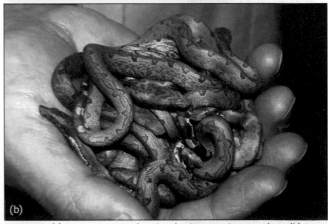

5.2 (a) A green tree python incubating eggs in a nest box. (b) A litter of Solomon Island boas at 2 weeks of age.

5.1 Providing reptiles with an environment that closely mimics their natural history offers the best chance for longevity and reproduction. An outdoor enclosure with a pair of yellow-footed tortoises in Florida, USA.

As a general rule, pythons, kingsnakes and ratsnakes are oviparous while garter snakes and American water snakes are viviparous. Viviparity is the general rule for boids and crotalids, with the notable exception of the Arabian sand boa and bushmasters. There are no known species of viviparous chelonians or crocodilians.

Parthenogenesis, the production of offspring from a single parent, has been well documented in whiptail lizards, geckos and the brahminy blind snake. Parthenogenesis has been documented under specific conditions in rattlesnakes, warty water snakes and garter snakes.

Inducing reproductive behaviour

Reproductive cycles

Continuous cycles

The majority of tropical zone reptiles come from habitats with minimal fluctuation in temperature or photoperiod (Figure 5.3a–b). These groups typically have a continuous reproductive cycle, where they are capable of fertile matings throughout the year. There is often some influence from minor shifts in temperature that occur between the wet and dry seasons. In some reptiles, one sex (typically male) may show a continuous cycle and the other sex (typically female) may show an associated cycle (see below).

Associated cycles

The majority of subtropical or temperate zone reptiles have an associated reproductive cycle, wherein sex hormone secretion and gonadogenesis stimulate copulation and egg or fetal development, with a final phase of gonadal regression before the next cycle of gonadogenesis. These reptiles come from environments with a long active season, and a predictable cycle of active and inactive seasons, and include the majority of pet trade reptiles (e.g. leopard gecko, bearded dragon, blue-tongued skink, ratsnakes, kingsnakes, milk snake) (Figure 5.3c). They typically require brumation (a more appropriate term for ectotherms *versus* mammalian hibernation) in order to become reproductively viable.

Dissociated cycles

Some reptiles have a dissociated cycle, wherein mating occurs at the start of the active season before gonadogenesis. Male reptiles inseminate using sperm produced during the prior active season, while females develop ova during the active season and store the acquired sperm until ovulation. A dissociated cycle is associated with a short active season and a predictable cycle of active and inactive seasons. The garter snake is a common pet reptile with a dissociated cycle.

Temperature manipulation

Many temperate reptiles do not breed unless they have brumated (Figure 5.3d–e). The pattern successful for temperate species of kingsnake, milk snake, ratsnake and pine or gopher snakes is readily adapted for many other reptiles.

Inducing brumation

In the northern hemisphere all adult reptiles should be in peak physical condition by the start of November. Any reptile that is underweight or has had a medical disorder within the past 3 months should be maintained at active season temperatures and fed instead of being brumated. Figure 5.4 shows a brumation protocol.

Many southern hemisphere temperate reptiles may not need extended brumation, and a 4–8 week period of cooling will suffice to induce breeding. Most tropical lowland reptiles will die if brumated but they do require minor nightly temperature drops to induce gonadogenesis. This can easily be achieved in species with a daytime preferred

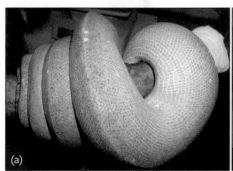
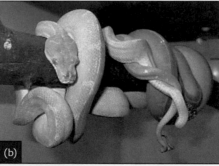
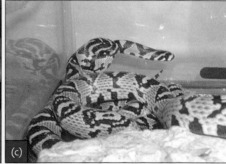
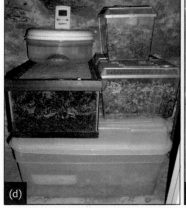
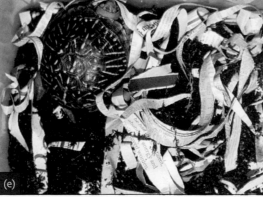

5.3 (a) Green tree pythons from South East Asia can be induced to cycle with minimal fluctuations in temperature and humidity. This is an example of a continuous reproductive cycle. Pictured is a female green tree python with preovulatory swelling occupying the midsection of the body. (b) Copulation in a compatible pair of green tree pythons. (c) Copulation in a compatible pair of Mandarin ratsnakes. This is an example of an associated reproductive cycle whereby gonadogenesis follows a period of brumation. Note the male biting the female. (d) A hibernaculum for temperate reptiles provides individual housing for each reptile in darkness where the temperature is monitored. (e) During brumation, a North American eastern box turtle is maintained on a combination of damp potting soil and shredded newspaper.

- Stop feeding on the last day in October
- Maintain at normal temperatures for about 2 weeks to allow gastrointestinal tracts to clear
- Weigh after the final defecation
- Turn off heat sources and supplemental lighting. Allow enclosure temperature to drop to around 10–12°C for the next 1–4 months, depending on species. A 3–4 month duration is typical for many North American colubrid snakes
- Keep the room dim or completely dark except when checking brumating reptiles, typically every other week. Clean and refill water bowls and give each reptile a close visual examination to assess health. Remove any reptile showing any abnormal signs, warm it to normal activity and give it a thorough health check
- Weigh the brumating reptiles at least once near the midpoint of brumation. Any reptile that has lost >7.5% of its bodyweight may need to be removed and returned to normal activity
- Around the first week of February or March, depending on the length of brumation targeted, warm the enclosures to normal active temperatures (i.e. 28–32°C hotspot during the day and 22–24°C hotspot at night) and resume the photoperiod
- Weigh all animals that same day. Any animal that has lost 10% or more from its prebrumation weight should be evaluated for medical conditions
- Feed breeding individuals frequent small meals in the first week after being removed from brumation. Thereafter, feed heavily to encourage gonadogenesis

5.4 A general brumation protocol. Requirements vary between species; for example, Mediterranean tortoises need a temperature of 4–7°C with a maximum duration of 3 months. The reader is advised to check other sources for species-specific details.

body temperature of 30–39°C by allowing the night-time temperature to drop by about 3–8°C for 6–12 weeks. A common mistake is to allow the temperature throughout the entire cage to drop; a hotspot should be available at all times for tropical reptiles, but the surrounding cage should reach the cooler temperatures. All other guidelines suggested for temperate reptiles apply to the tropical species.

Photoperiod manipulation

Some temperate species require photoperiod cues in addition to temperature cues. In general, 6–8 hours of daylight with a 16–18 hour night should be started at least 6 weeks before brumation. A photoperiod with 8–10 hours of daylight is appropriate upon emerging from brumation, gradually phasing into 14 hours of daylight in the middle of the active season. Tropical reptiles typically respond to a photoperiod with 12 hours of daylight throughout the year.

Other interacting factors

Some species show enhanced responses to manipulation of temperature and photoperiod if these changes are concurrent with changes in humidity and barometric pressure. Some that respond to photoperiod and temperature may also be induced to breed while being maintained at normal active temperatures and 12–14 hours daylight, but fed more frequently and with larger meals than normal. However, reproductive output and longevity may be decreased compared with hibernated reptiles of the same species.

Social factors

The presence of a suitable mate can have a profound impact on the reproductive cycle. For example, mature female leopard geckos rarely produce shelled eggs unless they have been exposed to a reproductively mature and sexually active male leopard gecko. This pattern is fairly widespread among oviparous snakes and lizards and, to a lesser extent, among chelonians and crocodilians.

If a female reptile produces small clutches, small eggs, poorly shelled or unshelled eggs, or fails to have fertile eggs or viable offspring despite mating, it is likely that the male was not in contact with the female at critical times prior to introduction for courtship and copulation. In some reptiles the males rely on cues from the females for gonadal development, just as females rely on cues from the males to trigger development.

Mating behaviour is generally triggered by the production of pheromones from specialized glands of sexually receptive females. Examples are the epidermal lipid glands in snakes, precloacal/femoral pores in lizards, mental/axillary/inguinal glands in chelonians, and Rathke's glands in sea turtles (Figure 5.5a–b). Pheromones, composed of lipids and fatty acids, are picked up by the male's tongue and transferred to the paired vomeronasal organs (Jacobson's organs), which are located in the roof of the oral cavity. Pheromones stimulate behavioural centres in the brain that initiate copulation (Figure 5.5c–d) (Raiti, 1995).

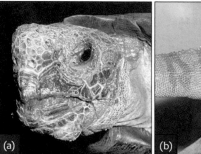
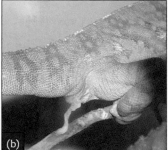
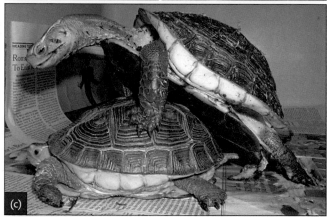
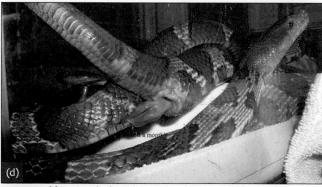

5.5 (a) During the breeding season, the mental glands of male North American gopher tortoises hypertrophy and produce pheromones that are important for agonistic behaviour and copulation. (b) A male veiled chameleon extruding semen on a branch in response to a receptive female; semen also contains pheromones. (c) Copulation in a pair of Asian box turtles. This species, in particular, should be closely monitored during courtship owing to the risk of the animals injuring each other. (d) Copulation in a pair of Chinese 100 flower snakes. A hemipenis has been inserted into the cloaca by the male to the left in the picture.

Social behaviours can inhibit ovarian or testicular cycles. Females may have their ovarian cycle inhibited if mated continually or if exposed to frequent male–male aggressive displays. After losing a combat, a male will often show reduced interest in breeding. Females of most garter snakes emerge from brumation with regressed ovaries that are only stimulated into activity by courtship with one or more males or by exogenous applications of oestrogen.

In highly social reptiles, neonates that are raised in isolation may not learn appropriate social signals to communicate effectively with rivals or mates, and may not be able to court successfully. Some reptiles, such as the shingleback skink, appear to be monogamous in the wild, and in captivity it may be difficult to provide the level of diversity of mate choice necessary to create this bond.

With the majority of colubrids common in the pet trade, best results are obtained when a male snake is introduced into the female snake's enclosure for breeding.

Inducing multiple egg clutches

The technique for inducing multiple clutching in oviparous species has been well documented for North American ratsnakes, kingsnakes and milk snakes (Figure 5.6).

Typically, the number of eggs produced decreases with each subsequent clutch and very few snakes are able to produce four clutches in a breeding season and still be healthy enough to enter brumation. The incidence of dystocia increases with each clutch in a season. Females that produce multiple clutches may not be reproductively active for as many years as females managed for single clutches. For these reasons, the authors discourage this practice.

- Feed a female snake just brought out of brumation small- to medium-sized meals at least three times a week so that her gastrointestinal tract is always in a digesting and absorbing state
- Continue feeding even if the snake is about to shed; although most females will only take favourite foods at this time
- Continue frequent feeding when she is obviously gravid, although she may only take smaller meals than previously. Patience and creativity are necessary to induce some snakes to take food items at these times, but these additional meals are essential for females to have the resources to produce second, third and even fourth clutches of eggs
- Continue the intense feeding schedule even after the first egg clutch has been laid
- If the female is still in good condition, introduce a male into her enclosure immediately after the eggs have been removed. Repeat this after each clutch is laid

5.6 A protocol for inducing multiple egg clutches in colubrid snakes.

Pre-nesting behaviours

Gravid females often bask frequently or spend more time in the cage's hotspot (Figure 5.7). Gravid viviparous snakes may bask in an upside-down position as a normal behaviour. The female may dig exploratory nest holes or scoop out shallow birthing pallets in the substrate. Many snakes shed their skin 7–14 days prior to oviposition. Females may become secretive and aggressive immediately prior to delivery. Most females lay eggs or give birth in the evening or very early morning.

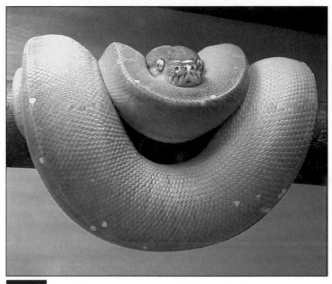

5.7 A gravid green tree python basking under a heat source.

Nesting or brooding environment

An appropriate oviposition site is essential or some reptiles may become egg-bound (see Chapter 20) (Figure 5.8a–c). If a nest box is used it needs to be large enough for the female to move around comfortably.

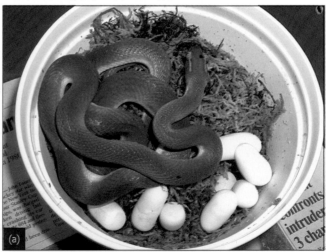

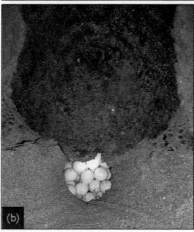

5.8 (a) A Namibian house snake with a clutch of eggs. Note the damp sphagnum moss placed in a container to encourage oviposition. (b) A loggerhead sea turtle ovipositing in the evening on a beach in Florida, USA. (continues) ▶

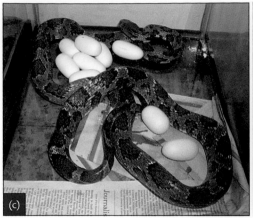

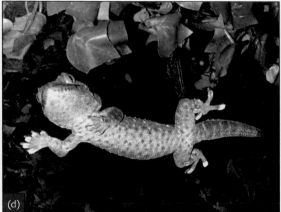

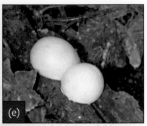

5.8 (continued) (c) This Chinese 100 flower snake oviposited despite the absence of a nest box. Dystocia due to retained eggs could have easily occurred. (d–e) This tokay gecko oviposited two eggs that adhered to a branch.

Panther and veiled chameleons need deep soil to construct their nests, and tolerate removal from their normal enclosure and placement within a 5 gallon bucket filled with lightly moistened garden soil. Large lizards may use large rubbish bins filled with moist sphagnum moss as nest boxes. Several species of gecko oviposit sticky eggs that adhere to a solid substrate (Figure 5.8d–e).

Many chelonians prefer to dig into the substrate and will stop nesting activity if picked up and placed in a new enclosure. However, several aquatic chelonians tolerate handling and will immediately start digging after being moved.

Some viviparous species like to use brood boxes during the later stages of gestation. It is important to provide several different brood boxes that have different thermal and humidity profiles, so that the female can choose the one that provides the most appropriate conditions to support gestation. Dystocia may result if a suitable brood box is absent.

Egg anatomy

The reptilian egg may have a brittle and calcareous or soft and leathery shell, depending on the taxon. Shell pores allow gas and water exchange and some mineral exchange. As a general rule, brittle eggs have minimal water loss to, or uptake from, the environment and have a fairly constant mass and volume throughout incubation. Soft eggs absorb water from the environment and often show substantial increases in volume and mass over the course of incubation, often with a slight decline just before hatching.

Some eggs may have calcium-based deposits as a part of normal anatomy, as is the case for indigo snakes, North American whipsnakes, racers and various Asian ratsnakes (Figure 5.9a). In other species, similar deposits develop if the eggs have been retained for too long in the female's shell gland. This extra calcification may lead to irregular contours and obscure the shell pores (Figure 5.9b–c). Often these abnormally heavily calcified eggs do not develop as the pores are constricted and impair embryonic respiration. In rare cases, the embryo within an overly calcified egg develops to a certain point and then dies.

Immediately beneath the shell is the chorion, the allantois and, finally, the amniotic membrane. The chorion fuses with the allantois, which stores the embryo's waste products such as uric acid. The fused chorioallantoic membranes develop blood vessels, which facilitate gaseous exchange with the environment and may modulate water exchange and mineral absorption to some

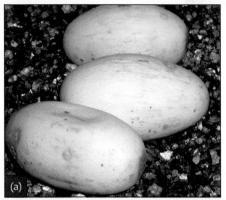

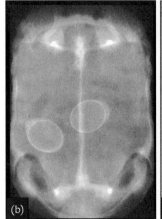

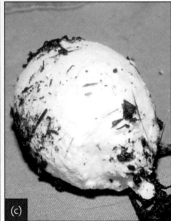

5.9 (a) The eggshells of Sulawesi black-tailed ratsnakes are very thick and possess calcified ridges. Hatching can be problematic owing to inability of neonates to slit the shells. (b) Dorsoventral radiograph of a red-footed tortoise with retained eggs. Note excessive calcium deposits on the shells. (c) Appearance of eggshell after induced oviposition.

degree. This chorioallantoic membrane becomes the placenta in viviparous reptiles. The amnion encloses the embryo in fluid and separates the embryo from the yolk and chorioallantoic membrane (Figure 5.10). The yolk sac is connected to the embryo via a yolk stalk. As the embryo develops, this yolk stalk fuses with the embryonic intestine. The embryo rests on the dorsal surface of the yolk, which is its food source. An air cell develops on the dorsal aspect of the eggshell.

Lizards and snakes typically oviposit eggs with advanced embryos, whereas chelonians and crocodilians lay eggs that have had few, if any, embryonic cell divisions.

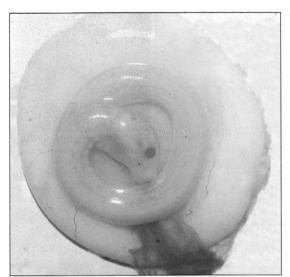

5.10 Appearance of a Solomon Island boa fetus at midterm. Note the non-pigmented fetus, yolk and vascularized chorioallantois.

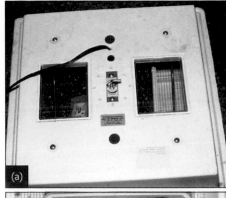

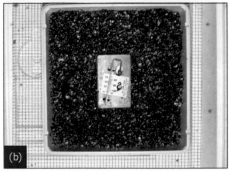

5.12 (a) A Styrofoam incubator with a thermostat works well for reptile eggs. (b) Vermiculite mixed 1:1 with water by volume is a commonly used substrate. Note the thermometer that would be located adjacent to the eggs.

Egg handling and incubation

Eggs should be removed from the nest, marked on their dorsal surface, weighed and then placed into an incubation box containing an appropriate incubation medium (Figure 5.11). Using an incubator ensures more efficient control of humidity and temperature, and reduces the risk of damage from adults (Figure 5.12). If eggs are not removed many snakes will stay coiled around them and refuse to eat.

Many reptile taxa have embryos that may die or suffer deformity if the egg is rotated or jostled during early to mid-development. Therefore, if an egg must be moved, it is essential not to rotate it around any axis. The egg should be reseated in the incubating medium with the appropriate side still in a dorsal position.

The incubator should be able to maintain the appropriate level of humidity and have a regular supply of fresh air that is free of volatile odours. Separate incubation boxes allow one incubator to support several microenvironments of differing relative humidity.

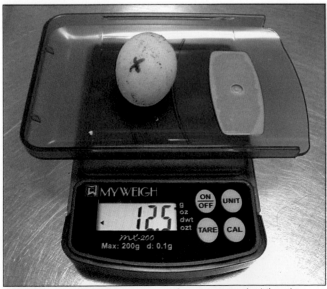

5.11 This spider tortoise egg weighs 12.5 g. Note the 'X' on the dorsal aspect of the egg. Pencil is preferred instead of felt-tipped markers.

The status of the eggs should be checked every 1–2 weeks. Opening the incubator door other than for planned air exchange should be avoided, as this typically causes a temperature drop and can interfere with incubation.

Incubation temperature

Most reptile eggs are incubated between 28 and 30°C (Figure 5.13). The incubator must be able to maintain a constant temperature with minimal fluctuation (±0.5°C). Some thermostats can raise or lower the temperature periodically, which may be a trigger for bringing some

Species	Egg incubation time (days)	Temperature range (°C)
Chelonians		
Snapping turtle	42–50	28–32
European pond turtle	52–65	28
Red-eared terrapin	54–80	28–29
Eastern box turtle	70–85	28–30
Asian box turtle	70–85	26–28
Horsfield's tortoise	60–75	28–32
Hermann's tortoise	85–100	30–33
African spurred tortoise	120–170	28–32
Leopard tortoise	140–155	28–32
Lizards		
Green iguana	60	25–30
Inland bearded dragon	65–115	28–32
Veiled chameleon	60–72	20 night-time low; 30 daytime high
Savannah monitor	200	29–30
Tegu	146–167	28–32
Leopard gecko	150–170	28–32
Snakes		
Colubrid snakes (e.g. corn snakes, kingsnakes, bullsnakes)	55–70	28–30
Pythons (Burmese, green tree, Children's)	55–65	28–32

5.13 Incubation times and temperature ranges for oviparous reptiles. (Data from Mattison (1986), Highfield (1996), Rogner (1997) and Gurley (2003))

eggs out of diapause or to control temperature-dependent sex determination. A maximum–minimum thermometer with an alarm is suggested so that the breeder is alerted to any untoward conditions that may develop.

Sex determination

Sex chromosomes determine the sex of snakes and viviparous lizards and possibly some chelonians – genotypic sex determination (GSD). In many other reptiles, the temperature at which eggs are incubated causes the development of either male or female gonads – temperature-dependent sex determination (TSD). There are currently three general patterns of TSD:

- Females develop at low incubation temperatures; males develop at high incubation temperatures. This pattern is found in alligators, the only crocodilian with this pattern, and in many lizard species
- Females develop at high incubation temperatures; males develop at low incubation temperatures. This pattern has been found to date in the majority of chelonians, excluding snapping turtles
- Females develop at either low or high incubation temperatures; mostly males develop at mid-range temperatures. The low and high temperatures are at the limit for successful incubation. Some females may develop in the intermediate ranges; the sequence of events that causes this is not well understood compared with other aspects of TSD. Snapping turtles, leopard geckos and many crocodilians fall into this category.

TSD is known for tuataras, crocodilians, chelonians and lizards. Unfortunately, the pattern of TSD is known for comparatively few species of reptiles. Within each pattern of TSD are critical or threshold temperatures, above or below which embryos develop into the different sexes, but the critical temperatures are known for very few species. Leopard geckos are an important pet trade species and have a well-documented pattern: only females develop at 26–28°C and 34–35°C while mostly males develop between 30.5 and 32.5°C.

Genetic and congenital traits

A number of genetically determined colour and pattern morphs have been developed in pet trade species but not all pattern morphs are genetically determined. It is common for neonates of a species with saddled or blotched patterns to show varying degrees of linear stripes if they were exposed to high temperatures during incubation. Scutellation abnormalities may be related to high incubation temperatures or may be heritable (e.g. scaleless water snakes). Other congenital abnormalities related to high incubation temperatures include extra carapacial or plastral scutes on the shells of chelonians, anophthalmia, missing digits, kinked tails and sterility (Figure 5.14).

Incubation media

Vermiculite, sphagnum moss, peat moss and perlite are commonly used alone or in combination for incubation media (Figure 5.15). Typically, the medium is moistened in a 1:1, 1:2 or 1:3 weight ratio of water to medium. As a general rule, moister media are needed for leathery eggs and drier media for brittle eggs. The humidity of the air surrounding the egg is important, and typically should be 50–95% relative humidity. Aged tap water or spring water should be used in the incubation box as distilled and reverse-osmosis deionized water have been linked to hatch-rate problems for leopard geckos.

Monitoring incubation

Figure 5.13 lists incubation times and temperature ranges for some commonly kept species.

Transillumination (candling)

Transillumination is performed by holding a bright light source (penlight) directly against the eggshell in a darkened room for the purpose of assessing initial fertility and continued viability of the embryo (Figure 5.16a–c). It should be done on the egg in situ, as rotational movement or abrupt motion may damage or kill the embryo.

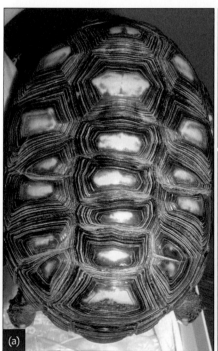
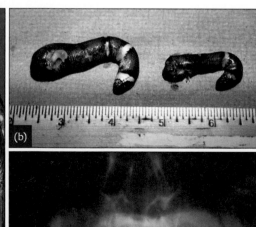
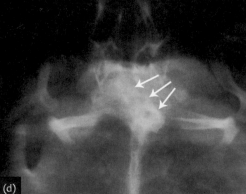
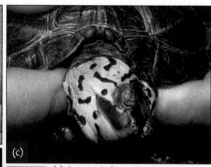

5.14 (a) Congenital supernumerary scutes in a red-footed tortoise. (b) Congenital caudal agenesis in Honduran milk snakes. (c) Congenital cervical agenesis in a juvenile diamondback terrapin. Note maximal extension of the neck. (d) A dorsoventral radiograph revealed the presence of three cervical vertebrae (arrowed) instead of the normal eight. Neck is in maximal extension.

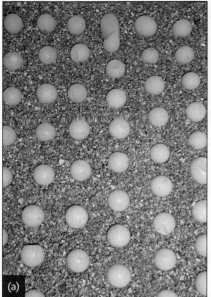

5.15 (a) Snapping turtle eggs incubating on a mixture of vermiculite and water; note the eggs are half buried in the substrate. (b) Chinese 100 flower snake eggs incubating on a plastic rack on top of shallow water. Note moistened peat moss surrounding the eggs. This set-up works well for eggs that require more humidity during incubation.

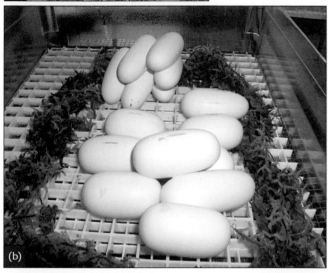

- Healthy fertile chelonian and crocodilian eggs appear translucent to white immediately upon laying and will glow a homogeneous yellow if candled at this point. Since most lizards and snakes lay eggs that are 20–50% developed, the initial candling may appear to show a more advanced stage than in chelonians and crocodilians.
- Within 1–7 days the yolk will drop and a blood spot will develop. After the yolk has dropped, a candled fertile egg appears slightly less yellow to clear on its upper half and a deeper yellow on its lower half. The blood spot can be detected as a small red blotch near the uppermost surface of the yolk in a round egg or at one end of the yolk in an elliptical egg. The blood spot may not be seen in some very large or thick-shelled eggs.
- As the embryo develops, the blood spot expands into a blood ring that has a distinct embryonic profile visible with the head oriented towards the dorsal surface of the egg.
- At a later stage an air cell appears in the upper half of the egg and blood vessels grow across the inner surface of the egg. The air cell is often still visible when the rest of the egg has become opaque.
- Crocodilian eggs and some chelonian eggs develop distinct chalky bands on the surface as embryonic membranes attach to its inner surface (Figure 5.16d).
- Soft-shelled eggs absorb water from the environment and grow considerably during development.

Eggs may grow completely opaque in the latter stages of incubation, which can make it difficult to assess visually whether an embryo is still viable.

Embryonic diapause

Some reptile embryos may not develop unless subjected to certain conditions or may develop to a certain point and then stop unless environmental cues stimulate activity. This feature, termed embryonic diapause, seems to be a trait that ensures the neonate hatches at the optimal time

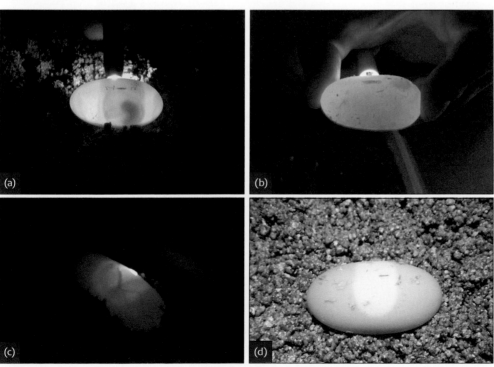

5.16 (a) Transillumination (candling) of a three-striped Asian box turtle at 72 hours; vasculature and embryo are clearly visible. (b) Transillumination of an infertile egg from the same clutch. (c) Transillumination of the egg of an Assam trinket snake; note the presence of vasculature at 48 hours. (d) 'Chalking' of a viable three-striped Asian box turtle egg at 48 hours.

of the year. Unfortunately, diapause is quite complicated and the exact parameters for successful incubation are not known for many species.

Infertile eggs

Infertile eggs may also develop the appearance of yolk drop but this usually happens weeks to months after the fertile eggs have all done so. This change is due to the decomposition and inspissation of the yolk and is usually accompanied by a noticeable foul smell (Figure 5.17).

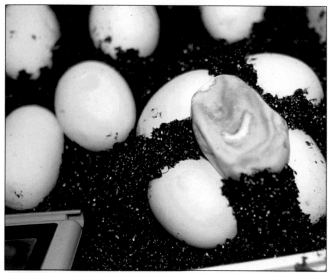

5.17 A necrotic infertile egg from a clutch of normal royal python eggs.

Incubation problems
Medium

Early embryonic death may happen if distilled or deionized water is used in the incubation medium.

Temperature

There are lethal temperatures above or below which eggs fail to hatch. Abnormal scutellation, anophthalmia, open coelomic cavity, neurological deficits and other deformities are associated with sublethal high temperatures, as may be some pattern abnormalities (see above).

Humidity

Embryos incubated under drier than ideal moisture tension (humidity) are typically smaller than other embryos and may have deformities of their extremities such as missing toes or feet. Embryos that are maintained in too moist an environment may die in the shell but otherwise have no pathological conditions detected.

Cracking

Brittle eggs with small cracks may hatch successfully if the underlying membranes are not torn. Repairs must stabilize the shell and prevent tears of the underlying membrane. Cyanoacrylate tissue glues, dental epoxy resins, candle wax and tape have been used to stabilize the shell pieces.

Hatching

Shortly before hatching, the outer calcareous layer of brittle eggshells may fall off in shards. Leathery eggs may darken and develop droplets of fluid on the shell. A day or two before hatching, leathery eggs may develop a wrinkled or collapsed appearance. As the embryo moves around it eventually slits the shell membranes with its egg tooth or claws (Figure 5.18). At this point, fluid may leak out of the egg and the neonate may breathe through the slit. It may take hours to days before the neonate leaves the shell, so the egg needs to be kept under relatively high humidity to prevent excessive drying, which can trap the infant in its egg.

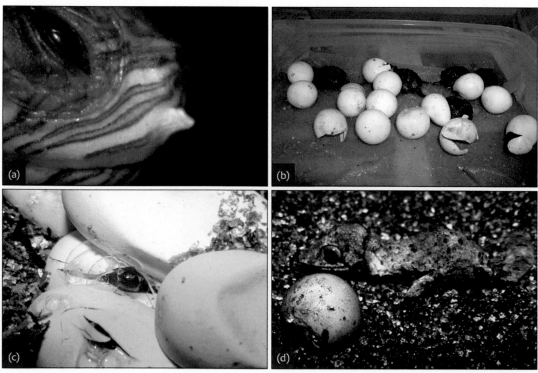

5.18 (a) Egg tooth (caruncle) just beneath the nostrils of a neonate red-eared slider. (b) Neonatal snapping turtles; note the pipping incisions. (c) Pipping Honduran milk snakes. (d) Neonatal leaf-tailed gecko; note the relatively small size of the egg compared with the camouflaged neonate.
(a, Courtesy of William Cermak)

The noise and movement of neonates may stimulate the rest of the clutch to 'pip', i.e. use the egg tooth to open the shell. Eggs should not be 'pipped' manually unless 2 days have elapsed since pipping times of other eggs in the same clutch and it is known that prolonged periods between hatches are unusual. A very small triangular window may be cut in the eggshell. If the neonate moves, stop! If there is no movement, the window may be extended slightly. It may take several days for some neonates finally to leave their eggshells (Figure 5.19).

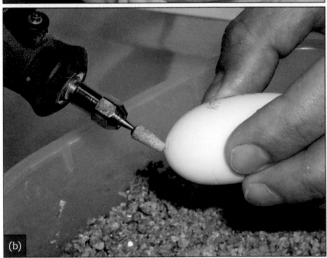

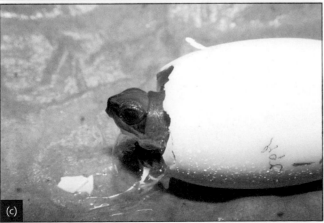

5.19 (a) Manual incisions to assist hatching in a clutch of Sulawesi black-tailed ratsnake eggs at 115 days. (b–c) Manual removal of eggshell fragments to assist hatching of a three-striped Asian box turtle at 87 days.

Live-bearers

Gestation period

The gestation periods of viviparous snakes vary among species (Figure 5.20) and are dependent upon surrounding conditions, particularly temperature. As with egg-laying reptiles, it is normal for pregnant reptiles to stop eating; however, adequate hydration and fat reserves are critical for successful gestation. Towards the end of gestation the fetuses are moved caudally in preparation for birth.

Viviparous	Gestation time (days)	Temperature range (°C)
Lizards (blue-tongued skink, prehensile-tailed skink)	180–240	28 with a basking area of 32.5
Colubrid snakes (water snakes, garter snakes)	90–100	24–29.5
Boas (common boa, tree boa, rainbow boa, rosy boa)	100–200	28 with a basking area of 32.5

5.20 Gestation times and temperature ranges for viviparous reptiles.

(Data from Mattison (1986) and Rogner (1997))

Dystocia

The diagnosis of dystocia is straightforward if a pregnant snake delivers only a portion of neonates during parturition. A snake with retained fetuses beyond 24 hours should receive veterinary care. Radiography or ultrasonography can be utilized to confirm the presence of retained fetuses and to determine viability (see Chapter 9).

The treatment of dystocia in viviparous reptiles can be problematic, particularly in snakes that carry a large number of fetuses (5–50) during pregnancy. Attention must first be given to correcting dehydration, followed by the administration of calcium/oxytocin. If parturition does not occur, surgical intervention is necessary – either salpingotomy (removal of fetuses only) or ovariosalpingectomy (removal of ovaries and oviducts with retained fetuses) (Figure 5.21).

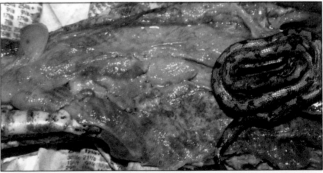

5.21 Sudden death of a pregnant Solomon Island boa due to salpingitis.

Neonatal husbandry

Parental care

Maternal care of neonates has been observed in a wide variety of reptiles. Nest and infant tending has been especially well documented in crocodilians. Female Burmese brown tortoises make large nest mounds of rotting vegetation and defend them from other animals. Some python species coil around their nests and can raise their body temperature several degrees by shivering, temporarily developing a modified form of endothermy, termed 'muscular thermogenesis', to support egg incubation. In captivity, most breeders prefer to remove python eggs and incubate them artificially to save the female's energy reserves. If females incubate the eggs they lose quite a bit of body mass in this process and are less likely to be able to regain sufficient weight for successful reproduction the following year.

There are some herbivorous reptiles that do not show any parental care but proximity of adults to their offspring neonates is important. Neonatal reptiles are born lacking the gastrointestinal bacteria, fungi and protozoans that have the enzymes necessary to break down cellulose into its component sugars. These reptiles need quickly to acquire the gut flora necessary to digest cellulose and do so by seeking out and licking or consuming fresh faeces of older animals. If the neonates do not have access to the appropriate faeces, establishment of an appropriate gut flora takes much longer to develop and this may slow their growth.

Single *versus* group rearing

Depending on the species, neonates may be raised singly or in groups. Monitor lizards are a good example of the impact of neonatal husbandry on adult behaviour. If monitor lizards are raised singly and introduced to others as adults, their first interactions are typically hostile and may result in severe injuries as neither monitor knows how to interpret and respond to the other monitor's behaviour. Group housing as neonates and juveniles prevents raising these 'social misfits' (Figure 5.22a).

A large enclosure with plenty of hiding places and visual barriers, and a mosaic of thermal, moisture and light environments are needed when group rearing reptiles (Figure 5.22b). Aggressive interactions between juveniles are often the result of being raised in an enclosure that is too small for the group size or is lacking sufficient hiding spots and visual barriers. If the enclosure concentrates essential resources (e.g. heat, light, food, water) in small areas, dominant specimens can prevent access by others. Food should always be offered under supervision and in excess, so that a few items are left over after every specimen has eaten (Figure 5.23).

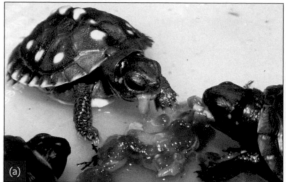

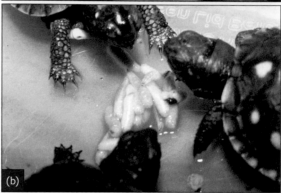

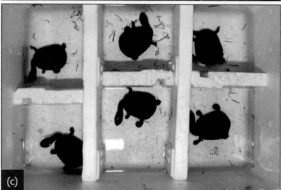

5.23 (a–b) Neonatal North American box turtles consuming thawed pinkies and dipteran larvae under close supervision; commonly, one individual seems to stimulate feeding behaviour in its clutchmates. This species is more carnivorous at a young age. (c) The safest method of food presentation is to separate neonates during feeding. Pictured are side-necked turtle neonates consuming bloodworms.

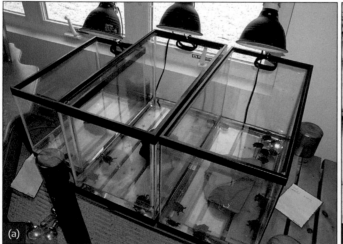

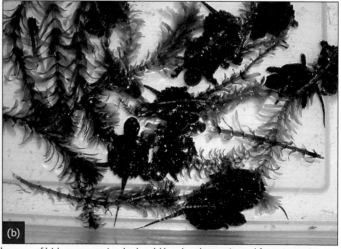

5.22 (a) Communal raising of neonate diamondback terrapins with an absence of hide areas; animals should be closely monitored for aggressive social interactions particularly during feeding. (b) Communal raising of neonate snapping turtles. Provision of anacharis supplies both food and a visual barrier; this is a more appropriate set-up than (a).

Captive propagation for release

Differential survivorship has been shown for snapping turtles that were incubated at different constant temperatures. Males produced from the low-threshold temperature and females produced from the high-threshold temperature had higher survivorship in an outdoor pond over males and females produced from the intermediate temperatures. This phenomenon may influence the choice of captive propagation programme to best support a reintroduction effort.

Neonates placed into a large and complex environment within days of birth are more likely to develop the behaviours necessary for life in the wild. Neonates that are raised in captivity under typical hobbyist conditions cannot subsequently develop behavioural maps of the environment that allow them to find and return to prey trails or food sources, water sources, or appropriate retreats. Any reintroduction programme must provide the appropriate postnatal environment to support complex behaviours.

Neonatal diseases

Neonatal reptiles are susceptible to all the infectious diseases of adult reptiles. There are no pharmacokinetic studies on drug distribution in neonatal reptiles. Allometric scaling of the dosage simply replaces one best guess with another, as the neonatal metabolic rates of most species of reptiles are unknown, and the data available are for reptiles that are maintained at, and acclimated to, a single temperature. Many metabolic rate studies have extremely small sample sizes that make statistical validation problematic. In consequence, the dosages used are the same as those published for adult reptiles. What follows is a description of maladies affecting neonate and juvenile reptiles.

Yolk sac retention and infection

It is relatively common to receive a call from a client concerned about a neonatal reptile's unabsorbed yolk sac. In many instances the neonate is normal and the client, who has been overly eager for the hatchling to emerge, has checked the egg once too often and provoked the neonate to leave the eggshell too early. The yolk sac may be swabbed with an antiseptic such as dilute povidone iodine or chlorhexidine solution but there are no data to suggest that this has any merit in preventing infections.

Neonatal susceptibility

Neonates that have emerged from the egg prematurely are more prone to develop yolk sac or generalized infections. Most incubation media are heavily contaminated with bacterial and fungal pathogens by the time the eggs are 'pipping'. If maternal nutrition and health were not optimal the neonate may be immunocompromised. Neonatal viviparous reptiles end up with yolk sac problems for similar reasons: premature birth; birth into a contaminated environment; or immune compromise as a result of maternal malnutrition or other health problems. Neonates resulting from hybridization attempts with different subspecies also appear to be at increased risk for yolk sac problems; these are prominent in prehensile-tailed skinks and Galapagos tortoises but also seen in some of the intergeneric hybrids such as jungle corn snakes.

Clinical signs

A normal hatching is accompanied by clear colourless odourless fluid dripping from the pipped eggshell. If a pipping egg has a foul or sweet smell, or if the fluid is anything other than clear and colourless, it is an indication that medical intervention is necessary. Odour and turbidity are signs of bacterial or fungal contamination; frequently, contaminated fluid has been swallowed and possibly inhaled by the hatchling, putting the neonate at high risk of localized or systemic infection.

A healthy but prematurely emerged neonate has an exterior yolk sac, where the yolk is bright yellow and homogeneous in colour and texture (like a 'sunny-side-up' runny fried chicken egg) (Figure 5.24a). In most instances, the youngster should be placed within a dark container lined with damp paper towels and the yolk will absorb and the skin or plastron will close over the umbilical gap within 24–96 hours (Figure 5.24b). The paper towel should be changed daily to reduce bacterial contamination.

If a recently pipped neonate has an exteriorized yolk sac and the material within the yolk sac is anything other than a homogeneous yellow, intervention is necessary. If a recently pipped neonate has a closed umbilicus but there is a firm mass palpable in the coelom, this suggests the presence of an infected yolk sac and again requires intervention. Unfortunately, at this point many neonates are also septic and die despite treatment. Potential problems with viviparous reptiles are similar. If the 'birth sac' has discoloured membranes, or a foul or sweet smell, the neonate has been heavily contaminated with bacteria or fungi.

The most common presentations for a neonatal snake with a retained yolk sac are: failure to complete its postnatal shed successfully; failure to eat within 30 days of birth; or palpation of a firm coelomic mass approximately 50–65% of its snout–vent length postcranially.

Maternal and paternal behaviour can suggest a problem in some viviparous lizards, such as prehensile-tailed skinks. If the neonatal skink is not healthy, the neonate is typically not attended by the parents and may be seen

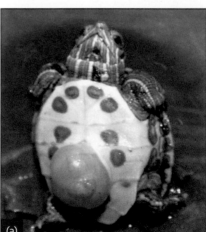

5.24 (a) A premature neonatal red-eared slider with unabsorbed yolk. It is critical to prevent desiccation and infection by keeping the turtle on a clean moist substrate such as paper towel while the yolk is being absorbed. (b) An open umbilicus in an albino hognose snake; a suture was used to oppose the skin. Note this is the same individual as in Figure 5.33.

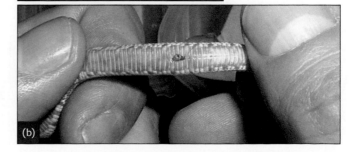

clearly in the enclosure rather than hiding like a normal neonate. If the yolk sac is not removed, the skink becomes dehydrated, its skin roughens and discolours, and a septic blush quickly develops (Figure 5.25).

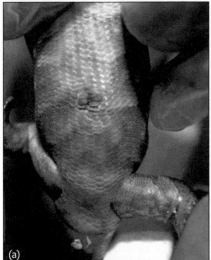

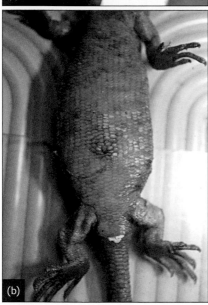

5.25 Neonatal prehensile-tailed skinks:
(a) individual with normal umbilicus;
(b) septic appearance due to yolk sac infection.
(Courtesy of Kevin M. Wright)

Treatment

Surgical intervention is mandatory in most cases. The majority of the yolk is internal in most cases and the external portion seen is a bubble off the thin yolk sac rather than the actual yolk stalk. Ligation of the external portion would rupture the yolk sac and create a chemical coelomitis in addition to introducing pathogens. Even if the external portion of the yolk sac were successfully ligated, a large amount of contaminated yolk would still be present in the remaining sac and would empty into the gastrointestinal tract to form a nidus of infection. Gentle retraction of the yolk sac off the skin or plastron allows the yolk stalk to be visualized. The yolk stalk can be ligated close to its intestinal attachment and the yolk sac excised (Figure 5.26).

It may be impossible to lift the yolk sac enough to visualize the yolk stalk. In this case, a paramedial incision is extended anteriorly and posteriorly from the umbilicus to exteriorize the yolk stalk's attachment to the intestine. This can be done even in chelonians, as the plastron is cartilaginous at this stage in life and may be easily cut. If the yolk sac remains intact, it is a simple matter to ligate the stalk at its base. Monofilament 3 to 3.5 metric (0 to 2/0 USP) suture material or stainless steel clamps should be used to ligate the yolk stalk. An aspirate of the excised yolk sac should be submitted for microbiological examination including anaerobic culture. A swab of the coelom should also be submitted for culture. Unfortunately, these cultures may not identify the causal agent.

The coelom should be flushed thoroughly with sterile saline or an antibiotic flush (e.g. 500 mg amikacin in 1 litre of saline). If the yolk sac has ruptured and spilled material into the coelom it is imperative to continue to flush until all yolk is removed. Any yolk left behind can evoke a chemical coelomitis. Closure of the coelom is by standard methods using non-absorbable monofilament sutures, or tissue glue may be used. Chelonians may pose a challenge during closure as the cartilaginous plastron does not close fully until after the yolk sac has been completely absorbed post-hatching. Horizontal mattress sutures should be placed across the gap and the opposing edges of the shell drawn together as closely as possible without putting so much tension on the edges that the suture material tears through the plastron. The remaining gap can be covered with epoxy (Figure 5.27);

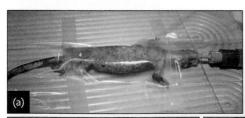

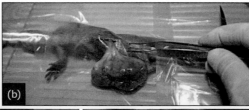

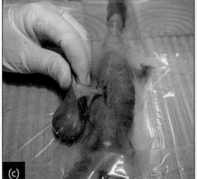

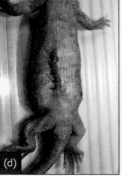

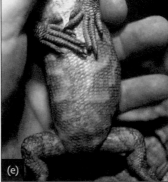

5.26 Omphalectomy in a prehensile-tailed skink with yolk sac infection. (a) The patient is anaesthetized. (b) The infected yolk sac has been exteriorized. (c) Ligation of the yolk sac at the point of attachment to the intestine. The sac is then excised and removed. (d) The skin has been closed using a horizontal mattress suture pattern. (e) Appearance several months after operation.
(Courtesy of Kevin M. Wright)

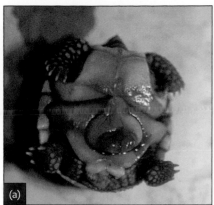
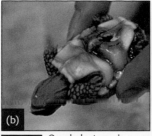
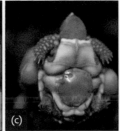
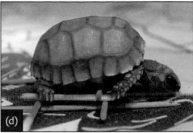

5.27 Omphalectomy in a neonatal yellow-footed tortoise with yolk sac infection. (a) The patient is prepared by scrubbing the surgical site with dilute povidone iodine or chlorhexidine. (b) After omphalectomy, the coelom is flushed and horizontal mattress sutures are placed across the suture site. (c) An epoxy resin patch covers the gap in the plastron to provide complete closure of the coelom. (d) The tortoise rests on a drying rack.
(Courtesy of Kevin M. Wright)

care should be taken not to contaminate the coelomic cavity. The sutures should be embedded in the epoxy so that it is firmly anchored to the plastron. The chelonian should then be placed in ventral recumbency on a platform that allows the epoxy to dry without becoming adhered to any other surface. The epoxy patch should be left in place for several months to ensure that the gap has healed appropriately. There is no rush to remove the patch and some patches have been left in place for more than 3 years without compromising the patient's health or growth.

Postoperative management

Hydration: The omphalectomized patient should be managed to ensure its hydration. Oral antibiotics (e.g. trimethoprim/sulfamethoxazole 15 mg/kg orally q24h, enrofloxacin 5–10 mg/kg orally q24h, or metronidazole 25 mg/kg orally q24h) should be administered to reduce the risk of any absorbed yolk causing gastroenteritis. A systemic advanced penicillin or cephalosporin (e.g. piperacillin 100 mg/kg i.m. or intracoelomically q24h, ceftazidime 20 mg/kg i.m. q72h) is recommended to combat systemic Gram-negative and anaerobic infections. Amikacin may be used in addition if necessary (e.g. 2.5 mg/kg i.m. or intracoelomically q72h).

Nutritional supplementation: Since the neonate has lost a large amount of stored nutrient by having the yolk removed, it is prudent to provide an oral formula that provides a lot of its energy through fat and has substantive stores of fat-soluble vitamins. Feline Clinical Care Liquid (Pet Ag) works well for carnivorous (insectivorous) reptiles and Canine Clinical Care Liquid (Pet-Ag) has been used successfully for herbivorous and omnivorous reptiles. The first tube feeding can be given approximately 48–72 hours postoperatively in herbivorous reptiles and 7–10 days postoperatively in carnivorous reptiles. Approximately 1 ml of formula per 50 g postoperative bodyweight should be given every 24–48 hours for a minimum of two treatments. After the initial feedings, the neonate may be offered normal food. Herbivorous reptiles will often start feeding within 10–14 days of surgery. Carnivorous reptiles, especially snakes, may not feed unless they are left undisturbed for 48–96 hours. If the neonate does not begin eating on its own it may need additional nutrient supplementation.

Prognosis

Omphalectomized reptiles appear to grow at the same rate as clutchmates and often catch up to their clutchmates' bodyweights within a year.

Fly strike

Hatching and neonatal reptiles need to be protected from flies. This is best accomplished with an airtight incubation box that is opened for air exchange twice a week for 15 minutes. If flies are noted in or around the incubator, sticky glue traps may be used to eliminate the pests. The presence of flies is correlated with dead or infertile eggs in the incubator, so a review of the incubation boxes is suggested to remove these eggs. Fly maggots can quickly invade 'pipping' eggs, eat through a neonatal reptile's unabsorbed yolk sac and penetrate into the coelom (Figure 5.28). Maggots should be flushed away with a warmed dilute solution of povidone iodine and saline. If maggots are suspected to have breached the coelom, surgery to remove the yolk sac and explore the coelom should be performed.

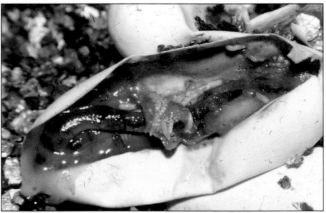

5.28 'Fly strike' afflicting a Honduran milk snake egg owing to premature death in the egg.

Gastrointestinal obstruction

Neonatal and juvenile herbivorous reptiles may develop gastrointestinal obstruction from hard vegetables such as carrots, sweet potatoes and broccoli stems. Hay and high-lignin-content leaves have also been found as gastrointestinal obstructions. Pebbles, gravel, sand, mulch, long-fibre sphagnum moss and bark chips may cause obstruction in young reptiles. Young reptiles will constantly taste items in their environment to determine edibility and may consume indigestible objects as part of this exploration.

Gastrointestinal obstruction is quickly fatal if uncorrected. A definitive diagnosis can be difficult to attain but should be suspected whenever a young reptile is anorexic and has had access to suspect food items or substrate. Corrective surgery needs to be performed quickly.

Cold stunning

Unfortunately, there is a black market in the USA for neonate reptiles such as the red-eared terrapin, which is legally farm-produced in massive numbers. In the Northeast (a region including the six New England states, New Jersey, and eastern parts of New York State and Pennsylvania), these reptiles are commonly sold illegally (at less than 10 cm) outdoors during the winter months. They present with respiratory (negative buoyancy) and neurological signs (ataxia). Slow restoration of body temperature, supportive alimentation and antibiotics are recommended; however, response to treatment is often unrewarding (Figure 5.29).

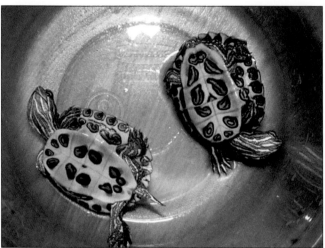

5.29 'Cold-stunned' neonatal red-eared sliders with torticollis and buoyancy problems.

Endoparasites

Captive bred and born neonate reptiles, mass-produced in facilities that have poor husbandry standards, are susceptible to numerous maladies including but not limited to endoparasitism. Affected neonates and juveniles demonstrate poor appetites, regurgitation, diarrhoea, intussusception and cloacal prolapse. Faecal analysis should routinely be part of the physical examination even with captive-born neonate animals (Figure 5.30) (see Chapter 24).

Nutritional secondary hyperparathyroidism

Motor paralysis and pathological fractures secondary to nutritional secondary hyperparathyroidism (NSHP) have been diagnosed in juvenile reptiles as young as 8 weeks of age and are discussed further in Chapter 22 (Figure 5.31).

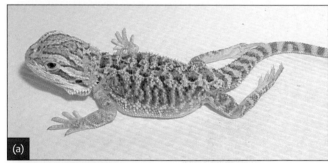

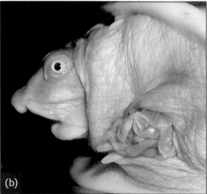

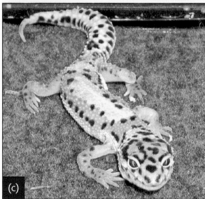

5.31 (a) A pathological fracture of the spine resulting in hindlimb paralysis in a bearded dragon with nutritional secondary hyperparathyroidism (NSHP). (b) Distortion of the maxillary and mandibular bones causing malocclusion in a flap-shelled turtle; also note curling of the edges of the carapace secondary to NSHP. (c) 'Swelling' of the extremities and plantigrade stance in a leopard gecko with NSHP.

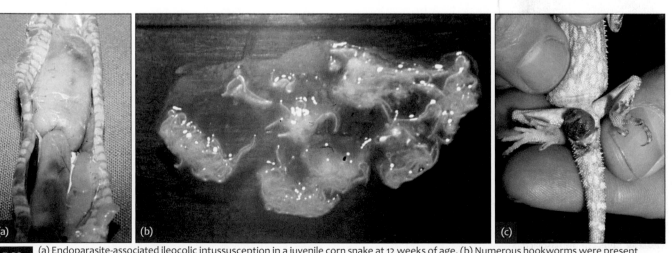

5.30 (a) Endoparasite-associated ileocolic intussusception in a juvenile corn snake at 12 weeks of age. (b) Numerous hookworms were present when the intussusception was opened. (c) Cloacal prolapse in a juvenile bearded dragon secondary to oxyurid infestation.

Prolapsed hemipenes

Rarely, male neonatal reptiles are born with prolapsed copulatory organs. The author [PR] has encountered this phenomenon in snakes and the organ usually returns to the respective sulcus within 24 hours, provided the reptiles are kept on moistened towel roll (Figure 5.32). A water-soluble lubricant can also be applied to the prolapsed tissues and gentle manipulation performed to encourage regression of the hemipenes into the sulci.

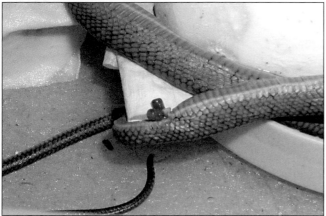

5.32 Prolapsed hemipenes in a neonate Sulawesi black-tailed ratsnake that has just emerged from its egg.

Blocked nasolacrimal duct

Blockage of the nasolacrimal duct appears to occur more commonly in neonate snakes than other reptiles (Figure 5.33). Most cases are unilateral and the condition is either present at birth or develops several days to weeks later. The affected eye appears swollen owing to build-up of secretions from the lacrimal and Harderian glands. Drainage of secretions normally occurs from the subspectacular

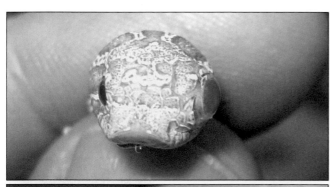

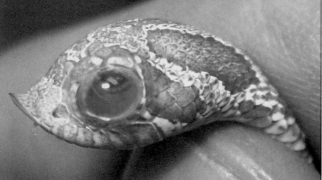

5.33 Pseudobuphthalmos of the left eye, secondary to a congenital defect of the nasolacrimal duct in a neonate albino hognose snake.

space into the lacrimal duct, which terminates in the roof of the oral cavity. Congenital malformation and/or inflammation of the duct due to oral infections are the most common causes. Repeated aseptic fine-needle aspiration of the distended subspectacular space can sometimes cause resolution of signs. See Chapter 16 for further treatment details.

Dysecdysis

Dysecdysis occurs with some frequency in neonate/juvenile squamates. Snakes and lizards such as bearded dragons and leopard geckos can shed every 2–3 weeks once they are consuming food and growing rapidly. Some snakes are born opaque and shed within 48 hours, which is normal. If the neonates are not provided with sufficient ambient humidity, retained sheds adhere to tail tips, toes and periocular tissues (Figure 5.34a–b). Cachectic leopard geckoes may not remove and ingest their shed skins (Figure 5.34c). Aquatic turtles (e.g. red-eared terrapin, river cooter) that are always in water and not provided with 'haul out' sites are prone to retained scutes (Figure 5.34d) (see Chapters 15 and 16 for further treatment details). In addition to dehydration, neurological disease may also contribute to dysecdysis.

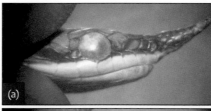

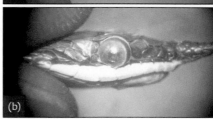

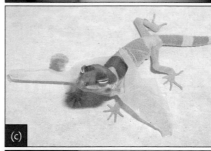

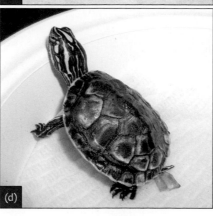

5.34 (a) Retained spectacle in a rhino ratsnake at 6 weeks of age, secondary to suboptimal ambient humidity.
(b) Appearance of the eye after placing the snake on moist paper towels for 12 hours and removal of the retained spectacle.
(c) Weakness and inability of a juvenile leopard gecko to remove its skin secondary to chronic diarrhoea.
(d) Dysecdysis in a neonatal river cooter that was constantly maintained in water. Note the edges of the retained scutes that are raised and discoloured; one shed scute lies in the water.
(a, b, Courtesy of William Cermak)

Starvation

Healthy neonatal reptiles normally possess adequate yolk reserves for sustenance until they are voluntarily feeding. Specific time schedules differ among taxa and are affected by factors such as seasonality, health of neonates at birth, presentation of appropriate food items and pertinent husbandry requirements. It should also be noted that it is unrealistic to expect that all captive-born neonates will not only survive but flourish. Natural selection has an important role to play in nature which is often ignored in captivity. Intensive inbreeding over time leads not only to congenital defects but also increased morbidity and mortality of neonates. It is safe to say that the sooner neonates begin to feed voluntarily, the better the chances of long-term survival. In general, it is easier to get lizards and chelonians to start feeding than snakes. Larger neonatal snakes (e.g. kingsnakes) usually present fewer problems associated with alimentation than neonates of smaller species (e.g. Solomon Island boas). Neonatal chameleons present unique issues owing to their diminutive size and requirement for 'pinhead' crickets. Some species of reptile change their prey preferences as they grow. For example, juvenile snakes may consume small lizards, insects and fish, prior to changing to birds and mammals as adults (Figure 5.35a).

A technique that works well with shy recalcitrant snakes is to place individuals with food in paper bags overnight (Figure 5.35b). The authors recommend weighing each neonate at birth. Although it can be problematic to know precisely when to initiate nutritional supplementation, a 10% decrease in weight is what the author [PR] uses as a guideline (Figure 5.35c). Stress for the neonate associated with tube feeding also has to be taken into account (Figure 5.35d) (see Chapter 22).

Trauma

Trauma due to cagemate aggression occurs commonly in neonate bearded dragons and aquatic turtles. These avoidable accidents occur due to normal establishment of social hierarchies. Presented trauma victims have missing toes, feet and tails (Figure 5.36a–b). Morbidity and mortality can be correspondingly high. Rough handling on the owner's part is another cause, such as forcibly removing chameleons from their perches (Figure 5.36c). Accidental dropping of reptiles during handling also occurs. Intramuscular injections should not be administered in the limbs of neonatal reptiles owing to the risk of radial palsy and subsequent muscle atrophy (Figure 5.36d) (see Chapter 21).

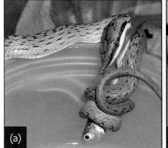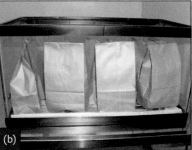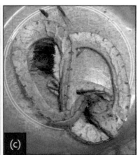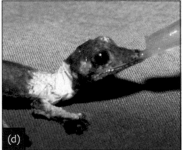

5.35 (a) Recalcitrant feeders such as this rhino ratsnake will often aggressively consume minnows as opposed to geckos and rodent pinkies. This probably represents an ontogenetic change in food preferences under natural conditions. (b) Placing individual snakes in paper bags for 24 hours with dead prey commonly stimulates a feeding response. (c) Severe cachexia and dehydration in this juvenile green tree python necessitated tube feeding. (d) The use of oral alimentation and a cooperative patient such as this anorexic leaf-tailed gecko greatly decreases recovery time.

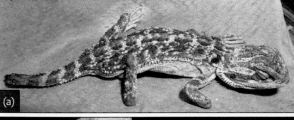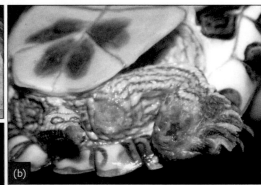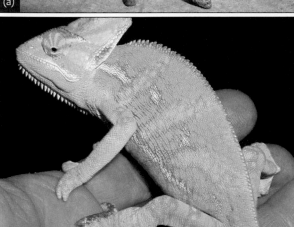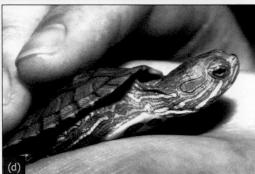

5.36 (a) A juvenile bearded dragon with severe injuries from aggressive conspecifics sharing a communal enclosure. (b) A juvenile red-eared slider with severe injuries from aggressive conspecifics sustained during feeding. (c) A juvenile veiled chameleon with a fractured tibia/fibula due to being pulled from its perch by the owner. (d) A hatchling red-eared slider with right radial palsy due to an intramuscular injection.

Hypovitaminosis A

Vitamin A deficiency does occur in neonate/juvenile reptiles after stored vitamin A supplies (yolk, liver) have been exhausted, coupled with a lack of ingested preformed vitamin A. Aquatic turtles, chameleons and leopard geckos seem to be prone to this problem. Blepharitis, blepharoedema and accumulation of ocular exudate due to squamous metaplasia of ocular glandular epithelial cells are the presenting signs (Figure 5.37). (For further information, see Chapters 4, 16 and 22.)

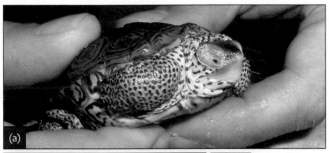

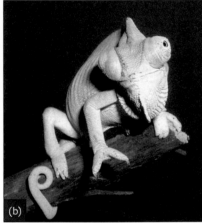

5.37 (a) Bilateral blepharoedema secondary to hypovitaminosis A in a juvenile diamondback terrapin. The turtle had been fed exclusively a pelleted diet that was deficient in vitamin A. (b) Bilateral periocular oedema in a juvenile veiled chameleon with early hypovitaminosis A.

Hypothiaminosis (hypovitaminosis B1)

Deficiency of vitamin B1 occurs in piscivorous reptiles that are fed exclusively on thawed fish. Thiamine is inactivated by the freezing process. Examples of affected reptiles are water snakes, garter snakes and turtles. The author [PR] has encountered thiamine-deficient diamondback terrapins exhibiting ataxia and motor paralysis by 3 months of age. Clinical signs consist of ataxia, incoordination and/or tremors (Figure 5.38). Diagnosis is based primarily upon dietary history and signalment. (See Chapters 4 and 22 for further information.)

Respiratory tract disease

Neonatal and juvenile reptiles appear to be more susceptible to respiratory tract diseases than adult reptiles. This can be caused by, for example, owners mistakenly 'hibernating' their turtles and tortoises, exposing them to suboptimal temperatures for prolonged periods of time (Figure 5.39a–b). Shipping of reptiles during the colder seasons is another common cause (Figure 5.39c) (see Chapter 18).

Chemical toxicity

Toxicity due to the use of vapour insect repellents containing organophosphates (18% dichlorvos) seems to have diminished; however, these products are still available.

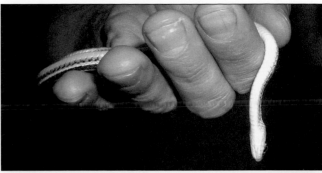

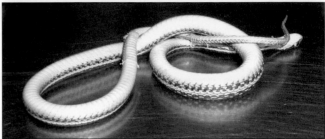

5.38 Ataxia and loss of righting reflex in a thiamine-deficient juvenile North American garter snake that was fed exclusively on thawed fish.

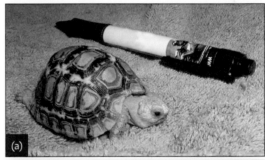

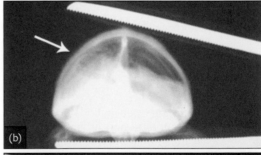

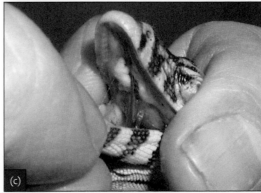

5.39 (a) Anorexia, dyspnoea, weakness and depression in a 5-month-old leopard tortoise. (b) Craniocaudal radiograph revealing infiltrates in the dependent portion of the right lung consistent with lower respiratory tract disease. (c) Accumulation of exudate in the right internal choana of a juvenile water monitor with an upper respiratory tract infection.

Organophosphate toxicity used to be commonly diagnosed in neonate and juvenile snakes from large reptile collections where mites were problematic (Figure 5.40). Permethrins, pyrethrins and carbamates, although not considered as toxic, are still potentially dangerous when inhaled at close proximity or ingested. Clinical signs (ataxia, paralysis) appear similar to those caused by organophosphates. Several juvenile spur-thighed tortoises (4 months of age) with motor paralysis presented to the author [PR] after exposure to ant traps which contained pyrethrins and carbamates. The signs eventually subsided over a period of several days after administration of parenteral parasympatholytics and soaks in balanced electrolyte solutions (see Chapter 21). Neonatal snakes maintained on cedar shavings are susceptible to irritation of mucous membranes of the nasal and oral cavities.

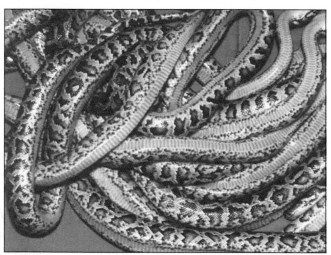

5.40 Ataxia and loss of righting reflex in hatchling Burmese pythons that were exposed to dichlorvos for the purpose of controlling a mite infestation.

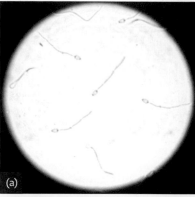
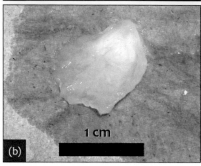

5.41 (a) Viable sperm cells from a Honduran milk snake. (b) A semen plug extruded by a female Asian ratsnake 24 hours prior to oviposition. The purpose of the plugs is to seal the oviducts after copulation.

Semen collection and artificial insemination

There have been numerous publications describing semen acquisition, semen storage and artificial insemination in various reptilian taxa (Figure 5.41). Semen collection is done during the breeding season and consists of either external massage of the cloacal area or intracloacal electrostimulation. Manual stimulation has been done mostly in snakes and small lizards, while the latter technique is used in large lizards and chelonians depending on the size of the reptile and probe. For example, a protocol developed for adult leopard tortoises (>3 years) consisted of anaesthetization with propofol followed by cloacal intromissions with an electro-ejaculator. Settings of 4–6 volts at 3-minute intervals resulted in successful collection of semen that averaged 0.26 ml in volume. Artificial insemination using fresh diluted and diluted refrigerated semen has been done successfully in corn snakes and other squamates (see Mattison et al. (1986) and Hoser (2008) for further details).

Acknowledgement

All photographs courtesy of Paul Raiti, except where noted.

References and further reading

Fahrig BM, Mitchell MA, Eilts BE, Paccamonti DL and Lock B (2006) Characterization and cooled storage of semen from corn snakes (Elaphe guttata). Proceedings of the Association of Reptilian and Amphibian Veterinarians Annual Conference, p. 99

Gurley R (2003) Keeping and Breeding Freshwater Turtles. Living Art Publishing, Ada, OK

Highfield AC (1996) Keeping and Breeding Tortoises and Freshwater Turtles. Carapace Press, London

Hoser R (2008) A technique for artificial insemination in squamates. Bulletin of the Chicago Herpetological Society 43(1), 1–9

Mattison C (1986) Snakes of the World. Facts on File Publications, New York

Mattson KJ, De Vries A, McGuire SM et al. (2007) Successful artificial insemination in the corn snake, Elaphe gutatta, using fresh and cooled semen. Zoo Biology 26(5), 363–369

Mitchell MA, Zimmerman D and Heggem B (2009) Collection and characterization of semen from green iguanas. Proceedings of the Association of Reptilian and Amphibian Veterinarians Annual Conference, p. 165

Mitchell MA, Zimmerman D and Heggem B (2009) Collection and characterization of semen from leopard tortoises. Proceedings of the Association of Reptilian and Amphibian Veterinarians Annual Conference, p. 166

Murphy JB, Adler K and Collins JT (1994) Captive Management and Conservation of Amphibians and Reptiles. Society for the Study of Amphibians and Reptiles, Ithaca, NY

Porter KR (1972) Reproductive adaptations of reptiles. In: Herpetology, pp. 378–436. WB Saunders, Philadelphia

Pough FH, Andrews RM, Cadle JE et al. (1998) Reproduction and life history. In: Herpetology, pp. 204–234. Prentice Hall, Upper Saddle River, NJ

Raiti P (1995) Reproductive biology of reptiles. Proceedings of the Association of Reptilian and Amphibian Veterinarians Annual Conference, pp. 101–105

Rogner M (1997) Lizards. 2 vols. Krieger, Malabar, FL, USA

Zug GR, Vitt LJ and Caldwell JP (2001) Reproduction and life histories. In: Herpetology, 2nd edn, pp. 107–153. Academic Press, San Diego

Chapter 6

Clinical examination

Aidan Raftery

A thorough clinical examination is very important in reptiles as in all species. The clinical examination will include collecting a history as well as the physical examination. Both are interwoven and something found on the physical examination may raise new questions of the history or *vice versa*. With every case it is important to go through and record all the findings from the history and the physical examination. It may be tempting to take a shortcut and home in on the presenting signs, but this may result in the treatment of secondary problems. For example, stomatitis and rectal prolapse are secondary conditions where a complete clinical examination and review of the husbandry is very important to identify the underlying problem.

First contact

Receptionists are usually the first members of the veterinary practice to make contact with the reptile owner. They should have training to allow recognition of urgent cases that need immediate care or refer to somebody within the practice who has the relevant knowledge to make triage decisions (see also Chapter 7). A specific protocol should be drawn up for organizing reptile appointments:

- Reptile consultations should only be scheduled for those veterinary surgeons (veterinarians) with the necessary knowledge
- The receptionist should be aware of which species the practice has the knowledge and equipment to handle
- A list of reptile specialists to whom unfamiliar species can be redirected should be available
- Owners should be requested to bring in:
  - Pictures of the home environment
  - A faecal sample
  - Husbandry records, if kept (see Chapter 3)
  - Any nutritional supplements used
  - Any home remedies that have been used.
- If this is a second opinion, the previous veterinary history should be obtained and presented to the veterinary surgeon as soon as possible.

Signalment

The signalment is usually recorded by the receptionist; however, the veterinary surgeon should check it as if it is inaccurate as this will affect the differential list.

Species

It is important to correctly identify the species owing to different environment requirements and disease susceptibilities. Both the common and scientific names of the species should be acquired. Many species have two or more common names and a common name may refer to more than one species. Knowing the scientific name will ensure that a proper identification has been made and the appropriate information is being relayed to the owner.

Age

Age is another key component of history taking. Unfortunately, the true age can often not be reliably ascertained. Without an accurate age it is not possible to identify which individuals are geriatric and which are relatively young for their species. Among reptiles there is a very wide range of longevity with many lizard species living into their 20s and many species of snake known to live into their 30s. Among chelonians many species are known for their extreme longevity with some species such as the Aldabran tortoise having been recorded living well beyond 100 years of age. Of course there are also species whose natural lifespan is very short. The carpet chameleon has a lifespan in the wild of 1–2 years and in captivity, even in the best conditions, these chameleons only live for an average of 2–3 years.

Gender

It is important to know whether the patient is male or female. Not only do conditions of the reproductive tract depend on gender but also behaviour can be influenced by gender. Gender-related conditions become more likely once the animal has reached sexual maturity. In many species, especially in juveniles, it can be very difficult to determine the gender by external characteristics. Refer to Chapters 1 and 5 for gender differentiation.

History

History taking can be divided into four separate categories:

- The reason for the visit
- Other body functional information
- Environment and diet and also any possible exposure to toxic/harmful materials
- Past medical history and also interactions with others.

A very important question is how long the animal has been in the client's care; if this is a very short time then greater effort will have to be made to collect more historical information. The origin of the animal also has a big influence on the interpretation of the history and the differential list. Wild caught and captive farmed animals may be carrying diseases and parasites endemic in those environments but not seen in captive-bred specimens.

Reason for presentation

The first step is always to clarify and record the reason for the examination. The client must describe the clinical signs they have observed and also signs observed by others. Record when the signs were first noticed and their progress. Identify if any treatment has been given and also the response to this treatment if relevant.

Bodily functions

The clinician can at this stage progress to ask about any other changes in bodily functions: food and water intake; breathing changes; any abnormal sounds; defecation (frequency and appearance); activity; locomotion; recent reproductive history; vision and hearing; changes in appearance; changes in habits; or unusual actions such as collapsing, seizures or scratching.

Husbandry review

A large number of problems presented are due, directly or indirectly, to incorrect or substandard husbandry. A thorough review of the husbandry is an essential part of the reptile clinical examination. Ideally, this can be accomplished most effectively at the client's premises where the environment can be seen; however, this is rarely possible, although most owners have pictures of their set ups on their cell phones which can be very useful. The clinician must be familiar with the current best practice for husbandry and nutrition for the species being examined. The husbandry review should cover:

- **Lighting:** photoperiod; UVB provision if required; position; 'life expectancy' of UVB source
- **Thermal provision:** heat sources; thermal gradient achieved; reliability of client's temperature readings; water temperature; night-time temperature; reliability of any temperature control system; ambient temperature; possibility of unplanned temperature spikes and troughs
- **Humidity:** hydrometer readings; means of generating humidity; water temperature; ventilation provided
- **Enclosure:** type (e.g. arboreal, terrestrial, semiaquatic); size; construction material; new or second-hand
- **Furnishings:** substrate; hides; plants (live or artificial); branches or rocks for climbing
- **Hygiene:** frequency and method of cleaning; disinfectants used
- **Nutrition:** food provided *versus* food consumed; feeding frequency; care of live insect food prior to feeding; supplements given; water provision
- **In-contact animals, including those in the same premises:** social structure; breeding history; quarantine protocols.

Refer to Chapter 3 for captive care and management and Chapter 4 for nutrition. At this stage also enquire about any possible exposure to harmful materials.

Past history

This is the last stage of history collection where information is gathered about any previous illness the animal may have had. If there is a history of previous illness collect as much information as possible about these past episode(s). If there was veterinary treatment then a copy of the clinical history should be obtained. Also, question whether any animals from the same group have had any illness. If yes, gather details as above including information on which age groups were affected and the sequence of the problem including any response to treatment. Additionally, attempt to acquire a copy of the clinical history if these animals were presented for veterinary treatment.

Use of questionnaires

History questionnaires, if used correctly, can be very valuable. A reptile clinical questionnaire should cover the signalment, source of the animal, in-contact animals, environment, husbandry practices and the nutrition provided for the animal, as well as the signs noticed by the owner that initiated the visit. If the owner has completed this prior to entering the consulting room, the clinician can use it to cover relevant areas in greater depth. It allows better use of consulting time and gives a good opportunity to evaluate the owner's level of knowledge. A sample questionnaire is shown in Figure 6.1.

Transportation

Reptiles should be transported to the surgery in secure containers. As a general rule, reptiles being transported should not be exposed to temperatures above 30°C or below 17°C. If the journey is short, a hot-water bottle or similar heat source within the container may suffice to keep the ambient temperature suitable. The heat source should be wrapped in a towel to ensure that there is no direct contact with the patient. In cold conditions an insulated box is required for transportation. Polystyrene boxes commercially made for this purpose are available, or insulated transport boxes can be improvised from cool boxes. These are also useful during hot conditions to try to prevent the temperature rising above the desired level. A thermometer should be placed in the container so that the temperature can be monitored. This is especially important during hot conditions. Containers must never be left in a car in the sun, as critical temperatures can be reached rapidly in that environment.

All animals should be transported singly. Snakes and larger lizards are best transported in cloth bags which are supported inside separate rigid containers with adequate ventilation. When a number of reptiles are transported together, the containers should be labelled to identify the animal within. The cloth bags must be free from holes and without loose threads in which the animal could become entangled and thereby injured. Small lizards and chelonians are usually transported in rigid boxes which are just slightly larger than the animal.

- **Chelonians** must be transported singly, inside a rigid box. They need to be in an upright position and cushioned to prevent undue movement and jarring, so that they will not end up upside down, which could be fatal in a dyspnoeic animal. Soft-shelled turtles need to be kept moist.

Reptile history form

Pet name/ID ....   Species ....   In present owner's care since ....

Colour ....   Date of birth/age ....   Sex: Male [ ] Female [ ] Unkown [ ]

Where did you obtain this animal? Breeder [ ] Pet shop [ ] Importer [ ] Other [ ] *please specify* ....

Enclosure/vivarium specifications

Type of enclosure: Arboreal [ ] Terrestrial [ ] Aquatic [ ]   Environment: Temperate [ ] Tropical [ ] Desert [ ]

Size of enclosure: Longest side ....   Shortest side ....   Height ....

Construction materials ....   Paint/varnish ....   Sealant ....

Interior fittings ....   Purchased ready-made [ ]   Substrate used ....

Temperature daytime range ....   Temperature night-time range ....   Basking temperature ....

Humidity level: Daytime ....   Night-time ....   Method provision: Spray [ ] Sprinkler [ ] Water bowl [ ]

Lighting equipment: Spot light [ ] Light bulb [ ] Fluorescent strip light [ ]

UVB light provision: Brand ....   When was it last renewed? ....   Day length ....

Distance from basking area ....

Diet/supplements

Diet ....

Amount of food normally offered ....   Amount eaten ....   Frequency of feeding ....

Method of providing drinking water: Bowl [ ] Spray [ ] Other [ ] *please specify* ....

How often is the water changed? ....   Vitamin/mineral supplements ....

How are supplements offered? ....   How often? ....

History

What signs prompted you to bring in this animal? ....

Other animals sharing the vivarium in the last 6 months ....

Other animals housed in the same room or visiting the room in the last 6 months ....

Please list any disease history of this animal ....

....

Please list the disease history of any in-contact animal(s) ....

Any other details that may be relevant ....

....

....

6.1   Example of a history questionnaire.

- **Lizards and snakes** should be first placed singly in cloth bags, sealed by knotting or twisting, folding and securely taping, which are then placed in rigid containers. Large lizards may need to be in sturdier bags made of a stronger material such as jute or canvas, as they may tear lighter fabrics.
- **Venomous snakes** are a special case. They must be transported clearly labelled as venomous and with accompanying documentation, and preferably antivenom, clearly detailing what to do in the case of envenomation (see Appendix 3).

Handling

Training and practice are required to become proficient in the use of restraint equipment for reptiles. Ideally, there should be more than one individual within the veterinary practice with reptile-handling skills.

Handling chelonians

Most chelonians are easy to handle and restrain (Figure 6.2a) but examination can be very difficult if they retreat into their shells. Care must be taken not to drop them, and two handlers are needed for larger specimens. Some species have functional hinges at the front and rear and can completely seal themselves into their shells; others are very strong and, if they have retreated into their shells, it is very difficult to extend the legs and head for examination. Sedation is needed in some of these cases. There is a risk of injury to the handler from fingers being trapped by the hinges, between the forelimbs or in the prefemoral fossae when a limb is suddenly withdrawn by one of the larger tortoises. Some of the turtle species can be very aggressive and are capable of inflicting a serious bite, their head being able to extend a surprising distance. In this case they should be grasped at the rear, usually at the femoral fossae, out of reach of their long necks (Figure 6.2b).

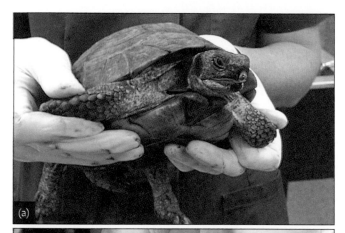

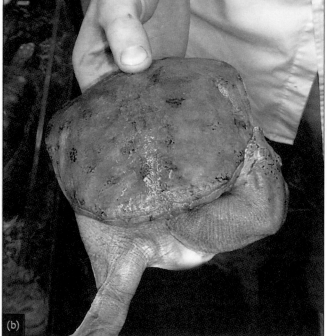

6.2 (a) Lifting a spur-thighed tortoise. (b) Aggressive species such as this soft-shelled turtle can be grasped at the caudal part of the carapace. Beware: the carapace can be very slippery.

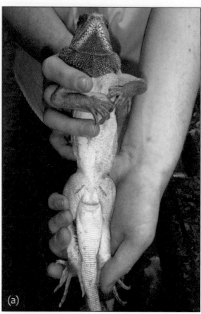

6.3 (a) Handling a water dragon. (b) Restraint of a veiled chameleon for examination of the vent region by gently controlling the limbs.

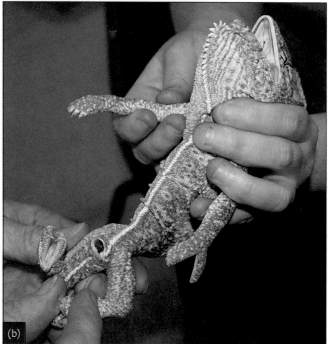

be difficult to catch and restrain owing to their speed and some geckos have skin that tears easily. These may be more safely caught and examined in a small net. Lizards must never be grasped by the tail as many species can shed their tails (autotomy); tail regrowth if it occurs (not all species regrow shed tails), takes several months and will not have the same coloration or scale pattern as the original.

Handling lizards

Feisty lizards are best captured initially with a towel, unless presented in a bag, in which case they can be restrained before being removed from the bag. One hand should restrain the pelvic limbs, keeping them stretched back parallel to the body, with the tail under one arm if the lizard is large, while the second hand restrains the upper body and head (Figure 6.3). Very small lizards can

Handling snakes

If presented in a bag for examination, snakes can be restrained before removal by grasping them just behind the head with all four fingers and thumb, while the second hand supports and restrains the snake's body about halfway along. *It must be remembered that snakes can, and do, bite through bags.* Snakes not presented in a bag can usually be caught by placing a towel over them first. More agile species can be held with snake tongs (Figure 6.4a) before grasping or bagging, or, by using a snake hook, they can be 'tubed' (Figure 6.4b–c). Snakes longer than 2 m should have at least two handlers restraining them (Figure 6.4d); larger snakes may need three or four handlers.

- Snakes should not be handled during ecdysis as the skin is easily damaged at this time.
- Snakes should not be held by the head or allowed to writhe about hold only by their neck as vertebral damage may result.
- Venomous snakes require special precautions. It must be remembered that even hatchlings are venomous and care must also be taken with dead specimens. The mouth should be taped shut prior to performing any post-mortem examination. Venomous snakes should only be seen by experienced reptile clinicians (see Appendix 3).

Snake/lizard tongs

Modern snake tongs, unlike the older versions, exert pressure over a wide area and are spring-loaded to prevent excessive force on the animal (Figure 6.4a). They are used to grasp the animal initially so that it can then be seized behind the head. Tongs can also be used to move cage furniture safely around the vivarium.

Snake hooks

These are used to allow capture and restraint (Figure 6.4b), especially of agile or dangerous snakes. The hooks should be light and easily cleaned. With the more agile species, care needs to be taken that they do not crawl up the handle to attack.

Snake restraining tubes

These plastic tubes are placed near to the snake's head and the snake encouraged to crawl two-thirds of the way into the tube. The snake and tube are then held simultaneously (Figure 6.4b–c). The ideal length is 60 cm and a range of diameters should be available. It is very important to choose the correct size of tube. If the tube is too wide the snake will be able to turn around, and if the tube is too short the snake may be able to stretch its body to strike out. If the tube is too narrow the snake will not be able to breathe. Tubes are especially useful for restraining and examining small to medium-sized aggressive snakes.

Physical examination

It is recommended that the clinician follows a structured clinical examination and that every patient is examined using the same sequential approach. The clinician must be familiar with what is normal for the species. It is advised that the aspiring reptile clinician make arrangements to examine as many healthy individuals as possible of the species that they are going to treat. It is only by being familiar with the normal that the clinician will be in a position to recognize the abnormal.

Observation

The animal should be observed before handling if possible. It is preferable to do this in its normal housing but this is rarely practical and in most cases it will have to be observed in its carrier or on the consulting-room table or

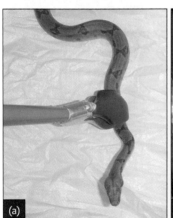
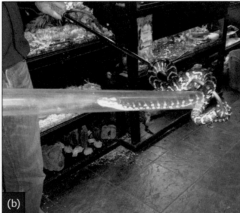
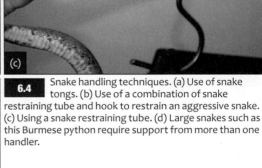
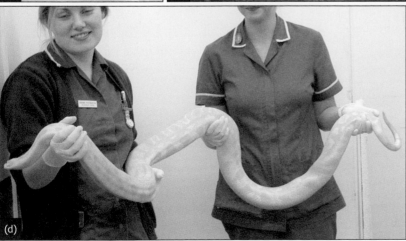

6.4 Snake handling techniques. (a) Use of snake tongs. (b) Use of a combination of snake restraining tube and hook to restrain an aggressive snake. (c) Using a snake restraining tube. (d) Large snakes such as this Burmese python require support from more than one handler.

floor. Degree of alertness, locomotion, stance and general attitude need to be observed and recorded. It is a good plan to take advantage of the time taken to collect the clinical history to observe the patient. This is also a good time for an assistant to weigh and take any other biometric measurements required for the record such as carapace length, width and depth in chelonians.

- The eyes of lizards and chelonians should be open, although many chelonians will withdraw into the relative safety of their shells.
- Monitor lizards and snakes should have active tongues, sampling the scent particles in the environment.
- A healthy reptile will have a normal alert body posture for the species. For example, iguanas should have a digitigrade stance (walking on their toes), whereas if not in full health the stance is often plantigrade (flat-footed). Allowances need to be made for the effect of any chilling that may have occurred as a result of inadequate transportation temperatures, as this will reduce metabolism and give a misleading impression of lethargy and weakness. If the head is out in chelonians, it should be held up and should not be resting on the ground. Nervous individuals will often have their head withdrawn inside the shell.
- Normal movement should also be observed before handling. Most species, even chelonians, ambulate with their bodies well above the ground. Aquatic turtles may have to be placed in water deep enough to encourage movement for observation.
- Record any limb lameness, weakness or any other abnormal motion observed, increased or decreased muscle tone, fasciculations, and spasm.
- The righting reflex should also be assessed (except for terrestrial chelonians). Poor righting reflexes may be due to severe weakness and not necessarily due to neurological disease (see Chapter 21).
- Observe respiration, including any sounds produced. Excessive rib movements and open-mouth breathing are signs commonly observed in dyspnoeic animals. However, agitated animals, especially snakes, may make hissing noises which may be mistaken for the effects of respiratory infections. Open-mouth gaping is usually (but not exclusively) a sign of lower respiratory tract pathology.
- Buoyancy changes to the aquatic and semiaquatic species are usually significant.

Measurements

Weighing is an extremely important part of the physical examination. The reptile patient should be weighed at every examination and, if hospitalized, should be weighed at the same time every day, ideally first thing in the morning before feeding and bathing. Allowances will have to be made for bladder contents, particularly in tortoises where up to 20% of their bodyweight can be due to bladder contents.

Other biometric measurements that can be recorded as a useful guide to the individual animal are detailed below under body condition. These measurements are most useful in the future as historical references to provide comparative information for that individual and include: total length; snout-to-vent length in lizards, snakes and crocodilians; and carapace length, carapace width and carapace height in chelonians.

Body condition

Body condition should be assessed.

Chelonians

Body condition in chelonians can be assessed by palpation, especially if the clinician has experience palpating normal individuals of the same species. Emaciation is appreciated by skinny bony limbs with baggy skin. These individuals are also weak and feel empty when picked up. Overweight individuals deposit fat in the prefemoral fossa and on either side of the neck. This can sometimes be mistaken for oedema.

Jackson's ratio has been used to assess the body condition of the Mediterranean spur-thighed tortoise and Hermann's tortoise. This ratio of bodyweight to carapace length can then be compared with 'normal' values. However, this method is no longer used as a gauge of health status. There are many reasons why normal healthy tortoises may vary from the 'normal' proposed by this method.

A formula has been devised for assessing the body condition of the Californian desert tortoise based on the carapace length (L), width at the widest part of the carapace (W) and maximum height from the bottom of the plastron to the top of the carapace (H) (Mader and Stoutenberg, 1998):

$$\text{Predicted bodyweight in grams} = 0.588\,(L \times W \times H) + 388$$

Animals weighing <90% of the predicted bodyweight are considered outside their normal range.

Carapace length, width (at the widest part) and height (from plastron bottom to top of carapace) are useful measurements in chelonians that can be recorded to provide a reference for the future for that individual (Figure 6.5).

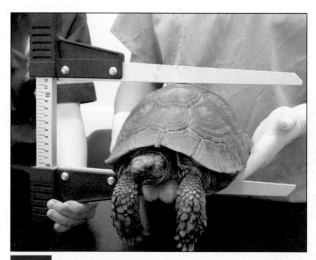

6.5 Measuring the carapace height.

Lizards

Obese lizards have a distended coelomic cavity with enlarged palpable fat-pads. The girth of the tail can be used as a measure of body condition in those species that store fat in their tails. When lizards become cachectic the bones of the pelvis become more prominent, the skin especially over the shoulders appears too big for the body, and the tail is shrunken and a triangular shape. In addition to bodyweight, total length (snout-to-tail tip) and snout-to-vent lengths can be recorded as a reference for the future.

Snakes

In obese snakes with increased fat deposition the last third of the body before the cloaca becomes obviously enlarged in some species. This often appears as lateral subcutaneous swellings that are not always symmetrical. Cachectic snakes that have lost sufficient muscle mass have a prominent dorsal spine and ribs, and the body shape appears more triangular in cross-section. Snakes can also have total length (snout-to-tail tip) and snout-to-vent lengths recorded in addition to bodyweight. However, it is difficult to make these measurements accurately in conscious snakes.

Clinical examination

Clinical examination generally commences at the head, working backwards along the body. However, it is sensible to perform non-invasive procedures first so that the patient is not stressed. For example, the head of a tortoise should be examined before the mouth is opened, as mouth opening may cause the animal to retract into its shell.

Rostrum or beak

Rostral areas should be checked for abrasions, tissue deficits and any other lesions. Rostral abrasions usually indicate trauma against a rough surface, lack of secure spaces for flighty individuals or reflective surfaces causing males to challenge their own image.

Only chelonians have a beak. It is a horny structure (the rhamphotheca) attached over the jaw bones. Tortoises are often seen with overgrown beaks (Figure 6.6). This can be secondary to trauma, internal disease or husbandry problems, (e.g. diets that do not provide normal wear). Deformities of the beak may require regular correction.

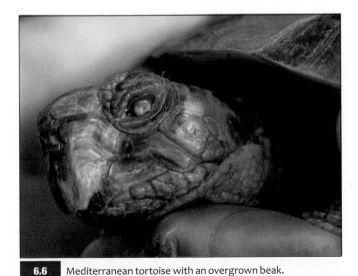

6.6 Mediterranean tortoise with an overgrown beak.

Nares

The external nares should be symmetrical and both openings should be patent. Using magnification and a light source, depending on the size and species, it is often possible to see a short way inside. There should not be any discharges visible, with the notable exception of some species of lizard that may have dried crystalline deposits due to salt excretion glands in the nasal cavities, (e.g. iguanids).

Pit organs

Pit organs are present in many species of snake. In most boas and pythons they are present as shallow pits along the upper lips and sometimes on the lower lips. Snakes of the Crotalinae (e.g. rattlesnakes) have a deep pit on each side of the head, just anterior to the eye. Pit organs allow snakes to detect infrared radiation. They are especially useful for hunting warm-blooded animals at night. Pit organs should be examined for any accumulations such as retained skin or parasitic ticks or mites.

Ears

In reptiles the hearing apparatus available for examination is limited. Snakes do not have external ears or tympanic membranes. The middle ears and Eustachian tubes are also missing. The inner ear is present and sound is transmitted via skin and bone, with the result that snakes hear low-frequency sounds best.

Tympanic membranes are present in lizards, chelonians and crocodilians. They should be examined for any changes, such as bulging of the tympanum, a visible fluid line behind it, retained skin shed over and around the tympanum or trauma to the area (Figure 6.7). Lizards, especially iguanas, can also be seen with otitis media, a bulging tympanic membrane being the main clinical sign, or occasionally with a fluid line visible through the tympanum. Normally there should be no fluid in the middle ear. Cryptosporidiosis should be included in the differential diagnosis for these signs in iguanas. Retained shed skin may predispose to secondary bacterial and fungal infections in the area.

Some lizards, e.g. inland bearded dragons and leopard geckos (Figure 6.8), possess short external ear canals. The ear canal should be examined carefully for any

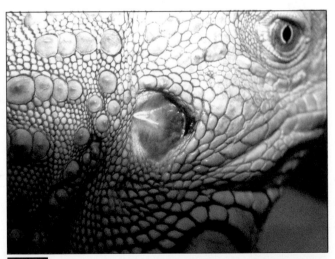

6.7 Trauma of the tympanic membrane in a green iguana.

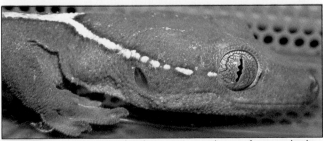

6.8 External ear canal and tympanic membrane of a normal palm gecko.

accumulations, such as retained skin. It is also an area where parasites may accumulate. Mites may cause inflammation leading to dysecdysis as the external ear canal in these species is one of their predilection sites.

Abscessation of the middle ear, causing bulging of the tympanic membrane, is commonly seen in aquatic chelonians, where pustular material may be seen exiting the auditory tube into the oropharyngeal area.

Eyes

The eyes are examined for any discharges or periocular swelling. Cachectic or dehydrated reptiles often have sunken eyes, while bulging eyes may be a result of retro-bulbar swelling, blepharitis or an enlarged eye. Care must be taken not to confuse the normal with a pathological condition. For example, megaglobus is normal in male leucistic Texas rat snakes.

Snakes and some species of skink and gecko have a spectacle covering the eye, and this should be examined for discoloration or bulging. If the nasolacrimal duct is blocked, fluid will build-up in the subspectacular space, i.e. the space between the spectacle and the cornea, and secondary infection may result. The spectacle is replaced at each ecdysis; it appears bluish prior to shedding while the replacement spectacle is forming behind. Sometimes an old spectacle is retained, giving it a wrinkled appearance. However, a non-retained spectacle may occasionally be wrinkled and it is important to distinguish between the two. Removal of a normal spectacle would expose the cornea, resulting in keratitis and permanent blindness.

The crevice between the spectacle and the skin should be inspected for mites in snakes and susceptible lizard species. This is a common place to find these parasites and their feeding habits in this area often lead to retained spectacles.

Blepharitis with swelling of the eyelids and conjunctival tissues is common in chelonians and lizards. Causes include bacterial, viral, fungal and parasitic infections and vitamin A deficiency.

Oral cavity

The mouth can be opened using a plastic card, wooden tongue depressor or rubber spatula. The first two are preferable as they are disposable and sterilization of the rubber spatula between patients is difficult. Care needs to be taken, especially in those species with acrodont teeth (agamids and chameleons; see below). Most reptiles have pleurodont teeth, i.e. they are replaced regularly throughout life. Some lizards will gape defensively if a finger is placed on their head, permitting an oral examination, so removing the need to use implements. Avian oral specula or atraumatic dental instruments may be used to open the beaks of chelonians (Figure 6.9).

Healthy oral mucous membranes are generally pale pink. Some species have pigmented membranes: some monitors and chameleons have melanotic mucous membranes; the yellowish mucous membranes of some species (e.g. bearded dragons) are a result of normal pigment and not jaundice.

When stomatitis is present, petechial haemorrhages and excessive salivation are seen initially (Figure 6.10). As stomatitis progresses, the mucosa of the mouth becomes oedematous and hyperaemic, and areas of ulceration may develop. In snakes and tortoises a white caseous material will start to accumulate and in tortoises this is commonly seen on the dorsal surface of the tongue.

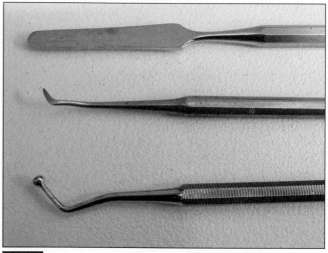

6.9 Instruments useful for oral examination in chelonians.

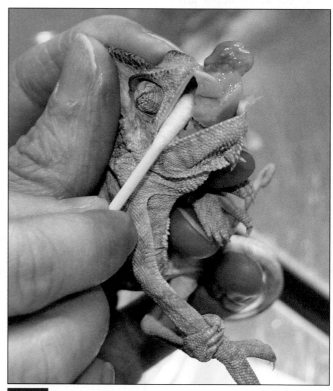

6.10 Veiled chameleon with severe stomatitis.

The roof of the mouth should be examined for areas of inflammation that may obstruct the nasolacrimal duct openings. The vomeronasal organs are present on the midline in this area. They are present in snakes and lizards but are poorly developed in chelonians and absent in crocodilians.

Chameleons have temporal glands and associated storage lakes at the commissures of their lips. These can become impacted and sometimes infected. On examination the area will be seen to be swollen, sometimes with a waxy yellow material or, if infected, a strong-smelling pustular material.

Many gecko species have endolymphatic calcium sacs, which are seen as swellings behind the ear and may form bulges into the oral cavity (Figure 6.11). These are visible as opaque areas on radiographs, are much more pronounced in reproductively active females and can occasionally become abscessed.

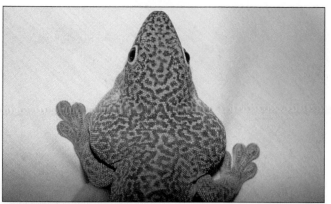

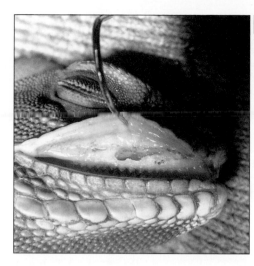

6.13 Water dragon with dental disease.

6.11 Female Standing's day gecko with cervical swellings caused by endolymphatic calcium sacs. Other causes of swellings could be bilateral abscesses.

Teeth: Chelonians do not have teeth; they have a horny beak, as discussed above. Most snakes have six rows of teeth: four in the upper jaw and two in the lower (Figure 6.12). Occasionally, one row may be lost traumatically, but there are no long-term ill effects.

Pleurodont teeth (all snakes and most lizards) rarely cause problems, as they are regularly replaced. However, lizards with acrodont teeth (agamids and chameleons) commonly develop dental problems. In addition to their teeth not being regularly replaced, species with acrodont teeth have only a thin layer of epithelium covering the narrow strip of jawbone adjacent to the teeth. It is in this area that plaque can build up if inappropriate diets are fed; diets composed of crickets and mealworms, which have relatively soft exoskeletons, and fruit are more likely to lead to plaque accumulation. This then mineralizes to form calculus, leading to periodontal disease and regression of the gum tissues. Changing the diet to incorporate more hard-bodied beetles and, where appropriate, greens and vegetables, dramatically reduces plaque build-up. During examination the lips should be elevated to fully visualize this area. In advanced cases, sections of maxilla and mandible may be missing, with their attached teeth, providing evidence of chronic disease (Figure 6.13). Any lesions should be probed under general anaesthesia to ascertain the depth of the lesion; samples should be harvested for bacterial and fungal culture and sensitivity testing.

Tongue and sheath: In chelonians the tongue is thick and fleshy with a rough surface and cannot be extended out of the mouth. Snakes and monitor lizards have a very active forked tongue that can be retracted into a sheath. It is seen just anterior to the glottis (Figure 6.14) and is used to investigate the environment and bring scent particles back to the vomeronasal organs. Most lizards have a fleshy tongue that can be extended to varying degrees from the mouth and often has a red tip that could be mistaken for an inflamed area (Figure 6.15). Chameleons have the most highly developed tongues, which are used in the capture of prey.

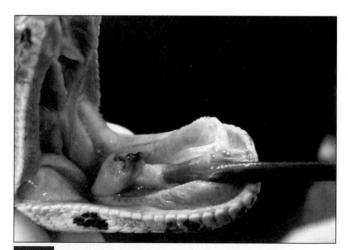

6.14 Examination of the tongue and its sheath in a snake.

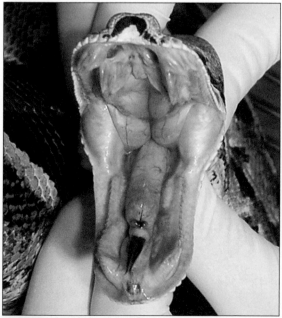

6.12 The common boa has rows of small teeth in the upper and lower jaws.

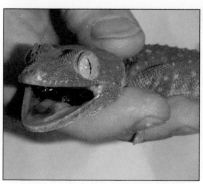

6.15 Tokay gecko showing normal red area at the tip of the tongue.

Tongues should be examined carefully for any wounds, abnormal swellings or scarring. A general anaesthetic is required to extend the tongues of snakes and monitor lizards fully to check for lesions and especially adhesions between the tongue and its sheath.

Loss of use of the tongue and its sensory function can be a cause of anorexia in snakes. This needs to be borne in mind when a lesion requiring amputation of the tongue is present, as these snakes often require life-long assisted feeding. Chameleons will also require life-long assisted feeding if they lose the use of their tongue. Paralysis of the tongue may be seen in chameleons affected by any disease process causing hypocalcaemia. In tortoises, glossitis is commonly seen with herpesvirus infection.

Glottis: The glottis is positioned on the floor of the oral cavity, just posterior to the tongue (see Chapter 1). It may be difficult to examine in lizards and chelonians because of its position. In these animals pushing the glottis anteriorly (with a finger just behind the mandible) while keeping the mouth wide open may allow good visualization. In snakes the glottis is easy to examine.

Breathing is a two-stage process, consisting of a brief ventilation cycle and a longer pause, during which the glottis is shut. Normally there are no discharges from the glottis. In cases of respiratory disease, serous mucoid or purulent discharges may be seen in the glottis and oral cavity. A lesion of the glottis may affect its ability to open and shut properly. Occasionally a foreign body, e.g. hair from mammalian prey, may become lodged around the glottis and cause dyspnoea.

External body surface

Skin: The entire body surface should be examined, including skin folds, especially in chelonians where lesions in the folds of skin around the limbs and cloaca may be difficult to see. The skin should be examined for:

- Wounds, e.g. bite wounds from prey
- Burns
- Blisters
- Scarring
- Swellings
- Signs of infectious disease or external parasites
- Signs of dysecdysis
- Colour change.

Large skin deficits often heal with scar tissue that is a lighter colour, while dead skin about to slough is often not very obvious as it may only appear to be slightly darker and less flexible than the surrounding skin.

Any swellings should be assessed for position, shape, size, consistency (hard or soft) and whether they are painful. Callipers should be used to measure them. Fine-needle aspirates or biopsy specimens may be needed to reach a diagnosis. The clinician should be familiar with normal anatomical swellings, such as the paired hemipenal bulges seen in some male snakes and lizards and the endolymphatic calcium stores seen in many mature female geckos (see Figure 6.11).

Retained skin of the extremities may form a stricture and cause avascular necrosis. This is very common in leopard geckos, causing loss of digit extremities (Figure 6.16). Missing digits or nails should be recorded.

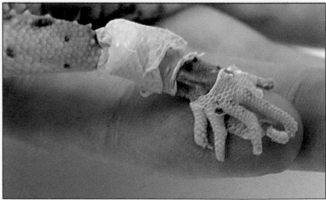

6.16 Leopard gecko with constricting bands of skin on toes and also round the distal radius and ulna.

Glands: Lizards have secretory glands on the ventral pelvic limb in the femoral area and/or in the pre- and post-anal areas, depending on species. These glands are usually better developed in males. They can become impacted in species from areas of high humidity when kept at below-optimal humidity levels, most often seen in green iguanas (Figure 6.17).

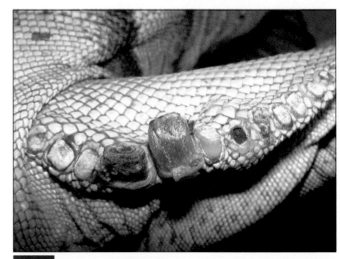

6.17 Femoral gland impaction in a green iguana.

Skeleton and muscle tone

The limbs and vertebral column should be palpated for any swellings that might indicate fractures, metabolic diseases of the bones, areas of osteomyelitis or tumours. Joints should be manipulated to ascertain the range of movement, and muscles assessed for tone and the presence of tetany that may be caused by nutritional and metabolic derangements or toxins.

Heart and lung sounds

The heart and lungs may be auscultated in lizards and snakes. Most lizards' hearts are positioned in the anterior thorax, and the stethoscope is best placed between the forelimbs, although in monitor lizards the heart is positioned more posteriorly. In snakes, the heart is in the anterior third of the body and can be located by palpation or by observing the cardiac thrill. Auscultation of the lungs is limited. Aggressive hissing noises must not be confused with abnormal lungs sounds. Chelonians are very difficult to auscultate owing to their shells.

Doppler blood-flow monitors are a much easier way to monitor the hearts of reptiles. Even in chelonians, monitoring the heart is easy with a Doppler monitor, by placing the probe in the cervicobrachial window, which is between the neck and the forelimb. Pencil probes are best for diagnostics, while flat probes are preferable for monitoring during anaesthesia (Figure 6.18).

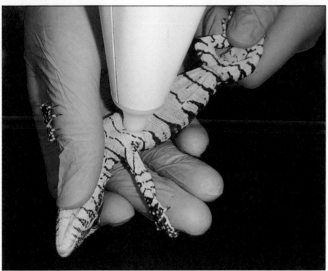

6.18 Monitoring the heart of a juvenile Nile monitor using a Doppler pencil probe.

Coelomic cavity palpation

The clinician should be familiar with the normal appearance of the species and be able to assess individual organs as to their size, normal position, shape and manoeuvrability.

Chelonians are difficult to palpate, but the prefemoral fossae provide 'windows' through which abnormal swellings such as retained eggs, uroliths and intestinal impactions may sometimes be palpable. Limited digital palpation of the cloaca can be accomplished via the vent in larger tortoises.

The coelomic cavity can be palpated in most lizards and snakes, but palpation must be gentle, especially in gravid females, as rough palpation can lead to ruptured ova with a resulting serious coelomitis. In smaller lizards and snakes a blunt-ended probe, such as a thermometer, can be used to palpate the distal coelom via the rectum. Care must be taken to ensure that no pressure is applied and that the probe is passed into the rectum.

In lizards the fat-pads should be identified and the gastrointestinal tract assessed for the presence of ingesta, gas and foreign bodies. It can sometimes be difficult to differentiate the gastrointestinal tract from ovarian follicles or eggs. Normal kidneys are not palpable in all species but are palpable when enlarged, e.g. enlarged liver in hepatic lipidosis. In green iguanas renomegaly is a common finding, as is the presence of large stores of fat in the paired lateral fat-pads in species such as Bosc/savannah monitors. In larger lizards limited digital palpation of the distal coelomic cavity can be accomplished through the cloaca.

In snakes the entire body should be palpated. The coelomic cavity is palpated ventrally between the ribs, through the ventral scales. This is very difficult in large strong snakes unless they are sedated. In the anterior third the heart is palpable, but in larger snakes this becomes more difficult. In healthy snakes ingesta within the gastrointestinal tract are often palpable in the caudal half of the body, depending on when the snake last fed. Sometimes the gall bladder is palpable just distal to the stomach, especially in anorexic individuals. In oviparous species eggs are often visible as swellings and are usually readily palpable, except in large snakes. Retained fetuses in viviparous species are more difficult to palpate. Ultrasonography may be necessary in these cases. Constipation is relatively common in snakes and is readily palpable. Single masses should be investigated by fine-needle aspiration, radiology and/or ultrasonography.

Transillumination

Some species of snake and lizard can be transilluminated. This uses a cold light to visualize internal structures. An endoscopic light source or an avian candling light can be used to transilluminate from the outside but a more specialized light is needed if it is to be introduced rectally. Leopard geckos and albino snakes can be transilluminated advantageously (Figure 6.19). Sometimes transillumination of the area of the tail just caudal to the vent can help with gender differentiation.

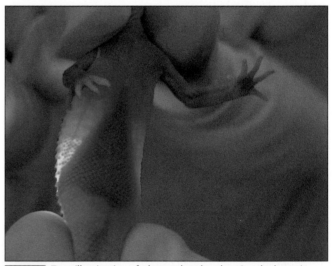

6.19 Transillumination of a leopard gecko, showing the hepatic shadow within the coelomic cavity.

Cloaca and tail base

The cloaca, the common opening for the gastrointestinal, reproductive and urinary tracts, should be investigated carefully. It can be probed with a blunt instrument or examined more closely with a speculum or endoscope, usually requiring sedation. The bladder, colon, oviduct, copulatory organs and cloacal tissue may prolapse into the cloaca. Inflammation or infection of the cloaca on its own is uncommon, but infection of the musk glands is common in snakes. This is often related to delayed emptying caused by another disease process. Cloacal uroliths are sometimes found, especially in the African spurred tortoise, caused by deficiencies in husbandry such as inappropriate diets.

Male snakes and lizards have paired hemipenes that are inverted one on each side of the tail base (see Chapters 1 and 5). In sexually mature animals these may be seen as paired bulges just distal to the vent opening. They can become impacted with accumulations of glandular secretions and shed skin, often progressing to abscessation.

Health and safety considerations

To ensure legal compliance, reference must be made to local health and safety legislation in the respective country.

When completing a risk assessment, the objective is to increase awareness of the hazards and to implement the best safe-operating practice, given the animal, its nature, the techniques and equipment being used, the environment, and the skills and number of people involved. An emergency procedure should also be incorporated, particularly when working with venomous snakes (see Appendix 3). The risk assessment should include:

- Description of the activity
- The procedure being followed
- For each hazard, identification of:
  - The potential risk, i.e. the likelihood of occurrence and the type of incident. This could be an injury, escape of the animal and damage it may cause, or other damage and injury resulting from the procedure failing
  - Who is at risk
  - The current controls
  - Whether the risk is as low as is reasonably practicable
  - Any further controls required to reduce the risk to as low as reasonably practicable.

Procedures should be reviewed regularly and following any significant changes (e.g. to equipment, drugs, working environment) or significant incident.

Zoonoses

Zoonoses should always be a consideration when recommending reptile ownership to a client. General hygiene precautions are given in Figure 6.20.

Salmonellosis is the most important reptile zoonosis. *Salmonella* spp. live in the intestinal tracts of carrier animals (mammals, birds and reptiles). Transmission is by the faecal–oral route (usually via contamination of food). The prevalence of salmonellosis in reptiles varies widely, depending on the species and the husbandry conditions. Salmonellosis in people, as in reptiles, can give rise to an inapparent infection, carrier state, enteritis, septicaemia or combination thereof. If a human case of salmonellosis is suspected to have arisen from a reptile then the serotype in both the human patient and the reptile should be identified. The elderly, infants and those with impaired immune

| 6.20 | General hygiene precautions for reptile owners. |

- Always wash hands with hot soapy water after handling any reptile, vivarium or vivarium accessory
- Do not keep reptiles in the kitchen, dining room or any food-preparation area
- Never eat, drink or smoke when handling reptiles or their vivaria
- Immune-compromised people and children under 5 years of age should avoid contact with reptiles
- Vivaria or their furnishings should never be cleaned in the kitchen sink, bathroom sink, shower or bath
- Always supervise children handling reptiles (their tendency to put things in their mouths puts them at greater risk)

systems are more at risk. Children under the age of 5 years are also at an increased risk, due to their propensity to put their fingers in their mouths.

Mycobacterial infections may cause cutaneous granulomas in handlers, gaining entry through small breaks in the skin. Immunocompromised people may be at a higher risk.

Pentastomiasis is the only parasitic zoonosis of importance (see Chapter 24).

Acknowledgements

The author wishes to thank Anthea Aggus MIOSH (Health and Safety Consultant) for help with the health and safety section.

References and further reading

Chitty J and Raftery A (2013) *Essentials of Tortoise Medicine and Surgery*. Wiley-Blackwell

Divers SJ (1999) Clinical evaluation of reptiles. *Veterinary Clinics of North America: Exotic Animal Practice* **2**, 291–331

Jackson OF (1980) Weight and measurement data on tortoises (*Testudo graeca* and *Testudo hermanni*) and their relationship to health. *Journal of Small Animal Practice* **21**, 409

Jacobson E (2007) *Infectious Diseases and Pathology of Reptiles: A Color Atlas and Text*. CRC Press, Boca Raton, FL

Mader DR and Divers SJ (2006) *Reptile medicine and surgery, 2nd edn*. Elsevier, St. Louis (MO)

Mader DR and Divers SJ (2014) *Current Therapy in Reptile Medicine and Surgery*. Elsevier, St. Louis (MO)

Mader DR and Stoutenberg G (1998) Assessing the body weight of the Californian desert tortoise *Gopherus agassizii* using morphometric analysis. *Proceedings of the Association of Reptilian and Amphibian Veterinarians Annual Conference* pp. 103–104

Mitchell MA and Shane SM (2001) *Salmonella* in reptiles. *Seminars in Avian and Exotic Pet Medicine* **10**, 25–35

Chapter 7

Emergency care

Michael Pees and Simon J. Girling

Although many emergency situations are similar for reptiles and mammals (e.g. trauma, toxicosis and septicaemia), the development and progression of clinical signs is often very different. Many, if not most, emergency situations in reptiles occur not as a result of an acute process, but rather as a result of chronic disease with acute end-stage decompensation. One reason for the insidious progress of disease, without the patient showing serious problems earlier in its development, is the ability of reptiles to tolerate disease processes and extreme dehydration, blood loss or malnutrition for longer periods than is possible for any comparable mammal. For example, in the case of hypoxia, as most reptiles require only low levels of oxygen consumption and can tolerate high carbon dioxide levels, with conditions such as lower respiratory tract disease (LRTD), early signs of disease are often not seen. As a consequence, reptiles are often presented at an advanced stage of disease when the compensation mechanisms fail and clinical signs become apparent. This problem is exacerbated by the fact that some owners do not check regularly the health status of their reptile, either because of the reptile's low activity cycles or due to a lack of knowledge. These circumstances emphasize the need for establishing a thorough history at presentation and for gathering as much information as possible on the husbandry conditions, as well as the course, and where possible, duration of the disease.

The first and most important aim of any emergency measure is stabilization of the patient and treatment of life-threatening conditions. In practice, however, this is often limited by a lack of knowledge regarding the physiological demands of reptiles and problems with diagnostic and therapeutic procedures. For instance, intravenous access is relatively straightforward in various mammalian species, but is a challenge or not achievable in many reptilian species. Further complications can arise due to the size of the reptile, as those regularly presented to practitioners may only be a few grams in weight. Finally, even with the administration of effective therapy, the reptile may be in such an advanced and debilitated stage of disease, that there is multi-organ failure with an inevitable fatal outcome. It should also be noted that, in some cases, the reptile presented as an emergency case may already be dead, as this is notoriously difficult to determine in many reptiles!

Despite these limitations, there are helpful and important diagnostic and therapeutic techniques available for first aid in reptiles. The aim of this chapter is to provide a brief review of these techniques and to outline the most important physiological conditions that need to be considered when presented with a reptile emergency. The essential points for the work-up of typical emergency situations are also considered.

Equipment

In the event of a reptile presenting as an emergency, some essential equipment should be on-hand, and a fully stocked crash or mobile cart (similar to one for mammals) can be invaluable. The contents of the crash cart should include:

- Drugs
- Mouth gags
- Speculums
- Breathing bags
- Endotracheal tubes of varying sizes
- Needles and syringes
- Intravenous catheters
- Fluid giving sets
- Alcoholic hand rub
- Antiseptic solutions
- Dressing materials (gauze, swabs, bandages and tape)
- Diagnostic equipment (swabs, slides, blood sampling equipment, sample pots, sterile tubes for lung washing)
- Infrared thermometer to measure body temperature.

Drug provision

Drugs that should always be available in the event of an emergency include:

- Appropriate infusion solutions
- Antimicrobial drugs (preferably broad acting, but effective particularly against Gram-negative bacteria)
- Drugs for stabilization of the circulatory system (e.g. hypovolaemic shock) and organ function
- Drugs for the treatment of (suspected) toxicosis.

In addition, even though there is limited information available on pain management in reptiles, it has been demonstrated that the use of analgesic and anti-inflammatory drugs can improve the general condition of the patient and should be considered. (NB: reptiles are covered by welfare legislation in the United Kingdom, European Union and United States and as such should be afforded analgesia; see Chapter 12). Figure 7.1 gives an overview of the most commonly used drugs in emergency medicine in reptiles.

Drug	Dosage recommendation	Comments
Aciclovir	80 mg/kg orally q8h	Chelonians: herpesvirus, high dosage necessary, side effects
Adrenaline (epinephrine)	0.5 mg/kg i.v., intraosseous; 1 mg/kg intratracheal diluted in 1 ml/100 g bodyweight	Asystole and recovery from anaesthetic
Allopurinol	10–20 mg/kg orally q24h	(Gout), reduces urate production but might be nephrotoxic
Atropine	0.1–0.2 mg/kg i.m. q24h	Organophosphate intoxication
Buprenorphine	0.005–0.02 mg/kg i.m. q24–48h	Most species analgesia
Butorphanol	0.4–1.0 mg/kg s.c., i.m. q12–24h	Opioid, analgesic
Calcium gluconate	40–100 mg/kg s.c., i.m. q24h	Hypocalcaemia, seizures
Carprofen	1–4 mg/kg i.m. q24h	Anti-inflammatory, analgesic, possible side effect gastric haemorrhage in iguanas (herbivorous reptiles)
Ceftazidime	20 mg/kg i.m. q72h	Broad-spectrum antibiotic, septicaemia, according to culture and sensitivity testing whenever possible
Dexamethasone	0.5–2 mg/kg i.m. q24h	Ultima ratio, trauma, brain swelling, side effect immunosuppression
Diazepam	1–2 mg/kg i.m., i.v. q12–24h	Seizures
Doxapram	4–12 mg/kg i.m., i.v., orally once	Respiratory stimulant
Diethylenetriamine penta-acetic acid (DTPA)	35 mg/kg i.m. q24h	Chelating agent, heavy metal intoxication
Ethylenediamine tetra-acetic acid (EDTA)	40 mg/kg i.m. q24h	Chelating agent, heavy metal intoxication
Enrofloxacin	10 mg/kg i.m., s.c. q24h	Broad-spectrum antibiotic, septicaemia, according to culture and sensitivity testing whenever possible
Furosemide	1–5 mg/kg i.m. q12–24h	Oedema, diuretic
Glycopyrronium (Glycopyrrolate)	0.01 mg/kg i.m., s.c.	Used for prolonged bradycardia but may not work in all species (e.g. green iguanas)
Meloxicam	0.1–0.5 mg/kg orally, s.c. q24h	Anti-inflammatory, analgesic
Methylprednisolone	1–5 mg/kg i.m. q12–24h	Ultima ratio, trauma, brain swelling, side effect immunosuppression
Vitamin B1 (complex)	1 mg/kg i.m., s.c. q48h	Central nervous system signs, usually as vitamin B complex, dosage following vitamin B1 concentration
Voriconazole	10 mg/kg i.m. q24h	Antifungal – effective against *Chrysosporium* anamorph of *Nanniziopsis vriesii* (CANV)

7.1 A list of relevant emergency/first aid drugs for use in reptiles.

Anaesthetic equipment

Anaesthetic equipment should include a volatile iso-flurane or sevoflurane system, in combination with a suit-able vent-ilation system. An automatic ventilation system, such as the small animal ventilator (Figure 7.2), is very effective not only during anaesthesia but also in cases of shock or circulatory depression. Uncuffed endotracheal tubes should be available in various sizes for intubation. A Doppler flowmeter can provide important monitoring information during anaesthesia. A digital thermometer with an external probe can be used to monitor the temperature of the patient during anaesthesia, and pulse oximeters and respirometers also provide useful information (see Chapter 12 for further information on monitoring during anaesthesia).

Diagnostic equipment

A small laboratory equipped for parasitological examina-tions and a basic cytology staining kit (e.g. Diff-Quik®) with a suitable microscope is mandatory.

Diagnostic imaging of emergency reptilian cases should at least include radiography and ultrasonography (see Chapter 9). Both techniques are extremely important for the diagnostic work-up of cases and are relatively easy to perform in most reptiles. In addition, endoscopy can be very helpful (see Chapter 10).

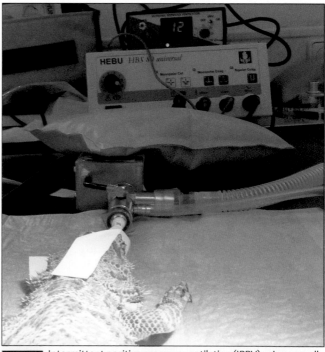

7.2 Intermittent positive pressure ventilation (IPPV) using a small animal ventilator in a bearded dragon. These devices can also be used in combination with 100% oxygen, as they provide forced ventilation of the lung.

Therapeutic equipment

For the treatment of small reptiles, insulin-gradated syringes and needles (25–27 G) should be used as they are less traumatic and allow exact drug dosages to be administered. Infusion pumps can also be used to administer fluids over a longer period of time (Figure 7.3).

Inpatient accommodation

It is essential that there is provision to accommodate reptiles as inpatients, so that optimal environmental conditions vital to recovery can be provided. Hospitalization also allows the veterinary surgeon (veterinarian) to regularly check the status of the reptile and to administer repeat treatments as necessary. Appropriate boxes or terrariums should be available, as well as ultraviolet B (UVB) bulbs, heating panels, heat lamps, thermostats and relative humidity gauges. A quarantine room is strongly recommended for cases with (suspected) contagious diseases. For further information on accommodation requirements for reptiles, see Chapter 3.

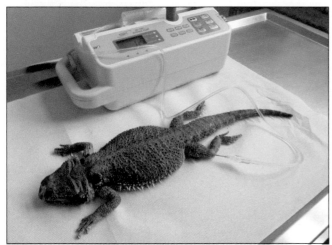

7.3 Infusion pumps can be used to slowly administer volumes up to 60 ml. Besides the intravenous or the intraosseous route, they can also be used with a needle placed subcutaneously in debilitated patients.

History and initial assessment

For information on conducting a thorough history and husbandry review, as well as how to perform a full clinical examination, see Chapter 6. With respect to an emergency case, the following points should always be checked with the owner as they are essential to determine an effective treatment for the individual reptile:

- Duration of ownership
- Presumed sex, age, reproductive history and hibernation (depending on species)
- Accommodation, including temperature management and humidity records (for both day and night)
- Nutrition, including food, feeding regimes and any food additives (e.g. vitamins, calcium)
- Recent medical history, including clinical observations and the success of administering any treatment.

The initial clinical assessment focuses on the general body and health condition of the reptile and any possible (hidden) emergency signs.

It should be noted that patient stabilization may be required prior to obtaining a detailed history from the owner. Immediate life-saving procedures may be necessary including:

- Resuscitation
- Applying direct pressure to bleeding tissue
- Gravity-assisted removal of fluids from the lower respiratory tract.

Bodyweight and condition

Assessment of bodyweight and condition helps to determine the chronicity of the disease process (Figure 7.4). An accurate bodyweight measurement is also necessary for any subsequent drug calculations. As with mammals, a reptile may be the 'correct' bodyweight for its age and species, but this may be due to retained fluid or neoplastic lesions, which is why an assessment of body condition should also be undertaken. This includes checking the muscles covering the epaxial area in snakes, the base of the tail and pelvis in lizards (and the tail itself in some species such as the leopard gecko where fat is stored), and the muscles of the antebrachium in chelonians. See Chapter 4 for more details.

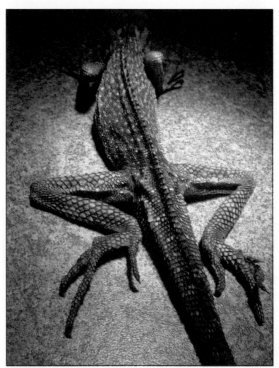

7.4 Emaciated mountain-horned dragon. Although the underlying disease is a chronic process, these patients are often presented in an emergency situation.

Core body temperature

Body temperature can be measured using a probe inserted into the cloaca, but it should be recognized that this may not be a true reflection of the reptile's core temperature. Alternatively, placing a temperature probe orally is possible, particularly in snakes. The measured core body temperature should be compared with preferred body temperature values, which are usually in the range of 32–36°C in most reptiles, and the environmental temperature adjusted as required. The maintenance of the preferred body temperature in reptiles is essential, especially in diseased animals. In hypothermic patients, active measures should be taken to increase the core body temperature slowly, including administering fluids warmed to the preferred body temperature intravenously, orally, intraosseously or via the cloaca (the intracoelomic route can also be used if other routes are not possible).

Hydration status

Hydration status should be assessed, where possible, when the reptile is at its preferred body temperature. The mucous membranes should be examined to assess dehydration. The oral mucous membranes should be moist; evidence of desiccation when touched suggests dehydration levels in excess of 7%. The presence of sunken eyes can also be a sign of dehydration. Collapse of the spectacle in snakes may indicate dehydration in excess of 5–7%. Prior correction of dehydration is strongly recommended particularly when antibiotics are used so as to support liver and kidney function.

Skin tenting to check for dehydration may not be as helpful in reptiles as it is in mammals, owing to the reduced elasticity of reptilian skin. However, skin tenting may be performed over the epaxial musculature in the caudal third of the body in snakes, over the thighs and base of the tail in lizards, and over the antebrachium in chelonians. Skin which takes longer than 2–3 seconds to return to its former position may indicate a level of ≥5% dehydration in the reptile being examined.

The heartbeat can be increased in cases of fluid loss (hypovolaemia); however, it can also be reduced due to circulatory collapse in advanced dehydration. It should also be noted that the heart rate is temperature-dependent and should be re-evaluated as the reptile is warmed. Oedema is often seen in cases of cardiac or renal failure (Figure 7.5).

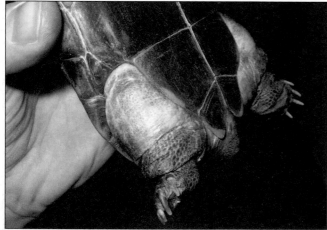

7.5 Oedema in a Chinese pond turtle, caused by renal insufficiency.

Signs of septicaemia

Systemic signs of septicaemia include reddish discolorations of the subcutis signifying ecchymoses. These are most evident in snakes on the ventral scales, and in chelonians on the plastron at the joints of scutes (Figure 7.6). This signifies a true emergency that requires immediate treatment using parenteral systemic broad-spectrum antibiotics effective against Gram-negative bacteria in particular (e.g. enrofloxacin). Petechiation of the mucous membranes (in the oral cavity and cloaca) is also suggestive of septicaemia, but may be associated with localized infection and inflammation.

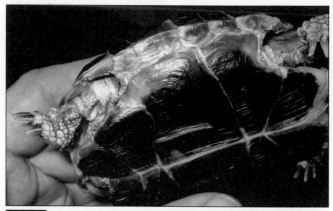

7.6 Septicaemia in a Russian tortoise.

Trauma and haemorrhage

Although some cases of trauma and blood loss are unmistakable (Figure 7.7), evidence of severe trauma and haemorrhage in other cases can be hidden (e.g. in the oral cavity or as internal bleeding), and so may be difficult to accurately assess. Reptiles are very resistant to the ill-effects of blood loss and can typically cope with a packed cell volume (PCV) as low as 10–12%. External bleeding may be halted using haemostatic powders or by wound closure and bandaging. With severe blood loss, volume substitution is essential (see below).

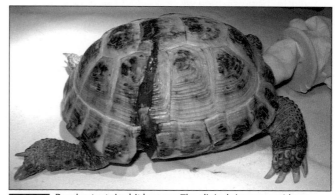

7.7 Russian tortoise hit by a car. The clinical signs are evident; however, some anamnestic information is still necessary to evaluate the reptile's individual situation.

Oral cavity

The mucosa of the oral cavity and glottis should be assessed for inflammatory reactions and petechiation suggestive of infection, as they are often seen with respiratory or intestinal diseases (Figure 7.8). Fluid emanating through the glottis is suggestive of LRTD and a sample should be collected for microbial culture and examined microscopically for nematode eggs or larvae. Further findings may include the presence of uric acid depositions in cases of visceral gout, trauma and foreign bodies.

Respiration and heartbeat

The rate and depth of respiration should be assessed. Open-mouth breathing is commonly associated with respiratory insufficiency, which can be caused by upper as well as lower respiratory disease. Respiration noises can also occur. These can be caused by disease, but may also be a part of a defence mechanism (e.g. hissing to scare off potential predators).

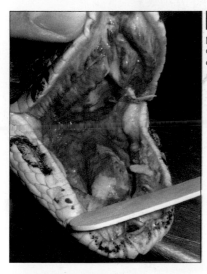

7.8 Severe stomatitis in a Burmese python. This condition is often seen with pneumonia or intestinal disease.

Ultrasonography can help to assess the heartbeat, and Doppler flowmeters can be used easily. In lizards, depending on the species, the transducer is placed either in the axillary region (agamids, iguanas) or on the chest (varanids) to visualize the heart (Figure 7.9). Alternatively, blood flow can be demonstrated by placing the Doppler probe over the ventral tail vein. In chelonians, the probe is placed cranially between the cervical region and the forelimb. In snakes, the probe is placed ventrally over the area of the heart. The heartbeat in snakes can also be seen on the ventral body surface when relaxed or anaesthetized.

Caudal coelomic cavity

The caudal coelomic cavity ('abdomen') should be palpated carefully, just cranial to the pelvis on either side of the lateral body wall, for swellings and palpable masses such as eggs, tumours, granulomas or foreign bodies. To some extent, this may be possible in chelonians by placing fingers in both inguinal areas simultaneously and balloting the coelomic contents. Alternatively, the chelonian may be placed on its side and fingers inserted into the dependent prefemoral fossa. Gravity will then make the palpation of objects such as eggs or bladder stones easier. In snakes, the forefinger may be gently pressed against the ventral body wall and run in a cranial to caudal direction down the length of the body. Snakes should be palpated for the presence of firm, immobile objects, which may indicate the presence of eggs, follicles, fetuses, neoplastic lesions, foreign bodies and granulomas, and

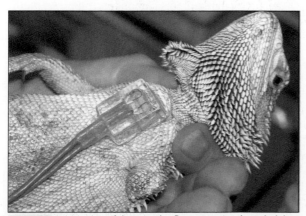

7.9 Positioning of the Doppler flowmeter in a bearded dragon. The device can be used easily to assess the heartbeat frequency in reptiles.

fluid-filled visci such as that found with enteritis, which can be associated with hyperalimentation, inappropriate ambient temperature extremes and parasitism (e.g. *Entamoeba invadens* infection).

First aid and resuscitation

The main focus of emergency supportive medicine is to supply oxygen to the body tissues. The 'airways, breathing, circulation' (ABC) rule, developed and refined in mammalian medicine to now focus on maintaining circulation in the first place (CAB), can be applied to reptilian medicine. Indeed, as reptiles can cope with significant levels of hypoxia, maintaining the circulation in the first instance followed by clearing the airways and restarting breathing (CAB) is an ideal approach to the critical care patient.

Oxygen supply

Any material in the oral cavity that can interfere with normal breathing must be removed. Foreign bodies are sometimes seen in the oral cavity of tortoises (e.g. stones and food particles), but other inflammatory material may also be present. Inflammatory material can be solid but most problems are caused by tenacious mucoid material, which is also present in the trachea. This is commonly seen in snakes and, to a lesser extent, chelonians with LRTD. As most reptiles do not have a diaphragm they are unable to cough, and so secretions can build up and block the trachea. The first measure is to remove the material from the tracheal opening. In cases with further material blocking the trachea itself, a tracheal wash followed by suction may be indicated.

Care should be taken not to deliver 100% oxygen to reptiles that are already breathing normally, as this can reduce the stimulus to breathe by reducing the partial pressure of carbon dioxide (PCO_2) and increasing the partial pressure of oxygen (PO_2). In cases of reduced or absent respiration, forced ventilation should be performed using one of several techniques:

- Intubation and forced ventilation using either a ventilation bag or an intermittent positive pressure ventilation (IPPV) device (see Figure 7.2 and Chapter 12)
- Gentle and rhythmic rib compression (lizards and snakes; in snakes this should be performed in the area of the air sac, not the lung)
- Rhythmic movements of the forelimbs (chelonians).

Assessment of oxygen levels in reptiles can be carried out by point-of-care analysers or via pulse oximetry. The latter may be applied to the cloacal area (if the reptile is large enough) or the tongue in chelonians and lizards (if sedated or anaesthetized). Pulse oximetry is inherently inaccurate in reptiles as commercial oximeters are calibrated to mammalian haemoglobin oxygen dissociation curves and reptilian haemoglobin is structurally different, therefore, absolute values are not to be relied upon. However, changing trends may be useful to assess progress in response to treatment. Normal blood gas levels in the conscious green iguana at 37°C have been published as: P_aO_2 81 mmHg (±10 mmHg) and P_aCO_2 42 mmHg (±9 mmHg) (Hernandez et al., 2011). There is some evidence that postprandial changes increase P_aCO_2 levels and increased body temperatures increase both P_aO_2 and P_aCO_2 levels in healthy animals within the preferred optimum temperature zone (Andrade et al., 2004).

Tracheal wash and suction procedure

A tracheal wash is performed using approximately 1–2 ml/kg of a sterile, warmed (30–34°C), isotonic (0.9%) saline solution and a flexible tube with several openings at the distal end.

- Disinfect the glottal opening using a dilute disinfectant (e.g. 0.01% povidone iodine).
- When the glottis opens during the respiratory cycle, gently advance the tube into the trachea (Figure 7.10).
- Flush the saline solution into the trachea.
- Immediately turn the patient upside down and suction the fluid back into the tube, while slowly retracting the tube from the trachea.
- Examine the sample collected for infectious agents and inflammatory cells.

This procedure is mainly used in snakes but can also be performed in lizards. In chelonians, it is important to remember that the trachea splits shortly behind the glottal opening, thereby making a flush difficult. Active suctioning using a suction device may be possible in larger species; however, for smaller species, the level of suction may be too strong and can result in tissue damage, and the size of the probe used with the suction device is often too large. In cases of unilateral disease, it is important to obtain a radiograph to confirm that the pulmonary wash tube is collecting material from the affected lung.

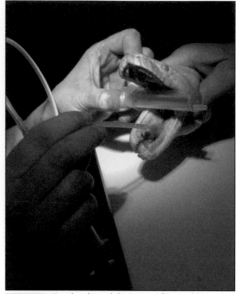

7.10 Tracheal wash being performed in a Burmese python. The material removed can be examined for the presence of infectious agents and inflammatory cells (see Figure 7.15).

Air sac cannulation of snakes

This procedure has been used most typically in snakes when the trachea is blocked (due to inflammation, foreign body or neoplasia) as many, similar to birds, have air sacs which communicate with the lungs. The technique preferably involves general anaesthesia and a surgical approach through the skin and body wall on the right side of the snake (most have only a right lung and air sac) at around 25–30% of the snout-vent length. The incision is made between the ribs at the ventral edge of the epaxial muscles and through the underlying thin air sac wall. A cut-down endotracheal tube or adapted avian air sac tube can be used and sutured in place to the skin surface. Once inserted the anaesthetic circuit can be connected to the air sac tube to maintain the anaesthesia while removal of the blockage to the trachea can be carried out. The tube may be left in place for several days but it needs to be inspected daily for any secretion build up which may occlude the tube.

Nebulization

This has been used to deliver medications (see Chapters 11 and 18) as well as allowing humidification of the air and so easing dyspnoea where thick respiratory secretions can build up. It has also been used to deliver bronchodilators such as aminophylline (25 mg/9 ml sterile saline solution) which may also help. This is not as effective in snakes whose elongated lung field means that the suspended droplets rapidly attach to the airway walls in the proximal lung field and so rarely reach the distal lung field. In chelonians and lizards, however, it works well. A nebulization chamber may be set up easily with a small vivarium or even, for smaller species, a small plastic container with airholes. Human nebulizers often quote a particle size of 1–5 μm as being essential – any larger the suspended particles do not reach the alveoli. In reptiles it is debateable whether the particle size needs to be that small as reptile airways are significantly larger. Nebulizing time is generally around 10–15 minutes, 2–4 times per day.

Fluid therapy

Fluid therapy is an essential and critical part of resuscitation and first aid procedures. However, due to the heterogeneous nature of reptiles, there is no general 'best choice' fluid that should be used. Basic blood values should be obtained to assess the nature (e.g. blood loss *versus* electrolyte loss) and degree of dehydration, with the haematocrit (PCV), total protein (TP), sodium (Na^+) and potassium (K^+) levels being of particular importance. When assessing these parameters, it should be remembered that accompanying disease processes might also influence the values and disguise the type of fluid loss.

Choice of fluids

Crystalloid fluids are the fluids of choice for reptiles and should be warmed to the preferred body temperature of the patient (approximately 32–36°C) prior to administration. There is some evidence that in reptiles (and probably amphibians) the isotonicity of the extracellular fluid is lower than that in mammals. Studies on non-marine reptiles suggest that isotonicity in many reptiles is 0.8%, rather than the 0.9% assumed in mammals (Jacobson, 1988). As many reptiles also demonstrate simple fluid loss, a number of crystalloid fluid combinations have been derived, including:

- Combination 1: one-third 5% glucose with 0.9% saline, one-third lactated Ringer's solution and one-third sterile water
- Combination 2: nine parts 5% glucose with 0.9% saline to one part sterile water.

However, further work by Guzman et al., (2011) indicates that plasma osmolality in corn snakes is higher than in mammals (mean value of 344.5 mOsm/kg). Guzman et al., (2011) showed that the osmolality could be calculated using the formula $(2 \times [Na^+ + K^+]) + ([Glucose (mg/dl)] / 18)$, although the simpler formula $(2 \times [Na^+ + K^+])$ agreed relatively closely. Bearded dragons have a similar osmolality to mammals (mean value of 295.4 mOsm/kg) (Dallwig et al.,

2010). Dallwig *et al.* (2010) showed that the osmolality in bearded dragons could be calculated using the formula (1.85 x [Na$^+$ + K$^+$]). Chelonians tend to have a slightly lower plasma sodium concentration and a higher pH. These differences demonstrate that the clinician should be aware that there is considerable variation in the fluid requirements of different reptile species. Controversy exists over the use of lactated mammalian fluids in reptiles, as the buffer agent (lactate) may add to the often high lactate levels in sick and active reptiles which produce significant amounts of lactate by anaerobic respiration.

In addition, the basic bloodwork values may also influence the composition of the crystalloid fluid to be administered:

- Increased sodium concentration – this indicates intracellular dehydration. In these cases, hypotonic solutions (free water and 5% dextrose solution) are indicated to restore the osmolality. As these solutions can also cause cell damage, they should be used carefully and only after proper rehydration of the vascular system
- Increased potassium concentration – this is often seen with kidney insufficiency and/or oliguria. In these cases, it is advisable to use crystalloid solutions without potassium (e.g. 0.9% sodium chloride solution). Potassium levels >5 mmol/l are associated with severe disease; levels >9 mmol/l are usually fatal.

Colloidal fluids and hypertonic saline: These may be used in mammals where profound hypovolaemia has occurred. Hydroxyethyl starches (HES) and dextrans are the most commonly used colloidal isotonic solutions with the former being favoured due to its larger molecular weight and therefore longer survival in the blood stream. There is little data on their usage in reptiles and large volumes in mammals are known to significantly prolong clotting times. They may be useful where rapid correction of fluid deficits in reptiles leads to a reduction in intravascular osmotic pressure and movement of water into the interstitial space, increasing interstitial space hydrostatic pressure and physical collapse of the lymphatic system. The lymphatic system is important for the return of fluid from the tissues to the cardiovascular system and is well-developed in reptiles which have a low blood pressure system (systolic pressures often around 60 mmHg). In these instances, colloids can help retain fluid in the circulation.

Hypertonic saline will rapidly draw fluid from the intracellular and interstitial spaces into the blood stream so rapidly reversing hypovolaemia. They are contraindicated where there is a sodium or chloride ion overload, cardiac disease, active haemorrhage and chronic dehydration and, combined with a lack of evidence of their safety or efficacy in reptiles, they are rarely used.

Routes of administration

The following routes can be used for fluid therapy administration:

- Enteral
- Subcutaneous
- Intracoelomic
- Intraosseous
- Intravenous.

The rate of fluid absorption is dependent on body temperature and cardiovascular function; hypothermic patients have a reduced rate of absorption, particularly if the fluid is administered enterally or subcutaneously. Thus, maintaining the reptile at its preferred body temperature is recommended. (The exception to this may be in cases of (suspected) head trauma, where a lower temperature may be indicated to reduce the risk of swelling and oedema, but this is an extrapolation from mammalian medicine.)

Enteral route: Enteral administration of fluids is normally performed via a stomach tube, but in some species dropping fluid into the mouth/placing fluid on to the tongue using a syringe can be tried. This route should not be used in cases with digestive tract dysfunction or severe dehydration (>7%). The technique for enteral administration of fluids is described in Chapter 11 (and can also be used for providing nutritional support and administering oral medications).

Subcutaneous route: Although absorption may be delayed in critically ill reptiles due to poor vascular perfusion, subcutaneous fluid administration is quite reliable and relatively easy to perform without causing too much stress to the patient (see Chapter 11). A total of 20 ml/kg can be injected at any one time and repeated up to 3-times daily. In weak patients, a subcutaneously placed catheter (Figure 7.11) can be considered as an alternative to other more invasive techniques.

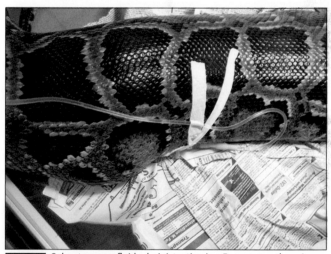

7.11 Subcutaneous fluid administration in a Burmese python. In debilitated reptiles, the subcutaneous route can also be used for constant infusions, e.g. using an infusion pump.

Intracoelomic route: The intracoelomic route provides better uptake of fluids than the subcutaneous route in dehydrated reptiles and the technique is easy to perform. In chelonians, the patient is restrained on its side with the hindlimb held caudally (Figure 7.12). The skin should be disinfected prior to needle insertion. The needle is inserted into the uppermost prefemoral area, aiming for the contralateral forelimb in a caudocranial direction. The urinary bladder should be checked prior to the procedure to ensure that it is not full, in order to avoid the inadvertent injection of fluids into the bladder. This can be determined using ultrasonography which should also be performed to check for space-occupying lesions (e.g. multiple follicles in reproductively active females) that should be avoided during the procedure.

In snakes, the needle should be inserted cranial to the vent, between the scales, 2–3 rows of lateral scales dorsal from the ventral body wall. The needle should be inserted between the ribs and the ventral body wall and slowly

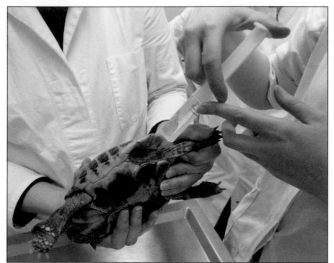

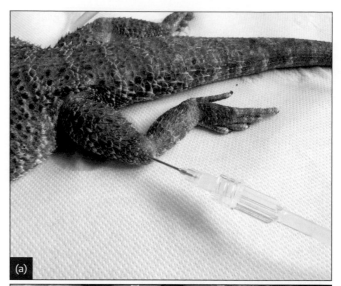

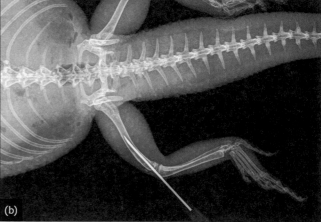

7.12 Fluid administration into the coelomic cavity in a tortoise. The tortoise needs to be held in an upside-down position to avoid puncture of the inner organs. Although this method provides rapid fluid resorption via the coelomic membranes, it is only suitable as long as there are no palpable masses in the femoral area.

7.13 (a) Placement of an intraosseous catheter into the tibia of a bearded dragon. (b) A radiographic image to ensure correct placement.

advanced until the bevel has just passed through the body wall. With the needle in this position there is no resistance to fluid injection.

In lizards, the preferred injection site is the right caudal quadrant of the ventral body wall, as this avoids the midline ventral abdominal vein. The lizard should be placed in dorsal recumbency with the head lowered to encourage the visceral organs to move away from the injection site. For this reason, intracoelomic injection is a stressful procedure in the conscious lizard and sedation may be appropriate. Alternatively, the lizard can be placed in lateral recumbency and fluids administered through the paralumbar fossa.

Intraosseous route: Intraosseous infusion allows access to the circulatory system. It is therefore useful in reptiles with collapsed peripheral vasculature due to advanced dehydration or blood loss, or where their peripheral vessels may be difficult to access due to the size of the patient. This route can also be used for the administration of colloid solutions. Whenever possible, local or general anaesthesia is required as intraosseous catheterization is a painful procedure.

In lizards, a long bone is used as the site for the intraosseous injection of fluids – typically the proximal tibia, the distal femur or the distal humerus. The skin should be disinfected prior to needle insertion. Use a sterile needle to first penetrate the bone prior to catheter placement; a radiograph is helpful to confirm correct placement (Figure 7.13). The catheter can be left in place for several days; however, wound infection is a common problem and the insertion site should be kept as sterile as possible using local disinfection and topical antibiotic ointments.

In chelonians, the best access is via the plastron–carapacial bridge, which connects the plastron to the carapace between the forelimbs and hindlimbs. A small hole is made in the shell caudally (either using an electric drill or a needle), and the catheter is inserted into the bridge in a cranial direction, parallel to the outer shape of the bridge. Misplacement of the catheter into the body cavity is possible and imaging techniques, such as contrast radiography, should be used to check positioning (see Chapter 9).

Intravenous route: Intravenous catheterization is an invasive procedure that may require anaesthesia and surgical preparation. There are several potential injection sites. In lizards, the cephalic or abdominal veins can be used. If the ventral abdominal vein is utilized then dressings over the catheter and/or suture of the catheter to the skin is advised to prevent dislodgement and consideration should be given to suturing the catheter to the skin. The cephalic vein requires access via a cut-down procedure in the region of mid-antebrachium. The ventral abdominal vein runs in the midline, just beneath the skin surface, and is accessible halfway down the body.

In chelonians and snakes, the jugular vein is commonly used. This vein is clearly visible in chelonians (see Chapter 8) but requires a cut-down procedure in snakes as the vein runs deep to the ribcage. Alternatively, in snakes, placement of an intracardiac catheter is possible using ultrasound guidance (Figure 7.14).

1. Sedate or anaesthetize the snake and place it in dorsal recumbency.
2. Locate the heart using ultrasonography.
3. Disinfect the skin prior to needle insertion.
4. Insert the needle/catheter between the ventral scutes and advance it towards the heart.
5. Advance the needle/catheter into the apex of the ventricle at a shallow 30-degree angle.
6. Suture the catheter to the skin, apply a needle port and flush with heparinized saline.

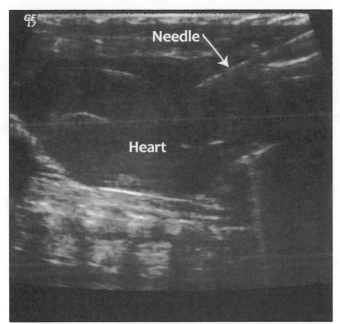

7.14 Ultrasound-guided puncture of the heart in a boa constrictor. Cardiac injection can deliver fluids and drugs into the circulatory system, but fluid accumulation in the pericardium can occur. There is acoustic reflexion due to the needle position (arrowed).

Fluid boluses can be administered via the intravenous route, and in relatively immobile or debilitated individuals a giving set can be attached to a syringe driver to provide a continuous-rate infusion. A possible side effect of this procedure is fluid accumulation in the pericardium if the catheter is not sited correctly within the ventricle. Another potential complication is haemopericardium, where blood leaks around a poorly placed catheter into the pericardial sac; serial ultrasound images can be obtained to assess the position of the catheter and the development of any cardiac tamponade; these complications, however, do tend to be rare.

Blood transfusion

There is little information available about the use of blood transfusions in reptiles. Some anecdotal reports demonstrate the feasibility of the technique using fresh blood from conspecific animals. It has been suggested that reptilian blood coagulates at a faster rate than mammalian blood, and this could interfere with the transfusion process. The use of a microfilter system for the prevention of embolic clots during transfusion has been tested in alligators and found to be effective without causing haemolysis (Nevarez *et al.*, 2011). Considering the current level of knowledge, blood transfusion is not recommended as a standard technique but only as a last resort.

Many reptiles have a normally low PCV, so determining when a blood transfusion is required can be difficult. Haematocrit levels <0.1 l/l (PCV of 10%) can be considered low; levels <0.05 l/l (PCV of 5%) should be considered critical and indicate that a blood transfusion is required. Blood groups are not described in reptiles. The blood donor should be the same species of reptile as the recipient. A blood volume of up to 2% bodyweight can be collected from a healthy reptile. Heparin can be used as an anticoagulant. If required, 1–2 ml of blood per kilogram bodyweight can be directly transferred from the donor to the recipient via an intravenous or intraosseous injection.

Diagnostic techniques

All emergency diagnostic techniques should aim to provide rapid, relevant information.

Haematology and biochemistry

Blood samples should be collected for haematology and biochemistry. Based on the clinical signs of the patient, the following parameters should be analysed: haematocrit (PCV), total protein (TP), albumin, creatine kinase (CK), aspartate aminotransferase (AST), glutamate dehydrogenase (GLDH), uric acid, calcium, phosphorus and glucose. In addition, blood samples can provide important information regarding organ function, blood and fluid deficits, and the presence of infectious processes such as septicaemia (identification of toxic heterophils, active monocytes or azurophils). For further information on sampling and result interpretation, see Chapter 8.

Parasitology

Although often a secondary finding, parasites can contribute to, or even cause, severe clinical signs in reptiles. For example, lungworms (*Entomelas* spp. in lizards and *Rhabdias* spp. in snakes) can cause verminous pneumonia or exacerbate an underlying cardiovascular condition such as dilated myopathy by resulting in inflammation and damage to the lung tissue, increasing post cardiac loading.

A faecal examination, preferably a Baermann flotation to detect lungworm ova and larvae, and other nematodes and protozoa, should be performed in all severely debilitated reptiles. If infection is suspected, swabs of tracheal mucus can be obtained and stained (using a standard staining solution such as Diff-Quik®). These swabs can then be examined for the presence of bacteria and fungi. Although this cannot replace microbiological culture, the results can be used to make a tentative diagnosis and institute treatment until laboratory results are available. Cytology can also be performed on any suitable sample (e.g. tracheal wash samples in cases of suspected inflammatory reactions in the lung; Figure 7.15).

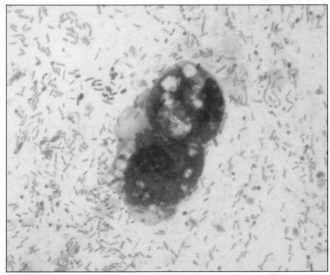

7.15 Tracheal wash sample from a Burmese python suffering from pneumonia, demonstrating bacteria as well as inflammatory cells.
(Courtesy of Dr. V Schmidt, Leipzig)

Diagnostic imaging

Radiography and ultrasonography can be performed relatively easily in reptiles and provide useful information about a range of common problems that can cause emergency situations, including trauma, dystocia and circulatory collapse due to cardiac failure, pericardial effusion or ascites. For further information on ultrasound diagnosis of cardiovascular collapse see Chapter 19. Both techniques can be undertaken without anaesthesia in most cases, thereby minimizing stress to the patient.

Radiography can demonstrate fractures, and radiodense structures, such as eggs and cystic foreign bodies, as well as the presence of space-occupying lesions caused by soft tissue masses. Ultrasonography can be used to investigate these soft tissue masses further, enabling differentiation between neoplastic processes, inflammatory reactions, fluid accumulations (Figure 7.16) and follicular stasis. If required, ultrasound-guided fine-needle aspirates can be collected for further examination.

Other imaging modalities such as computed tomography (CT) and endoscopy can also be extremely helpful (e.g. for surgical planning following shell trauma in chelonians; Figure 7.17), but are not first-line diagnostic techniques and tend to be performed once the reptile is stable.

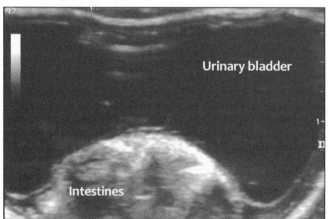

7.16 Ultrasonogram of a tortoise, demonstrating a massively filled urinary bladder. A needle can be used to quickly remove fluid if this is impacting on respiration as a fluid-filled viscus.

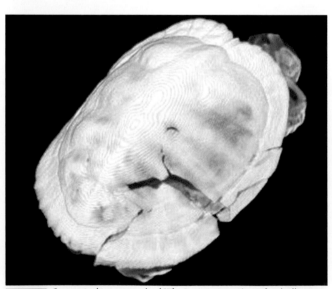

7.17 Computed tomography (CT) 3D-recontruction of a shell fracture in a turtle. CT is extremely helpful when planning surgical intervention in these cases.

Hospitalization and monitoring

Accommodation

Suitable accommodation should be provided for all reptile patients. Reptiles should be housed on dedicated wards (i.e. not on mammalian wards) and the cages should be arranged so that patients are unable to see one another. This helps to minimize stress, which can influence the recovery of reptilian patients (particularly chameleons). The temperature and humidity in the vivarium or terrarium should be monitored using a maximum/minimum thermometer and a hydrometer, respectively. A rough guide for humidity is approximately 30% for desert species and >60% for tropical species. For heating, overhead basking lamps are preferred to underfloor heating, especially in chelonians and weak reptiles that may be unable to move. The environmental temperature should be maintained at the patient's preferred body temperature. In the author's opinion, exposure to natural sunlight is beneficial. Where this is not possible, a suitable UV source should be provided (UVA can act as an appetite stimulant and UVB is important in regulating vitamin D3 in many lizards and chelonians; see Chapter 4). (Bathing reptiles in shallow warm water for approximately 20–30 minutes can also help to provide fluids, as well as stimulate intestinal and metabolic activity.) For further information on accommodation requirements for reptiles, see Chapter 3.

Nutritional support

Nutritional support is essential for all emergency patients and there are various commercial preparations available based on the feeding behaviour of the reptile (herbivore, omnivore or carnivore) (see Useful websites below). Other preparations that are not specifically designed for reptiles are also available but should only be used temporarily to provide nutritional support. Before initiating nutritional support it is important that the patient be fully rehydrated and any electrolyte imbalances corrected. Once rehydrated, food, in the first instance, should be provided in a suitable container; however, if the reptile is unwilling or unable to feed independently, assisted-feeding may be necessary. Smaller lizards may accept feeding via a syringe placed directly into the mouth. For other species, such as chelonians and snakes, that will not tolerate this type of assisted-feeding, a feeding tube may need to be placed. In chelonians, placement of an oesophagostomy tube is preferred for long-term assisted-feeding, as this is less stressful for the patient (Figure 7.18). For a description of placing a pharyngostomy tube see Chapter 13.

In acute cases, it is essential to provide nutrition as soon as possible, once dehydration has been addressed, in order to prevent collapse of the intestinal lining and removal of the barrier to bacteria in the gut. In chronic cases of anorexia, before significant volumes of food are provided, the patient should be fully rehydrated and any electrolyte imbalances corrected. If this is not achieved, then re-feeding syndrome may occur when food is provided. Re-feeding syndrome occurs because during the time the patient is not eating, there is a slow leaching of potassium and phosphate ions from the intracellular space into the extracellular space to replace those lost from the body. If a large meal is fed, the influx of nutrients results in a rapid uptake of potassium and phosphate ions back into the intracellular space, along with glucose. This results in hypokalaemia and hypophosphataemia, leading to cardiac arrhythmias and potentially heart failure and death.

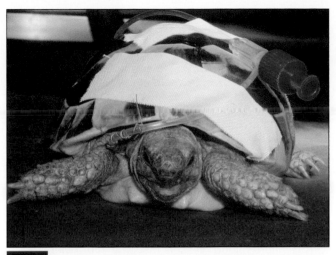

7.18 Gastric feeding tube in a Hermann's tortoise.

Monitoring

Basic monitoring includes a daily general examination and recording of bodyweight, food and water intake, and urination and defecation. It is worth noting that faeces production may not occur for several days. Trends in bodyweight should be evaluated during the whole period that the reptile is hospitalized. Continued weight loss is interpreted as a poor clinical sign. Continuous weight gain, especially in chelonians and lizards, when correlated to the amount of food and water provided is also a cause for concern. It may indicate constipation/obstipation or fluid retention (due to ascites or an obstructed or atonic urinary bladder). This can lead to pressure being exerted on the other internal organs, such as the lungs, resulting in dyspnoea. Ultrasonography can be used to check for the presence of an atonic or obstructed urinary bladder (commonly seen in chelonians; see Figure 7.16) and ascites. In these cases, further food and fluid provision should be tailored to the clinical situation to reduce the risk of severe side effects such as lung compression and circulatory collapse. The cause of the obstruction (e.g. calculi or refluxed eggs in females) should be identified and removed. Atonic urinary bladders are generally associated with spinal trauma, kidney failure or severe debilitation. Spinal radiography or computed tomography scanning is therefore recommended to ascertain the level of the injury in conjunction with neurological assessment (see Chapters 9 and 21).

Emergency situations

Traumatic injuries

Traumatic injuries are a common problem in reptiles and can involve both the skeletal system and central nervous system (CNS). The first step in the management of these cases is control of the haemorrhaging to prevent further blood loss. Suitable compression bandages, sutures and even electrocautery should be considered. Any fluid losses should be compensated (see above).

The next step is thorough wound debridement, starting with the removal of any foreign bodies. Contaminated areas can be flushed with a sterile 0.9% saline solution (using a needle and syringe), if needed. Care should be taken not to flush the debris deeper into the wound or create a high-pressure jet stream that could damage potential granulation tissue. Once the debris has been removed, the wound should be disinfected using a suitable solution (0.05% chlorhexidine or 0.01–0.02% povidone iodine). Following cleaning, the wound should be closed using either sutures (monofilament suture material should always be used in contaminated wounds) or by maintaining an environment which will promote secondary intention healing. The latter, often involves dressings which prevent drying of the wound, yet also prevent maceration of tissues, is recommended. A number of such dressings are available to the veterinary surgeon and generally involve a hydrocolloid gel trapped inside the dressing with a semi-permeable membrane to allow water movement from wound to dressing and *vice versa*. These dressings may be bandaged on to the wound or, in species such as snakes where a dressing rarely stays on the reptile, they may be sutured in place. The use of sterile porcine derived xenografts sutured over the wound have also been reported as a means of protecting a granulation bed where primary intention closure is not feasible (Alworth *et al.*, 2011).

The administration of corticosteroids may be considered in acute trauma cases, to prevent CNS oedema and aid stabilization. The use of methylprednisolone and dexamethasone (administered intramuscularly or intravenously up to twice a day) has been reported. Due to the possible immunosuppressant effects, consideration should also be given to the use of broad-spectrum antimicrobial drugs (e.g. ceftazidime or enrofloxacin). Systemic antimicrobial therapy is recommended in cases where perforation of the coelomic cavity has occurred, due to the risk of infection. Thorough irrigation and flushing of the contaminated cavity with warmed (34–36°C) 0.9% sterile saline followed by repair of any perforations or damage to the internal organs is also required.

In the warmer months, reptile wounds are susceptible to myiasis (chelonians are affected most often). Prevention of myiasis is important and covering the hospital cage with an anti-fly gauze may be beneficial.

Hypothermia and hyperthermia

Hypothermia often occurs in reptiles that have been housed or transported in inadequate conditions, or following a sudden change in weather (in animals kept outdoors). Clinical signs of hypothermia include apathy, reduced reflexes, frostbite, CNS signs (such as circling and head tilt) and ocular damage (e.g. cataracts and corneal ulceration). There is a significant risk of secondary infection due to immunosuppression in these cases and skin infections, septicaemia and even pneumonia can occur. Including an infrared thermometer on the crash cart to measure body temperature may be advantageous.

Management of these cases focuses on raising the core body temperature of the reptile by 2–3°C per day until its preferred body temperature is reached (Norton, 2005). This can be achieved by administering warm (34–35°C) fluids and maintaining an appropriate environmental temperature within the cage. Nutritional support should only be provided once the patient has been warmed to its preferred body temperature, otherwise food will not be digested properly and microbial fermentation in the gut may occur. In cases with pneumonia, diarrhoea or septicaemia, antimicrobial therapy may also be indicated.

Hyperthermia in reptiles mainly occurs following over-exposure to the sun or because the temperature in the vivarium/terrarium is inappropriate (malfunction in the heat source or its regulation). There is also the risk of hyperthermia when shipping reptiles during the summer months. Reptiles have limited compensation mechanisms for elevations in body temperature, e.g. increased respiration frequency and behavioural changes, and problems arise primarily when reptiles are confined to improper captive conditions. Elevations in body temperature can quickly lead to a fatal outcome. Increased activity may be seen initially (probably because the reptile is searching for a cool hiding place), followed by apathy and then coma. The reptile may demonstrate open-mouth breathing and the skin often becomes hyperaemic.

Initial therapy involves quickly cooling down the patient using water (e.g. by placing in a lukewarm bath or sprinkling with lukewarm water). Systemic fluids should be administered slowly to prevent oedema formation. In cases of suspected brain/CNS oedema, corticosteroids can be considered. The reptile should be placed in a cage at the lower end of the preferred optimum temperature zone (POTZ). Management of thermal burns typically involves the use of hydrocolloid or porcine xenograft dressings as skin deficits can be large and difficult to close by primary intention. Secondary Gram-negative bacterial (e.g. *Pseudomonas* or *Aeromonas* spp.) infections are commonplace and so systemic antimicrobial therapy suitable for this includes third generation cephalosporins, penicillins and fluoroquinolones.

Drowning

Drowning is seen occasionally in lizards and snakes but most often in chelonians. However, as many reptiles are able to survive for relatively long periods of time without oxygen (e.g. some chelonians that have been submerged underwater for approximately 24 hours have successfully recovered) (Fago and Jensen, 2015), this condition does not have the extremely poor outcome that is associated with mammals.

The first step in the management of these cases is removal of fluid from the lungs. For this procedure, the reptile must be positioned with the head/tracheal opening towards the ground. The fluid is then either sucked out using a syringe/pump or removed using manual ventilation. Following removal of most or all of the fluid, respiratory stimulation can be attempted using doxapram (5 mg/kg s.c., i.m., orally). Preferably, 100% oxygen should be used to perform IPPV in these instances, but an AmbuBag® may be used with room air in emergency situations. Any fluid removed from the airways/lungs should be submitted for microbial culture and sensitivity testing. Antimicrobial treatment is indicated in all cases, as the source of water is usually contaminated. Diuretics such as furosemide and hydrochlorothiazide have also been used to facilitate removal of inhaled fluid. However, these often cause increased stress on the renal system and take time to work and so their use in these situations is debateable. Removal of excess fluids and IPPV are therefore preferred.

Septicaemia

Septicaemia is a common problem in reptiles and is often caused by immunosuppression. Clinical signs include apathy, anorexia and petechial haemorrhage into the scales or plastron (see Figure 7.6). Clinical pathology will show an elevation in acute phase proteins (globulins) and potentially elevation of organ specific leakage or damage enzymes according to organs affected (e.g. AST in the case of the liver). In addition, haematology will often show an elevated leucocyte count, although chronic sepsis often presents with leucocyte depletion. Analysis of the leucocytes by blood smear microscopy is therefore recommended. This can give valuable information on the disease state by identifying the cell types, for example, increased monocytes or azurophils in snakes suggests chronicity of infection and increased heterophils may indicate acute infection. The activity of the leucocytes can also be identified (e.g. the stages of death of heterophils – so called 'toxicity' and the presence of phagocytosed bacteria in circulating monocytes or azurophils). For more information see Chapter 8. In addition, the mucous membranes sometimes become red–purple. A malodour from the mouth may also be perceptible. Disseminated intravascular coagulation (DIC) can occur in advanced cases and the prognosis is poor. Preceding DIC is the systemic inflammatory response syndrome (SIRS) where blood vessels become more permeable, inflammatory proteins are released and inflammatory cells sequestered to the site of the infection. The result is a decrease in the circulating blood fluid volume and decreased tissue perfusion. This can lead to multiple organ failure which can be exacerbated by infection and damage of organs directly. This leads to an increase in the circulating fibrinogen levels (and other acute phase proteins) and a hypercoaguable state (seen with end-arteriole disease and necrosis of digits, tail tips, dorsal spines in lizards etc.). If this progresses to the point of fibrinogen depletion then DIC can be seen with haemorrhages most easily seen under the skin (better visualized on the less pigmented ventrum of the reptile) and on the mucosa of the mouth and cloaca. Due to the low blood pressure system of the reptile in general, hypotension with septic shock is not reported in the literature and so is not reliable as a clinical indicator.

Culture of an aseptically collected blood sample often reveals the presence of Gram-negative bacteria, which are the predominant organisms in the reptile gut, but anaerobic bacteria and fungi may also be recovered. Immediate broad-spectrum antimicrobial and fluid therapy is essential, and should focus on antibiotics effective against Gram-negative bacteria (e.g. ceftazidime and enrofloxacin). Once the culture and sensitivity test results are available, treatment can be adjusted as required.

Circulatory collapse

Circulatory collapse is often the result of severe dehydration and hypovolaemia. Heart disease, such as dilated cardiomyopathy (commonly seen in snakes) and atherosclerosis (seen in varanids and some chelonians), may also play a role. In addition, chronic disease processes such as liver disease and chronic kidney disease can lead to hypoalbuminaemia and fluid accumulation in the coelomic cavity. In these cases, the use of colloidal solutions as indicated above, or small boluses of hypertonic saline (7.2%, 1–2 ml/kg) may temporarily provide clinical stabilization. However, both techniques have limited duration of activity and so the cause of the hypoalbuminaemia needs to be identified and if possible corrected. Plasma or blood transfusions in reptiles have been reported and may also be used as therapy (Nevarez et al., 2011). Blood groups in reptiles appear weakly immunogenic but the donor and the recipient should be the same species.

Clinical signs include apathy, dehydration and ascites with subcutaneous oedema. The diagnostic work-up should include ultrasonography to assess ascites and cardiac function, and blood biochemistry to assess organ function, TP, albumin and electrolytes. In cases of mineralized atherosclerosis, radiography can sometimes demonstrate radiodense vessels.

Initial treatment focuses on appropriate rehydration in cases of hypovolaemia. There are limited reports on the use of cardiac drugs in reptiles for the treatment of cardiac insufficiency. However, in the authors' experience, the administration of angiotensin-converting enzyme (ACE) inhibitors (enalapril at a dose of 1–5 mg/kg orally q24h), diuretics (hydrochlorothiazide at a dose of 1 mg/kg i.m. q24h) and furosemide (at a dose of 1–4 mg/kg i.m. as required) over a prolonged period of time, demonstrated some success in cases of atherosclerosis and were well tolerated in iguanas.

When hypoalbuminaemia is present, hypertonic saline (1–5 ml/kg bolus as required) can be used to draw fluid out of the tissues and into the circulation. Alternatively, colloids may be administered to support the circulation, but the cause of the hypoalbuminaemia should be identified and addressed wherever possible.

Central nervous system signs

With the exception of trauma and some toxicoses, most cases demonstrating CNS signs are the result of chronic processes rather than acute disease. Causes include infectious diseases (such as acanthamoebiasis – although this is extremely rare in clinical practice), inclusion body disease (IBD; caused by an arenavirus) and metabolic disorders (e.g. hypocalcaemia or hypoglycaemia). It should also be noted that thiaminase toxicity can cause seizures and tetany in piscivorous reptiles maintained exclusively on thawed fish. In addition to the CNS, other body systems may also be involved and signs of respiratory disease (due to ferlavirus infection and IBD in snakes), dystocia (resulting from hypocalcaemia) and trauma affecting the musculoskeletal system may be seen. The diagnostic work-up should therefore include radiography, haematology and blood biochemistry, as well as further tests based on the clinical signs and the history obtained from the owner. For more information see Chapter 21.

Seizures

In cases of acute seizures, diazepam can be administered as an initial treatment. However, it should be recognized that this is only a palliative measure and that successful treatment of the underlying condition is required in the longer term (see Chapter 21).

Toxicosis

Most cases of toxicosis in reptiles are due to the ingestion of toxic substances. These substances include: plants, for example, cannabis intoxication with sedation, bradycardia and seizures in green iguanas (Girling and Fraser, 2009); heavy metals, for example, lead poisoning in chelonians with non-regenerative anaemia and renal failure (Chitty, 2003); pyrethrins, with seizures, collapse and death at high exposure and thyroid dysfunction (hypothyroidism) at low exposure (Chang et al., 2018) and both effects are more lethal when the reptile is kept at higher environmental temperatures (Talent, 2005); and organophosphates, with seizures, loss of righting reflex and death (Norton, 2005). Iatrogenic toxicosis can also occur, usually as a result of a lack of knowledge on the impact of drugs used in human and mammalian medicine on reptiles. For example, ivermectin toxicosis at doses therapeutic in other reptiles

(0.2 mg/kg) is seen in chelonians due to the high number of gamma-aminobutyric acid (GABA) receptors in the CNS and so ivermectin should not be used at all in these species (Teare and Bush, 1983). At doses >0.2 mg/kg ivermectin can also cause paralysis in other reptile species (Gibbons et al., 2013). Metronidazole can also cause toxic effects at higher doses particularly in indigo and kingsnakes at doses >40 mg/kg) with liver failure and terminal seizuring being most commonly seen. Fenbendazole has been associated with bone marrow suppression and intestinal damage in reptiles at 50 mg/kg and above (Neiffer et al., 2005).

The diagnosis is mainly based on a thorough history. In cases where toxicosis is suspected, it can be rewarding to ask the owner to check the home environment of the reptile where the reptile is regularly allowed out of its vivarium, in particular to assess the evidence of exposure e.g. damage to woodwork paints (often lead-based) on skirting boards; exposure to environmental pyrethrin insect control products. Radiography and blood biochemistry are helpful in cases of suspected heavy metal intoxication. Lead is not used for any physiological process, so any level of lead is abnormal. Toxicosis has been reported at levels >1.2 μmol/l (Chitty, 2003). Initial treatment consists of fluid therapy to support liver and kidney function. In cases of suspected heavy metal toxicosis, the author has found use of chelating agents such as diethylenetriaminepentaacetic acid (DTPA) and ethylenediaminetetraacetic acid (EDTA) at a dose of 20–50 mg/kg to be effective. General supportive therapy with vitamins (vitamin C and E) is often helpful. However, vitamin A must not be administered parenterally to chelonians as toxicity can occur (at doses >10,000 IU/kg epithelial sloughing and multi-organ failure may be seen).

References and further reading

Alworth LC, Hernandez SM and Divers SJ (2011) Laboratory reptile surgery: Principles and techniques. *Journal of the American Association for Laboratory Animal Science* **50(1)**, 11–26

Andrade DV, Brito SP, Toledo LF and Abe AS (2011) Seasonal changes in blood oxygen transport and acid-base status in the tegu lizard, *Tupinambis merianae*. *Respiration Physiology and Neurobiology* **140(2)**, 197–208

Chang J, Hao W, Xu Y et al. (2018) Stereoselective degradation and thyroid endocrine disruption of lambda-cyhalothrin in lizards (*Eremias argus*) following oral exposure. *Environmental Pollution* **232**, 300–309

Chitty JR (2003) Lead toxicosis in a Greek tortoise (*Testudo graeca*). *Proceedings of the Association of Reptilian and Amphibian Veterinarians*, pp. 101

Dallwig RK, Mitchell MA and Acierno MJ (2010) Determination of plasma osmolality and agreement between measured and calculated values in healthy adult bearded dragons (*Pogona vitticeps*). *Journal of Herpetological Medicine and Surgery* **20(2–3)**, 69–73

Fago A and Jensen FB (2015) Hypoxia tolerance, nitric oxide, and nitrite: lessons from extreme animals. *Physiology (Bethesda)* **30(2)**, 116–126

Gibbons PM, Klaphake E and Carpenter JW (2013) Chapter 4 Reptiles In: *Exotic Animal Formulary*, ed. JW Carpenter, pp. 83–182. Saunders Elsevier, St Louis, Missouri, USA

Girling SJ and Fraser MA (2011) Cannabis intoxication in three green iguanas (*Iguana iguana*). *Journal of Small Animal Practice* **52(2)**, 113–116

Guzman DSM, Mitchel, MA and Acierno M (2011) Determination of plasma osmolality and agreement between measured and calculated values in captive male corn snakes (*Pantherus (Elaphe) guttatus guttatus*). *Journal of Herpetological Medicine and Surgery* **21(1)**, 16–19

Hartzler LK, Munns SL, Bennett AF and Hicks JW (2006) Metabolic and blood gas dependence on digestive state in the Savannah monitor lizard (*Varanus exanthematicus*): an assessment of the alkaline tide. *Journal of Experimental Biology* **209(6)**, 1052–1057

Hernandez SM, Schumacher J, Lewis SJ, Odoi A and Divers SJ (2011) Selected cardiopulmonary values and baroreceptor reflex in conscious green iguanas (*Iguana iguana*). *American Journal of Veterinary Research* **72(11)**, 1519–1526

Jacobson ER (1988) Use of chemotherapeutics in reptile medicine In: *Exotic Animals*, ed. ER Jacobson and GV Kollias Jr, pp. 35–48. Churchill Livingstone Inc NY

Krautwald-Junghanns ME, Pees M, Reese S and Tully T (2011) *Diagnostic imaging of exotic pets: birds, small mammals, reptiles*. Schlütersche Verlagsgesellschaft mbH & Co.KG, Hanover

Mader DR (2006) Emergency and critical care. In: *Reptile Medicine and Surgery, 2nd edn*, ed. DR Mader, p 533. Saunders Elsevier, St Louis, Missourie, USA

Maclean B and Raiti P (2014) Emergency care. In: *BSAVA Manual of Reptiles, 2nd edn*, ed. SJ Girling and P Raiti, pp. 63–70. BSAVA Publications, Gloucester, UK

Neiffer DL, Lydick D and Doherty D (2005) Hermatologic and plasma biochemical changes associated with fenbendazole administration in Hermann's tortoises (*Testudo hermanni*). *Journal of Zoo and Wildlife Medicine* **36(4)**, 661–672

Nevarez JG, Cockburn J, Kearney MT and Mayer J (2011) Evaluation of an 18-micron filter for use in reptile blood transfusions using blood from American alligators (*Alligator mississippiensis*). *Journal of Zoo and Wildlife Medicine* **42(2)**, 236–240

Norton TM (2005) Chelonian Emergency and Critical Care. *Seminars in Avian and Exotic Pet Medicine* **14(2)**, 106–130

Talent LG (2005) Effect of temperature on toxicity of a natural pyrethrin pesticide to green anole lizards (*Anolis carolinensis*). *Environmental Toxicological Chemistry* **24(12)**, 3113–3116

Teare JA and Bush M (1983) Toxicity and effiicacy of ivermectin in chelonians. *Journal of the American Veterinary Medical Association* **183**, 1195–1197

Useful websites

Website for commercially available feeding preparations
Lafeber:
www.emeraid.com
Oxbow Animal Health:
www.oxbowanimalhealth.com
Hills Pet nutrition:
www.hillspet.co.uk

Chapter 8

Diagnostic sampling and laboratory tests

Nicole Stacy, Darryl Heard and Jim Wellehan

Accurate collection, handling, processing and submission of appropriate diagnostic specimens are powerful diagnostic tools and essential components of reptile medicine. This chapter describes sampling techniques and laboratory tests in chelonians (turtles and tortoises), lizards, snakes and crocodilians. The reader is referred to Chapter 24 for parasitology techniques.

Blood samples

Collection

- Use the smallest needle size appropriate to the species and sample volume. In medium to small reptiles the most common needle size range is 22–27 G.
- Calculate the maximum safe blood volume before collection. Reptilian total blood volume is approximately 5–8% of bodyweight. In a healthy normovolaemic animal, 10% of the blood volume can be collected safely, i.e. 0.5–0.8% of bodyweight (g).
- Collect blood samples as soon as possible after the animal is restrained or anaesthetized to minimize effects of restraint or sedation on haematological and biochemical analytes.

Chelonians

Blood collection in chelonians can be challenging because of the shell and the ability of chelonians to retreat and protect vulnerable vascular sites. Some, especially aquatic turtles and terrapins, will bite during venepuncture. It may therefore be necessary to anaesthetize these animals for sample collection. Blood collection sites include:

- Jugular vein
- Occipital sinus (spinal vein)
- Subcarapacial vein
- Brachial vein
- Femoral vein
- Dorsal and ventral coccygeal veins
- Heart
- Carotid artery.

Jugular vein: The external jugular veins are very superficial and located on the lateral neck. They are more dorsal than those of mammals and lie at the level of the auricular scale (Figure 8.1). An assistant or the venepuncturist gently

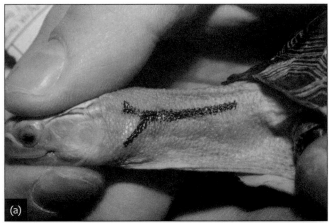

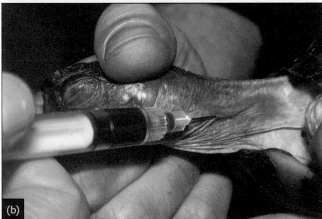

8.1 (a) Location of the jugular vein in a Chinese box turtle.
(b) Venepuncture of the jugular vein in an Eastern box turtle.
(Courtesy of Paul Raiti)

extends the head and neck for appropriate exposure of the jugular vein. This may only be possible in very ill or anaesthetized animals. Caution to avoid cervical spinal trauma is merited. Applying pressure at the thoracic inlet distends the vessel to facilitate visualization. A Q-tip is useful for this purpose because it does not impair visualization of the vessel. If the animal is anaesthetized and intubated, positive pressure ventilation will also dilate the jugular vein. Turning the animal into a lateral position and tilting the neck may also be helpful. Large Galapagos and Aldabran tortoises may extend their head and neck in response to neck rubbing or being hosed with water, allowing access to the jugular veins.

Occipital sinus: The occipital sinus (spinal vein) lies dorsal to the spinal cord and is approached from behind the partially flexed skull (Figure 8.2) (Martinez-Silvestre *et al.*, 2002). A small-gauge needle is inserted perpendicularly to the skin and gently advanced until blood is identified in the syringe. Care needs to be taken to avoid advancing too deeply and entering the spinal canal. This site is rarely used except in anaesthetized or recently dead animals.

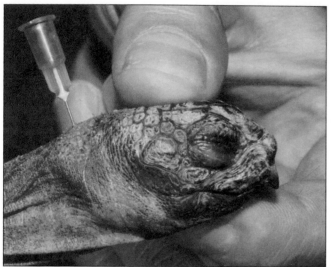

| 8.2 | Venepuncture of the occipital sinus in an Aldabran tortoise. |

(Courtesy of Paul Raiti)

Subcarapacial vein: The subcarapacial vein is located in the midline below the anterior aspect of the carapace (Figure 8.3). The needle is inserted where the skin joins the shell and advanced caudally until blood is aspirated. The vessel is usually located just above the posterior cervical vertebrae. This technique may require a long needle. The vessel closely approximates the spinal canal. If clear liquid is observed, in addition to the possibility of lymph, it may be cerebrospinal fluid.

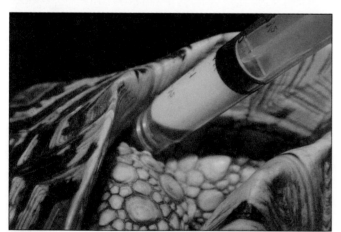

| 8.3 | Venepuncture of the supravertebral (subcarapacial) vein of a leopard tortoise for propofol administration. |

(Courtesy of Paul Raiti)

Brachial vein: The brachial vein is a plexus of vessels at the flexor surface of the elbow. This site is particularly useful in large chelonians, especially tortoises. The animal is gently placed in dorsal recumbency and the leg extended forward either by the veterinary surgeon (veterinarian) or by an assistant. The junction of the biceps tendon and the radius forms a 'V' into which the needle is inserted.

The needle is directed at an acute angle into the notch in small tortoises (Figure 8.4) or at a perpendicular angle in large tortoises. Tilting the tortoise so that the leg used for venepuncture is dependent may facilitate blood collection.

Femoral vein: The femoral vein is located on the ventral aspect of the pelvic limb, adjacent to the femur. Venepuncture is performed near the junction of the limb with the plastron, while the chelonian is in dorsal recumbency. This site is not commonly used, owing to limb movement and small blood volume.

Dorsal coccygeal vein: The dorsal coccygeal vein is accessed most easily in giant tortoises and snapping turtles (Figure 8.5). It is located in the dorsal midline above the vertebrae. Large tortoises are gently turned on their back, causing them to curl their tail over and allow access to the dorsal midline surface. The skin must be cleaned thoroughly because of the often heavy faecal contamination of this area. The sample-taker should proceed with

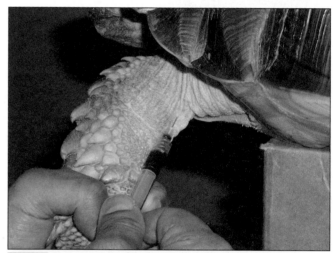

| 8.4 | Venepuncture of the brachial vein in an African spurred tortoise. |

(Courtesy of Paul Raiti)

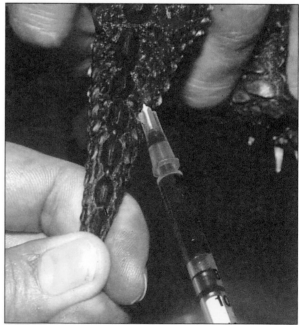

| 8.5 | Venepuncture of the dorsal coccygeal vein in a common snapping turtle. |

(Courtesy of Paul Raiti)

caution as these animals may kick. This vessel extends under the shell and can sometimes be accessed by placing the needle in the midline and directing anteriorly under the posterior edge of the carapace.

Heart: Cardiac puncture is used in small juvenile tortoises, in which the plastron is still soft, and in soft-shelled turtles. A regular or spinal needle is passed through the plastron at the junction of the humeral and pectoral scutes (Figure 8.6). This site should only be used on anaesthetized animals and is typically used in terminal procedures.

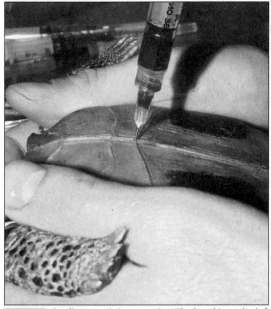

8.6 Cardiocentesis in a tortoise. The head is to the left. (Courtesy of Paul Raiti)

Carotid artery: The carotid artery can be visualized in some tortoise species (e.g. Hermann's tortoise) and may be used for blood collection for blood gas analysis. It is located on the lateral surface of the neck, ventral to the jugular vein, and covered by muscle. Care must be taken to ensure good haemostasis after collection to prevent haematoma formation.

Lizards

Blood collection sites include:

- Ventral coccygeal vein
- Ventral abdominal vein
- Brachial plexus
- Jugular vein
- Heart.

Ventral coccygeal vein: The ventral coccygeal vein is the most convenient blood collection site. The vessel lies along the midventral aspect of the vertebral bodies, partly protected by the ventral spinous processes. The needle should be of sufficient length to reach the vertebral body but of an appropriate diameter relative to the vessel. For a medium to large lizard, the author [DH] will use a 2.5–3.8 cm (1–1.5 inch) 25 G needle attached to a 3 ml syringe. Alternatively, in small lizards a 1.3 cm (0.5 inch) 27 G needle attached to a 0.5–1 ml syringe is used. A 25 G butterfly catheter attached to a syringe may also be used.

The vessel is approached either from the ventral midline or laterally (Figure 8.7). Some lizard species

(e.g. shingleback and blue-tongued skinks) have tough semicalcified ventral scales that inhibit the insertion of a needle through the scales at this site. In these species the needle is inserted between the scales. It is often helpful to hold the animal vertically with the tail down; it may be useful to hold large lizards on an open kennel cage door.

For the *ventral approach*, the lizard is placed in either dorsal or sternal recumbency. Sternal recumbency is preferred for large lizards that are difficult to restrain. In these animals the tail is either draped over the edge of a table or gently dorsiflexed. The needle is inserted in the midline and advanced until the vertebral body is contacted. The needle may be either inserted at a 45-degree angle to the vertebrae, to facilitate passage between the ventral spinous processes, or perpendicularly. The needle should be introduced sufficiently caudally to the cloaca to avoid the hemipenes in males. Once the vertebral body is contacted, a slight negative pressure is applied to the syringe and the needle slowly retracted until blood flow occurs (Figure 8.7a). If blood does not flow the needle position is reassessed and adjusted.

The *lateral approach* allows the lizard to remain in sternal recumbency and requires a shorter needle. The needle is introduced from the lateral tail surface just below the identified transverse vertebral processes (Figure 8.7b). It is directed at a 90-degree angle to intersect the vertebral body. When the needle makes contact with bone it is 'walked' ventrally until it contacts the vein. A slight negative pressure is maintained in the syringe during this process.

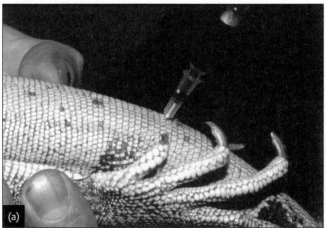

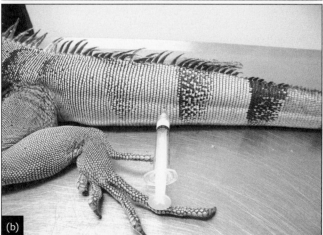

8.7 Venepuncture of the ventral coccygeal vein in a green iguana: (a) ventral approach; (b) lateral approach. The syringe contains propofol. (Courtesy of Paul Raiti)

Ventral abdominal vein: The ventral abdominal vein is accessed in the midline of the caudal abdomen immediately under the skin. It may be used in small lizards, but has the disadvantages of uncontrolled haemorrhage if lacerated, or contamination of the abdomen with intestinal contents if the bowel is penetrated. The abdomens of geckos and other small lizards may be transilluminated to visualize the ventral abdominal vein, as well as the heart.

Brachial plexus: Blood can be collected in some lizards from the brachial area of the forelimb (Figure 8.8).

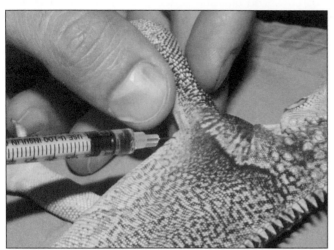

8.8 Venepuncture of the brachial plexus in a green iguana.
(Courtesy of Paul Raiti)

Jugular vein: The jugular vein is highly variable in location between squamate species. Ultrasonography-guided venepuncture may be possible if Doppler ultrasonography is available. This site is perhaps most commonly used in green iguanas, where it has been described as a 'blind stick' midway between the ear and the point of the shoulder.

Heart: The heart can be used as a site for blood collection although this is done reluctantly because of potential injury and haemorrhage. In lizards the cardiac position is highly variable; in some (e.g. iguanas and skinks) the heart is located between the shoulders but in others (e.g. monitors and chameleons) it is located almost mid-abdomen. The cranial heart is accessed either through the thoracic inlet or between the ribs. When available, a Doppler flow detection monitor or ultrasonography is used to define cardiac location (Figure 8.9). This site should only be used on anaesthetized animals and is typically used in terminal procedures.

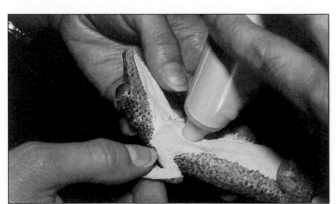

8.9 Use of a blood-flow Doppler probe to locate the heart in a leaf-tailed gecko.
(Courtesy of Paul Raiti)

Snakes

Blood collection sites include:

- Ventral coccygeal vein
- Heart
- Palatine vein
- Vertebral sinus.

Ventral coccygeal vein: The coccygeal vein is approached from the ventral tail (Figure 8.10) as described for lizards. Rattlesnakes that possess active muscular tails appear to have large ventral coccygeal vessels. However, even large snakes of other species may have relatively small coccygeal vessels, making blood collection difficult. Boas and pythons have small ventral coccygeal vessels. Small-gauge needles and accurate controlled movement of both the needle and syringe are essential for successful collection in all species. Resting the tail, as well as one's hands, on a table will facilitate blood collection, as will holding the animal's body vertically with the tail down.

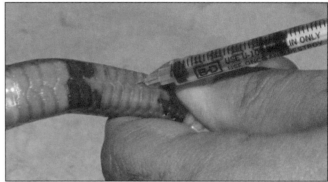

8.10 Venepuncture of the ventral coccygeal vein in a Honduran milk snake.
(Courtesy of Paul Raiti)

Heart: The position of the snake heart varies between species. It is closer to the middle of the body in aquatic snakes than in terrestrial or arboreal snakes, which have hearts typically 15–20% of the body length from the head (Figure 8.11). In wide-bodied animals, the heart may lie on either the right or the left side of the coelomic cavity. In small snakes and non-constrictors, the heart is the first round palpable structure caudal to the head. However, it is more difficult to palpate the heart in large constrictors, especially if the snake is obese. Anaesthesia with an inhalant anaesthetic may be necessary to provide adequate relaxation for cardiac venepuncture. Placing a snake in dorsal recumbency and angling a light source to create a

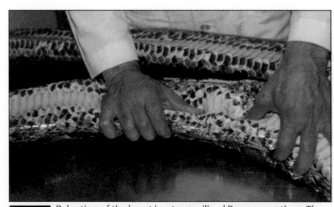

8.11 Palpation of the heart in a tranquilized Burmese python. The head is to the left.
(Courtesy of Paul Raiti)

reflected area on the ventral scales will usually allow visualization of scale movement above the heart. In constrictors, placing the animal in ventral recumbency and visualizing the scales from below will have the same effect. Alternatively, the heart can be identified with either a Doppler flow detection apparatus or ultrasound machine.

Once located, the heart is gently stabilized by placing a thumb below the apex of the ventricle and applying a slight cranial pressure. It may be useful to also stabilize from cranial to the heart with an index finger. The needle is introduced cranially into the ventricle, at 45 degrees, while a slight negative pressure is applied until blood flow is attained (Figure 8.12). The flow is pulsatile and the negative pressure should be released intermittently to allow cardiac chamber filling. As with other venepuncture sites, the needle should be placed with accuracy and control to prevent cardiac laceration and excessive haemorrhage. When performed appropriately this procedure has low morbidity or mortality; the most common complication is haemopericardium.

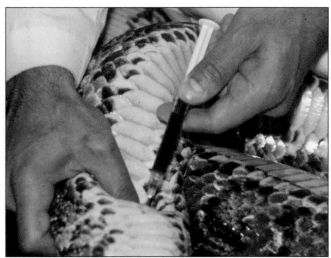

8.12 Cardiocentesis in a Burmese python.
(Courtesy of Paul Raiti)

Palatine vein: The palatine vein may be used for collection of blood from large snakes. The vessels lie on the medial surface of the palatine dental arcade and the teeth may injure the venepuncturist. Further, the vessels have minimal surrounding tissue to contribute to haemostasis, and haematoma formation is common. These vessels should only be used in anaesthetized large snakes and, even then, with great care to avoid being bitten.

Vertebral sinus: The vertebral sinus may sometimes be accessed in snakes by placing the animals in ventral recumbency and draping the caudal third of the body over the edge of the table. This causes ventral flexion of the spinal column, opening up the dorsal spaces between spinous processes. A small-gauge needle is then carefully inserted through one of these spaces to enter the sinus.

Sample processing and submission

Anticoagulation

Reptilian blood samples submitted for haematological analysis are best anticoagulated with heparin. Calcium EDTA has been associated with haemolysis in some reptile species (especially chelonians). For this reason and because clot formation is unpredictable in reptiles, lithium heparin is the preferred anticoagulant in reptiles. Plasma samples are obtained by collecting blood into syringes containing heparin or by placing a whole-blood sample into a heparinized tube. It should be noted that injectable heparin is generally sodium heparin, which may falsely increase the concentration of sodium in the sample if added in a significant volume. Therefore, all visible droplets of injectable heparin should be thoroughly expelled prior to venepuncture.

Blood film

Since delay in processing (>24 hours) can cause alterations in leucocyte morphology (i.e. granulocyte degranulation or cell degeneration), blood samples submitted to a laboratory for analysis should be accompanied by air-dried unstained blood films prepared immediately after collection. Proper technique is essential for preparation of a good quality blood film, as reptile blood cells are larger in size and thus rupture more easily than mammalian blood cells during blood film preparation. Details of blood smear techniques and staining can be found in the *BSAVA Manual of Canine and Feline Clinical Pathology*. After staining the blood films with a Romanowsky-type stain, such as Wright–Giemsa, the smears can be evaluated.

Plasma

Since heparin is the most frequently used anticoagulant in reptile medicine, blood biochemical evaluation is performed using plasma. The use of plasma is advantageous with small sample volumes: an aliquot of whole blood can be removed from the sample for haematological analysis and the remainder of the sample centrifuged to harvest plasma. Heparinized plasma samples can be centrifuged immediately after processing for haematology, which avoids prolonged contact of cells with plasma. The plasma colour after centrifugation should be reported, e.g. normal, haemolysis, biliverdinaemia.

Lymphodilution

Many vessels used for blood collection in reptiles are in close proximity to lymph vessels. Normal lymph contains small well-differentiated lymphocytes and variable concentrations of biochemical analytes, depending on location. Since lymph is dissimilar to blood, excessive contamination may affect haematological and plasma biochemical values (i.e. decreased packed cell volume (PCV), white blood cell (WBC) count, total protein, potassium, chloride). The heart and jugular veins seem to be the sites least likely to be contaminated by lymph.

Haematology

The main components of reptilian haematology are PCV, WBC quantification, plasma colour and blood film evaluation for WBC differential and blood cell morphology. Circulating reptile blood cells include erythrocytes, thrombocytes, granulocytes (heterophils, eosinophils, basophils) and mononuclear cells (lymphocytes, monocytes, azurophils/azurophilic monocytes). In the sections below, the morphological description of cells refers to Wright–Giemsa staining unless otherwise stated. Details on laboratory methods, morphological description, leucogram responses in disease and additional images pertaining to reptile haematology are referred to elsewhere in the literature (Strik *et al.*, 2007).

White blood cell count and estimate

Since all blood cells are nucleated in reptiles, automated haematology analysers cannot be used in reptile haematology. Current available methods are manual and include WBC counts by haemocytometer (i.e. with Natt–Herrick's; available as Natt-Herricks-TIC®, Bioanalytic GmbH, Germany) and WBC estimates from a well prepared blood film with even cell distribution using the following formula as for avian haematology (Campbell and Coles, 1986; Weiss, 1984):

$$\text{WBC estimate/}\mu l = (\text{average \# of cells in 10 fields}) \times (\text{objective power})^2$$

Confirming the WBC count by an estimate from the blood film is recommended as a control for the manual count. It is important to be aware of the imprecision of manual counts. In mammals, there are reported 30% coefficients of variation for manual compared with 5% for automated methods. This demonstrates the importance of consistency in laboratory methods for comparing and monitoring trends in the individual patient. The absolute counts of each WBC type per microlitre are obtained by multiplication of the relative counts (percentage) of each leucocyte type by the total WBC concentration. Only the absolute counts per microlitre should be used for interpretation of the leucogram and not the differential leucocyte percentages.

Reference intervals are not readily available for many reptile species and those that are published in the veterinary literature should be used cautiously, since studies vary notably in analytical and statistical methods, size of reference study group and inclusion criteria. These published studies may prove useful as a baseline for interpretation of the reptilian haemogram, if applicable. Extrinsic and intrinsic factors need to be correlated with blood work results and any relevant clinical findings in the patient. Monitoring haemogram trends can be very useful in the individual reptile patient for diagnosis, treatment and prognosis.

Erythrocytes

Normal mature reptilian erythrocytes are ellipsoid in shape, have eosinophilic cytoplasm and contain a dark purple nucleus with clumped chromatin (Figure 8.13).

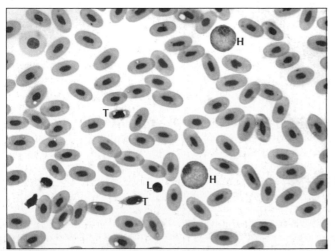

8.13 Mature erythrocytes (some with small distinct basophilic inclusions or clear punctate vacuoles) in a blood film from a ball python. H = heterophil; L = lymphocyte; T = thrombocyte. (Wright–Giemsa stain; original magnification X100)

Immature forms: Polychromatophilic erythrocytes and rubricytes are rounder and often smaller compared with mature erythrocytes and have polychromatophilic to dark basophilic cytoplasm that contains a larger nucleus (higher nucleus to cytoplasm ratio) with coarse chromatin. Healthy reptiles have <1% polychromatophils or rubricytes in the peripheral circulation (Figure 8.14); thus, mild anisocytosis and polychromasia are normal for healthy non-anaemic reptiles. Evidence of erythroid regeneration in response to anaemia include one or more of the following: increased anisocytosis and polychromasia, mitotic figures, binucleation, basophilic stippling and synchronous appearance of immature erythroid precursors back to rubricytes and even rubriblasts (Figure 8.15). In early regeneration, only rubricytes or rubriblasts may be seen admixed with mature erythrocytes in circulation, and may be misinterpreted as abnormal. For example, immature erythroid precursors can be misidentified as large lymphocytes, which will lead to misinterpretation of the leucogram. It is important to identify accurately these cells and interpret the morphological changes in the erythroid cell line in context with the PCV and physical examination findings. Reticulocyte counts are not routinely evaluated in reptile haematology.

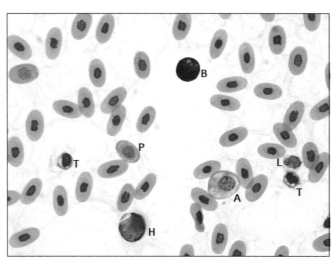

8.14 Blood film from a blood python: mature erythrocytes. A = azurophil; B = basophil; H = heterophil; L = lymphocyte; P = polychromatophil; T = thrombocyte. (Wright–Giemsa stain; original magnification X100)

Anaemia

Causes of anaemia in reptiles are similar to those in birds and mammals (haemorrhagic, haemolytic or decreased red blood cell (RBC) production). PCV and morphological evaluation of erythrocytes upon blood film evaluation are most useful in the laboratory assessment of whether a reptile patient has a regenerative or non-regenerative anaemia. Erythroid regeneration is best interpreted in the context of clinical history and duration and degree of anaemia of the individual patient.

Inclusions: One to multiple variably sized small basophilic cytoplasmic inclusions and/or clear, distinct punctate vacuoles can be seen in erythrocytes of healthy chelonians and other reptile species. They have been identified to represent degenerated organelles and are not known to have clinical significance (Alleman et al., 1999). Multiple fine dust-like basophilic cytoplasmic inclusions consistent with basophilic stippling can be seen as part of the erythroid regenerative response (see Figure 8.15a).

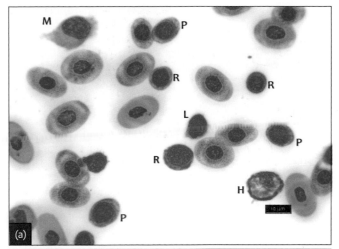

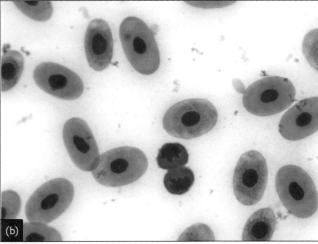

8.15 (a) Blood film from an anaemic green turtle (PCV 12%) with synchronous erythroid regeneration. H = heterophil; L = lymphocyte; M = monocyte; P = polychromatophil; R = rebricyte (increased polychromasia, basophilic stippling). (Wright–Giemsa stain; original magnification X200). (b) Blood film from a Kemp's ridley sea turtle with anaemia (PCV 17%) and erythroid regeneration (polychromasia, basophilic stippling and mitotic figure). (Wright–Giemsa stain; original magnification X500)

Haemogregarine parasites, such as *Haemogregarina*, *Hemolivia*, and *Hepatozoon*, are the most common blood parasites observed in reptiles, although other parasites, such as trypanosomes and filarial worms, may also be seen (Figure 8.16b–c). For additional reading, the authors refer to Telford's *Hemoparasites of the Reptilia* (2008).

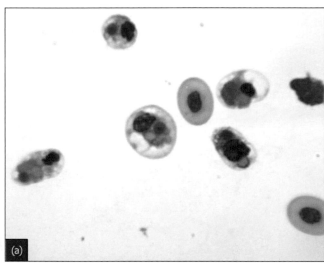

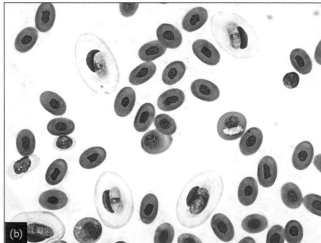

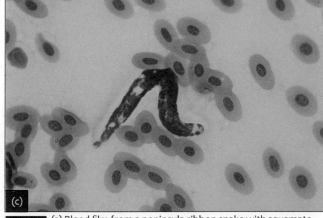

8.16 (a) Blood film from a peninsula ribbon snake with squamate erythrocytic virus (SEV) infection (crystalline inclusions and purple granular aggregates within erythrocytes). (Wright–Giemsa stain; original magnification X500). (b) Blood film from an indigo snake with intraerythrocytic haemogregarines (*Hepatozoon* sp.). (Wright–Giemsa stain; original magnification X200). (c) A filarial worm in the blood of a monitor lizard. Possible genera include *Foleyella, Piratuboides, Oswaldo, McDonadus*. (Wright–Giemsa stain; original magnification X1000)

Square to rectangular or hexagonal clear crystalline inclusions have been observed in erythroid cytoplasm and nuclei of apparently healthy animals in several species. Such inclusions investigated by transmission electron microscopy in rhinoceros iguanas appeared to be similar to haemoglobin crystals, which can also be observed in mammals (Harr *et al.*, 2001). These inclusions have not been associated with clinical disease in published reports of reptiles.

Viral inclusions may also be present in erythrocytes. Erythrocytic iridoviruses, which are likely to represent a istinct genus in the family Iridoviridae, form purple granular cytoplasmic inclusions that vary in staining intensity and may be associated with severe anaemia (Wellehan *et al.*, 2008) (Figure 8.16a). Rhabdoviruses reportedly can form pale blue cytoplasmic inclusions in the erythrocytes of squamates (Wellehan *et al.*, 2012). Transmission electron microscopy is needed for virus visualization, and polymerase chain reaction (PCR) with sequencing of products will provide a definitive diagnosis of viral infection. Inclusion body disease inclusions have been documented in erythrocytes, thrombocytes and leucocytes of boas and pythons.

Thrombocytes

Thrombocytes are the counterpart of mammalian platelets and are essential for haemostasis. They are round, oval to elliptical or fusiform in shape and have a small round condensed nucleus with a small quantity of colourless or pale blue cytoplasm. Thrombocytes can have clear vacuoles that stain positively with periodic acid–Schiff (PAS) consistent with glycogen, and/or pink to purple granules. Thrombocytes can be difficult to distinguish from lymphocytes (see Figures 8.13 and 8.17). Heparinized samples often display thrombocyte clumping, which can be very helpful in this differentiation. The clumping in heparinized samples prevents accurate quantitation of thrombocytes by haemocytometer or blood-film estimate. Their number

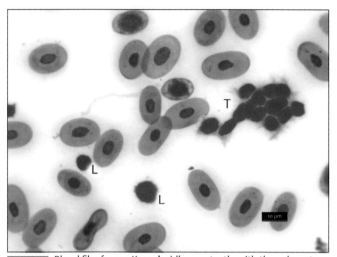

8.17 Blood film from a Kemp's ridley sea turtle with thrombocyte clump (T) and lymphocytes (L). (Wright–Giemsa stain; original magnification X200)

can only be subjectively assessed and reported as decreased, normal or increased by blood film evaluation. If there is concern for thrombocytopenia, sample collection and handling errors (i.e. difficult blood withdrawal, clotted sample, delay in processing) should be ruled out before making that interpretation.

Heterophils

Heterophil nuclei in most reptiles are round (see Figures 8.13–8.15a), but some lizard species can have bi- or multilobed nuclei. The heterophil cytoplasm is filled with distinct fusiform pink to bright orange coloured granules. Delay in processing can cause degranulation. Most reptilian heterophils do not stain positively with benzidine peroxidase as mammalian heterophils do, indicating that they rely on oxygen-independent mechanisms to defend against microorganisms. Heterophils of snakes and some lizard species stain variably positive for peroxidase. The difference in oxidative burst may be the reason that reptiles respond to bacterial infection with granuloma formation. Morphological assessment and quantitation of heterophil toxicity and left-shifting (Figure 8.18) are valuable features for the clinician for diagnosis, monitoring of patients and prognosis. Heterophil toxicity is characterized and quantified from mild (cytoplasmic basophilia, mild vacuolation or degranulation, if delay in processing can be excluded), to severe (increased vacuolation, abnormal granulation and/or nuclear pleomorphism), on a scale of 1+ to 3+. The degree and severity of heterophil toxicity provide clinically useful information (for example, see Figure 8.18a: 2+/all). Heterophil toxicity is a non-specific finding and can be observed with inflammation, various infections, tissue necrosis, some drugs or metabolic derangements. Degranulation and/or vacuolation in the absence of other features of toxicity may indicate storage artefact.

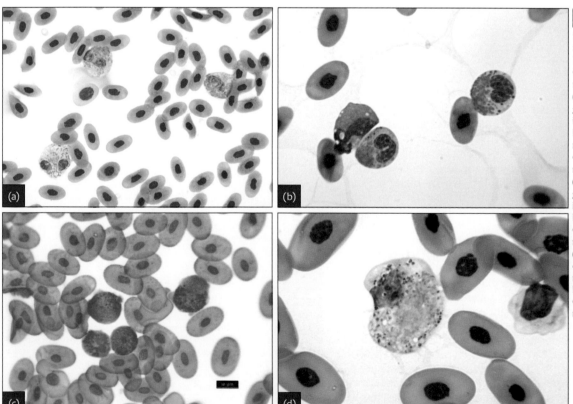

8.18 (a) Blood film from a green iguana with moderately toxic heterophils. (Wright–Giemsa stain; original magnification X200). (b) Blood film from a green iguana with two immature, mildly toxic heterophils and a monocyte. (Wright–Giemsa stain; original magnification X500). (c) Blood film from a green turtle with four immature, toxic heterophils. (Wright–Giemsa stain; original magnification X500). (d) Blood film from a caiman lizard with a markedly toxic heterophil. (Wright–Giemsa stain; original magnification X1000)

Eosinophils

Eosinophils of reptiles typically display variable numbers of eosinophilic granules in clear or faintly blue cytoplasm with a round nucleus. Several species of lizard, such as iguanas, tegu lizards and rainbow lizards, have blue-green round granules in their eosinophils, which are referred to as green eosinophils (Figure 8.19).

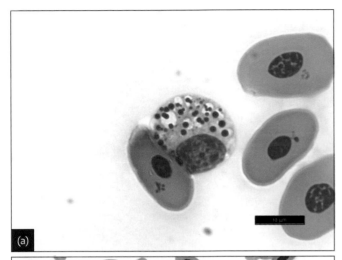

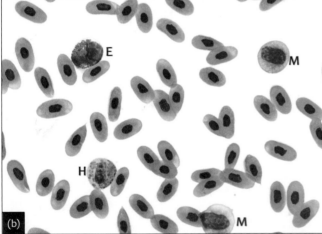

8.19 (a) Green turtle eosinophil. (Wright–Giemsa stain; original magnification X1000). (b) Blood film from a green iguana: E = green eosinophil; H = left-shifted heterophil; M = azurophilic monocyte. (Wright–Giemsa stain; original magnification X200)

Basophils

Basophils in reptiles have round nuclei and are generally packed with round metachromatic (purple) granules that often obscure visualization of the nucleus (Figure 8.20). Degranulated basophils can be observed with delay in processing. Many reptile species have large numbers of basophils and the percentage may vary greatly, for example, freshwater turtles reportedly have up to 65% basophils. Unlike in mammals, the inflammatory response to bacterial or other pathogens can manifest in basophilia, especially in species that have high resting numbers.

Lymphocytes

Lymphocytes of reptiles are very similar in morphology to lymphocytes of mammals (see Figures 8.13 and 8.17). The main challenge in reptile haematology is the differentiation of small lymphocytes and thrombocytes, since misidentification of these two cell types in the haemocytometer and upon blood-film examination can lead to significant laboratory error. Reactive lymphocytes and/or plasma cells can be observed with antigenic stimulation. Reactive lymphocytes can be larger and thus more immature, have more, darker, basophilic cytoplasm and possibly a few dust-like granules or distinct vacuoles (Figure 8.21). When these cells are observed in the circulation of a patient with other evidence of inflammatory disease, their presence is most consistent with inflammation rather than neoplasia.

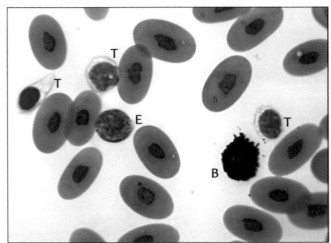

8.20 Blood film from a rainbow boa: B = basophil; E = eosinophil; T = thrombocyte. (Wright–Giemsa stain; original magnification X500)

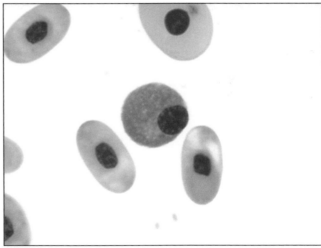

8.21 Blood film from a gopher tortoise: plasma cell. (Wright–Giemsa stain; original magnification X1000)

Monocytes

Monocytes of reptiles are similar in morphology and function to mammalian monocytes. Their blue cytoplasm may contain a variable number of clear heterogeneously sized vacuoles, dependent on activity (see Figure 8.18b). Phagocytosed debris, melanin or even infectious organisms, such as *Chlamydia* or *Mycobacterium* spp., may be observed. Erythrophagia (Figure 8.22) may indicate intravascular haemolysis and warrant consideration of blood culture as additional diagnostic test, if delay in processing can be excluded.

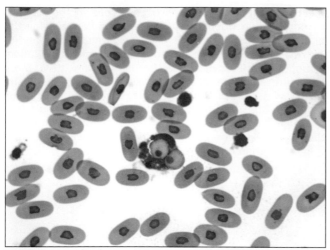

8.22 Blood film from a pine snake: monocyte with two phagocytosed erythrocytes and a small amount of globular dark basophilic–black pigment suggestive of haemosiderin. (Wright–Giemsa stain; original magnification X200)

Azurophilic monocytes/azurophils

Azurophilic monocytes/azurophils have round nuclei and light-blue to clear cytoplasm containing dust-like purple to pink granules (see Figures 8.14 and 8.19b). In contrast to other reptilian species, azurophils of snakes and some lizards (iguana, rainbow lizard, gila monster) stain variably positive with peroxidase. Because of this cytochemical staining characteristic and since acute inflammatory responses in snakes are characterized by a rapid response of azurophils in the peripheral circulation, the authors recommend differentiation of azurophils as a separate cell line in the leucocyte differential of squamates (snakes and lizards). In chelonians and crocodilians, azurophilic monocytes should be combined with monocytes.

Blood biochemistry

As in reptile haematology, the interpretation of reptilian biochemistry results needs to take into account a number of intrinsic and extrinsic factors of the particular reptile species, including age, sex, nutrition, reproductive status, temperature and season, as well as laboratory methods. Additional complicating factors are that studies on biochemical analyte variations in disease are limited in reptile medicine and that some assay techniques (e.g. bile acids) have not been validated for use in reptiles. While reference intervals for chemistry analytes have been reported in some reptile species, the methodology of published studies needs to be considered when comparing results. Reference ranges for haematology and plasma biochemistry of some reptile species are given in Figure 8.23. For a more detailed compilation and additional information see, Fudge (2000), Carpenter et al. (2001) and Mader and Divers (2014). When using reptile reference ranges for evaluation of a clinical case, it is important to remember that many of these published values have been obtained from a small sample size and possibly, in some studies, from animals with unknown health status. Many clinicians use clinical decision intervals or individual trends, if available.

Assessment and reporting of plasma colour is very helpful clinically, since haemolysis or lipaemia can interfere with many analytes. Green plasma may be normal in some (e.g. king cobra, with greenish yellow plasma colour) or it may indicate biliverdinaemia in other species (e.g. chelonians), in which it has been associated with starvation, haemolysis, or liver disease.

Since small sample volume is often an issue in reptile patients, the most useful analytes in the reptilian chemistry panel include total protein, glucose, uric acid, magnesium, creatine kinase (CK), calcium (Ca), phosphorous (P), electrolytes and, if sufficient volume is available, protein electrophoresis.

Parameter	Spur-thighed tortoise			Hermann's tortoise			Green iguanas			Red-eared terrapin	Royal python
	Winter	Spring	Summer	Winter	Spring	Summer	Males	Females	Juveniles		
Haematology											
PCV (l/l)	0.32 (0.24–0.45)	0.34 (0.28–0.42)	0.28 (0.2–0.35)	0.33 (0.25–0.45)	0.38 (0.32–0.45)	0.29 (0.2–0.38)	0.34 (0.29–0.38)	0.38 (0.33–0.44)	0.38 (0.30–0.47)	0.29 (0.25–033)	0.18 (0.20–0.28)
RBC (x 10¹²/l)	0.76 (0.54–0.96)	0.82 (0.65–1.08)	0.67 (0.46–0.84)	0.83 (0.64–1.28)	0.96 (0.73–1.36)	0.67 (0.47–0.87)	1.3 (1.0–1.7)	1.4 (1.2–1.8)	1.4 (1.3–1.6)	(0.3–0.8)	
Hb (g/dl)	9.3 (7.1–13.0)	10.1 (8.8–12.8)	9.1 (6.5–12.2)	10.1 (8.6–13)	11.3 (9.5–12.8)	9.3 (6.5–12.2)	8.6 (6.7–10.2)	10.6 (9.1–12.2)	9.6 (9.2–10.1)	8.0	6.7 (3.4–8.8)
MCV (fl)	416 (350–444)	423 (365–492)	427 (403–463)	402 (350–432)	408 (331–442)	426 (417–444)	266 (228–303)	270 (235–331)		(310–1000)	
MCH (pg)	124 (105–148)	126 (90–160)	137 (125–153)	124 (101–138)	122 (85–143)	137 (127–146)				(95–308)	
MCHC (g/dl)	29.8 (25.4–34.4)	29.8 (24.5–33.3)	32.2 (29.2–35.0)	31.1 (28.6–34.4)	29.8 (25.5–32.6)	32.2 (30.4–33.1)	25.1 (22.7–28)	27.9 (24.9–31)		31	
WBC (x 10⁹/l)	8.5 (5.4–12.8)	5.1 (1.5–13.0)	7.1 (5.5–12.5)	10.8 (7.5–14)	7.7 (2–13)	9.8 (6–12.5)	15.1 (11.1–24.6)	14.8 (8.2–25.2)	16.3 (8–22)		12.2 (4.6–38.2)
Heterophils (%)	66 (42–83)	63 (12–83)	58 (34–80)	66 (12–83)	63 (12–83)	58 (34–80)	24	21	13		62 (40–82)
Lymphocytes (%)	33 (15–58)	24 (12–50)	41 (20–64)	33 (15–58)	24 (12–50)	41 (20–64)	64	67	79		14 (1–49)
Monocytes (%)	0.4 (0–2)	2 (0–10)	0.7 (0–0.2)	0.4 (0–2)	2 (0–10)	0.7 (0–2)	9	8	2.4		0.6 (0–2)
Eosinophils (%)	0.6 (0–2)	11 (0–30)	0.3 (0–5)	0.6 (0–2)	11 (0–30)	0.3 (0–5)	0.7	0.7	1.8		
Basophils (%)							2.7	3.4	3.1		1 (0–4)
Azurophils (%)											17 (7–34)

8.23 Reference values (mean, with range in parentheses, where available) for haematology and plasma biochemistry in a range of reptiles. A:G ratio = albumin:globulin ratio; BUN = blood urea nitrogren: Hb = haemoglobin; MCH = mean corpuscular haemoglobin; MCHC = mean corpuscular haemoglobin concentration; MCV = mean corpuscular volume; PCV = packed cell volume; RBC = red blood cell; WBC = white blood cell. (continues) ▶

Parameter	Spur-thighed tortoise			Hermann's tortoise			Green iguanas			Red-eared terrapin	Royal python
	Winter	Spring	Summer	Winter	Spring	Summer	Males	Females	Juveniles		
Biochemistry											
Alkaline phosphatase (IU/l)	Range 61–211			Range 196–425			39 (14–65)	59 (22–90)		21 (81–343)	106 (63–145)
Alanine aminotransferase (IU/l)							32 (4–76)	45 (5–96)		202 (0–420)	14 (3–22)
Aspartate aminotransferase (IU/l)	Range 18–222			Range 19–103			33 (19–65)	40 (7–102)	41 (13–72)		33 (1–77)
BUN (mmol/l)	10 (3–15)	113 (105–124)	1 (0–2)	9 (4–14)	103 (58–140)	1 (0–2)				22	
Uric acid (µmol/l)	Range 35–244			Range 125–577			161 (89–345)	214 (54–399)	196 (47–339)	59	214 (107–297)
Cholesterol (mmol/l)	2.3 (1.7–3.6)	1.95 (1–3)	2.7 (1.8–4)	2 (1.2–2.5)	1.9 (1.4–2.3)	3.1 (1.3–4.7)	4.16 (2.12–5.53)	6.59 (5.28–8.97)			
Glucose (mmol/l)	0.6 (0.4–0.8)	13.3 (6.4–5.9)	1.5 (0.8–2.2)	0.6 (0.5–0.7)	13.8 (6.7–22)	1.5 (0.9–2.1)	9.2 (3.9–13.5)	9.4 (5.8–14.3)	15.1 (7.3–18.6)	3.7 (1.1–6.3)	1.6 (1.4–1.8)
Calcium (mmol/l)	Range 2–2.29 (up to 10 in egg-producing females)			Range 2.7–3.5 (up to 10 in egg-producing females)			2.82 (2.15–3.52)	3.12 (2.69–3.49)	3.57 (3.02–5.79)	3.49 (3.49–3.74)	3.4 (2.8–3.8)
Phosphorus (mmol/l)	Range 0.45–1.7			Range 1.7–3.3			1.71 (1.03–2.45)	2.03 (0.90–3.00)	2.49 (1.39–2.90)	1.29 (1.19–1.39)	0.98 (0.74–1.7)
Potassium (mmol/l)	Range 3.9–4.8 (lower in winter)			Range 4.5–5.0 (lower in winter)			4.0 (2.8–6.1)	3.6 (2.0–5.8)		6.3 (4.3–8.3)	
Sodium (mmol/l)	Range 130–150 (higher in winter)			Range 130–144 (higher in winter)			157 (152–162)	163 (156–172)		137 (133–140)	
Chloride (mmol/l)	Range 103–118 (higher in winter)			Range 96–115 (higher in winter)			119 (115–124)	121 (113–129)		102 (97–107)	
Total protein (g/l)	80 (63–103)	82 (65–126)	80 (65–118)	73 (51–92)	89 (71–112)	87 (74–103)	54 (44–65)	61 (49–76)	50 (42–61)	5.3 (4.0–6.5)	52 (43–59)
Albumin (g/l)	Range 5–18			Range 7–28			20 (13–30)	24 (15–30)	23 (22–30)		
Globulin (g/l)	Range 8–21			Range 10–26			35 (25–44)	38 (28–52)	27 (22–30)		
A:G ratio							0.6 (0.4–0.9)	0.7 (0.3–1.0)	0.8 (0.7–0.9)		

8.23 (continued) Reference values (mean, with range in parentheses, where available) for haematology and plasma biochemistry in a range of reptiles. A:G ratio = albumin:globulin ratio; BUN = blood urea nitrogren: Hb = haemoglobin; MCH = mean corpuscular haemoglobin; MCHC = mean corpuscular haemoglobin concentration; MCV = mean corpuscular volume; PCV = packed cell volume; RBC = red blood cell; WBC = white blood cell.

Plasma proteins

The most accurate method of total protein measurement in reptiles is the biuret method in combination with plasma protein electrophoresis for quantitation of albumin and globulin fractions. The assessment of protein dyscrasias is similar to that in mammals and birds, with increased concentrations observed with dehydration and inflammatory disease *versus* hypoproteinaemia, which is often observed with conditions of decreased protein synthesis (e.g. malbsorption/maldigestion) or increased loss from vascular space (e.g. loss of blood or plasma, nephropathy, enteropathy).

Glucose

Glucose concentrations can vary significantly by species, body condition and environmental temperature in reptiles, and can be artifactually decreased with delayed separation of plasma from blood cells. While hypoglycaemia may be associated with maldigestion, malabsorption, starvation or possibly septicaemia, differentials for hyperglycaemia include iatrogenic administration, glucocorticoid excess, gastric neuroendocrine carcinoma in bearded dragons (Ritter *et al.*, 2009) and, rarely, diabetes mellitus.

Kidney

Unlike in mammals, the primary nitrogenous excretory product depends on the reptile's environment. Terrestrial animals mainly excrete uric acid and urate salts, while aquatic turtles and crocodilians excrete variable proportions of urea, ammonia and, in some species, uric acid. Blood uric acid in reptiles does not correlate well with the severity of renal disease, since uric acid is primarily eliminated by tubular secretion, and thus blood concentrations are not related to the glomerular filtration rate. Increased uric acid concentrations can be observed postprandially in carnivorous reptiles, and with advanced stages of renal disease, or gout. Since magnesium increases only with iatrogenic administration or decreased urinary excretion, it is helpful in the assessment of kidney function in reptiles.

Muscle

Creatine kinase is the most sensitive and specific enzyme measurable in reptilian plasma and is consistent with muscle injury, which may result from trauma, intramuscular injections, exertion, catabolic conditions, restraint or infectious causes.

Calcium and phosphorus

Protein-bound calcium increases significantly in female reptiles during folliculogenesis compared with times of non-reproductive state. The calcium–phosphorus ratio should, however, remain unchanged in these animals (Fudge, 2000). In most reptile species, circulating calcium concentrations are greater than those of phosphorus. The concept of the calcium–phosphorus ratio does not readily apply to growing marine turtles in captivity. Inversion of the calcium–phosphorus ratio is suggestive of renal disease in iguanas and other terrestrial species. Properly handled samples for measurement of ionized calcium have been proven useful in reptile medicine. Disorders associated with calcium and phosphorus metabolism can be associated with diet and husbandry (i.e. dietary deficiency, over-supplementation) and increases in both may be seen with osteolysis. Hypercalcaemia with normal phosphorus concentration may be associated with granulomatous disease. Marked hypercalcaemia and hyperphosphataemia are often present in otherwise healthy captive eastern indigo snakes (Drew, 1994).

Electrolytes

Sodium and chloride can be very useful in the assessment of the hydration status in reptile patients. Potassium alterations often indicate changes in diet, disorders in acid–base balance, or possibly renal or gastrointestinal disease. *In vitro* haemolysis or cell leakage of potassium because of prolonged contact of erythrocytes with plasma may cause falsely increased potassium concentrations and should be excluded before considering causes of hyperkalaemia.

Liver

The lack of tissue specificity of alanine aminotransferase (ALT), lactate dehydrogenase (LDH), alkaline phosphatase (ALP) and aspartate aminotransferase (AST) in terrestrial and aquatic reptiles presents a significant diagnostic limitation for the clinician in the assessment of liver disease in reptiles. These enzymes completely lack tissue specificity and indicate non-specific tissue injury (Ramsay and Dotson, 1995; Wagner and Wetzel, 1999; Anderson *et al.*, 2013). Bilirubin is not useful, since reptiles lack biliverdin reductase and excrete biliverdin instead. The University of Georgia, Athens, USA, offers an assay for the measurement of biliverdin concentrations. Commercially available bile acids are not validated in reptiles, but reptile-specific assays may be available in some laboratories in the UK.

Endocrinology

When submitting samples for endocrinological analysis, it is important that the laboratory is familiar with reptile samples. It is also useful to submit control samples from apparently healthy animals of the same species for comparison. Samples submitted may be either plasma or serum.

- Hypothyroidism has been described in tortoises that have been fed excessive amounts of goitrogenic plants, such as cabbage, broccoli and bok choi.

- Thyroid-adenoma-induced hyperthyroidism was reported in a green iguana (Hernandez-Divers *et al.*, 2001). The affected animal had an elevated total T4 value of 30.0 nmol/l compared with clinically healthy iguanas (3.81 ± 0.84 nmol/l).
- Persistent hyperglycaemia and suspected diabetes mellitus have been reported in the green iguana (blood glucose 259–700 mg/dl, 14.2–38.5 nmol/l; Crocker and Miller, 2002), a Chinese water dragon (blood glucose 734 mg/dl, 44.01 nmol/l; Heatley *et al.*, 2001), and various turtles (blood glucose 360–830 mg/dl, 19.8–45.6 nmol/l; Frye, 1999). Hyperglycaemia has been associated with gastric neuroendocrine carcinomas in bearded dragons (Ritter *et al.*, 2009).

Tissue samples

Collection techniques, sample handling and processing

Biopsy

Biopsy samples collected for histopathology, culture, electron microscopy, polymerase chain reaction (PCR) or other molecular diagnostic testing can be very useful for diagnosis. The biopsy samples may be carefully imprinted on a glass slide for cytological evaluation, which can be useful for preliminary diagnostic information and/or for guidance for additional diagnostic testing. Histological interpretation is dependent upon preservation of normal cell and tissue architecture, and the biopsy sample should be of sufficient size to allow interpretation. When possible, multiple samples should be collected. Obvious overlying necrotic tissue may need to be removed to allow collection of a diagnostic sample. The transition area between a lesion and apparently healthy tissue should also be sampled. Surgical biopsy techniques are illustrated in Chapter 13. The most common fixative for biopsy samples is 10% buffered formalin. However, other solutions may be required depending on the type of lesion and suspected cause. When gout is thought to be present, some tissue samples should be placed in alcohol fixative, since uric acid crystals will dissolve in buffered formalin.

Samples for PCR and culture should be collected aseptically and placed in sterile sealed containers. The samples should be refrigerated or frozen if a delay in processing is anticipated. If a virus or other infectious agents are suspected, frozen tissue provides a valuable substrate for possible further testing. PCR may also be performed on tissue from paraffin blocks that have been stored for several years, provided that they did not spend excessive time in formalin before paraffin embedding, although there is a significant loss in sensitivity and false negatives are common. Storage in formalin is not recommended for tissue intended for PCR, since storage in formalin for more than 2 weeks cross-links DNA to the point where PCR is likely to be unsuccessful.

If electron microscopy is indicated, tissue can be placed in 2.5% glutaraldehyde at a 1:10 ratio.

Tissue imprints, scrapings and discharge

Tissue imprints are made by either touching a tissue or biopsy sample to a glass slide or by touching the slide to the lesion after removal of excess blood. The tissue is then gently touched to the slide in multiple places in a regular pattern. After preparation of the tissue imprint, the biopsy sample should be placed in buffered formalin for histopathological evaluation.

A scrape of a mass, organ or lesion should be performed in the active parenchymal area. Necrotic regions as well as organ or mass capsules generally yield non-informative samples and should be avoided. The region of interest can be scraped with the blunt or sharp edge of a scalpel blade and the sample gently spread on to a glass slide. If the smear is thick, a second slide should be placed gently on top and a pull preparation created. Tissue discharge (e.g. nasal discharge) can be carefully sampled with a moistened cotton swab that is gently rolled on the slide. The cytological preparations are air-dried, stained and ready for immediate evaluation.

Fine-needle aspiration

A tissue aspirate is obtained by inserting a cannula (a hypodermic needle or a catheter) into the tissue of interest (Figure 8.24). A syringe is used to provide suction. The accumulated aspirate is then gently expressed on to a slide. The authors prefer to use an 18 or 20 G hypodermic needle attached to a 6 or 12 ml syringe. Negative pressure is repetitively generated in the syringe by pulling on the plunger while the needle is directed within the lesion. If an excessive amount of blood is collected, the needle is withdrawn and a new needle and syringe applied. Even if no tissue appears to have been collected in the syringe, the needle is disconnected, the plunger drawn back and reconnected, any trapped material in the needle blown directly onto the slide and then spread with a second slide.

A stab technique works well for most masses, especially fibrous and vascular masses. The mass is palpated and held between the pointer and the thumb. The bevel of a 20 G needle is placed through the epidermis and redirected several times through the mass, taking care not to stab the stabilizing fingers. The needle is attached to a syringe charged with air and the sample is expelled on to a glass slide. A pull preparation is then made using a second slide.

Aspirates can also be obtained through the side port of an endoscope using a flexible cannula. Ultrasonography facilitates the accurate placement of the needle within the tissue of interest.

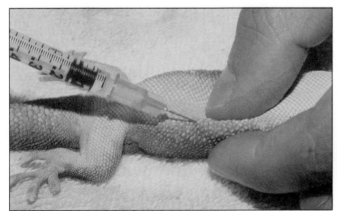

8.24 Fine-needle aspiration for cytology and bacterial culture/ sensitivity testing in a day gecko.
(Courtesy of Paul Raiti)

Cavity washes and coelomic fluid

Cavity washes are used to collect samples from the coelomic cavity. Sterile isotonic solutions best preserve cytological integrity and prevent tissue injury. In some patients, coelomic fluid may be obtained directly without cavity washing being necessary. Ideally, coelomic fluid should be processed by preparing direct and concentrated smears (i.e. centrifugation of fluid as for urine sediment, removal of a drop of sediment and preparation of sediment smears). Total protein measurement in the context of cellular components and WBC count of the fluid allow for characterization of the coelomic fluid and assessment of underlying disease, and provide guidance for additional testing (Figure 8.25).

Concentrated samples (sediment smear or cytospin preparation) from washes should be prepared as soon as possible after collection and can be cytologically evaluated for the presence of cellular material and infectious agents. Cultures, special stains (e.g. Gram stain for bacteria, acid fast for *Mycobacterium* spp., Gomori methenamine silver (GMS) stain or PAS for fungi) and parasitological evaluation can be helpful to identify the latter.

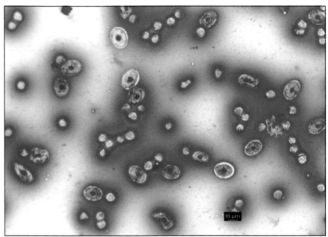

8.25 Loggerhead sea turtle: direct smear of coelomic fluid with proteinaceous background, total protein of 3.5 g/dl, 35,000/μl WBC estimate (heterophils) consistent with exudate; infectious agents were absent. (Wright–Giemsa stain; original magnification X100)

Tracheal or lung wash: A tracheal or lung wash is performed when respiratory disease is suspected. To obtain an uncontaminated sample, the trachea is intubated with a sterile endotracheal tube and a sterile catheter passed through it into the respiratory tract (Figure 8.26). Chemical immobilization may be necessary for endotracheal tube placement. Approximately 1–5 ml/kg of isotonic fluid is

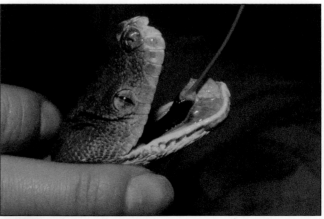

8.26 Performing a lung wash in a green tree python with pneumonia. A sterile flexible catheter is placed through the glottis and into the distal trachea.
(Courtesy of Paul Raiti)

then introduced, the animal is manipulated to wash the fluid around the lung, and fluid is then aspirated. This may have to be repeated a few times to obtain a diagnostic sample. Positioning the animal to allow gravity to assist fluid flow will facilitate good sample collection. The most useful diagnostic material is often obtained from the distal portion of the catheter and should not be discarded. If mucus is retrieved from the endotracheal tube after its removal, direct smearing of the material on to a glass slide for cytological evaluation may also provide useful diagnostic information.

Gastric wash: Gastrointestinal (GI) washes are performed using a catheter of appropriate length. Gastric washes may require longer tubes in snakes because the stomach extends over half the length of the body from the head. The wash is performed similarly to a tracheal wash but the fluid volume may be increased.

Cloacal wash: Cloacal washes are often performed when a reptile has not defecated recently or a sample is required for parasitic examination. A cloacal wash is used to collect faecal material from the cloaca and lower colon (see Chapter 17). There is a sphincter between the colon and cloaca; a wash may, therefore, not truly reflect the material in the lower colon. A flexible urinary catheter of appropriate diameter is carefully inserted into the cloaca/colon and an isotonic electrolyte solution infused and aspirated. In snakes and some lizards, there is a large ventral scale that acts as a flap to protect the cloaca. This flap needs to be carefully elevated before a catheter can be directed cranially into the cloaca. The specimen is then concentrated (sediment smear or cytospin) as for other washes, air-dried, stained and can be evaluated by light microscopy. One drop of the sediment may also be examined for the presence of motile protozoans and parasite ova (Figure 8.27). If a wash needs to be shipped to a diagnostic laboratory, submission of freshly prepared unstained direct and/or sediment smear preparations can be very helpful to avoid artefacts of delay in processing, such as cellular degeneration or bacterial overgrowth.

Cerebrospinal fluid

Reptiles do not have the subarachnoid space from which mammalian cerebrospinal fluid (CSF) samples are collected. Although rarely indicated and weighing the benefits and risks of this procedure, fluid may be collected from the subdural space, which is located between the pia-arachnoid layer – that lines the surface of the brain and spinal cord – and the dura mater. As the spinal cord extends to the very end of the tail tip in reptiles, CSF samples are best collected at the junction between the occiput and the first cervical vertebra. Many reptiles are too small for any sample to be collected.

The site is cleaned with appropriately diluted chlorhexidine. A hypodermic needle (attached to a 2 ml syringe) is inserted midline at 90 degrees to the skin surface and advanced slowly. A slight 'give' in the resistance to the insertion of the needle is felt when entering the subdural space and CSF starts to flow freely. The three fluid types encountered in the occipital sinus are lymph, blood and CSF; thus, the risk for contamination of CSF with lymph or blood is very high. Care should be taken to avoid excessive retraction of the syringe plunger as this will result in damage to the underlying nervous tissue. CSF samples should be processed and examined immediately since cellular deterioration can rapidly alter sample quality.

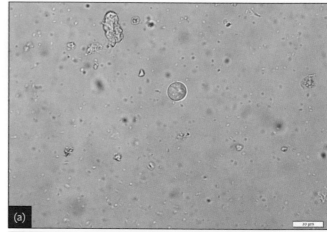

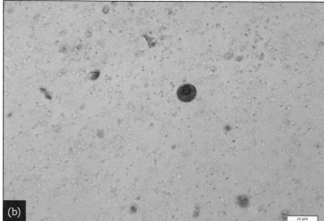

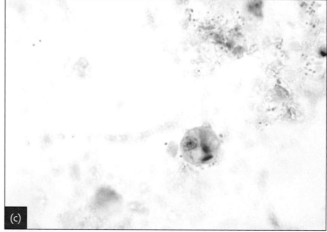

8.27 (a) Crested gecko: *Entamoeba invadens* cyst in a faecal wet mount. (b) Crested gecko: cyst in a faecal wet mount stained with iodine. (c) Crested gecko: cyst in a faecal direct smear (trichrome stain).
(Courtesy of Dr Heather Walden and Toni McIntosh, University of Florida, USA)

Bone marrow

Bone marrow is rarely collected from live reptiles. Aspiration is generally not possible owing to the fibrous nature of reptilian bone. If indicated, a biopsy may be performed using a Jamshidi needle. A 16 G needle is suitable in most moderately sized reptiles. Although bone marrow can be collected from bones of the appendicular skeleton of lizards, it is difficult to obtain in snakes and chelonians from this site. An additional consideration is that adult reptiles may have very little active bone marrow. Bone marrow in adult chelonians may only be present in some portions of the flat bones or margin of the carapace. Examination and staining are similar to that for mammalian samples.

Faeces

Faecal samples are examined for the presence of protozoans, parasitic ova, larvae (see Chapter 24), inflammatory cells, abnormal bacteria and fungi. Excretions from the reptile cloaca often contain a mixture of urine, urates and faeces. Faecal excretion is intermittent in many reptiles and GI transit time can be up to 3 weeks or more in large tortoises. The frequency of excretion is primarily dependent upon species, diet and temperature.

A small specimen is ideal for faecal examination. A wet mount can be prepared by placing a small amount of faeces on the slide, mixing it with an isotonic solution and covering it with a coverslip. For cytological preparations, a moistened cotton swab can be used for fluid or firm faecal samples to prepare thin direct faecal smears.

Urine

Chelonians and some lizards (e.g. green iguana) possess bladders. In these animals, the ureters do not empty directly into the bladder but close to the area where the bladder neck connects to the cloaca. Urine samples may be collected by cystocentesis, potentially using ultrasonography to identify the bladder. Samples collected by cystocentesis should not be treated as aseptic. Interpretation of reptile urinalysis can be difficult if urine is admixed with renal, intestinal or reproductive excretions.

Normal reptile urine is clear to light yellow with a white to light yellow urate component. Specific gravity is lower than in mammalian species. Since both the bladder and cloaca modify urine, it is not a direct product of the kidneys. Normal urine sediment is composed of uric acid precipitates, sloughed squamous epithelial cells, <5 white and <5 red blood cells per 40X field, and low quantities of (predominantly Gram-negative) bacteria. Motile and non-motile protozoans are occasionally observed in low numbers in normal reptilian urine. Many of these are believed to be intestinal commensals or contaminants; however, some protozoans, such as *Entamoeba invadens*, *Monocercomonas* and *Hexamita* spp., may be true pathogens.

The majority of urinary waste excreted is composed of a white to light yellow colloidal suspension (urates) made up of small spherical conglomerates that range in diameter from 0.5–15 μm. The urate precipitate is composed of uric acid, sodium and/or potassium, and protein. This precipitate is not measured in the specific gravity of the urine supernatant. Needle-shaped uric acid crystals may be observed in normal urine. Uric acid crystals polarize and can be chemically tested using the murexide test: a drop of concentrated nitric acid is added to the crystals and heated to evaporation; a drop of ammonia is then added; if uric acid is present, the liquid will turn pale purple.

Sampling for toxicological analysis and infectious agents

Toxicology

The diagnosis of heavy metal toxicosis requires whole-blood and/or tissue-level assays. It is recommended that a veterinary toxicologist be contacted to determine appropriate sample submission based on possible suspected toxins. As for endocrine samples, a laboratory familiar with animal samples should be used, and samples from apparently healthy animals of the same species may be required for comparison. Reptiles appear very resistant to some toxins and the clinical significance of blood or tissue concentrations cannot necessarily be compared with clinical effects as in mammals. Organophosphate poisoning and iatrogenic drug toxicities are discussed in Chapter 7.

Lead

Lead poisoning occurs due to ingestion of fishing sinkers, pieces of metal, hunting pellets and other lead-containing objects (Borkowski, 1997; Chitty, 2003). Clinical features of lead toxicity in reptiles are less well documented than in mammals, and crocodilians appear to be able to deal with lead levels that would be rapidly fatal in a mammal. High blood lead levels have been reported in a common snapping turtle (3.6 ppm; normal <0.6 ppm; Borkowski, 1997) and a spur-thighed tortoise (1.89 μmol/l; avian normal <1.2 μmol/l; Chitty, 2003), although the correlation with clinical signs was limited. Treatment consists of removal of lead from the digestive tract and chelation with sodium calcium edetate (10–40 mg/kg i.m. q24h, tapering the dose as blood lead levels decrease).

Plants and insects

Ingestion of toxic plants has been reported. Azalea (*Rhododendron* spp.) poisoning has been described in green iguanas (Rossi, 1995). Clinical signs consisted of tachypnoea, dermal blackening and emesis.

Acute death has been reported in inland bearded dragons that ingested fireflies (*Photinus* spp.) (Glor et al., 1999). Fireflies contain cardiotoxic lucibufagins.

Cytology and histopathology

Light microscopic evaluation of cytology and/or biopsy specimens can be very helpful to categorize a lesion into one or more of the following cytological categories: inflammation; haemorrhage; cyst; neoplasia or mixed cell population, and to identify infectious agents. If microorganisms are absent, then the type of inflammation may provide guidance for additional diagnostic testing, such as culture, special stains, parasitological evaluation or molecular diagnostics. For examples, see Figure 8.28.

Virology

Appropriate samples will vary depending on the suspected virus. It is important to determine which type of sample needs to be processed for the question to be answered by viral diagnostics.

- Virus isolation or PCR will give information regarding the presence of virus but these tests require virus in the sample submitted. The choice of sample for these tests is therefore crucial. For example, in a patient with a viral infection that is not viraemic at the time of sample collection, test results on blood will be negative. This does not imply that the virus is absent in the tissues of the patient.
- It is critical that products of PCR testing have their identities validated. Sequencing is one acceptable method for this purpose. Binding of a specific probe, as in a TaqMan® real-time PCR, is also an acceptable method. Other techniques, such as sole use of

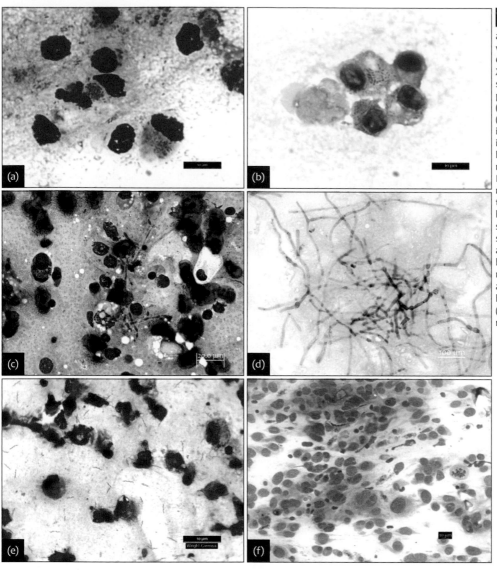

8.28 (a) Gopher tortoise, swab of nasal discharge: heterophils and mononuclear inflammatory cells with phagocytosed bacilli. (Wright–Giemsa stain; original magnification X1000) (b) Gram-stained slide of the same preparation as in Figure 8.25 with presence of Gram-negative bacilli. (Original magnification X1000) (c) Loggerhead sea turtle: lung lesion imprint with histiocytic and heterophilic inflammation and branching septate hyphae. (Wright–Giemsa stain; original magnification X100) (d) Preparation of Figure 8.28c with GMS (Gomori's methenamine silver) stain. (e) Gopher tortoise, nasal discharge direct smear: heterophilic inflammation and spirilliform bacteria. The bacteria stained positive with Warthin–Starry and were identified as *Helicobacter* sp. by PCR. (Wright–Giemsa stain; original magnification X100) (f) Bearded dragon: anaplastic sarcoma with mild heterophilic inflammation on eyelid. (Wright–Giemsa stain; original magnification X100)

electrophoresis for product size, or SYBR® Green real-time PCR for indication of some kind of amplification, do not validate the product and should be avoided.

- Consensus PCR is now available for most reptilian viruses, and all of those listed below, for example at the University of Florida in the USA, Laboklin GmbH in Germany, and Murdoch University in Australia. It is important to keep in mind that any PCR product obtained by consensus PCR needs to be sequenced to confirm the identity of the amplified virus and to detect potential contamination. Samples for PCR should be handled similarly to culture samples, for example on a cotton swab, cooled and with shipment overnight. Note that viral transport media may interfere with PCR.
- For virus isolation, the virus needs to be viable and thus the sample needs to be collected and stored in a manner that prevents inactivation of the virus.
- Serological testing gives evidence that an animal has had a humoral immune response to a virus, but does not give information on whether the virus is currently present. Serology does not assess cellular immune responses, which is the more clinically relevant branch of the acquired immune system for detecting active infection with viruses. It is also important to consider

whether the patient has had time to develop a humoral response to a virus, since this may take several weeks in reptiles and a serological response may be absent in acute infections.

Herpesviruses

Herpesviruses have been associated with hepatitis, stomatitis and neurological disease in tortoises; fibropapillomatosis and tracheitis in marine turtles; stomatitis and hepatitis in lizards; and poor venom production in snakes. Many herpesviruses have a latent stage in nervous tissue. To date, all known reptilian herpesviruses are in the subfamily Alphaherpesvirinae.

Performing a biopsy of affected fresh tissue is recommended, although swabs of oral lesions yield appropriate samples. Consensus PCR that works on all known reptile herpesviruses is available. Concurrent histopathology of biopsy specimens is essential; however, not all herpesvirus infections result in large numbers of classic intranuclear inclusions. Virus neutralization for tortoise anti-herpesvirus 1 and 3 antibodies is available at Laboklin GmbH. If virus culture is to be attempted, herpesviruses are not very tolerant of multiple freeze/thaw cycles, so it is recommended that biopsy samples be shipped refrigerated in viral transport media as soon as possible for culture.

Paramyxoviruses

Paramyxoviruses have been associated with pneumonia and neurological disease in squamates and tortoises. The most studied paramyxoviruses of non-avian reptiles are in the genus *Ferlavirus*; more recently, the highly divergent Sunshine virus has been documented in pythons (Hyndman *et al.*, 2012). As the clinical course of these diseases is often rapid and fatal, samples are frequently taken post-mortem. For diagnosis in a live animal, lung washes and buffy coats are recommended. Consensus PCR that works on all known ferlaviruses, as well as a separate assay for Sunshine virus, are available. Haemagglutination inhibition is available for detection of antibodies to ferlaviruses at Laboklin GmbH in Germany, and the University of Florida, Texas A&M University, and the University of Tennessee in the USA. However, there are at least four different genotypes of ferlaviruses, and cross-reactivity of antibodies is limited; this is likely to be one factor contributing to the poor concordance between laboratories using different isolates (Allender *et al.*, 2008). Given this complication, as well as the usual greater clinical interest in knowing whether virus is present rather than whether there has been a historic exposure to a ferlavirus, PCR-based testing is strongly recommended over serology. Concurrent histopathology of tissue specimens is essential. If virus culture is to be attempted, paramyxoviruses, like herpesviruses, are not very tolerant of multiple freeze/thaw cycles, so it is recommended that biopsy samples for culture be shipped refrigerated in viral transport media as soon as possible.

Reoviruses

Reoviruses in the genus *Orthoreovirus* have been associated with pneumonia and neurological disease in snakes. If pursuing a diagnosis in a live animal, lung washes and buffy coats are recommended. Consensus PCR that works on all known orthoreoviruses is available. Reoviruses are very tolerant of freezing, thus it is recommended that biopsy samples for culture be shipped frozen. To detect exposed animals, serum neutralization is available for ophidian reovirus at Laboklin GmbH in Germany.

Arenaviruses

Inclusion body disease in snakes has been strongly associated with a novel clade of arenaviruses (Stenglein *et al.*, 2012). If pursuing a diagnosis in a live animal, buffy coats are recommended. Consensus PCR that works on all known snake arenaviruses is available. Immunostaining can be performed at the University of Florida.

Nidoviruses

Nidoviruses in the subfamily Torovirinae are strongly associated with significant respiratory disease in a variety of pythons and boas (Stenglein *et al.*, 2014). If pursuing a diagnosis in a live animal, lung washes or oesophageal swabs are recommended. Consensus PCR that works on all known snake nidoviruses is available at the University of Florida.

Adenoviruses

Adenoviruses have been associated with hepatitis, stomatitis and enteritis in lizards, snakes, turtles/tortoises and crocodilians. The known adenoviruses of squamates are in the genus *Atadenovirus*, and most known adenoviruses of turtles/tortoises are in the proposed genus *Testadenovirus*, but a virus in the genus *Siadenovirus* caused a major mortality event in tortoises (Rivera *et al.*, 2009). Performing a biopsy of affected tissue is recommended. Many adenoviruses are shed enterically, so cloacal swabs are a good less invasive sample. Consensus PCR that works on all known adenoviruses is available. TaqMan® assays have been developed at the University of Florida for more rapid and less expensive quantitative detection of agamid adenovirus 1 (from bearded dragons), Sulawesi tortoise adenovirus 1 and Box turtle adenovirus 1. Virus neutralization testing is available at Laboklin GmbH in Germany.

Poxviruses

Poxviruses have been associated with skin lesions in lizards, tortoises and crocodilians. Performing a biopsy of affected tissue is recommended. Consensus PCR that works on all known poxviruses of vertebrates is available. Poxviruses are tolerant of freezing, so it is recommended that biopsy samples be shipped frozen for culture.

Iridoviruses

The family Iridoviridae currently consists of five genera, although a clade of intraerythrocytic iridoviruses characterized from squamates is likely to represent a sixth genus (Wellehan *et al.*, 2008). Species of the genus *Iridovirus* infect insects, although they have also been found to infect squamates. The genus *Ranavirus* infects fish, amphibians and reptiles, causing significant epizootics, with destruction of multiple tissues, including spleen and bone marrow. Consensus PCR that works on all known erythrocytic iridoviruses is available. TaqMan® assays for ranaviruses are available at multiple institutions, including the University of Florida.

Bacteria

Many infectious microorganisms of reptiles grow best at lower temperatures than do those of mammals. Hence, samples may need to be cultured at different temperatures. Additionally, many if not all bacterial identification kits for laboratories are developed around organisms likely to be found in mammals or birds. If an identification appears unusual, it is appropriate to question the result with a microbiologist. The country's national diagnostic laboratory is a good source of information.

Both aerobic and anaerobic bacteria are common causes of disease in reptiles. They are also a normal part of the fauna of the GI and upper respiratory tracts, as well as the skin. Consequently, a sample culture alone is insufficient to make a causal association, and results need to be correlated with histopathology or cytology. Samples commonly submitted for bacterial culture include swabs from body orifices or lesions (Figure 8.29), cavity washes, tissue aspirates, blood cultures and biopsy samples. Many bacteria have not been successfully cultured, and for organisms such as *Chlamydia* spp., *Mycoplasma* spp. and *Mycobacterium* spp., special culture requirements or consensus PCR and sequencing-based diagnostics should be considered.

Sample handling and transport media

Whenever possible, culture specimens are collected prior to initiating antimicrobial therapy. All specimens should be transported in clean, tightly sealed leak-proof containers. Aspirates of lesions are preferable to swabs owing to a

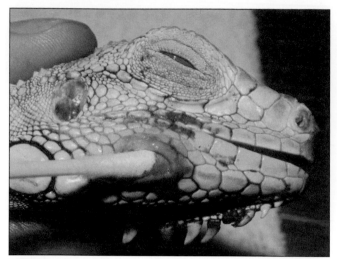

8.29 Collecting a swab sample for bacterial culture and sensitivity testing from the capsule of a granuloma, after debridement, in a green iguana.
(Courtesy of Paul Raiti)

lesser degree of contamination. If swabs are to be used, mini-tip culturettes may enable the practitioner to swab the area of interest more precisely.

Selection of appropriate transport media is essential for useful culture results. Less fastidious organisms, such as pseudomonad and coliform bacteria, are relatively hardy and can be expected to survive overnight transport at room temperature on a standard collection swab such as Stuart's or Amies transport medium. For non-coliform bacteria, Amies is preferable. Anaerobic samples should be placed immediately into anaerobic transport media such as thioglycollate agar. More fastidious organisms may require specific transport media.

Samples for *Mycoplasma* should immediately be placed into a mycoplasma culture broth such as SP4 or Frey's. As mycoplasmas lack cell walls, they are highly susceptible to desiccation. If the sample is taken with a swab, chances for successful culture are greatly improved by pre-moistening swabs in sterile mycoplasma broth. Many mycoplasmas are slow growing, and it may take up to several weeks to obtain culture results. Concurrent serology and/or PCR are recommended if mycoplasmal disease is suspected. Samples for serology should be shipped refrigerated or frozen in tightly sealed leak-proof containers.

Mycobacterial or actinomycete cultures are often most successful from biopsy samples. Tissue samples may be sent directly to the laboratory in a sterile sealed container. Mycobacteria are very slow growing and culture results may take up to several months. Concurrent histology with acid-fast and/or GMS staining is recommended if mycobacterial or nocardial disease is suspected, respectively.

Chlamydia spp. cultures require specialized transport media. If the sample is taken with a pre-moistened swab, chances for successful culture are greatly improved. Concurrent PCR is recommended if disease associated with *Chlamydia* spp. is suspected.

Blood culture

A blood culture is indicated when an animal is suspected of being septicaemic. Bacteraemia is more common in healthy reptiles than in mammals or birds, but blood culture can be useful for identification of pathogenic microorganisms. The skin at the venepuncture site should be aseptically prepared. The needle should be changed and the bottle wiped with alcohol before transferring the sample into the blood culture bottle. Paediatric blood culture bottles are available and require smaller sample volumes (e.g. 0.1–0.3 ml). While it is ideal to sample the volume recommended by the manufacturer of blood culture bottles, collecting the recommended volume may be contraindicated by the size of smaller patients. In such cases, culture of a smaller sample size is often successful. Anaerobic bacteria are frequently cultured from the blood of apparently healthy lizards, making interpretation in ill animals difficult. Bacteria may require incubation at ambient temperature and for a longer time period compared with mammalian cultures. Discussion of such special growth requirements with the microbiology laboratory can be helpful and may increase the chance of growing reptile-specific organisms.

Fungal culture

Fungi are classified in a nomenclature inconsistent with the rest of biology. There are separate genus and species names for asexual anamorph stages and sexual teleomorph stages of the same organism, resulting in multiple species names and paraphyletic taxa. The anamorph species *Blastomyces dermatitidis* and *Histoplasma capsulatum* are in different genera, but the corresponding teleomorphs, *Ajellomyces dermatitidis* and *Ajellomyces capsulatus*, are congeneric. Since the publication of the *BSAVA Manual of Reptiles, 2nd edition* in 2004, fungal diseases initially mislabelled as the *Chrysosporium* anamorph of *Nannizziopsis vriesii* have been shown to be diverse organisms, including *Nannizziopsis guarroi* and *Ophidiomyces ophiodiicola*. Fungal cultures can be very successful from biopsy samples. Samples may be sent directly to the laboratory in a sterile sealed container. In cases with suspicion of fungal pneumonia where performing biopsy via bronchoscopy is not an option, fungal culture of a pulmonary wash may be of use. When fungal skin infection is suspected, the skin is cleaned with alcohol and allowed to dry; a biopsy sample is then taken and embedded in culture medium. Reptiles are often infected with unusual fungal species not commonly encountered in many diagnostic laboratories, so it is important to work with a laboratory with expertise in this area. Concurrent histology with special staining and/or PCR is recommended if fungal disease is suspected.

Parasitic protozoa

Cryptosporidium, a genus of coccidian parasites that infects many orders of vertebrates, is a significant concern in reptiles. Since reliable morphological species identification is not possible, *Cryptosporidium* species have been characterized using DNA-sequence-based techniques. Phylogenetic analyses have revealed two major clades of *Cryptosporidium*: one with tropism for the intestine, and the other with tropism for the stomach (Griffin *et al.*, 2010). In most cases, *Cryptosporidium* spp. cause gastrointestinal disease, but extra-enteric infections including aural polyp-associated infections have been reported in green iguanas. Gastric species are best diagnosed using gastric washes or biopsies and intestinal species are best diagnosed using intestinal biopsies or faeces. Differentiating species infecting reptiles from 'pass-throughs' from prey animals is critical. Consensus PCR and sequencing are available at the University of Florida.

Systemic intranuclear coccidiosis is a major problem in tortoises, with a high fatality rate, and lesions are found in diverse organs. Both consensus PCR and sequencing as well as a TaqMan® assay are available at the University of Florida (Alvarez *et al.*, 2013).

References and further reading

Alleman AR, Jacobson ER and Raskin RE (1999) Morphologic, cytochemical staining and ultrastructural characteristics of blood from Eastern diamondback rattlesnakes (*Crotalus adamanteus*). *American Journal of Veterinary Research* **60**, 507–514

Allender MC, Mitchell MA, Dreslik MJ *et al.* (2008) Measuring agreement and discord among hemagglutination inhibition assays against different ophidian paramyxovirus strains in the Eastern massasauga (*Sistrurus catenatus catenatus*). *Journal of Zoo and Wildlife Medicine* **39(3)**, 358–361

Alvarez WA, Gibbons PM, Rivera S *et al.* (2013) Development of a quantitative PCR for rapid and sensitive diagnosis of an intranuclear coccidian parasite in Testudines (TINC), and detection in the critically endangered Arakan Forest Turtle (*Heosemys depressa*). *Veterinary Parasitology* **193**, 66–70

Anderson ET, Socha VL, Gardner J *et al.* (2013) Tissue enzyme activities in the Loggerhead sea turtle (*Caretta caretta*). *Journal of Zoo and Wildlife Medicine* **44(1)**, 6–69

Borkowski R (1997) Lead poisoning and intestinal perforations in a Snapping turtle (*Chelydra serpentina*) due to fishing gear ingestion. *Journal of Zoo Animal Medicine* **28**, 109–113

Campbell TN and Coles EH (1986) Avian clinical pathology. In: *Veterinary Clinical Pathology, 4th edition*, ed. EH Coles, pp. 279–301. WB Saunders, Philadelphia

Carpenter JW, Mashima TY and Rupiper DJ (2001) *Exotic Animal Formulary, 2nd edition*. WB Saunders, Philadelphia

Chitty JR (2003) Lead toxicosis in a Greek tortoise (*Testudo graeca*). *Proceedings of the Association of Reptilian and Amphibian Veterinarians* p. 101

Crocker C and Miller D (2002) Persistent elevated blood glucose in the iguana (*Iguana iguana*): a case study. *Proceedings of the Association of Reptilian and Amphibian Veterinarians* pp. 7–9

Drew M (1994) Hypercalcemia and hyperphosphatemia in Indigo snakes (*Drymarchon corais*) and serum biochemical reference values. *Journal of Zoo and Wildlife Medicine* **25**, 48–52

Frye FL (1999) Spontaneous autoimmune pancreatitis and diabetes mellitus in a Western pond turtle, *Clemmys m. marmorata*. *Proceedings of the Association of Reptilian and Amphibian Veterinarians* pp. 103–105

Fudge AM (2000) *Laboratory Medicine: Avian and Exotic Pets*. WB Saunders, Philadelphia

Girling SJ and Raiti P (2004) *BSAVA Manual of Reptiles, 2nd edn*. BSAVA Publications, Gloucester

Glor R, Means M, Weintraub MJH *et al.* (1999) Two cases of firefly toxicosis in Bearded dragons, *Pogona vitticeps*. *Proceedings of the Association of Reptilian and Amphibian Veterinarians* pp. 27–29

Griffin C, Reavill DR, Stacy BA, Childress AL and Wellehan JFX (2010) Cryptosporidiosis caused by two distinct species in Russian tortoises and a Pancake tortoise. *Veterinary Parasitology* **170(1–2)**, 14–19

Harr KE, Alleman AR, Dennis PM *et al.* (2001) Morphologic and cytochemical characteristics of blood cells and hematologic and plasma reference ranges in Green iguanas. *Journal of the American Veterinary Medical Association* **218**, 915–921

Heatley JJ, Johnson A, Tully T and Mitchell M (2001) Persistent hyperglycemia in a Chinese water dragon, *Physignathus cocincinus*. *Proceedings of the Association of Reptilian and Amphibian Veterinarians* pp. 207–211

Hernandez-Divers SJ, Knott CD and Macdonald J (2001) Diagnosis and surgical treatment of thyroid adenoma-induced hyperthyroidism in a Green iguana (*Iguana iguana*). *Journal of Zoo and Wildlife Medicine* **32**, 465–475

Hyndman TH, Marschang RE, Wellehan JFX and Nicholls PK (2012). Isolation and molecular characterization of Sunshine Virus, a novel paramyxovirus found in Australian snakes. *Infection, Genetics, and Evolution* **12(7)**, 1436–1446

Johnson JH and Benson PA (1996) Laboratory reference values for a group of captive Ball pythons (*Python regius*). *American Journal of Veterinary Research* **57**, 1304–1307

Lawrence K (1986) Seasonal variations in haematological data from Mediterranean tortoises (*Testudo graeca* and *T. hermanni*) in captivity. *Research in Veterinary Science* **40**, 225–230

Lawrence K (1987) Seasonal variation in blood biochemistry of long term captive Mediterranean tortoises (*Testudo graeca* and *T. hermanni*). *Research in Veterinary Science* **43**, 379–383

Mader DR and Divers SJ (2014) *Current Therapy in Reptile Medicine and Surgery*. Elsevier Saunders, St. Louis, MI

Martinez-Silvestre A, Perpinan D, Marco I and Lavin S (2002) Venipuncture technique of the occipital venous sinus in freshwater aquatic turtles. *Journal of Herpetological Medicine and Surgery* **12**, 31–32

Morgan RV (1994) Lead poisoning in small companion animals: an update (1987–1992). *Veterinary and Human Toxicology* **36**, 18–22

Quesada RJ, Aitken-Palmer C, Conley K and Heard DJ (2010) Accidental submeningeal injection of propofol in Gopher tortoises (*Gopherus polyphemus*). *Veterinary Record* **167(13)**, 494–495

Ramsay EC and Dotson TK (1995) Tissue and serum enzyme activities in the yellow rat snake (*Elaphe obsoleta quadrivitatta*). *American Journal of Veterinary Research* **56**, 423–428

Redrobe S and MacDonald J (1999) Sample collection and clinical pathology of reptiles. *Veterinary Clinics of North America Exotic Animal Practice* **2**, 709–730

Ritter JM, Garner MM, Chilton JA *et al.* (2009) Gastric neuroendocrine carcinomas in Bearded dragons (*Pogona vitticeps*). *Veterinary Pathology* **46(6)**, 1109–1116

Rivera S, Wellehan JFX, McManamon R *et al.* (2009) An epizootic in Sulawesi tortoises (*Indotestudo forstenii*) caused by a novel Siadenovirus. *Journal of Veterinary Diagnostic Investigation* **21(4)**, 415–426

Rossi J (1995) Azalea, *Rhododendron* sp., toxicity in a Green iguana, *Iguana iguana*. *Bulletin of the Association of Reptilian and Amphibian Veterinarians* **5**, 4–5

Stenglein MD, Jacobson ER, Wozniak EJ *et al.* (2014) Ball python nidovirus: a candidate etiologic agent for severe respiratory disease in Python regius. *mBio* **5(5)**, e01484-14

Stenglein MD, Sanders C, Kistler AL *et al.* (2012) Identification, characterization, and *in vitro* culture of highly divergent arenaviruses from Boa constrictors and annulated Tree boas: candidate etiological agents for snake inclusion body disease. *mBio* **3(4)**, e00180-12

Strik NI, Alleman AR and Harr KE (2007) Circulating inflammatory cells. In: *Infectious Diseases and Pathology of Reptiles*, ed. ER Jacobson, pp. 167–218. CRC Press, Boca Raton, FL

Telford SR (2008) *Hemoparasites of the Reptilia*. CRC Press, Boca Raton, FL

Villiers E and Ristić J (2016) *BSAVA Manual of Canine and Feline Clinical Pathology, 3rd edn*. BSAVA Publications, Gloucester

Wagner RA and Wetzel R (1999) Tissue and plasma enzyme activities in juvenile Green iguanas. *American Journal of Veterinary Research* **60**, 201–203

Wellehan JFX, Pessier AP, Archer LL *et al.* (2012) Initial sequence characterization of the rhabdoviruses of squamate reptiles including a novel rhabdovirus from a Caiman lizard (*Dracaena guianensis*). *Veterinary Microbiology* **158**, 274–279

Wellehan JFX, Strik NI, Stacy BA *et al.* (2008) Characterization of an erythrocytic virus in the family Iridoviridae from a Peninsula ribbon snake (*Thamnophis sauritus sackenii*). *Veterinary Microbiology* **131(1–2)**, 115–122

Weiss DJ (1984) Uniform evaluation and semiquantitative reporting of hematologic data in veterinary laboratories. *Veterinary Clinical Pathology* **13**, 27–31

Chapter 9

Non-invasive imaging

Paul Raiti

A thorough physical examination of reptiles can be challenging owing to the exoskeleton of chelonians, thick dermis of many lizards and strong muscle tone of snakes. Consequently, diagnostic imaging is an important aspect of the health evaluation of reptiles. This chapter describes the four types of non-invasive imaging techniques that are used for reptiles:

- Radiography
- Ultrasonography
- Computed tomography (CT)
- Magnetic resonance imaging (MRI).

Radiography

Radiography is the primary non-invasive imaging technique used in reptile medicine. Veterinary surgeons (veterinarians) should keep a set of radiographs of normal reptiles as an aid in interpretation.

General guidelines

Equipment

Although analogue X-ray machines have the capacity to produce high quality radiographs of reptiles, they are gradually being replaced by digital units that possess several advantages such as enhanced image detail and lower radiation exposure. Digital software permits brightness, contrast and colour to be adjusted. The reverse-contrast option is an added benefit for radiographic interpretation (Figure 9.1). Neither film nor chemicals are needed. There is immediate image availability and internet transfer if required. Additionally, images and duplicate copies can be archived easily. Digital dental X-ray units are beneficial for imaging diminutive reptiles, depending upon patient and sensor sizes (Figure 9.2). High-speed blue-sensitive film is recommended for analogue units.

Views

- Dorsoventral (DV) views are taken as for other species.
- Horizontal views (lateral and cranial–caudal) are recommended because organs are maintained in their normal positions; hence, image artefacts are minimized. The cassette is positioned perpendicularly to the X-ray beam and in physical contact with the

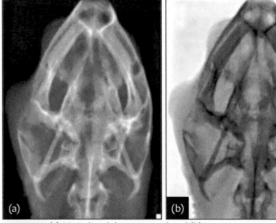

9.1 (a) Digitalized dorsoventral and (b) reverse-contrast radiographs of a red-eared terrapin with an aural abscess. Soft-tissue swelling and lysis of the left squamosal bone is visible.

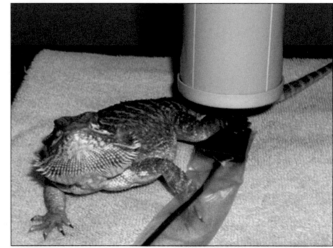

9.2 A dental X-ray unit being used to radiograph the foot of a bearded dragon. Note the sensor enclosed in a protective transparent sleeve that is positioned under the foot.

reptile. Horizontal views are not necessary for snakes owing to internal fibrous adhesions holding organs in position. Older X-ray units may not have this capacity; accordingly, vertical views are used.
- Larger snakes and lizards need opaque identification markers placed on sections of their bodies to ensure continuity of successive radiographs.

BSAVA Manual of Reptiles, third edition. Edited by Simon J. Girling and Paul Raiti. ©BSAVA 2019

Immobilization

The physical immobilization techniques for chelonians, lizards and snakes are summarized in Figure 9.3.

Chelonians can usually be positioned for DV views with minimal physical restraint; however, retraction of the head and limbs may compromise interpretation depending upon which organ system is being investigated. Propofol and alfaxalone are two examples of short-acting anaesthetics that are appropriate for immobilization. For horizontal lateral and cranial–caudal (CC) views, chelonians can be physically immobilized by being placed on raised platforms that are smaller than their plastrons, so that the extremities do not touch the X-ray table (Figure 9.4).

Active lizards such as green iguanas are restrained by placing a ball of cotton wool over each eye and securing them to the globes by wrapping cohesive tape around the head. This technique commonly inactivates many lizards by stimulation of the vago-vagal response whereby the application of pressure to the eyes causes a decrease in heart rate and blood pressure. For the horizontal lateral view, the lizard's forelimbs should be extended cranial to the body and taped to each other. Likewise, the hindlimbs are extended caudally and taped to the tail. This provides immobilization and prevents image artefacts. Do not tape the tails or extremities of active diminutive lizards to the cassette for DV views. Some species of day gecko can exfoliate their skin, while others such as leopard geckos and juvenile green iguanas are capable of caudal autotomy. These reptiles should be restrained in radiolucent containers.

Snakes are restrained in plastic radiolucent tubes of appropriate diameter and length; however, image artefacts due to body contractions can occur. Intractable reptiles such as monitor lizards and large pythons may require complete anaesthesia.

Reptile group	Techniques
Chelonians	Place on a raised platform with limbs hanging over edges for lateral horizontal and cranial–caudal views
Lizards	Apply cotton pledgets over orbits and wrap with cohesive bandage. Forelimbs can be secured to each other and hindlimbs secured to the tail. Use aquaria or plastic containers for active diminutive specimens
Snakes	Use plastic restraint tubes or snake bags

9.3 Summary of physical immobilization techniques for radiography.

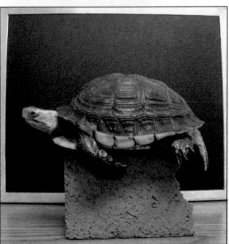

9.4 For a horizontal lateral radiograph, this Chinese box turtle is immobilized on a raised platform. The X-ray plate is behind the turtle.

Normal radiographic anatomy
Chelonians

The DV view is used to examine the skeletal, digestive and urogenital systems (Figure 9.5). The skull, appendicular bones, and pectoral and pelvic girdles should be distinctly visible with prominent cortices. Large aquatic turtles, such as the common snapping turtle and mata mata that create suction to ingest prey, possess well developed hyoid bones (Figure 9.6). The lungs, which are located in the dorsal coelomic cavity just beneath the plastron, are best

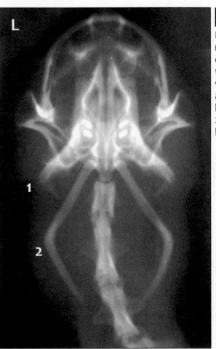

9.5 Dorsoventral radiograph of a normal gravid eastern box turtle. 1 = humerus; 2 = acromion; 3 = coracoids; 4 = vertebral column; 5 = pubis; 6 = obturator foramen; 7 = ischium; 8 = femur; 9 = egg; 10 = plastral hinge.

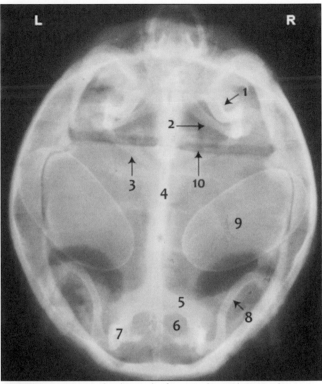

9.6 Dorsoventral radiograph of the skull of a normal mata mata turtle illustrating the well developed hyoid apparatus. 1 = first branchial horn; 2 = second branchial horn.

evaluated on the lateral and CC views. They are not normally visible on the DV view owing to superimposition by bone and coelomic viscera. Small amounts of ingesta and gas are normal findings in the gastrointestinal (GI) tract.

On the lateral view the visceral organs are visible below the lungs (Figure 9.7). The heart is normally not visible unless there is severe cardiomegaly or metastatic mineralization of the systemic arteries. The hepatic silhouette is visible just beneath the lungs and the GI tract lies caudal to the liver. The kidneys are located in the dorso-caudal aspect of the coelomic cavity and are normally not visible unless there is significant renomegaly or metastatic mineralization. The ovaries, oviducts and urinary bladder are normally not visible.

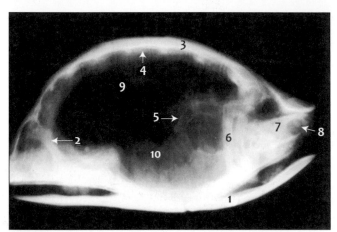

9.7 Left lateral radiograph of a normal Malayan box turtle. 1 = plastron; 2 = ilium; 3 = carapace; 4 = vertebral column; 5 = cervical vertebrae; 6 = scapula; 7 = skull; 8 = orbit; 9 = lungs; 10 = viscera.

Lizards

The DV view allows examination of the skeletal, respiratory, digestive and urogenital systems (Figure 9.8). The skull, extremities, pectoral/pelvic girdles and lateral coccygeal processes should be distinctly visible. Superimposition of the hyoid bones occurs on the DV view; hence, these structures should also be evaluated on a lateral view. The hyoid apparatus is well developed in lizards with dewlaps. In herbivorous lizards the large caecum commonly obscures other organs due to distension with ingesta. Superimposition by the expanded lungs can provide negative contrast to help outline the liver and intestines. Adipose tissue is located along the lateral and ventral aspects of the caudal coelomic cavity. In obese animals it may obscure other organs. The lungs are not always clearly visible owing to the cycle of breathing and superimposition by coelomic viscera.

The lateral view allows examination of the skeletal, respiratory, cardiovascular, digestive and urogenital systems (Figure 9.9). Some female geckos store calcium in specialized structures called endolymphatic sacs, which lie in the cervical area and are easily seen on radiographs (Figure 9.10). The cardiac shadow is visible either in the cranial coelomic cavity, partially superimposed by the scapulae (iguanids and agamids), or in the mid-coelomic cavity just cranial to the liver (varanids). Two aortas exit cranially from the single ventricle and fuse into one descending aorta. In lizards the triangular hepatic shadow is distinct, with the base located on the floor of the coelomic cavity. In green iguanas and bearded dragons the kidneys are not visible because they are located within the pelvic canal. In monitor lizards the kidneys are located cranial to the pelvis.

The reproductive tract is normally not visible unless there is ovarian activity or gravidity/pregnancy. The urinary bladder (when present) is usually not visible owing to superimposition by the fat bodies. Sexually mature male mangrove, green tree and Gould's monitors and *Heloderma* spp., can be sexed radiographically due to calcification of the hemibacula of the hemipenes.

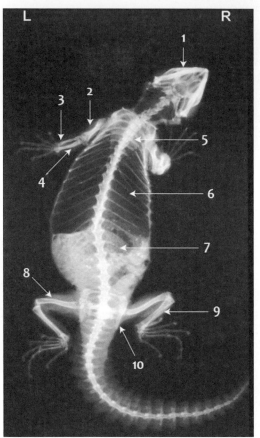

9.8 Dorsoventral radiograph of a normal spiny-tailed lizard. 1 = mandible; 2 = humerus; 3 = radius; 4 = ulna; 5 = heart; 6 = lung; 7 = intestines; 8 = femur; 9 = tibia; 10 = ischium.

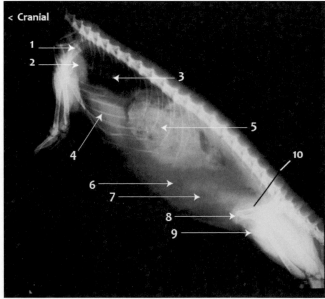

9.9 Right lateral radiograph of a normal green iguana. 1 = trachea; 2 = heart; 3 = lungs; 4 = liver; 5 = stomach with ingesta; 6 = small intestine; 7 = fat deposits; 8 = pubis; 9 = ischium; 10 = ilium.

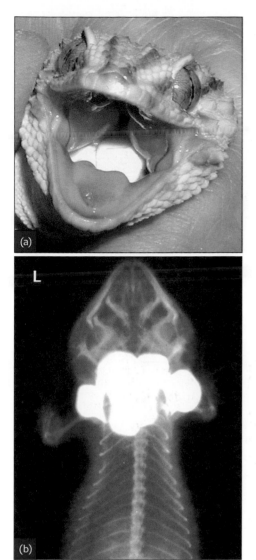

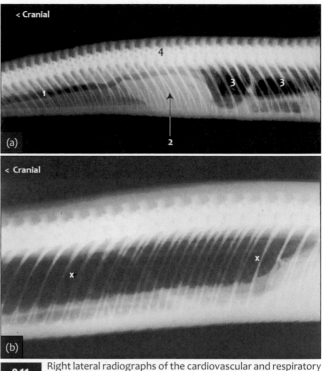

9.11 Right lateral radiographs of the cardiovascular and respiratory systems of a normal common boa: (a) 1 = trachea; 2 = heart; 3 = lung; 4 = spine and ribs; (b) X = air sac.

9.10 (a) The calcified endolymphatic sacs are easily visualized in this defensive female Moorish gecko on physical examination. (b) Note the radiopaque deposits of calcium on a dorsoventral radiograph of the same gecko.

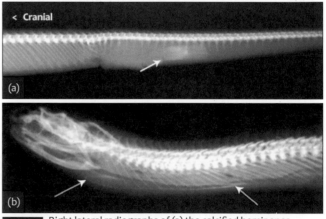

9.12 Right lateral radiographs of (a) the calcified hemipenes (arrowed) and (b) hyoid apparatus (arrowed) of a normal adult indigo snake. Note the trachea (radiolucent stripe) coursing just dorsal to the hyoid bones.

Snakes

On the DV view the skull and ribs are distinctly radiopaque. On the lateral view the trachea is seen as a radiolucent stripe extending from the skull to the cardiac shadow. The lungs and air sac(s) are visible from the cardiac shadow to the caudal third of the snake (Figure 9.11). The intestines are visible due to the presence of gas and ingesta. The coelomic cavity ends with the last pair of ribs. The lateral view permits examination of the skeletal, cardiovascular, respiratory, digestive and urogenital systems. The reproductive tract is normally not visible unless there is ovarian activity or gravidity/pregnancy. The kidneys, which are located in the caudal third of the body, are normally not visible unless there is either significant renomegaly or metastatic mineralization. Boas and pythons possess calcified pelvic remnants that are visible near the last pair of ribs. Sometimes the hemibacula of the hemipenes in mature male snakes calcify and are visible in the base of the tail (Figure 9.12a). In some snakes the hyoid apparatus is visible (Figure 9.12b).

Common radiographic findings in reptiles
Abscesses and granulomas

These discrete soft-tissue swellings are usually bacterial or fungal in origin and are commonly subcutaneous in location. Granulomas appear radiographically as soft-tissue densities that are indistinguishable from other masses such as neoplasms and cysts (Figure 9.13). Trauma and subsequent introduction of microorganisms through breaks in the integrity of the dermis are common in reptiles. Over time the immune system 'walls off' the infective area; hence, the term granuloma or fibriscess. Sepsis also plays a significant role in the formation of granulomas throughout the body. Granulomas have been identified in all organ systems, and when located intracoelomically are best evaluated by ultrasonography.

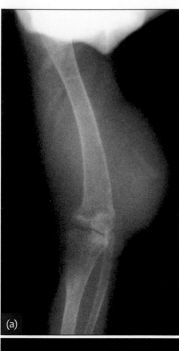

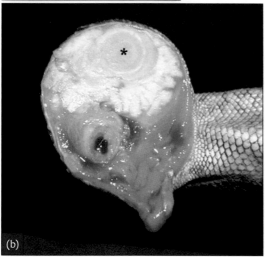

9.13 (a) Dorsoventral radiograph of soft-tissue swelling of the right femur of a green iguana. (b) Transverse view of the encapsulated granuloma (*) from the same iguana after euthanasia.

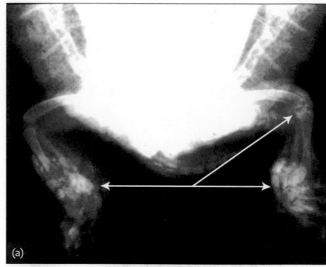

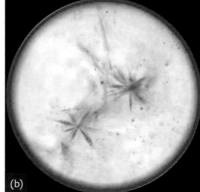

9.14 (a) Dorsoventral radiograph of a red-eared terrapin with polyarticular gout. Note the mixed pattern of lysis and mineralized proliferative changes of the stifle and both hock joints. (b) Needle-like urate crystals aspirated from the affected stifle joint.

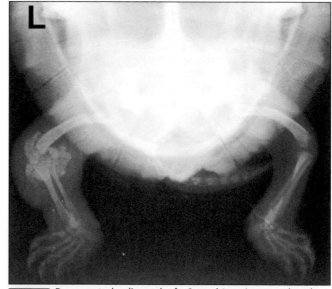

9.15 Dorsoventral radiograph of a Central American wood turtle with articular and periarticular mineralized opacities of the left stifle joint. A diagnosis of calcinosis circumscripta was based upon biopsy of the affected joint.

Articular gout: In reptiles, gout develops secondary to renal disease and hyperuricaemia. When uric acid crystals deposit in joints the condition is referred to as articular gout. Visceral gout occurs when uric acid crystals are deposited in soft tissues. Articular gout occurs most commonly in chelonians and lizards. Radiographically, articular gout is characterized by a mixed pattern of osteolysis and proliferative densities in and around the affected joints (Figure 9.14a). Diagnosis is by arthrocentesis to identify the needle-shaped urate crystals (Figure 9.14b).

Calcinosis circumscripta: Calcinosis circumscripta or dystrophic calcification is the deposition of calcium salts in damaged or non-vital tissues. Trauma is probably the most common cause in reptiles. In contrast to metastatic mineralization (see below), it is not associated with an active systemic disease process. Calcium salts are deposited in small nodules in the skin, subcutaneous tissues and joint capsules. Previously, the term pseudogout has been used when the calcium salts are deposited periarticularly. The affected joint(s) can appear radiographically similar to articular gout (Figure 9.15); however, calcium hydroxyapatite crystals are typically present. Aspiration or biopsy of the affected joint is necessary to differentiate articular

gout and calcinosis circumscripta. Sometimes, both urate and calcium crystals can be identified in aspirates of chronically affected joints.

Cellulitis: Cellulitis is the inflammation of subcutaneous tissue usually associated with bacterial infections or trauma. The radiological sign is diffuse soft-tissue swelling (Figure 9.16). Onset can be acute with no discernible history.

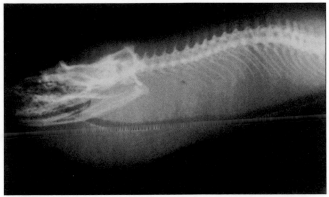

9.16 Right lateral radiograph of a Burmese python with severe soft-tissue swelling of the cervical area that was associated with a bacterial infection. Note the trachea (radiolucent stripe) and calcified tracheal rings.

Congenital defects

Congenital skeletal defects such as dicephalus, vertebral agenesis, scoliosis, kyphosis and lordosis have been reported in reptiles. Scoliosis is the abnormal lateral curvature of the spine on the DV view. Kyphosis is the abnormal dorsal curvature of the spine on the lateral view (Figure 9.17). Many of these abnormalities are thought to be due to improper incubation temperatures during embryogenesis.

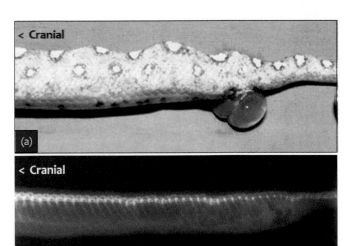

9.17 (a) Deformities of the caudal spine of a juvenile chondropython with a prolapsed cloaca. (b) Right lateral radiograph of the same snake. Note multiple DV curvatures of the axial skeleton consistent with kyphosis.

Constipation

Constipation and occasionally obstipation are seen in reptiles that are dehydrated and maintained at suboptimal temperatures. Hyperalimentation coupled with inactivity are additional inciting factors. Constipation occurs more commonly in reptiles that have relatively slow metabolisms, such as boid snakes and tortoises. It is also encountered in juvenile lizards and chelonians which are hypocalcaemic. Radiographs reveal large dense faecal masses in the dilated colon (Figure 9.18).

Degenerative joint disease

Osteoarthritis is a degenerative joint disease defined as inflammation of the joint(s) and surrounding tissues. Acute trauma and chronic mechanical stress are the most

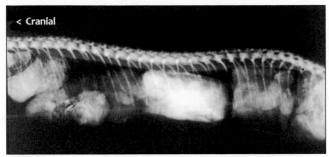

9.18 Right lateral radiograph of a Burmese python with faecal retention. Note the presence of multiple irregularly shaped radiopaque densities containing foreign material within the large intestine. The snake had been maintained at suboptimal temperatures.

common causes. Osteoarthritis is relatively common in geriatric reptiles, particularly lizards such as green iguanas and the larger monitors. Arthritis of bacterial origin (osteomyelitis) is discussed below. In lizards, such as the green iguana, the elbow joints and lumbar and coccygeal vertebrae are the most commonly affected sites. Arthritis of the appendicular joints is characterized radiographically by distended joint capsules, osteophyte formation and subchondral changes (Figure 9.19a). Affected joints of the long bones can appear radiographically similar to articular gout and calcinosis circumscripta. In lizards and snakes, vertebral osteoarthritis often progresses to ankylosing spondylopathy characterized by the formation of bony bridges fusing multiple vertebrae to each other (Figure 9.19b). This condition can be difficult to differentiate radiographically from vertebral osteomyelitis (see below). Ankylosing spondylopathy has been attributed to various aetiologies such as vitamin deficiencies, lack of exercise, immune-mediated disease, viruses and bacteria.

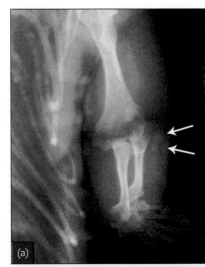

9.19 (a) Dorsoventral radiograph of the right elbow joint of a geriatric green iguana. Note extensive periarticular osteophyte formation and joint swelling (arrowed). (b) Right lateral radiograph of a geriatric green iguana with ankylosing spondylopathy. There is new bone formation on the ventral margins of multiple coccygeal vertebrae. Note fractures of the dorsal vertebral process and body of a coccygeal vertebra below the radiopaque marker.

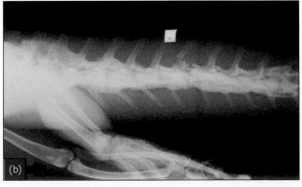

Ovarian follicular development

Active ovaries are only radiographically visible in squamates. Due to the presence of the chelonian's extensive exoskeleton, ultrasonography is required for visualization of the ovaries. In lizards, preovulatory follicles are radiographically visible as circular soft-tissue densities that can fill the coelomic cavity (Figure 9.20a). In snakes, follicles are visible as linear circular soft-tissue densities located approximately midway down the body length (Figure 9.20b–c).

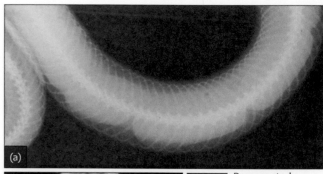

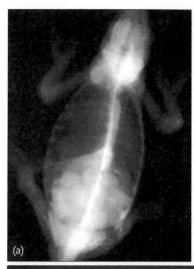

9.20 (a) Preovulatory follicular development in a juvenile veiled chameleon. Soft-tissue spherical densities are present in the caudal coelom. Note the generalized rarefied skeletal anatomy consistent with nutritional secondary hyperparathyroidism. (b) An emerald tree boa with distension of its mid-body due to enlarging ovaries. (c) Right lateral radiograph of the same snake with soft-tissue spherical densities consistent with follicular development.

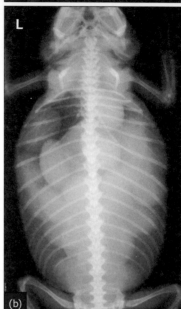

9.21 Dorsoventral radiographs of normal gravid reptiles: (a) indigo snake; (b) bearded dragon; (c) calcified fetal skeletons during late-stage pregnancy in a crocodile lizard.

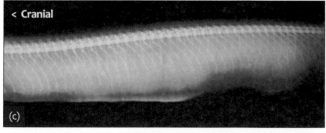

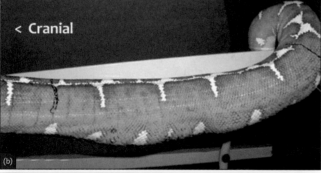

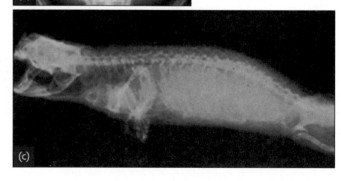

Gravidity/pregnancy

Chelonian eggs are the most calcified of reptile eggs and are easily visualized on DV radiographs (see Figure 9.5). To date, there has been no evidence that exposure to X-rays is harmful to viable eggs. Squamate eggs are less calcified but are still visible with radiography (Figure 9.21a–b). Eggs should be counted, with locations and relative sizes noted and shells should be checked for deformations. Egg diameters should be compared with pelvic canal diameter. Abnormally large eggs may have to be decompressed prior to administration of prokinetics (see Chapter 20). Fetal skeletons of squamates are radiographically visible towards the end of gestation (Figure 9.21c).

Dystocia

A diagnosis of dystocia is based upon clinical signs and radiography. Clinical signs can include but are not limited to lethargy, weakness and sometimes tenesmus that may be preceded by the passage of eggs several days or weeks earlier. Anorexia is common during gestation and is not a reliable indicator of dystocia unless it is acute in onset. Radiographically, chelonians' eggs that are pathologically retained are characterized by excessive mineralization of the shells (Figure 9.22a). This feature is less apparent in lizards and snakes, which normally have poorly calcified shells. The radiographic appearance of eggs that are abnormally large, misshapen or fractured should alert the clinician to dystocia (Figure 9.22b). Other causes, particularly with chelonians, include fractured pelvises and/or spinal trauma with hindlimb paralysis. Occasionally, ectopic eggs are located free within the coelomic cavity or urinary bladder, because of either trauma or inappropriate use of prokinetics.

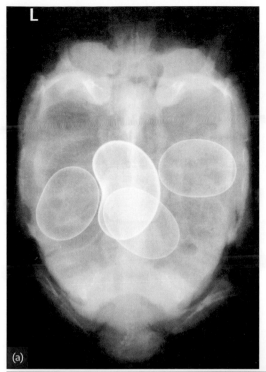

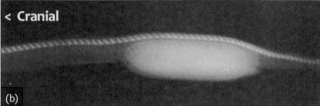

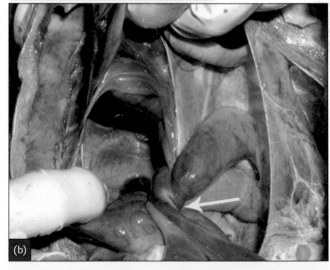

Ileus

In reptiles, ileus (paralysis of the intestine) is usually mechanical in origin. Examples of causes of mechanical ileus are foreign bodies, intramural masses, intussusceptions, mesenteric volvuli, torsions, strictures and large urinary calculi (Figure 9.24). Strictures are usually due to ingested sharp material which has traumatized the gastrointestinal wall. The radiographic signs consist of accumulations of gas and fluid orad to the obstruction site; however, the absence of these signs does not rule out an obstruction. Functional ileus is the occurrence of intestinal stasis in the absence of an actual obstruction. Causes of functional ileus include electrolyte and mineral (hypocalcaemia) imbalances, severe gastroenteritis, drugs and general anaesthesia.

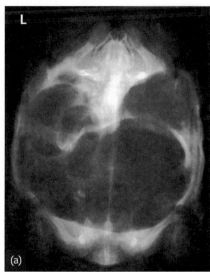

9.24 (a) Dorsoventral radiograph of a leopard tortoise that presented with anorexia of 3-weeks' duration. The small and large intestines are dilated with excessive amounts of gas consistent with ileus. (b) Necropsy revealed a mesenteric volvulus (arrowed).

9.22 (a) Dorsoventral radiograph of a gravid red-footed tortoise. In addition to normal eggs, there is a large comma-shaped egg that has been retained as evidenced by excessive mineralization of its shell. (b) Right lateral radiograph of a gravid kingsnake with an excessively large retained egg.

Oesophagitis/gastroenteritis

Inflammation of the intestinal tract is characterized by anorexia, emesis, diarrhoea and increased frequency of defecation. Chronically affected reptiles commonly lose weight. Plain X-ray films often reveal pockets of intestinal fluid and gas; however, radiographs can also be normal in appearance. Positive-contrast studies best enable the clinician to evaluate the intestines (see below). In affected reptiles, the contrast agent moves quickly through the GI tract due to hypermotility of the intestines. Irregularities of the mucosal pattern and filling defects can be visualized (Figure 9.23). In reptiles, enteritis is commonly associated with parasitism (amoebiasis, trichomoniasis, cryptosporidiosis) or neoplasia.

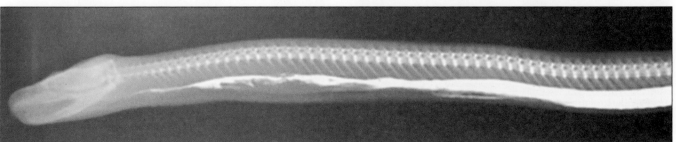

9.23 Right lateral radiograph of a diamond python with oesophagitis. The snake had been force-fed by the owner several times and began regurgitating shortly thereafter. A barium swallow revealed filling defects of the proximal oesophagus consistent with oesophageal erosions.

Positive-contrast radiography of the gastrointestinal tract: The gut transit time varies considerably in reptiles, particularly in chelonians, and is affected by species, hydration status, body size, core body temperature, season and diet. Omnivorous turtles have relatively short GI transit times of approximately 48–96 hours owing to their shorter intestinal length and diminutive caeca. Conversely, herbivorous tortoises are hindgut fermenters with large caeca and possess relatively slower GI transit times, averaging from several days to several weeks. The use of a 30–50% strength barium sulphate suspension (e.g. Liquid Polibar, E-Z-EM, 5–10 ml/kg) administered by stomach tube is useful in identifying the presence of radiolucent foreign bodies, intraluminal masses, nematodes and displacement of bowel loops by extraluminal space-occupying lesions. Barium transit slows markedly once it reaches the colon. This is because of absorption of water, which increases the viscosity of barium. Total transit time can be up to 2 weeks in large tortoises. Radiographs are usually taken immediately; at 30 minutes; and at 1, 3, 12, 24, 48 and 96 hours (or more) after barium administration (Figure 9.25). In the author's experience, correction of dehydration deficits prior to administration of contrast medium, rather than the use of prokinetic drugs (metoclopramide, cisapride), decreases gut transit time. The use of barium-impregnated polyethylene spheres also administered via stomach tube is indicated for confirming suspected obstruction, and these may be safer to use than liquid contrast agents, particularly when regurgitation is present.

Iodinated contrast agents are classified as either ionic or non-ionic. Both types have been used in reptiles. Iodide solutions are the contrast agents of choice when there is the possibility of a ruptured bowel. These agents possess the advantage of having a significantly shorter gut transit time than barium; however, mucosal detail is generally not outlined as well. Iodinated contrast agents are particularly useful in identifying alimentary obstructions. Since ionic iodide compounds are hypertonic and excreted by glomerular filtration, it is important to check renal function and hydration status prior to administration. When 37% meglumine diatrizoate (7.5 ml/kg at 21.5°C) was administered via stomach tube to Hermann's tortoises, the gut transit time was 3–8 hours. Oral dosages have been calculated by using the formula of volume of contrast agent (ml) = 2% bodyweight (kg). Another ionic iodide the author has used

orally in adult reptiles is the intravenous preparation of 50% sodium diatrizoate solution at 10.0 ml/kg (Figure 9.26). Iohexol, a non-ionic iodinated contrast agent (525–700 mg/kg) is a 'safer' alternative to an ionic iodide for positive gastrointestinal contrast, owing to its lower osmolality and reduced stress on renal function.

Retrograde positive-contrast studies are indicated to rule out obstructions of the lower intestinal tract. Contrast agents administered through lubricated rubber catheters or ball-tipped stainless steel feeding tubes (Figure 9.27) that are inserted into the cloaca work well. While it is theoretically possible for contrast to enter the ureters or oviducts, the author has not encountered this situation. Sedation of the reptile may be required.

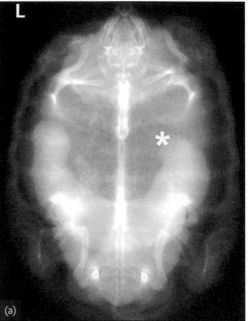

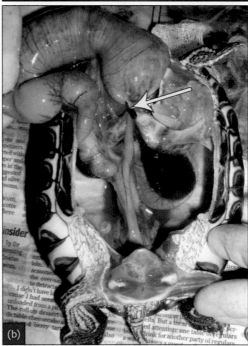

| 9.26 | (a) Dorsoventral radiograph of a 50% sodium diatrizoate contrast study of a red-eared terrapin that presented with vomiting of 2-weeks' duration and a prolapsed penis. There is stasis of contrast in the transverse colon 14 days post administration (*). (b) Necropsy revealed a stricture of the descending colon, presumably due to ingestion of a sharp foreign object (arrowed). |

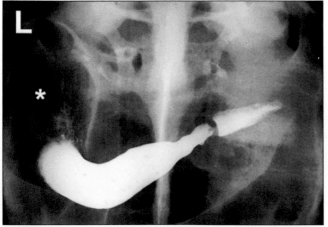

| 9.25 | Dorsoventral radiograph of a double-contrast study of the stomach and duodenum of a normal African spurred tortoise. Note the presence of gas in the gastric lumen (*) and smooth outline of contrast in the fundus. In the small intestine the barium has a 'brush' appearance due to the presence of villi. There is a peristaltic wave in the proximal duodenum. |

Ultrasonography

Ultrasonography is used routinely in reptiles and complements radiography. Ultrasound examination is non-invasive; does not expose the patient or personnel to ionizing radiation; permits excellent visualization of soft tissues; and only occasionally requires the use of sedation, particularly in larger snakes and chelonians. The ability to perform repetitive examinations over time and the portability of ultrasonography equipment for field use are additional assets. Figure 9.39 defines some terms used.

Terms	Interpretation
Anechoic	Black: areas where there is no reflection of the ultrasound beam, e.g. fluid-filled structures (gall and urinary bladders, cardiac chambers, blood vessels, previtellogenic follicles, ascites)
Echoic or echogenic	Bright: areas representing reflected ultrasound waves
Homogeneous	Consisting of a uniform echogenicity throughout
Heterogeneous	Consisting of a non-uniform echogenicity throughout
Hyperechoic	Possessing greater echogenicity (i.e. brighter) than another structure
Hypoechoic	Possessing less echogenicity (i.e. darker) compared with another structure
Isoechoic	Possessing the same echogenicity as another structure
Transducer (probe)	Scan head that produces and receives ultrasound waves

9.39 Terms used in ultrasound imaging and interpretation.

Indications

- Examination of soft tissues of the coelomic cavity and extremities (Figure 9.40).
- Examination of periocular, intraocular (Figure 9.41) and retrobulbar tissues.
- Sex determination of monomorphic species.
- Staging of reproductive cycles of females (Figure 9.42).
- Confirmation of gravidity or pregnancy.
- Identification of intracoelomic fluid, gastrointestinal foreign bodies (Figure 9.43) and radiolucent cystic calculi.

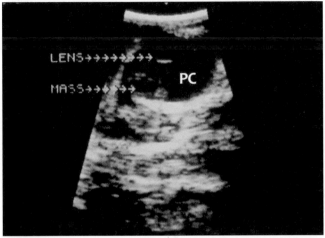

9.41 Ultrasonographic image of a hyperechoic mass attached to the posterior globe in an asymptomatic adult green iguana. This was suspected to be a hyaline remnant or blood vessel. PC = posterior chamber.

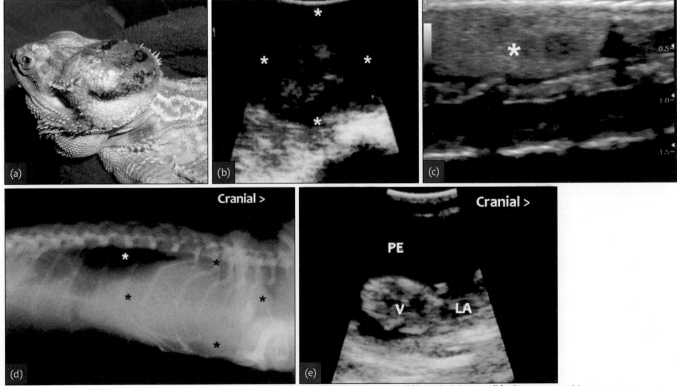

9.40 (a) Gross appearance of a soft-tissue mass that gradually developed on a 2-year-old bearded dragon. (b) Ultrasonographic appearance revealing a heterogeneous mass consisting of a central core of hyperechoic material surrounded by anechoic fluid (*). The diagnosis was an aneurysm. (c) Ultrasonographic appearance of the gastric neuroendocrine carcinoma shown in Figure 9.33a–b. Note the homogeneous appearance to this solid mass (*) and shadows produced by the ribs. (d) Left lateral radiograph of an adult bearded dragon that presented with anorexia and dyspnoea. A soft-tissue opacity in the cranial coelom (black *) is causing a mass effect on the lungs (white *). (e) Ultrasonography revealed cardiomegaly secondary to pericardial effusion (PE). Note the presence of anechoic fluid surrounding the heart. LA = left atrium; V = ventricle.
(c, Courtesy of Bruce Levine)

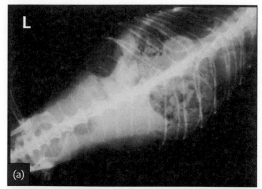

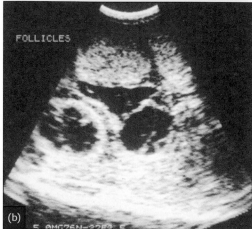

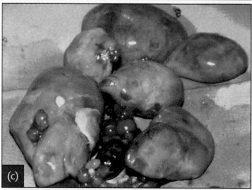

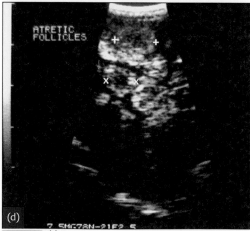

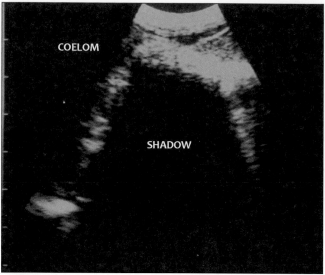

9.43 Ultrasonographic appearance of a plastic foreign body in the stomach of a green iguana. Note the distal shadow caused by the inability of the ultrasound waves to penetrate the object.

9.42 (a) Dorsoventral radiograph of an anorexic adult female iguana with opacification of the caudal coelom, which is producing a mass effect upon the intestines. (b) Ultrasonographic appearance of irregularly shaped preovulatory follicles in various stages of development from the same lizard. Note that some contain anechoic fluid while others possess hyperechoic contents. Oophoritis was diagnosed. (c) Postsurgical appearance of the excised necrotic ovaries. (d) Ultrasonographic appearance of atretic follicles in a green iguana. Note multiple irregularly shaped hyperechoic structures marked with calipers.

Limitations

- The presence of bone (including dermal bone) prevents penetration of ultrasound waves. Air (lungs, gas in intestines) produces distal reverberations (see Figure 9.54c).
- Reptiles <5 cm in diameter require a stand-off pad for adequate examination of organs.
- During ecdysis, snakes and lizards are difficult to examine due to interference from the unshed epidermis.
- The size and frequency of the transducer can impose limitations on the usefulness of ultrasound techniques in diminutive reptiles.

Technique

Most reptiles are imaged while in ventral recumbency. Manual restraint is usually adequate for lizards and snakes. Chelonians may require chemical immobilization so that the extremities can be extended to permit placement of the transducer in the appropriate fossa. Ultrasound coupling gel should be allowed at least 5 minutes of contact time on the skin of squamates in order to penetrate the air interface between the scales and transducer.

Selection of an appropriate transducer is based upon the dual goals of tissue penetration and production of an image of high resolution. In the author's experience, a 7.5 MHz transducer which penetrates soft tissues to a depth of approximately 5 cm is the most commonly used type in reptiles. A 5.0 MHz transducer is used when deeper penetration (10 cm) is required. Structures should always be viewed in longitudinal (sagittal) and cross-section (transverse) to provide a three-dimensional image.

Knowledge of regional anatomy determines where the transducer is placed (Figure 9.44). The imaging windows are most restricted in chelonians, because of their extensive exoskeleton. There are four windows – two cervical (mediastinal) and two inguinal (prefemoral) – that provide access for examining the coelomic cavity. With lizards and snakes, the transducer is placed against the lateral coelomic wall; ribs produce distinct shadow artefacts. The transducer can also be placed on the ventral midline with the reptile in dorsal recumbency (Figure 9.45).

Reptile group	Transducer location	Patient position	Organs or systems evaluated
Chelonians	Cervical (between neck and either forelimb)	Ventral recumbency	Heart, thyroid, liver, gall bladder
	Inguinal (cranial to either hindlimb)	Ventral recumbency	Urogenital, gastrointestinal, liver, cardiac apex
Lizards	Lateral cranial chest	Ventral recumbency	Heart
	Lateral body wall	Ventral or dorsal recumbency	Liver, gall bladder, gastrointestinal, urogenital
Snakes	Cranial quarter	Ventral recumbency	Heart
	Cranial third	Ventral recumbency	Liver
	Mid-body	Ventral recumbency	Stomach, gall bladder, small intestine, splenopancreatic
	Caudal third	Ventral recumbency	Urogenital, small intestine, fat deposits
	Caudal quarter	Ventral recumbency	Fat deposits, kidneys, colon, cloaca
	Ventral tail base	Dorsal recumbency	Hemipenes, scent glands

9.44 Ultrasonography protocol for reptiles.

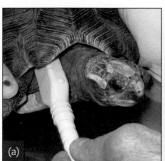
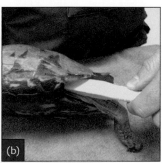
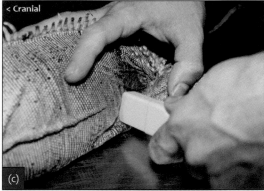
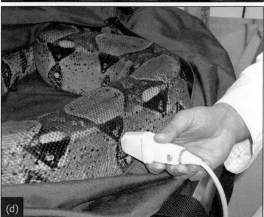

9.45 Ultrasound transducer placement. (a) Placing the transducer on the right cervical window of chelonians permits visualization of the thyroid gland, heart, liver and gall bladder. (b) To visualize organs in the caudal coelomic cavity (kidneys, urinary bladder, ovaries, testes, gastrointestinal tract) the transducer is placed on either inguinal window. (c) Placement of the transducer against the caudal lateral coelomic wall of lizards permits visualization of the urogenital and gastrointestinal systems. (d) Snakes are imaged by placing the transducer against the lateral or ventral coelomic wall.

Chelonians

Heart

The three-chambered heart is located between the hepatic lobes and is best examined through the right or left cervical fossa. Cardiac contractions are readily apparent. Both atria and ventricle are visible as anechoic chambers surrounded by echogenic cardiac muscle (Figure 9.46; see Chapter 19). The atrioventricular valves are hyperechoic compared with the myocardium. The pericardial sac appears as a hyperechoic band surrounding the heart. Small amounts of anechoic pericardial fluid are normally present. The pulmonary arteries, aortic arches, thyroid gland and vena cavae are also visible. Metastatic mineralization of vasculature is characterized by hyperechoic accentuation of the intimal linings of arteries. Mediastinal masses can also be identified through the cervical fossae (Figure 9.47).

Gastrointestinal tract

The liver can be examined through either the cervical window or the inguinal pockets. The vasculature (hepatic veins, portal veins, caudal vena cava) appears as anechoic stripes with echogenic walls. The anechoic gall bladder is readily identified in the right hepatic lobe (Figure 9.48).

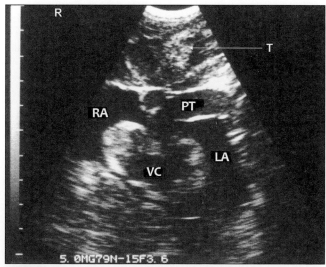

9.46 Normal ultrasound image of the chelonian heart through the right cervical window. LA = left atrium; PT = pulmonary trunk; RA = right atrium; T = thyroid gland; VC = ventricular chamber.

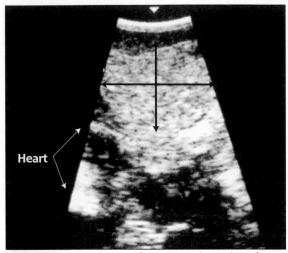

9.47 Ultrasound image of a mediastinal granuloma (cross-arrowed) in a Chinese box turtle. The spherical encapsulated homogeneous mass was just cranial to the heart and visualized through the left cervical window.

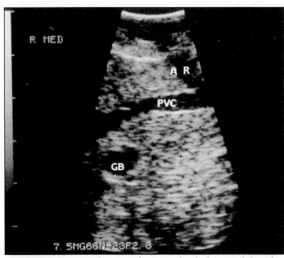

9.48 Ultrasound image of a normal right hepatic lobe of a chelonian acquired through the right cervical window. GB = gall bladder; PVC = posterior vena cava.

The liver has a hyperechoic capsule. Gout tophi appear as discrete hyperechoic intensities that do not produce distal shadowing (Figure 9.49). The stomach is located ventral to the left hepatic lobe and usually contains a combination of gas and fluid. The gastric and small intestinal walls possess a hypoechoic layer (mucosal lining) which aids in their identification.

Urogenital tract

Through the left and right inguinal pockets the ultrasonographer is able to view the cardiac apex, stomach, liver, intestines, ovaries, urinary bladder and sometimes the kidneys, depending upon the conformation of the carapace. Vitellogenic follicles appear as clusters of spherical echogenic densities. The fluid-filled urinary bladder can significantly enhance the appearance of any follicles present (Figure 9.50). The oviducts are visible as coiled linear hyperechoic structures (Figure 9.51). Eggs possess hyperechoic rims. Testes can be difficult to image due to their relatively small size; they are located cranioventral to the kidneys and are hyperechoic compared with the kidneys.

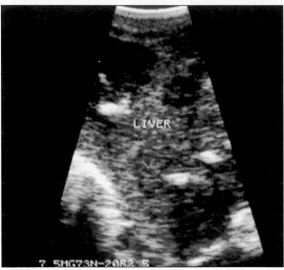

9.49 Ultrasound image of the left hepatic lobe of a chelonian acquired through the left cervical window. Note the hyperechoic densities devoid of shadows within the liver parenchyma; differentials include fibrosis, granulomas or visceral gout; biopsy revealed gout tophi.

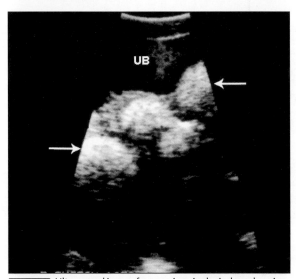

9.50 Ultrasound image from an inguinal window showing vitellogenic follicles in a diamondback terrapin. The urinary bladder (UB) has enhanced the appearance of the hyperechoic spherical follicles (arrowed).

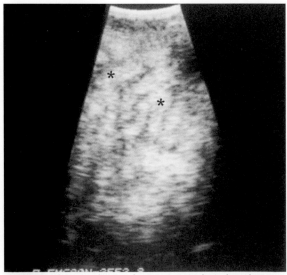

9.51 Ultrasound image from an inguinal window showing the hyperechoic plicated oviduct (*) in an impressed tortoise.

The urinary bladder lies cranial to the pelvis. Urates are visible as hyperechoic densities that freely move within the bladder lumen when pressure is applied by the transducer. Cystic calculi produce distinct distal shadows. Adequate visualization of the kidneys depends upon size of the inguinal fossa and conformation of the shell. The dome-shaped carapaces of tortoises can make renal ultrasonography challenging. The transducer must be angled dorsocaudally in the inguinal pockets owing to the kidneys' location in the retrocoelomic space. Normal kidneys are triangular in shape, with a hypoechoic hilus and hyperechoic capsule (Figure 9.52). Renal vasculature appears as hypoechoic stripes within the parenchyma. Magnetic resonance imaging and computed tomography provide the best visibility.

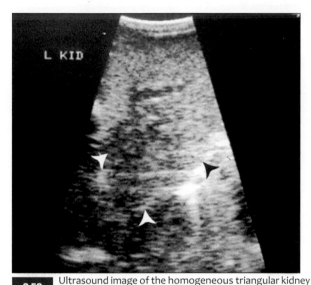

9.52 Ultrasound image of the homogeneous triangular kidney (arrowheads) of a yellow-footed tortoise. Note the hypoechoic vasculature. The image was visualized through the left inguinal fossa.

Lizards

Heart

The heart varies in position depending on the species being examined. In iguanids and agamids, the heart is located within the pectoral girdle and is viewed by placing the transducer immediately caudal to either humerus. In varanids the heart is located more caudally between the liver lobes. Small amounts of anechoic pericardial fluid are normally present. Reptiles with visceral gout can have urate tophi which are visible as an increased echo intensity of the pericardium (Figure 9.53a). Calcium deposits of vascular linings are visible as hyperechoic stripes (Figure 9.53b).

Gastrointestinal tract

The liver is bilobed and occupies the cranial half of the coelomic cavity. The right lobe contains the caudal vena cava and gall bladder (Figure 9.54a–b). Occasionally, accumulations of bile salts (biliary sand) can be visualized as speckles that move when disturbed by motion. Hepatomegaly and changes in parenchymal structure may also be identified (Figure 9.54c). The stomach is dorsal to the left hepatic lobe. The pancreas, spleen and small intestine are caudal to the liver. The large intestine is caudal to the right hepatic lobe. The large intestine and cloaca are located between the kidneys and contain gas, urates and faeces (Figure 9.55).

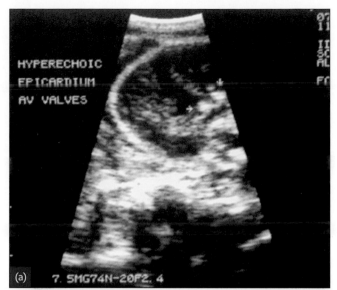

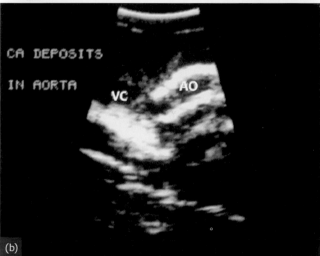

9.53 (a) Ultrasonographic appearance of increased echogenicity of the epicardial lining and atrioventricular valves of the heart, due to deposition of urate crystals in a green iguana. (b) Hyperechoic changes to the intimal linings of the aorta and endocardium of a green iguana (see Figure 9.32) diagnosed with metastatic mineralization. AO = aorta; VC = ventricular chamber.

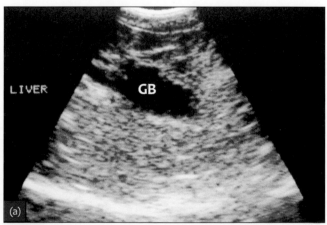

9.54 (a) Ultrasonographic appearance of the normal liver of a savannah monitor. Note the homogeneous appearance of the parenchyma and the gall bladder (GB) containing anechoic bile. (continues) ▶

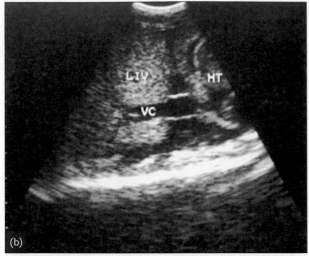

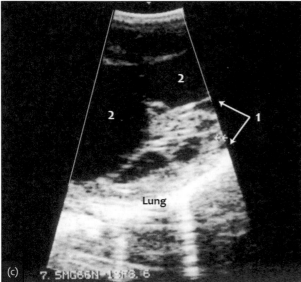

Urogenital tract

The gonads lie between the liver and urinary bladder. Ovaries and testes become visible as sexual maturity develops. It can be difficult to image inactive ovaries because of their small size (Figure 9.56a). However, active ovaries are easily imaged due to the presence of enlarging follicles clustered like grapes (Figure 9.56b). Yolk coelomitis due to ruptured follicles can also be identified (Figure 9.56c). Eggs possess hyperechoic rims (Figure 9.57). In viviparous lizards (e.g. blue-tongued skinks), fetuses are identified by echo-intense signals surrounded by anechoic fluid and membranes. In the later stages of gestation the skeletons and cardiac contractions become visible.

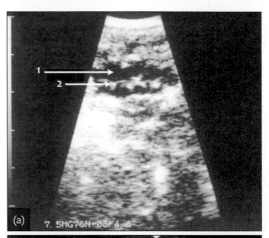

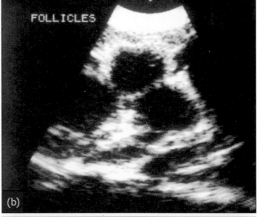

9.54 (continued) (b) Normal ultrasound image of the caudal vena cava (VC) exiting the liver and entering the right atrium of a green iguana; note the echogenic walls of the vena cava. HT = heart; LIV = liver. (c) Ultrasound image of a biliary duct carcinoma in a savannah monitor. The liver parenchyma (1) has been displaced by anechoic cavitations (2) that are lined with neoplastic cells. Note the presence of hyperechoic distal reverberations due to air from the lung.

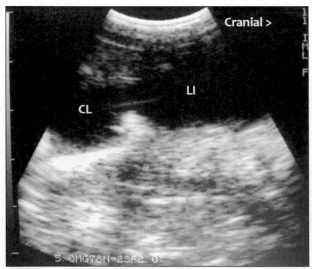

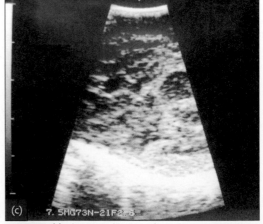

9.55 Normal ultrasound image of the terminal part of the large intestine (LI) and cloaca (CL) of a savannah monitor. Both organs contain anechoic fluid. Note the dorsal hyperechoic mucosal fold partially separating the cloaca from the large intestine.

9.56 (a) Ultrasound image of a quiescent ovary in a green iguana. The cortex (1) contains small anechoic follicles. The echogenic medulla (2) contains connective tissue and blood vessels. (b) Ultrasound image of an active ovary containing enlarged anechoic vitellogenic follicles in a green iguana. (c) Ultrasound image of egg yolk coelomitis in a green iguana. The hyperechoic exudate prevents visualization of other organs.

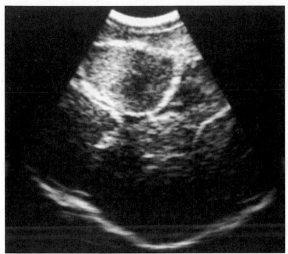

9.57 Ultrasound image of a gravid green iguana. Note the irregular shapes of the hyperechoic shell membranes of the eggs.

In green iguanas it is easier to visualize the testes during the breeding season when there is gonadal hypertrophy. If inactive gonads are not visible through the flanks, the male lizard is placed in dorsal recumbency with the transducer placed on the linea alba. After locating the aorta, which appears as a pulsating anechoic stripe, the transducer is moved laterally to image the gonads, which straddle the aorta (Figure 9.58). In sexually monomorphic lizards such as Gila monsters and prehensile-tailed skinks, the hemipenes can be identified by placing the transducer against the ventral tail base. The hemipenes appear as elongated heterogeneous structures that are hypoechoic compared with the surrounding muscle tissue (Figure 9.59).

The urinary bladder lies cranial to the pelvis. Some lizards, such as monitors and bearded dragons, possess a cloacal bladder (urodeum) instead of a urinary bladder. The kidneys are variable in location depending upon the species. In monitor lizards and chameleons they lie cranial

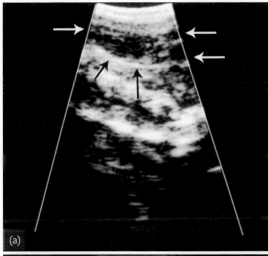

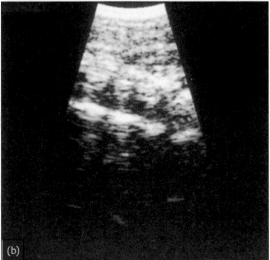

9.59 (a) Ultrasound image of the tail base of a male prehensile-tailed skink. The heterogeneous structure (arrowed) is the hemipenis. (b) Note the absence of this structure in the tail base of a conspecific female.

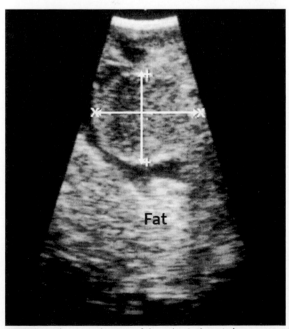

Fat

9.58 Ultrasound image of the spherical testis (cross-arrowed) in a green iguana. There is a small amount of anechoic fluid surrounding the testis, which is normal. Note that the testis possesses a hyperechoic capsule and is less echogenic than the surrounding fat.

to the pelvis; in the green iguana and bearded dragon they are recessed within the pelvis. Placing the transducer against the sublumbar fossa and directing the beam caudally towards the pelvic inlet permits visualization of the kidneys in iguanids (Figure 9.60a).

The kidneys are hyperechoic compared with the liver and possess hyperechoic capsules. Each renal vein is visible as an anechoic stripe. In the green iguana and bearded dragon the caudal poles of the kidneys can be visualized when the transducer is placed against the lateral base of the tail with the beam directed cranially towards the pelvic outlet. In green iguanas and bearded dragons with renomegaly the kidneys protrude into the coelomic cavity and are easily visualized (see Figure 9.37b). Metastatic mineralization is characterized by focal hyperechoic densities that produce distal shadows (Figure 9.60b).

In chelonians and lizards, the bilateral fat-pads extend cranially from the pelvis. In cachectic animals fat deposits are reduced in size and may even be absent. Reptilian adipose tissue is hyperechoic compared with other coelomic organs and is divided into lobes by hyperechoic septae (Figure 9.60c). In obese animals adipose tissue extends to the heart and can significantly interfere with imaging of the coelomic cavity.

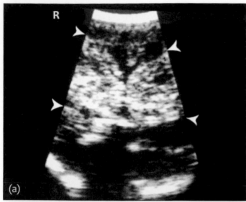

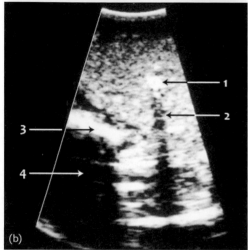

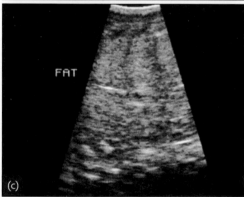

9.60 (a) Ultrasound image of the cranial poles of the kidneys (arrowheads) of a green iguana in ventral recumbency. There is increased echogenicity to the renal parenchyma due to urate infiltration. The probe has been placed on the sublumbar area and angled caudally towards the pelvic inlet. (b) Ultrasound image of metastatic calcification in the kidney of a green iguana: 1 = mineralized deposit; 2 = shadow created by calcium phosphate complex; 3 = ischium; 4 = shadow created by bone. (c) Adipose tissue of a well nourished royal python. Note the hyperechoic septum separating two fatty lobes.

Snakes

Heart

The heart is located in the cranial third of the body. Due to the tubular shape of the body, the heart is somewhat elongated compared with other reptiles. Contractions are easily visualized.

Gastrointestinal tract

The single-lobed cylindrical liver begins at the apex of the heart and extends half the length of the snake. It is homogeneous in appearance and possesses a hyperechoic

capsule. The large hepatic vein is visualized as an anechoic stripe with echogenic walls. The caudal vena cava can be visualized as it exits the liver before entering the right atrium of the heart. The anechoic gall bladder is caudal to the liver and in well nourished animals is surrounded by fat (Figure 9.61). It is located approximately halfway down the body length and is a convenient anatomical marker for the ultrasonographer. The splenopancreas is adjacent or just caudal to the gall bladder and can be difficult to image. The stomach is dorsal to the liver. The linear intestinal tract is surrounded by fat which obscures its visualization. Luminal contents consist of a mixture of fluid and gas (Figure 9.62). The colon and cloaca lie between the kidneys and vent. Luminal contents consist of gas, urates and faeces, which can interfere with image quality. The lung(s) lie dorsal to the heart and liver and may affect image quality due to reverberation artefacts. The air sac in boids is extensive and its air content also causes reverberation artefacts.

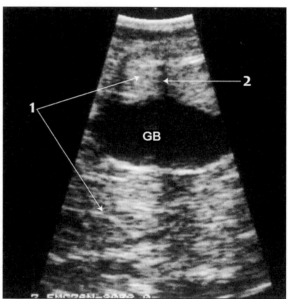

9.61 Ultrasound image of the anechoic gall bladder (GB) filled with bile in a royal python: 1 = fat; 2 = rib shadow.

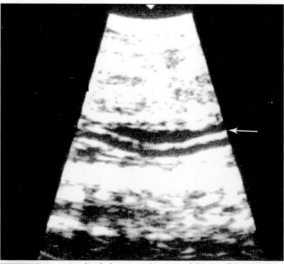

9.62 Longitudinal ultrasound image of the small intestine in a Solomon Island boa. The hyperechoic stripe is the lumen, which contains chyme. In this picture, the walls of the intestine are anechoic.

Urogenital tract

The gonads are caudal to the gall bladder. Follicles appear as linear spherical echogenic densities (Figure 9.63a). Ovarian masses can also be identified (Figure 9.63b). Eggs possess hyperechoic rims, which are the shell membranes (Figure 9.63c). During the initial stages of pregnancy fetuses are identified by the development of the anechoic amnion within the yolk sac. Towards the latter stages of pregnancy, fetuses are identified by their echogenic curvilinear skeletons, cardiac contractions and body movements (Figure 9.63d). The testes are fusiform in shape and are difficult to image because of the presence of coelomic fat and intestinal contents. The hemipenes can be imaged at the base of the tail and appear as elongated heterogeneous structures.

The kidneys lie caudal to the gonads, with the right kidney cranial to the left. They are hyperechoic compared with the liver and hypoechoic compared with the fat bodies. The unique swirl-like anatomy of the renal parenchyma coupled with the presence of the renal vein enables the ultrasonographer to identify these organs (Figure 9.64).

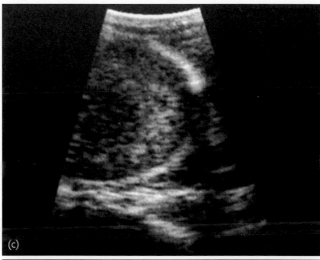

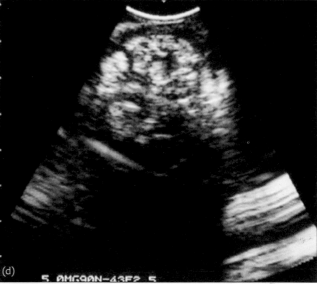

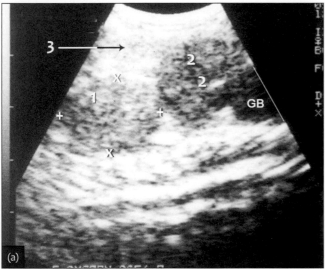

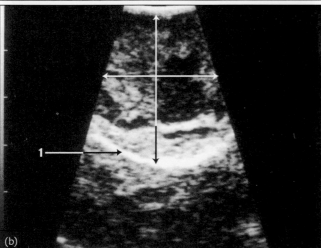

9.63 (continued) (c) Ultrasound image of an Asian ratsnake egg; note the hyperechoic shell membranes surrounding hypoechoic yolk. (d) Ultrasound image of Solomon Island boa fetuses; note the distal shadowing created by the fetuses.

9.63 (a) Ultrasound image of two homogeneous vitellogenic follicles (1 and 2) in a Solomon Island boa. As follicles develop, they increase in echogenicity due to yolk formation. Compare the relative echogenic characteristics of the follicles, fat (3) and gall bladder (GB). (b) Ultrasound image of an ovarian tumour (cross-arrowed) of mixed (heterogeneous) echogenicity in a corn snake: 1 = capsule of tumour. (continues) ▶

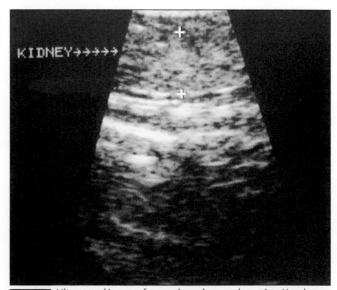

9.64 Ultrasound image of normal renal parenchyma in a Honduran milk snake. Note the more heterogeneous appearance compared with the kidney of a yellow-footed tortoise in Figure 9.52.

Computed tomography

Computed tomography (CT) produces transverse X-ray images of slices (tomographs) of bone and tissue. Unlike conventional radiography, the visualization of organs is not limited by overlying structures such as soft tissue and bone. CT provides excellent detail of lungs, bone, parenchymal calcification and acute central nervous system haematoma formation. Normal chelonian lungs appear as radiolucent air-filled cavities divided by septations consisting of pulmonary vasculature and smooth muscle (Figure 9.65a). Bone shows excellent contrast, demonstrating

cortical thickness and density. The trabeculae of medullary cavities are also visualized. Soft tissues do not emit high-contrast signals; however, preovulatory follicles and dystrophic calcification are easily defined (Figure 9.65b–c). CT is limited by its low soft-tissue contrast and number of scanning planes. Chemical immobilization with propofol (see Chapter 12) can be used owing to the short scanning time in CT.

Modern CT software permits tomographs to be built by stacking axial slices. The software then cuts slices through the tomographs in a different plane. Multiplanar reconstruction enables organs to be visualized in three dimensions (Figure 9.66).

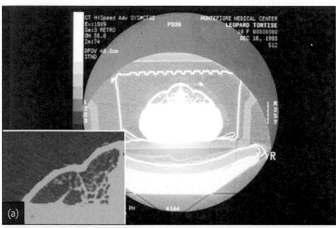

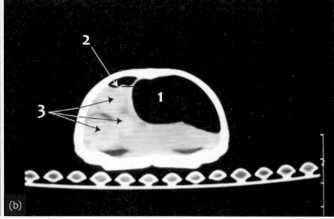

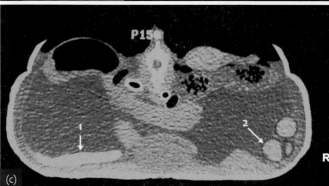

9.65 (a) Transverse CT image of the lungs of a leopard tortoise. Note the reticular pattern of normal lung parenchyma (inset). (b) Transverse CT image demonstrating unilateral folliculogenesis in a musk turtle that had buoyancy problems: 1 = normal lung; 2 = lung with compression due to follicles; 3 = vitellogenic follicles. (c) Transverse CT image of a leopard tortoise with hepatic dystrophic mineralization (1) and vitellogenic follicles (2).

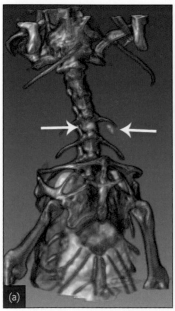
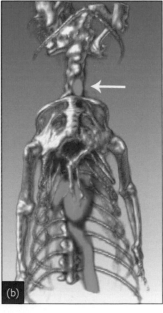

9.66 (a) Single photon emission computerized tomographic (SPECT) image of a 1 miCi technetium scan at 15–45 minutes of a normal leopard gecko, with thyroxine of 6.05 nmol/l. Technetium mimics iodine; note the normal bilateral thyroid glands (arrowed) ventral to the cervical vertebrae. (b) SPECT image of a 1 miCi technetium scan at 15–45 minutes in a hyperthyroid leopard gecko, with thyroxine of 64.35 nmol/l. The single midline focus of increased uptake is thought to be the overactive thyroid gland (arrowed); the contralateral gland is not visible because of negative feedback and atrophy.

(Courtesy of Thomas Boyer, Seth Wallack, Ann Bettencourt and Mario Bourdon)

Magnetic resonance imaging

The physics of magnetic resonance imaging (MRI) is based upon the fact that the nucleus of the hydrogen atom, which contains one proton, makes up approximately 70% (in water) of all living tissue. The positively charged protons possess angular momentum (spin). When a powerful magnetic field is applied to these protons, they orientate themselves like tiny magnets. As a radio wave of a specified pulse is then sent through the magnetic field, the protons tilt. When the radio wave ceases, the protons return to their original positions (relaxation) emitting radio signals which can then be used to produce an image.

T1 and T2 weighting are terms that refer to radio signal manipulation of the relaxation times that selectively enhances the contrast of different tissues. T1 weighting is used to enhance organ parenchyma, permitting visualization of lesions such as diffuse organ enlargement, granulomas and tumours. T2 weighting is used to enhance vascular flow and inflammatory or oedematous changes in soft tissue. Virtually all internal organs can be imaged with MRI owing to the many choices of slice orientation (Figures 9.67 and 9.68). MRI is also extremely sensitive to iron owing to the magnetic properties of this element. In human medicine MRI is used to monitor haemorrhaging (>72 hours) and to assess ferritin deposition in the geriatric brain (Mazziotta and Gilman, 1992). MRI is superior to CT in evaluating soft-tissue diseases owing to its intrinsic high tissue contrast. MRI, like CT, also provides excellent visualization of the lungs. MRI has low sensitivity to calcium; hence, it is inferior to CT for bone examination. The disadvantages of MRI are high cost, slow rate of data acquisition (approximately 60 minutes for a typical scan) and high sensitivity to motion artefacts. Accordingly, chemical immobilization is required. MRI cannot be performed on reptiles with metal implants.

Figure 9.69 summarizes and compares the non-invasive imaging techniques described in this chapter.

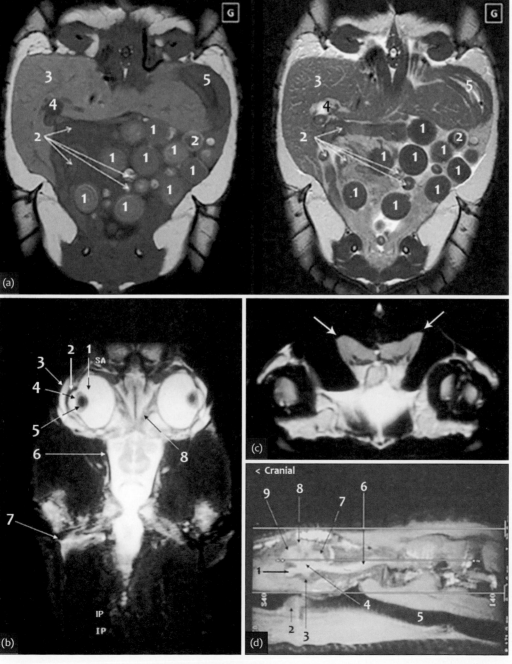

9.67 (a) Axial T1- and T2-weighted magnetic resonance (MR) images of an adult female red-eared terrapin: 1 = developing follicles; 2 = loops of intestine; 3 = liver; 4 = gall bladder; 5 = stomach. (b) Coronal T1-weighted MR image of the head of an Asian water monitor at the level of the orbits: 1 = vitreous humour; 2 = cornea; 3 = eyelid; 4 = aqueous humour; 5 = lens; 6 = forebrain; 7 = auditory canal; 8 = optic nerve. (c) Transverse T1-weighted MR image of the kidneys (arrowed) of an adult impressed tortoise. (d) Sagittal T1-weighted MR image of the head of an Asian water monitor at the level of the brain: 1 = olfactory bulbs; 2 = glottis; 3 = pituitary gland; 4 = diencephalon; 5 = trachea; 6 = spinal cord; 7 = cerebellum; 8 = pineal gland; 9 = cerebrum. (a, Courtesy of Noemie Summa; c, d, Courtesy of Robert Wagner)

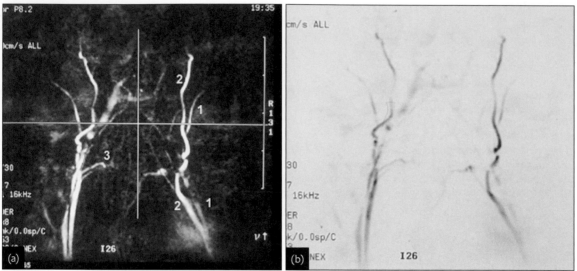

9.68 (a) Coronal T1-weighted magnetic resonance (MR) image of the head of a water monitor with gadolinium contrast enhanced angiography. The contrast agent was injected into the coccygeal vein and images were taken approximately 2 minutes later: 1 = external carotid artery; 2 = internal carotid artery; 3 = caudal cerebral artery. (b) Reverse-contrast MR image of the same reptile.
(Courtesy of Robert Wagner)

Parameter	Radiography	Ultrasonography	Computed tomography (CT)	Magnetic resonance imaging (MRI)
Indications	Evaluation of bone, calcified tissue, lungs, enlarging follicles in squamates, eggs, cystic calculi and some types of foreign bodies	Evaluation of soft tissues	Evaluation of lungs, calcified tissue and bone	Evaluation of all soft tissues, lungs and medullary cavities of long bones
Advantages	Availability; low cost; chemical restraint not usually required; quick results	No exposure to ionizing radiation; chemical restraint not usually required; excellent penetration of fluid; portability for field use	Production of multiple X-ray images that are not limited by overlying soft tissue or bone	No exposure to ionizing radiation; ability to provide many types of slice orientations (transverse, sagittal, coronal)
Limitations	Difficult to penetrate fluid, osteoderms of lizards and exoskeletons of chelonians; diminutive reptiles require specialized equipment such as mammographic and dental units	Cannot penetrate bone or air; reptiles in active shed are refractory to ultrasonography; diminutive reptiles require specialized equipment such as stand-off pads and higher frequency transducers (10 MHz); steep learning curve for performing technique and interpreting images	Availability and cost; poor soft-tissue contrast; requires many scanning planes, which are limited to transverse sections; requires chemical restraint	Availability and cost; poor cortical bone contrast; long time required to acquire data (1 hour minimum for standard scan); requires chemical restraint owing to high sensitivity to motion artefacts; cannot be utilized in reptiles with metal implants

9.69 Summary and comparison of non-invasive imaging techniques.

Acknowledgements

The author would like to thank William Cermak for his assistance with the imaging pictures, and Exotic DVM magazine where several of the ultrasound images were first published.

References and further reading

Bennett RA, Divers SJ, Schumacher J *et al.* (1999) Roundtable: anaesthesia. *Bulletin of the Association of Reptilian and Amphibian Veterinarians* **9(4)**, 20–28

Boyer TH, Wallack S, Bettencourt A and Bourdon M (2010) Hyperthyroidism in a leopard gecko (*Eublepharis macularius*) and radioiodine (I–131) treatment. *Proceedings of the Association of Reptilian and Amphibian Veterinarians Annual Conference*, p. 53

DeShaw B, Schoelnfeld A, Cook RA and Haramati N (1996) Imaging of reptiles: a comparison study of various radiographic techniques. *Journal of Zoo and Wildlife Medicine* **27**, 364–370

Divers SJ and Lawton M (2000) Spinal osteomyelitis in a green iguana, *Iguana iguana*: cerebrospinal fluid and myelogram diagnosis. *Proceedings of the Association of Reptilian and Amphibian Veterinarians Annual Conference*, p. 77

Frye FL (1991) *Biomedical and Surgical Aspects of Captive Reptile Husbandry*. Krieger, Malabar, FL

Gomez JA (1974) The gastrointestinal contrast study. *Veterinary Clinics of North America* **4(4)**, 805–842

Helmick KE, Bennett RA, Ginn P *et al.* (2000) Intestinal volvulus and stricture associated with a leiomyoma in a green turtle (*Chelonia mydas*). *Journal of Zoo and Wildlife Medicine* **31**, 221–227

Hernandez-Divers SJ, Strunk A, Frank PM *et al.* (2002) Scintigraphic imaging of a Horsfield's tortoise (*Testudo horsfieldi*) with multifocal bacterial and fungal Infections, and plastron necrosis. *Proceedings of the Association of Reptilian and Amphibian Veterinarians Annual Conference*, pp. 103–104

Holland MF, Hernandez-Divers S and Frank PM (2008) Ultrasonographic appearance of the coelomic cavity in healthy green iguanas. *Journal of the American Veterinary Medical Association* **233**, 590–596

Isaza R, Garner M and Jacobson E (2000) Proliferative osteoarthritis and osteoarthrosis in 15 snakes. *Journal of Zoo and Wildlife Medicine* **31**, 20–27

Jacobson ER (1993) Snakes. *Veterinary Clinics of North America Small Animal* **23**, 1179–1212

Kealy JK and McAllister H (2005) *Diagnostic Radiology and Ultrasonography of the Dog and Cat*. Elsevier Saunders, St Louis, MO

Lawton MPC (1997) Hands-free, non-chemical restraint of Iguanidae for radiography. *Proceedings of the Association of Reptilian and Amphibian Veterinarians Annual Conference*, pp. 1–4

Levine BS (2011) Gastric endoneurocrine carcinoma (somatostatinoma) in a bearded dragon, *Pogona vertices*. *Proceedings of the Association of Reptilian and Amphibian Veterinarians Annual Conference*, p. 149

Mador DR (2006) *Reptile Medicine and Surgery*. WB Saunders, Philadelphia

Mazziotta JC and Gilman S (1992) *Clinical Brain Imaging: Principles and Applications*. FA Davis, Philadelphia

McArthur S, Wilkinson R and Meyer J (2004) *Medicine and Surgery of Tortoises and Turtles*. Iowa State Press, Ames, IA

Meyer J (1998) Gastrografin as a gastrointestinal contrast agent in the Greek tortoise (*Testudo hermanni*). *Journal of Zoo and Wildlife Medicine* **29**, 183–189

Morgan JP (1974) Systematic radiographic interpretation of skeletal diseases in small animals. *Veterinary Clinics of North America: Small Animal Practice* **4(4)**, 611–626

Morris PJ (1997) Ultrasound imaging for sex determination in lizards. *Proceedings of the North American Veterinary Conference*, [on CD-ROM]

Morris PJ and Alberts AC (1996) Determination of sex in white-throated monitors (*Varanus albigularis*), Gila monsters (*Heloderma suspectum*), and beaded lizards (*H. horridum*) using two-dimensional ultrasound imaging. *Journal of Zoo and Wildlife Medicine* **27**, 371–377

Morris PJ and Henderson P (1998) Gender determination in mature Gila monsters (*Heloderma suspectum*) and Mexican beaded lizards (*Heloderma horridum*), by ultrasound imaging of the ventral tail. *Bulletin of the Association of Reptilian and Amphibian Veterinarians* **8(4)**, 4–5

Norton TM, Spratt J, Behler J and Hernandez K (1998) Medotomidine and ketamine anesthesia with atipamizole reversal in private free-ranging gopher tortoises, *Gopherus polyphemus*. *Proceedings of the Association of Reptilian and Amphibian Veterinarians Annual Conference*, pp. 25–28

Nyland TG and Mattoon JS (1995) *Veterinary Diagnostic Ultrasound*. WB Saunders, Philadelphia

Raiti PR (1999) Transcoelomic ultrasonography of the reptile reproductive tract. *Exotic DVM* **1(6)**, 27–32

Raiti PR and Haramati N (1997) Magnetic resonance imaging and computerized tomography of a gravid leopard tortoise (*Geochelone pardalis*) with metabolic bone disease. *Journal of Zoo and Wildlife Medicine* **28**, 189–197

Redrobe S (1997) Aspects of ultrasonography of chelonia, lizards and snakes. *Proceedings of the Association of Reptilian and Amphibian Veterinarians Annual Conference*, pp. 127–130, 179–186

Romer AS (1997) *Osteology of the Reptiles*. Krieger, Malabar, FL

Rubel A, Kuoni W and Augustiny N (1990) Endoscopic and imaging techniques. *Seminars in Avian and Exotic Pet Medicine* **3(3)**, 156–161

Rubel GA, Isenbugel E and Wolvekamp P (1991) *Atlas of Diagnostic Radiology of Exotic Pets*. WB Saunders, Philadelphia

Sainsbury AW and Gilli C (1991) Ultrasonographic anatomy and scanning technique of the coelomic organs of the Bosc monitor (*Varanus examanthematicus*). *Journal of Zoo and Wildlife Medicine* **22(4)**, 421–433

Schildger BJ, Casares M, Kramer M *et al.* (1994) Technique of ultrasonography in lizards, snakes, and chelonians. *Seminars in Avian and Exotic Pet Medicine* **3(3)**, 147–155

Schildger BJ, Tenhu H, Kramer M *et al.* (1999) Comparative diagnostic imaging of the reproductive tract in monitors: radiology-ultrasonography-coelioscopy. Advances in monitor research II. *Mertensiella* **11**, 193–211

Schilliger L, Dominique T, Pouchelon JL *et al.* (2006) Proposed standardization of the two-dimensional echocardiographic examination in snakes. *Journal of Herpetological Medicine and Surgery* **16**, 76–87

Silverman S and Janssen JL (1996) Diagnostic imaging. In: *Reptile Medicine and Surgery*, ed. DR Mader, pp. 258–263. WB Saunders, Philadelphia

Snyder PS, Shaw NG and Heard DJ (1999) Two-dimensional echocardiographic anatomy of the snake heart (*Python molurus bivattatus*). *Veterinary Radiology and Ultrasound* **40**, 66–72

Taylor SK, Citino S, Zdziarski JM and Bush RM (1996) Radiographic anatomy and barium sulfate transit time of the gastrointestinal tract of the leopard tortoise (*Testudo pardalis*). *Journal of Zoo and Wildlife Medicine* **27**, 180–186

Tenhu H, Schildger B, Kuchling G and Thompson G (1999) Ultrasonographic examination and anatomy of monitors (*Varanus gouldii*, *V. indicus* and *V. griseus*) (Sauria: Varanidae). Advances in monitor research II. *Mertensiella* **11**, 181–187

Zwart P (1992) Urogenital system. In: *BSAVA Manual of Reptiles*, ed. PH Beynon *et al.*, pp. 117–127. BSAVA, Gloucester, UK

Chapter 10

Diagnostic and surgical endoscopy

Stephen J. Divers

A definitive diagnosis is important to maximize treatment success, but reptile cases are frequently mismanaged simply because of a failure to identify a specific problem and provide precise treatment. Definitive diagnosis relies upon the demonstration of a host pathological response (by histopathology, less reliably cytology or using paired rising antibody titres) and the causative agent (by microbiology, parasitology or toxicology). There are few reliable serological tests available for reptiles, and those that are available require a minimum of 6–9 weeks to demonstrate the necessary two-fold increase in titres. It is therefore clear that tissue samples offer the most expedient means to a diagnosis, and endoscopy offers a minimally invasive ante-mortem method to collect such material. Previously plagued by vague medical histories, non-pathognomonic physical examinations, indistinct diagnostic images and less than conclusive clinical pathology results, many clinicians have discovered that diagnostic endoscopy offers an unparalleled ability to facilitate an accurate diagnosis and improve case outcome.

Owing to space restrictions, preference has been given to those species and procedures that are most commonly performed in zoological practice. Furthermore, to reduce the number of journal citations, some references have been reduced to major reviews that contain the more detailed sources. More detailed publications on reptile endoscopy and endosurgery are available to the interested practitioner (Divers, 2014ab).

Prior to the 1990s, there were only sporadic reports of reptile endoscopy. The majority of earlier reports described the use of endoscopy to examine or retrieve foreign objects from the gastrointestinal tract, along with case descriptions of coelioscopy, bronchoscopy and urogenital endoscopy. More recently, further development and reviews of single- and multiple-entry techniques have been made expanding endoscopic applications in the Reptilia (Divers, 2014ab). In particular, validation of endoscopy procedures in chelonians (e.g. hepatic and renal biopsy, neonate gender identification, oophorectomy and orchidectomy), lizards (e.g. hepatic and renal biopsy) and snakes (e.g. pulmonoscopy and lung biopsy) have helped confirm the safety and diagnostic value of this approach (Hernandez-Divers, 2004; Hernandez-Divers *et al.*, 2004, 2005b, 2007, 2009a; Stahl *et al.*, 2008). Given the often small and fragile nature of small reptile pets, the continued development of minimally invasive endoscopy appears assured in these taxa.

Equipment

Endoscopy equipment for the reptile practitioner has been recently reviewed (Divers, 2014ab). See Figure 10.1 for basic equipment recommendations.

Rigid endoscopy tower
• Documentation cart with two fixed shelves and single drawer (any appropriate cart can be used as long as it is mobile and the equipment secure)
• Electrical CO_2 insufflator, 0–10 l/min, digital display; medical grade CO_2 cylinder
• TelePak (all in one unit; endoscopic video unit including single-chip standard-definition camera (PAL/NTSC), hybrid xenon or LED light source, air insufflation pump, digital image/video processing, USB/SD memory; colour LCD monitor): or separate equipment items (nova xenon light source, 175 W; light guide cable, 3.5 mm x 230 cm; veterinary video camera III (PAL/NTSC), soakable and gas sterilizable, with control unit; colour monitor)
Standard (2.7 mm) rigid endoscopy system
• Hopkins telescope, 2.7 mm x 18 cm, 30 degrees
• Operating sheath for 2.7 mm telescope, 4.8 mm (14.5 Fr) with 1.7 mm (5 Fr) instrument channel
• Examination and protection sheath for 2.7 mm telescope, 3.5 mm outside diameter
• Biopsy forceps, 1.7 mm (5 Fr)
• Grasping forceps, 1.7 mm (5 Fr)
• Scissors, 1.3 mm (4 Fr)
• Injection needle with outer tube, 0.7 mm
Additional equipment
• Miniature straightforward telescope, 1 mm × 20 cm, 0 degrees
• 100 cm x 3 mm flexible bronchofibrescope with 1.2 mm working channel
• 110 cm x 5.9 mm video gastroscope with 2 mm working channel
• Hopkins telescope, 1.9 mm x 14 cm, 30 degrees, with integrated sheath and 1 mm (3 Fr) instrument channel
• Grasping forceps, 1 mm (3 Fr)
• Biopsy forceps, 1 mm (3 Fr)

10.1 Equipment for diagnostic endoscopy. This list represents a basic entry-level system, with additional equipment that is commonly utilized indicated as well. There is an extensive assortment of equipment and instrumentation options available (including high-definition camera systems), and practitioners are advised to try equipment at conferences or trade shows, or request in-practice demonstrations before purchase.

Single-entry rigid endoscopy equipment

Single-entry procedures are technically easier and less invasive than multiple entries that require additional access ports and instrument triangulation. Modern rod-lens

BSAVA Manual of Reptiles, third edition. Edited by Simon J. Girling and Paul Raiti. ©BSAVA 2019

telescopes, invented by Professor Hopkins, utilize long rods of glass and smaller air spaces. The advantages of the rod-lens system are:

- Greater light transmission
- Better image resolution
- Wider field of view
- Greater image magnification.

The system centres on a 2.7 mm Hopkins telescope with 30-degree oblique view (Figure 10.2). The 30-degree oblique not only enables a straight-ahead view but, by simply rotating the telescope around its longitudinal axis, a much greater field of vision can be obtained. Recently, this telescope underwent a revision and the field of view has been significantly increased. The 2.7 mm Hopkins telescope is typically used in conjunction with a 3.5 mm protection sheath, or a 4.8 mm operating sheath, which provides two ports for gas insufflation or fluid infusion/irrigation, and an operating channel (Figure 10.2). The operating channel permits the use of 1.7 mm (5 Fr) flexible instruments. A smaller 1.9 mm telescope with integrated operating sheath is also available, and accommodates 1 mm (3 Fr) flexible instruments.

Multiple-entry rigid endoscopy equipment

Endoscopy research and procedural development at the University of Georgia have resulted in the evolution of a multiple-entry endosurgical system for reptiles and other exotic species. This minimally invasive surgical system has been based upon human paediatric laparoscopy and encompasses:

- 2.7 mm Hopkins telescope within a 3.5 mm protective sheath (which can be inserted through a 3.9 mm cannula)
- 3.5 mm trocars and 3 mm instruments
- Monopolar and bipolar radiosurgery for haemostasis.

One or two additional entries are made into the coelom using trocars that possess valves to prevent loss of intra-coelomic CO_2 pressure. The 3.5 mm trocars provide numerous 3 mm instrument options including various forceps, scissors, palpation probes, irrigation/suction probes and radiosurgery devices (Figure 10.3). Minimally invasive surgery generally requires the use of a second surgical assistant to hold the telescope, while the primary surgeon operates the instruments. However, there are endoscope clamps and holding devices commercially available that can remove the need for an assistant (Divers, 2014c).

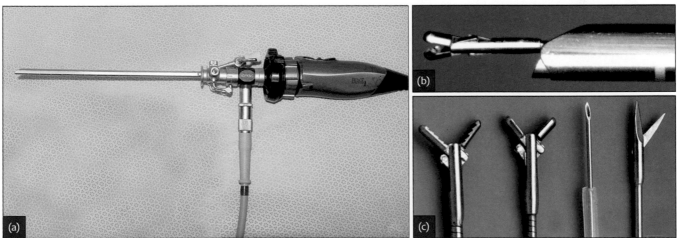

10.2 A 2.7 mm telescope system. (a) 2.7 mm telescope housed within a 4.8 mm operating sheath, connected to a light cable and an endovideo camera. (b) 1.7 mm biopsy forceps inserted down the instrument channel and emerging directly in front of the telescope. (c) A variety of 1.7 mm instruments can be used through the operating channel, including (from left to right) retrieval forceps, biopsy forceps, remote injection/aspiration needle, and single-action scissors.
(© SJ Divers, University of Georgia)

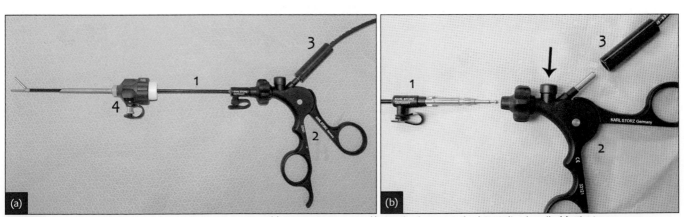

10.3 Human paediatric 3 mm laparoscopy equipment. (a) A 3 mm instrument (1) attached to a standard CLICKline handle (2). The instrument, attached to a radiosurgery unit via a connector on the handle (3), has been inserted through a 3.5 mm graphite/plastic cannula with insufflation port (4). (b) Instrument (1) and handle (2) can be quickly exchanged by pressing on the release button (arrowed).
(© SJ Divers, University of Georgia)

Light sources

There are two major types of light source available, the cheaper tungsten–halogen and the more expensive rare-earth xenon. The more powerful and better quality xenon sources are preferred for video endoscopy (Figure 10.4). The light source is connected to the endoscope via a flexible fibre-optic cable.

Cameras and documentation

Video cameras greatly improve endoscopy ergonomics, decrease surgery time, reduce surgeon fatigue and improve procedural success (Figure 10.4). The camera, attached to the eyepiece of the telescope, relays the image to a monitor that is positioned in front of, and angled towards, the endoscopist (Figure 10.5). The use of a camera also facilitates the recording of images and video. Digital video recorders, image-capture devices and colour printers can be used to document findings for publication, as well as for client and staff education. Camera costs vary dramatically depending upon offered features, with the more expensive units offering computer interface, programmable camera head buttons, parfocal zoom, multiple imaging chips and high definition (1920 x 1080 pixels). However, for practical purposes, the single-chip standard-definition cameras (800 x 640 pixels) are perfectly functional.

Mobile units

The Tele Pack Vet X system combines a hybrid xenon or LED light source, endovideo camera and 15" colour liquid crystal display with digital image/video capture and storage into a portable unit that is well suited for working in the field or when space is at a premium (Figure 10.6). An even more mobile (and less expensive) option is the battery-powered LED light source and C-Cam system (Figure 10.7). The LED battery light source is waterproof, fully immersible for cleaning and disinfection, and lasts approximately 2 hours. The C-Cam offers both S-video and USB outputs for connection to an external monitor, video printer, capture device or laptop computer.

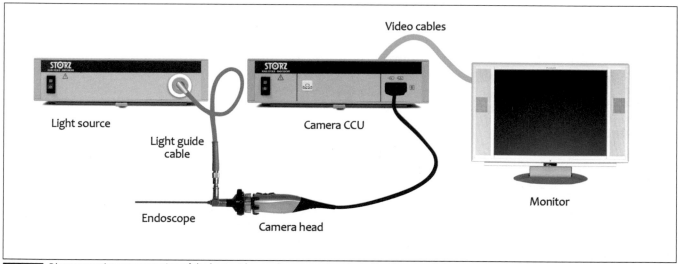

10.4 Diagrammatic representation of the basic video-endoscopy system including the essential components: a light source, camera and monitor.
(© Karl Storz GmbH & Co. KG)

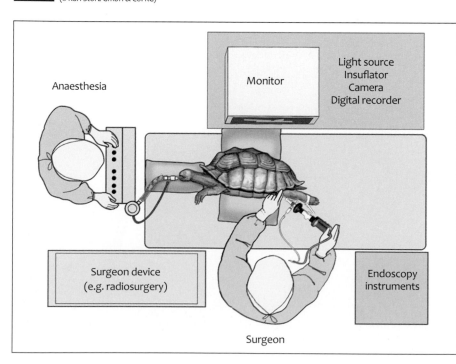

10.5 Correct ergonomic room layout for endoscopy. Note that the monitor and endoscopy equipment are facing the surgeon, with instruments close to the surgeon's superior (in this case, right) hand.
(© K Carter, University of Georgia)

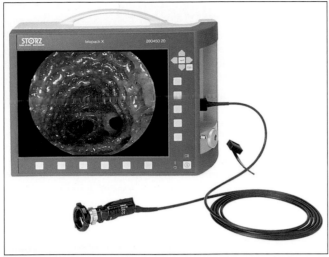

10.6 Tele Pack Vet X. This mobile unit comprises a standard-definition camera, hybrid xenon light source and air insufflation, and can be used with both rigid and flexible endoscopes.
(© Karl Storz GmbH & Co. KG)

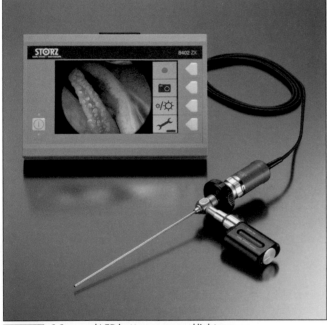

10.7 C-Cam and LED battery-powered light source.
(© Karl Storz GmbH & Co. KG)

Gas insufflation

Insufflation is essential to provide the lens–organ distance required for visceral visualization. For gastrointestinal endoscopy, air is used; however, for coelioscopy medical-grade carbon dioxide is preferred. Dedicated CO_2 insufflators, connected to a sheath or trocar port via a flexible gas line, provide precise control and maintain a constant coelomic pressure. For most reptiles a CO_2 flow rate of 0.2–1.0 l/min and a coelomic pressure of 2–5 mmHg are suitable. The higher insufflation pressures used in mammals will result in severe respiratory and cardiovascular compromise in most reptiles. Careful communication between the endoscopist and anaesthetist is required to ensure that adequate ventilation is achieved during prolonged procedures. For short procedures lasting less than 25 minutes (e.g. gender identification) ventilation is of minor concern.

An endoscopic air source (on some light sources and the Tele Pack Vet X) or an aquarium air pump can be used for crude air insufflation. They are not designed for creating a pneumocoelom, and in addition to the risks associated with air emboli, such air sources are not automatically controlled or adjusted to maintain desired patient pressures. The air pump is connected to one of the sheath ports, while the second port acts as an outflow valve. Crude insufflation control is achieved by partial closure of the outflow port or by using a finger to partially occlude this outflow port.

Fluid infusion and irrigation

When performing endoscopy within a hollow structure (e.g. bladder, cloaca, stomach) warmed sterile fluid infusion and irrigation (e.g. lactated Ringer's or sterile saline) often provides better clarity than air insufflation, and certainly provides improved mucosal detail. Warm (28–30°C) fluid bags are suspended above the endoscopy table and connected to one of the sheath ports using an intravenous infusion set. A second infusion set connects the other sheath port to a collection receptacle under the table. By turning the port valves on and off, the ingress and egress of fluid can be controlled by the endoscopist to maintain a clean field of view.

Radiosurgery and laser

As the complexity of endoscopic procedures increases, so does the requirement for accurate haemostasis. The modern Surgitron 4.0 MHz dual frequency radiosurgery unit (Ellman International Inc.) can be connected to various endoscopy instruments that permit both monopolar and bipolar radiosurgery. The more expensive CO_2 and diode lasers can also be used, but more stringent human health regulations relate to their use. Although the flexible quartz fibres used with diode lasers can be easily introduced into operating channels of most flexible and rigid endoscopes, the more rigid nature of CO_2 probes makes them less versatile. However, a CO_2 laser probe has been developed specifically for the 2.7 mm telescope and 4.8 mm sheath. The diode laser has unparalleled haemostatic ability, being able to seal blood vessels up to 2 mm in diameter; however, the CO_2 laser has the advantage of reduced penetration and collateral damage (Hernandez-Divers, 2002; Hernandez-Divers et al., 2009b). From both economical and most practical perspectives, there is little to challenge the superiority of radiosurgery for endoscopic applications, but whatever device is used, foot-pedal activation is vital to allow the endoscopist precise hands-free control.

Flexible endoscopy equipment

Flexible ureterocystoscopes and bronchoscopes (≤3 mm) are most useful for respiratory endoscopy in snakes or gastrointestinal endoscopy in small species where the 2.7 mm telescope is insufficient in length. Larger video gastroscopes (5.9 and 7.9 mm by 1.2–1.5 m) provide excellent image quality, and permit both air and fluid irrigation for larger reptiles. Some Karl Storz cameras and light sources are now compatible with both rigid and flexible endoscopes, and therefore, for the first time, the private practitioner can invest in just a single endoscopy camera and light source that will permit both rigid and flexible endoscopy.

Equipment care, storage and preparation

The monitor, light source, camera, digital still/video recorders, insufflator and CO_2 cylinders are best stored on a mobile cart or tower (Figure 10.8). Scopes, sheaths, trocars and instruments should be cleaned using a neutral pH enzymatic cleaner and suitable brushes, rinsed with distilled or deionized water, and dried before storage in approved instrument containers. It is essential to use properly sterilized equipment to prevent postoperative infection. Autoclaving is certainly practical for modern telescopes that are manufactured to be autoclavable, but permanent damage will result if they are not. The two most commonly used options are gas sterilization (e.g. ethylene oxide or hydrogen peroxide) and cold sterilization (e.g. 2% glutaraldehyde solution). Endoscope equipment should not be soaked in any solution for more than 30 minutes, and sterile water is used to rinse off residual glutaraldehyde before patient use. Always follow the endoscopy manufacturer's recommendations regarding cleaning and disinfection, and practitioners should expect detailed instructions from their suppliers.

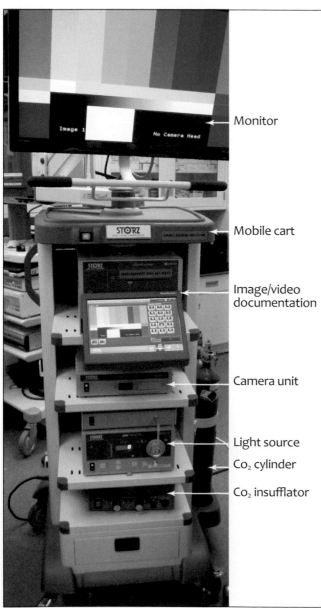

Monitor

Mobile cart

Image/video documentation

Camera unit

Light source
CO_2 cylinder
CO_2 insufflator

10.8 Endoscopy tower capable of both rigid and flexible endoscopy. (© SJ Divers, University of Georgia)

Diagnostic endoscopy

General anaesthesia is recommended for all endoscopy procedures. Certain examinations (e.g. buccal cavity and cloaca) may be possible in the conscious or sedated patient using a mouth gag or other appropriate restraint, but complete immobilization is preferred to avoid risking damage to equipment, patient or staff.

Some consideration should be given to the design and layout of the operating room. In general, the endoscopy cart/tower should be positioned directly in front of the primary surgeon with instruments close to hand (see Figure 10.5). Although an assistant is often useful, the author trains veterinary surgeons (veterinarians) to perform diagnostic techniques as single-surgeon procedures because this is often the reality in private practice. At the other end of the spectrum, both private and institutional referral practices are investing in dedicated endoscopy operating-room systems. Such systems (e.g. OR-1 use ceiling booms to support endoscopy equipment and integrate centralized control to manage endoscopic and peripheral devices. This system permits viewing; display; documentation; and communication from video and other data sources in and out of the operating room, including teleconferencing, resident teaching, telesurgery, and networking with hospital systems like PACS (picture archiving and communication system), HIS (hospital information system) or RIS (radiology information system).

The general handling technique when using the rigid telescope is to support the base of the telescope, eyepiece and camera with the superior hand, while the terminal end of the telescope and sheath are held by the thumb and forefinger of the inferior hand. Handling the telescope in this fashion provides fine control without tremor (Figure 10.9).

Oral and upper gastrointestinal endoscopy

For oral approaches to the buccal cavity and upper gastro-intestinal (GI) tract, sternal or dorsal recumbency with head and neck extended is required. It is helpful to have the reptile positioned close to the table edge so that the light guide cable is not in contact with the table surface.

The rigid telescope–sheath system can be used to examine the buccal cavity, oesophagus and stomach of small lizards, crocodilians and chelonians (Figure 10.10a–b). Flexible endoscopes are required for almost all snakes and larger reptiles of other orders and left lateral recumbency tends to permit better evaluation down to the proximal small intestine in some cases (Figure 10.10c–d). Air is generally used to dilate the intestine, which provides good exposure for detecting gross lesions and foreign bodies. Warm saline irrigation provides superior clarity especially when examining for mucosal detail, and tracheal intubation is essential to avoid aspiration of irrigation fluid. Whether air or fluid is used, it is important to gently dilate the tract as the telescope is advanced to avoid damage and laceration to the intestinal wall. Oesophagoscopy can be useful to help place, verify position of and evaluate issues associated with an oesophagostomy tube.

Cloacoscopy (lower gastrointestinal and urogenital systems)

The reptile can be positioned in dorsal or ventral recumbency with the tail extended to expose the vent. Rigid telescopes and warm saline irrigation are preferred for

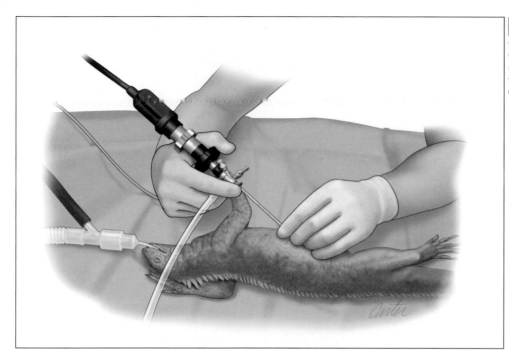

10.9 Standard two-handed endoscopy technique. Note that the superior hand supports the weight of the telescope–sheath–camera unit while the thumb and forefinger of the inferior hand control the tip.
(© K Carter, University of Georgia)

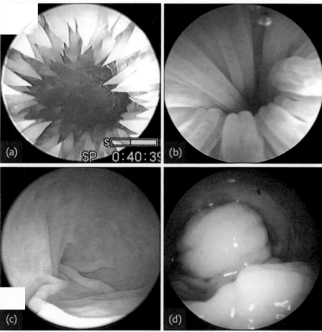

10.10 Upper GI tract. (a) Air-dilated oesophagus of a loggerhead sea turtle, demonstrating papillae characteristic of most sea turtles. (b) Saline-irrigated oesophagus of a green iguana. (c) Air-dilated stomach of a savannah monitor. (d) Air-dilated stomach of a corn snake, demonstrating a leiomyoma at the pylorus.
(© SJ Divers, University of Georgia)

cloacoscopy, and permit examination of the proctodeum, urodeum and coprodeum. Detailed appraisal of the cloacal mucosa, urogenital papillae, and, when present, the urethral opening and oviductal openings is possible (Figure 10.11). With practice, the endoscope can be directed through the urethra into the thin-walled bladder in chelonians and certain lizards. It is also possible to enter the distal oviducts of female reptiles, especially if they are reproductively active or suffering from oviductal disease. More recently, neonate gender identification by indirectly observing the gonads through the bladder wall has been suggested (Selleri *et al.*, 2013). This technique has the advantage of avoiding entry into the coelomic cavity but, because examination is through a membrane, may not be as sensitive or reliable as direct coelioscopic visualization (Hernandez-Divers *et al.*, 2009a). In addition, more recent research has demonstrated major safety issues (perforation) for transbladder gender identification in at least one species (Proença and Divers, 2014).

Pulmonoscopy (upper and lower respiratory systems)

Depending upon the size of the reptile, a 2.7, 1.9 or 1.0 mm endoscope can be used to examine the upper respiratory tract of most lizards, chelonians and snakes (Figure 10.12a–b). It is always preferable to protect the 1.9 and 2.7 mm rigid telescopes with a sheath but the increased diameter may be prohibitive. Rigid telescopes of sufficient length can usually be directed into the lungs of lizards by careful manipulation of the lizard's head, neck and body (Figure 10.12c). For larger reptiles, especially most snakes, fine-diameter flexible endoscopes will permit a deeper examination, including the lungs via a glottal approach (Figure 10.12d). The reptile is positioned in sternal recumbency, with head and neck extended. A mouth gag is recommended to guard against a lightly anaesthetized reptile from biting down on the endoscope. The endoscope should be gently inserted into the glottis and then driven under direct visual control to avoid damaging the mucosa. Complete tracheal occlusion for several minutes is well tolerated by anaesthetized reptiles. Although there is no need to provide intermittent ventilation, it can be helpful to dilate the lungs to provide better visualization.

A transcutaneous approach to the lungs of snakes has also been described (Jekl and Knotek, 2006; Stahl *et al.*, 2008). This involves a mini-coeliotomy approximately 40–50% from snout to vent, on the right side (or left/right side for boas and pythons because they have two lungs). Following a 1 cm skin incision, and blunt dissection through an intercostal space, the lung is identified as it is ventilated, grasped, secured and punctured using a

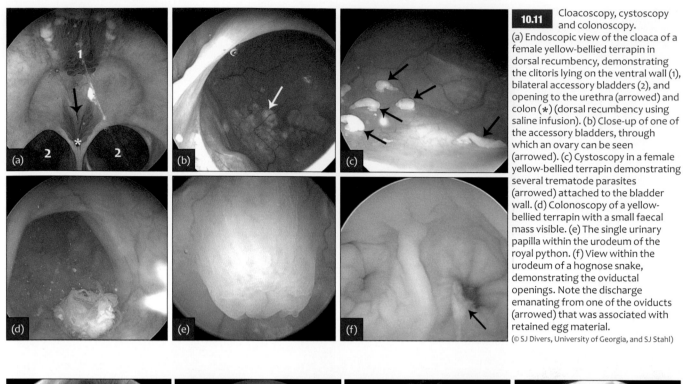

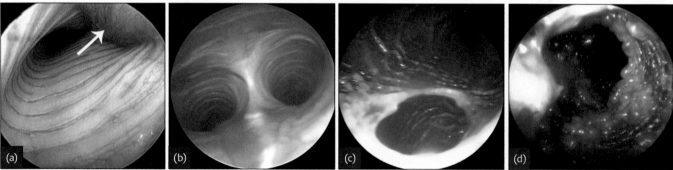

10.12 Transglottal pulmonoscopy. (a) Royal python trachea with obvious dorsal ligament (arrowed). (b) Tracheal bifurcation and primary bronchi in a green iguana. (c) Compartmentalized lung in a panther chameleon. (d) Granulomatous pneumonia due to *Mycobacterium* spp. in a royal python.
(© SJ Divers, University of Georgia)

scalpel blade or mosquito haemostats before insertion of the telescope (Figure 10.13a). In larger boids, a flexible endoscope can be inserted and advanced craniad and caudad to examine most of the unilateral pulmonary system. Lung and skin are closed as separate layers using single sutures. This technique has been thoroughly evaluated in royal pythons, where the surgical approach and visualization of the distal portion of the trachea; primary bronchus; intrapulmonary bronchus; cranial lung lobe; and faveolar, semisaccular and saccular lung regions were considered excellent (Figure 10.13b–e) (Stahl *et al.*, 2008). This study also evaluated faveolar biopsy specimens collected using 1.7 mm biopsy forceps and concluded that the diagnostic quality of specimens that were shaken from biopsy forceps into physiological saline solution before fixation in 10% formalin was superior to those manually removed from the biopsy forceps using a moistened cotton-tipped applicator. Re-evaluation of the same snakes a year later confirmed complete healing of the previous entry and biopsy sites with no clinically apparent deleterious effects.

A tracheal approach to the chelonian lung can be particularly challenging because of the narrow trachea and meandering primary bronchi. It is possible in larger species (e.g. sea turtles) using fine flexible endoscopes, but generally not in smaller specimens. Two alternative approaches to the chelonian lung have been developed (Divers, 2014a). The first requires a 5 mm temporary osteotomy in the carapace over the suspected lesion, pinpointed by radiography, computed tomography (CT) or magnetic resonance imaging (MRI) (Figure 10.14a). The pleuropulmonary membrane is punctured using a sharp trocar or mosquito haemostats while the animal is held at maximal inspiration. Leakage of anaesthetic gases confirms entry into the lung, and additional anaesthetic gas scavenging should be positioned close to the pneumotomy site. The sheathed telescope can be inserted into the lung for examination (Figure 10.14b–c). Following endoscopy the osteotomy can be temporarily maintained with a catheter and injection cap to permit intrapneumonic therapy. Alternatively, the osteotomy can be closed using the same epoxy or acrylic compounds that are employed for plastronotomy or shell repair. The covering can be removed after 8–12 weeks. A second method involves a surgical approach to the caudolateral lung via a craniodorsal prefemoral incision. Following a small craniodorsal prefemoral coeliotomy, the caudolateral aspect of the ventral lung is identified during ventilation. While at maximal ventilation, stay sutures are placed to hold the lung close to the prefemoral area,

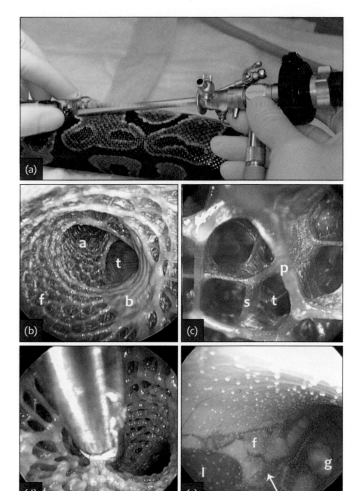

and a small stab incision is made through an avascular window into the lung (Figure 10.15a). The telescope is then inserted and the examination can proceed (Figure 10.15b–c). Upon withdrawal, the lung must be sutured to avoid post-operative pneumocoelom. This can often be most easily accomplished by using one (or both) of the stay sutures in a circumferential manner.

Coelioscopy

Precise positioning for coelioscopy depends upon the type of reptile, the structure(s) of particular interest and the preferences of the endoscopist (Hernandez-Divers et al., 2005a; Divers, 2010, 2014a). The entry site is aseptically prepared and draped, and adhesive clear plastic drapes are preferred because they permit better visualization of the patient.

Chelonians

- Generally performed in front of the pelvic limb through the prefemoral fossa.
- CO_2 insufflation is not essential, but often helpful.
- Single entry permits examination of most organs, including liver and kidneys.
- It is important to remove CO_2 before single suture and/or tissue adhesive closure of skin.

The most useful coelioscopic approach in tortoises, turtles and terrapins is via the left or right prefemoral fossa with the animal supported in lateral recumbency (Divers et al., 2010; Divers 2014a). Right-handed surgeons will generally find it easier to enter the left prefemoral fossa, and left-handed surgeons the right. In general, unless diagnostic imaging or organ asymmetry dictates a left or right approach, the surgeon's preference can prevail. A large bladder can hinder coelioscopy and chelonians should be encouraged to urinate prior to surgery. This can be achieved by bathing the animal, or by gentle digital manipulation of the cloaca prior to premedication and anaesthesia.

The pelvic limb is retracted and taped caudad to expose the prefemoral fossa (Figure 10.16). In chelonians with a well developed plastron hinge (e.g. box turtles), it is wise to place a wedge between the caudal plastron and carapace to maintain exposure. Following aseptic

10.13 Royal python transcutaneous pulmonoscopy. (a) Sheathed 2.7 mm telescope inserted through the lateral body wall and introduced into the lung of a research python that has not been draped for photographic purposes. (b) View of the cranial lung demonstrating the distal trachea (t), intrapulmonary bronchus (b), anterior lung lobe (a) and the faveolar lung tissue (f). (c) Close-up view of the faveolar region demonstrating the primary (p), secondary (s) and tertiary (t) septae of the anterior vascular lung. (d) Lung biopsy using the 1.7 mm biopsy forceps. (e) View of the thin transparent caudal air sac through which the caudal edge of the liver (l), fat body (f), gastrointestinal tract (g) and caudal vena cava (arrowed) can be seen.
(© SJ Divers, University of Georgia)

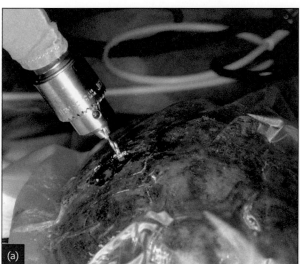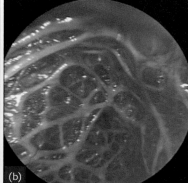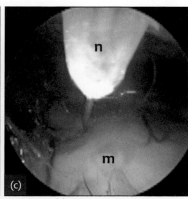

10.14 Chelonian transcarapacial pulmonoscopy. (a) Drilling a 5 mm temporary osteotomy through the carapace of a spur-thighed tortoise to access the lung. (b) Normal view of the chelonian lung through the temporary osteotomy. (c) Fine-needle aspiration (n) of a pulmonary mass (m) within the lung of a juvenile loggerhead sea turtle.
(© SJ Divers, University of Georgia)

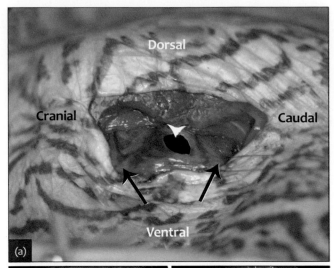

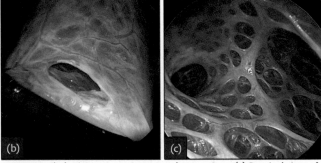

10.15 Chelonian transcutaneous pulmonoscopy. (a) Surgical view of the prefemoral fossa of a map turtle following a mini-coeliotomy incision. Two fine stay sutures (arrowed) have been placed to elevate the lung to the skin incision, and a small stab incision has been made through an avascular window of the lung (arrowhead).
(b) Endoscopic view of the surface of the lung held by stay sutures, following stab incision. (c) Endoscopic view from within the lung of a chelonian.
(© SJ Divers, University of Georgia)

preparation, a small (4 mm) craniocaudal skin incision is made in the centre of the prefemoral fossa. The subcutaneous fat and connective tissues are bluntly dissected using straight haemostats down to the coelomic aponeurosis (formed by the broad tendinous portions of the transverse and oblique abdominal muscles), being careful to remain cranial to the sartorius muscle of the pelvic limb, and ventral to the iliacus muscle that lies between the femur and ventral surface of the ilium. The coelomic aponeurosis is penetrated by advancing the sheath and obturator (or straight haemostats) towards the midpoint of the cranial rim of the carapace. Some force is often required, and it is important to direct the telescope craniad, and not ventrad (which increases the risk of damage to the bladder or intestinal tract). With the telescope tip positioned within the coelom, passive or active insufflation creates a pneumocoelom to aid visualization.

The dark red-brown to tan-yellow liver is the most obvious organ to use for orientation (Figure 10.17a). The heart is ventral to the liver and partially obscured by a prominent pericardium (Figure 10.17b). The stomach is most prominent on the left, while the small intestinal tract, pancreas, right liver lobe, gall bladder and, less easily, the spleen are visible on the right (Figure 10.17c–d). The colon, gonads, oviducts (in females), bladder and kidneys can be viewed from either side. The bladder is situated in the most dependent area, while the ovaries and oviducts of reproductively active females can occupy much of the coelom (Figure 10.18a). The male testes, yellow to brown in colour, are situated in the caudodorsal coelom, and the vas deferens and epididymis can often be identified (Figure 10.18b). The kidneys are retrocoelomic, residing behind the coelomic membrane, but they are closely associated with the male testes, which aids identification. In females with pigmented coelomic membranes, it can be challenging to locate the kidneys (Figure 10.18c–d).

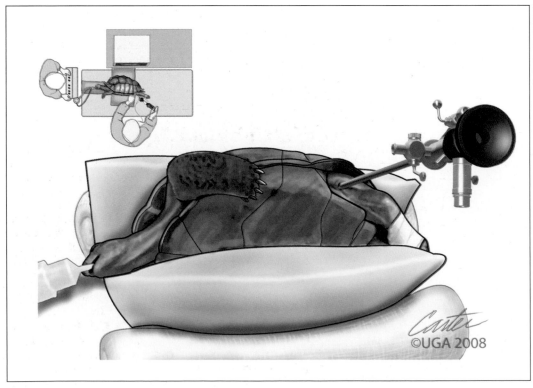

10.16 Operating room layout and positioning for a left prefemoral approach (in front of the left pelvic limb) in order to access the chelonian coelomic cavity.
(© Kip Carter, University of Georgia)

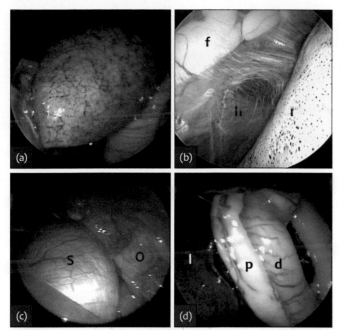

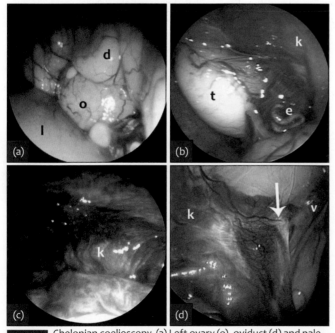

10.17 Chelonian coelioscopy, left prefemoral approach. (a) Normal liver in a female radiated tortoise. (b) Heart (h) and pericardial fat (f) behind the coelomic membrane of a yellow-bellied terrapin. Note the pale liver (l) within the coelomic cavity. (c) Stomach (s) and oviduct (o) in a red-footed tortoise. (d) Liver (l) and pancreas (p), with closely associated duodenum (d) in a male red-eared terrapin.
(© SJ Divers, University of Georgia)

10.18 Chelonian coelioscopy. (a) Left ovary (o), oviduct (d) and pale liver (l) in a female spur-thighed tortoise (left prefemoral approach). (b) Left testis (t), epididymis (e) and kidney (k) in a male red-eared terrapin (left prefemoral approach). (c) Enlarged left kidney (k) behind a pigmented coelomic membrane but protruding into the coelom in a female leopard tortoise (left prefemoral approach). (d) Normal right kidney (k) clearly visible behind a transparent coelomic membrane, adrenal (arrowed) and renal (v) vein in a female yellow-bellied terrapin (right prefemoral approach).
(© SJ Divers, University of Georgia)

An objective evaluation of coelioscopy of freshwater turtles including visceral biopsy has been published (Divers *et al.*, 2010). This study evaluated the ability of the 2.7 mm telescope to visualize the coelomic viscera of red-eared and yellow-bellied terrapins, and perform diagnostic biopsies on liver and kidney. Ease of entry and organ visualization were satisfactory to excellent for all observed structures, except the spleen, which could only be reliably located from the right side.

Recently, saline-infusion coelioscopy has been shown to be accurate for identifying gender in hatchling and neonate chelonians before gender identification by external means is possible or reliable (Hernandez-Divers *et al.*, 2009a). Such approaches are invaluable to breeders and conservationists involved in head-start programmes because gender bias is a real concern due to temperature-dependent gender determination in most chelonians. To date, these techniques have been used to identify gender in hundreds of neonates (6–18 months of age), including Chinese box turtles, radiated tortoises, Bolson tortoises, Hermann's tortoises, desert tortoises, Galapagos tortoises and Aldabran tortoises (Figure 10.19).

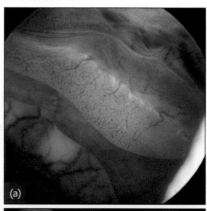

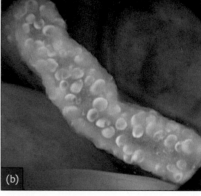

10.19 Neonate chelonian gender identification using a 1.9 mm telescope and saline infusion. (a) Immature testis in a male radiated tortoise weighing 70 g. (b) Immature ovary in a female Chinese box turtle weighing 20 g.
(© SJ Divers, University of Georgia)

Lizards

- Often performed with the lizard in dorsal or lateral recumbency depending upon body conformation, primary structures of interest and the surgeon's preference.
- CO_2 insufflation is essential.
- Lateral entry permits examination of most organs, including liver, gonads and kidneys.
- It is important to remove CO_2 before single-suture closure of skin.

Given the relatively small size of most pet lizards, a single entry point, either in a paramedian or paralumbar area, will usually permit examination of many, if not all, of the coelomic structures of interest. Research in green iguanas concluded that endoscope entry, insufflation and general coelomic visualization were straightforward and safe (Hernandez-Divers *et al.*, 2004). There was no significant difference in visualization of lung, liver, pancreas, small intestine, large intestine, ovary, oviduct, testis, epididymis, vas deferens, bladder, fat body or kidney from either left or right lateral approaches. However, a left lateral approach to the heart, stomach and spleen, and a right lateral approach to the gall bladder and right adrenal gland were favoured. A left paralumbar approach is described and is generally preferred by right-handed surgeons unless anatomy, physical examination or other diagnostic tests dictate a right approach.

The iguana is positioned in right lateral recumbency, with the left pelvic limb taped caudad against the tail base. The entry area is bordered craniad by the ribs, dorsad by the lateral processes of the spine, caudad by the pelvic limb and ventrad by the pelvic and abdominal veins (Figure 10.20). Aseptically, a 4 mm skin incision is made in the centre of the defined area. The skin and underlying muscle are grasped and elevated away from the coelomic viscera and the sheath and obturator (or straight haemostats) are gently forced through the thin muscular wall and into the coelomic cavity. It is wise to temporarily cease ventilation until the telescope has been introduced into the coelom, thereby reducing the possibility of damage to an inflated lung. By making a small skin incision with blunt entry into the coelom, the sheath will be tight fitting and insufflation gas leakage will be minimal. Once in place the obturator is removed and replaced with the telescope. Once inserted and following creation of a pneumocoelom, it may be necessary to gently touch the tip of the telescope against a serosal membrane to clean the terminal lens of condensation or tissue fluid. If there is fat or blood on the lens, it may be necessary to remove the telescope, leaving the sheath *in situ*, and clean with sterile damp gauze before continuing. Do not persist with a dirty lens; poor vision is the endoscopist's enemy that will reduce surgical ability and increase procedure time far more than the time required to clean the telescope.

Upon left paralumbar entry into the iguanid, the first organ to note is the large brown liver lying in the mid-ventral coelom (Figure 10.21a). Advancing the telescope craniad will reveal the heart at the cranioventral aspect of the coelom, close to the cranial coelomic inlet (Figure 10.21b). There are no diaphragmatic, postpulmonary or longitudinal membranes in the iguanids. These membranes do exist to a greater or lesser extent in other species, especially tegus and monitors. Minor perforation of these membranes by the telescope will not cause any harm, but care is required not to damage viscera in the process. These membrane penetrations do not need to be repaired. Dorsal to the heart and extending from coelomic inlet to mid-coelom are the paired lungs (Figure 10.21b–c). Lung ventilation will be substantially reduced during insufflation and careful communication with the anaesthetist is required to balance inspiration and insufflation pressures. Caudal to the lungs, in the mid-coelom, is the stomach (Figure 10.21d), with the spleen, an elongated dark red organ in iguanas, situated close behind (Figure 10.22a). Careful examination deep to the stomach and spleen may reveal the splenic limb of the pancreas.

The gonads are located just caudal to the spleen either side of dorsal midline (Figure 10.22a–c). Rigid endoscopy can be utilized to determine the gender of reptiles, even at a very early age. This is extremely useful in monomorphic species of lizard (e.g. blue tongue skinks, prehensile-tailed skinks, monitor lizards, gila monsters and beaded lizards) and has proven to be of value for breeders, as well as providing feedback on reproductive activity and disease. The testis is usually ovoid and smooth, and size often varies dramatically with season. The immature or inactive ovary appears as a cluster of small fluid-filled vesicles. As the ovary matures and becomes active, some of the follicles will enlarge as they fill with yolk, and appear yellow to orange in colour.

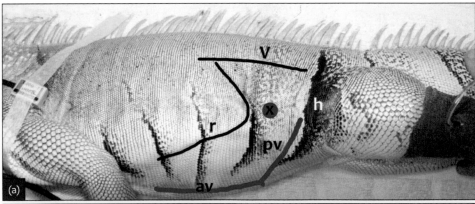

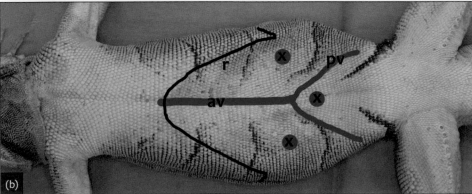

10.20 Telescope entry sites for coelioscopy in lizards. (a) For a lateral entry into the coelom, the general entry point (x) is bordered craniad by the last rib (r), dorsad by the lateral processes of the lumbar vertebrae (v), caudad by the musculature of the hindlimb (h), and ventrad by the ventral abdominal (av) and pelvic (pv) veins. (b) For a ventral approach to the coelom, insertion points (x) may be in the midline behind the anastomoses of the lateral pelvic veins (pv), or lateral to the ventral abdominal vein (av), caudal to the last rib (r) and cranial to the pelvic veins (pv). (© SJ Divers, University of Georgia)

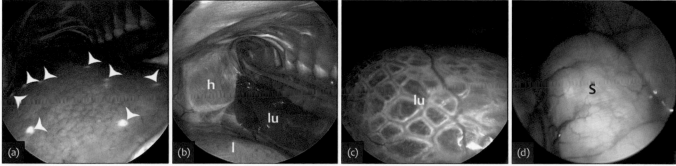

10.21 Left coelioscopy in the green iguana. (a) Ventral surface of the left liver lobe demonstrating multiple small granulomas (arrowheads). (b) Heart (h), liver (l) and deflated left lung (lu). (c) Inflated lung (lu) – note the absence of any postpulmonary membrane in iguanid lizards. (d) Stomach (s).
(© SJ Divers, University of Georgia)

Dorsal to the gonads are the adrenal glands, lying adjacent to the renal veins (Figure 10.22a–b). The vas deferens of males and oviducts of females are also visible and can be followed caudally to the pelvic inlet (Figure 10.22c–d). It is more difficult, but nevertheless always possible, to examine the normal kidneys of healthy iguanas even though they reside largely within the pelvic canal (Figure 10.22d). Moving ventrally from the pelvic inlet, the endoscopist will encounter the bladder and fat body.

On the right side, the heart is partially obscured by the ascending or caudal vena cava (Figure 10.23a). The pancreas is easier to locate via a right approach, residing close to the midventral region, caudal to the liver and gall bladder, and intimately associated with the duodenum (Figure 10.23b–c). A left paralumbar approach will reveal the small intestine and terminal colon; however, a right approach will provide access to the large sacculated colon (Figure 10.23d).

Snakes

- Coelioscopy is less commonly performed in snakes.
- CO_2 pneumocoelom is essential and visualization can be more difficult to achieve.
- Targeted approach permits restricted examination of limited viscera.
- Liver evaluation and biopsy are possible via a pulmonoscopy approach and through the caudal air sac membrane.

Snakes are less commonly subjected to coelomic endoscopy because:

- They have more diffuse coelomic fat
- It is impossible to examine all the major organs via a single approach
- Visualization, despite insufflation, is generally more difficult.

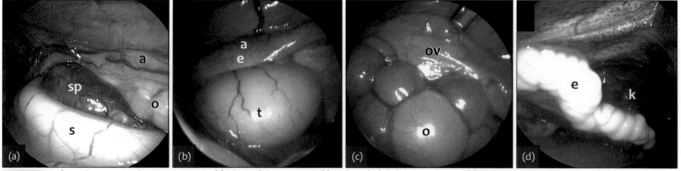

10.22 Left coelioscopy in the green iguana. (a) View of the stomach (s), spleen (sp), left adrenal gland (a) and immature left ovary (o). (b) Left testis (t), closely associated epididymis (e), and adrenal gland (a). (c) Mature left ovary (o) and oviduct (ov). (d) Left kidney (k) and epididymis (e), at the pelvic inlet.
(© SJ Divers, University of Georgia)

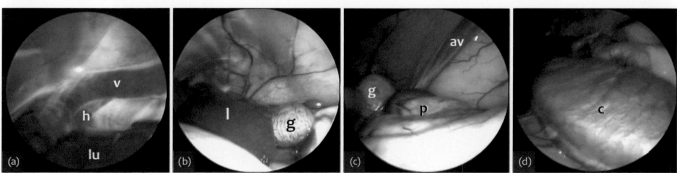

10.23 Right coelioscopy in the green iguana. (a) Heart (h) partially obscured by the caudal vena cava (v) and right deflated lung (lu). (b) Liver (l) and gall bladder (g). (c) Pancreas (p) situated caudal to the gall bladder (g). The ventral abdominal vein is also visible (av). (d) Large sacculated colon (c).
(© SJ Divers, University of Georgia)

However, if a targeted endoscopic approach to a single coelomic region is required, lateral positioning and entry between the first and second rows of lateral scales is suggested. In larger snakes, the telescope is inserted between the ribs, through the intercostal musculature. In smaller snakes, the telescope is directed through the coelomic musculature, just ventromedial to the ribs. A recently developed technique for liver biopsy entails access via the pulmonoscopy approach to the serpentine air sac. From within the air sac it is possible to visualize and perform a biopsy of the liver (Figure 10.24). Obviously, CO_2 insufflation is contraindicated and lung insufflation is maintained by anaesthesia.

Sampling techniques

In reptiles, a variety of pathologies may be appreciated endoscopically, often with surprisingly few clinicopathological or discernible radiographic or ultrasonographic changes. Ongoing studies at the University of Georgia appear to indicate a superiority of endoscopic biopsies over ultrasonography-guided aspirates for the diagnosis of experimentally induced liver disease in iguanas (Hernandez-Divers et al., 2007; Schnellbacher and Divers, unpublished data). In addition, ultrasound-guided liver biopsies in snakes and iguanas have resulted in significant morbidity and mortality.

When an abnormal structure or pathological lesion is observed, endoscopic biopsy can be performed under direct visual control (Figure 10.25a–b). Biopsy samples can be harvested from most organs and, in general, any abnormal soft-tissue structure (although aspiration should precede biopsy when dealing with potentially fluid-filled structures). In order to insert and manipulate the instruments it is necessary to change from a two-handed hold to a one-handed grip of the rigid endoscope. The previous thumb and forefinger support of the sheath tip is adjusted so that the inferior hand takes the entire weight of the sheath–telescope–camera system. The thumb is slid up the shaft of the sheath, and the fingers are curled over the top to encircle the sheath. With the sheath grasped in a fist-like grip with further support by the thumb to prevent rotation, the superior hand can be used to manipulate an instrument down the operating channel (Figure 10.25c). This can only be performed using a correctly sheathed telescope – damage will occur to an improperly sheathed or unsheathed telescope due to bending and fracture of the glass rods.

The 1.7 mm grasping forceps are useful for manipulating tissues, debridement and retrieving foreign objects, including parasites. The fine aspiration/injection needle can be used for the aspiration of fluid from cystic structures where biopsy may be contraindicated owing to post-sampling leakage. The remote injection needle can

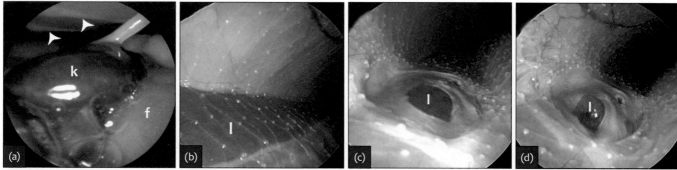

10.24 Snake coelioscopy. (a) Left lateral approach, 82% snout to vent, revealing the caudal pole of the left kidney (k), fat body (f) and ribs (arrowhead) in a boa constrictor. (b) Ball python liver (l) viewed from within the air sac of the right lung. (c) The air sac and serosal membranes have been incised to expose the liver parenchyma (l). (d) View of the liver (l) following biopsy using 1.7 mm forceps.
(© SJ Divers, University of Georgia)

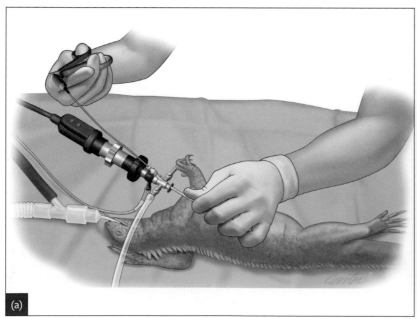

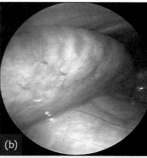

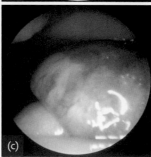

10.25 Biopsy. (a) Diagram illustrating the technique used to support the camera–sheath–telescope with the inferior hand, while the superior hand can manipulate instruments within the channel of the operating sheath. (b) Enlarged liver in a green iguana due to bacterial hepatitis. (c) Enlarged kidney in a veiled chameleon due to glomerulonephritis.
(© SJ Divers, University of Georgia)

also be used for targeted drug administration. The 1.7 mm biopsy forceps are used to harvest tissue samples for histopathology and microbiology in patients as small as 30 g. The small sample size usually permits the collection of several biopsy samples for multiple laboratory tests, and the use of serial biopsies to monitor disease progression over time. To take a tissue sample, the biopsy forceps are inserted down the operating channel and into the middle of the field of view (Figure 10.26). It is much easier to advance and manipulate the sheath–telescope–instrument as a single device than to try to keep the sheath–telescope still and independently move the biopsy forceps back and forth. With the biopsy forceps held open, the sheath–telescope–instrument is advanced to the tissue of interest and, when tissue enters the biopsy cup, the handle is released. These instruments are delicate and the biopsy handle is only required to open the biopsy jaws. The handle's spring mechanism is often sufficient to perform a soft-tissue biopsy with minimal manual pressure, as long as the instrument is sharp. Clamping down on the handle will damage the forceps and increase biopsy crush artefact. Some organs may be protected by a more fibrous membrane. The fixed blade of the scissors is inserted at a shallow angle through the membrane, and the sheath–telescope–scissors are advanced as a single unit, cutting the membrane as it proceeds (Figure 10.26c). The scissors can then be replaced by the biopsy forceps to take a sample through the capsular incision (Figure 10.26d). This technique has been validated for the collection of diagnostic kidney and liver samples from lizards and chelonians, and lung biopsy samples from snakes (Hernandez-Divers, 2004; Hernandez-Divers *et al.*, 2005b, 2007; Stahl *et al.*, 2008; Divers *et al.*, 2010).

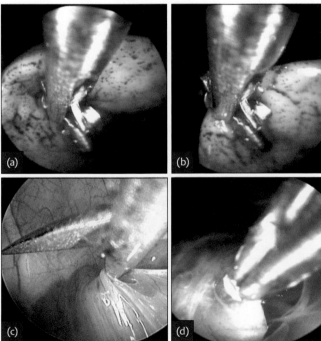

10.26 Liver and kidney biopsy in chelonians. (a) The biopsy forceps are positioned under, and used to elevate, the caudal edge of the liver. (b) The sheath–telescope–forceps is withdrawn slightly until the edge of the liver falls into the open biopsy jaws, and a biopsy sample is collected. (c) The fixed blade of the single-action scissors is inserted through the coelomic membrane over the kidney. (d) The biopsy forceps can then be inserted through this incision to collect a biopsy sample from the kidney. (© SJ Divers, University of Georgia)

Minimally invasive endosurgery

Recent advances in minimally invasive endosurgery have been possible by expanding the diagnostic system already described with the addition of 3 mm human paediatric laparoscopy instrumentation (Figure 10.27). Orchidectomy, oophorectomy (immature) and mass/cyst resection, as well as an assortment of endoscope-assisted procedures including oophorectomy (mature), enterotomy, enterectomy and cystotomy have become possible (Divers, 2014b). While true intracorporeal procedures (i.e. endosurgery completed within the coelom) are outside the purview of this general practice review, it is important to appreciate that they are provided by some referral centres. Endosurgical orchidectomy techniques for the green iguana, red-eared terrapin and desert tortoise have been developed (Innis *et al.*, 2013; Proença *et al.*, 2014) (Figure 10.28). In addition, endosurgical oophorectomy of immature Galapagos tortoises has also been described (Knafo *et al.*, 2011).

While intracorporeal endosurgery requires additional specialized equipment and a more highly developed surgical skill set, the reptile practitioner can certainly undertake endoscope-assisted procedures using the 2.7 mm system. Endoscope-assisted procedures utilize endoscopy to identify and exteriorize an organ or tissue of interest (often bladder, reproductive tract or intestinal tract) through a small prefemoral incision, thereby avoiding a major coeliotomy or plastronotomy. The actual surgical procedure is then performed using traditional techniques outside of the coelom. An excellent and practical example is endoscope-assisted oophorectomy in mature chelonians, which has proven to be safe and effective for sterilizing and treating reproductive disease in several species (Innis *et al.*, 2007; Knafo *et al.*, 2011; Divers, 2014b). With the chelonian in dorsal recumbency, a unilateral, prefemoral coeliotomy is performed, typically 2–3 cm in size (large enough to exteriorize the largest follicle). The telescope is inserted through the coeliotomy site, and used to identify the ipsilateral ovary (Figure 10.29a–b). Using the telescope to guide a pair of

- Coagulating dissecting needle[a]
- Monopolar coagulation needle[a]
- Bipolar forceps[a]
- Radiosurgery polypectomy snare, 1.7 mm (5Fr)[a]
- 3.5 mm x 5 cm trocar with leaf valve
- 3.5 mm x 5 cm trocar with stopcock and auto valve
- 3 mm grasping/dissecting forceps, plastic handle without racket
- 3 mm grasping forceps, plastic handle without racket
- 3 mm dissecting and grasping forceps, plastic handle without racket
- 3 mm dissecting and grasping forceps, plastic handle with racket
- 3 mm dissecting and biopsy forceps, plastic handle without racket
- 3 mm Babcock's with racket handle
- 3 mm scissors, plastic handle without racket
- Distensible palpation probe
- Palpation probe
- Irrigation/suction cannula
- Two-way stopcock
- Endoscope mechanical holding arm
- Equipment case suitable for safe storage and sterilization of the above equipment

10.27 Additional equipment required for entry-level endosurgery. Note that this list represents a selection of items that the author has found useful. However, there is a huge assortment of instruments available, and practitioners are advised to try equipment at conferences or trade shows or request in-practice demonstrations before purchase. [a] Separate radiosurgery unit required (e.g. 4.0 MHz Surgitron, Ellman International).

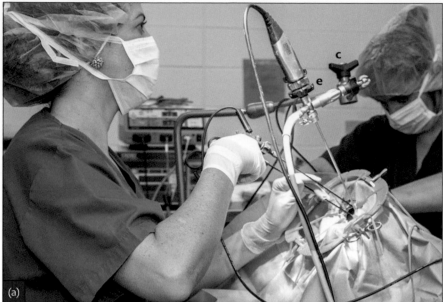

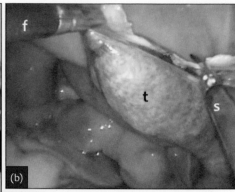

10.28 Endoscopic orchidectomy via the left prefemoral fossa in a chelonian. (a) A mechanical holding arm (c) supports the endoscope and camera (e), which permits the surgeon to, (b) utilize 3 mm grasping forceps (f) and monopolar scissors (s) to dissect the testis (t) free.
(© LM Proenca and SJ Divers, University of Georgia)

10.29 Endoscope-assisted oophorectomy in a terrapin. (a) Following a prefemoral surgical approach to the coelom, the telescope (t) and forceps (f) are introduced and used to locate the ipsilateral ovary. (b) Endoscopic view of the several ovarian follicles (o) associated with the ipsilateral ovary. The closely associated bladder (b) and colon (c) are also visible. (c) Atraumatic 3 mm forceps (f), or long haemostats, are used to grasp the interfollicular tissue to avoid rupturing a follicle. (d) Gently, the ovary is retracted towards the prefemoral incision using the forceps (f). (e) Once the ovary is partially exteriorized the forceps and telescope are placed to one side and gentle digital retraction is used to exteriorize the entire ovary. (f) The ovarian ligament and associated vasculature are ligated before resecting the ovary free. The endoscope and forceps are then reinserted into the coelom to locate the contralateral ovary, which is removed in a similar fashion. A final endoscopic evaluation is performed to ensure adequate haemostasis and that all ovarian tissue has been removed. The coelom is closed in a routine manner.
(© SJ Divers, University of Georgia)

atraumatic forceps, the interfollicular tissue is grasped and the ovary gently elevated out of the prefemoral incision (Figure 10.29c–e). Once exteriorized, the ovarian vessels and mesovarian ligament are ligated, and the ovary dissected free (Figure 10.29f). For those species with large prefemoral fossae, it is generally possible to remove the contralateral ovary through the same prefemoral incision. Those species with very small fossae, voluminous bladders or large intestines may require a bilateral prefemoral approach. Similar endoscope-assisted procedures have been undertaken for the removal of retained eggs, bladder calculi and gastrointestinal foreign bodies. There appear to be significant reductions in surgical morbidity and improved recovery with these endoscopic procedures, compared with traditional coeliotomy and plastronotomy approaches.

Training and proficiency

Proficiency at endoscopy is not innate but the application of three-dimensional colour imagery combined with hand–eye coordination is something that we humans can do well. Interested veterinary surgeons are strongly encouraged to seek practical hands-on instruction at a dedicated endoscopy teaching facility, and courses are regularly offered at the conference of the Association of Reptilian and Amphibian Veterinarians and at the University of Georgia. Once trained, it is important to practice regularly, especially if caseload is initially low. To this end, practitioners are encouraged to keep endoscopy equipment non-sterile to encourage use with fresh cadavers. Indeed, many clients may be more accepting of an endoscopic (cosmetic) necropsy examination over a full necropsy of a beloved pet. Such a service also provides the veterinary surgeon with the ability to practice endoscopy without risk.

Summary

The benefits of endoscopy include visualization; inspection and sampling procedures; gender determination of juvenile or monomorphic species; therapies, including foreign-body removal; assessing response to treatment by serial examinations; and minimally invasive endoscopic surgery. Practical experience is essential to become competent with the basic techniques that are simple to learn and will quickly open doors to ante-mortem diagnoses that were previously elusive. Furthermore, continued development of endoscopic surgery in exotic species promises to reduce surgical morbidity, and holds considerable benefits to our small and delicate exotic patients. The endoscope is an essential tool for any veterinary surgeon dealing with reptiles (or any exotic species) on a regular basis.

Acknowledgments

Thanks to the dedicated technicians Carol McElhannon, Ashley Schuller and Nia Chau, and residents Drs Johanna Meija-Fava, Rodney Schnellbacher, Laila Proença, Izidora Sladakovic and my colleague Dr Joerg Mayer for their assistance and support. Mr Kip Carter (Educational Resources, University of Georgia) prepared Figures 10.5, 10.9, 10.16 and 10.25c, and Dr Scott Stahl (Stahl Exotic Animal Veterinary Services) kindly provided Figure 10.11f. Thanks also to Dr Christopher Chamness and Dan Mahon (Karl Storz Veterinary Endoscopy America Inc.) for their continued support of endoscopy research and development, and for providing Figures 10.4, 10.6 and 10.7.

Equipment for diagnostic endoscopy

All equipment used by the author clinically was purchased by (and not donated to) the Veterinary Teaching Hospital, University of Georgia. The author does not endorse or receive any payment from any particular manufacturer; however, Karl Storz is the sole source of equipment used by the author. Therefore, unless otherwise stated, all endoscopy equipment described in this chapter was manufactured by Karl Storz. Similar items are available from other manufacturers, and internet or second-hand bargains are certainly available; however, the general practitioner should be cognisant of variable compatibility and quality issues before making any capital investment.

References and further reading

Divers SJ (2010) Reptile diagnostic endoscopy and endosurgery. *Veterinary Clinics of North America: Exotic Animal Practice* **13**, 217–242

Divers SJ (2014a) Diagnostic endoscopy. In: *Current Therapy in Reptile Medicine and Surgery*, ed. DR Mader and SJ Divers, pp. 154–178. Elsevier, St Louis, MO

Divers SJ (2014b) Endoscope-assisted and endoscopic surgery. In: *Current Therapy in Reptile Medicine and Surgery*, ed. DR Mader and SJ Divers, pp. 179–196. Elsevier, St Louis, MO

Divers SJ (2014c) Video telescopic operating microscope: a recent development in reptile microsurgery. In: *Current Therapy in Reptile Medicine and Surgery*, ed. DR Mader and SJ Divers, pp. 213–216. Elsevier, St Louis, MO

Divers SJ, Stahl SJ and Camus A (2010) Evaluation of diagnostic coelioscopy including liver and kidney biopsy in Freshwater turtles (*Trachemys scripta*). *Journal of Zoo and Wildlife Medicine* **41**, 677–687

Hernandez-Divers SJ (2002) Diode laser surgery: principles and application in exotic animals. *Seminars in Avian and Exotic Pet Medicine* **11**, 208–220

Hernandez-Divers SJ (2004) Endoscopic renal evaluation and biopsy of Chelonia. *Veterinary Record* **154**, 73–80

Hernandez-Divers SJ, Hernandez-Divers SM, Wilson GH *et al.* (2005a) A review of reptile diagnostic coelioscopy. *Journal of Herpetological Medicine and Surgery* **15**, 16–31

Hernandez-Divers SJ, Stahl S, Hernandez-Divers SM *et al.* (2004) Coelomic endoscopy of the green iguana (*Iguana iguana*). *Journal of Herpetological Medicine and Surgery* **14**, 10–18

Hernandez-Divers SJ, Stahl S, Stedman NL *et al.* (2005b) Renal evaluation in the green iguana (*Iguana iguana*): Assessment of plasma biochemistry, glomerular filtration rate, and endoscopic biopsy. *Journal of Zoo and Wildlife Medicine* **36**, 155–168

Hernandez-Divers SJ, Stahl SJ and Farrell R (2009a) An endoscopic method for identifying sex of hatchling Chinese box turtles and comparison of general *versus* local anesthesia for coelioscopy. *Journal of the American Veterinary Medical Association* **234**, 800–804

Hernandez-Divers SJ, Stahl SJ, McBride M *et al.* (2007) Evaluation of an endoscopic liver biopsy technique in green iguanas. *Journal of the American Veterinary Medical Association* **230**, 1849–1853

Hernandez-Divers SJ, Stahl SJ, Rakich PM *et al.* (2009b) Comparison of CO_2 laser and 4·0 MHz radiosurgery for making incisions in the skin and muscles of green iguanas (*Iguana iguana*). *Veterinary Record* **164**, 13–15

Innis CJ, Feinsod R, Hanlon J *et al.* (2013) Coelioscopic orchiectomy can be effectively and safely accomplished in chelonians. *Veterinary Record* **172**, 526

Innis CJ, Hernandez-Divers S and Martinez-Jimenez D (2007) Coelioscopic-assisted prefemoral oophorectomy in chelonians. *Journal of the American Veterinary Medical Association* **230**, 1049–1052

Isaza R, Ackerman N. and Schumacher J (1993) Ultrasound-guided percutaneous liver biopsy in snakes. *Veterinary Radiology and Ultrasound* **34**, 452–454

Jekl V and Knotek Z (2006) Endoscopic examination of snakes by access through an air sac. *Veterinary Record* **158**, 407

Knafo SE, Divers SJ, Rivera S *et al.* (2011) Sterilisation of hybrid Galapagos tortoises (*Geochelone nigra*) for island restoration. Part 1: endoscopic oophorectomy of females under ketamine-medetomidine anaesthesia. *Veterinary Record* **168**, 47

Proença L and Divers SJ (2015) Comparison between coelioscopy *versus* cloacoscopy for gender identification in immature turtles (*Trachemys scripta*). In *Proceedings of the 2nd International Conference on Avian, Herpetological and Exotic mammal medicine*, Paris (France), p. 356

Proença LM, Fowler S, Kleine S *et al.* (2014). Single surgeon coelioscopic orchiectomy of desert tortoises (*Gopherus agassizii*) for population management. *Veterinary Record* **175(16)**, 403–410

Selleri P, Girolamo ND and Melidone R (2013). Cystoscopic sex identification of posthatchling chelonians. *Journal of the American Veterinary Medical Association* **242(12)**, 1744–1750

Stahl SJ, Hernandez-Divers SJ, Cooper TL *et al.* (2008) Evaluation of transcutaneous pulmonoscopy for examination and biopsy of the lungs of ball pythons and determination of preferred biopsy specimen handling and fixation procedures. *Journal of the American Veterinary Medical Association* **233**, 440–445

Specialist contacts and useful websites

Karl Storz Veterinary Endoscopy America Inc., 1 South Los Carneros Road, Goleta, CA 93117, USA

Karl Storz Veterinary Endoscopy (UK) Ltd, 415 Perth Avenue, Slough, Berkshire, SL1 4TQ, UK

Surgitron 4.0 MHz dual frequency radiosurgery unit, Ellman International Inc., 400 Karin Lane, Hicksville, NY 11801, USA

AccuVet Lasers at LuxarCare LLC, 16932 Woodinville-Redmond Rd NE, 11818 North Creek Parkway North, Suite 100, Bothell, WA 98011, USA

Association of Reptilian and Amphibian Veterinarians:
www.arav.org

University of Georgia:
www.vet.uga.edu/ce/calendar

Chapter 11

Therapeutics and medication

Sid Knotek

The class Reptilia is made up of between 8000 and 9000 different species of varying shapes, sizes and physiological idiosyncrasies. For ease of explanation in this chapter reptiles will be divided into three groups: snakes; lizards; and chelonians (tortoises and turtles) and the information will adopt a practical approach to choosing the most appropriate method of drug administration for treating disease. Detailed dose rates for individual medications are summarized in Appendix 2: Formulary; anaesthetics and analgesic drugs may also be found in Appendix 2 and in Chapter 12.

Methods of administering medication

When choosing the most appropriate method of administering medication in reptiles, the following criteria need to be considered:

- The particular medical problem and its ramifications
- Actual health status of the patient
- The safety of the selected administration procedure for staff and the patient, in case of repeated applications
- Pharmacokinetics and pharmacodynamics of the drug, so that the effective level of the active ingredient is achieved quickly and for the required period of time (if relevant information is obtainable)
- Information on the previous use of the drug in the same species or related groups of reptiles
- Possible interactions with other medications used in the patient
- Risks of side effects due to the medication and the means of minimizing this risk
- Market availability of the drug (or different forms of the same active ingredient)
- The necessity to administer the treatment, including application of the medication, by professional staff.

Bearing in mind these criteria, it should be noted that in the majority of cases the initial treatment is performed at the veterinary clinic. However, if home medication is necessary it may be possible to instruct and train experienced owners to safely administer the prescribed drugs at home.

Topical administration
Skin

Before using topical medications, it is often necessary to modify the conditions in the terrarium, especially by elimination of all forms of substrate that could adhere to the treated skin. The ideal substrate for the treatment period is clean paper, and a cardboard box can serve as an appropriate form of shelter (Figure 11.1). For cases where in-water topical or bathing medication is required it is important to limit alternative water reservoirs in the terrarium (we may, for example, temporarily empty all pools) and the water is provided for the patient in small bowls or by mist spraying appropriate to the species (e.g. chameleons).

The skin should be cleaned before applying any drug; remove any dirt including older remnants of epidermis that were not shed previously. Especially in snakes during the sloughing cycle a short bath in lukewarm water is recommended, and by gently pressing on the skin, old parts of

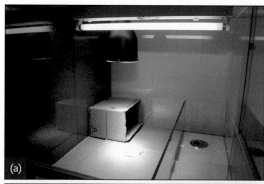

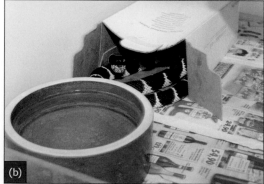

11.1 (a) The enclosure with clean paper substrate for a terrestrial reptile during the treatment period; (b) a cardboard box can serve as an appropriate form of shelter.

BSAVA Manual of Reptiles, third edition. Edited by Simon J. Girling and Paul Raiti. ©BSAVA 2019

the epidermis can be removed. Application of the drug directly onto the skin is mainly used during repeated treatments of superficial lesions and in topical or systemic therapy against ectoparasites. Despite the fact that reptile skin has a very specific anatomical structure and it is very resistant to penetration by solutions and other medication formulations, there is documented information about successful administration of antiparasitic drugs in the form of a spot-on preparation (emodepsid/praziquantel or imidacloprid/moxidectin, Brames, 2008; Schilliger *et al.*, 2009; Chitty and Raftery, 2013; Gibbons, 2014). The skin may also be more permeable, particularly in snakes, immediately after a slough has occurred.

For localized skin lesions, topical application of creams and ointments may be effective. They can be administered either directly on to the skin without any protection, or applied with a light bandage dressing for added protection (turtle carapaces, limbs of lizards and chelonians, and tails of lizards and snakes). Bandages placed on snake skin need to be fixed securely. This can mean using adhesive tape or elastic bandages or even suturing certain dressings to the skin itself.

Eyes

Eyes are covered by a transparent scale (brielle) in snakes and certain species of lizards (notably some geckos) thus preventing the use of topical eye medications for ocular problems in these species without removing a portion of the spectacle (see Chapter 16). Commercially formulated ophthalmic solutions and ointments with antimicrobial medications are available for use (Figure 11.2) and in patients with acute inflammatory conditions administration of ophthalmic ointments is an option. However, as *Pseudomonas* spp. bacteria are commonly part of the

normal bacterial flora in even healthy reptiles, extreme care should be taken to look for the development of melting ulcers particularly if the preparation contains corticosteroids. In general, therefore, these preparations should be avoided and antibiotic-only preparations used in preference; however, if a corneal stain is negative, then eye preparations containing a steroid are commonly very useful in reducing ocular inflammation.

Oral cavity

In patients where stomatitis is the primary disease, or it is a sign of a systemic disease, the first step in the course of treatment should include aggressive removal of necrotic lesions from the oral mucosa, which are often contaminated with food or substrate particles. In cases where abscesses or more severe lesions are discovered, surgical resection is advisable. The patient requires anaesthesia in the majority of cases or the use of local anaesthetic and analgesic medication. The effective topical treatment in the oral cavity can be achieved by rinses with heavily diluted disinfecting agents (0.05% chlorhexidine, 0.01% povidone iodine or F10® 1:250–500). The main emphasis, however, should be placed on systemic therapy once adequate debridement has been achieved.

Nostrils

The shape and patency of nostrils are of particular interest during examination of reptiles. In some iguanid and agamid lizards, nasal secretions from salt-excreting nasal glands are a normal finding. Especially in snakes (although not exclusively) the nostrils can be covered by old epidermis due to incomplete shedding. The most effective method to open the passages is based on a combination of gradually increasing the pressure exerted on the nasal cavity (Figure 11.3) and irrigating with sterile saline solution accompanied by suction of the blocking material. This procedure must be followed with repeated rinses of the nostrils with dilute disinfecting agents or antimicrobial ophthalmic solutions if infected, or sterile saline if not (Figure 11.4). If long-term topical application of solutions into the nostrils is recommended due to infection, a syringe can be used to administer the drug (0.3–0.5 ml) or alternatively the drug can be administered via a latex intravenous catheter, in preference to using a pipette.

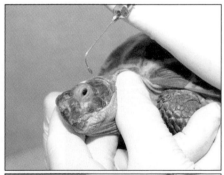

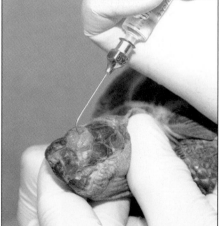

11.2 Using an ophthalmic needle to flush the eye of a Greek tortoise. Flushing can be done using either saline or an antibiotic solution depending on the situation and which disease is being treated. Anaesthesia, even local, is not necessary for this procedure.

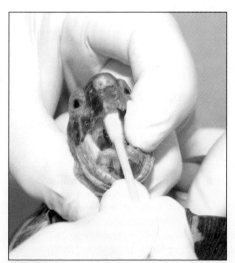

11.3 The most effective method to make the chelonian nostrils patent before flushing is by gradually increasing the pressure exerted on the rostral part of the soft palate.

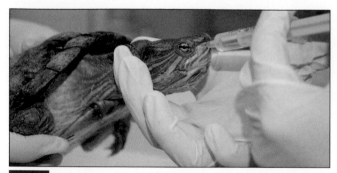

11.4 Using sterile saline to rinse the nostrils of a red-eared terrapin.

Cloaca

Local application of creams containing active ingredients (antiparasitics, antibiotics, antimycotics, anti-inflammatory drugs) into the reptile cloaca can be a useful adjunct to a systemic treatment (Innis, 1995) (Figure 11.5). Cloacal mucosa effectively absorbs variable substances and therefore a lavage with a low concentration of disinfectant solution (0.05% chlorhexidine, 0.01% povidone iodine or F10® 1:250) can be administered as a local treatment for cloacitis. However, absorption across the cloaca, can be unreliable as some animals void – as a reflex – any material inserted.

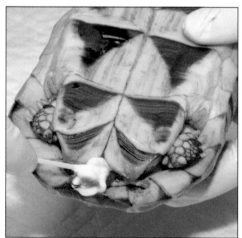

11.5 Topical administration of EMLA cream on the cloaca of a marginated tortoise.

Wounds

Wounds are relatively common in reptiles. When microbial agents are present in the wound, the lesions tend to become encapsulated and the formation of closed and walled-off granulomas ensue, requiring surgical treatment. In addition, systemic antimicrobial drug therapy and local administration of antimicrobials directly into the lesion can aid recovery. In the first stage of surgical therapy, local lavage with dilute disinfectants – 0.01% povidone iodine or F10® 1:250, is performed. Chlorhexidine solution is not effective against many Gram-negative organisms such as *Pseudomonas* spp. and needs to be used with care as there is some association with toxic reactions in reptiles. However, the author reports that he has not seen toxic reactions when using low concentrations of chlorhexidine solution. Therapy may be altered accordingly when the results of microbial testing are available. Medications in the form of powdered or heavily oil-based creams are, in these cases, inappropriate because they become wet and inactive (powders) and they limit the healing process (oils).

Systemic administration

The purpose of systemic drug administration is to achieve effective medication levels in the blood quickly and then maintain them for successful treatment. When considering the appropriate location for systemic drug administration, the important role the kidneys' play and their connection to blood circulation should not be underestimated. Unfortunately, iatrogenic kidney failure can be a sequel to insufficient rehydration of the patient during administration of nephrotoxic drugs (Figure 11.6). Aminoglycoside antibiotics, potentiated sulphonamides, tetracyclines and toltrazuril are all potentially nephrotoxic. The renal portal system (see Chapter 1) is the reason why drugs, particularly those removed by, or toxic to, the kidneys are in most cases injected into the frontal third of the body in snakes and into the forelimbs in chelonians and lizards. Fluid therapy using conventional infusion solutions (sterile saline, Ringer's solution or lactated Ringer's solution) can be administered subcutaneously with relative safety into the caudal region of the body (e.g. lateral skin in snakes, popliteal skin fold in chelonians and subcutaneous tissue of the pelvic limbs in lizards. (Figure 11.7).

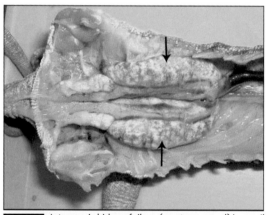

11.6 Iatrogenic kidney failure (gout, arrowed) in a veiled chameleon caused by administration of high doses of the nephrotoxic drug toltrazuril.

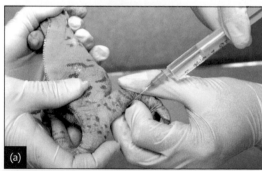

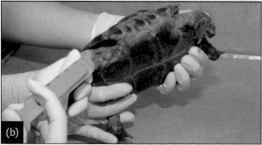

11.7 Fluid therapy infusions consisting of sterile saline, Ringer's solution or lactated Ringer's solution being administered subcutaneously in (a) the pelvic limb in a chameleon and (b) the prefemoral fossa in a Greek tortoise.

Oral administration

Oral administration of tableted medications is often unsuccessful. Tablets will not dissolve, reptiles will not actively swallow them and besides, they usually stick to the animal's oral mucosa and are eventually spat out. If a drug has to be administered orally, it is preferable to use a fine elastic tube, or a small syringe (without a needle) inserted deep into the oesophagus ensuring adequate lubrication with K-Y jelly or water. The end of a tube that will be inserted into the oral cavity and oesophagus or stomach can be blunted easily by holding the end briefly over a lighter flame and then applying pressure between thumb and forefinger (Figure 11.8). This rounds-off the tube end making it slightly wider. A syringe may be applied to the luer fitting end of the tube. Alternatively, avian crop tubes may be used to gavage liquid medications. In reptiles that swallow whole prey, and assuming they are still eating, tablets can be inserted into the body cavity of the prey item for ease of administration so making them an option. A similar technique can be used in herbivores by hiding tablets in the food but is clearly more difficult, making liquid formulations preferable.

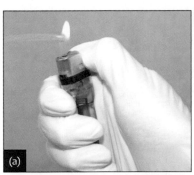

11.8 The end of a tube for insertion into the oral cavity and oesophagus is made blunt by (a) holding the tube briefly over a lighter flame. (b) After pressing the end of the tube gently between the fingers it becomes rounded and slightly wider.

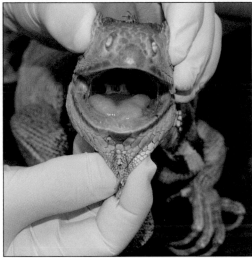

11.9 The mouth of an adult iguana can be opened by gently pulling the skin of the ventral dewlap at the same time as applying gentle pressure on both corners of the mouth.

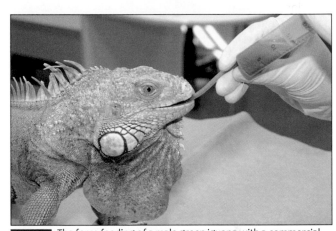

11.10 The force feeding of a male green iguana with a commercial herbivorous reptile diet.

Lizards: If it proves difficult to open the oral cavity in skinks, monitor lizards and some geckos, a flat plate with blunt edges can be used as a mouth gag. The plate is used to apply pressure repeatedly on the margins of the oral cavity without trying to prise the jaws open. This step must be done with great care to avoid injury or fracture of teeth or damage to the mandible. Once the oral cavity is open, a professional avian mouth gag or opened forceps should be placed between the jaws. In lizards with large dewlaps (iguanas, basilisks, anoles and chameleons), the skin of the ventral dewlap can be pulled gently and, at the same time, a pressure should be applied on both corners of the mouth (Figure 11.9). The skin must be pulled very slowly to avoid damage to the skin and hyoid apparatus. A short elastic tube is inserted into the caudal oral cavity. The jaws and head can then be released and the syringe plunger gently pushed. The lizard starts swallowing spontaneously, which is apparent by its regular tongue movements (Figure 11.10). Tubes from infusion sets or cat/rabbit feeding tubes are usable in many lizards. In larger lizards, or in situations where the animal could bite the tube off, stronger tubes such as foley catheters should be used;

alternatively, the tube may be protected by a commercial plastic gag. For very small volumes of liquid, the use of a latex intravenous catheter inserted midline at the labial notch, may allow oral administration with minimal stress and without having to prise the jaws apart.

Chelonians: In chelonians, administration of drugs by oesophageal or pharyngostomy tube is the most effective method, particularly if it is necessary for tubing to be performed on a regular basis (see Chapter 13). If oesophageal/stomach tubing is required on only one occasion, it may be facilitated by using a firm and flat plate inserted between the margins of the upper and lower jaw, and slowly rotated (Figure 11.11). Alternatively, the veterinary surgeon (veterinarian) can insert a forefinger into the corner of the mouth which does not possess the keratinized beak. The neck is held in an extended position and the tube is gently inserted along the midline into the distal oesophagus (Davies and Klingenberg, 2004); however, if the tube passes through the caudal oesophageal sphincter then there is the possibility of regurgitation with subsequent oesophageal irritation and the risk of aspiration pneumonia. When drugs are administered, only small volumes of the fluid (2–3 ml/kg) should be used to minimize the risk of regurgitation. However, if the procedure is being performed to ensure rehydration or assisted feeding (Figure 11.12), the dose may need to be higher. If this is the

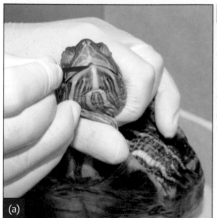

11.11 A technique for opening the mouth of chelonians. (a) A firm, flat plate is inserted between the margins of the upper and lower jaw. (b) The plate is slowly rotated until (c) the mouth is finally open.

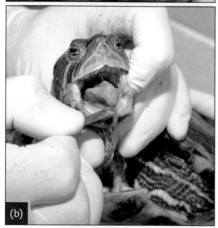

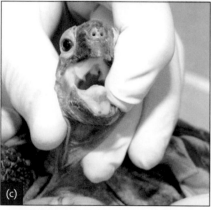

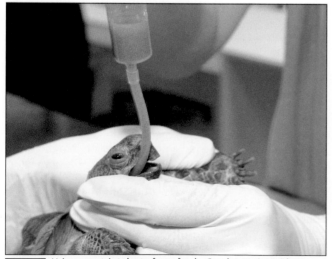

11.12 Using a gastric tube to force feed a Greek tortoise with a commercial herbivorous reptile diet.

case, the volumes administered should be below 50% of the maximum stomach capacity to avoid regurgitation. The suggested maximum volume for gavage administration in chelonians is 5–15 ml/kg.

Snakes: The jaws of most snakes can be opened easily but it will probably be necessary to have an assistant on-hand to restrain the snake. After the jaws are opened, forceps can be used as a mouth gag (Figure 11.13). When inserting the tube, the cranial part of the snake's body is held in a vertical position so that the head is uppermost and care must be taken not to snag the tube on the animal's teeth. The tube is inserted as deep as possible to the oesophagus; in many adult snakes it is impossible to insert the tube into the stomach. In snakes, a safe volume to be delivered via an oesophageal tube ranges from 15–30 ml/kg. For very small volumes of liquid, the use of a latex intravenous catheter inserted midline at the labial notch may allow oral administration with minimal stress and without having to open the mouth.

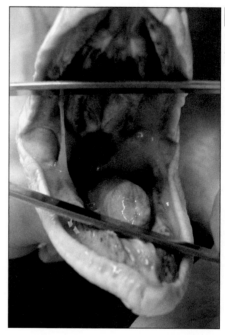

11.13 Using forceps as a mouth gag once the jaws of a snake have been opened.

Oesophagostomy tube

Oesophagostomy tubes are used for repeated application of food or drugs via the digestive tract with minimal stress to handler and reptile. This is particularly important for practice with larger *Geochelone*, *Stigmochelys*, *Chelenoidis* or *Cuora* chelonians that retract their head vigorously. Oesophagostomy tubes should also be used in semi-aquatic chelonians whose aggressive behaviour during repeated manual fixation of the head and neck might lead to injury of the handler.

The tube must be sufficiently long so that it reaches the caudal part of the oesophagus when the patient's neck is extended. Analgesia and general anaesthesia must be induced prior to surgery.

The catheter is pulled out from the oral cavity, and its end is turned back and inserted (using the haemostat) into the caudal oesophagus (Figure 11.14). The loose end of the tube is fixed to the carapace by adhesive tapes and elastic bandages (Figure 11.15).

(For a more detailed description of the insertion of a pharyngostomy tube see Chapter 13).

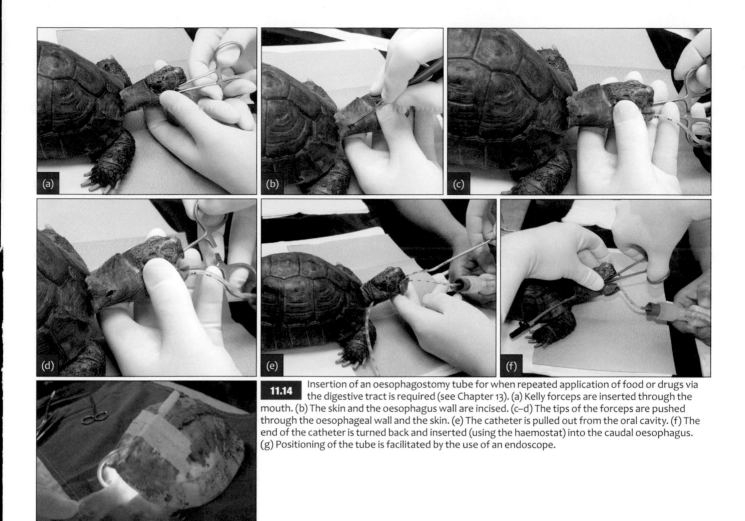

11.14 Insertion of an oesophagostomy tube for when repeated application of food or drugs via the digestive tract is required (see Chapter 13). (a) Kelly forceps are inserted through the mouth. (b) The skin and the oesophagus wall are incised. (c–d) The tips of the forceps are pushed through the oesophageal wall and the skin. (e) The catheter is pulled out from the oral cavity. (f) The end of the catheter is turned back and inserted (using the haemostat) into the caudal oesophagus. (g) Positioning of the tube is facilitated by the use of an endoscope.

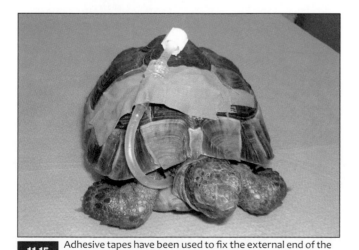

11.15 Adhesive tapes have been used to fix the external end of the oesophagostomy tube to the carapace of this Greek tortoise.

Subcutaneous injections

Some species of reptiles (for example, skinks and many snakes) have relatively inelastic dorsal skin, thus making it difficult to ensure the drug has been administered to the desired location. However, skin on the lateral body walls is markedly elastic in the majority of snakes and therefore this location can be used for subcutaneous administration of larger volumes of solutions (Figure 11.16). Prior to skin puncture, the site should be mechanically cleaned and properly disinfected with a dilute disinfectant such as povidone iodine. In chelonians, most medications can be applied into the areas of loose skin between the neck and thoracic limbs (Figure 11.17) or in the inguinal region in front of the pelvic limbs. When administering subcutaneous drugs in lizards (even in small and young lizards), it is preferable to use the thoracic limbs (Figure 11.18), although loose skin at the caudal aspect of the pelvic limbs represents a safe place for fluid (non-nephrotoxic) injections. In severely dehydrated lizards, the preferred subcutaneous application site might be skin on the sides of the body (agamas, iguanas). The volume of subcutaneous administration can reach up to 1% of the patient's bodyweight. It is desirable to administer larger volumes of medications with several injections at different sites of the body. It should be noted that irritant injections (e.g. fluoroquinolones) may result in a localized discoloration of the skin. This is usually transient but occasionally permanent, and sometimes localized skin sloughing may occur; therefore, intramuscular administration of fluoroquinolones is recommended.

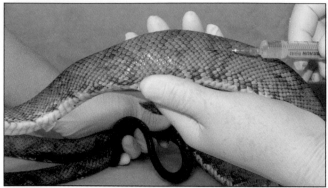

11.16 The subcutaneous administration of drugs into the dorsal musculature in a snake.

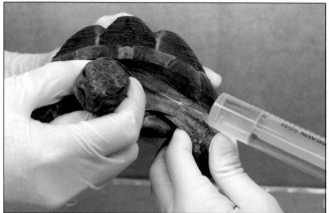

11.17 Most medications in chelonians can be administered into the areas of loose skin between the neck and thoracic limbs.

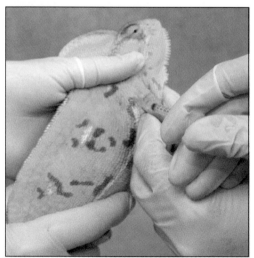

11.18 The subcutaneous administration of drugs into the thoracic limb of a veiled chameleon.

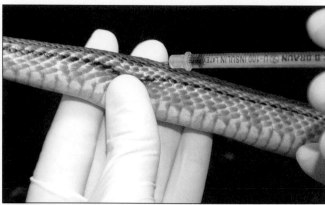

11.19 The intramuscular administration of drugs into the dorsal epaxial musculature in a four-lined snake.

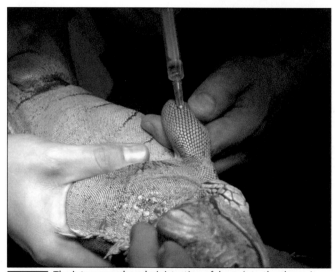

11.20 The intramuscular administration of drugs into the thoracic limb of a male green iguana.

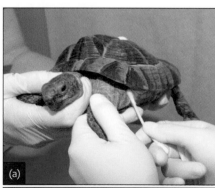

11.21 The intramuscular administration of a drug into the muscles of the thoracic limb in a Greek tortoise. (a) Always disinfect the skin with povidone iodine solution before (b) administering the drug.

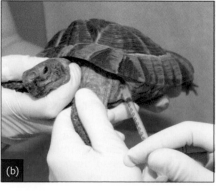

Intramuscular injection

Intramuscular injection is the most frequently used route of administration for small volumes of drugs in reptiles. Ideally, snakes should be injected into the dorsal epaxial musculature (Figure 11.19). As discussed above, the first third of the body should be used in preference where renal clearance or nephrotoxic drugs are an issue. Chelonians and lizards should be injected into the muscles of the thoracic limbs (Figures 11.20 and 11.21). The location choice for injection of those drugs not actively cleared by the kidneys or those that are non-nephrotoxic, is the pelvic limbs (*m. quadriceps* or gluteal musculature) or at the root of the tail. However, avoid the tail in those species demonstrating autotomy e.g. day geckos and iguanids, or which use the tail as a fat deposition site, which is the case for many geckos such as the leopard gecko. Patients weighing less than 100 g should not be given more than 0.15–0.2 ml of solution into one application site. In very small lizards it is difficult to recognize whether the solution was injected strictly into the muscle or also into the subcutis. In a well-hydrated reptile, this does not seem to make a significant difference to the uptake of the drug.

Intracoelomic injection

The intracoelomic injection route is useful particularly when it is necessary to administer larger volumes of isotonic or hypotonic fluid. Due to the risk of mechanical damage to soft organs in the coelom, the patient must be appropriately positioned prior to the injection. Snakes should be fixated on their right side and injected from the left into the caudal quarter of the body in the ventrolateral area. Lizards are fixated in lateral or dorsal position and injected on their ventral surface, caudally and paramedially (to avoid the ventral midline abdominal vein) by applying mild pressure. The needle should be positioned at a shallow angle (30 degrees) towards the skin of the ventral abdomen, from caudal to cranial and the puncture depth should be shallow to reduce the risk of damage to underlying viscera.

Chelonians are treated in a similar way. The puncture should be proximal to the pelvic limb with the chelonian placed on its side to encourage the urinary bladder to fall away from the injection site. The needle must be inserted through the loose skin proximal to the hindlimb which should be drawn caudally to keep it out of the way. The insertion will need to penetrate the body wall and therefore is a deeper insertion than for squamates, with the needle angled from caudal to cranial in the direction of the contralateral forelimb.

Intravenous injection

The intravenous route of administration is only suitable for medium-sized and larger patients with accessible vessels of sufficient size. Chelonians should be injected into the dorsal tail vein (*vena coccygea dorsalis*), jugular veins (*vena jugularis*), *sinus cervicalis*, subcarapacial plexus (Figure 11.22) and occipital sinus (*sinus occipitalis dorsalis*). An intravenous catheter is rarely used in chelonians because it requires a surgical approach (Mitchell 2006). The larger limb vessels, *vena femoralis* or *vena brachialis*, are used less often.

Lizards can be injected into the ventral tail vein (*vena coccygea ventralis*) (Figure 11.23) and abdominal vein. If using the jugular veins (*vena jugularis*) or cephalic veins (*vena cephalica*), the skin has to be incised first in a sterile fashion to find the vein meaning the reptile requires chemical immobilization and analgesia.

Snakes are usually injected into the ventral tail vein (*vena coccygea ventralis*) (Figure 11.24). Small amounts of medicinal solution may be slowly injected into the palatine veins (*venae palatinae*) in a sedated or anaesthetized snake (Figure 11.25). Prior to injection into the jugular veins, the skin has to be incised to find the vein that will be catheterized, meaning the reptile requires chemical immobilization and analgesia. The intracardiac route, although not technically intravenous, has been used in snakes also – see below.

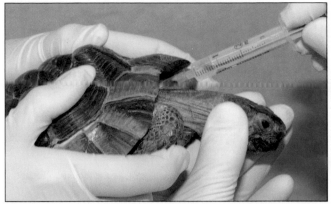

11.22 The intravenous route of administration into the subcarapacial (subveretebral) plexus in a Greek tortoise.

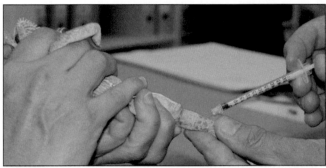

11.23 The intravenous route of administration into the ventral tail vein in a veiled chameleon.

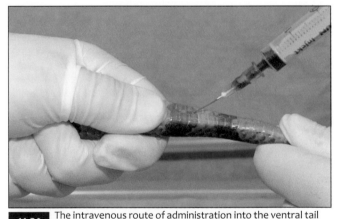

11.24 The intravenous route of administration into the ventral tail vein in a king snake.

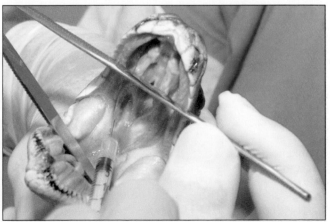

11.25 Small amounts of medicinal solution may be slowly injected into the palatine veins (*venae palatinae*) in a sedated or anaesthetized boid snake.

Intraosseous injection/catheterization

All solutions for intravenous injections can also be successfully and safely administered by the intraosseous route (Chitty and Raftery, 2013). In order to avoid infection of a bone, antibiotics should be administered topically or systemically and the skin over the insertion site surgically prepared thoroughly prior to needle insertion. In lizards, the distal femur is the most suitable site for catheterization (Figure 11.26). Correct positioning of the catheter is checked by gently aspirating a drop of blood or marrow from the bone. In chelonians, catheterization of long bones can be maintained only for the duration of a surgery unless the distal femur is used and the relevant hindlimb taped to the caudal carapace to prevent its retraction into the shell and dislodgement of the catheter. Indwelling catheters may be inserted into the carapace bone marrow, particularly in the caudal plastrocarapacial pillar or cranial part of the plastron (epiplastron). A small hole is drilled in the plastron-carapacial pillar to be able to insert intraosseous catheters in adult chelonians due to the thickness of the shell (Figure 11.27). After the bone is catheterized, the needle (intraosseous infusion needle, Cook® Critical Care; or large diameter hypodermic needle) is fixated by tissue glue or epoxy cement that is normally used to treat carapace fractures (Figure 11.28). The catheter should be attached to a syringe pump and placed in such a manner as to avoid its damage when the patient moves (Figure 11.29).

Intracardial injection

Considering the poor accessibility of peripheral vessels and lack of an intraosseous route in snakes, the intra-cardial route of administration should be considered as an alternative, particularly for fluid administration in cases of acute hypovolaemia. The heart of most snakes is located in the cranial third of their body (approximately 20–25% of the 'snout-to-vent' length) and its position can be identified visually by palpation or by using a Doppler blood pressure ultrasonography machine. The snake generally requires chemical immobilization prior to catheterization. This also facilitates placing the snake in dorsal recumbency for insertion of the needle. After the heart is fixated manually to minimize its free movement, the needle is inserted caudal to the apex of the heart between the ventral scutes, at a shallow 30 degree angle in a cranial manner so entering the ventricle (Figure 11.30). Due to the specific anatomy of lizards and chelonians, safe intra-cardial access in these species is even more difficult than in snakes. The chelonian heart can be localized by the use of a Doppler probe (Chitty and Raftery, 2013). Intracardial

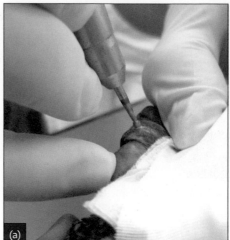

11.27 The intraosseous route of administration in an adult chelonian. (a) After disinfecting the shell, a hole was drilled into the epiplastron. (b) Through this drill hole an intraosseous catheter can be inserted.

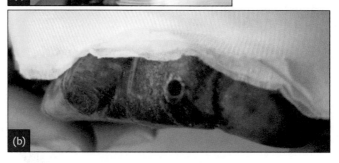

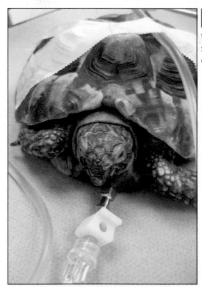

11.28 The inserted needle in the tortoise in Figure 11.27, is secured with tissue glue or cement.

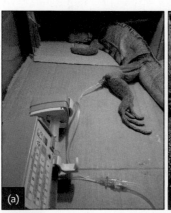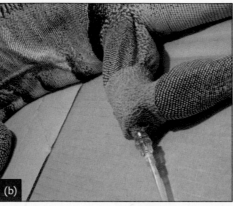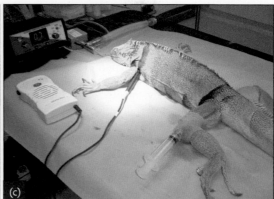

11.26 (a–c) The intraosseous route of administration into the distal femur in a green iguana.

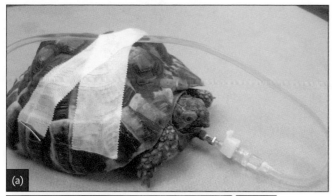

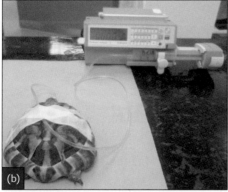

11.29

An intraosseous catheter (a) for fluid therapy in a tortoise. (b) Connected to a small infusion pump for continuous fluid therapy.

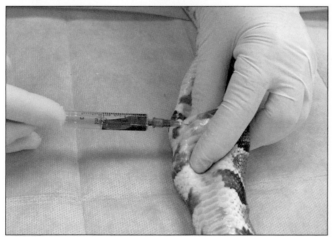

11.30 The intracardial route of drug administration in a manually restrained ball python. The snake is placed on its back and the needle is inserted via the ventral approach.

injection through the plastron at the junction of pectoral and humeral scutes can be used for euthanasia in young or small chelonia.

Intra-articular application

Information about direct application of drugs into the joint space in reptiles is limited. However, debriding the affected joint followed by lavage of the affected area with sterile saline solution (0.9% sodium chloride (NaCl)) or, alternatively, saline plus antibiotic solution, are effective orthopaedic procedures.

Implants

Deep wounds affecting bones may benefit from the use of antibiotic-impregnated polymethylmethacrylate (AIPMMA) beads (Divers and Lawton, 1999). Mixing of the active

ingredient (usually antibiotics, e.g. clindamycin) with PMMA bone cement matrix leads to bead formation. After consequent sterilization in ethylene oxide, the beads can be placed directly into the disinfected wound where they are deposited for a period of time spanning several months to years (Tobias *et al.*, 1996). Apart from preparation of AIPMMA beads at the clinic, commercial products are also available. For example, GENTA-COLL® HD CONE (Resorba, Germany) is a fine sponge impregnated with gentamicin (Figure 11.31). Gentamicin-impregnated bone cement is also widely available for veterinary orthopaedic procedures. It can be divided easily into smaller parts and then placed into the wound. Other implants used in reptiles include electric transponders (microchips) used in veterinary practice for clear identification of animals particularly those CITES listed (Figure 11.32) and hormonal implants (in particular, commercially available implants with a gonadotrophin-releasing hormone (GnRH) agonist such as deslorelin. The purpose of using hormonal implants was to manage the ovarian activity in captive female reptiles. These reptiles suffer from persistent ovarian follicles and egg binding disease (POFS and POES) and this was an attempt at trying to stop their ovarian activity. In many species this proved unsuccessful. The problem of hormonal implants with mammalian GnRH is their very limited use in clinical practice. Both microchips and hormonal implants are administered subcutaneously by attached applicators (Figure 11.33).

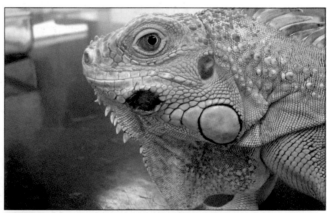

11.31 A fine sponge impregnated with gentamicin has been placed into the wound in a male green iguana.

Reptile	Microchip administration and location
Chelonians	Subcutaneously in left hindlimb (intramuscularly in thin-skinned species) Subcutaneously in the tarsal area in giant species
Crocodilians	Anterior to nuchal cluster. Or the craniolateral tail – this is particularly good for hatchlings of smaller species (where anterior to the nuchal cluster would be difficult) that should be chipped within a few days of birth, as is the case for CITES species. It also has the advantage that if the crocodile is big, the chip can be read away from the sharp end
Lizards	Lateral aspect of left femoral area, over quadriceps muscle, or subcutaneous on caudal half of left flank if too small or legs too skinny or absent
Snakes	Left flank, anterior to cloaca. In this position the microchip is less likely to interfere with ingestion of very large prey or with handling. It is also much safer for the handler if dealing with venomous species and probably easier to implant, mainly in smallest species where fingers can get in the way

11.32 British Veterinary Zoological Society guidelines for implanting microchips in reptiles.

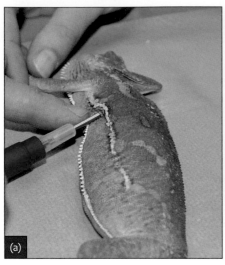

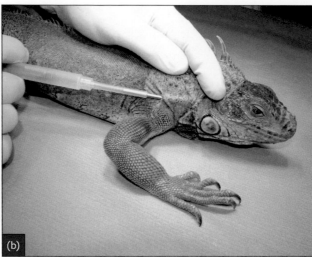

11.33 Implant administration: (a) electric transponder (microchip) used in the left-hand side of a female veiled chameleon; (b) GnRH implant administered in the right-hand side of a green iguana. A skin suture is not necessary as surgical glue can be used to close the small hole in the skin.

Catheterization

Intratracheal catheterization

Direct access to the trachea with the use of a speculum or forceps is relatively easy in snakes and larger lizards (only light sedation is required), but more complicated in chelonians. Tracheal structure in chameleons is especially complicated due to its curved shape and the presence of a small accessory air sac. Procedures such as catheterization of the trachea, bronchial or tracheal lavage are mainly used for diagnostic purposes and to establish airway patency in snakes rather than for administration of medications.

Catheterization of air sacs

Air sacs represent an important part of the respiratory tract of snakes. Medications can be applied directly to the lower respiratory tract in snakes by introducing a catheter into the air sac using an endoscope to guide insertion and then securing it in place by suturing it to the skin dorsolaterally (Jekl and Knotek, 2006). Irritant medications (disinfectants) should not be administered via this route as they can severely damage the delicate mucosa in the respiratory tract.

Nebulization

The principle of nebulization is to provide inhalation of medications in a natural way (Raiti, 2002). Active ingredients (e.g. antibiotics or antifungal drugs, bronchodilators and mucolytic drugs) are dissolved in a sterile solution of water for injection or electrolytes (0.9% NaCl) and then made into an aerosol that is piped into the nebulizing chamber formed by a plastic box or a smaller glass terrarium. Effective nebulization is dependent upon several factors such as the particle size of the drug and the presence of disinfectant which can cause irritation, etc. (Lightfood, 2001). Only drugs that are manufactured for nebulization are truly considered effective agents. A 1:250 dilution of F10® has been reported to be very effective for treatment of upper and low respiratory tract disease in reptiles (Chitty, 2004). While the optimum size of the droplets for nebulization in reptiles has been suggested to be less than 5 μm, which means specialist nebulization equipment is needed, Chitty (2004) suggested a positive effect despite the size of droplets using

standard portable nebulizers; this may reflect the more open and areolar nature of reptile lungs when compared with the narrower, alveolar lung structure of mammals. On the other hand, Raiti (2002) suggested, not surprisingly, that nebulization may be ineffective in reptiles with consolidated lungs. Respiratory infections caused by *Aspergillus* spp. can be treated effectively with itraconazole or amphotericin B nebulization. Chelonians and lizards seem to benefit particularly from nebulization therapy, although it is generally less effective in snakes due to the elongated lung and air sac.

Application of drugs in the cloaca, colon and urinary bladder

Although the mucosa of the cloaca and distal intestine absorb active substances well, this route of administration for specific drugs is not commonly used in reptiles (Figures 11.34 and 11.35). Catheterization of the distal intestine or the urinary bladder of larger chelonians can be performed manually (by a forefinger) or using an endoscope. This procedure requires patient sedation in large reptile species. Fluids (5–10 ml/kg) are administered slowly by applying even pressure. The percloaca method has been used to administer anthelmintics such as fenbendazole to chelonians that are difficult to administer orally; however, there is the possibility of the medication being defecated from the patient soon after medication.

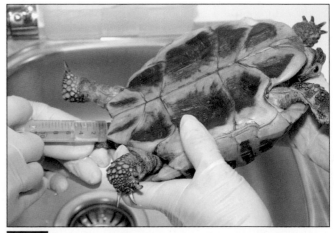

11.34 Flushing the cloaca with saline in a Hermann's tortoise.

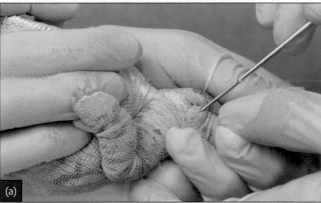

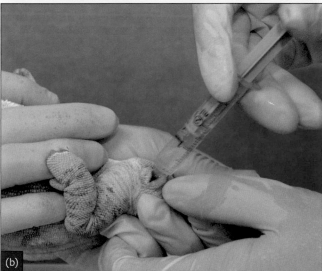

11.35 The gentle massage and subsequent opening of the cloaca in a female veiled chameleon using (a) a stainless steel probe, in order to (b) flush the cloaca with saline solution. This can be done either to relieve constipation or to rehydrate the patient.

Fluid therapy

Stabilization of patients in a critical condition, rehydration of dehydrated patients suffering from a chronic disease, or the support of renal function during prolonged anaesthesia, requires an effective method of fluid supply. In patients in critical and life-threatening conditions, the most effective method of administering fluids, as with mammals, is the application of solutions directly into the circulation. Recommended sites of application include large veins for intravenous catheters or cavities of long bones for intraosseous catheters. Intraosseous fluid therapy is performed by catheterization of long bones (femur, tibia). Parenteral administration of fluids is often performed once or twice a day, according to the patient's condition, by bolus fluid administration, splitting the daily requirements into 4–6 doses. Fluids may be applied continuously by syringe driver or infusion pump where the species will tolerate drip tubing and is sufficiently large enough for the small fluid rates to be within the delivery range of the device. The volume of administered fluids is best calculated according to the patient's bodyweight and degree of dehydration. However, in clinical practice, mildly dehydrated patients are usually rehydrated by assuming a rate of 20 ml/kg (10–30 ml/kg) of crystalloid fluid daily. Some authors recommend adjusting osmolality of administered fluids

e.g. by adding up to 10% of water (sterile water for injection) to classic infusion solutions (such as physiological saline or Ringer's solution). Some studies, however, suggest that the isotonic mammalian solutions do not have to be diluted (Guzman *et al.*, 2011). On the other hand this has been studied in a few select species and any form of extrapolation should be made with caution.

The advantage of enteral fluid therapy is that it supports intestinal motility, dilutes intestinal content and enhances activity of intestinal microflora. Chelonians and some lizards have a large thin-walled bladder, which is an outpouching of the cloacal mucosa. It has been suggested that this bladder (and probably the wall of the urodeum in species lacking a defined bladder), rather than being simply a storage organ as in mammals, may provide an important part of the fluid and electrolyte homeostatic mechanisms. After voiding urine many reptiles, if soaked in a warm bath, will aspirate fluid back into the cloaca and bladder from the environment. This can involve a considerable volume of liquid (up to 300 ml in a 1.5 kg Testudo tortoise) (Davies and Klingenberg, 2004). The urinary bladder can first be emptied by massaging the bladder through a cloaca or by its catheterization, and lavaged with water or saline to remove toxins. In large chelonians and iguanas, the finger of the veterinay surgeon can be situated almost in the urinary bladder – the sphincter is opened and the urine is released. In small chelonians and lizards – catheterization of the bladder is possible or cloacal massage is enough for stimulating the urination and defecation. Once the bladder is empty, it can be filled with isotonic sterile fluids which may be absorbed across the wall of the urinary bladder, or may be flushed into the cloaca and from there back into the terminal rectum where again water may be reabsorbed. Similarly beneficial hydrating effects have been observed after regular bathing (soaking) of reptiles in lukewarm water (once or twice a day for 20–30 minutes) where fluid may be taken up per cloaca and so from there into the urinary bladder or terminal rectum and so absorbed. In reptiles that have no urinary bladder (snakes and some lizards), the cloaca (urodeum) has a similar function but clearly has a very small capacity in comparison. Enteral fluid administration can also be achieved via the oral route using rubber or stainless steel tubes. In all cases of enteral fluid therapy, whichever route of administration is being used, the fluid should be warmed to the reptile's preferred body temperature prior to administration.

Drug dose determination

Reptiles are ectothermic vertebrates whose body temperature is largely, yet not completely, influenced by ambient temperature. In nature, reptiles seek an environment that allows them to maintain their preferred body temperature (PBT) (Figure 11.36). At its PBT, a reptile's enzymatic process and metabolism is allowed to function optimally, an important consideration when administering medications. It is important therefore to try to ensure their environment provides a preferred optimal temperature zone (POTZ) into which the reptile can move to vary its own body temperature, so maintaining its PBT (Figure 11.37). Prior to any therapy, patients have to be kept under conditions that enable them to reach their PBT. This acclimatization period can last up to several days in large chelonians after hibernation, or several minutes or hours in small reptiles. In general, higher temperatures accelerate

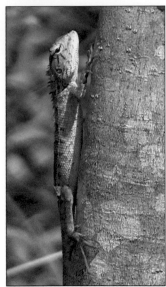

11.36 This small agamid lizard climbing a tree in Indonesia is seeking a suitable environment to maintain its preferred body temperature.

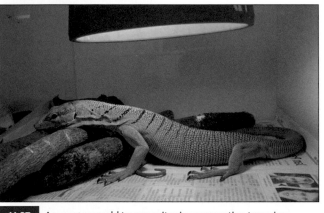

11.37 A young emerald tree monitor in a quarantine terrarium.

metabolic processes and thus may support faster onset of a drug's effect. On the other hand, too high temperatures can have an adverse impact such as heat stress, dehydration and collapse. Suboptimal temperatures may delay the onset of the drug effect or significantly limit the drug's activity as well as immune system function (Figure 11.38). Moreover, it is necessary to respect certain limitations of hospitalized patients. The capacity of apathetic, debilitated or injured reptiles (with multiple fractures) to move naturally in a terrarium may be significantly limited. The PBT of such patients therefore needs to be ensured by the terrarium heating system alone.

Metabolic status of reptiles can be established by measuring the patient's cloacal temperature and heart rate. At suboptimal temperatures, the heart rate would be slower. The normal heart rate of reptiles can be calculated according to the following formula:

$$S = 34 \times (H)^{-0.25}$$

where S = heart rate, H = bodyweight in kg, 34 = a constant derived from optimum cloacal temperature.

As small reptiles (or young) and large reptiles have a significantly different metabolic rate, they have to receive different doses of drugs at different intervals. In clinical practice this knowledge is very important when treating extremely small or large reptile patients. In such situations, the metabolic scaling method is highly recommended (for an example see Girling and Fraser, 2009).

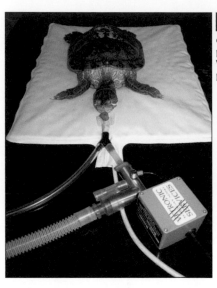

11.38 A red-eared terrapin kept on an electric heating pad during anaesthesia. Warm water heating pads can also be used.

Metabolic (allometric) scaling

It is generally accepted that energy requirements as well as the speed of metabolic processes in reptiles are 8–10 times lower per kilogram bodyweight when compared with most birds or mammals (Pokras *et al.*, 1992). Small and young reptiles have higher heart rates and density of hepatocytes in the liver and a faster flow of blood through the circulatory system and relative glomerular filtration in the kidneys than larger, older reptiles (Pokras *et al.*, 1992). It follows that a large adult reptile patient requires a lower dose of a drug than a small young specimen of the same species.

The method of allometric scaling is needed for dosing a novel drug for a novel species. Considering the huge weight differences between adult and young snakes, lizards and some chelonians, the administered doses of drugs, and intervals between individual doses, should be different. Details of the metabolic scaling method including the limitations and applications of allometric scaling, was highlighted by Mayer *et al.* (2006) and mentioned by Innis *et al.* (2017). They concluded that much more research on physiology and pharmacokinetics in reptiles is needed. For detailed information see dedicated studies (Pokras *et al.*, 1992; Sedgwick and Borkowski, 1996, Mayer *et al.*, 2006). Pharmacokinetic studies in specific reptile species gives the most accurate information on drug dosing.

Selected pharmaceuticals – overview of dosage

Antiviral agents

Aciclovir

Aciclovir inhibits the incorporation of thymidine into viral DNA. When used *in vitro* aciclovir significantly reduces replication of herpesviruses isolated in the cases of clinical stomatitis in reptiles. For the purpose of oral administration, dissolved tablets of aciclovir (80 mg/kg q24h) can be used (Klingenberg 1996; Gaio *et al.*, 2007). The oral use of aciclovir in chelonians should be used very carefully because high doses of aciclovir (70–80 mg/kg daily) can have side effects including swelling of the mucosa (Schumacher, 1996). Aciclovir in the form of 5%

ointment applied to the affected mucosa proved success-ful in the therapy of early viral stomatitis or dermatitis of chelonians (Frye, 1991; Rossi, 1995; Marschang *et al.*, 1997, Origgi and Jacobson 2000).

Valaciclovir

The mechanism of action of valaciclovir (esterified form that is converted to aciclovir after being administered orally) would be similar to aciclovir in the treatment of chelonian iridovirus infections (Allender *et al.*, 2013). It is proposed that dosage of valaciclovir of 40 mg/kg orally q24h may be effective in the treatment of herpesvirus in tortoises (Allender *et al.*, 2013).

Antibacterial agents

The majority of bacterial infections in reptiles are caused by Gram-negative bacteria such as *Pseudomonas*, *Aeromonas*, *Klebsiella*, *Proteus*, *Providencia*, *Citrobacter*, *Salmonella*, *Serratia*, *Arizona* and *Morganella* spp. (Holt 1981; Wilkinson 2004). Although these bacteria are often detected in healthy reptiles, they may cause disease in animals debilitated by stressful conditions or viral infec-tions (Kauffman 1997). Antibiotics should always be selected according to the laboratory results of microbial culture and sensitivity testing to antibiotics that are asso-ciated with the least risk of renal or hepatic damage. In particular, nephrotoxic antibiotics (e.g. aminoglycosides) should be used with great caution and care should be taken to maintain the hydration status (Mader, 1991; Klingenberg, 1996).

Fluoroquinolones

Fluorinated quinolones are bactericidal and inhibit the syn-thesis of bacterial DNA. They are active in low concentra-tion and very quickly reach effective levels in reptiles' blood (within several hours after application) but their effects rely on achieving a peak dose rather than maintain-ing a constant level in the body. Fluoroquinolones are well distributed in an organism and easily penetrate the affected tissues (Spörle *et al.*, 1991; Klingenberg 1996). They are eliminated particularly through the kidneys; cipro-floxacin is eliminated also in bile. They are highly active against Gram-negative and many Gram-positive micro-organisms, but only partially effective against anaerobes; enrofloxacin is only poorly effective against anaerobic bacteria. In general, fluoroquinolones must not be admin-istered to gravid females or young animals, due to the risk of damage to cartilage and impaired growth of bones which, although such adverse effects have not been confirmed yet in reptiles, are extrapolated from their adverse effects in mammals. Injection site reactions of drugs such as enrofloxacin are not uncommon and may result in discoloration of skin and localized skin sloughing in some cases.

Ciprofloxacin: Ciprofloxacin is available as a solution for intravenous injection. Intramuscular application of this drug may cause damage to tissues. In veterinary practice, reptiles can be given ciprofloxacin tablets orally at a dose of 10 mg/kg q48–72h (Klingenberg and Backner, 1991; Klingenberg, 1996; Divers, 1998). Similar precautions apply to the use of ciprofloxacin as they do to the use of enrofloxacin (see below).

Enrofloxacin: Enrofloxacin has been proven to have reliable activity against bacteria *Pasteurella* (*P. testudinis*),

Pseudomonas, *Klebsiella*, *Salmonella*, *Citrobacter* and *Mycoplasma* spp.. Subcutaneous application of this product may lead to local damage to tissues and forma-tion of gelatine-like subcutaneous oedema. The affected site is painful to the touch; ulceration and depigmentation of the skin may be observed. In such cases, higher doses (each dose above 5 mg/kg of enrofloxacin) should be applied by deep intramuscular injections to multiple sites and the drug should be diluted with sterile saline (Klingenberg, 1996). The dose depends on the treatment protocol of bacteria (5 mg/kg i.m. q12h for *Pseudomonas* sp. and *Citrobacter* sp., q24h for other bacterial infec-tions, Raphael *et al.*, 1994). The dose of 10 mg/kg intra-muscularly q24h proved effective in the treatment of tortoises suffering from runny nose syndrome (rhinitis, conjunctivitis, stomatitis, tracheitis, Spörle *et al.*, 1991). The most common treatment protocol for reptiles is 5–10 mg/kg i.m. q24–48h (Funk and Diethelm 2006; Carpenter *et al.* 2014).

Marbofloxacin: Pharmacokinetics and dose regimen of marbofloxacin for reptiles have been published (Coke *et al.*, 2006; Mitchell, 2006; Lai *et al.*, 2007). Marbofloxacin is currently the drug often used as the first choice in the treatment of bacterial infections in reptiles (snakes, lizards, tortoises and terrapins) (Funk, 2000; Davies and Klingenberg, 2004; Diethelm, 2005). Marbofloxacin is bactericidal against a broad range of Gram-negative and Gram-positive organisms including *Pseudomonas* sp., *Klebsiella* sp. and *Corynebacterium* sp. (Gibbons, 2014). The subcutaneous application of marbofloxacin (10 mg/kg q24–48h) does not cause any local damage to tissues or formation of subcutaneous oedema. Marbofloxacin can be administered orally to snakes, lizards and chelonians (10 mg/kg q24–48h, Coke *et al.*, 2006). Pharmacokinetics studies determined that 2 mg/kg i.m. q24h is appropriate for treatment in red-eared terrapins (Lai *et al*, 2007).

Danofloxacin: Pharmacokinetics of danofloxacin after intravenous, intramuscular and subcutaneous administra-tion to chelonians has been published (Marin *et al.*, 2008). It is active against Gram-negative and Gram-positive bacteria (Gibbons, 2014). The dose of 6 mg/kg i.m. q48h has been recommended for the treatment of mycoplas-mosis in tortoises (Gibbons *et al.*, 2012).

Aminoglycosides

Aminoglycosides are highly active against Gram-positive and Gram-negative bacteria. Historically, the two most commonly used aminoglycosides were gentamicin and amikacin. These bactericides bind to ribosomes and inhibit bacterial proteosynthesis; they are eliminated from the body by glomerular filtration. Aminoglycosides have nephrotoxic and, possibly, neurotoxic effects (ototoxic and cardiotoxic effects have been reported as well). Currently in clinical practice, aminoglycosides are used only against Gram-negative bacteria that are resistant to other anti-biotics. Gentamicin is rarely used systemically today as it is highly nephro- and ototoxic. Amikacin is preferred as it is less nephrotoxic and has a broader spectrum of activity. In general, fluid therapy is essential when using aminoglycosides to ensure adequate hydration and avoid renal damage.

Gentamicin: Data about gentamicin dosage in reptiles are derived from studies in turtles, snakes and crocodiles (Raphael *et al.*, 1985; Jacobson *et al.*, 1988; Michaels,

1988; Hilf *et al.*, 1991). It has been proven that the half-life of the active substance decreases with increasing body temperature of the patient (Michaels, 1988). In aquatic turtles kept in aquariums at 26°C, gentamicin blood levels decreased to half after 32 hours. In snakes (*Pituophis melanoleucus*) the same decrease in antibiotic level was observed as late as 82 hours after dosing (Michaels, 1988). Today, gentamicin tends to be used topically or as a constituent of AIPMMA beads, where its effects can be somewhat confined to a local area so reducing its systemic side-effects.

Amikacin: It has been demonstrated that at favourable ambient temperatures (i.e. higher values within the POTZ), amikacin is effective and does not induce renal pathologies in reptiles (Mader *et al.*, 1985; Caliguri *et al.*, 1990; Johnson *et al.*, 1997). When compared with gentamicin, amikacin is, in reptiles, much more effective against *Pseudomonas* spp. bacteria. In addition, it has a lower nephrotoxic effect. Therapeutic levels of amikacin in reptile blood ranges from 2–10 μg/ml. The dose of amikacin for reptiles ranges from 2.5–5 mg/kg i.m. q24–72h (Jacobson *et al.*, 1988; Caliguri *et al.*, 1990; Johnson *et al.*, 1997). Today amikacin is not the drug of choice because it has limited ability to penetrate infected tissues compared with fluoroquinolones.

Other aminoglycosides: Netilmicin administered intramuscularly has somewhat lower nephrotoxic and ototoxic effects than gentamicin, yet it is less effective against *Pseudomonas* spp. bacteria. Tobramycin has lower nephrotoxic impact and higher therapeutic effect against pseudomonades when compared with gentamicin (Ross and Marzec, 1984). Framycetin (framomycin) is used to treat infections of the oral cavity or cloaca and is usually applied topically as a cream. Paromomycin is used in reptiles for the treatment of amoebiasis and cryptosporidiosis. It was found that treatment with 100 mg/kg q24h for 7 days prevented shedding of *Cryptosporidium* spp. as did a dosage of 360 mg/kg q48h for 10 days. (Grosset *et al.*, 2011). Paromomycin can be nephrotoxic. It is hypothesized that systemic absorption across the intestinal mucosa when it is compromised may occur more readily. This potential toxicity should be considered in reptiles with intestinal diseases (McArthur, 2004).

Penicillins

Penicillins induce painful reactions at the injection site. When they are used as a long-term therapy, they may cause hepatopathies (Klingenberg, 1996). Traditional penicillins such as penicillin, ampicillin or amoxicillin are effective in the treatment of staphylococcal infections in reptiles. Semi-synthetic penicillins (SSPs), carbenicillin, piperacillin, mezlocillin and ticarcillin are broad-spectrum antibiotics with very good activity against infections caused by *Pseudomonas* and *Aeromonas* spp. bacteria. However, as they are potentially nephrotoxic (resulting in tubular damage), concurrent fluid therapy is always necessary.

Carbenicillin: Carbenicillin is highly active against Gram-negative pathogens, particularly pseudomonal infections. A disadvantage of common use of this antibiotic in veterinary practice is the risk of resistance to antibiotics and a considerably large volume of the drug that has to be injected. Moreover, it is strongly irritating to the skin and muscles. Carbenicillin is eliminated primarily through the kidneys. This antibiotic was tested in pharmacokinetic trials performed with Colubridae and Boidae snakes (*Boiga*

dendrophila, *Lampropeltis getulus*, *Python reticulatus*, *Pantherophis guttatus*, *Pantherophis obsoletus*). Effects of placement of the injection site on carbenicillin pharmacokinetics has been investigated in the carpet python (Holz *et al.*, 2002). Therapeutic concentrations of the antibiotic in blood were achieved after the application of unexpectedly high doses (Klingenberg, 1996). Increase of carbenicillin concentration in the blood of tortoises *Testudo graeca* and *T. hermanni* during the course of treatment was explained by the apparent reservoir function of the urinary bladder. This enables recycling of the antibiotic in the patient's body and needs to be taken into consideration when using carbenicillin (Lawrence *et al.*, 1986). The recommended dose of carbenicillin for reptiles ranges from 200–400 mg/kg s.c. or i.m. q24–48h (Lawrence *et al.*, 1984, 1986; Holz *et al.*, 2002).

Piperacillin: Piperacillin is highly active against Gram-negative pathogens (*Pseudomonas* spp. particularly) and certain Gram-positive bacteria (*Streptococcus* spp.) and anaerobes. Sensitivity testing confirmed that this antibiotic shows very good activity against pathogens causing respiratory infections of reptiles (*Pseudomonas aeruginosa*, *Aeromonas hydrophilia*, *Providencia rettgeri*, *Proteus mirabilis*, *Escherichia coli*, *Morganella morganii*, *Alcaligenes odorans*) (Hilf *et al.*, 1991b). Piperacillin is administered to reptiles intramuscularly, in doses of 50–200 mg/kg q24–48h.

Cephalosporins

Cephalosporins are broad-spectrum bactericidal antibiotics with minimal side effects. Parenteral administration of cephalosporins in clinical practice with reptiles kills pathogens by disrupting the synthesis of bacterial cell walls in a similar fashion to the penicillin family (Klingenberg, 1996). The nucleus of cephalosporins is 7-aminocephalosporanic acid. Based on antimicrobial spectrum, resistance to beta-lactamases and pharmacological properties, cephalosporins are classified into the following four groups:

- The use of first-generation cephalosporins such as cefalotin, cefazolin, cephalexin and cefadroxil has been reported by various authors. They are effective in the therapy of staphylococcal and streptococcal infections which, as they are rather rare in reptiles, makes their use limited
- Second-generation cephalosporins (cefamandol, cefuroxime, cefoxitin, cefotetan, cefaclor, cefuroxime axetil) represent a breakthrough in the treatment of Gram-positive infections, having a broader spectrum of activity, and are effective against certain Gram-negative bacteria (e.g. *Salmonella* spp. and *Citrobacter* spp.)
- Third-generation cephalosporins have been used in reptiles most often over the last few years. These antibiotics feature excellent tissue penetration, resistance to beta-lactamases and strong activity against Gram-negative microorganisms (*Proteus* spp., *Providencia* spp., *Citrobacter* spp. and others). An independent subgroup of third-generation cephalosporins are antipseudomonal cephalosporins that are active against 90% of pseudomonal strains (ceftazidime, cefoperazone, cefsulodin (Lawrence *et al.*, 1984)
- Out of the fourth-generation cephalosporins, cefepime and cefpirome seem to be most promising for treatment of reptiles suffering from antibiotic resistant bacterial infections.

Side effects of cephalosporins at the injection site include pain and systemically, possible nephrotoxic effects in patients with pre-existing renal problems, and hepatopathy. Ceftazidime also shows good activity against anaerobes. Today, it is one of the antibiotics that is most suitable for the treatment of infections caused by *Enterobacteriaceae* bacteria in reptiles and is used at a dosage of 20 mg/kg q72h (Innis *et al.*, 2012). It is a human preparation and as such unlicensed in reptiles/veterinary medicine. Care should therefore be taken in its responsible use to avoid resistance developing which will have wider implications for human health as well as reptile health. Unlike ceftazidime which is eliminated through the kidneys (Stamper *et al.*, 1999), cefoperazone is eliminated largely in the liver (Lawrence *et al.*, 1984). Cefalotin and cefaloridine are not active against *Pseudomonas* bacteria, but are useful in the treatment of infections induced by *Klebsiella*, *Enterobacter* and *Proteus* microorganisms. Ceftiofur at a dosage of 5 mg/kg i.m. q24 is used in lizards as the most effective drug for treatment of *Devriesea agamarum* infection in captive lizards (Hellebuyck *et al.*, 2009). Other reptiles are treated with ceftiofur at a dosage of 2.2–5 mg/kg i.m. q24–48h (turtles, snakes) (Stein, 1996; Benson *et al.*, 2003).

Chloramphenicol

Chloramphenicol is a bacteriostatic antimicrobial that binds to ribosomes of bacteria and inhibits the synthesis of bacterial proteins. It has been indicated largely for the therapy of chelonian septicaemic cutaneous ulcerative disease (SCUD), caused by, among others, *Citrobacter freundii* and salmonellosis in reptiles. Chloramphenicol has been used in veterinary practice with reptiles, and plasma concentrations of chloramphenicol in snakes have been investigated (Clark *et al.*, 1985). However, as its effect is primarily bacteriostatic, bactericidal activity is seen only after the administration of higher doses. The main risks of its application include damage to bone marrow in water snakes (Jacobson, 1993) and a significant impact on intestinal microflora (sterile gut syndrome – SGS). It is not currently available in veterinary medicine and is used with caution in human medicine owing to its potentially fatal bone marrow suppression in humans.

Tetracyclines

Tetracyclines are seldom used. They are primarily bacteriostatic antibiotics with a broad spectrum of activity. Side-effects include teratogenic effect during gravidity, neurological disorders, nausea, vomiting, calcium binding and fatty degeneration of the liver. Tetracycline could be useful in the treatment of infections caused by *Klebsiella*, *Staphylococcus*, *Mycoplasma* and *Chlamydia* spp. bacteria. *Salmonella* and *Pseudomonas* spp. bacteria are resistant to tetracyclines. The recommended dosage of tetracycline for reptiles is 10 mg/kg orally q24h (Jacobson *et al.*, 1983; Funk and Diethelm, 2006).

Macrolides, lincosamides and azalides

Lincosamides are bacteriostatic antibiotics active against Gram-positive and anaerobic microorganisms. They are easily absorbed from the intestine (lincomycin 40%, clindamycin 90–100%) and penetrate bones. A clarithromycin dose of 15 mg/kg orally q48–72h is particularly effective in the treatment of mycoplasmal and chlamydial infections (Johnson *et al.*, 1998; Wimsatt *et al.*, 1999). Clarithromycin pharmacokinetics and practical use of per rectum deposition of clarithromycin in the desert tortoise have been published (Wimsatt *et al.*, 1999, 2008). Tylosin is reported to be useful in the treatment of respiratory infections as it has good activity against *Mycoplasma* spp. but it does cause significant muscle necrosis at injection sites, which should be borne in mind if using parenterally.

Potentiated sulphonamides

Potentiated sulphonamides have a very broad spectrum of activity against both Gram-negative and Gram-positive aerobic bacteria. Sulphonamides commonly used in reptiles include sulfadimidine, sulfadimethoxine, sulfadiazine and sulfaquinoxaline. Trimethoprim used in combination with sulphonamides (sulfadiazine or sulfamethoxazole) is a preparation with a very broad spectrum of activity. In reptiles it is used intramuscularly or orally in doses from 10–30 mg/kg q24–48h (Vree *et al.*, 1986; Jacobson, 1993; Klingenberg, 1996; Stein, 1996). In veterinary practice, the sulphonamides sulfadiazine (75 mg/kg orally the first day and then 45 mg/kg q24h for 5 days) and sulfamethazine (50 mg/kg orally q24h for 3 days) can be used for the treatment of coccidia (Carpenter *et al.*, 2014).

Metronidazole

Metronidazole is used in reptiles to treat anaerobic bacterial infections induced by *Bacteroides*, *Fusobacterium*, *Clostridium* and *Peptostreptococcus* spp. bacteria. Metronidazole is metabolized in the liver and eliminated through the kidneys. Nausea, apathy, loss of muscle tone, stargazing and other signs of metronidazole intoxication have been reported very rarely. Doses >40 mg/kg daily should be avoided in kingsnakes and indigo snakes as these species appear particularly sensitive to the side effects of metronidazole (Jacobson *et al.*, 1983; Jacobson, 1993). In American king snakes, complications and death were observed after being dosed at 100 mg/kg (Jacobson, 1993). None of these complications are seen when metronidazole is used at doses <40 mg/kg. Doses of 20 mg/kg orally q24h for at least one week are recommended (Bodri *et al.*, 2006; Kolmstetter *et al.*, 1998; Kolmstetter *et al.*, 2001). For treatment of the amoebiasis and infections caused by flagellated protozoans the dosages are 20–40 mg/kg orally q24h for 2–5 days (Carpenter *et al.*, 2014). From the author's practical experience as well as published reports (Mitchell, 2006) it is indicated that doses around 100 mg/kg are very dangerous or even fatal in adult boid snakes. The animals died within 3 days after showing signs of CNS damage (loss of muscle tone with stargazing (Figure 11.39), and spasms). Very low doses of metronidazole have been used by reptile keepers to increase appetite in anorexic reptiles – around 12.5 mg/kg, but exact clinical studies have not been published yet.

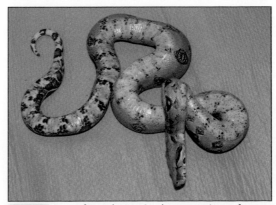

11.39 Loss of muscle tone in a boa constrictor after metronidazole intoxication.

Polypeptide antibiotics

Polypeptide antibiotics are effective against most of the *Enterobacteriaceae* bacteria but are not active against *Proteus* spp.. In high doses they could damage renal epithelium and may have a neurotoxic effect; therefore, polypeptide antibiotics, bacitracin and polymyxin B are used only for local treatment of superficial wounds or as ingredients of ophthalmological ointments and eye drops (Pokras *et al.*, 1992).

Combinations of antibacterial products

In clinical practice, antibiotic treatment of reptiles has often to be started before the pathogen is reliably identified and its susceptibility to antibiotics established. If a combination of antimicrobials is used to cover the broadest possible spectrum of pathogenic bacteria, the so-called four-quadrant approach to antibiosis targeted on Gram-positive, Gram-negative, aerobic and anaerobic bacteria should be taken. Bactericidal and bacteriostatic antibiotics should not be combined. Antibiotics should also be chosen based on an assessment of the risk of damage to the patient's organs (liver, kidneys, etc.). If multiple different antibiotics are to be given by injection they should not be mixed and should be injected at separate sites. This is the only way to avoid adverse interaction or inactivation of drugs that occur before or immediately after application. Adverse effects may also be caused by the fact that antibiotics contain different preservatives, which can interact or create unfavourable conditions for the antibiotic activity. A possible choice to treat effectively Gram-negative aerobic and anaerobic bacterial infection includes a combination of drugs such as marbofloxacin and metronidazole, amikacin and metronidazole for example.

Antifungal agents

The main disadvantage of many antimycotics is that often they have to be administered over long periods of time to ensure effective treatment. The risk of adverse effects (hepatotoxicity or nephrotoxicity) of any treatment lasting weeks or even months is high.

Polyene antibiotics (amphotericin B, nystatin) are efficacious fungicides that treat yeast and fungal infections. As they are not absorbed from the digestive tract or the respiratory tract they may be administered orally to treat gastrointestinal mycoses, nebulized or administered into airways for respiratory infections (Hernandez-Divers, 2001). However, they should not be used to treat systemic mycoses due to their nephrotoxicity. Nystatin has been used successfully to treat intestinal candidiasis in reptiles (100,000 IU/kg orally q24h for 10 days) (McArthur, 2004).

Imidazoles and triazoles

Imidazole and triazole antimycotics inhibit the cytochrome systems involved in the synthesis of ergosterol in fungal cell membranes, causing increased cell wall permeability and allowing leakage of cellular contents, ultimately leading to the destruction of the fungi. Imidazoles include clotrimazole and miconazole that are commonly used in chelonians for the superficial topical treatment of mycotic infections of the shell (*Candida albicans*). Triazoles such as itraconazole, ketoconazole, enilconazole and fluconazole have been used in reptiles for the systemic therapy of severe mycoses that include respiratory infections – aspergillosis, coccidiomycosis, blastomycosis, cryptococcosis, etc. (Girling and Fraser, 2009). They have also been used successfully for the treatment of gastrointestinal candidiasis and skin infections including dermatophytosis. Triazoles may be administered orally in cases of systemic mycoses of reptiles, as they are absorbed from the digestive tract (Page *et al.*, 1991). Long-term triazole therapy, however, may lead to complications such as inappetence or hepatopathy. Ketoconazole is a commonly used antimycotic in reptiles; tablets are dissolved and the suspension is administered via an oesophageal tube (15–30 mg/kg orally q24h for 2–4 weeks). Ketoconazole shampoo may be used to treat superficial mycoses (author's personal experience). Ketoconazole is, however, ineffective in treating either *Aspergillus* spp. or the *Chrysosporium* anamorph of *Nannizziopsis vriesii* (CANV) infections and has more severe hepatic side effects than itraconazole. Fluconazole and itraconazole have a broad spectrum of activity, fewer side effects and are better absorbed than ketoconazole. Fluconazole is available as an injection in some countries (Wilkinson, 2004). In recent years, voriconazole has been shown to be effective in the treatment of mycoses of reptiles (Innis *et al.*, 2008). Voriconazole treats aspergillosis and extensive skin mycoses, as well as a promising option for the treatment of CANV and other *Chrysosporium* spp. (Van Waeyenberghe *et al.*, 2010, Schmid-Ukaj *et al.*, 2014). The recommended dosages are 5–10 mg/kg orally q24h, for many weeks/months). Itraconazole has also been shown to be effective in some cases against CANV as well as other severe systemic infections, but it is more hepatotoxic than voriconazole.

Griseofulvin

Griseofulvin is a fungistatic drug that inhibits cell division of fungi. Generally, griseofulvin is not used in clinical practice to treat reptiles due to its hepatotoxic and possibly teratogenic effect, as well as its limited antifungal range.

Other antimycotic agents

Superficial mycoses like *Fusarium incarnatum* can be treated with ointments or solutions such as dilute povidone iodine (Rose *et al.*, 2001). Povidone iodine is usually used in the form 0.05% solution or it is diluted approximately in a ratio of 1:10. This concentration is suitable for baths, i.e. repeated treatment of larger body surfaces. Also, it is used for wound rinsing e.g. after surgical removal of abscesses.

Solutions of potassium permanganate have been proven to be useful as well. High-concentration solutions (1:100–200) may be used for the therapy of superficial mycoses; low-concentration solutions (1:500–1000) are suitable for baths or rinses of the oral cavity in the incipient stage of stomatitis.

Mycotic infections causing damage to aquatic turtle shells (*Candida* spp.) can be treated by any of the methods that are used in aquarist fish medicine practice: malachite green (solution of 2 mg/l of water for shell lavages) in particular can be useful.

Antiparasitic agents

Parasites are among the most commonly reported causal agents of pathogenic processes in reptiles. Despite the fact that there are a number of approaches to the use of antiparasitic products in individual groups of reptiles, the therapy of parasite infestation in these animals is on no account easy. Many of the previous findings should be revised, for the following three reasons:

- Some traditional products are not currently commercially available
- Clinical experience indicates that certain parasites are demonstrating resistance to classic antiparasitics such as levamisole and metronidazole (Gibbons, 2014)
- Increasing information is available showing the risks of adverse effects of antiparasitics on the patient's health.

The overview below has been developed with respect to the above mentioned reasons. If there is more than one antiparasitic protocol available, the most often used is described here.

Antiprotozoal agents

Metronidazole: Metronidazole is used for the treatment of infections caused by flagellates (especially *Hexamita* spp., *Trichomonas* spp.) and amoebas. The therapy of flagellate intestinal infection usually requires a limited number of metronidazole doses. High metronidazole doses of around 100 mg/kg orally cause fatalities even after a one-dose application. Metronidazole is toxic in indigo snakes and some kingsnakes (Davies and Klingenberg, 2004). The risk of fatal intoxication is considerable in large and heavy reptiles particularly snakes (see Metronidazole in antibacterial treatment). Metronidazole doses for big snakes (>10 kg bodyweight) should be calculated by the metabolic scaling method. Alternatively, veterinary surgeons may decide to use empirically lower doses ranging from 20–40 mg/kg orally q24h. Contraindications in reptiles include debilitation, gravidity or liver failure. Early signs of metronidazole poisoning comprise lethargy, weakness, vomiting and diarrhoea. Advanced intoxication causes neurological signs and leads to death. Pharmacokinetics of metronidazole in ten red-eared terrapins after intracoelomic bolus administration (deep through the prefemoral fossa) (20 mg/kg) has been published (Innis *et al.*, 2007).

Toltrazuril: Toltrazuril is mainly used as a coccidiocidal agent. *Isospora* spp. coccidia are commonly detected in veiled chameleons or various species of agamids including the inland bearded dragon. Toltrazuril is available in a concentrated form for commercial poultry and must be diluted prior to use owing to its high alkalinity. After adding water to create the standard dilution as for poultry use (25 ppm or 0.025 mg/ml), it is administered in two doses of 5–15 mg/kg orally 2–3 weeks apart. Although toltrazuril is very effective against *Isospora* spp. coccidia, it does not treat other severe coccidiosis infections such as those caused by *Choleoeimeria* spp.; this is because *Choleoeimeria* spp. is localized in liver and gall bladder. Toltrazuril treatment needs to be combined with active rehydration/fluid support to prevent kidney damage.

Ponazuril: Ponazuril, triazine drug, can also be used as a coccidiocidal agent in lizards. The dose of 30 mg/kg orally q48h twice, was published as a successful treatment of coccidiosis in bearded dragons (Bogoslavsky, 2007; Mitchell, 2008).

Trimethoprim/sulphonamide: Trimethoprim in combination with sulphonamides blocks biochemical processes associated with folic acid and para-amino benzoic acid (PABA) in coccidia. Drugs from this group are contraindicated in patients with confirmed renal failure and should not be used in dehydrated and debilitated reptiles as they are nephrotoxic. If hydration of the patient is ensured, potentiated sulphonamides can be used with care at similar dosages as used for bacterial infections (see above).

Chloroquine: Chloroquine is used in the treatment of blood parasites such as *Hepatozoon* spp.; however, it is questionable whether the unicellular parasites present in blood cells are clinically significant in the majority of cases. In practice, a high prevalence of intra-erythrocytic parasites in aquatic and semiaquatic turtles living in natural biotopes has been observed with anaemia. Intracellular parasites are often found in royal pythons imported from Africa. Stein (1996) reported its use in chelonians as three 125 mg/kg doses of chloroquine every 48 hours; however, the effect of such therapy was not clearly demonstrated. In fact, parasite counts in the peripheral blood of most imported reptiles gradually decrease without any treatment.

Anthelmintics

Adult nematodes or cestodes, as well as their developmental stages including eggs, are commonly found parasitizing mainly the digestive but also the respiratory tract of wild-caught reptiles. Coprological examination or microscopic analysis of sputum taken from the upper airways of imported reptiles makes it possible to detect the eggs of parasitic worms. It should be noted though, that captive bred reptiles are commonly parasitized, and those parasites with a direct life-cycle may rapidly reach high concentrations within the reptile (see Chapter 24).

Benzimidazole group: The products that have been commonly used in veterinary medicine to kill parasitic worms include albendazole, fenbendazole, mebendazole and thiabendazole (Holt, 1981: Innis, 1995; Klingenberg, 1996). Fenbendazole inhibits the ability of worms to utilize and process glucose obtained from the host, which explains the gradual and slow onset of its therapeutic effect causing paralysis of adult worms. This is one reason why it is often recommended that patients should receive fenbendazole for several consecutive days or the dosage should be repeated (Giannetto *et al.*, 2007). The ovicidal effect of benzimidazoles is based on their capacity to sterilize female worms. Fenbendazole is the most often used benzimidazole for the treatment of parasitic worm infections in reptiles. It is applied in the form of oral solutions or suspensions (Neiffer *et al.*, 2005). In several clinical cases, repeated application of high fenbendazole doses (>60 mg/kg) decreased the appetite of tortoises (author's personal observation) while another veterinary surgeon did use 100 mg/kg divided over 3 days with good results (P. Raiti – personal communication). It was not proved that adverse effect resulted from the application of fenbendazole; however, it is known that fenbendazole has radiomimetic effects, which can cause intestinal and bone marrow damage in mammals and therefore its use at high dosages (>60 mg/kg) in reptiles should be viewed with caution. Alvarado (2001) reported a case of fenbendazole toxicity in Fea's viper, but the dose was extremely high (> 500 mg/kg). Albendazole has been shown to have a teratogenic effect and embryotoxic effect in mammals; therefore, albendazole cannot be recommended for the treatment of gravid reptile females (Davies and Klingenberg, 2004).

Levamisole: Levamisole inhibits the worms' ability to metabolize carbohydrates, induces paralysis of the nervous system leading to elimination from the host. It can be used in doses 5–10 mg/kg s.c. (Mitchell, 2006). The advantage of this imidazothiazole anthelmintic is that it may be injected as well as administered orally, making it easier to dose; however, levamisole has a relatively narrow range of safety and so is not used widely in reptile medicine. After levamisole treatment when dosed higher than 10 mg/kg, reptiles show signs such as muscular tremors, salivation, convulsive head motions and irritability.

Pyrantel: Pyrantel has a similar mode of activity as levamisole. It is a depolarizing neuromuscular blocking agent, leading to paralysis of the parasite. This mechanism is often likened to a hundredfold effect of acetylcholine. A dose of 5 mg/kg orally, repeated in 14 days has been suggested for the treatment of endoparasites (Meredith, 2015); however, potential toxicity of pyrantel and contraindications of its use in reptiles is also similar to levamisole and so it is rarely used.

Ivermectin: Ivermectin is a veterinary product that belongs to the avermectin anthelmintics. It is active against both nematodes and ectoparasites (arthropods) but not cestodes or trematodes. Various forms of ivermectin application are used in practice; peroral, topical and injectable preparations. Ivermectin increases the release of gamma-aminobutyric acid (GABA) on presynaptic neuronal endings resulting in paralysis of the parasite. Ivermectin is commonly used in a broad spectrum of reptiles and its positive antiparasitic effects include the capacity to penetrate most organs and tissues of the host. The ivermection dose used is 0.2 mg/kg i.m. and the treatment is repeated in 2 weeks.

Chelonians are known to be very susceptible to ivermectin and other avermectins resulting in paralysis and fatalities, which means they should never be used in this group of reptiles. Clinical signs of avermectin toxicity in chelonians include depression, stiffness of the neck and limbs, muscular tremors and ataxia (Teare and Bush, 1983). The animals suffer from spasms and paralysis and usually die. Ivermectin toxicity has also been suggested in some snakes and lizards (king snakes, skinks or chameleons) but this was not proved by any experimental study and toxicity may have been associated with anaphylaxis due to the death of large helminth burdens.

Praziquantel: Praziquantel is a cestocide that increases cell membrane permeability of susceptible worms, resulting in loss of intracellular calcium and paralysis. This allows the parasites to be phagocytosed or digested. It may be administered orally or by subcutaneous or intramuscular injection. Praziquantel is effective against tapeworms and trematodes. Praziquantel should be used with caution in reptiles – the patient's bodyweight must be established accurately and an optimum dose calculated accordingly (5–8 mg/kg orally once for chelonians; 5–10 mg/kg orally once in snakes; 5–30 mg/kg orally once for lizards; Wilkinson, 2004). Imported patients that are very often debilitated and dehydrated first of all need to be stabilized and rehydrated. It has been reported that praziquantel administered in doses above 20 mg/kg caused neurological signs in royal pythons (Davies and Klingenberg, 2004).

Ectoparasiticides

Many substances that were previously used to kill ectoparasites in reptiles may be toxic for certain groups of reptiles when applied in higher doses, or even harmful for

veterinary staff when used in very high concentrations. As far as new products are concerned, relatively few have been shown to be effective and safe in reptiles; therefore, they must be used very carefully.

Fipronil: Fipronil is a widely used insecticide that belongs to the phenylpyrazole chemical family. It disrupts the insect central nervous system by blocking the passage of chloride ions through GABA receptors and glutamate–gated chloride (GluCl) channels. Although it is usually applied in the form of a spray, spot-on and shampoo formulations are available as well. Fipronil spray (2.5 mg/ml) is successfully used to kill mites (particularly on snakes) and to treat internal surfaces of mechanically cleaned terrariums. When applying fipronil spray on the reptile body, the patient's head must initially be covered with a drape for protection. When safe to do so the drape is removed and a fipronil treated swab is used to carefully treat the patient's head between and around the eyes and the skin below the mandible towards the neck. Then the snake is placed in a plastic box for 20 minutes. The box in which the patient was transported to the clinic should be disposed of or thoroughly mechanically cleaned and sprayed with fipronil and washed with water before reuse. After the patient is treated with fipronil it is placed in another clean box. Fipronil spray should be applied at least twice or on three occasions every 2–3 weeks. Care must be taken especially in snakes immediately post slough because the skin is more permeable. In the author's practice, neurological signs such as depression and salivation were observed after the application of fipronil spray in royal pythons. In all these cases, fipronil was applied by the owner, so it cannot be ruled out that the spray was applied inappropriately (e.g. sprayed directly to the head, nostrils, oral cavity or eyes).

Ivermectin: Ivermectin is used to kill mites, ticks and other blood sucking insects. It can be applied environmentally to kill off the host stages of the snake mite (*Ophionyssus natricis*) by spraying a mixture of 10 mg of 1% ivermectin solution and 1 litre of water. Dissolution of ivermectin may be enhanced by adding 2 parts of propylene glycol to 1 part of ivermectin. If the final solution is protected from light, it may be stored for 30 days. The spray is applied at 2–3 week intervals for at least 2 months, which corresponds with the duration of development of snake mite adults from their eggs. Both the patient and environment must be treated and the terrarium should be repeatedly and carefully cleaned to physically remove both live and dead mites. Paper is an ideal terrarium substrate during the treatment process. Subcutaneous injection is another effective route of administration. If necessary, ivermectin (0.2–0.3 mg/kg) is injected in two or three doses 2–3 weeks apart. This application method proved successful in the author's practice with large snakes (pythons, boas) and lizards (green iguana, desert monitor). However, the risk of intoxication cannot be ruled out in small lizards and snakes if accurate weights are not recorded and ivermectin doses suitably titrated. Some veterinary surgeons prefer administering ivermectin orally to reptiles; however, sufficient reliable data that would support or disprove this method is not currently available. Efficacy and safety of topical administration of 'spot-on' preparations of ivermectin in reptiles is even more difficult to appraise. Skin thickness and permeability varies markedly between species and different ages of the same species making this route of administration unreliable. **Ivermectin must not be used in chelonians.**

Pyrethrins and permethrins: It should be noted that pyrethrins and permethrins have the potential to be toxic to reptiles. Both natural pyrethrins and synthetic pyrethroids influence the exchange of ions on the membranes of synapses and affect GABA receptors and ATPase transport of nerve stimuli. When used in higher concentrations, pyrethrins and pyrethroids (cyfluthrin, deltamethrin and permethrin) may be toxic to reptiles as well as having a potentially adverse effect on veterinary staff (Davies and Klingenberg, 2004). Toxicity signs in reptiles include hypersalivation, restlessness, dyspnoea, impaired reflexes (e.g. pupillary reflex), restricted motility, or paralysis, and the reptiles die due to respiratory failure. Small reptiles with permeable skin (leopard gecko, anoles lizards) may show higher susceptibility to permethrin, cypermethrin, flumethrin and deltamethrin. Flumethrin strips that are placed in terrariums to kill mites (*Ophionyssus natricis*) were successfully used in snakes. The strips were placed in the terrarium in such a manner as to avoid their direct contact with snakes' mucosae (they were for instance placed in a finely perforated protective box; DeNardo and Wozniak, 1997). In comparison with dichlorvos-impregnated strips (Frye 1991), those with flumetrin are not cut into small pieces. After spraying the empty terrarium with 0.1% solution, all surfaces need to be thoroughly rinsed and dried to remove residues.

Vitamins

Vitamins act in basic metabolic processes as biocatalysts (*vita* = life). In reptiles, certain vitamins are produced by fermentation activity of intestinal microflora; other vitamins or their precursors must be received in the diet. Vitamins are classified in various groups, most often according to their solubility in fats (lipophilic – A, D, E, K) or water (hydrophilic – C and the complex of B vitamins).

Vitamin A: Vitamin A is a combination of A1 retinol and A_{2-3}-dehydroretinol (40% efficacy of retinol) and is contained particularly in carotene. Herbivorous reptiles obtain beta-carotene from the flowers and fruits of plants. Beta-carotene is split in the intestinal wall by the enzyme carotenase into two molecules of vitamin A. Carnivorous reptiles require pre-formed vitamin A in their diet. Hypovitaminosis A is most often observed in aquatic omnivorous/carnivorous terrapins (e.g. *Trachemys scripta elegans*). At birth, these terrapins have supplies of vitamin A that are sufficient only for a few weeks of life. The clinical signs of hypovitaminosis A include bilateral oedema of the eyelids, pale colour of the mucosa of the mouth cavity (anaemia), anorexia and apathy. Hypovitaminosis A can be present also in captive chameleons and leopard geckos that are fed with crickets kept on a diet with low levels of beta-carotenes or vitamin A. Natural sources of beta-carotene include aquatic plants; or in the visceral organs (principally the liver) of rodents and other small vertebrates. Treating hypovitaminosis A may be by 1000–2000 IU/kg administered orally q7d. If subcutaneous injection of vitamin A is used care must be taken because of the high risk of iatrogenic hypervitaminosis A, which results in skin hyperkeratosis with full skin-thickness sloughing and bleeding (Figure 11.40). Parenteral doses of 7000–10,000 IU/kg administered only once may result in skin sloughing in chelonians. Oral vitamin A is a natural route of administration and is not associated with the risk of visceral injuries and less likely to result in toxicity. The health state of reptiles can be improved by feeding them with new-born mice, fish meat, earthworms, commercial

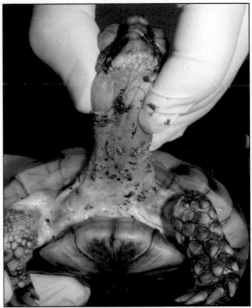

11.40 Iatrogenic hypervitaminosis A with hyperkeratosis, full skin-thickness sloughing and bleeding in a marginated tortoise.

feeds (containing preformed vitamin) and aquatic plants, as well as providing a suitable vitamin A supplement if necessary.

Vitamin B complex: Vitamins of the B group are necessary for a wide range of functions within the body and may be helpful in supporting debilitated reptiles.

Vitamin B1 (thiamine, aneurin): Vitamin B1 is a component of many significant tissue enzymes. It is readily available in the fruits and vegetables making up the diet of herbivorous reptiles and is found in the form of free thiamine or thiamine diphosphate. In herbivores, vitamin B1 deficiency may result from long-term antibiotic treatment (especially from antibiotics administered orally), which negatively influences synthesis of thiamine by intestinal bacteria. In carnivores, deficiencies are more likely to be seen, particularly in those animals exclusively fed thawed salt-water fish (e.g. many water or garter snakes in captivity), as the thiamine is destroyed during the freezing process. This is a similar problem in herbivores fed exclusively thawed vegetables. Thiamine deficiency results in peripheral neuritis and cardiomyopathy, but the most important is the necrosis of the brain (cerebrocortical necrosis). Adverse effects of hypovitaminosis B1 include neurological signs, incoordination, blindness, spasms, paralysis or opisthotonus. Treatment of thiamine deficiency includes administration of vitamin B1 daily with doses of 50–100 mg/kg orally or parenterally. Prevention is based on providing a 'proper' diet, e.g. vegetables and plants (dandelion flower) for herbivores and fresh fish meat (or mice) for carnivorous reptiles. Vitamin B mixtures (known on the market as B-complex) are often used in veterinary practice to stimulate non-specifically the active metabolism of patients.

Vitamin B2 (riboflavin): Flavin enzymes play an important role in retinal biochemical processes. Riboflavin deficiency results in peripheral neuropathy in chickens (weakness and paralysis) and skeletal and soft tissue abnormalities have been described in the offspring of rats and mice fed a riboflavin-deficient diet. In reptiles, scientific based information dealing with riboflavin deficiency is unavailable.

Vitamin B6 (pyridoxine, adermin): Vitamin B6 is present as a complex of three forms – pyridoxal, pyridoxol and pyridoxamine – that act as coenzymes in amino acid metabolism. Pyridoxine deficiency may cause blood, skin, and nerve changes. Clinical reports dealing with riboflavin deficiency in reptiles are not presently available.

Vitamin B7 (biotin): Biotin may bind to avidin from albumen eaten by reptile species living on raw unfertilized eggs (monitor lizards, beaded lizards, egg-eating snake – *Dasypeltis scabra*). Biotin-avidin interaction may lead to a relative biotin deficiency resulting in keratin damage and myasthenia that should be treated by enriching the diet with biotin products. Prevention of this deficiency is based on the feeding of small rodents, birds and/or fertilized eggs.

Vitamin B12 (cyanocobalamin, aquacobalamin and nitrito-cobalamin): Vitamin B12 participates in the metabolism of amino acids and ribonucleotides. It is necessary for erythropoiesis and may act as appetite stimulants in lizards (in doses of 0.05 mg/kg i.m. q24h).

Vitamin C1 (L-ascorbic acid): This is involved in oxidation–reduction processes by mutual conversion to vitamin C2 (dehydro-L-ascorbic acid). Vitamin C1 is synthetized in the gut of healthy reptiles. Deficiency of ascorbic acid in snakes may cause skin ruptures and bleeding of the oral cavity (Frye, 1991; Carpenter *et al.*, 2014). Vitamin C is administered to support non-specific stimulation of the immune system. The recommended doses of vitamin C1 (as a part of stomatitis treatment) in reptiles are 10–20 mg/kg i.m. q7d.

Vitamin D3 (calciol, cholecalciferol): This is necessary for the metabolism of calcium and phosphorus as it facilitates the absorption, distribution and excretion of these minerals within the organism. Moreover, it has an impact on the development of the skeleton and locomotor system. Precursors of vitamin D3 are naturally acquired in the diet. Gradual conversion of cholesterol to 1,25-dihydroxycholecalciferol has been studied in green iguanas. This process is controlled by thyroid and parathyroid hormones (see Chapter 4 for more information). Vitamin D3 deficiency may lead to structural defects of the skeleton, spasms and paralysis. Long-term high levels of circulating parathyroid hormone will eventually lead to renal failure. The optimum calcium to phosphorus ratio in the blood plasma of reptiles is 1.5–2:1. Nutritional secondary hyperparathyroidism is the most common form of metabolic bone disorder (MBD) seen in captive reptiles presenting in veterinary practice and although recommended treatment protocols have been published the author has found that the best treatment is based on the use of high quality UV (UVB) radiation. The recommended dose of vitamin D3 is 200 (100–1000) IU/kg orally in weekly intervals (Barten, 1993, 1996; Boyer, 1997; Stahl, 1998, Funk and Diethelm, 2006; Carpenter *et al.*, 2014).

Vitamin E: The tocopherols (alpha-, beta-, gamma-tocopherols) are significant antioxidants of lipids, unsaturated fatty acids and lipophilic vitamins. Deficiency of dietary tocopherol may cause fatty degeneration of the liver, liver steatitis and muscular dystrophy in lizards, snakes and crocodiles (Larsen *et al.*, 1983; Dierenfeld, 1989; Fraser and Girling, 2004). Treatment may be managed by changing the diet and providing vitamin E supplementation. The diet should reduce the levels of fats by feeding lean meat and insects rich in vitamin E (include shellfish and crustaceans for semiaquatic species), and increase the tocopherol levels by including a wider variety of fruits and vegetables (e.g. spinach, vegetable oils, broccoli, herbs such as oregano etc.) for omnivores and herbivores. The suggested dose of vitamin E supplementation in reptile diets is 1 UI/kg orally q24h (Calvert, 2004).

Vitamin K (vitamin K1 phylloquinone and vitamin K2 farnoquinone): These vitamins are synthesized in the intestine by the gut bacteria. Vitamin K is important for the production of prothrombin and other blood clotting factors. Deficiency of vitamin K has not been documented in reptiles. Supplementation of vitamin K may be considered in reptiles with bleeding and chronic liver diseases.

Minerals

Calcium: Dietary calcium deficiency may lead to impaired development of the skeleton in reptiles and will be exacerbated by vitamin D3 deficiency and an inverse calcium to phosphorus ratio. Young animals show signs of calcium deficiency; motor weakness, lethargy, constipation, anorexia and tetany in lizards. Late onset signs of calcium deficiency include saddle-shaped deformations of the carapace in chelonians, swollen joints in lizards and fibrous osteodystrophy of long bones. Reptiles may show hypocalcaemic collapse/tetany and their pelvic limbs become paralyzed. Others may show fine muscular fasciculation. The author has seen cases of cloacal prolapse in reptiles with calcium deficiency (checked by monitoring the ionized calcium levels in peripheral blood; Figure 11.41). Prevention of dietary calcium deficiency is based on supplementing the diet with foodstuffs that are rich in calcium or at least show favourable calcium/phosphorus (cuttlefish, sepia bone, egg shell or commercial supplements in powdered form). If recommended oral doses of calcium glubionate (1 ml/kg q12h) are administered, overdose should not occur unless the animal receives excessive doses of vitamin D3. For the treatment of hypocalcaemic tetany, calcium gluconate with at a dose of 100 mg/kg i.m. q6h is recommended.

Iodine: Chemical links between iodine and thyroglobulin produce iodized thyronines (triiodothyronine (T_3) and thyroxine (T_4)), which circulate in the blood and participate in regulative functions of the thyroid gland that control basic metabolic processes (stimulation of proteosynthesis, release of thermal energy and regulation of oxidative processes). Secondary iodine deficiency was recorded in

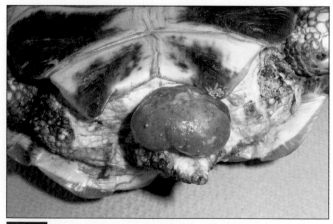

11.41 Cloacal prolapse in a Horsfield's tortoise with hypocalcaemia.

herbivorous lizards and giant chelonians fed with brassicas/goitrogens – kale, broccoli, cabbage (Frye and Dutra, 1974; Frye, 1991). Medical management of giant chelonians suffering from hypothyroidism with the use of iodine has been published (Norton et al., 1989). Dried kelp or kelp tablets as a source of iodine have been recommended by Donoghue and Langenberg (1996).

Oxytocin

Oxytocin is used to stimulate parturition in reptiles (see Chapter 20). Very good results were achieved in chelonians that received doses of 1.5–10 IU/kg i.m.. In practice, moderate doses (5–6 IU/kg i.m.) proved most effective. Overdose with oxytocin may induce spasms and rupture of oviduct walls. Efficacy of oxytocin can be enhanced by injecting calcium in advance (e.g. calcium gluconate) especially in patients suffering from calcium deficit. Oxytocin stimulation may be repeated after 24 hours using half the previous dose. Oxytocin is less efficacious in snakes and lizards and should not be used in weak and dehydrated females with a high number of eggs in the oviduct, such as chameleons, due to the risk of obstructive dystocia developing. In these situations surgical treatment can be recommended.

Non-steroidal anti-inflammatory drugs

Non-steroidal anti-inflammatory drugs (NSAIDs) are used as analgesics and for anti-inflammatory properties (Sladky, 2014). It is imperative to consider the possible adverse effects of NSAIDs on the gastric mucosa, kidney function and blood coagulation (Wellehan and Gunkel, 2004, Tuttle et al., 2006). Meloxicam and carprofen appeared to be safe for green iguanas. Neither carprofen (2 mg/kg i.m. q24h) nor meloxicam (0.2 mg/kg i.m. q24h) induced gastric mucosa bleeding and ulceration, nor clinically important changes in haematological parameters (Trnkova et al., 2007). Pharmacokinetics data on NSAIDs in green iguanas have been published (Tuttle et al., 2006; Divers et al., 2010) and NSAIDs are used widely in reptile clinical practice (Sladky, 2014) (see also Chapter 12).

Opioids

Opioid receptors are expressed in reptiles, but the scientific based knowledge about the optimal opioid use (drugs, dosages, frequency) in reptile patients is in its infancy. Experimental evaluation of analgesic properties of opioids in reptiles is limited to only one laboratory based results (with the use of thermal stimulus, Sladky et al., 2007, 2008, 2009). In clinical practice with reptiles, morphine, butorphanol, buprenorphine, fentanyl and tramadol have been used for pain management with different antinoxious effects (Sladky, 2014) (see also Chapter 12). For further drug and dosage information see the Formulary in Appendix 2.

References and further reading

Allender MC, Mitchell MA, Yarborough J et al. (2013) Pharmacokinetics of a single oral dose of acyclovir and valacyclovir in North American box turtles (Terrapene sp.) Journal of Veterinary Pharmacology and Therapeutics 36, 205–208

Alvarado TP (2001) Fenbendazole overdose in four Fea's vipers. Proceedings of the Association of Reptilian and Amphibian Veterinarians, 35–37

Barten SL (1993) The medical care of iguanas and other common pet lizards. Veterinary Clinic of North America: Small Animal Practice 23, 1213–1249

Barten SL (1996) Diseases of the green iguana (Iguana iguana). Proceedings of the North American Veterinary Conference, 811–814

Benson KG, Tell LA, Young LA et al. (2003) Pharmacokinetics of ceftiofur sodium after intramuscular or subcutaneous administration in green iguana (Iguana iguana). American Journal of Veterinary Research 64, 1278–1282

Bodri M, Rambo TM, Wagner RA et al. (2006) Pharmacokinetics of metronidazole administered as a single oral bolus to red rat snakes, Elaphe guttata. Journal of Herpetological Medicine and Surgery 16, 15–19

Bogoslavsky BA (2007) The use of ponazuril to treat coccidiosis in eight inland bearded dragons (Pogona vitticeps). Proceedings of the Association of Reptilian and Amphibian Veterinarians, New Orleans, 8–9

Boyer TH (1996) Metabolic bone disease. In: Reptile Medicine and Surgery, ed. DR Mader, pp. 385–392. WB Saunders, Philadelphia

Brames H (2008) Efficacy and tolerability of Profender in reptiles: spot-on treatment against nematodes. Exotic DVM 10, 29–34

Burgmann PM, McFarlen J and Thiesenhausen K (1993) Causes of hypocalcaemia and metabolic bone disease in Iguana iguana. Journal of Small Exotic Animal Medicine 2, 63–68

Calvert I (2004) Nutritional problems. In: BSAVA Manual of Reptiles, 2nd edn, ed. SJ Girling and P Raiti, pp. 289–308. BSAVA Publications, Gloucester, UK

Caliguri R, Kollias GV, Jacobson E et al. (1990) The effects of ambient temperature on amikacin pharmacokinetics in gopher tortoises. Journal of Veterinary Pharmacology and Therapeutics 13, 287–291

Carpenter JW, Klaphake E and Gibbons PM (2014) Reptile formulary and laboratory normal. In: Current therapy in reptile medicine and surgery, ed. DR Mader and SJ Divers, pp. 382–410. Saunders Elsevier, St. Louis

Chitty J (2004) Respiratory system. In: BSAVA Manual of Reptiles, 2nd edn, ed. SJ Girling and P Raiti, pp. 230–242. BSAVA Publications, Gloucester, UK

Chitty J and Raftery A (2013) In: Essentials of tortoise medicine and surgery, p. 338. Wiley Blackwell, Chichester

Clark CH, Rogers ED and Milton JL (1985) Plasma concentrations of chloramphenicol in snakes. Journal of the American Veterinary Association 46, 2654–2657

Coke RL, Isaza R, Koch DE et al. (2006) Preliminary single-dose pharmacokinetics of marbofloxacin in ball pythons (Python regius). Journal of Zoo and Wildlife Medicine 37, 6–10

Davies RR and Klingenberg RJ (2004) Therapeutics and medication. In: BSAVA Manual of Reptiles, 2nd edn, ed. SJ Girling and P Raiti, pp. 115–130. BSAVA Publications, Gloucester

De Nardo D and Wozniak EJ (1997) Understanding the snake mite and current therapies for control. Proceedings of the Association of Reptilian and Amphibian Veterinarians Conference, 137–147

Dierenfeld ES (1989) Vitamin E deficiency in zoo reptiles, birds and ungulates. Journal of Zoo and Wildlife Medicine 20, 3–11

Divers SJ (1996) Empirical doses of antimicrobial drugs commonly used in reptiles. Exotic DVM 1, 23

Divers SJ and Lawton MPC (1999) Antibiotic-impregnated polymethylmethacrylate beads as a treatment for osteomyelitis in reptiles. Proceedings of the Association of Reptilian and Amphibian Veterinarians Conference, 145–147

Divers SJ, Papich M, McBride M et al. (2010) Pharmacokinetics of meloxicam following intravenous and oral administration in green iguanas (Iguana iguana). American Journal of Veterinary Research 71, 1277–1283

Diethelm G (2005) Reptiles. In: Exotic Animal Formulary, 3rd edn, ed. JW Carpenter, pp. 55–131. Elsevier Saunders, St. Louis

Donoghue S and Langenberg J (1996) Nutrition. In: Reptile Medicine and Surgery, ed. DR Mader, pp. 148–174. WB Saunders, Philadelphia

Fraser MA and Girling SJ (2004) Dermatology. In: BSAVA Manual of Reptiles, 2nd edn, ed. SJ Girling and P Raiti, pp. 184–197. BSAVA Publications, Gloucester, UK

Frye FL (1991) Biomedical and surgical aspects of captive reptile husbandry, p. 637. Krieger Publishing Company, Malabar, Florida, USA

Frye FL and Dutra FR (1974) Hypothyroidism in turtles and tortoises. Veterinary Medicine, Small Animal Clinician 69, 990–993

Funk RS (2000) A formulary for lizards, snakes, and crocodilians. Veterinary Clinics of North America: Exotic Animal Practice 3, 333–358

Funk RS, Diethelm G (2006) Reptile formulary. In: Reptile Medicine and Surgery, 2nd edn, ed. DR Mader, pp. 1119–1139. Saunders Elsevier, St. Louis

Gaio C, Rossi T, Villa R et al. (2007) Pharmacokinetics of acyclovir after a single oral administration in marginated tortoises, Testudo marginata. Journal of Herpetological Medicine and Surgery 17, 8–11

Giannetto S, Brianti E, Poglayen G et al. (2007) Efficacy of oxfendazole and fenbendazole against tortoise (Testudo hermanni) oxyurids. Parasitology Research 100, 1069–1073

Gibbons PM (2014) Therapeutics. In: Current therapy in reptile medicine and surgery, ed. DR Mader and SJ Divers, pp. 57–69. Saunders Elsevier, St. Louis

Gibbons PM, Klaphake EA and Carpenter JW (2012) Reptiles. In: Exotic animal formulary, 4th edn, ed. JW Carpenter, pp. 83–182. Elsevier, St. Louis

Girling SJ and Fraser MA (2009) Treatment of Aspergillus species infection in reptiles with itraconazole at metabolically scaled doses. Veterinary Record 165, 52–54

Grosset C, Villeneuve A, Brieger A et al. (2011) Cryptosporidiosis in Juvenile Bearded Dragons (Pogona vitticeps): Effects of Treatment with Paromomycin. Journal of Herpetological Medicine and Surgery 21, 10–15

Guzman DSM, Mitchell MA and Acierno M (2011) Determination of plasma osmolality and agreement between measured and calculated values in captive male corn snakes (*Pantherus [Elaphe] guttatus guttatus*). *Journal of Herpetological Medicine and Surgery* **21**, 16–19

Hellebuyck T, Pasmans F, Haesebrouck F *et al.* (2009) Designing a successful antimicrobial treatment against *Devriesea agamarum* infections in lizards. *Veterinary Microbiology* **139**, 189–192

Hernandez-Divers SJ (2001) Pulmonary candidiasis caused by *Candida albicans* in a Greek tortoise (*Testudo graeca*) and treatment with intrapulmonary amphotericin B. *Journal of Zoo and Wildlife Medicine* **32**, 352–359

Hilf M, Swanson D and Wagner R (1991) A new dosing schedule for gentamicin in blood pythons (*Python curtus*): a pharmacokinetic study. *Research in Veterinary Science* **50**, 127–130

Hilf M, Swanson D, Wagner R *et al.* (1991) Pharmacokinetics of piperacillin in blood pythons (*Python curtus*) and *in vitro* evaluation of efficacy against aerobic Gram-negative bacteria. *Journal of Zoo and Wildlife Medicine* **22**, 199–203

Holt PE (1981) Drugs and dosages. In: *Diseases of the Reptilia*, ed. JE Cooper and OF Jackson, 2, pp. 551–583. Academic Press, London

Holz P, Burger JP, Pasloske K *et al.* (2002) Effect of injection site on carbenicillin pharmacokinetics in the carpet python (*Morelia spilotes*). *Journal of Herpetological Medicine and Surgery* **12**, 12–16

Innis C (1995) In my experience: per-cloacal deworming of tortoises. *Bulletin of the Association of Reptilian and Amphibian Veterinarians* **5**, 4

Innis CJ, Harms CA and Manire CA (2017) Therapeutics. In: *Sea Turtle Health and Rehabilitation*. eds. CA Manire, TM Norton, BA Stacy, CJ Innis, Harms CA, pp. 497–526. J. Ross Publishing, Jupiter, Florida, USA

Innis C, Ceresia ML, Merigo C *et al.* (2012) Single-dose pharmacokinetics of ceftazidime and fluconazole during concurrent clinical use in cold-stunned Kemp's ridley turtles (*Lepidochelys kempii*). *Journal of Veterinary Pharmacology and Therapeutics* **35**, 82–89

Innis C, Papich M and Young D (2007) Pharmacokinetics of metronidazole in the red-eared slider turtle (*Trachemys scripta elegans*) after single intracoelomic injection. *Journal of Veterinary Pharmacology and Therapeutics* **30**, 168–171

Innis C, Young D, Wetzlich S *et al.* (2008) Plasma voriconazole concentrations in four red-eared slider turtles (*Trachemys scripta elegans*) after a single subcutaneous injection. *Proceedings of the 15th Annual Conference of the Association of Reptilian and Amphibian Veterinarians*, 72

Jacobson ER (1993) Antimicrobial drug use in reptiles. In: *Antimicrobial therapy in veterinary medicine*, ed. JF Prescott and JD Baggot, pp. 543–552. Iowa State University, Ames

Jacobson ER (1993) Snakes. *Veterinary Clinics of North America: Small Animal Practice* **23**, 1179–1212

Jacobson ER (1999) Bacterial infections and antimicrobial treatment in reptiles. *Proceedings of the North American Veterinary Conference*, 771–774

Jacobson ER, Brown MP, Chung M *et al.* (1988) Serum concentration and disposition kinetics of gentamicin and amikacin in juvenile American alligator. *Journal of Zoo Animal Medicine* **19**, 188–194

Jacobson ER, Kollias GV and Peters LJ (1983) Dosages of antibiotics and parasiticides used in exotic animals. *Compendium on Continuing Education for the Practising Veterinarian* **5**, 315–324

Jekl V and Knotek Z (2006) Endoscopic examination of snakes by access through an air sac. *Veterinary Record* **158**, 407–410

Johnson JD, Mangone B and Jarchow JL (1998) A review of mycoplasmosis infections in tortoises and options for treatment. *Proceedings of the Association of Reptilian and Amphibian Veterinarians Conference*, 89–92

Johnson JH, Jensen JM, Brumbaugh GW *et al.* (1997) Amikacin pharmacokinetics and the effects of ambient temperature on the dosage regimen in ball pythons (*Python regius*). *Journal of Zoo and Wildlife Medicine* **28**, 80–88

Kauffman GE (1997) Pharmacology, pharmacodynamics and drug dosing. In: *The Biology, Husbandry and Health Care of Reptiles, Vol III*. The Health Care of Reptiles, ed. L Ackerman, pp. 803–821. TFH Publications, Neptune, USA

Klingenberg RJ and Backner B (1991) The use of ciprofloxacin, a new antibiotic, in snakes. *Proceedings of the 15th International Symposium of Captive Propagation and Husbandry*, 127–140

Klingenberg RJ (1996) Therapeutics. In: *Reptile Medicine and Surgery, 1st edn*, ed. DR Mader, pp. 299–321. WB Saunders, Philadelphia

Kolmstetter CM, Frazier D, Cox S *et al.* (1998) Pharmacokinetics of metronidazole in the green iguana, *Iguana iguana*. *Bulletin of the Association of Reptilian and Amphibian Veterinarians* **8**, 4–7

Kolmstetter CM, Cox S and Ramsay EC (2001) Pharmacokinetics of metronidazole in the yellow rat snake, *Elaphe obsoleta quadrivitatta*. *Journal of Herpetological Medicine and Surgery* **11**, 4–8

Lai OR, Laricchiuta P, Putignano C *et al.* (2007) Pharmacokinetics, pharmacokinetic/pharmacodynamics integration and dose regimen of marbofloxacin on red-eared slider (*Trachemys scripta elegans*). *Proceedings of International Zoo and Wildlife Research* **43**, 273–275

Larsen RE, Buergelt C, Cradeilhac PT and Jacobson ER (1983) Steatitis and fat necrosis in captive alligators. *Journal of the American Veterinary Association* **183**, 1202–1204

Lawrence K, Muggleton PW, and Needham JR (1984) Preliminary study on the use of ceftazidime, a broad-spectrum cephalosporin antibiotic in snakes. *Research in Veterinary Science* **36**, 16

Lawrence K, Palmer GH and Needham JR (1986) Use of carbenicillin in two species of tortoise (*Testudo graeca* and *T. hermanni*). *Research in Veterinary Science* **40**, 413

Lightfoot T (2001) Nebulization therapy in tortoises pneumonia. *Exotic DVM* **2**, 5

Mader DR (1991) Antibiotic therapy. In: *Biomedical and Surgical Aspects of Captive Reptile Husbandry*, ed. FL Frye, pp. 621–633. Krieger Publishing Company, Malabar, Florida

Mader DR, Conzelman GM and Baggot JD (1985) Effects of ambient temperature on the half-life and dosage regimen of amikacin in the gopher snake. *Journal of the American Veterinary Association* **187**, 1134–1136

Marin P, Baynon A, Fernandez-Varon E *et al.* (2008) Pharmacokinetics of danofloxacin after single dose intravenous, intramuscular and subcutaneous administration to loggerhead turtles (*Caretta caretta*). *Diseases of Aquatic Organisms* **82**, 231–236

McArthur S (2004) Problem-solving approach to common diseases of terrestrial and semi-aquatic chelonians. In: *Medicine and Surgery of Tortoises and Turtles*, ed. S McArthur, R Wilkinson and J Meyer, pp. 309–377. Blackwell Publishing, Oxford

Marschang RE, Gravendyck M and Kaleta EF (1997) Herpesviruses in tortoises: investigation into virus isolation and the treatment of viral stomatitis in *Testudo hermanni* and *T. graeca*. *Journal of Veterinary Medicine B* **44**, 385–394

Mayer J, Kaufman G and Pokras M (2006) Allometric scalling. In: *Reptile Medicine and Surgery, 2nd edn* ed. DR Mader, pp. 419–427. WB Saunders, Philadelphia

Meredith A (2015) In: *BSAVA Small Animal Formulary 9th edn • Part B: Exotic Pets*, ed A Meredith, p 252. BSAVA, Gloucester, UK

Michaels SJ (1988) Update on pharmaceuticals useful in reptile and amphibian medicine. *Proceedings of the 13th International Symposium of Captive Propagation and Husbandry*, 37–60

Mitchell MA (2006) Therapeutics. In: *Reptile Medicine and Surgery, 2nd edn*, ed. DR Mader, pp. 631–664. WB Saunders, Philadelphia

Mitchell MA (2008) Ponazuril. *Journal of Exotic Pet Medicine* **17**, 228–229

Neiffer DL, Lydick D, Burks K *et al.* (2005) Hematologic and plasma biochemical changes associated with fenbendazole administration in Hermann's tortoises (*Testudo hermanni*). *Journal of Zoo and Wildlife Medicine* **36**, 661–672

Norton TM, Jacobson ER, Caligiuri R and Kollias GV (1989) Medical management of Galapagos tortoise (*Geochelone elephantopus*) with hypothyroidism. *Journal of Zoo and Wildlife Medicine* **20(2)**, 212–216

Origgi FC, Jacobson ER (2000) Diseases of the respiratory tract of chelonians. *Veterinary Clinics of North America: Exotic Animal Practice* **3**, 537–549

Page CD, Mautino M, Derendorf H and Mechlinski W (1991) Multiple-dose pharmacokinetics of ketoconazole administered orally to gopher tortoises (*Gopherus polyphemus*). *Journal of Zoo and Wildlife Medicine* **22**, 191–198

Pokras MA, Sedgwick CJ and Kaufman G (1992) Therapeutics. In: *Manual of Reptiles 1st edn*, ed. PH Beynon, MPC Lawton and JE Cooper, pp. 194–213. BSAVA, Cheltenham, UK

Raiti P (2002) Administration of aerosolised antibiotics to reptiles. *Exotic DVM* **4**, 87–90

Raphael BL, Clark CH and Hudson R (1985) Plasma concentration of gentamicin in turtles. *Journal of Zoo Animal Medicine* **16**, 136–139

Raphael BL, Papich M and Cook RA (1994) Pharmacokinetics of enrofloxacin after a single intramuscular injection in Indian star tortoises (*Geochelone elegans*). *Journal of Zoo and Wildlife Medicine* **25**, 88–94

Ross RA and Marzec G (1984) *The Bacterial Diseases of Reptiles*, p. 114. Institute for Herpetological Research. Stanford, CA

Rossi J (1995) Practical reptile dermatology. *Proceedings of the North American Veterinary Conference*, 648–649

Schilliger L, Betremieux O, Rochet J *et al.* (2009) Absorption and efficacy of a spot-on combination containing emodepside plus praziquantel in reptiles. *Revue De Medecine Veterinaire (Toulouse)* **160**, 557–561

Schumacher J (1996) Viral diseases. In: *Reptile Medicine and Surgery, 1st edn*, ed. DR Mader, pp. 224–234. WB Saunders, Philadelphia

Spörle H, Göbel T and Schildger B (1991) Blood levels of some anti-infectives in the Hermann's tortoise (*Testudo hermanni*). *Proceedings of the 4th International Colloquium on Pathology and Medicine of Reptiles and Amphibians*, 120–128

Sladky K (2014) Analgesia. In: *Current therapy in reptile medicine and surgery*, ed. DR Mader and SJ Divers, pp. 217–228. Saunders Elsevier, St. Louis

Sladky KK, Miletic V, Paul-Murphy J *et al.* (2007) Analgesic efficacy and respiratory effects of butorphanol and morphine in turtles. *Journal of American Veterinary Medical Association* **230**, 1356–1362

Sladky KK, Kinney ME and Johnson SM (2008) Analgesic efficacy of butorphanol and morphine in bearded dragons and corn snakes. *Journal of American Veterinary Medical Association* **233**, 267–273

Sladky KK, Kinney ME and Johnson SM (2009) Effects of opioid receptor activation on thermal antinociception in red-eared slider turtles (*Trachemys scripta*). *American Journal of Veterinary Research* **70**, 1072–1078

Stahl SJ (1998) Common diseases of the green iguana. *Proceedings of the North American Veterinary Conference*, 806–809

Stamper MA, Papich MG, Lewbart GA *et al.* (1999) Pharmacokinetics of ceftazidime in loggerhead sea turtles (*Caretta caretta*) after single intravenous and intramuscular injections. *Journal of Zoo and Wildlife Medicine* **30**, 32–35

Stein G (1996) Reptile and amphibian formulary. In: *Reptile Medicine and Surgery, 1st edn*, ed. DR Mader, pp. 465–472. WB Saunders, Philadelphia

Teare JA and Bush M (1983) Toxicity and efficacy of ivermectin in chelonians. *Journal of the American Veterinary Association* **183**, 1195–1197

Tobias KMS, Schneider RK and Besser TE (1996) Use of antimicrobial impregnated polymethyl metacrylate. *Journal of the American Veterinary Association* **208**, 841–845

Trnkova S, Knotkova, Z, Hrda A *et al.* (2007) Effect of non-steroidal anti-inflammatory drugs on the blood profile in the green iguana (*Iguana iguana*). *Veterinarni Medicina* **52**, 507–511

Tuttle AD, Papich M, Lewbart GA *et al.* (2006) Pharmacokinetics of ketoprofen in the green iguana (*Iguana iguana*) following single intravenous and intramuscular injections. *Journal of Zoo and Wildlife Medicine* **37**, 567–570

Van Waeyenberghe L, Baert K, Pasmans F *et al.* (2010) Voriconazole, a safe alternative for treating infections caused by the *Chrysosporium* anamorph of Nannizziopsis vriesii in bearded dragons (*Pogona vitticeps*). *Medical Mycology* **48**, 880–885

Vree TB, Vree JB and Nouws JFM (1986) Acetylation and hydroxylation of sulfadimidine by the turtle *Cuora amboniensis*. *Journal of Veterinary Pharmacology and Therapeutics* **9**, 330–332

Wilkinson R (2004) Therapeutics. In: *Medicine and Surgery of Tortoises and Turtles*, ed. S McArthur, R Wilkinson and J Meyer, pp. 465–485. Blackwell Publishing, Oxford

Wimsatt J, Johnson J, Mangone BA *et al.* (1999) Clarithromycin pharmacokinetics in the desert tortoise (*Gopherus agassizii*). *Journal of Zoo and Wildlife Medicine* **30**, 36–43

Wimsatt J, Tothill A, Offerman CF *et al.* (2008) Long-term and per rectum diposition of clarithromycin in the desert tortoise (*Gopherus agassizii*). *Journal of the American Association for Laboratory Animal Science* **47**, 41–45

Chapter 12

Anaesthesia and analgesia

Mads F. Bertelsen

Sedation and anaesthesia are essential components of veterinary care of reptiles, and in most cases are relatively straightforward. Sedation may be employed to facilitate handling and to enhance the quality or safety of diagnostic procedures, while anaesthesia is indispensable to enable surgery and other painful or invasive procedures. Although the field of reptilian anaesthesia has seen a radical evolution over the past decades, controlled clinical studies and solid pharmacokinetic data are still comparably scarce. Generally speaking, reptiles make rewarding anaesthetic subjects: they are rather tough, life-threatening anaesthetic complications are rare, and spur of the moment decisions are rarely necessary.

Anatomy and physiology

Reptiles are ectothermic vertebrates with relatively low metabolic rates. Several anatomical and physiological features differ from those of mammals and may have implications for anaesthetic management. Chapter 1 provides an overview, but certain relevant characteristics are discussed here.

Cardiovascular system

The incomplete ventricular separation of non-crocodilian reptiles (and the foramen of Panizza in the crocodilians) creates the potential for intracardiac mixing or shunting of blood. This may occur as a left-to-right (L–R) shunt or a right-to-left (R–L) shunt. A L–R shunt results in oxygenated pulmonary venous blood re-entering pulmonary circulation, while a R–L shunt results in a fraction of deoxygenated systemic venous blood bypassing the lungs and returning into systemic circulation, resulting in alveolar-to-arterial gradients for respiratory gases.

The extent and direction of shunting is highly dependent on the degree of functional separation, determined by evolutionary adaptations. At one extreme, aquatic turtles have large intracardiac shunts, while boas, pythons and varanid lizards only exhibit low-grade shunting.

As a result of functional intrapulmonary venous admixture and R–L intracardiac shunting, the systemic arterial blood of reptiles may have gas tensions considerably different from the gas within the lung. The consequence may be that induction and recovery from inhalational anaesthesia are slower and less predictable than in mammals and birds. Variation in shunting may also account

for sudden changes in anaesthetic depth experienced in reptiles maintained on inhalational agents.

A renal portal system exists in chelonians and some squamates (Holz et al., 1997b; Benson and Forrest, 1999), but appears to only minimally affect pharmacokinetics of drugs injected in the hindlimbs (Holtz et al., 1997a); however, when possible, the injection of nephrotoxic or renally excreted drugs into the hindquarters of a reptile should be avoided.

Respiratory system

The glottis is located at the base of the tongue, quite rostrally in the oral cavity. The glottis is closed during most of the respiratory cycle, opening only during inspiration and expiration. The trachea of snakes and lizards has incomplete cartilaginous rings, while that of chelonians and crocodilians has complete tracheal rings.

Reptiles, most notably freshwater turtles, are remarkably resistant to ambient hypoxia. While green iguanas can breath-hold for up to 4.5 hours, certain chelonians may survive complete environmental anoxia for hours or days at their normal body temperatures, and weeks to months at very low temperatures. An increase in body temperature, however, leads to increased metabolic oxygen consumption and consequently to increased ventilation.

Vascular access sites

While it may be a challenge to gain vascular access in certain reptiles, with patience and practice it is mostly achievable. This author's preferred sites are listed in Figure 12.1. Indwelling catheters may be placed in the jugular, cephalic, femoral or abdominal veins using cutdown techniques. During anaesthesia, a butterfly needle can often be taped in place in the ventral tail vein of lizards to allow continuous intravenous access. Fluids and

Species	Vascular access sites
Turtles	Supravertebral, jugular vein, dorsal tail vein
Tortoises	Jugular vein, supravertebral, brachial plexus, dorsal tail vein
Lizards	Ventral tail
Snakes	Ventral tail, heart, palatine veins
Crocodilians	Occipital sinus, ventral tail

12.1 Reliable vascular access sites for drug administration, listed in order of preference.

certain drugs may also be administered by the intraosseous route. Intraosseous catheterization may be performed in the humerus, femur or tibia following local analgesia of the cannulation site. In chelonians, cannulation of the bridge between the plastron and carapace is possible, but may be difficult. In snakes, cardiac puncture appears to result in only minor damage to the myocardium; however, as cardiac tamponade has been documented, and the procedure is likely stressful in the conscious snake, this author sees cardiac injections as a last resort.

Pre-anaesthetic considerations

History and physical examination

Obtaining a thorough history and assessing the patient's physical status will aid in decision-making around the choice of anaesthesia and supportive care. Bodyweights vary markedly, and an accurate weight must be obtained prior to administering drugs to the reptilian patient (Figure 12.2). The hydration status of the subject should be assessed, and severe abnormalities corrected. If time, budget and facilities allow, a blood sample for packed cell volume (PCV), complete blood count (CBC) and a plasma biochemistry profile may be useful. In this author's experience, the most important parameter is plasma total protein, as regular doses of protein-bound drugs such as propofol may lead to clinical overdosing in severely hypoproteinaemic patients.

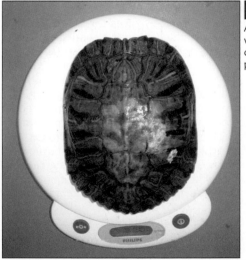

12.2 An accurate weight should be obtained for all patients.

Acclimatization

Following transport to the clinic, patients should be allowed to acclimatize before anaesthetic induction. It is of particular importance that the body temperature is within the preferred range. See Supportive care below.

Fasting

If possible, it is recommended to fast animals 24–48 hours prior to anaesthesia to avoid complications arising from live invertebrate prey items in the stomach or impaired pulmonary function due to compression. Particularly in tortoises, a full stomach may compromise lung expansion. Large carnivorous reptiles may require to be fasted for several days due to slow digestion times.

In snakes feeding infrequently, massive increases in oxygen consumption follow feeding, and heart as well as liver weight increases due to hypertrophy. The effect of these changes on drug metabolism is unknown, but the variability in response to anaesthetic drugs in certain reptiles may be partly due to these mechanisms. This unpredictability, as well as the potential for pulmonary compression by the full gastrointestinal tract mentioned above, might increase the risk of anaesthetic complications; therefore, elective procedures should be avoided in recently fed animals.

Supportive care

Maintaining body temperature

The metabolic rate of reptiles is highly temperature dependent. This means that the effective anaesthetic dosage and the induction and recovery time all depend on body temperature, and that maintaining the animal's body temperature constant and within the preferred optimum zone is crucial (Preston *et al.*, 2010; Kischinovsky *et al.*, 2013; Shepard *et al.*, 2013). This may be achieved through the use of heating pads, circulating water blankets, water bottles, bean bags, etc. A body temperature of 25–30°C for temperate species and 30–35°C for tropical species during induction, anaesthesia and recovery will be appropriate, and most dosage recommendations are based on this. In general, increasing the temperature by 10°C will reduce recovery time by 50%, but will also increase the dosage required for achieving anaesthesia.

Endotracheal intubation

Owing to the large oral cavities and rostral position of the glottis, lizards and snakes are easily intubated. In chelonians, the oral cavity is smaller and the tongue fleshier, but the glottis can still be visualized at the bottom of the mouth, immediately caudal to the tongue (Figures 12.3 and 12.4). A non-cuffed endotracheal tube of appropriate size is inserted and taped in place, ensuring airway patency and allowing positive pressure ventilation, either manually or using mechanical ventilators (Figure 12.5). Larger squamates may have a cuffed tube placed as they have C-shaped rings of cartilage, whereas chelonians

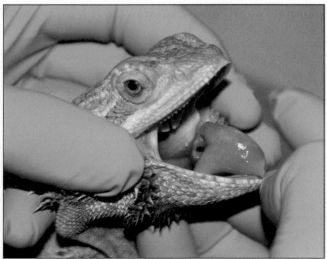

12.3 In lizards and turtles the glottis is located immediately caudal to the fleshy tongue, seen here in a bearded dragon.

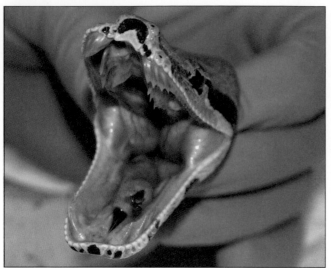

12.4 In snakes the glottis is located far rostrally, just above the tongue, seen here in a boa constrictor.

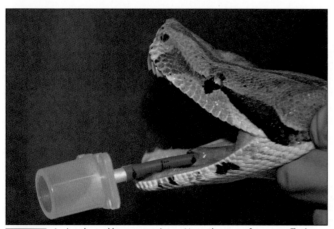

12.5 An intubated boa constrictor. Note the use of an uncuffed tube.

have complete O-rings of cartilage, making them unsuitable candidates for cuffed tubes because of the possibility of pressure necrosis and stricture formations. Snakes and some lizards may be intubated awake following the application of topical analgesics to the glottis, as the absence of a diaphragm means there is no cough reflex. In crocodilians, a valve-like structure separating the oral cavity from the pharynx must be displaced dorsally to gain access to the glottis.

Endotracheal tubes are commercially available down to 1 mm internal diameter, but for the smallest subjects, over-the-needle intravenous catheters (12–19 G) may be used. Some form of mouth gag, which could simply be a piece of rubber tubing or a piece of a syringe, depending on the size of the subject, may be used to prevent the animal from biting on the tube. This is particularly important in larger chelonians.

In small reptiles, taping the animal, the endotracheal tube and the breathing system to the table, a board or a tongue depressor may prevent tube displacement and injury.

Mechanical ventilation

Anaesthetized reptiles may experience long periods of apnoea without deleterious effects due to their low metabolic rates and resilience to hypoxaemia. However, mechanical ventilation is recommended during deep or prolonged anaesthesia. Apart from preventing hypoxaemia and hypercapnia, ventilation ensures delivery and removal of inhalational anaesthetics.

Following endotracheal intubation, mechanical ventilation may be achieved by simply manually 'bagging' the animal or by means of a ventilator of appropriate size. When artificially ventilating reptiles, the larger tidal volume and lower minute ventilation compared with mammals must be taken into consideration, and the machine should be set so that it visibly moves the chest (or forelimbs of chelonians), while avoiding over-inflation of the lungs. A rough estimate would be no more than one-third chest diameter increase in squamates if manually ventilating. Although shunting may make values inaccurate, capnography can be used to monitor the level of ventilation but should be used with caution. A minute ventilation of 50–75 ml/kg and a frequency of 0.5–4 breaths/minute will be adequate in most species, and specialized equipment may be necessary to avoid over-ventilation (Bertelsen *et al.*, 2015).

Fluid therapy

As the intercellular osmolality of reptiles is generally lower than in mammals, it has been suggested that fluids of lower osmolalities be used, such as saline or Ringer's solution diluted with 5–10% water (Mader and Rudloff, 2006). Some texts, however, suggest that reptile extracellular fluids are isotonic in relation to mammals, making broad assumptions difficult (Guzman *et al.*, 2011).

Fluids may be administered intravenously, subcutaneously, intracoelomically or intraosseously. During longer procedures, this author routinely gives 25–50 ml Ringer's solution per kg bodyweight subcutaneously or intracoelomically. Refer to Chapter 11 for general recommendations.

Monitoring physiological function

Most monitoring modalities known from domestic species may be applied to reptiles. Body temperature should be monitored with a cloacal thermometer or temperature probe (Figure 12.6). Make sure that the device is able to measure temperatures lower than mammalian ranges; most standard rectal thermometers are not.

Heart rate and rhythm may be monitored using electrocardiography (ECG) or Doppler flow detection units. In snakes, the heart rate may usually be determined by visual inspection of the ventral scales approximately 25% of the snake's length from the head, while in many lizards and some chelonians the heart rate may be visually observed in the jugular groove. Blood pressure may be measured invasively only following cut-down procedures,

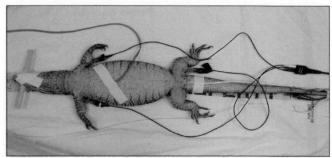

12.6 An anaesthetized monitor lizard monitored using a cloacal temperature probe, Doppler flow probe, electrocardiography and capnography.

limiting usefulness to research settings. Commercially available oscillometric devices applied to the limbs or tail appear to have limited value, but may provide trend information. Respiration may be assessed visually and in intubated animals mainstream or sidestream capnography provides some useful information. However, cardiac shunting and dilution as a consequence of excessive sampling rates of the devices used may give rise to erroneous readings and so this form of monitoring should be used with caution.

The use of pulse oximetry in reptiles remains controversial, as values obtained may not correlate with measured arterial oxygenation, potentially due to differences in haemoglobin structure compared with mammalian haemoglobin. However, if monitored continuously, pulse oximetry may provide trends to assess oxygenation over time.

Arterial blood gas analysis can provide valuable information on oxygenation and acid–base status. Although cost-effective portable equipment for analysis is increasingly available, the difficulty of obtaining arterial blood samples reduces relevance in the clinical setting. Venous blood samples are readily available and may partly reflect arterial values, as tissue metabolism is very low during anaesthesia. Again, intracardiac shunting may confuse results, particularly in chelonians.

Monitoring depth of anaesthesia

The clinical signs associated with induction of general anaesthesia in reptiles are fairly consistent. Generally, muscle relaxation starts in the cranial part of the body, and then moves backwards so that tail tone is lost last. The righting reflex is typically lost just prior to loss of tail tone. The palpebral reflex (cannot be measured in snakes because of the spectacle) should be lost at surgical anaesthesia, whereas the corneal reflex (see note regarding snakes above), as well as the 'tongue-retraction reflex' in snakes and varanids, typically persist at the surgical plane. Loss of these reflexes may indicate excessive anaesthetic depth. Animals retain the ability to react to painful stimuli even after the loss of righting reflex and tail tone, and the response to toe or tail pinching should be evaluated before deciding that surgical anaesthesia has been achieved (Figure 12.7).

Progressive depth of anaesthesia	Sign (loss of ...)	Stage
	Forelimb tone	Induction
	Hindlimb tone	
	Neck tone	
	Righting reflex	
	Jaw tone	Sedation
	Toe pinch	
	Tail tone	Surgical plane
	Bauchstreich reflex	
	Palpebral reflex	
	Vent pinch	
	'Tongue-retraction reflex' (snakes, varanids)	Excessive depth
	Corneal reflex (in those with eyelids)	

12.7 Assessing anaesthetic depth. Typical sequence of loss of muscle tone and reflexes, with correlation to stages of anaesthesia.

Inhalant anaesthetics

As in other species, the advantages of inhalational anaesthetics include superior control of anaesthetic depth, wide safety margins, excellent muscle relaxation, fast recovery and 'built-in' oxygen supplementation. For these reasons, inhalational anaesthesia is commonly used for induction and maintenance of reptiles with the notable exception of chelonians, in which induction with inhalants is slow and unpredictable resulting from a marked tendency to breath-hold. One should remember that the analgesic effects of inhaled drugs are incomplete, and limited to the administration period. Generally, due to breath-holding, intracardiac shunting and slow circulatory time, induction as well as recovery times tend to be longer and more variable than in mammals and birds.

Anaesthetic potency

Minimum alveolar concentration or minimum anaesthetic concentration (MAC) is the standard measure of potency of inhalational anaesthetic agents. MAC is defined as the anaesthetic concentration that prevents gross purposeful movement in 50% of an anaesthetized population subjected to a supramaximal noxious stimulus, traditionally a surgical incision (Quasha et al., 1980). The value permits comparison of anaesthetic agent potency, as well as standardization and comparison of various depths of anaesthesia as multiples of MAC. Other terms, essentially equivalent to MAC, sometimes reported in birds and reptiles include minimum anaesthetic dose, effective dose 50 and minimum infundibular concentration. Generally, MAC for a given agent varies little across mammalian species and the limited number of reports available indicates that the same applies to reptiles.

As MAC only 'accounts for' 50% of the population, vaporizer settings of 1.3 MAC are recommended to achieve surgical anaesthesia. As a likely consequence of R–L intracardiac shunting, the equilibrium between inhaled substances and the body occurs more slowly in reptiles than in mammals. Consequently, effective MAC decreases over time in iguanas and probably other reptiles, indicating that inhaled gas levels should be decreased towards the end of longer procedures.

Equipment

Inhalant anaesthetics are delivered by agent-specific vaporizers using oxygen or a mix of oxygen and nitrous oxide as the carrier gas. Standard anaesthetic machines fitted with non-rebreathing (Bain's) or circle systems are used, and for smaller patients, laboratory animal equipment, such as mini-Bain's mini-circles, Mapleson C, etc., has great potential. Regular small-animal face masks, as well as masks made from plastic bottles or syringe cases, work well.

Owing to low metabolic rates, oxygen consumption is low (<1 ml/kg/min) and flow rates may be reduced compared with mammalian standards. The flow rate is often determined by the performance of flow meters and vaporizers, and rates of 250–1000 ml/min will be appropriate for most reptiles encountered in practice.

Induction

Apart from chelonians where inductions may be prohibitively prolonged as a result of breath-holding, mask induction is generally feasible in most reptiles. An easier approach is to induce animals in chambers or plastic bags filled from a vaporizer at maximal setting, or simply by adding a small volume of the concentrated agent on a piece of cotton wool (e.g. approximately 1 ml isoflurane/l chamber volume). With this approach, close attention should be paid to the clinical signs, as inductions may be quite rapid and toxic levels could be reached if animals are left too long. Some authors feel that administration of analgesics such as morphine and buprenorphine 30–60 minutes prior to elective anaesthesia has an anaesthetic sparing effect, but there is currently no published information to substantiate this claim.

Inhalation anaesthetics

Early inhalants such as chloroform, methoxyflurane and ether, as well as the newer halothane, are considered obsolete in the clinical setting, and currently only two agents are regularly used by reptilian practitioners: isoflurane and sevoflurane. A third inhaled drug, nitrous oxide, may be used as an adjunct agent. A list of drugs is given in Figure 12.8.

Drug	Minimum alveolar concentration (MAC)	Induction dose	Maintenance dose
Isoflurane	1.5–2%	4–5%[a]	2.5%[bc]
Sevoflurane	2.5%	6–8%[a]	3.5%[bc]

12.8 Drugs used for inhalation anaesthesia. [a] Higher concentrations may be achieved if drug is introduced directly into chamber or plastic bag; monitor animals closely. [b] Lower if other drugs are given, due to synergy. [c] With longer procedures, decrease by 10–50% over time.

Isoflurane

Isoflurane is used extensively in reptiles. In lizards and snakes, the time to initial relaxation and loss of righting reflex when breathing 5% is typically 4–9 minutes, while the time to complete relaxation may be up to 20 minutes depending on the species (Bertelsen et al., 2005b). With direct intubation of conscious snakes followed by mechanical ventilation with 5% isoflurane, rapid induction may be achieved and, as mentioned, the same applies to inductions using higher inspired concentrations by adding isoflurane directly to the induction chamber or bag. The addition of 50–66% nitrous oxide may speed up inductions slightly. At low isoflurane concentrations animals continue breathing, but at levels adequate for surgical anaesthesia mechanical ventilation is usually necessary.

Isoflurane causes a moderate (approximately 25%) reduction in heart rate and a severe reduction in respiratory rate compared with values in manually restrained animals. However, values in manually restrained subjects are significantly higher than in undisturbed animals. A dose-dependent reduction in systemic blood pressure is observed during anaesthesia. In a research setting, seven mechanically ventilated iguanas were subjected to up to 9.2% isoflurane without detectable ill effects, suggesting a very wide margin of safety (Mosley et al., 2003b).

The MAC at 30–35°C has been reported to be 1.9 ± 0.59% in ratsnakes (Maas and Brunson, 2002), 1.8 ± 0.3% to 2.1 ± 0.6% in iguanas (Mosley et al., 2003a; Barter et al., 2006) and 1.54 ± 0.17% in varanids (Bertelsen et al., 2005c), indicating that vaporizer settings of 2–2.5% will be appropriate to maintain surgical anaesthesia in most subjects. As mentioned above, MAC has been reported to decrease over time in iguanas, indicating that inhaled gas levels should be decreased towards the end of lengthy procedures (Barter et al., 2006).

Recovery time depends on the depth and duration of anaesthesia, and is relatively short (2–12 minutes) following brief anaesthetic events at low anaesthetic depth, but may last up to an hour following deep prolonged anaesthesia.

Sevoflurane

Induction times using sevoflurane are slightly shorter than with isoflurane. In lizards induced with 8%, the time to initial relaxation and loss of righting reflex is around 6 minutes, while the time to complete relaxation is approximately 11 minutes (Bertelsen et al., 2005b). However, there are considerable species variations in ease of induction as a sole agent, with some species showing more resilience. As for isoflurane, direct intubation of the conscious animal followed by mechanical ventilation with the drug, or induction using higher concentrations in a bag or chamber, leads to faster inductions.

Clinically, in reptiles examined so far, there is little or no difference between anaesthetic induction times and side effects with sevoflurane and isoflurane. Sevoflurane causes a moderate reduction in heart rate and a severe reduction in respiratory rate compared with values in manually restrained animals, and the haemodynamic effects of sevoflurane are similar to those with isoflurane (Hernandez-Divers et al., 2005).

The MAC at 30–35°C has been reported to be 2.42 ± 0.57% in ratsnakes (Maas and Brunson, 2002), 2.51 ± 0.46% in varanids (Bertelsen et al., 2005a) and 3.1 ± 1.0% in iguanas (Barter et al., 2006), indicating that vaporizer settings of 3–3.5% will be appropriate to maintain surgical anaesthesia in most subjects. In a study of monitor lizards, the co-administration of 66% nitrous oxide resulted in a 25% reduction in sevoflurane MAC (Bertelsen et al., 2005a), and similar reductions are likely to occur in other species and with other inhalants.

After light-level anaesthesia, sevoflurane will result in faster recoveries than isoflurane, but following prolonged deep anaesthesia, the difference is marginal.

Nitrous oxide

Nitrous oxide (N_2O) may be used as a supplemental anaesthetic (at 50–66% with oxygen) during induction with inhalational agents, resulting in marginally shorter induction times. Two-thirds N_2O with one-third oxygen delivered with sevoflurane reduces sevoflurane requirement (MAC) by approximately 25% (Bertelsen et al., 2005a). Apart from reducing the concentration of the primary agent, which may improve cardiopulmonary function, the use of N_2O is likely to provide improved analgesia over delivery in 100% oxygen. As in other species, N_2O should be used cautiously in cases where compartmentalized gas is present, such as gastric dilatation, as N_2O will equilibrate to and distend these areas.

Injectable anaesthetics

General anaesthetics
Propofol

Provided vascular access can be gained, propofol is this author's agent of choice for anaesthetic induction. Administered intravenously or intraosseously at dosages of 5–10 mg/kg, propofol will cause induction in 1–5 minutes (Figures 12.9 and 12.10). Propofol administered

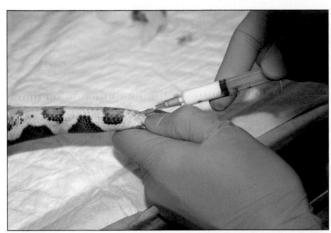

12.9 Anaesthetic induction with propofol injected into the tail vein of a boa constrictor.

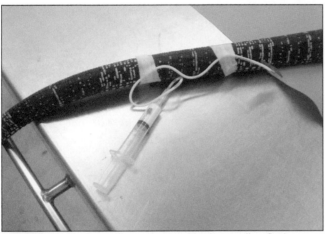

12.10 A butterfly needle may be taped in place to allow fluid administration or bolus top-up of propofol into the ventral tail vessels.

perivascularly is ineffective, but does not cause tissue damage. Several cases of accidental submeningeal injection have been reported following attempts to inject propofol into the supravertebral sinus in tortoises, so extreme care that injections are actually intravenous should be exerted if this route is to be used. In aquatic turtles this does not appear to be a concern, and indeed the supravertebral sinus is this author's preferred injection site in these species.

In all reptiles investigated, propofol causes marked respiratory depression. The respiratory depression is dose dependent and appears to be affected by the speed of administration – low doses given slowly cause less apnoea than high doses administered at once. In lizards and snakes a slight decrease in heart rate is observed (Bennett *et al.*, 1998; Anderson *et al.*, 1999), while in chelonians heart rate may remain stable (Ziolo and Bertelsen, 2009).

The dosage necessary for induction depends heavily on body temperature, species and the level of anaesthesia required.

In aquatic turtles at 20°C, 10 mg/kg results in superficial anaesthesia lasting approximately 60 minutes, while 20 mg/kg provides a surgical plane lasting for 2–30 minutes and a total anaesthesia time of approximately 90 minutes (Ziolo and Bertelsen, 2009). In snakes and lizards, 5 mg/kg results in 20–30 minutes of anaesthesia, while longer recovery times are seen following 10 mg/kg dosage (Bennett *et al.*, 1998; Anderson *et al.*, 1999). For most terrestrial species, a dose of 5–10 mg/kg given

slowly is appropriate for short procedures or to allow intubation. For longer procedures, this author prefers intubation and maintenance by isoflurane or sevoflurane. However, provided stable intravascular access can be provided, anaesthesia can be maintained by continuous propofol infusion at rates of 0.1–0.4 mg/kg/min (see Bennett *et al.*, 1998).

Only limited analgesia is provided by propofol, so for surgical procedures, local analgesics and/or supplementary analgesia (such as low-dose ketamine or alpha-2 agonists) are required.

Alfaxalone

The steroid anaesthetic alfaxalone is highly insoluble in water and historically was formulated in combination with alfadalone and the solubilizing agent cremophor. This formulation was discontinued as cremophor was associated with allergic reactions in domestic animals. More recently, alfaxalone has been successfully solubilized with 2-hydroxypropyl-beta-cyclodextrin. When given intravenously, alfaxalone has similar effects to propofol and is an excellent induction agent. Induction time is rapid, and in lizards a surgical plane of anaesthesia lasting for 5–15 minutes is achieved using 5 mg/kg i.v. (Knotec *et al.*, 2011a; 2011b).

The major distinguishing feature of alfaxalone is that, unlike propofol, alfaxalone is effective when administered intramuscularly (i.m.) or subcutaneously (s.c.). Via this route, two to four times the intravenous dose is necessary, and induction times are longer, typically 4–10 minutes. In iguanas, 10 mg/kg i.m. provides light sedation, 20 mg/kg provides a level of sedation suitable for minor procedures or for endotracheal intubation and supplementation with inhalational anaesthesia, and 30 mg/kg provides an anaesthetic plane suitable for surgical procedures of limited duration (up to 40 minutes) (Bertelsen and Sauer, 2011). In red-eared sliders, 10 mg/kg i.m. results in heavy sedation, while 20 mg/kg provides anaesthesia of approximately 20 minutes' duration, appropriate for induction of inhalational anaesthesia or for brief surgical procedures (Kischinovsky *et al.*, 2013).

In tortoises, 10–20 mg/kg i.m. provides heavy sedation and allows intubation (Hansen and Bertelsen, 2013). As would be expected, smaller individuals require higher dosages. In an unpublished study in leopard geckos, 30–40 mg/kg of alfaxalone i.m. was required to achieve heavy sedation (Hydeskov and Bertelsen, unpublished data), and 50 mg/kg i.m. is likely to be required for a surgical level. In theory, continuous rate infusion with alfaxalone should be possible, but the challenges are the same as those mentioned for propofol.

In all species investigated, alfaxalone causes an initial dose-dependent depression of respiration.

As with propofol, the analgesic properties of alfaxalone are limited, and supplementary analgesia such as local infiltration or systemic low-dose ketamine or an alpha-2 agonist should be provided for painful procedures.

Ketamine

Ketamine hydrochloride has been used extensively in reptiles, either alone or in combination with various sedatives, including xylazine, medetomidine and midazolam. Effects are highly species dependent and large individual variation is also observed.

Used alone, recommended dosages range from 10–50 mg/kg for sedation to 55–90 mg/kg for surgical anaesthesia, while yet higher doses (100–220 mg/kg) have occasionally been reported (Glenn *et al.*, 1972; Harding, 1977; Arena *et al.*, 1988). The time to peak effect following intramuscular injection is approximately 30 minutes. The problems with using ketamine as a sole agent in reptiles are poor muscle relaxation and extended recovery periods. Reported recovery times range from 6 hours at 20 mg/kg to several days at dosages above 50 mg/kg (Glenn *et al.*, 1972).

In reptiles, moderate ketamine dosages are associated with stable to slightly increased heart rates, mild hypertension and respiratory depression, the latter peaking at 30–60 minutes. At increasing dosages ketamine will induce apnoea and bradycardia.

Ketamine may be combined with sedatives such as benzodiazepines and alpha-2 agonists for better muscle relaxation, a reduction in required dose and shorter recovery times. The main combinations are ketamine + medetomidine and ketamine + midazolam. Refer to the appropriate sections below.

Zolazepam/tiletamine

The potent cyclohexamine tiletamine, combined with the benzodiazepine zolazepam, has found some use in reptile anaesthesia, but very little published information exists. The onset of effects is faster than with ketamine, while cardiopulmonary effects are likely to be similar to those produced by ketamine. In iguanas, 10 mg/kg resulted in a brief period of excitement followed by good muscle relaxation (Mauthe von Degerfeld, 2004). Despite its long duration of action and variable effects, low dosages (2–5 mg/kg) may be useful for sedation prior to handling or intubation, particularly of larger animals.

Sedatives

Sedative and tranquilizing drugs such as benzodiazepines and alpha-2 agonists may be used in reptiles, but studies to document their effects are lacking. Because of the difficulty in accessing the vascular system and airways in chelonians there has been much more focus on the use of these drugs in turtles and tortoises, mostly in combination with ketamine, e.g. midazolam (Bienzle and Boyd, 1992; Holz and Holz, 1995; Alvez-Júnor *et al.*, 2012), xylazine (Holz and Holz, 1995; Santos *et al.*, 2008) and medetomidine (Sleeman and Gaynor, 2000; Greer *et al.*, 2001; Dennis and Heard, 2002; Chittic *et al.*, 2002; Knafo *et al.*, 2011).

Alpha-2 agonists

Only a few reports exist on the use of xylazine in reptiles, but the more potent medetomidine is commonly used in combination with ketamine for anaesthetic induction in chelonians. In tortoises, 0.1 mg/kg medetomidine combined with 10 mg/kg ketamine i.m. provides sedation allowing minor procedures and endotracheal intubation, but responses are variable (Sleeman and Gaynor, 2000; Greer *et al.*, 2001; Dennis and Heard, 2002; Chittic *et al.*, 2002; Knafo *et al.*, 2011).

Cardiopulmonary effects include hypertension and respiratory depression. Effects of medetomidine may be reversed through intramuscular administration of 0.5 mg/kg atipamezole. Intravenous administration has resulted in marked hypotension. Very high dosages of medetomidine (0.5 mg/kg) have been reported to induce sedation in juvenile estuarine crocodiles, but cardiopulmonary effects were not evaluated.

Dexmedetomidine may be replaced for medetomidine at half the dosage. So far there is nothing to indicate that it is superior to medetomidine in reptiles; but the same theoretical considerations apply as in other species – namely that while both isomers together contribute to undesirable circulatory effects, the D-form alone has sedative properties, making dexmedetomidine as efficient but half as toxic as medetomidine. As in other species, atipamezole reverses the effects of alpha-2 agents.

Benzodiazepines

Of the benzodiazepines, midazolam is the most relevant, as it is effective when administered intramuscularly and is available in relatively concentrated formulations. However, only very limited information is available on the use of midazolam: in chelonians, 2 mg/kg midazolam combined with 10–20 mg/kg ketamine i.m. provides sedation allowing minor procedures (Bienzle and Boyd, 1992; Alvez-Júnior *et al.*, 2012). As in other species midazolam may be added to other drug combinations to obtain additional sedation and muscle relaxation and effects may be reversed with flumazenil.

Neuromuscular blocking agents

Neuromuscular blocking agents, which immobilize animals without affecting consciousness, have little use in clinical medicine except in allowing non-painful manipulation of large crocodilians.

Gallamine has been used extensively for immobilization of Nile crocodiles. A dose of 1–4 mg/kg i.m. will render animals immobile in 20–30 minutes. The effect lasts for 12–24 hours, but recovery in approximately one hour may be achieved through the intramuscular administration of 0.03–0.06 mg/kg neostigmine. While safe and well tested in Nile crocodiles, gallamine has caused death in false gharials and American alligators.

Brief immobilization of box turtles and giant Amazon turtles with 0.25–0.5 mg/kg rocuronium allowed endotracheal intubation in 10–15 minutes, and recovery occurred 1–2 hours after 0.07 mg/kg i.m. of neostigmine.

Recommended protocols

It is difficult to give precise recommendations on protocol selection, as the protocol to select depends on the situation as well as the experience of the anaesthetist. However, provided that intravenous access can be gained, intravenous induction with propofol or alfaxalone is the induction method preferred by this author. If intravenous access is not readily achieved, chamber or bag induction with isoflurane or sevoflurane is a convenient option in non-chelonian species. An alternative is intramuscular administration of alfaxalone or ketamine combined with medetomidine and/or midazolam. See Figure 12.11 for recommended protocols.

For any species, and after any induction, this author prefers maintenance with isoflurane or sevoflurane delivered by endotracheal tube.

Pre-anaesthetics are not commonly used; for large and aggressive patients, injection with low doses of ketamine (e.g. 5 mg/kg i.m., s.c.) or tiletamine/zolazepam (e.g. 3 mg/kg i.m., s.c.), combined with medetomidine (e.g. 0.1 mg/kg i.m., s.c.) or midazolam (e.g. 2 mg/kg i.m., s.c.), may be used to allow safe handling. Dosages of commonly used drugs are presented in Figure 12.12.

Taxon	Induction
Turtle	5–20 mg/kg propofol i.v.
	5–15 mg/kg alfaxalone i.v.
	20–30 mg/kg alfaxalone i.m., s.c.
Tortoise	5–12 mg/kg propofol i.v.
	4–10 mg/kg alfaxalone i.v.
	15–20 mg/kg alfaxalone i.m., s.c.
	10 mg/kg ketamine + 0.1 mg/kg medetomidine i.m., s.c.
Small lizard	20–40 mg/kg alfaxalone i.m., s.c.
	Chamber/bag induction with iso/sevo
Large lizard	3–10 mg/kg propofol i.v.
	5 mg/kg alfaxalone i.v.
	Mask induction with iso/sevo
	5–15 mg/kg ketamine and 0.1–0.15 mg/kg medetomidine i.m., s.c.
Venomous snake	Chamber induction with iso/sevo
	5–10 mg/kg propofol i.v.
Small snake	Chamber induction with iso/sevo
	5–10 mg/kg propofol i.v.
	Direct intubation and ventilation with iso/sevo
Large snake	3–8 mg/kg propofol i.v.
	Mask or chamber induction with iso/sevo
	Direct intubation and ventilation with iso/sevo
	Premedicate with 5–10 mg/kg zoletil i.m., or 10 mg/kg alfaxalone i.m., s.c. and continue with one of the above
	5–10 mg/kg ketamine and 0.1–0.15 mg/kg medetomidine i.m., s.c.

2.1 Selected protocols for anaesthetic induction. For longer procedures, endotracheal intubation and maintenance with isoflurane or sevoflurane is recommended. iso = isoflurane; sevo = sevoflurane; zoletil = zolazepam/tiletamine.

Drug	Dosage (mg/kg)	Route	Reversal agent
Propofol	3–20	i.v.	None
Alfaxalone	3–10 20–40	i.v. i.m., s.c.	None
Midazolam	1–2	i.m., s.c.	Flumazenil (0.1–0.2 mg/kg)
Medetomidine	0.05–0.15	i.m., s.c.	Atipamezole (0.3–0.5 mg/kg)
Dexmedetomidine	0.03–0.08	i.m., s.c.	Atipamezole (0.1–0.3 mg/kg)
Ketamine	10–40	i.m., s.c.	None
Zolazepam/ tiletamine	5–10	i.m., s.c.	Flumazenil for zolazepam

2.12 Selected anaesthetic and sedative drugs.

Recovery

Generally, recovery times in reptiles are prolonged compared with birds and mammals. Body temperature critically affects speed and quality of recovery, so animals should be kept warm. If mechanical ventilation has been used, animals should be gradually weaned off ventilation. The easiest way to do so is by manually ventilating every 5 minutes using an Ambu-bag or similar to allow build-up of CO_2 (Figure 12.13). Periods of apnoea of 5–10 minutes are unlikely to cause deleterious effects. As hyperoxia may

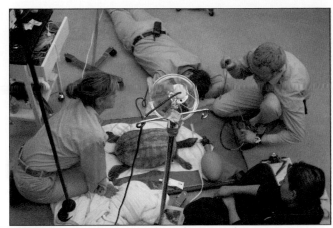

12.13 Recoveries may be prolonged owing to slow metabolism, sluggish circulation, intracardiac shunting, hypothermia and hypoventilation. Maintaining body temperature and assisting ventilation as required are important.

decrease the ventilatory drive in reptiles and possibly promote R–L shunting, recovery in room air (21% oxygen) as opposed to 100% oxygen has been proposed; however, clinical studies have failed to demonstrate such a difference (Bertelsen et al., 2005b; Churgin et al., 2015). There is some evidence to validate the use of epinephrine for increasing heart rate and consequently decreasing post-surgical recovery time in selected reptiles (Goe et al., 2016); however, this author is of the opinion that more research is necessary before this can be recommended clinically. When animals are consistently breathing on their own, they can be left to recover unassisted.

Analgesia

Since the turn of the millennium, a fair amount of attention has been given to reptilian pain perception and analgesia (Mosley, 2011). Despite these efforts, reptilian analgesia is still a controversial subject, and solid recommendations are hard to give. Despite the lack of documentation, analgesia should be part of any anaesthetic regimen that involves potentially painful procedures. Opioids, non-steroidal anti-inflammatory drugs (NSAIDs) and local analgesics are the most relevant candidates for successful treatment (see below), and suggested dosages of selected drugs are given in Figure 12.14. Multimodal analgesia, combining low dosages of ketamine, opioids and alpha-2 agonists, has not been investigated systematically in reptiles, but appears effective in this author's experience, and should be considered as a supplement to protocols with poor inherent analgesia, such as inhaled agents, propofol and alfaxalone.

Drug	Dosage (mg/kg)	Route
Meloxicam	0.1–1	orally, s.c.
Methadone	3–5	s.c.
Morphine	1–5	s.c.
Fentanyl	12.5 µg/h	t.d.*
Tramadol	5–25	orally, s.c.
Hydromorphone	0.5	s.c.

12.14 Selected analgesic agents. Effects of NSAIDs have not been scientifically demonstrated. *t.d. = transdermal patch.

Opioids

Significant interspecies differences appear to exist when it comes to opioids. The mu-receptor opioid morphine (5 mg/kg i.m.) has been shown to cause a latency of the tail-flick response in anoles (Mauk *et al.*, 1981). Similarly, morphine (10–20 mg/kg) increased thermal withdrawal latency in red-eared sliders and bearded dragons, but appears to be ineffective in corn snakes at dosages up to 40 mg/kg (Sladky *et al.*, 2007, 2008). In the species where it does work, morphine is associated with severe respiratory depression, but another mu-receptor opioid, tramadol (10–15 mg/kg orally, s.c.) appears to have similar effects on thermal withdrawal latency in turtles with much less respiratory depression (Baker *et al.*, 2011). Another mu-receptor opioid, hydromorphone (0.5 mg/kg i.m.), also increased thermal withdrawal time in sliders (Mans *et al.*, 2012). In contrast, the predominant kappa-receptor opioid butorphanol appears to be ineffective in bearded dragons, iguanas and red-eared sliders, and only at extreme dosages (20 mg/kg) increased thermal withdrawal latency in corn snakes (Sladky *et al.*, 2007, 2008). In ball pythons, butorphanol (10 mg/kg i.m.) caused sedation, but failed to reduce the reaction to the injection of an irritant (Williams *et al.*, 2015). These differences are probably associated with species differences in expression of the different classes of opioid receptors, making extrapolation to other species very difficult (Sladky *et al.*, 2009).

Recently, the use of transdermal patches of fentanyl have shown promise in several snake species (see Figure 12.14).

Non-steroidal anti-inflammatory drugs

In contrast to opioids, NSAIDs would be expected to behave much the same across species, and although the role of the cyclo-oxygenase system in reptiles has not been studied, clinical evidence supports the efficacy of NSAIDs in reptiles and they are widely used with no ill effects. A pharmacokinetic trial of meloxicam in iguanas showed excellent bioavailability following oral administration, and suggested that administration of meloxicam at a dose of 0.2 mg/kg i.v. or orally results in plasma concentrations >0.1 µg/ml for approximately 24 hours (Divers *et al.*, 2010). Furthermore, daily administration of high doses (5 mg/kg) for 12 days did not induce histological changes in gastric, hepatic or renal tissues (Divers *et al.*, 2010). Meloxicam (0.3 mg/kg i.m.) had no obvious effect on the postoperative physiological stress response in ball pythons (Olesen *et al.*, 2008). However, even the saline-treated control group showed only minimal measurable physiological response to surgery, questioning the validity of the model. This author routinely uses meloxicam at 1 mg/kg s.c. once, and 0.2–0.5 mg/kg daily orally or subcutaneously.

Local analgesia

Local analgesics (e.g. lidocaine) have probably been under utilized in the past. For surgical pain, local analgesia is simple, effective and hard to beat. Simple infiltration may be used, as may nerve blocks, e.g., around a limb or tail. To avoid cardiotoxicity, dosages of local analgesics should not exceed 4 mg/kg; so, in small subjects, it may be beneficial to dilute the drugs (e.g. 1:10 in sterile saline) prior to administration. Although not investigated in reptiles, bupivacaine is expected to have significantly longer duration of activity than lidocaine.

Intrathecal anaesthesia with lidocaine has been employed in larger chelonians to facilitate hindlimb or cloacal surgery (Rivera *et al.*, 2011). A dorsal approach between the spinal processes was employed.

As in any species, pre-emptive/preoperative analgesia offers intraoperative as well as postoperative analgesia, and is likely to reduce the amount of anaesthetic needed. As circulation is already reduced compared with mammals, the use of lidocaine formulations which include adrenaline/noradrenaline (epinephrine/norepinephrine) should be avoided to prevent potential local ischaemia.

Acknowledgements

Drs Stephen Divers and Sid (Zdenek) Knotek are thanked for helpful suggestions to this chapter.

References and further reading

Alves-Júnior JR, Bosso AC, Andrade MB, Werther K and Santos AL (2012) Association of midazolam with ketamine in giant Amazon river turtles *Podocnemis expansa* breed in captivity. *Acta Cirurgica Brasileira* **27(2)**, 144–147

Anderson N, Wack R, Calloway L, Hetherington T and Williams J (1999) Cardiopulmonary effects and efficacy of propofol as an anesthetic agent in brown tree snakes, *Boiga irregularis*. *Bulletin of the Association of Reptilian and Amphibian Veterinarians* **9**, 9–15

Arena P, Richardson K and Cullen L (1988) Anaesthesia in two species of large Australian skink. *Veterinary Record* **123**, 155–158

Baker BB, Sladky KK and Johnson SM (2011) Evaluation of the analgesic effects of oral and subcutaneous tramadol administration in red-eared slider turtles. *Journal of the American Veterinary Medical Association* **238**, 220–227

Barter LS, Hawkins MG, Brosnan RJ, Antognini JF and Pypendop BH (2006) Median effective dose of isoflurane, sevoflurane and desflurane in green iguanas. *American Journal of Veterinary Research* **67**, 392–397

Bennett RA, Schumacher J, Hedjazi-Haring K and Newell SM (1998) Cardiopulmonary and anesthetic effects of propofol administered intraosseously to green iguanas. *Journal of the American Veterinary Medical Association* **212(1)**, 93–98

Benson KG and Forrest L (1999) Characterization of the renal portal system of the common green iguana (*Iguana iguana*) by digital subtraction imaging. *Journal of Zoo and Wildlife Medicine* **30(2)**, 235–241

Bertelsen MF, Buchanan R, Jensen HM *et al.* (2015) Assessing the influence of mechanical ventilation on blood gases and blood pressure in rattlesnakes. *Veterinary Anaesthesia and Analgesia* **42(4)**, 386–393

Bertelsen MF, Mosley CA, Crawshaw GJ, Dyson DH and Smith DA (2005a) Anesthetic potency of sevoflurane with and without nitrous oxide in mechanically ventilated Dumeril monitors. *Journal of the American Veterinary Medical Association* **227**, 575–578

Bertelsen MF, Mosley CA, Crawshaw GJ, Dyson D and Smith DA (2005b) Inhalation anesthesia in Dumeril's monitor (*Varanus dumerili*) with isoflurane, sevoflurane and nitrous oxide: effects of inspired gases in induction and recovery. *Journal of Zoo and Wildlife Medicine* **36**, 62–68

Bertelsen MF, Mosley CA, Crawshaw GJ, Dyson D and Smith DA (2005c) Minimum alveolar concentration of isoflurane in mechanically ventilated Dumeril monitors. *Journal of the American Veterinary Medical Association* **226**, 1098–1101

Bertelsen MF and Sauer CD (2011) Alfaxalone anaesthesia in the green iguana (*Iguana iguana*). *Veterinary Anaesthesia and Analgesia* **38(5)**, 461–466

Bienzle D and Boyd CJ (1992) Sedative effects of ketamine and midazolam in snapping turtles (*Chelydra serpentine*). *Journal of Zoo and Wildlife Medicine* **23**, 201–204

Chittick EJ, Stamper MA, Beasley JF, Lewbart GA and Horne WA (2002) Medetomidine, ketamine and sevoflurane for anesthesia of injured loggerhead sea turtles: 13 cases (1996–2000). *Journal of the American Veterinary Medicine Association* **221(7)**, 1019–1025

Churgin SM, Sladky KK and Smith LJ (2015). Anesthetic induction and recovery parameters in bearded dragons (*Pogona vitticeps*): comparison of isoflurane delivered in 100% oxygen *versus* 21% oxygen. *Journal of Zoo and Wildlife Medicine* **46(3)**, 534–539

Dennis PM and Heard DJ (2002) Cardiopulmonary effects of a medetomidine–ketamine combination administered intravenously in gopher tortoises. *Journal of the American Veterinary Medicine Association* **220(10)**, 1516–1519

Divers SJ, Papich M, McBride M *et al.* (2010) Pharmacokinetics of meloxicam following intravenous and oral administration in green iguanas (*Iguana iguana*). *American Journal of Veterinary Research* **71**, 1277–1283

Glenn J, Straight R and Snyder C (1972) Clinical use of ketamine hydrochloride as an anesthetic agent for snakes. *American Journal of Veterinary Research* **33**, 1901–1903

Goe A, Shmalberg J, Gatson B and Wellehan JFX (2016) Epinephrine or GV-26 electrical stimulation reduces inhalant anaesthetic recover time in common snapping turtles (*Chelydra serpentine*). *Journal of Zoo and Wildlife Medicine* **47(2)**, 501–507

Greer LL, Jenne KJ and Diggs HE (2001) Medetomidine–ketamine anesthesia in red-eared slider turtles (*Trachemys scripta elegans*). *Contemporary Topics in Laboratory Animal Science* **40(3)**, 9–11

Guzman DSM, Mitchell MA and Acierno M (2011) Determination of plasma osmolality and agreement between measured and calculated values in captive male corn snakes (*Pantherus (Elaphe) guttatus guttatus*). *Journal of Herpetological Medicine and Surgery* **21(1)**, 16–19

Hansen LL and Bertelsen MF (2013). Assessment of the effects of intramuscular administration of alfaxalone with and without medetomidine in Horsfield's tortoises (*Agrionemys horsfieldii*). *Veterinary Anaesthesia and Analgesia* **40(6)**, e68–75

Harding K (1977) The use of ketamine anaesthesia to milk two tropical rattlesnakes (*Crotalus durissus terrificus*). *Veterinary Record* **100**, 289–290

Hernandez-Divers SM, Schumacher J, Stahl S and Hernandez-Divers SJ (2005) Comparison of isoflurane and sevoflurane anesthesia after premedication with butorphanol in the green iguana (*Iguana iguana*). *Journal of Zoo and Wildlife Medicine* **36**, 169–175

Holz P, Barker IK, Burger JP, Crawshaw GJ and Conlon PD (1997a) The effect of the renal portal system on pharmacokinetic parameters in the red-eared slider (*Trachemys scripta elegans*). *Journal of Zoo and Wildlife Medicine* **28(4)**, 386–393

Holz P, Barker IK, Crawshaw GJ and Dobson H (1997b) The anatomy and perfusion of the renal portal system in the red-eared slider (*Trachemys scripta elegans*). *Journal of Zoo and Wildlife Medicine* **28(4)**, 378–385

Holz RM and Holz P (1995) Electrocardiography in anaesthetized red-eared sliders (*Trachemys scripta elegans*). *Research in Veterinary Science* **58(1)**, 67–69

Kischinovsky M, Duse A, Wang T and Bertelsen MF (2013) Intramuscular administration of alfaxalone in red-eared sliders (*Trachemys scripta elegans*): effects of dose and body temperature. *Veterinary Anaesthesia and Analgesia* **40(1)**, 13–20

Knafo SE, Divers SJ, Rivera S *et al.* (2011) Sterilisation of hybrid Galapagos tortoises (*Geochelone nigra*) for island restoration, Part 1: endoscopic oophorectomy of females under ketamine–medetomidine anaesthesia. *Veterinary Record* **168(2)**, 47

Knotec Z, Hrda A, Kley N and Knotkova Z (2011a) Alfaxalone anesthesia in veiled chameleon (*Chameleo calyptratus*). *Proceedings of the American Association of Reptile and Amphibian Veterinarians Annual Conference,* pp. 179–181

Knotec Z, Hrda A and Trnkova S (2011b) Alfaxalone anesthesia in green iguanas (*Iguana iguana*). *Proceedings of the Annual Meeting of the European College of Zoological Medicine,* p. 68

Maas A and Brunson D (2002) Comparison of anesthetic potency and cardiopulmonary effects of isoflurane and sevoflurane in colubrid snakes. *Proceedings of the American Association of Zoo Veterinarians,* pp. 306–308

Mader DR and Rudloff E (2006) Emergency and critical care. In: *Reptile Medicine and Surgery, 2nd edition,* ed. DR Mader, 2006, pp. 533–548. Elsevier, Philadelphia

Mans C, Lahner LL, Baker BB, Johnson SM and Sladky KK (2012) Antinociceptive efficacy of buprenorphine and hydromorphone in red-eared slider turtles (*Trachemys scripta elegans*). *Journal of Zoo and Wildlife Medicine* **43**, 662–665

Mauk MD, Olson RD, LaHoste GJ and Olson GA (1981) Tonic immobility produces hyperalgesia and antagonizes morphine analgesia. *Science* **213**, 353–354

Mauthe von Degerfeld M (2004) Personal experiences in the use of association tiletamine/zolazepam for anaesthesia of the green iguana (*Iguana iguana*). *Veterinary Research Communications* **28(S1)**, 351–353

McFadden MS, Bennett RA, Reavill DR, Ragetly GR and Clark-Price SC (2011) Clinical and histologic effects of intracardiac administration of propofol for induction of anesthesia in ball pythons (*Python regius*). *Journal of the American Veterinary Medical Association* **239**, 803–807

Mosley G (2011) Pain and nociception in reptiles. *Veterinary Clinics of North America: Exotic Animal Practice* **14**, 45–60

Mosley CA, Dyson D and Smith DA (2003a) Minimum alveolar concentration of isoflurane in green iguanas and the effect of butorphanol on minimum alveolar concentration. *Journal of the American Veterinary Medical Association* **222**, 1559–1564

Mosley CA, Dyson D and Smith DA (2003b) The cardiac anesthetic index of isoflurane in green iguanas. *Journal of the American Veterinary Medical Association* **222**, 1565–1568

Mosley CA, Dyson D and Smith DA (2004) The cardiovascular dose-response effects of isoflurane alone and combined with butorphanol in the green iguana (*Iguana iguana*). *Veterinary Anaesthesia and Analgesia* **31**, 64–72

Olesen MG, Bertelsen MF, Perry SF and Wang T (2008) Effects of preoperative administration of butorphanol or meloxicam on physiologic responses to surgery in ball pythons. *Journal of the American Veterinary Medical Association* **233**, 1883–1888

Preston DL, Mosley CAE and Mason RT (2010) Sources of variability in recovery time from methohexital sodium anesthesia in snakes. *Copeia* **2010(3)**, 496–501

Quasha A, Eger EI and Tinker J (1980) Determination and applications of MAC. *Anesthesiology* **53**, 315–334

Rivera S, Divers SJ, Knafo SE *et al.* (2011) Sterilisation of hybrid Galapagos tortoises (*Geochelone nigra*) for island restoration, Part 2: phallectomy of males under intrathecal anaesthesia with lidocaine. *Veterinary Record* **168(3)**, 78

Santos AL, Bosso AC, Alves-Júnior JR *et al.* (2008) Pharmacological restraint of captivity giant Amazonian turtle Podocnemis expansa (*Testudines, Podocnemididae*) with xylazine and propofol. *Acta Cirurgica Brasileira* **23(3)**, 270–273

Shepard MK, Divers S, Braun C and Hofmeister EH (2013) Pharmacodynamics of alfaxalone after single-dose intramuscular administration in red-eared sliders (*Trachemys scripta elegans*): a comparison of two different doses at two different ambient temperatures. *Veterinary Anaesthesia and Analgesia* **40(6)**, 590–598

Sladky KK, Kinney ME and Johnson SM (2008) Analgesic efficacy of butorphanol and morphine in bearded dragons and corn snakes. *Journal of the American Veterinary Medical Association* **233**, 267–273

Sladky KK, Kinney ME and Johnson SM (2009) Effects of opioid receptor activation on thermal antinociception in red-eared slider turtles (*Trachemys scripta*). *American Journal of Veterinary Research* **70**, 1072–1078

Sladky KK, Miletic V, Paul-Murphy J *et al.* (2007) Analgesic efficacy and respiratory effects of butorphanol and morphine in turtles. *Journal of the American Veterinary Medical Association* **230**, 1356–1362

Sleeman JM and Gaynor J (2000) Sedative and cardiopulmonary effects of medetomidine and reversal with atipamezole in desert tortoises (*Gopherus agassizii*). *Journal of Zoo and Wildlife Medicine* **31(1)**, 28–35

Williams CJ, James LE, Bertelsen MF and Wang T (2016) Tachycardia in response to remote capsaicin injection as a model for nociception in the ball python (*Python regius*). *Veterinary Anaesthesia and Analgesia* **43(4)**, 429–434

Ziolo MS and Bertelsen MF (2009) Effects of propofol administered via the supravertebral sinus in red-eared sliders. *Journal of the American Veterinary Medical Association* **234(3)**, 390–393

Chapter 13

Surgery: principles and techniques

Stephen J. Divers

In general, performing surgery on a reptile patient should be approached with the same principles as those used for domestic animals. However, there are some specific anatomical considerations, as well as unique aspects of patient preparation, positioning and equipment, with which the reptile clinician should be familiar. The complexity and vastness of reptile surgery in over 8000 species necessitates the incorporation of only the most important factors and frequently performed procedures. Much detailed information has been omitted and cross-reference to other parts of this manual as well as other texts on reptile anatomy, physiology, husbandry, anaesthesia and surgery is required (Mader, 2006b; Mader and Divers, 2014). Sections on wound healing, anaesthesia, and intra- and postoperative support are included in Chapters 12 and 15.

Equipment

Instrumentation

It can be challenging to maintain a prepackaged 'reptile surgery pack' that is applicable for a wide variety of species and procedures (Figure 13.1). For truly giant reptiles, including giant tortoises and crocodilians, the use of stronger large-animal instruments is recommended. Likewise, for reptiles weighing 5–50 kg, most small-animal instruments are appropriate. However, most patients are less than 5 kg in size, and the majority are less than 1 kg. For these smaller reptiles, microsurgical instruments are often required (Figure 13.2).

Microinstruments, which are not merely miniaturized versions of standard instruments, but rather balanced instruments with fine small tips, are the optimum instrumentation for small reptiles (Figure 13.3). Since microinstruments can be costly, other viable options include cheaper ophthalmological instruments. Standard iris scissors, tenotomy scissors, Castroviejo needle holders, and Colibri forceps can be very useful. One of the most important considerations in surgery is exposure. Plastic self-retaining retractors (e.g. the Lone Star® retractor) can be adjusted to fit different sizes of incisions and do not compromise the ventilation of these patients (Figure 13.4). Smaller versions of standard abdominal retractors such as paediatric Balfour retractors, Haight baby rib spreaders, etc. can also be utilized, but are significantly heavier. Eyelid retractors can be useful for retracting coelomic incisions in small lizards and snakes.

A variety of surgical drills and saws should also be available. Autoclavable or gas-sterilizable models are preferred. For general orthopaedic work, the Stryker drill offers excellent control and versatility, even for the smallest of patients (Figure 13.5a). The oscillating sagittal saw attachment to the air-powered 3M mini-driver provides fine control and reduced tissue trauma compared with rotating saws (Figure 13.5b). The VI MiniDriver® and MaxiDriver® systems appear to be comparable, offer sagittal saw as well as pin and wire driver attachments, and are commercially available in Europe. Small versions of suction tips, rongeurs, elevators and bone-holding clamps are also useful.

Epoxy resins (e.g. Enviroset® 5 minute epoxy, Environmental Technologies Inc.) or low-temperature veterinary acrylics (e.g. Technovite® 8100 MG kit, APEF acrylic packs) may be used for chelonian plastron closures and shell repairs. A two-polymer orthopaedic putty (Veterinary Instrumentation Ltd) is also a very useful aid to external fixation.

- Plain ophthalmic fine thumb forceps
- Adson ½ forceps, very fine
- Small scissors (top sharp tip, bottom blunt tip)
- Castroviejo retractor
- Small suture scissors
- Derf needle holder
- Strabismus scissors
- Four curved ophthalmic mosquito forceps
- 20 small gauze sponges
- 20 cotton-tipped applicators
- Clear plastic adhesive drape
- Vetrap 2 inches
- No. 15 scalpel blade
- Lone Star® retractor

13.1 A suggested standard reptile surgery pack.

- Mini Gelpi retractor
- Avian/exotic or eyelid retractor
- K-wire pin driver vice
- Doolen avian bone-holding device
- Stevens tenotomy scissors
- Two balanced microscissors
- Doolen avian spay hook
- Extra delicate mosquito forceps, straight
- Extra delicate mosquito forceps, curved
- Sontec curved tying forceps
- Ring-tipped thumb forceps with holes
- Two spring bulldog clamps
- Lone Star® retractor

13.2 A suggested reptile microsurgery pack.

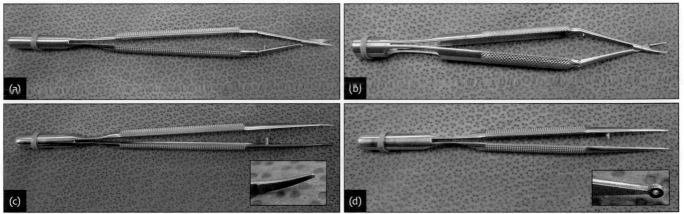

13.3 A selection of small and microsurgical instruments commonly used in exotic animal surgery: (a) straight microscissors with round handle and counterbalanced; (b) micro needle holders with round handle and counterbalanced; (c) curved microforceps with platform tips and round handle and counterbalanced; (d) straight microforceps with 2 mm ring tips and round handle and counterbalanced.
(© SJ Divers)

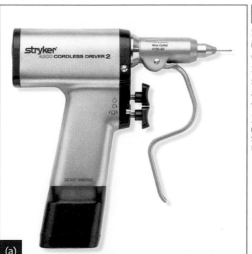

13.4 The Lonestar® retractor incorporates an adjustable plastic ring to which elastic stays with hooks are attached. This retractor is extremely versatile and works well with a variety of species and surgical procedures.
(© SJ Divers)

A selection of intramedullary pins, miniature fixator pins, aluminium/carbon fibre clamps and titanium/carbon fibre support rods can be used with larger reptiles (IMEX Veterinary Inc., Veterinary Instrumentation Ltd, UK). A lightweight tubular fixation system, FESSA (Fixateur Externe du Service de Santé des Armées), is small and lightweight, and incorporates a pin clamping mechanism that is preferred for external fixation. The system is available in 6 and 8 mm tube diameters, with ranges in length from 31 mm (3.0 g) to 97 mm (12.2 g), and permits the placement of multiple pins close together in small fragments (Figure 13.6a). For internal fixation, small locking compression plates are preferred because they facilitate fixed-angle constructs and do not rely on plate–bone compression for stability, which is a frequent cause of cortical fractures when using conventional plates and screws (Figure 13.6b).

13.5 Surgical saws: (a) Stryker 4200 Cordless Driver 2; (b) oscillating sagittal saw attachment to the air-powered 3M mini-driver.
(a, Courtesy of Stryker Instruments Inc.; b, © SJ Divers)

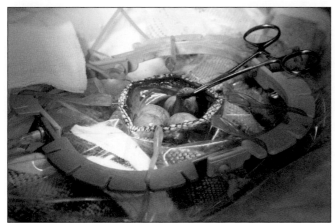

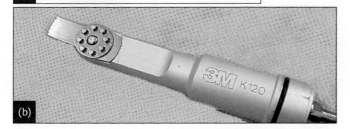

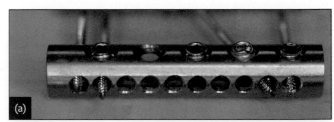

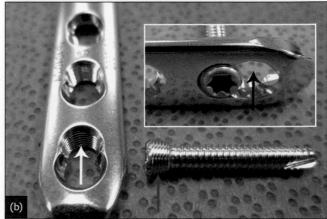

13.6 Orthopaedic implants. (a) FESSA bar with four mini-IMEX pins secured using low-profile screws. (b) Small locking plate and screw. The screw thread (red arrow) engages the plate (white arrow) as shown in the inset, thereby preventing compression of the bone to the plate. Alternatively the screw could be inserted through the adjacent aperture (black arrow) to create compression between the plate and bone.
(© SJ Divers)

Modern rapidly absorbed suture materials (particularly poliglecaprone 25) are recommended for short-term internal soft-tissue applications, and antibiotic-impregnated options are now available. Polyglactin 910 has been associated with greater inflammation and is not recommended (Govett *et al.*, 2004). Polydioxanone lasts for several months, but for permanent internal durability nylon is required. Monofilament nylon and polydioxanone are favoured for skin suturing, although wire may be necessary for crocodilians and shell repairs.

Magnification and illumination

Proper lighting is an obvious requirement for surgery. However, it becomes even more important in small patients, and surgical lights should be focused with variable power settings. Most reptile patients that present for surgical care are significantly smaller than mammalian patients; therefore, some degree of magnification is recommended, and often essential. There are a variety of magnification systems available. Operating microscopes (e.g. M501, Leica Microsystems (UK) Ltd) are powerful, but can be prohibitively expensive for the private practitioner, although second-hand models are frequently available. Headband- or frame-mounted operating loupes (X2–X4 magnification) with a dedicated halogen or xenon light source are affordable, versatile, comfortable and simple to use (Surgitel, General Scientific Corporation) (Figure 13.7). The VITOM (video telescope operating monitor) system allows practitioners to use their rigid endoscopy tower for operating microscopy (Divers, 2014b). The basic system involves an articulated arm that holds a telescope above the surgical field, with the image relayed to the endoscopy monitor (Figure 13.8). An 11 cm 0-degree telescope at 25 cm from the surgical site provides a 7–10 cm field of view at X4–X8 magnification; however, the standard 2.7 mm telescope can also be used in a similar fashion.

Haemostasis and surgical devices

A healthy reptile, depending on species, can generally tolerate between 0.4 and 0.8 ml of blood loss per 100 g bodyweight. Patients in need of surgery are often compromised and diagnostic blood samples may have been collected prior to surgery. Therefore, the amount of intraoperative blood that a reptile can afford to lose may be considerably less. Careful consideration must be given to evaluating, documenting and reducing haemorrhage intraoperatively.

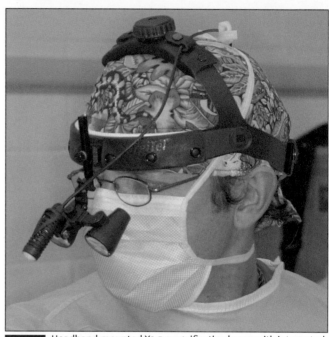

13.7 Headband-mounted X2.5 magnification loupe with integrated light source.
(© SJ Divers)

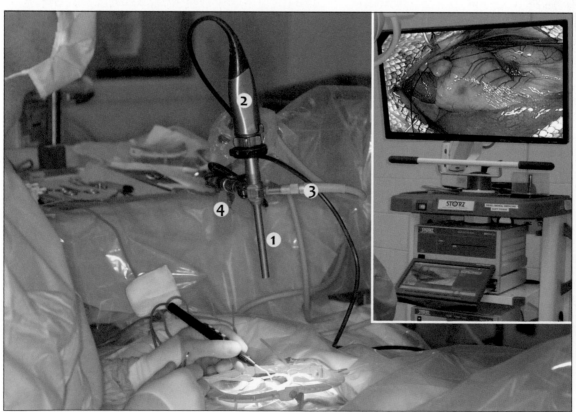

13.8 Video-telescope-operating microscopy. The operating telescope (1) with camera (2) and light cable (3) attached, and supported above the surgical site by a mechanical arm (4), provides a large magnified image on the endoscopy monitor (inset).
(© SJ Divers)

Gauze and swabs

To allow the surgeon to apply localized pressure to a small vessel and keep track of blood loss, cotton-tipped spears or applicators are less traumatic and more manageable in small confined spaces than standard gauze squares. A blood-soaked cotton-tipped applicator may hold 0.25–0.50 ml of blood.

Vascular clips

Hemoclips® (Weck Closure Systems, Teleflex) are a convenient and effective way to clamp vessels (Figure 13.9). Weck closure systems utilize autoclavable applicators and clips of various sizes – the medium and small sizes are most useful. The application of vascular clips is faster than standard suture ligatures, and therefore their use significantly decreases operating time.

Radiosurgery

Radiosurgery utilizes high-frequency radio waves to cause focal thermal tissue damage. Unlike electrocautery, radiosurgery maintains a cooler electrode, and offers superior accuracy and reduced collateral damage that rivals laser incisions. The 4.0 MHz dual-radiofrequency Surgitron® (Ellman International Inc.) offers monopolar/bipolar applications with foot-pedal/finger switch control for cut, coagulate, haemostasis, fulgurate and bipolar modes. Monopolar cutting needles are typically used for dissection, and bipolar forceps for sealing blood vessels (Figure 13.10). Figure 13.11 compares the relative collateral damage effects caused by 4.0 MHz radiosurgery and CO_2 laser.

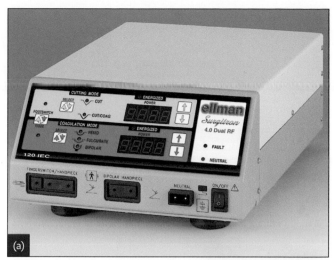

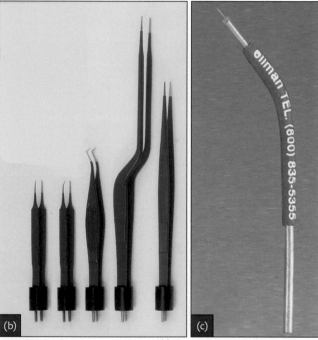

13.10 Radiosurgery equipment: (a) the 4.0 MHz Surgitron® dual-frequency radiosurgery base unit; (b) bipolar forceps; (c) monopolar cutting electrode.
(Courtesy of Ellman International Inc.)

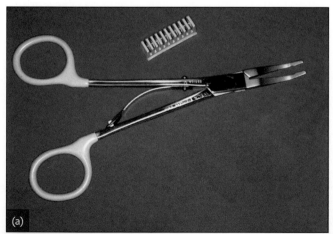

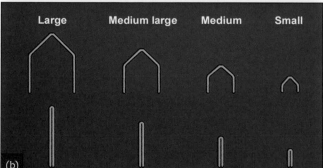

13.9 (a) Medium vascular clip cartridge containing 10 clips and an applicator (Hemoclips®, Weck). (b) Four different available sizes of vascular clips.
(© SJ Divers)

Tissue	4.0 MHz radiosurgery	CO_2 laser
Skin	307 ± 94 µm	386 ± 108 µm
Muscle	18 ± 7 µm	91 ± 15 µm

13.11 Comparison of lateral collateral coagulative damage caused by 4.0 MHz radiosurgery and CO_2 laser in iguanid lizards.
(Data from Hernandez-Divers et al., 2009)

Laser (light amplification by the stimulated emission of radiation)

The CO_2 laser (10,600 nm) is probably the most commonly used veterinary laser and offers bloodless dissection comparable to radiosurgery (Accuvet®). In contrast, the diode lasers (980 nm) are less expensive and can seal blood vessels up to 2 mm in diameter, but tend to produce more collateral damage. Both types of laser require enhanced human safety precautions, including a sealed windowless surgery room and the use of protective glasses specific for the wavelength of laser being used.

Fluoroscopy

A fluoroscopy C-arm (OEC 9800 Plus Mobile C-arm, GE Healthcare) is an expensive but useful device that permits radiographic imaging during surgery. It is particularly useful for the intraoperative assessment of orthopaedic repairs and the placement of surgical implants.

Intraoperative temperature maintenance

Maintaining patient temperature is essential for similar reasons to mammals. In addition, reduced body temperature in reptiles results in considerable increases in recovery and healing time. Warm-water-circulating blankets and/or forced-air devices offer the most effective means of maintaining patient temperature (Figure 13.12).

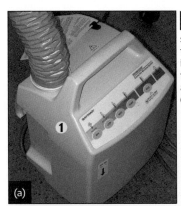

13.12 The Bair Hugger is a forced-air heating system for maintaining patient temperature. (a) The heat unit (1) is positioned under or adjacent to the table, and is (b) connected to an air blanket (2) under this lizard.
(© SJ Divers)

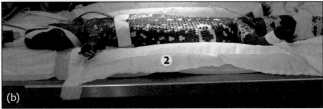

Patient preparation

Prior to surgery a pre-anaesthetic evaluation should be completed, and followed by appropriate premedication, induction, intubation, catheterization and application of intraoperative monitoring devices (see Chapter 12).

Patient positioning

Precise patient positioning will depend upon the species and the nature of the surgery (Figure 13.13). Some careful consideration should be given to:

- Ensuring that head and neck position does not interfere with ventilation
- Avoiding excessive compression of the head, limbs or coelom to prevent pressure necrosis, visceral rupture or hypoventilation of the lungs
- Avoiding extreme and prolonged hyperextension or hyperflexion of any joint
- Ensuring that the surgical site is easily accessible and does not require surgeon positioning that will result in fatigue
- The use of sandbags, vacuum beanbags, foam supports and adhesive tapes to maintain patient position.

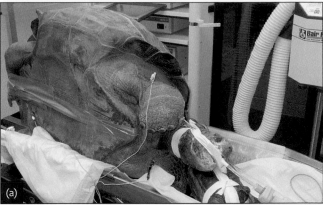

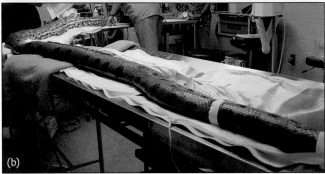

13.13 Patient positioning: (a) a large tortoise held in lateral recumbency using a V-trough operating table; (b) a large anaconda supported using multiple tables.
(© SJ Divers)

Surgeon ergonomics

Rather than assuming contorting positions, the surgeon must dedicate some time to planning factors such as patient positioning and table height. The ideal posture for the surgeon involves sitting with a straight back, and a slightly flexed neck. In addition, when performing microsurgery, the arms and wrists should rest on a padded support on the surgical table. In most cases, utilizing sandbags or similar objects to support the wrist allows the surgeon optimal motor control when incising or suturing delicate tissues. Poor positioning will quickly lead to surgeon fatigue, reduced surgical ability and increased patient morbidity. During microsurgery, surgeons should follow the 20-20-20 rule to reduce fatigue – every 20 minutes look at something 20 feet away for 20 seconds.

Presurgical preparation

Aseptic surgery should be performed in an appropriately clean and sterile operating room by surgeons wearing surgical masks, hats, sterile gloves and gowns. The surgical site should be aseptically cleaned using standard chlorhexidine or povidone iodine surgical scrubs, and a toothbrush is particularly useful for cleaning scaled skin. Dousing with alcohol is not recommended because of increased evaporative heat loss; however, a final alcohol wipe will ensure a dry grease-free area to which adhesive drapes will readily adhere.

Traditional cloth drapes can be heavy and hinder animal observation for anaesthetic monitoring. Transparent adhesive drapes have several advantages (Figure 13.14), including better visualization and monitoring of the patient, maintenance of a waterproof barrier, ability to be secured without towel clamps and being lightweight.

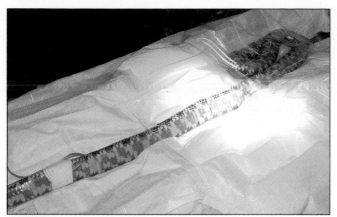

13.14 This kingsnake has been positioned on a forced-air heating blanket, and a sterile adhesive drape has been applied. Note the focused illumination of the surgical site.
(© SJ Divers)

Soft-tissue procedures

Integumental surgery

Reptile skin is often tougher than that of domesticated mammals, and incisions may have to circumvent large scales, osteoderms or other highly keratinized structures. Skin incisions should be made between scales whenever possible, thus making most surgical wounds scalloped. Incising through large scales is often more difficult, can cause permanent damage to the scales, and lead to post-healing dysecdysis. In some cases using a guarded scalpel incision technique is important to avoid inadvertent damage to deeper structures.

Skin suturing

When reptile skin is incised, it has a tendency to invert. Therefore, everting suture patterns (e.g. horizontal or vertical mattress) are recommended to ensure opposition of tissue without future dysecdysis (Figure 13.15). The skin suture materials are usually non-absorbable and strong. The most common materials used include polypropylene, nylon and polydioxanone. Wire suture may be required for repairs involving shell and crocodilian skin. Staples have also been advocated as they cause mild eversion of the skin. Reptile skin is inelastic and tension across suture

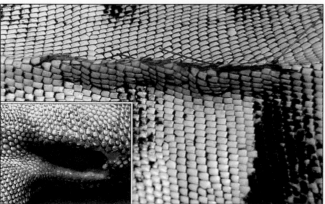

13.15 Routine coeliotomy skin closure in a green iguana using monofilament nylon in an everting horizontal mattress pattern. Inset – open surgical wound following abscess removal in a giant day gecko; note the inverting wound edges.
(© SJ Divers)

lines frequently results in dehiscence. Given the length of time it takes for reptile wounds to heal, suture removal should be delayed until 6–8 weeks postoperatively. Ecdysis may lead to the premature loss of skin sutures that were placed too superficially.

Central line catheters and other therapeutic implants

A variety of surgical implants have been utilized in reptiles, including intra-arterial telemetry devices to monitor blood pressure, vascular access devices, intrapulmonary catheters in chelonians, and osmotic pumps for long-term drug administration (Hernandez-Divers, 2002a; Chinnadurai *et al.*, 2010; Gibbons, 2014). While some of these techniques may be too specialized for general practice, the use of biluminal or triluminal central line catheters in larger reptiles has proven to be effective and practical for facilitating repeated intravenous administration of drugs, as well as for blood collection and transfusions (Pardo and Divers, 2016). Central line placement in most reptiles requires sedation or light anaesthesia with lidocaine infiltration, and a surgical cut-down procedure (Figure 13.16). The catheter should be flushed two to three times daily to prevent fibrin blockages, and the catheter–skin interface should be inspected and cleaned daily. With proper care, the central line catheter can remain functional for weeks to months in outpatients, and greatly simplifies serial blood collection, examinations and procedures.

Soft-tissue wounds

Wounds, usually infected, are frequent presentations, and, given the caseous nature of the reptilian inflammatory response, simple flushing is rarely, if ever, enough and surgical debridement is typically required. Reptiles have the capacity to recover from horrific injuries, although repeated veterinary attention and long-term owner compliance are key, as healing may take many months (Figure 13.17). Following medical stabilization and wet–dry bandage applications, sharp dissection is employed to remove all adherent necrotic debris and infected tissue, which should then be submitted for histopathology and microbiology (Figure 13.18). The maintenance of topical medications, dressings and bandages can be challenging in some cases. In lizards and chelonians, as long as the head, limbs and cloaca are unhindered, such dressings are well tolerated (Figure 13.19). Vacuum-assisted wound closure techniques have gained popularity, particularly in chelonians, and certainly appear to reduce infection and speed recovery (see Shell repair section below, and Figure 13.60) (Marin *et al.*, 2014). In small snakes, the use of adhesive dressings on the dorsum and non-spermicidally lubricated condoms has proven effective (Frye, 1993). In larger boids, conventional tie-in dressings have been used to manage extensive wounds (Pavletic, 2009) (Figure 13.20). Allogeneic and xenogeneic grafts have been used in reptiles. There is little information on autogeneic skin grafts in reptiles, probably owing to the difficulties associated with harvesting inelastic skin, and post-harvest defect closure. Successful xenogeneic skin grafts using porcine small-intestinal submucosa (Biosist®, Cook Veterinary Products) have been reported in reptiles (see Figure 13.61) (Divers and Lawton, 2000). Spectacle ulceration, skin and shell trauma were successfully treated using this material; however, the greatest challenge was postoperative graft management and maintaining a moist environment for the first 7–10 days.

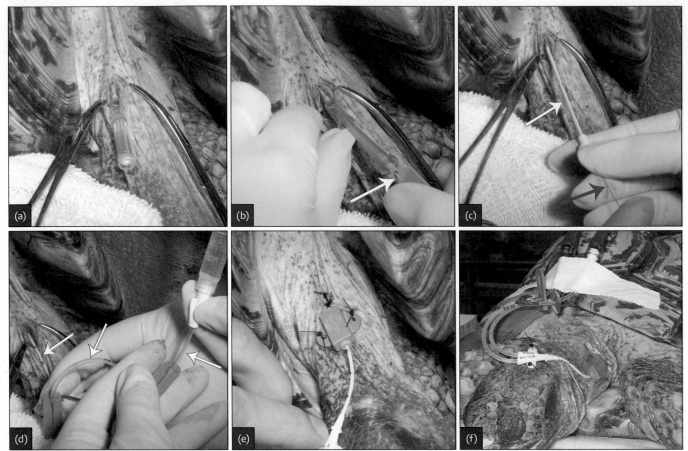

13.16 Biluminal central line placement in the left jugular of a leopard tortoise. In all images, the head is positioned at the bottom of the image with the cranial rim of the carapace to the left and cranial plastron to the right. (a) Following a surgical cut-down procedure to identify the vessel, a 20 G intravenous catheter has been temporarily placed into the jugular. (b) The catheter-pack sterile wire (arrowed) has been threaded through the intravenous catheter and advanced into the vein. (c) While the position of the wire (red arrow) is maintained, the intravenous catheter is removed and replaced by a dilator (white arrow), which slightly enlarges the opening in the vein. (d) While maintaining the wire in place, the dilator is removed and the silicone central catheter (arrowed) is threaded over the wire, and into the vein. The wire is then removed, and the catheter flushed and capped. (e) A blue plastic support is placed over the catheter close to the insertion point, and used to secure the catheter to the skin using sutures. (f) The catheter is additionally secured to the head using sutures, and finally the two ports are taped to the cranial carapace. The catheter insertion site is covered with a transparent adhesive dressing.
(© SJ Divers)

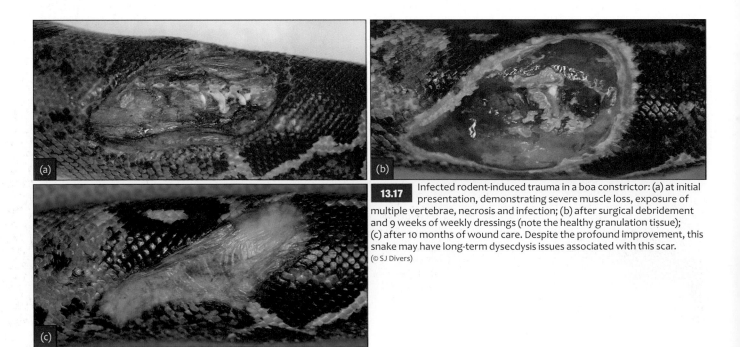

13.17 Infected rodent-induced trauma in a boa constrictor: (a) at initial presentation, demonstrating severe muscle loss, exposure of multiple vertebrae, necrosis and infection; (b) after surgical debridement and 9 weeks of weekly dressings (note the healthy granulation tissue); (c) after 10 months of wound care. Despite the profound improvement, this snake may have long-term dysecdysis issues associated with this scar.
(© SJ Divers)

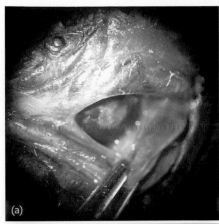

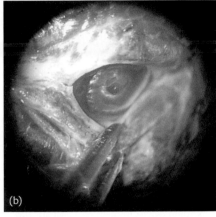

13.23 Focal corneal infection in a Hermann's tortoise: (a) initial presentation of a focal accumulation of bacteria and leucocytes on the cornea; (b) following corneal debridement, further treatment includes topical antimicrobial therapy and, if deemed necessary, a third eyelid flap procedure.
(© SJ Divers)

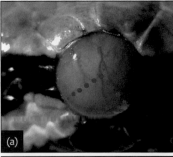

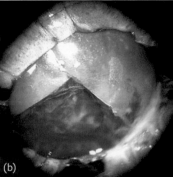

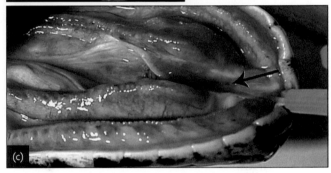

13.24 Subspectacular abscess treatment in a Burmese python. (a) Initial presentation with distension of the subspectacular space and neovascularization of the spectacle. The recommended 90-degree wedge resection in the most dependent aspect of the spectacle is indicated (blue dotted line). (b) Intraoperative view following wedge resection and flushing. Note that the cornea is now visible and exposed. (c) View of the opening to the lacrimal duct (arrowed) that has been catheterized for retrograde flushing.
(© SJ Divers)

Subspectacular abscess

Blockage of the lacrimal duct in snakes (and lizards that possess spectacles) results in fluid accumulation between the spectacle and the cornea (Figure 13.24a). Often this fluid becomes infected and inspissated. A wedge of 45–90 degrees is removed from the ventral aspect of the spectacle (Figure 13.24a–b) (Maas *et al.*, 2010). The caseous material is removed for cytology and microbiology, and the subspectacular space thoroughly flushed with sterile saline. The patency of the lacrimal duct must be assured. It is generally easier to catheterize the buccal opening of the duct as it emerges close to the cranial margin of the palatine teeth, and flush retrograde (Figure 13.24c). The spectacle wedge incision is left open and topical ophthalmic medication is recommended for the first 7 days, by which time the subspectacular space and normal wetting of the corneal surface are re-established beneath a proteinaceous plaque (Maas *et al.*, 2010). Germinal epithelium of the spectacle is repaired by 3 weeks, with complete spectacle healing by 3 months.

Conjunctivoralostomy

In snakes (and lizards that possess spectacles) with persistent lacrimal duct blockage that fails to respond to spectacular wedge resection, a conjunctivoralostomy can be performed. At the medial canthus edge of the spectacle, a 30-degree incision allows the introduction of a needle that is forced from the inferior fornix of the subspectacular space through the roof of the mouth, to emerge between the palatine and maxillary teeth. Silastic tubing is threaded through the needle, and the needle removed. The tube is sutured to the roof of the buccal cavity and to the periocular skin to maintain patency. The tube is removed 4–6 weeks postoperatively.

Enucleation and evisceration

Removal of the globe is required where irreversible ocular damage, prolapse or pain persist (Figure 13.25a). In snakes (and lizards that possess spectacles), a circular incision is continued around the entire spectacle, which is then removed. The eye is then grasped with forceps, gently elevated, and dissected free from its attachments. The optical vessels are ligated using a small vascular clip and a curved applicator, although sutures can be used. The ocular deficit is left open and topical ophthalmic antibiotics should be used to prevent infection. Healing typically takes 4–6 weeks, and most snakes do well following surgery. As an alternative, the globe may be eviscerated, leaving the sclera and bony ossicles. The advantage of evisceration is that the globe does not collapse and result in a sunken appearance. In chelonians, crocodilians and most lizards it is possible to close the orbit by tarsorrhaphy (Figure 13.25b). In small reptiles, a small radiosurgery loop or CO_2 laser can be used to eviscerate the globe.

Cloacal organ prolapse

Various organs have been reported to prolapse through the vent, including phallus/hemipenes, oviduct, cloaca, colon and bladder (see Chapters 17 and 20). It is vital that the precise nature of any prolapse is identified, as treatment options vary dramatically. Endoscopic examination of the cloaca and associated organs is worthwhile (see Chapter 10).

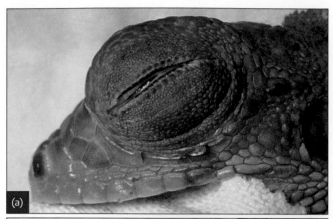

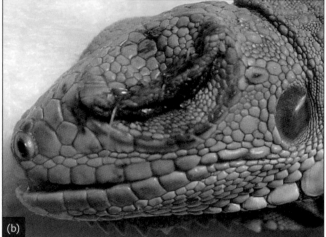

13.25 Enucleation in a green iguana: (a) original presentation of panophthalmitis; (b) collapse of the globe following enucleation and tarsorrhaphy.
(© SJ Divers)

Phallus and hemipenes

The phallus (because it contains no urethra) of a crocodilian or chelonian is a single organ and is usually retracted into the cranioventral cloaca. Snakes and lizards possess paired hemipenes that retract into the ventral tail, caudal to the cloaca (see Chapters 1 and 20). Phallus/hemipenis prolapse is a common condition of reptiles. If the prolapsed tissue appears viable, the oedema should be reduced using concentrated sugar or salt solutions before the structure is cleaned, lubricated and gently replaced. The lizard/snake hemipenes should be replaced caudally from the vent, while the crocodilian/chelonian phallus should be replaced cranially into the urodeum of the cloaca. Two simple interrupted sutures can be placed across the 'long axis' margins of the vent to prevent immediate recurrence for 5–10 days. A purse suture should not be utilized, as it is likely to deform the slit-like opening of the vent and damage local structures including urogenital openings. It is important that suture placement allows for normal urination and defecation. If the tissue appears necrotic, amputation is the treatment of choice. The reptilian copulatory organ does not contain a urethra; therefore, mattress sutures or circumferential ligatures can be placed at the base and the organ safely resected (Figure 13.26). Obviously this procedure will compromise future breeding, although snakes and lizards with a single remaining hemipenis can still reproduce. Animals often benefit from systemic and local antibiotics given the proximity of the surgical site to the lower gastrointestinal tract.

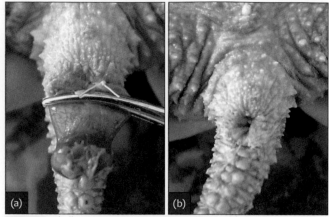

13.26 Phallus amputation in a snapping turtle: (a) prolapsed phallus clamped, and mattress sutures placed along the base in preparation for removal; (b) view of the vent immediately following amputation, with the small stump retracted into the cranioventral cloaca.
(© SJ Divers)

Cloaca and colon

Prolapse of the cloaca and distal colon are not uncommon (Figure 13.27). However, they are often treated inappropriately by replacement and purse-string sutures without due regard for the underlying cause (e.g. obesity, organomegaly, constipation, dystocia, intestinal parasitism, secondary nutritional hyperparathyroidism, cloacitis, colitis). Minor prolapses can be replaced and two simple interrupted sutures can be placed near the edges of the vent to prevent recurrence. More severe prolapse is treated by transcutaneous cloaco- or colopexy (Figure 13.28). Uncommonly, this procedure will fail and a coeliotomy is required to anchor the colon to the last one to three ribs using nylon.

In cases of severe cloacal and colonic necrosis, resection and end-to-end anastomosis are essential; however, a combination of cloacal and coeliotomy approaches may

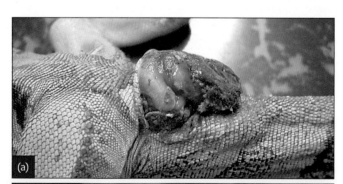

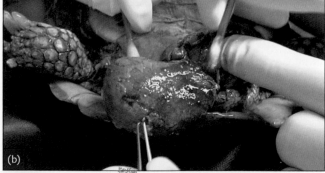

13.27 Cloacal prolapse: (a) presentation of cloacal prolapse in a green iguana; (b) cleaning a cloacocolonic prolapse in a spur-thighed tortoise in preparation for surgical replacement.
(© SJ Divers)

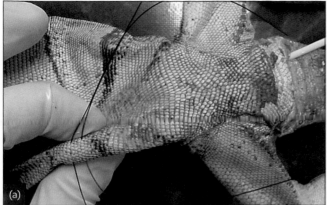

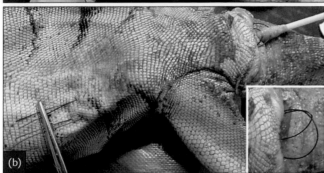

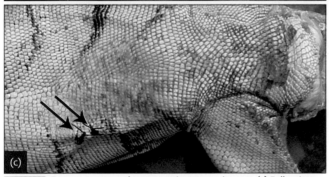

13.28 Transcutaneous cloacopexy in a green iguana. (a) Following replacement of the viable prolapsed tissue and aseptic skin preparation of the caudolateral coelom, a large lubricated cotton-tipped applicator is inserted into the cloaca, and tented against the ventrolateral body wall. Two to three simple interrupted polydioxanone sutures are placed through the skin and cotton-tip. (b) The suture ends are left long and held by haemostats. The cotton-tipped applicator, carrying the sutures, is removed from the cloaca. The cotton is teased away from the sutures (inset). (c) After pulling the sutures back into the cloaca with the haemostats, they are tied (arrowed). The cloacocolonic wall is now sutured to the body wall and a fibrous adhesion generally develops over the next 4–8 weeks.
(© SJ Divers)

be required. Great care is needed to identify and preserve the openings of the ureters and oviducts within the urodeum. Postsurgical stricture following colon prolapse and replacement has been reported, but was subsequently corrected following transverse closure of a longitudinal enterotomy incision at the site of stricture (Lloyd, 2003).

Oviduct

The prolapsed oviduct can appear plicated (normal appearance) or grossly swollen and oedematous. Correction usually requires both a coelomic and a cloacal approach. Even if the prolapse is fresh and viable, replacement per cloaca is unlikely to correct the internal malposition. In many cases, severe pathology is discovered on coeliotomy, and an ovariosalpingectomy is often required.

Bladder

Bladder prolapse may be reduced after aspiration and collapse. The bladder is thin walled and fragile and will not tolerate excessive handling. A combination of coeliotomy and cloacal approaches may be required. A severely necrotic bladder can be partially resected or even removed as the ureters empty into the urodeum of the cloaca and not the bladder. However, the long-term effects of a lack of postrenal bladder modification of urine have not been documented, and such animals are likely to have less tolerance to water restriction in the future.

Coeliotomy

Surgical coeliotomy provides access to most of the major internal organs and is therefore useful for a range of surgical procedures, including exploration and biopsy. The technique is simplest to perform in the uncompartmentalized coelom of most lizards, but more difficult in snakes with diffuse fat bodies and multiple fascial planes, and in chelonians and crocodilians owing to their bony integument and/or compartmentalized coelomic cavities. The visceral organs of small reptiles are delicate and friable, necessitating gentle handling.

Chelonians

Depending upon the species and the surgical site or organ of interest, there are two major approaches; transplastron and prefemoral. The traditional transplastron coeliotomy approach requires a temporary osteotomy through the plastron, while the prefemoral approach is a soft-tissue technique that involves entry into the coelom in front of a pelvic limb. Figure 13.29 compares transplastron and prefemoral coeliotomy.

Transplastron procedure	Prefemoral procedure
Technically more demanding, requiring shell-cutting equipment	Technically easier to perform with standard surgical instrumentation
Longer operational times	Shorter operational times
Provides extensive surgical access to all major organs	Provides more variable surgical access; better in aquatic species with large prefemoral fossae
Likely to be more painful postoperatively	Likely to be less painful postoperatively
Longer healing times of 12–18 weeks	Shorter healing times of 4–8 weeks

13.29 Comparison between transplastron and prefemoral coeliotomy in chelonians.

Transplastron coeliotomy: With the chelonian supported in dorsal recumbency, and following aseptic preparation, the cranial, caudal and two lateral plastron incisions are planned, taking into careful consideration the regional anatomy below the plastron (Figure 13.30).

- Consider the degree of access required to perform the required procedure (e.g. bladder stone or foreign body removal). Access cannot be easily enlarged so ensure that the initial cuts are of sufficient size.
- Appreciate the position of the heart at the midline intersection of the pectoral and abdominal scutes (species dependent).
- Appreciate the position of the two parallel abdominal veins running caudocranially below the plastron.

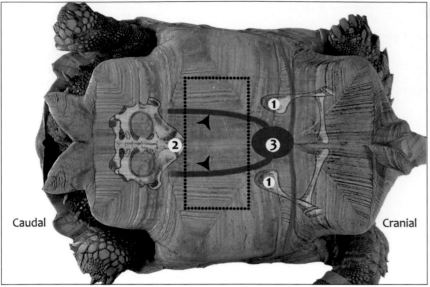

13.30 Transplastron coeliotomy in chelonians. View of the ventrum of a generic chelonian illustrating the positions of the clavicles (1), cranial rim of the pelvis (2), heart (3) and paired abdominal veins (arrowheads). The approximate locations of plastron hinges in *Testudo* spp. (green line) and *Terrapene* spp. (blue line) are also shown. The four proposed osteotomy incisions are indicated (black dotted lines). (© SJ Divers)

- Appreciate any plastron hinges (if present, often between the abdominal and femoral scutes, or the pectoral and abdominal scutes) and remember to maintain their functionality during shell repair.
- Appreciate the increasing thickness of the plastron as it forms the plastrocarapacial bridge laterally.

An oscillating sagittal saw couples accuracy with reduced collateral damage and minimal soft-tissue trauma (Figure 13.31a). Rotating saws can be used but are less forgiving on soft tissues, and over-scoring at the corners occurs with larger blade diameters. The saw is held at 45 degrees to bevel the shell incisions. The two lateral cuts are made first, and a 25 G needle is used to ensure that the cuts are full-shell thickness. The caudal cut and, finally, the cranial cut are made in a similar fashion. Penetration of the shell over the heart is generally made last. Using a periosteal elevator or scalpel handle, the cranial edge of the plastron segment is lifted to expose the muscle attachments (Figure 13.31b).

Staying as close to the plastron segment as possible, blunt dissection separates the plastron osteotomy segment from the underlying soft tissues. The paired abdominal veins are sometimes very closely associated with the plastron and it may be necessary to strip away the periosteum of the flap to preserve these vessels. The caudal soft-tissue attachments can be left intact, as the plastron flap is reflected caudally, and covered with moistened sterile gauze. Depending upon the circumstances, several variations are possible regarding entry into the coelom, including incisions between the abdominal veins (Figure 13.32a), lateral to the abdominal veins, and even ligation and transection of one abdominal vein to permit an L-shaped flap for removing large structures. An elastic ring retractor often improves exposure (Figure 13.32b). Ligation of both abdominal veins is not recommended, as circulatory disturbance is likely to be significant.

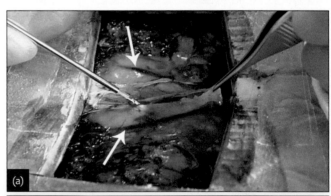

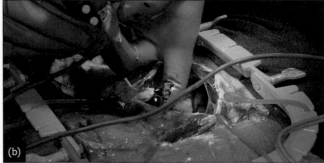

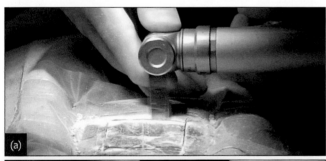

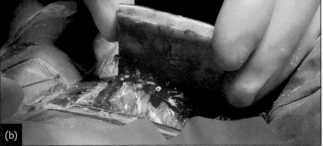

13.31 Transplastron coeliotomy in chelonians: (a) using an air-powered oscillating saw to cut through the plastron; (b) the plastron flap is elevated and the muscle attachments dissected free. (© SJ Divers)

13.32 Transplastron coeliotomy in chelonians: (a) midline incision between the abdominal veins (arrowed); (b) ring retractor and elastic stays improve access as a liver biopsy is performed. (© SJ Divers)

A two-layer closure is routine. The coelomic membrane is closed in a simple continuous pattern using absorbable suture material (Figure 13.33a). Three or four stabilizing sutures (usually polydioxanone, but wire can be used for giant species) can be placed through drilled holes to anchor the bony section to the plastron (Figure 13.33b). The incision line can be filled with sterile antibiotic to prevent the repair material from seeping below the shell. The plastron section is replaced and secured using epoxy resin or acrylic, either at four points or around the entire bony incision line. The shell is carefully cleaned with an alcohol swab to remove any grease, before epoxy resin or an acrylic (e.g. polymethyl methacrylate) is used to seal the area (Figure 13.33c). It is helpful to use masking tape to protect adjacent areas, particularly hinges, before applying the repair material. Any excess repair material can then be easily removed along with the tape, thereby creating a clean finish (Figure 13.34a). The healing process depends directly upon the quality of the repair. Accurate reduction of the bony section and the plastron will improve the chances of first or second intention healing. However, in many cases the plastron flap becomes a sequestrum that

provides temporary protection to the new bone developing beneath. The plastron heals in around 12 weeks; however, the covering is usually left in place for 6–12 months before removal (Figure 13.34b). Radiography is seldom helpful in the assessment of healing because radiolucent lines tend to persist after healing.

Prefemoral coeliotomy: Prefemoral coeliotomy provides limited lateral access to the coelom. However, when requiring a lateral approach to the coelom of certain species that have a large prefemoral fossa, the prefemoral approach may be more appropriate (Figure 13.35). With the chelonian in lateral to dorsal recumbency, the pelvic limb is secured caudad to expose the prefemoral fossa. Following aseptic preparation, a craniocaudal incision is made in the middle of the fossa. Blunt dissection cranial to the sartorius and ventral to the iliacus muscles reveals the coelomic aponeurosis of the transverse and oblique abdominal muscles. This coelomic aponeurosis is fibrous and some force may be required to breach the membrane. Elastic stays and a ring retractor improve surgical exposure. Muscle and skin closure are routine. Bilateral surgery may be required if contralateral structures cannot be visualized or exteriorized through a single prefemoral incision (e.g. gonadectomy).

Lizards

Most lizards are placed in dorsal recumbency, but some laterally compressed species (e.g. chameleons) are often placed in left or right lateral recumbency (Figure 13.36). The head and body are supported, and the legs are secured with tape. Following aseptic preparation, there are two major approaches to the coelom of most lizards, paramedian and midline. For either approach it is important to

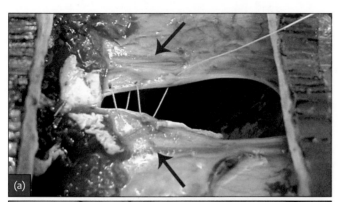

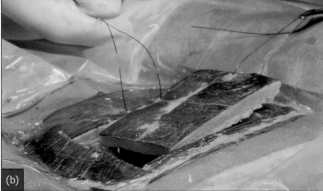

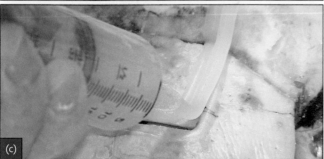

13.33 Transplastron coeliotomy in chelonians: (a) routine closure of the coelomic membrane using absorbable sutures in a simple continuous pattern; (b) absorbable suture placed through predrilled holes in the plastron flap and shell in preparation for flap reposition; (c) application of low-temperature polymethyl methacrylate (Technovite®) by syringe.
(© SJ Divers)

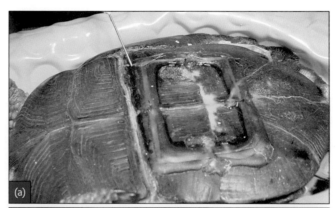

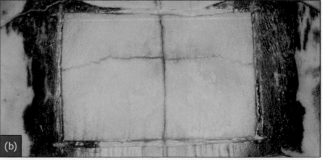

13.34 Transplastron coeliotomy in chelonians. (a) Final repair with the incision and sutures buried beneath the repair material. (b) View of the plastron of a spur-thighed tortoise that underwent transplastron coeliotomy 12 weeks earlier. The plastron flap had become a sequestrum and, following removal, new bone can be seen filling the entire area. It is recommended to leave this sequestrum flap in place for 6–12 months to provide additional protection.
(© SJ Divers)

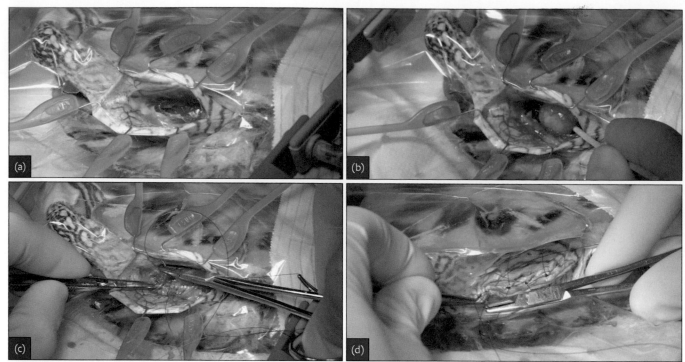

13.35 Prefemoral coeliotomy in a red-eared terrapin in dorsal recumbency: (a) following prefemoral skin incision, a ring retractor and elastic stays have been placed, and the coelomic musculature can be seen; (b) following blunt dissection through the musculature, part of the left ovary can be seen; (c) following the intracoelomic procedure, the musculature is closed using a continuous pattern; (d) finally, the skin is closed in a routine manner.
(© SJ Divers)

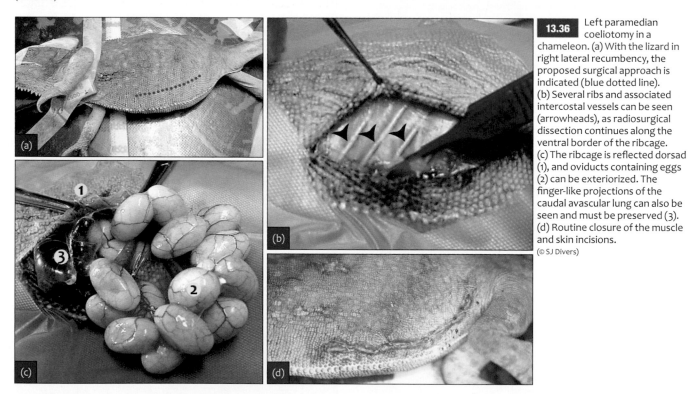

13.36 Left paramedian coeliotomy in a chameleon. (a) With the lizard in right lateral recumbency, the proposed surgical approach is indicated (blue dotted line). (b) Several ribs and associated intercostal vessels can be seen (arrowheads), as radiosurgical dissection continues along the ventral border of the ribcage. (c) The ribcage is reflected dorsad (1), and oviducts containing eggs (2) can be exteriorized. The finger-like projections of the caudal avascular lung can also be seen and must be preserved (3). (d) Routine closure of the muscle and skin incisions.
(© SJ Divers)

appreciate the ventral vasculature and particularly the location of the ventral abdominal vein (Figure 13.37a).

A paramedian approach involves a craniocaudal incision made parallel to, but lateral from, the ventral midline (Figure 13.37a–c). The abdominal musculature is thin and easily incised by radiosurgery, CO_2 laser or blunt dissection using cotton-tipped applicators. Sharp incision using scalpel or scissors results in increased haemorrhage. The coelomic membrane is very thin and is easily breached using cotton-tipped applicators; care is required to identify a distended bladder and avoid accidental rupture upon entry into the coelom. In small lizards, there is no need to suture the coelomic membrane or thin abdominal musculature, only the skin need be closed. Coeliotomy closure in larger lizards should be in two layers, with the muscle closed using a simple continuous pattern with absorbable sutures. Skin closure is routine. The advantage of this technique is clear avoidance of the large midline abdominal vein (Figure 13.37d); however, incision through abdominal musculature may produce more postoperative discomfort.

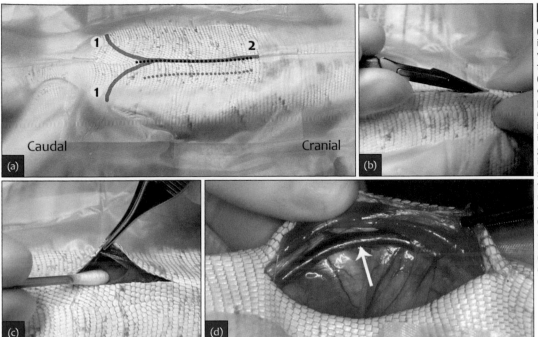

13.37 Coeliotomy in the green iguana.
(a) Ventrum of an iguana illustrating the paired pelvic veins (1), anastomosing to form the large abdominal vein (2). Possible coeliotomy entry can be made using a paramedian (blue dotted line) or midline (black dotted line) incision. (b) Paramedian skin incision made using a reversed guarded scalpel blade to avoid inadvertent damage to deeper structures. (c) Dissection through the thin abdominal musculature using cotton-tipped applicators. (d) Exposure of the coelom and visualization of the ventral midline abdominal vein (arrowed).
(© SJ Divers)

The midline incision should be started caudal to the anastomosis of the paired pelvic veins, where they join to form the midline abdominal vein (see Figure 13.37a). This requires an incision started at, or caudal to, the umbilical scar and extended craniad. Careful incision through the skin and underlying linea alba reveals the abdominal vein, which should be preserved and gently retracted laterally. A simple continuous pattern, using absorbable suture material, is used to close the linea alba, and skin closure is routine. The advantages of this technique are equal accessibility to both sides of the coelom and less muscle trauma; however, greater surgical skill is required to preserve the abdominal vein.

Whichever technique is used, the incision may have to extend from the xiphoid process to just cranial to the pelvis to provide sufficient exposure for certain procedures. Indeed, access to the cranial coelom often requires incision through the sternum. Elastic stays and ring retractors are useful to achieve appropriate exposure in many species. In lizards, the urinary bladder (if present), colon or fat bodies may obstruct visualization of other visceral structures, and need gentle manipulation and retraction using cotton-tipped applicators.

Snakes

The elongated nature of snakes makes it impossible to make a single coeliotomy incision to view all major organs. Therefore, it is vital that the precise surgical site is accurately determined ahead of time using anatomy references, palpation, clinical pathology and diagnostic imaging (McCracken, 1999). A permanent marker is used to mark the surgical site on the snake and on tape on the table (see Figure 13.39c). Ideally, the incision is made between the second and third rows of lateral scales, although incision between the first and second rows is also acceptable (Figure 13.38). Care is taken to incise between the scales whenever possible. This ensures that the incision is positioned laterally and off the floor when the recovered snake is mobile. Radiosurgery, CO$_2$ laser or blunt dissection is continued through the muscle layer, just ventral to the ribs.

Entry into the coelom is made ventral to the ribs and associated musculature. It is often necessary to navigate through multiple fascial layers, and extensive fat bodies can hinder visualization (Figure 13.38b). Elastic stays and ring retractors can greatly aid visualization (Figure 13.39a). A two-layer closure is routine, with the muscle layer closed using absorbable sutures in a continuous pattern (Figure 13.39b). Skin closure is routine, with the knots positioned on the dorsal side of the incision (Figure 13.39c).

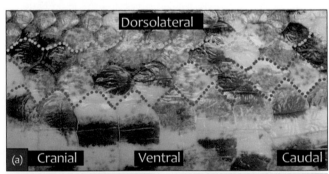

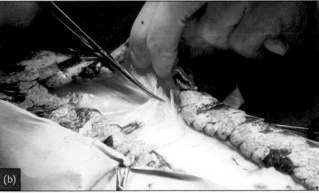

13.38 Coeliotomy in a green anaconda. (a) Initial skin incision can be made between the first and second (blue dotted line) or second and third (green dotted line) rows of lateral scales. Incision through the large ventral scutes or between the large ventral scutes and the first row of lateral scales (red dotted line) is not advised. (b) Subcutaneous dissection to gain access to the coelom.
(© SJ Divers)

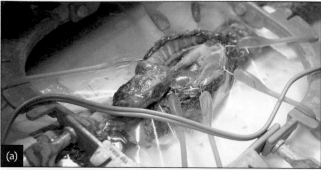

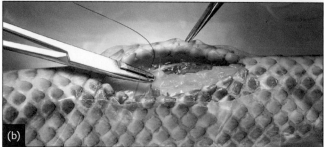

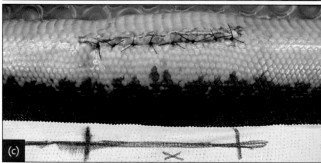

13.39 Coeliotomy in snakes. (a) Entry into the coelom just ventral to the ribs to permit exteriorization of a large mass, with a ring retractor used to improve visualization (corn snake). (b) Closure of the coelomic musculature using absorbable poliglecaprone 25 suture material in a continuous pattern (kingsnake). (c) Routine skin closure using nylon sutures in an everting horizontal mattress pattern. Note the marked tape adjacent to this Kenyan sand boa that helped indicated the required approach.
(© SJ Divers)

Crocodilians

The thick osteoderm integument of crocodilians makes coeliotomy difficult. It is generally easier to make an incision directly over the organ of interest rather than make a standard ventral approach in the hope of assessing most organs. For example, for gastrotomy, a craniocaudal incision is made in the ventrolateral body wall midway between the pectoral and pelvic limbs on the left side.

Urogenital surgery

Reproductive disease is common in captive reptiles and represents one of the common reasons for surgical treatment (Mader *et al.*, 2006). However, given the continued improvements in anaesthesia and surgical (especially endoscopic) techniques, sterilization should continue to gain in popularity and help to reduce the incidence of disease.

Orchidectomy and vasectomy

Orchidectomy is most often performed on lizards. Although there is debate over the effectiveness of castration to reduce behavioural problems, it may still be recommended to prevent breeding or as a treatment for reproductive disease.

In lizards, the testes are generally located adjacent to the dorsal renal veins and adrenal glands, in the mid to caudal coelom. The testes are suspended by a short mesorchium from the dorsal body wall, within which the testicular artery and veins are located. The left adrenal gland is positioned between the left testis and left renal vein, and care must be exercised to identify and preserve the gland during orchidectomy. The right adrenal is below the renal vein and is therefore less likely to be damaged. It is easier to use vascular clips to ligate the vessels, rather than sutures, and then dissect the testes free distal to the vascular clips (Figure 13.40). Endoscopic castration is also possible (see Chapter 10).

In snakes, orchidectomy is less commonly performed. Testis location varies with family but the surgery is straightforward following a targeted coeliotomy. Vasectomy has been reported in the garter snake (Zwart *et al.*, 1979). The technique requires a 5 cm incision from the 45th to 40th ventral scale (from the cloaca). The ducti deferentes are located on either side of the intestinal tract, and a 3 cm segment is excised from each duct.

Orchidectomy is more difficult in chelonians owing to the caudodorsal location of the testes and intimate relationship with the kidneys. Recently, endoscopic and endoscope-assisted procedures have been described in several species (see Chapter 10).

Oophorectomy (or ovariectomy)

With the advent of improved techniques, oophorectomy should, size permitting, be considered for any non-breeding lizard or chelonian in order to prevent the common

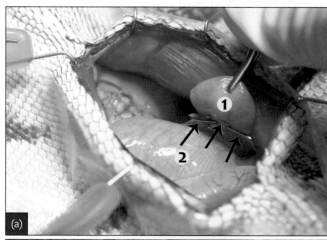

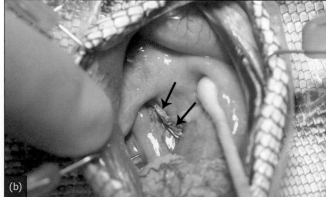

13.40 Orchidectomy in the green iguana: (a) elevation of the left testis (1) with vascular clips applied to the mesorchium (arrowed); the colon (2) is also visible; (b) following resection of the testis, the vascular clips (arrowed) can be seen resting on the renal vein.
(© SJ Divers)

presentations of dystocia and other reproductive diseases. In snakes, routine sterilization of females is more controversial and seldom recommended because of the extensive surgical exposure required to perform oophorectomy (e.g. an incision extending for 20–25% of the snout-to-cloaca length would be required to expose both ovaries). Nevertheless, unilateral oophorectomy has been performed as a treatment for ovarian neoplasia.

In female lizards that are not reproductively active the ovaries are generally small. They are located adjacent to the dorsal renal veins and adrenal glands in the mid to caudal coelom. The application of vascular clips along the mesovarium ligates the associated vasculature and permits the safe dissection of the ovary (Figure 13.41a). It is not necessary to remove the oviducts if they are normal. In cases of preovulatory follicular stasis, the active ovaries are considerably enlarged and immediately obvious upon entering the lizard's coelom as they resemble clusters of yellow–orange grapes. Each ovary is elevated to expose the suspensory ligament, containing three to eight large vessels that branch off the aorta and renal veins. Vascular clips (or sutures) are used to ligate these vessels before the ovary is dissected free (Figure 13.41b). The oviducts are usually small and involuted and do not need to be removed unless diseased.

Oophorectomy in chelonians should routinely be performed as part of dystocia surgery to prevent future breeding (unless an endangered species where future breeding potential is of paramount importance); transplastron or prefemoral coeliotomy is required. The chelonian ovaries originate close to the ventrolateral aspect of the kidneys, but in mature females they are large and extend into the central coelom. The mesovarium is extensive and great care is required to ensure that the entire ovary has been isolated before haemostasis and dissection proceed (Figure 13.42). Recently, endoscope-assisted (mature females) and endoscopic (immature females) techniques have been described (Divers, 2014a). These techniques enable a practitioner to offer routine oophorectomy, via a soft-tissue prefemoral approach in many chelonians (see Chapter 10).

Salpingotomy and salpingectomy

In most pet chelonians and lizards, bilateral ovariosalpingectomy is recommended. In cases of postovulatory egg stasis or dystocia, the oviducts full of eggs or fetuses are immediately obvious upon entry into the coelom (Figure 13.43). The large numerous blood vessels that supply each oviduct must be ligated with sutures or vascular clips. Vascular clips and radiosurgery greatly reduce surgery time

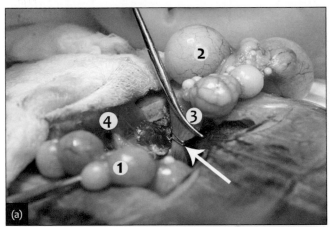

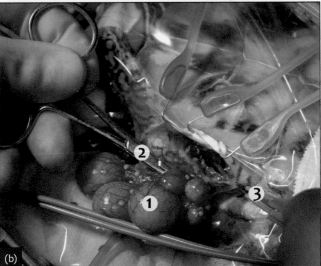

13.42 Oophorectomy in chelonians. (a) Transplastron oophorectomy in a box turtle. Both left (1) and right (2) ovaries have been exteriorized, with a haemostat clamped on the right mesovarium (3) and a vascular clip applied (arrowed). Note the muscle attachments to the caudal margin of the plastron flap (4). (b) Left prefemoral coeliotomy in a red-eared terrapin. The left ovary (1) has been exteriorized and the mesovarium clamped using a haemostat (2). Following vascular clip ligation of the major vessels, the mesovarium is transected using bipolar radiosurgery (3).
(© SJ Divers)

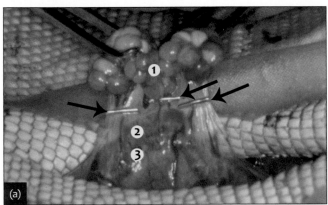

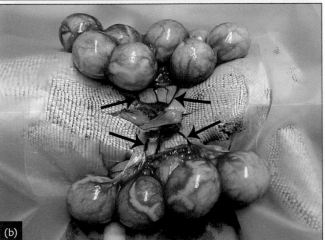

13.41 Oophorectomy in the green iguana. (a) Elevated right ovary (inactive) (1) revealing the ovarian ligament and associated vessels that have been ligated with vascular clips (arrowed). Below the clips, the renal vein (2) and left adrenal gland (3) can be seen. (b) Exteriorized active ovaries owing to preovulatory follicular stasis. Note the massive enlargement of both ovaries and the mesovarian vessels (arrowed).
(© SJ Divers)

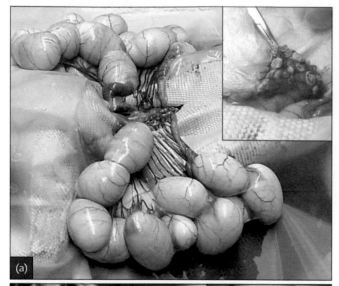

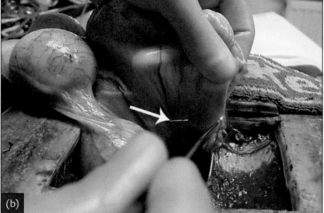

13.43 Salpingectomy in lizards and chelonians. (a) Exposure of both oviducts containing eggs in a green iguana. Inset – the ovaries are anatomically separate from the oviducts and involuted; however, it is critical that they are removed following salpingectomy.
(b) Exteriorization of an oviduct containing eggs following a transplastron coeliotomy in an African spurred tortoise. A vascular clip (arrowed) has been applied to ligate several vessels, and the mesovarium is being dissected using a 980 nm diode laser.
(© SJ Divers)

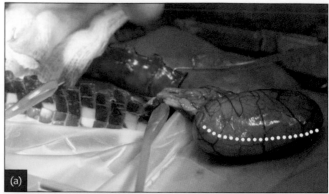

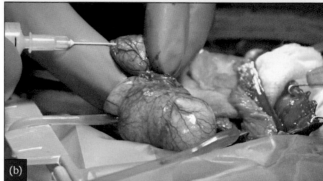

13.44 Reproductive surgery in an endangered Guatemalan beaded lizard. (a) A retained egg is obvious within the exteriorized oviduct. The proposed salpingotomy incision in order to remove the egg is indicated (white dotted line). The incision is subsequently closed using fine absorbable suture material. (b) Ovocentesis in the same lizard to resolve preovulatory follicular stasis but retain reproductive capability.
(© SJ Divers)

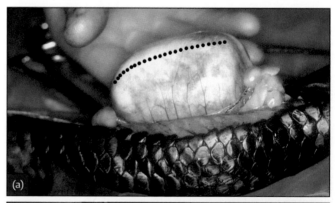

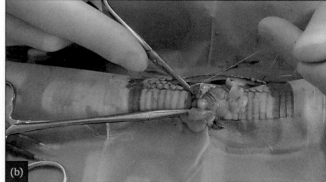

13.45 Salpingotomy in snakes. (a) Following coeliotomy in this endangered indigo snake, an egg retained within the oviduct has been exteriorized. The proposed salpingotomy incision is indicated (black dotted line). (b) Following egg removal in this corn snake, the thinly walled oviduct is closed using fine suture material.
(© SJ Divers)

and several vessels can often be clamped with a single clip. The oviducts are ligated close to their insertion with the cloaca, using a circumferential transfixing ligature, and removed. In most lizards the ovaries are often small and involuted, lying close to the renal veins. In chelonians they often remain large. Their removal is essential, however, if future folliculogenesis, ovulation and egg coelomitis are to be avoided (see Oophorectomy above). Single or multiple salpingotomy incisions can be made to remove the eggs or fetuses or unilateral ovariosalpingectomy can be performed in an effort to maintain future breeding capacity (Figure 13.44). However, maintenance of reproductive capacity in the face of disease requires additional skill (McArthur and Hernandez-Divers, 2003; Mader *et al.*, 2006).

Salpingectomy is not routinely performed in snakes owing to the extensive length of the serpentine reproductive tract. Instead, single or multiple coeliotomy and salpingotomy incisions are created, with efforts made to manipulate more cranial and caudal eggs or fetuses out of the same incision (Figures 13.45 and 13.46) (Mader *et al.*, 2006). Nevertheless, in cases of neoplasia or severe infection, such extensive exposure and salpingectomy may be indicated (Figure 13.47).

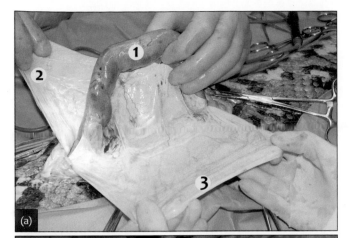

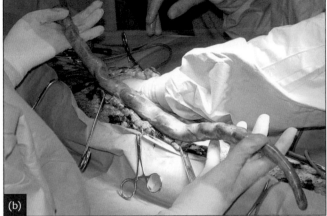

13.46 (a) Removal of an ectopic mummified fetus (1) from between the normal right (2) and left (3) oviducts in a green anaconda. (b) The complete fetus following removal.

(© SJ Divers)

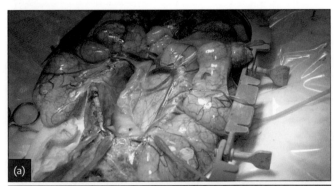

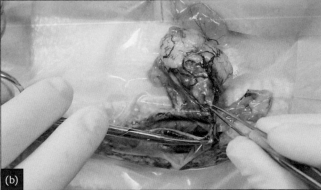

13.47 Salpingectomy in snakes. (a) In this timber rattlesnake, severe bacterial salpingitis necessitated major surgical exposure and salpingectomy. (b) In this corn snake, a granulosa cell tumour involving the oviduct required ovariosalpingectomy.

(© SJ Divers)

Cystotomy

Bladder stones are common in lizards and chelonians, and may reach gigantic sizes (Mader, 2006a). In addition, eggs may also be found within the bladder of chelonians that were previously induced to lay with intramuscular oxytocin. The sudden expulsion of multiple eggs into the cloaca may cause some to fall through the urethra and into the bladder. Following coeliotomy, the bladder is located in the caudo-ventral coelom and stay sutures are often used to prevent coelomic contamination by non-sterile urine (Figure 13.48). Aspiration of fluid contents is recommended prior to incision. Scalpel incision permits the stone (or egg) to be

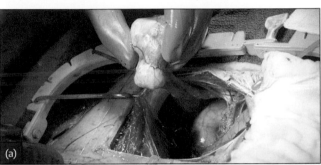

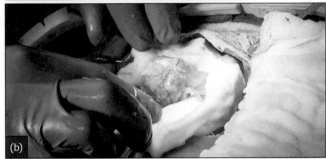

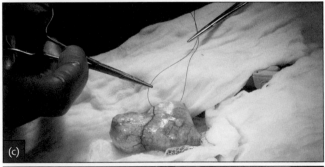

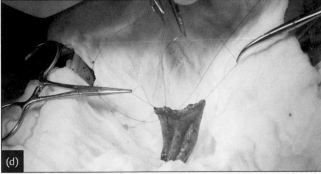

13.48 Cystotomy and urolith removal in a desert tortoise: (a) elevation of the urolith within the thinly walled bladder; (b) packing the coelom with moistened sterile gauze is recommended as bladder contents are seldom sterile in chelonians; (c) stay sutures are placed at either end of the cystotomy incision to help keep the bladder elevated and to assist with closure; (d) following the removal of the urolith, the stay sutures are elevated and assist with two-layer closure of the thinly walled bladder.

(© SJ Divers)

removed. The bladder should be flushed with sterile saline and closed in two layers using fine absorbable suture material. Some stones may be removable by non-invasive cystoscopic or lithotripsy techniques.

Gastrointestinal surgery

Devenomation

Removal of normal venom glands from venomous snakes is not recommended and is illegal in most countries. There can be no guarantee that a devenomated snake will be safe, and postsurgical human bites create considerable liability.

Oesophagostomy tube placement

It is often difficult to impossible to repeatedly administer oral medications to shy or intractable chelonians. The surgical placement of an oesophagostomy tube provides an oral route for fluids, nutrition and medications that can be utilized for up to several months. Surgical placement requires sedation or anaesthesia, although critical patients may only require physical restraint and local infiltration of lidocaine. A soft feeding catheter (of sufficient diameter to permit food material to pass) is premeasured from the cranial rim of the plastron to the junction of the pectoral and abdominal scutes, and marked with a permanent marker. Small-diameter tubes are prone to blockage and so larger tubes are preferred (e.g. for a 1–2 kg tortoise a 12 F or 4 mm tube is appropriate). Tubes made of silicone are often toler-ated for longer than those made of other forms of plastic or rubber. It is important that the tube enters the oesophagus in the caudolateral neck to avoid removal by the forelimbs.

Curved haemostats are introduced into the oesoph-agus and tented against the caudolateral neck. A small incision is made through the aseptically prepared skin,

over the point of the haemostats, so that the instrument's closed jaws can be forced through the oesophagus and out through the skin incision (Figure 13.49a). Beware of the dorsolateral jugular vein and the ventrolateral carotid artery. The end of the feeding catheter is grasped, pulled through the incision into the lumen of the oesophagus, and redirected down towards the stomach. The feeding tube is advanced into the stomach, to the predetermined mark on the tube. Correct placement should be verified by endo-scopy or radiography using a small amount of barium administered via the tube (Figure 13.49b). A butterfly tape is placed around the tube, close to its exit from the neck, and sutured to the dorsolateral aspect of the caudal neck. Alternatively, a Chinese finger-trap suture can be used (Figure 13.49c). In chelonians, the tube should also be attached to the carapace, cut to length, and capped with a three-way tap or other stopper (Figure 13.49d). Oesophagostomy tubes should be flushed at least once daily to maintain patency, while the tube–skin interface should be cleaned daily. Incorrect placement can result in subcutaneous or epicoelomic deposition of material and abscessation. Upon tube removal, the oesophagostomy site contracts and heals by second intention.

Gastrotomy, gastrectomy, enterotomy and enterectomy

Gastrointestinal tissues, particularly the large intestine, are often thin and friable in reptiles and call for the use of fine suture material and atraumatic forceps and needles. Foreign-body removal, resection–anastomosis and anasto-mosis for colorectal atresia have been successfully per-formed in reptiles (Frye, 1994a; Divers, 1996; Latimer and Rich, 1998; Helmick et al., 2000; Lloyd, 2003). In general, fine sutures and standard intestinal closure techniques are used (Figure 13.50). The mesentery that suspends the

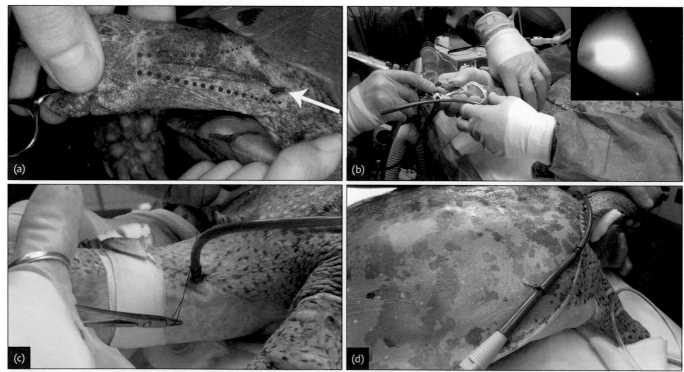

13.49 Oesophagostomy tube placement in chelonians. (a) The positions of the left dorsolateral jugular vein (blue dotted line) and ventrolateral carotid artery (red dotted line) are shown, and avoided by the haemostat jaws (arrowed) exiting the caudolateral neck in this spur-thighed tortoise. (b) The correct placement of the tube is verified using endoscopy in this soft-shelled turtle. Inset – intraluminal view of the red rubber feeding tube. (c) The tube is secured using a Chinese finger-trap suture in this soft-shelled turtle. (d) The capped tube is also attached to the carapace, usually with tape, but in aquatic soft-shelled turtles, sutures can be used.
(© SJ Divers)

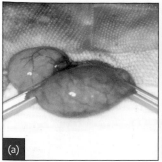
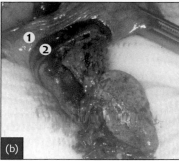
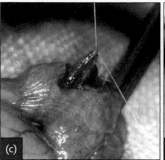
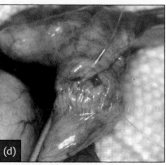

13.50 Enterotomy in a bearded dragon with intestinal foreign body and partial obstruction unresponsive to medical therapy. (a) The exteriorized intestinal viscus is isolated using atraumatic paediatric bowel clamps and sterile gauze. (b) Craniocaudal enterotomy incision permits the removal of the foreign body and associated digesta. Note that both the serosa (1) and mucosa (2) are clearly visible. (c) Following removal of the contaminated material and gauze, and using clean instruments, the mucosa is closed using absorbable antibiotic-impregnated (triclosan) poliglecaprone 25 suture material in a simple interrupted pattern. (d) The serosal layer is closed using a simple continuous pattern. Alternatively, a single-layer closure is also acceptable. The intestinal tract and entire coelom are flushed with sterile saline before routine coeliotomy closure.
(© SJ Divers)

gastrointestinal tract is also variable and may prevent exteriorization through the coeliotomy incision. For example, in chelonians gastrointestinal exteriorization via transplastron access is rarely possible, and a prefemoral approach may be more rewarding. Packing the coelom with sterile gauze and copious irrigation before coeliotomy closure are recommended.

Respiratory surgery

Tracheal obstructions in royal pythons due to chondromas and their surgical correction have been described (Diethelm *et al.*, 1996; Drew *et al.*, 1999). Resection and anastomosis appear most common, although endoscopic debridement and laser ablation have also been successful. In most lizards and snakes, the lack of a functional diaphragm enables the surgeon to directly approach and enter the lungs for the purposes of debridement, resection and parasite removal. In chelonians, access to the lungs generally requires a dorsal osteotomy through the carapace, although endoscope-assisted procedures can be performed via a prefemoral approach.

Oncological surgery

Large neoplasms involving liver, kidney and reproductive tract are not uncommon and can require extensive surgical access (Hernandez-Divers and Garner, 2003; Mauldin and Bone, 2006).

Surgical biopsy

Lack of pathognomonic signs, coupled with variability in clinical pathology, makes the submission of biopsy samples for histopathology and microbiology of paramount diagnostic importance (Figures 13.51 and 13.52). Sample collection techniques include:

- Fine-needle aspiration
- Endoscopic biopsy (see Chapter 10)
- Incisional biopsy
- Tru-cut® biopsy
- Excisional biopsy.

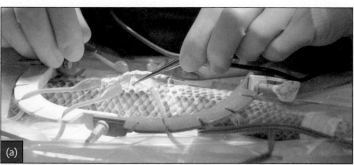
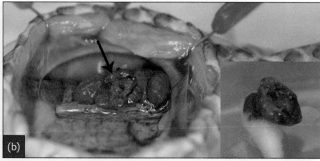

13.51 Coeliotomy and renal biopsy in a kingsnake. (a) Coeliotomy approach and a ring retractor to improve visualization. (b) Intraoperative view of the kidney following renal biopsy (arrowed). Inset – excised renal biopsy sample.
(© SJ Divers)

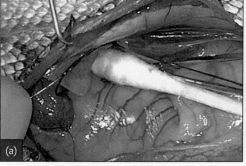
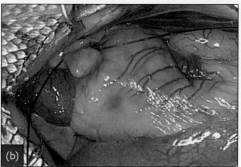

13.52 Coeliotomy and liver biopsy (guillotine method) in a small bearded dragon: (a) intraoperative view of the coelom and placement of a suture loop over the caudal aspect of the left liver lobe; (b) the suture is tightened, taking care not to cut through the tissue, and the distal tissue is sharply dissected free.
(© SJ Divers)

Orthopaedic procedures

Tail amputation

Amputation is indicated when presented with a necrotic or diseased tail that fails to respond to medical management. The site of amputation must be proximal to all abnormal tissue, and radiography is advisable. In lizards that perform autotomy, tail amputation can be most easily accomplished by simply snapping and twisting the tail through a fracture plane of a coccygeal vertebra (Figure 13.53). The muscle strands are trimmed and local antiseptic can be applied to the open wound. Even though autotomy is a natural phenomenon, anaesthesia and aseptic preparation are mandatory.

More substantial tails that do not lend themselves to autotomy (e.g. proximal amputation of some lizards, all snakes, chelonians and crocodilians), will require a more detailed approach. The surgeon should ensure that sufficient skin is preserved for closure once the soft tissues and vertebrae have been transected (Figure 13.54).

Digit and limb amputation

Digits are commonly traumatized and infected and, if osteolysis is evident, amputation of the affected digit but preservation of the remaining limb is favoured (Figure 13.55). If disease has progressed to include the carpus or tarsus, complete or partial limb amputation should be performed. Partial amputation preserves a stump that a small lizard may continue to use for ambulation. Stump trauma and infection are common complications in larger reptiles and chelonians and can be avoided by complete amputation through the scapulohumeral or coxofemoral joints (Figure 13.56). Postoperative complications tend to increase as animal size increases, so careful evaluation is required before amputating the limb of a giant monitor or chelonian. The skin incision should include a large skin flap to permit closure. The soft tissues are best transected using radio or CO_2 laser surgery; although the position of major blood vessels may be unknown, a proximal tourniquet will reduce haemorrhage until major vessels are identified and ligated using vascular clips or sutures. A prosthesis (wheel on hard surfaces or castor on grass or soil) may be provided to assist with ambulation in chelonians.

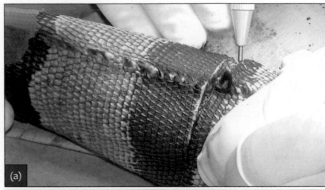
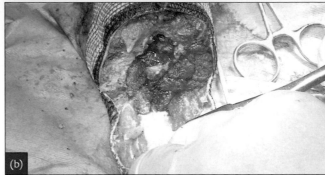
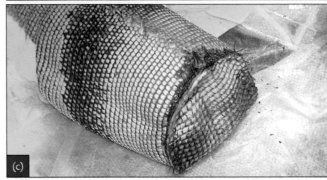

13.54 Proximal tail amputation in a green iguana. (a) Incising the dorsal skin of the proximal tail using a CO_2 laser. (b) The surgical dissection continues through the tail musculature and vertebra, ensuring that a large ventral skin flap is preserved. (c) This ventral flap is lifted over the exposed musculature and spine and sutured to the dorsal skin margin using simple interrupted sutures.
(© SJ Divers)

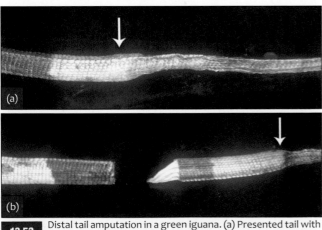

13.53 Distal tail amputation in a green iguana. (a) Presented tail with distal avascular necrosis. The margin between visibly normal and abnormal tissue is marked (arrowed). (b) Following aseptic preparation, the tail is amputated by snapping and twisting the caudal tail cranial to the beginning of the necrosis (arrowed) to ensure that all diseased tissue is removed. The muscle strands of the proximal tail have been trimmed.
(© SJ Divers)

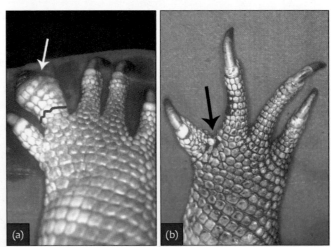

13.55 Digit amputation in a Bosc monitor. (a) Preoperative view of the left forelimb illustrating the planned incision (red line) between the scales at the proximal base of digit two (arrowed). (b) Following amputation, two mattress sutures close the defect (arrowed), and any excess skin is trimmed.
(© SJ Divers)

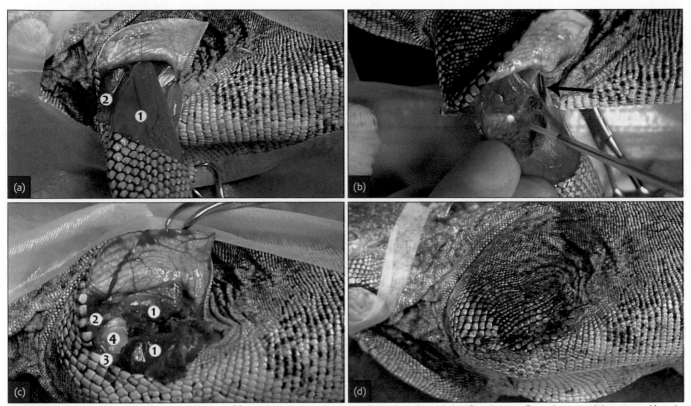

13.56 Forelimb amputation in a green iguana. (a) Initial skin incision creates a large dorsolateral skin flap that is reflected to reveal the triceps (1) and brachialis (2) muscles. (b) The musculature is transected, the humerus disarticulated and the limb removed, taking care to ligate the major vessels and nerves (arrowed). (c) The transected muscle bellies of the triceps (1), biceps (2) and coracobrachialis (3) are sutured over the exposed glenoid fossa (4). (d) The lateral skin flap is sutured over the defect using horizontal mattress sutures, and any excess skin is trimmed and discarded.
(© SJ Divers)

Fracture repair

Fractures are common in lizards (owing mainly to secondary nutritional hyperparathyroidism (SNHP) predisposing to pathological fractures), chelonians (predation and trauma) and crocodilians (intraspecific aggression) (Mitchell, 2002; Mader *et al.*, 2006). The need for medical stabilization will usually supersede immediate surgery, and in such cases limbs should be temporarily immobilized against the body/tail or inside the shell to prevent further damage.

External coaptation

Radiography is essential and multiple views may be required. General anaesthesia is required for fracture manipulation as well as repair, and often for simple splinting. Fractures involving the digits can be immobilized using a ball bandage. A cotton-wool ball is placed in the centre of the plantar/palmar aspect. The digits are curled around the ball and taped in position, encasing the entire foot and lower limb in the bandage. Small lizards and crocodilians with fractures of the radius, ulna, tibia or fibula (especially if secondary to SNHP) are best treated using external coaptation (Figure 13.57). Forelimbs are extended and strapped to the lateral body wall, while pelvic limbs are strapped to the tail base. The inclusion of a small splint (e.g. wooden tongue depressor or fibreglass strut) between limb and body/tail helps prevent movement. Alternatively, a large syringe case can be placed over the entire limb and bandaged in place.

Fractures of the femur and humerus can be treated in a similar manner but reduction and healing are usually less perfect owing to movement at the scapulohumeral or coxofemoral joints. Better healing can be expected if a Hexcelite or thermal polymer plastic cast is used to immobilize the pectoral or pelvic girdle (Figure 13.57c). It is important to keep any caste as lightwieght as possible. Healing typically takes 6–18 weeks, but physical and radiographic re-evaluations should be performed before removing support materials. Callus formation is often not readily appreciated on radiographs as initial healing may be by fibrous union.

Internal fixation

A variety of internal fixation techniques can be used to manage fractures in reptiles as long as bone quality is adequate. The reptile's overall nutritional and health status must be critically assessed, as bones affected by secondary nutritional hyperthyroidism will not support internal or external fixation. Bone plates (especially locking plates), intramedullary pins and cerclage wire are available for long-bone fractures in lizards, crocodilians and chelonians (Mitchell, 2002; Mader *et al.*, 2006) (Figure 13.58). In general, placement of these devices follows the same general principles as in mammalian patients.

External fixation

Modern carbon-fibre and FESSA tubular external fixator systems are extremely strong and lightweight, and are suitable for larger animals. They can be used in reptiles following general surgical principles. It is usually impossible to use them for limb repairs in chelonians owing to

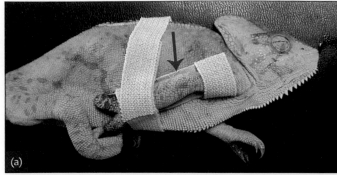

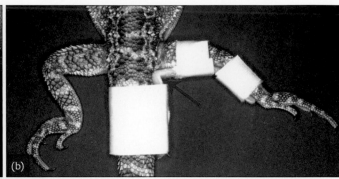

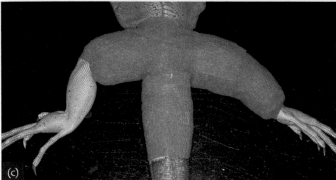

13.57 External coaptation for fracture repairs in lizards. (a) Closed ulnar fracture in a Yemen chameleon immobilized by strapping the forelimb to the lateral body wall. Note the wooden splint (arrowed) that prevents bending of the fracture site. (b) Femoral fracture in a bearded dragon immobilized using a thermal plastic splint (arrowed) moulded to the caudal pelvic limb and tail base, and secured using adhesive tape. The splint prevents movement of the coxofemoral joint, which is essential for immobilization of the femoral fracture site. (c) Right femoral and right pelvic fractures in a green iguana immobilized using a Hexcelite cast that extends from the right tarsus to the left stifle. This splint immobilizes the pelvis and both the right stifle and coxofemoral joints.
(© SJ Divers)

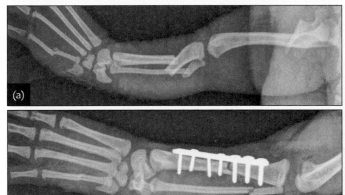

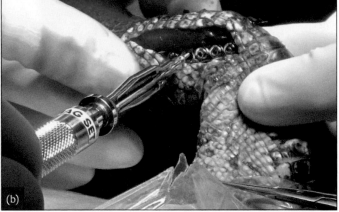

13.58 Internal fixation in an alligator: (a) radiograph of the right pelvic limb demonstrating fractures of the tibia, fibula and the metatarsal of digit five; (b) intraoperative view of the placement of a locking bone plate on to the tibia; (c) postoperative radiograph demonstrating adequate reduction of the tibial and fibular fractures.
(© SJ Divers)

the close proximity of the shell. However, small external fixators have been used to repair chelonian mandibular fractures (Figure 13.59).

Shell repair

Shell fractures are common in chelonians and a detailed review of recent advances and techniques is available (Fleming, 2014). They can be caused by a variety of traumatic events, including dog attacks and high falls. When the chelonian is first presented, the clinician should assess the wound and determine whether the shell fracture extends into the coelomic cavity, and whether the wound is infected. Infected wounds with extensive communication with the coelomic cavity and visceral trauma carry the worst prognosis. Separate surgeries may be required to manage the coelomic defect and then repair the shell.

If the trauma occurred immediately prior to presentation, then irrigation and primary repair can often proceed.

If the trauma occurred within 6–12 hours, the wound is assumed to be contaminated but not infected. The wound can be irrigated with an antiseptic solution, rinsed with physiological saline and closed, although delay for 1–3 days is often advisable to ensure no infection develops. If it has been longer than 12–24 hours, the wound is assumed to be contaminated and infected. In this case, the wound is irrigated with antiseptic solution and managed as an open wound. Covering the wound with a sterile bandage minimizes further contamination. Standard wet-to-dry bandaging will assist in the removal of debris over several days, and both systemic and local antimicrobial agents should be considered following the submission of material for microbiological culture. Extensive surgical debridement may be required and vacuum-assisted wound closure has been of proven value in managing chelonian shell wounds (Figure 13.60) (Marin et al., 2014).

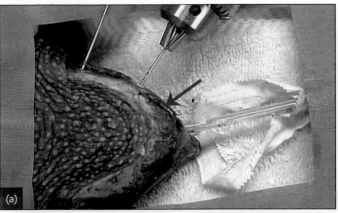

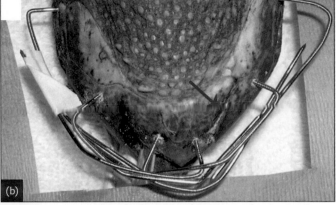

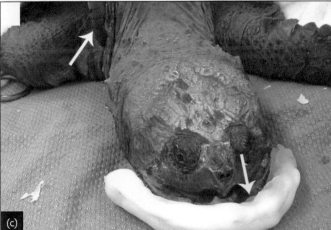

13.59 Mandibular fracture (red arrows) repair in a snapping turtle: (a) multiple positive-profile pins are placed into the mandible; (b) the ends of the pins are bent along the long axis of the mandible to add strength to the external fixator; (c) acrylic material has been placed over the pins to complete the rigid external fixation (yellow arrow). Note the placement of an oesophagostomy tube (white arrow) to facilitate nutritional support during healing.
(© SJ Divers)

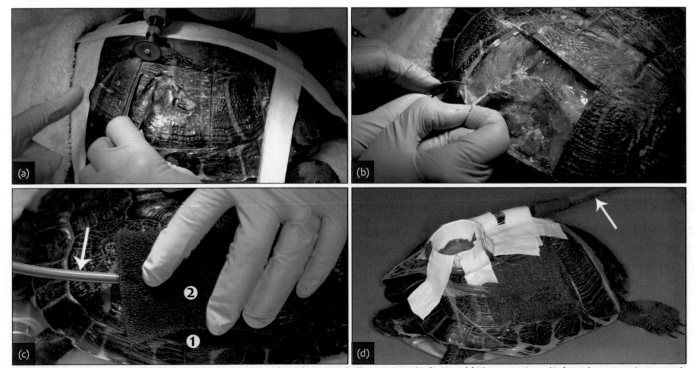

13.60 Vacuum-assisted wound closure in an aquatic turtle with severe shell necrosis and infection. (a) The necrotic and infected carapace is resected using a rotary saw. (b) Additional debridement of the underlying soft tissues is performed. (c) A non-adherent mesh wound covering is applied, followed by the first layer of sterile open-cell foam (1), a fenestrated sterile tube (arrowed), and the second layer of foam (2); an occlusive adhesive drape covers the wound and incorporates the surrounding normal shell to ensure an air-tight seal. (d) The wound drainage tube is connected to a vacuum line (arrowed), and once negative pressure is applied the foam collapses as shown.
(© SJ Divers)

Radiography, or better still, computed tomography is used to assess whether the bony portion of the shell has been affected (rather than just the keratinized scutes). Since the margins of the scutes do not match those of the underlying bony plates, fractures of the bony shell, scapulae or ilia can be missed. Once the clinician is satisfied that there is no longer infected tissue within the wound (this process may take days to a week or more), shell repair can be completed. Displaced fractures are reduced using either screws and wire, or plates (Figure 13.61). Another, inexpensive technique is the use of cable ties and plastic bases to reduce shell fractures (Figure 13.62). The advantages of this approach are reduced costs, the variety of cable ties available to suit different animal sizes and the ability to directly monitor the shell for evidence of healing or complications. The positions of the plastic bases are determined and the shell scored or sanded to aid adhesion. A small amount of baking soda is placed on the shell and a plastic mount gently pushed on. Cyanoacrylate glue (thin modelling type, not gel) is then dripped around the plastic base. The cyanoacrylate glue seeps under the base and forms an instant concrete bond with the shell. A cable tie is then inserted through one base, across the fracture and through a second base. The cable tie is secured using a second cable tie base, and pressure is applied to reduce the fracture. The ends of the cable ties are trimmed. Once healed, the plastic bases are easily removed using a small osteotome.

Covering the external fixator (whether it be plates, screws/wire or cable ties) with fibreglass or acrylic is not essential, and has both advantages and disadvantages. The main benefit is an immediate waterproof seal (which can otherwise take several days to achieve), but when covered it is difficult to impossible to monitor or medicate the site, and for this reason is generally not performed by the author. Once the bone fragments are aligned, the shell is cleaned with alcohol to remove any greasy debris or algae. Light sanding can also help generate a strong bond

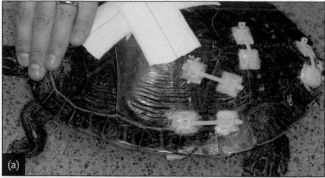

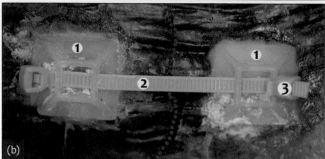

13.62 Cable-tie fracture repair in an aquatic turtle. (a) Aquatic turtle with a simple fracture of the caudolateral carapace (red dotted line) that has been repaired using cable ties and plastic bases. (b) Close-up view illustrating the position of the plastic bases (1) across the fracture site (red dotted line). One cable tie (2) has been placed through both bases and secured using the base of a second cable tie (3). (© SJ Divers)

between shell and repair material. Large defects can be bridged with autoclaved fibreglass patches or car-repair aluminium mesh. Small crevices are filled with sterile antibiotic to prevent repair material from penetrating below the shell. Masking tape can be used to protect adjacent areas. Epoxy resin (e.g. Enviroset®) or acrylic (e.g. Technovite®) are commonly used materials according to the manufacturer's instructions. Repair material is applied to cover the deficit and allowed to harden. The repair provides additional immobilization and ensures waterproofing of the defect. Aquatic turtles are typically 'dry docked' for only 24 hours if the repair is waterproof.

These shell repairs should be considered as a splint; as they may prevent proper growth of the shell, especially in juveniles, they should be removed following healing. Most shell repairs are left in place for 6–12 months, although uncomplicated healing of reduced fractures typically takes only 12 weeks.

Miscellaneous orthopaedic procedures

Joint injuries resulting in ligament rupture and luxation are best approached in a similar way to domestic animals. Stifle luxation and cranial cruciate rupture in the tortoise have been successfully repaired using an over-the-top technique and autograft of the lateral vastus muscle (Hernandez-Divers, 2002b) (Figure 13.63). Less favourable results have been obtained following surgery for coxofemoral luxation in lizards (Barten, 1996; Coke, 1999).

Osteomyelitis is a common problem of reptiles that often requires limb amputation. However, the radical debridement of diseased bone using drills and burrs, coupled with the implantation of antibiotic-impregnated polymethyl methacrylate beads, has proved successful on numerous occasions (Divers and Lawton, 1999) (Figure 13.64). Beads are generally removed from joints once infection has resolved. There is no need to remove beads embedded within bone.

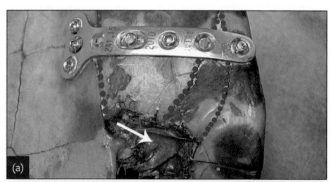

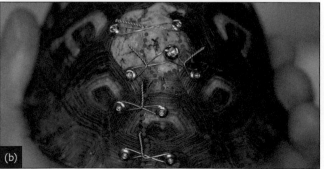

13.61 Fractured-shell repairs in chelonians. (a) A T-plate and screws have been used to stabilize the comminuted plastron fracture (red dotted line) in this aquatic turtle. Note the porcine small intestinal submucosal graft (Biosist®) (arrowed) that has been used to fill a defect. (b) Screws and cerclage wire have been used to repair the carapacial fracture (red dotted line) in this box turtle. (© SJ Divers)

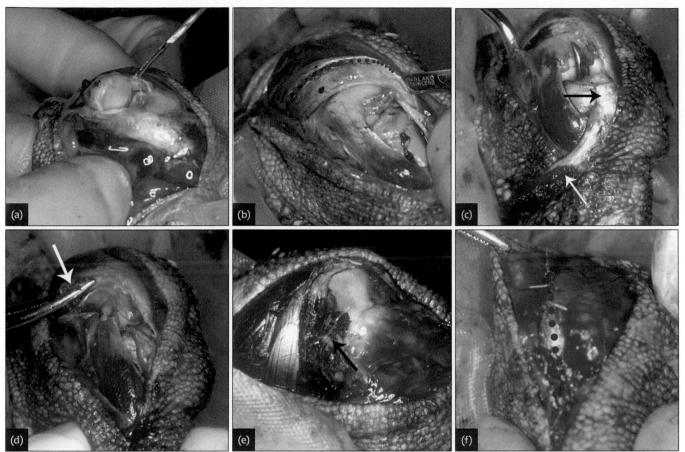

13.63 Stifle luxation and cranial cruciate repair in a spur-thighed tortoise. (a) Arthrotomy incision to expose the stifle joint for removal of the cruciate remnant and flushing of the joint. (b) Incision along the cranial aspect of the lateral vastus muscle (red dotted line) to create an autograft. (c) Elevation of the lateral vastus graft from its proximal origin (white arrow) but remaining attached to its insertion at the tibial tuberosity (black arrow). A small cruciate hook has been passed through the intercondylar space of the joint. (d) The graft, drawn through the joint space, is held over the lateral femoral condyle (arrowed). (e) The autograft is sutured to the periosteum on the lateral surface of the lateral femoral condyle using four simple interrupted absorbable monofilament polydioxanone sutures (arrowed). (f) Closure of the joint capsule with lateral imbrication (blue dotted line) to improve joint stability. Closure of the superficial fascia and skin were routine.
(© SJ Divers)

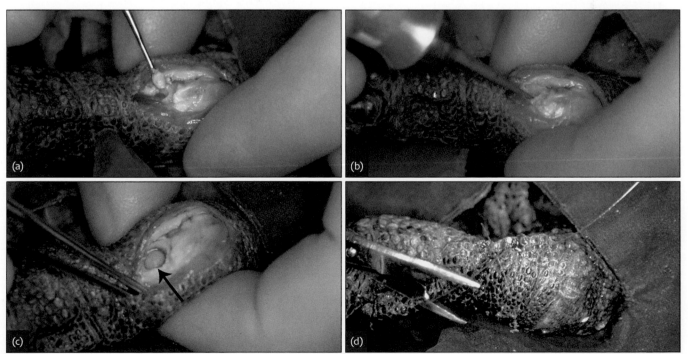

13.64 Surgical implantation of antibiotic-impregnated polymethyl methacrylate (AIPMMA) beads in a tortoise with proximal tibial osteomyelitis: (a) curette debridement of the caseous lesion from the proximal tibia; (b) further debridement using an orthopaedic burr to ensure removal of all necrotic and infected material; (c) placement of a single AIPMMA bead (arrowed) into the tibial defect; (d) routine closure of the subcutaneous fascia and skin.
(© SJ Divers)

Intra- and postoperative care

Details of intra- and postoperative care, including analgesia, are given in Chapter 12. Reptiles should not be discharged until fully recovered from anaesthesia, typically the day after surgery. Rechecks should be scheduled at 1 and 8 weeks following surgery to check for postsurgical complications and suture removal, respectively (Figure 13.65). Reptiles that have had upper gastrointestinal surgery should be fasted for two feeding cycles, and then fed a gradually increasing plane of nutrition. Small lizards and chelonians can often be fed 5–7 days postoperatively, and larger snakes 3–4 weeks postoperatively. Snakes with sutures should only be fed small prey items that will not substantially increase their girth.

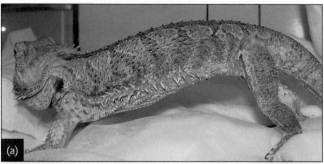

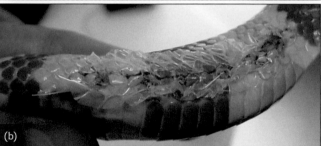

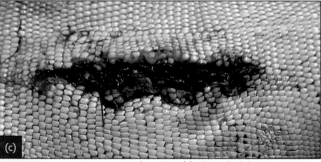

13.65 Postoperative care of reptiles. (a) A bearded dragon following coeliotomy. This abnormal posture, believed to be associated with ventral coeliotomy pain, resolved shortly after the administration of analgesics. (b) Localized dysecdysis around the suture line is to be expected and will resolve upon suture removal. (c) Infected coeliotomy wound in a green iguana. In this case, postoperative hygiene was poor and wound infection necessitated a second procedure 1 week after the initial surgery. Thanks to improvements in hygiene, the iguana recovered uneventfully.

(© SJ Divers)

Efforts have been made to provide UK distributors for equipment and supplies used by the author. While the author endorses no particular company, an internet review indicated that Veterinary Instrumentation Ltd (www.veterinary-instrumentation.co.uk) appears to provide many of the products (or viable alternatives) cited in this chapter.

References and further reading

Barten SL (1996) Treatment of chronic coxofemoral luxation by femoral head and neck excision arthroplasty in a white-throated monitor (*Varanus albigularis*). *Bulletin of the Association of Reptilian and Amphibian Veterinarians* **6**, 10–13

Baxter JS and Meek R (1988) Cryosurgery in the treatment of skin disorders in reptiles. *Herpetological Journal* **1**, 227

Chinnadurai SK, DeVoe R, Koenig A *et al.* (2010) Comparison of an implantable telemetry device and an oscillometric monitor for measurement of blood pressure in anaesthetized and unrestrained green iguanas (*Iguana iguana*). *Veterinary Anaesthesia and Analgesia* **37**, 434–439

Coke RL (1999) External skeletal fixation of bilateral sacroiliac luxations in a savannah monitor, *Varanus exanthematicus*. *Bulletin of the Association of Reptilian and Amphibian Veterinarians* **9**, 4–7

Diethelm G, Stauber E, Tillson M *et al.* (1996) Tracheal resection and anastomosis for an intratracheal chondroma in a ball python. *Journal of the American Veterinary Medical Association* **209**, 786–788

Divers SJ (1996) Constipation in snakes with particular reference to surgical correction in a Burmese python (*Python molurus bivittatus*). *Proceedings of the Association of Reptilian and Amphibian Veterinarians Annual Conference*, Tampa, FL, pp. 67–69

Divers SJ (2014a) Endoscope-assisted and endoscopic surgery. In: *Current Therapy in Reptile Medicine and Surgery*, ed. DR Mader and SJ Divers, pp. 179–196. Elsevier, St Louis

Divers SJ (2014b) Video telescopic operating microscope: a recent development in reptile microsurgery. In: *Current Therapy in Reptile Medicine and Surgery*, ed. DR Mader and SJ Divers, pp. 213–216. Elsevier, St Louis

Divers SJ and Lawton MPC (1999) Antibiotic-impregnated polymethylmethacrylate beads as a treatment for osteomyelitis in reptiles. *Proceedings of the Association of Reptilian and Amphibian Veterinarians Annual Conference*, Columbus, OH, pp. 145–147

Divers SJ and Lawton MPC (2000) Biosist skin grafts in reptiles. *Proceedings of the Association of Reptilian and Amphibian Veterinarians Annual Conference*, Reno, NV, pp. 151–152

Done LB (1996) Neoplasia. In: *Reptile Medicine and Surgery*, ed. DR Mader, pp. 125–141. WB Saunders, Philadelphia

Drew ML, Phalen DN, Berridge BR *et al.* (1999) Partial tracheal obstruction due to chondromas in ball pythons (*Python regius*). *Journal of Zoo and Wildlife Medicine* **30**, 151–157

Fleming GJ (2014) New techniques in chelonian shell repair. In: *Current Therapy in Reptile Medicine and Surgery*, ed. DR Mader and SJ Divers, pp. 205–212. Elsevier, St Louis

Frye FL (1993) Use of a condom as an occlusive bandage in snakes: a new wrinkle on an old resource. *Journal of Small Exotic Animal Medicine* **2**, 13–14

Frye FL (1994a) Colo-rectal atresia and its surgical repair in a juvenile amelanistic Burmese python (*Python molurus bivittatus*). *Journal of Small Exotic Animal Medicine* **2**, 149–150

Frye FL (1994b) Diagnosis and surgical treatment of reptilian neoplasms with a compilation of cases 1966–1993. *In Vivo* **8**, 885–892

Gibbons PM (2014) Therapeutics. In: *Current Therapy in Reptile Medicine and Surgery*, ed. DR Mader and SJ Divers, pp. 57–69. Elsevier Saunders, St Louis

Gould D and McLellan G (2014) *BSAVA Manual of Canine and Feline Ophthalmology, 3rd edn*. BSAVA Publications, Gloucester

Govett PD, Harms CA, Linder KE *et al.* (2004) Effects of four different suture materials on the surgical wound healing of loggerhead sea turtles, *Caretta caretta*. *Journal of Herpetological Medicine and Surgery* **14**, 6–11

Helmick KE, Bennett RA, Ginn P *et al.* (2000) Intestinal volvulus and stricture associated with a leiomyoma in a green turtle (*Chelonia mydas*). *Journal of Zoo and Wildlife Medicine* **31**, 221–227

Hernandez-Divers SJ (2002a) Pulmonary candidiasis due to *Candida albicans* in a Greek tortoise (*Testudo graeca*) and treatment using intrapneumonic amphotericin B. *Journal of Zoo and Wildlife Medicine* **32**, 352–359

Hernandez-Divers SJ (2002b) Diagnosis and surgical repair of stifle luxation in a spur-thighed tortoise (*Testudo graeca*). *Journal of Zoo and Wildlife Medicine* **33**, 125–130

Hernandez-Divers SJ, Knott CD and MacDonald J (2001) Diagnosis and surgical treatment of thyroid adenoma-induced hyperthyroidism in a green iguana (*Iguana iguana*). *Journal of Zoo and Wildlife Medicine* **32**, 465–475

Hernandez-Divers SJ, Stahl SJ, Rakich PM *et al.* (2009) Comparison of CO_2 laser and 4.0 MHz radiosurgery for making incisions in the skin and muscles of green iguanas (*Iguana iguana*). *Veterinary Record* **164**, 13–15

Hernandez-Divers SM and Garner MM (2003) Neoplasia of reptiles with an emphasis on lizards. *Veterinary Clinics of North America: Exotic Animal Practice* **6**, 251–273

Latimer KS and Rich GA (1998) Colonic adenocarcinoma in a corn snake (*Elaphe guttata guttata*). *Journal of Zoo and Wildlife Medicine* **29**, 344–346

Lloyd CG (2003) Surgical management of colon prolapse and subsequent stricture in a Mediterranean spur-thighed tortoise, *Testudo graeca*. *Journal of Herpetological Medicine and Surgery* **13**, 10–13

Maas AK, Paul-Murphy J, Kumaresan-Lampman S *et al.* (2010) Spectacle wound healing in the royal python (*Python regius*). *Journal of Herpetological Medicine and Surgery* **20**, 29–36

McArthur S and Hernandez-Divers SJ (2003) Surgery. In: *Medicine and Surgery of Tortoises and Turtles*, ed. SM McArthur, R Wilkinson and J Meyer, pp. 403–464. Blackwell, Oxford

McCracken HE (1999) Organ location in snakes for diagnostic and surgical evaluation. In: *Zoo and Wildlife Medicine Current Therapy 4*, ed. ME Fowler and RE Miller, pp. 243–248. WB Saunders, Philadelphia

Mader DR (2006a) Calculi: urinary. In: *Reptile Medicine and Surgery, 2nd edition*, ed. DR Mader, pp. 763–771. WB Saunders, Philadelphia

Mader DR (ed.) (2006b) *Reptile Medicine and Surgery, 2nd edition*. WB Saunders, Philadelphia

Mader DR, Bennett RA, Funk RS *et al.* (2006) Surgery. In: *Reptile Medicine and Surgery, 2nd edition*, ed. DR Mader, pp. 581–630. Elsevier, St Louis

Mader DR and Divers SJ (eds) (2014) *Current Therapy in Reptile Medicine and Surgery*. Elsevier, St Louis

Marin ML, Norton TM and Mettee NS (2014) Vacuum-assisted wound closure in chelonians. In: *Current Therapy in Reptile Medicine and Surgery*, ed. DR Mader and SJ Divers, pp. 197–204. Elsevier, St Louis

Mauldin GN and Bone LB (2006) Oncology. In: *Reptile Medicine and Surgery, 2nd edition*, ed. DR Mader, pp. 299–322. WB Saunders, Philadelphia

Mitchell MA (2002) Diagnosis and management of reptile orthopedic injuries. *Veterinary Clinics of North America: Exotic Animal Practice* **5**, 97–114

Pardo M, and Divers SJ (2016) Jugular central venous catheter placement through a modified seldinger technique for long-term venous access in chelonians. *Journal of Zoo and Wildlife Medicine* **47(1)**, 286–290

Pavletic M (2009) *Atlas of Small Animal Wound Management and Reconstructive Surgery, 3rd edition*. Wiley-Blackwell, England

Zwart P, Dorrestein GM, Stades FC *et al.* (1979) Vasectomy in the garter snake (*Thamnophis sirtalis radix*). *Journal of Zoo Animal Medicine* **10**, 17–21

Useful contacts

3M mini-driver:
Conmed (Linvatec) UK Ltd, 73/74 Shrivenham Hundred
Business Park, Swindon, SN6 8TY, UK

4.0-MHz dual radiofrequency Surgitron®:
Ellman International Inc., 400 Karin Lane, Hicksville, NY 11801, USA

Adhesive surgical drape:
Veterinary Specialty Products, 10504 79th St, Shawnee, KS 66214, USA

CO_2 and diode lasers:
Lumenis (UK) Ltd, 385 Centennial Ave, Elstree,
Borehamwood WD6 3TJ, UK

Enviroset® 5 minute epoxy:
Environmental Technology, Inc., PO Box 365, Fields Landing,
CA 95537, USA

Fracture repair equipment:
IMEX® Veterinary Inc., 1001 McKesson Drive,
Longview, Texas 75604, USA

Lone Star® retractor:
CooperSurgical, Inc., 95 Corporate Drive,
Trumbull, CT 06611, USA

M501 operating microscope:
Leica Microsystems (UK) Ltd, Larch House,
Woodlands Business Park,
Breckland, Linford Wood, Milton Keynes MK14 6FG, UK

OEC 9800 Plus Mobile C-arm:
GE Medical Systems Ltd., Amersham Place, Little Chalfont,
Buckinghamshire HP7 9NA, UK

Stryker drill:
Stryker Corporation, 2825 Airview Boulevard, Kalamazoo,
MI 49002, USA

Surgitel loupes:
General Scientific Corporation, 77 Enterprise Drive,
Ann Arbor, MI 48103, USA

DP Medical Systems Ltd, 15A Oakcroft Road,
Chessington, KT9 1RH, UK

Technovite® 8100 MG kit:
Energy Beam Sciences, 29B Kripes Road,
East Granby, CT 06026-9669, USA

Veterinary Instrumentation Ltd,
Broadfield Road,
Sheffield, S8 0XL, UK
(A UK supplier of many of the US products mentioned, including sagittal saws, mini-driver, epoxy putty, adhesive drapes, operating loupes, FESSA external fixators, locking bone plates, small external fixator pins, vascular clips, staplers, microsurgical instruments, etc.)

Weck Closure Systems:
Teleflex Medical, 3015 Carrington Mill Boulevard,
Morrisville, NC 27560, USA
Teleflex Medical Europe Ltd., IDA Business and Technology Park,
Dublin Road, Athlone, Co Westmeath, Ireland
(Ethicon Ligaclips are a viable alternative)

Chapter 14

Euthanasia and post-mortem examination

John E. Cooper

Captive and free-living reptiles may need to be killed for a variety of reasons. In the case of reptiles kept in captivity for companionship or private study, or wildlife 'casualties', euthanasia is usually justified in order to prevent suffering (Cooper and Jackson, 1981; Cooper, 1989a). Animals maintained in research laboratories may be culled at the end of an experiment. Free-living (sometimes farmed or ranched) reptiles intended for food will be slaughtered before processing. In all cases the killing should be performed as humanely as possible.

The post-mortem examination (necropsy) of reptiles that die or have to be euthanased is an important part of disease diagnosis (Frye, 1984, 1991; Cooper, 1986; Mader and Divers, 2014) and/or health monitoring (Cooper, 1989b). It also plays a part in legal cases, including those relating to charges of causing 'unnecessary suffering' (Cooper and Cooper, 1998, 2007, 2013). It is often a necessary component of investigating unexplained morbidity and mortality in free-living reptiles (Cooper and Laurie, 1987; Cooper and Davies, 1997).

Euthanasia

The term 'euthanasia' (Greek) means 'good death' and implies that killing is carried out with a minimum of pain or distress to the animal. This is a requirement for humanitarian reasons (Mader, 2006) but can also be important when veterinary investigations are to be carried out post-mortem on the body of the reptile.

Special considerations

Reptiles and other ectothermic animals can present a number of challenges when they have to be killed. Some of these relate to the anatomy of the species – for instance, the inaccessibility of certain blood vessels – while others concern particular physiological features, such as the ability of aquatic chelonians and crocodilians to hold their breath for prolonged periods. Of most relevance, however, is the fact that reptiles (and most other ectothermic vertebrates) are able to tolerate hypoxia for considerable periods of time without incurring the irreversible effects to the central nervous system (CNS) that are shown by (endothermic) mammals and birds. This means that a reptile may survive, even if respiration has ceased and cardiac function has been much impaired.

The CNS of a reptile that has been decapitated may continue to receive – and probably to be aware of – painful stimuli. Recognition of this trait in reptiles followed unrelated experimental studies on tortoises and led to public discussion about the way such animals were killed (Cooper et al., 1984). Decapitation and certain other physical methods of killing reptiles were critically reassessed during the 1980s (Cooper et al., 1989) and recommendations were made as to how these animals might be killed with a minimum of pain and distress.

Subsequently, the subject has been addressed by a number of authors and committees/working groups (see, for example, Frye, 1991; Close et al., 1996, 1997; American Veterinary Medical Association, 2001; British Veterinary Zoological Society, 2003; Ewert et al., 2004; Mader, 2006; Expert Panel, 2013).

Techniques

Techniques used for euthanasia of reptiles depend upon a combination of factors:

- Practicability: is the appropriate equipment or agent available? Can this technique be carried out simply in the confines of a small consulting room or within sight or hearing of the public? Is the veterinary surgeon (veterinarian) familiar with the technique and competent in its use?
- Safety of the veterinary surgeon, staff who may be assisting, the owner(s) or the public (Figure 14.1): both physical dangers and the possibility of spread of pathogens (zoonoses) – see later – need to be considered and form part of a risk assessment. There are legal implications – both criminal and civil (Cooper, 1987)
- Welfare of the animal: is unnecessary pain, discomfort, excitement or stress likely? Parameters for assessing the welfare of reptiles were given in Cooper and Williams (1995) and the use of new criteria continues to be explored
- Aesthetic aspects: is the method acceptable to both the veterinary surgeon and to any observers?
- The needs once the animal is dead: the brain may, for example, be required for pathological examination or the intact carcase may need to be returned to the owner or to a museum or reference collection (see later).

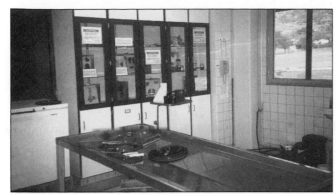

14.1 A system is required whenever animals are euthanased or examined after death. In this post-mortem room, hygiene is strict and a colour code – red to indicate infection or contamination – is used to minimize the risk of spread of pathogens.

Hypothermia

Immobilization of reptiles by cooling is considered inappropriate and probably inhumane, even if combined with other physical or chemical methods of euthanasia. Quick freezing of deeply anaesthetized animals can, however, be acceptable. In the laboratory, dropping an animal into liquid nitrogen at minus 196°C – a very extreme form of freezing, far removed from a domestic freezer – may be appropriate for animals of less than 40 g bodyweight (i.e. less than 1 cm in diameter) as liquid nitrogen freezes an entire body of that size instantaneously.

Chemical methods

These involve the use of agents by inhalation or injection (see below). Using inhalant agents (isoflurane, halothane, methoxyflurane, ether), the animal can be placed in a closed receptacle containing cotton wool or gauze soaked in an appropriate amount of the anaesthetic, or the agent can be introduced from a vaporizer. The latter method may be associated with a longer induction time. The agent is inhaled until respiration ceases and death ensues.

As mentioned earlier, many reptiles are capable of holding their breath and reverting to anaerobic metabolism: as a result, they can survive long periods of anoxia. Because of this, induction of anaesthesia and time to loss of consciousness may be greatly prolonged when inhalants are used. Death in some species, especially chelonians, may not occur even after prolonged inhalant exposure, and therefore euthanasia by inhalation is not considered by some to be an acceptable method for euthanasia of reptiles (Expert Panel, 2013).

Agents by injection (barbiturate, tricaine methane sulfonate, T-61 (embutramide, mebenzonium iodide and tetracaine hydrochloride) and others) can in theory be administered by various routes (e.g. intravenous, intraperitoneal, intrapulmonic, intramuscular, subcutaneous, intracardiac, oral, rectal). Sodium pentobarbitone (pentobarbital) is an effective and humane method of euthanasia in reptiles. The intravenous route can be used by well trained personnel and results in rapid death. Where an intravenous injection is difficult, the intraperitoneal route may be used but is slower acting. Intracardiac injection should only be used on a fully anaesthetized animal as it appears to be painful. Intramuscular or subcutaneous injections should not, as a general rule, be employed as they are often not effective and may, too, cause pain.

The 'fish anaesthetic' tricaine methanesulfonate (TMS, MS-222) may be administered by various routes. This is an expensive means of euthanasia and, as there is little information on the humaneness of the method, it was not considered acceptable for reptiles by the (Swiss) Expert Panel (2013).

T-61 (embutramide, mebenzonium iodide and tetracaine hydrochloride) (not available in the United Kingdom) should only be injected intravenously and slowly as it is otherwise painful. The animal must be sedated prior to administration.

Some authors recommend the intramuscular injection of ketamine as premedication a few minutes prior to intravenous injection of sodium pentobarbitone; however, ketamine should not be used as a sole agent for euthanasia.

The key point in killing reptiles humanely is that the brain has to be destroyed by either chemical or mechanical methods.

Some recommended chemical and physical methods for the euthanasia of reptiles are given in Figure 14.2. For completeness, techniques are included that are generally more applicable to larger reptiles kept in zoos or for commercial purposes than they are to companion animals. The reader is also referred to the literature listed at the end of this chapter.

Type	Method	Acceptability
Chemical	Overdose of pentobarbital or other injectable anaesthetic agent	Intravenous access may be difficult. Premedication with ketamine (100 mg/kg i.m.) may assist (see text)
	Overdose of isoflurane or other volatile anaesthetic agent (or certain gases) by inhalation	Induction and onset of anaesthesia may take a long time if the animal holds its breath (see text)
Physical	Concussion (striking animal's head with hard object or on a surface), followed by exsanguination and destruction or fixation of brain	Requires skill to be performed accurately. Causes damage that may hamper necropsy
	Stunning with captive-bolt pistol, followed by exsanguination etc.	Mainly for large crocodilians. Positioning of the stunner requires knowledge of anatomy. Some safety considerations
	Destruction of brain with free bullet	Mainly for large crocodilians. Usually effective, quick and humane. Requires anatomical knowledge and training, appropriate bullet for size of the animal and adherence to legislation. Minimizing the distance between the animal and marksman will reduce any margin for error in terms of hitting the brain. Can be combined with spinal severance and pithing
	Freezing with liquid nitrogen	Small reptiles (up to 40 g). Ensure rapid whole-body immersion
	Cervical dislocation	Must be performed rapidly and correctly, and only in some species (<200 g). Usually an emergency procedure – for instance, road casualties or under field conditions. Must be followed by another procedure (e.g. pithing) to ensure death

14.2 Methods of euthanasia for reptiles.

It is important for veterinary staff involved in (or who may be consulted about) euthanasia of reptiles to be fully aware of methods that are *not* acceptable (see earlier). Those listed in British Veterinary Zoological Society (2003) remain on the proscribed list:

- Freezing
- Drowning
- Overdose of anaesthesia by non-ideal route (including intracoelomic, intramuscular, gaseous) without pithing
- Use of muscle relaxants without inducing anaesthesia
- Trauma, other than cranial trauma sufficient to induce complete and instantaneous loss of brainstem activity (e.g. shooting, captive bolt, massive blunt trauma).

To these can be added (Expert Panel, 2013) exsanguination, cooling/supercooling, heating (hyperthermia) and suffocation.

Signs of death

It is important to be sure that the reptile is dead before its body is discarded or it is subjected to necropsy. Partly for the reasons alluded to earlier, reptiles can survive and recover from methods of euthanasia that would prove rapidly fatal in a mammal or a bird. A 'dead' snake placed in a refrigerator, for example, may – as a result of reduced oxygen demand – survive chemical euthanasia and 'come back to life'.

Signs of death in reptiles include a combination of total immobility, lack of detectable respiratory activity (no spontaneous breathing; larynx open, flaccid and unresponsive to touch), absence of heartbeat (Doppler waves, ultrasonography, electrocardiography) and total abolition of reflexes (such as righting, limb withdrawal, cornea/third eyelid response). Certain organ systems of reptiles continue to function for some time after brain death (destruction): for example, the heart may continue to beat for some hours – ideal for collecting a post-mortem blood sample but disconcerting when removing tissues for histopathological investigation.

Reptiles that are deeply anaesthetized, very ill or even just hypothermic will usually have few, if any, outward signs of activity; they can appear dead by the criteria above but subsequently regain consciousness after metabolizing the anaesthetic or being warmed.

Confirmation of death in a reptile is sometimes only possible on the basis of signs of autolysis. In order to ensure that the animal is dead – and on welfare grounds – it is recommended (*once the animal is fully unconscious*) that pithing or freezing is performed.

Pithing (physical destruction of the brain tissue) can be carried out in most species through the oral cavity. This method does not involve crushing the skull and is therefore also cosmetically acceptable. A metal instrument such as a dental scaler can easily be introduced through the roof of the mouth and then inserted into the cranial vault to destroy the brain. In chelonians a hypodermic needle attached to a syringe can be inserted through a nostril and from there into the brain directly by advancing it in a straight line. The advantage of using a syringe is that negative pressure can be rapidly and repeatedly applied to the neural tissue thus facilitating its destruction.

The alternative to the oral route is to insert a sharp metal rod or probe through the foramen magnum into the base of the brain to ensure rapid brain destruction.

Destruction of the proximal spinal cord, using a thin rod, is also recommended, when this is feasible – thus minimizing the risk that the animal might perceive pain via its spinal cord (Kusuma *et al.*, 1979).

Post-mortem examination

Material from reptiles intended for necropsy can consist of whole carcases, parts of the body (for special, especially legal, investigations), and eggs or embryos. Post-mortem samples should not be referred to as 'biopsies' as they do not come from a live animal.

Submission of material

Correct submission and reception of material are most important. There are both legal considerations (see later) and practical aspects. Every effort should be made to minimize the delay between the animal's death and the post-mortem examination. See Figures 14.3 and 14.4 for suggested submission forms.

Pre-necropsy considerations

The traditional purpose of the post-mortem examination has been to ascertain the cause of death of an individual reptile or of groups of reptiles. However, there are other reasons for carrying out a necropsy (Figure 14.5). The veterinary surgeon must be aware of these categories and the different approaches required, and plan accordingly.

Another consideration is whether only one reptile needs to be examined or whether there is a colony problem – or a 'die-off' in a free-living population – in which case a whole group of animals may be available for necropsy. The approach may differ (see below).

The person planning the examination must also remember that others may lay claim to a carcase, or part of it; this also can influence how the necropsy is carried out and/or the fate of all or part of the body. For example: an owner may want an animal's carcase returned; museum curators and taxidermists may require the body for mounting or for preparation of a skeleton or study skin; or, in legal and insurance cases, the carcase may be needed by the police, as evidence, and/or by 'experts' – including pathologists who have been called by the prosecution/defence and wish to do a second examination (Cooper and Cooper, 2007).

The condition of the carcase, in terms of autolysis or predation, will influence how thorough a necropsy can be. It is a mistake to think that a partly decomposed or mutilated body is 'unsuitable for post-mortem examination'. Useful information can be gleaned from the most unpromising of specimens. Having said this, the practitioner should become familiar with signs that suggest that autolysis is underway and be aware that some tests, such as bacteriology and histopathology, may be of limited value. A foetid smell and visible lysis or sloughing of tissues are clear-cut indications of decomposition. More subtle ones include bile staining of the ventral abdomen, especially of snakes and lizards (Figure 14.6), and the collapse and discoloration of eyes. All such changes are temperature-dependent, emphasizing the need for herpetologists to check their charges regularly and to remove dead animals promptly, especially from heated vivaria. Careful storage of the carcase by the veterinary surgeon prior to necropsy is the next stage.

In legal cases it may be necessary to determine when death occurred and this can be assisted by an understanding of the changes that take place as a dead reptile decomposes. A useful reference to post-mortem interval determination is Cooper (2012).

Submission form – dead reptiles

Name and contact details of person presenting the animal ....

....

....

Species (if known).. Age (if known)..

Sex (if known)... Time in possession of person presenting the reptile ....

If a captive reptile:

Origin: Captive-bred/Purchased/Other .... If Other, give details ....

....

Other animals kept at same premises..

Summary of management system ....

Diet... Supplements..

Source and storage of diet (food)..

Date and time of death..

Clinical signs ('symptoms') observed before death – give details ....

....

....

Specific comments on feeding ....

Specific comments on defecation..

Specific comments on sloughing (where appropriate) ....

Any treatment given before death (and when)..

Comments on factors that may (or may not) be relevant to the reptile's death (e.g. changes in management, disease in other animals on the premises)

....

....

Other information that may be relevant (if appropriate, add photographs, drawings of vivarium, etc.)...........................

....

....

If a wild (free-living) casualty:

Date and time of recovery..

Location of recovery (with grid reference or GPS reading if available)...

Circumstances of recovery (including any relevant observations at the time)..

....

....

....

Name... Signature..

Date... Time..

14.3 A suggested submission form. This form is designed for either a captive reptile or a wildlife casualty that needs a post-mortem examination and/or laboratory tests.

Submission form – eggs of reptiles

To: Name of laboratory .... Date of submission of sample ....

Name of person submitting the egg(s): ....

Details of egg(s): ....

Species (common name) .... Species (scientific name) ....

If from a group of reptiles, the number involved, and whether they are all of the same, or mixed, species: ....

....

....

Reason for submitting the egg(s) ....

Previous breeding history (tick)

Eggs or young produced successfully ☐   Copulation observed but no eggs or young produced ☐   Not known ☐

Any other relevant background information, e.g. history of ill health, diseases ....

....

....

....

Date and time when egg was collected   Date .... Time ....

Method of storage since egg was taken   Ambient (environmental) temperature ☐ Refrigerator (+4°C) ☐   Frozen ☐

Fixed in formalin ☐   Alcohol ☐   Other ....

Reason for submitting samples ....

....

....

....

Contact details of person submitting sample:

Name ....

Address ....

....

Phone (day).. Phone (night) ....

E-mail .... Fax ....

Name of veterinary surgeon: ....

Address ....

....

Phone (day) .... Phone (night) ....

E-mail .... Fax ....

Any other relevant information (if appropriate); attach copies of daily record sheets, previous laboratory reports, any other information.

....

....

....

14.4 A suggested submission form for reptile eggs.

Purpose	Category	Comment
To determine the cause of a reptile's or an embryo's death or the failure of an egg to hatch	Diagnostic	Routine techniques needed
To ascertain the cause of ill health or failure to thrive (not necessarily the cause of death)	Diagnostic/health monitoring	Routine – but detailed examinations and laboratory tests may be needed to detect non-lethal changes (Cooper, 1986, 1989b)
To provide background information on supposedly normal reptile, e.g. on presence or absence of lesions, macroparasites, microparasites or other factors, such as fat reserves or carcase composition	Health monitoring	As above. Must be methodical if information is not to be missed. Follow established protocols (Woodford, 2001)
To provide information for a legal case or similar investigation, e.g. on circumstances of death or the possibility that the reptile suffered pain or distress while it was alive	Forensic/legal	Can be very different from the categories above. The approach depends upon the questions that are being asked. There must be a proper 'chain of custody' and all material *must* be retained (Cooper and Cooper, 1998, 2007)
For research purposes, e.g. removal of tissue samples, such as testes, or examination of organs, such as oviducts, in order to assist biologists or others	Investigative	Depends upon the requirements of the research worker

14.5 The main categories of post-mortem examination.

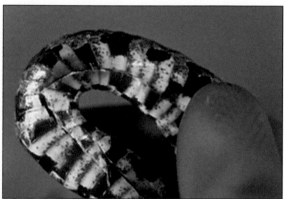

14.6 Green staining (bile) on the integument of a snake, indicative of post-mortem change.

Important tips

- Think and consult before starting the post-mortem examination.
- Be prepared to retain the carcase and portions of it: once discarded, they are unlikely to be recoverable.
- Never assume that a specimen cannot be examined on account of autolysis or damage.

Requirements for a necropsy

In order to be able to carry out a satisfactory post-mortem examination of a reptile, the practitioner needs to have:

- Knowledge of the normal anatomy of reptiles and (in the case of eggs) of basic embryology
- Awareness of the common causes of morbidity and mortality in reptiles (see References and further reading)
- Access to appropriate literature – books, articles and websites. In the UK the Royal College of Veterinary Surgeons Library can help with this and will carry out comprehensive searches if needed. Requesting reprints or PDF attachments from authors of papers will not only help in the acquisition of original material

but also provide contact with colleagues in the same field
- Adequate equipment and facilities, including those necessary for health and safety reasons. Important items are listed in Figure 14.7
- A methodical approach, including the use of standard forms that permit rapid analysis and meaningful comparison of findings (Figures 14.8 and 14.9)
- A willingness to consult suitably qualified or experienced colleagues for advice. Particularly in legal cases – or when an unusual or rare species is to be examined – it may be wise to solicit the help of a specialist pathologist, preferably one with experience of the class Reptilia. Knowledgeable herpetologists are also a valuable source of information, and collaboration between veterinary surgeons and those who keep or study reptiles is necessary, as emphasized repeatedly in the past (Cooper and Laurie, 1987; Cooper, Bloxam and Tonge, 1998).

Essential

- Post-mortem examination table
- Instruments
- Protective clothing
- Incinerator, macerator or other means of disposal
- Refrigerator, freezer
- Balance/scales
- Disinfectants
- Sterilizer or autoclave
- Bottles and fixatives
- Bone forceps, saws and pneumatic drills to facilitate examination of chelonians

Useful additions

- Protective hood or flow cabinet
- X-ray machine
- Container for head of venomous species

Special precautions

- Adequate drainage, disinfection and ventilation
- Dowsing carcase in disinfectant may reduce risk of airborne infection although hood or flow cabinet is preferable

14.7 Equipment for post-mortem examination of reptiles. Some requirements may be a legal responsibility under health and safety legislation. Care must be taken with venomous species.

Post-mortem examination form for reptiles

Species .... Reference No ....

Date of submission .... Origin ....

Relevant history/circumstances of death ....

....

....

....

....

Request – diagnosis (cause of death/ill health), health monitoring, forensic investigation/research

Any special requirements re. techniques to be followed, fate of body/samples ....

....

....

Submitted by .... Date ....

Received by .... Date ....

Measurements

Snout–vent (SV) .... Vent–tail tip (VT) .... Bodyweight (Mass) ....

(Chelonians) Body length .... Condition score ....

Condition score: Obese or fat/good/fair or thin/poor ....⎫

State of preservation: Good/fair/poor/marked autolysis ....⎬ *A number ('score') can be used for these*

Storage since death: Refrigerator/ambient temperature/frozen/fixed ....⎭

External observations (including ectoparasites, skin condition, shell lesions, evidence of sloughing) ....

....

....

....

Macroscopic evaluation on opening the body (including position and appearance of organs, lesions)..........

....

....

....

Alimentary system .... Musculoskeletal ....

Cardiovascular .... Respiratory ....

Urinary .... Reproductive ....

Nervous system ....

This section can be expanded as necessary – subheadings can be inserted, including checklist of organs and tissues

Other samples taken

....Bact Paras Hist DNA Cytology Other (e.g. serology)

....Bact Paras Hist DNA Cytology Other (e.g. serology)

....Bact Paras Hist DNA Cytology Other (e.g. serology)

....Bact Paras Hist DNA Cytology Other (e.g. serology)

....Bact Paras Hist DNA Cytology Other (e.g. serology)

....Bact Paras Hist DNA Cytology Other (e.g. serology)

....Bact Paras Hist DNA Cytology Other (e.g. serology)

14.8 A suggested post-mortem examination form for dead reptiles. (continues) ▶

Laboratory findings ....
....
....
Date .... Initials .... Reported to whom ....

Preliminary report (based on gross findings and immediate laboratory results, e.g. cytology) ....
....
....
Reported to .... Date .... Time ....

Final report (based on all available information) ....
....
....
....

Fate of carcase / tissues   destroyed/frozen/fixed in formalin (other)/retained for reference collection/sent elsewhere
....
....
PM examination performed by .... Date .... Time ....
Reported by .... Date ....

14.8   (continued) A suggested post-mortem examination form for dead reptiles.

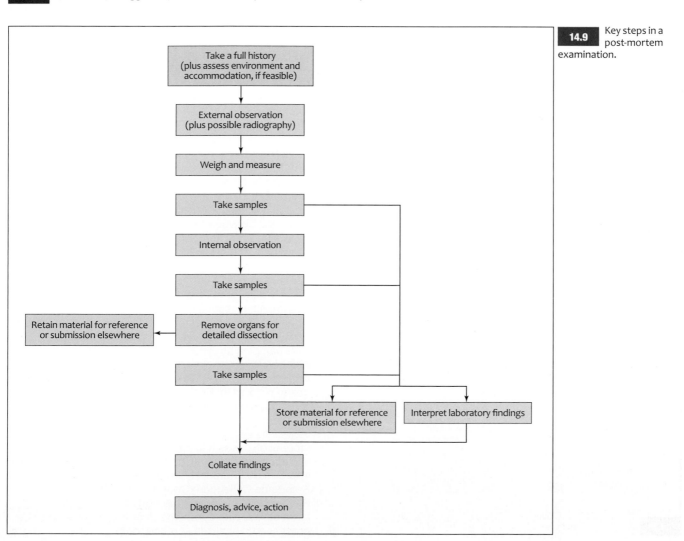

14.9 Key steps in a post-mortem examination.

Performing the necropsy

The post-mortem examination must be *systematic*, even if time is short and the veterinary surgeon plans only to perform a rudimentary investigation prior to seeking further help and/or sending off samples. The key steps in any post-mortem examination of a reptile are depicted in Figure 14.9; Figure 14.10 gives a protocol for examination of eggs.

An abbreviated approach to post-mortem examination, which has proved ideal for busy practitioners, is given below. This technique can also prove useful when a group of reptiles is examined; it ensures that the same investigations are carried out on all animals and that appropriate samples are saved.

1. Plan to carry out the necropsy as soon as possible. If there is any delay, chill the carcase at +4°C. Avoid freezing as this damages tissues (Figure 14.11) and hampers histopathological examination. Fixation avoids this but renders other tests, such as microbiology, useless.
2. On reception of the specimen, record the history and give the animal a unique reference number – always good practice; essential if legal action is possible.
3. Examine the animal externally – record any parasites, lesions or abnormalities. The orifices – mouth and cloaca (Figure 14.12) – need careful investigation (Cooper and Sainsbury, 1994). Check chelonians carefully for nasal discharge. Radiography is often overlooked once an animal is dead but can be of great

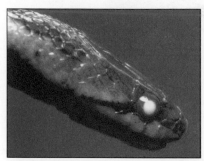

14.11 Freezing and thawing can have a variety of adverse effects, both macroscopically and microscopically. The opacity in the eye of this snake is attributable to freezing.

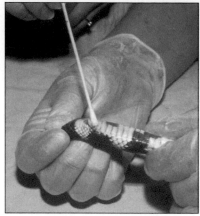

14.12 Swabs from the skin or orifices should be taken early on in the examination. Here, a cloacal swab is taken from a kingsnake.

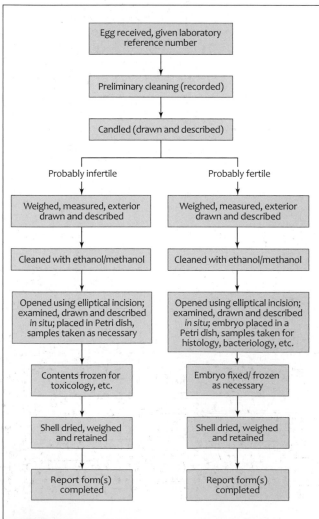

```
Egg received, given laboratory
reference number
        ↓
Preliminary cleaning (recorded)
        ↓
Candled (drawn and described)
        ↓
   ┌────────────┴────────────┐
Probably infertile        Probably fertile
```

Probably infertile	Probably fertile
Weighed, measured, exterior drawn and described	Weighed, measured, exterior drawn and described
Cleaned with ethanol/methanol	Cleaned with ethanol/methanol
Opened using elliptical incision; examined, drawn and described *in situ*; placed in Petri dish, samples taken as necessary	Opened using elliptical incision; examined, drawn and described *in situ*; embryo placed in a Petri dish, samples taken for histology, bacteriology, etc.
Contents frozen for toxicology, etc.	Embryo fixed/ frozen as necessary
Shell dried, weighed and retained	Shell dried, weighed and retained
Report form(s) completed	Report form(s) completed

14.10 Suggested protocol for post-mortem examination of reptile eggs.

value (Figure 14.13). It can reveal skeletal and other lesions that are relevant to the animal's death or to the health of the colony or group from which it came (Cooper and West, 1988).

4. Weigh and record standard measurements: snout-to-vent and vent-to-tail tip distances or, in chelonians, a 'shell' length (often also a width) and compilation of a Jackson's ratio or its equivalent (see Chapter 4). An animal's bodyweight (mass) without a measurement is of very limited value.
5. Open the reptile and examine the internal organs (Figures 14.14–14.16). Record any lesions or abnormalities, and whether or not the stomach and other parts of the digestive tract contain food. Interpretation of gross findings requires a knowledge of what is normal (see later) – and there can be important variations between different species. Nothing should be touched until the organs have been observed and described. The latter is most important and can help to distinguish ante-mortem from post-mortem changes.
6. Remove and fix in buffered 10% formalin, samples of major organs (e.g. lung, liver, kidney etc.) plus any abnormalities (see later).
7. Open portions of intestine and look with the naked eye or hand lens for lesions and parasites.
8. Take samples as required for laboratory investigation (see below).
9. After examination, save the reptile in the refrigerator, frozen or fixed in 10% buffered formalin. A general rule is that carcases can be kept in the fridge (+4°C) for up to 5 days but should be frozen/fixed thereafter, especially when rare species are involved. In legal ('forensic') cases it is important to retain all material including wrappings (Cooper and Cooper, 2013). Where appropriate, material should be deposited in a Reference Collection (Cooper *et al.*, 1998).
10. Record how and where the body and samples have been saved, with a reminder that they may need to be processed/discarded at a later date.

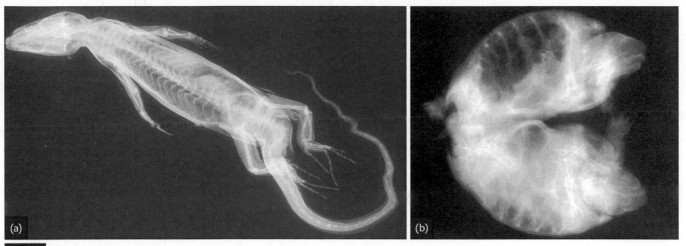

14.13 Post-mortem radiography may be valuable. (a) Skeletal abnormalities in a Round Island skink. (b) Conjoined ('Siamese twin') leopard tortoises.

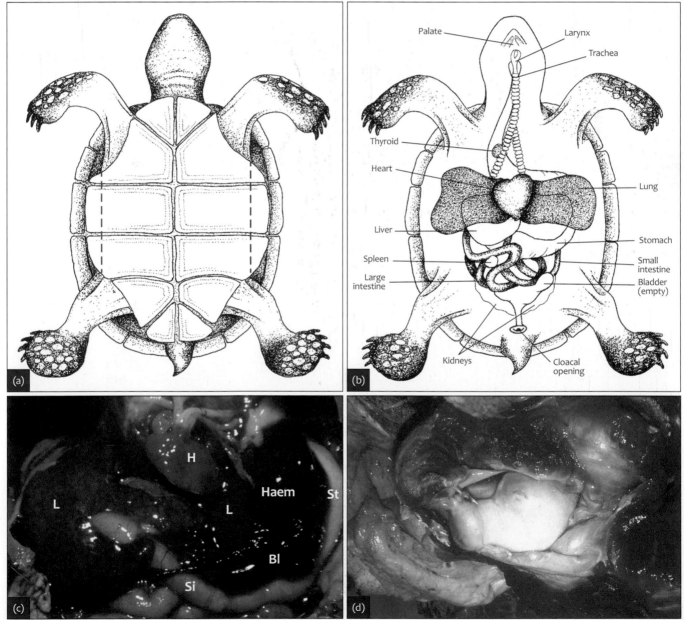

14.14 Chelonian necropsy. (a) Ventral view, showing the position of the initial incision in the bridge between plastron and carapace. (b) Ventral view following removal of the plastron, showing the main organs visible in the body cavity. (c) Massive liver trauma in a painted turtle that fell from a third-storey flat (apartment): Bl = blood from liver; H = heart; Haem = haematoma; L = liver; Si = small intestine; St = stomach. (d) Because of a known history, this joint of a giant tortoise was dissected to investigate possible arthritic change.
(c, Courtesy of Paul Raiti)

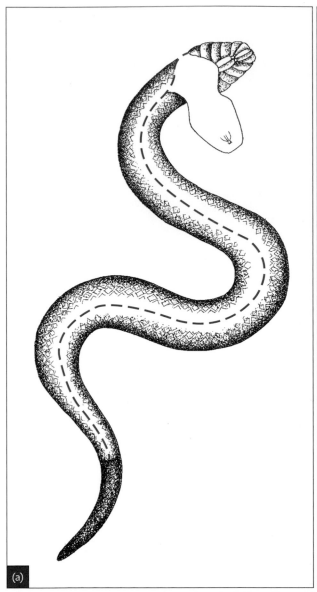

(a)

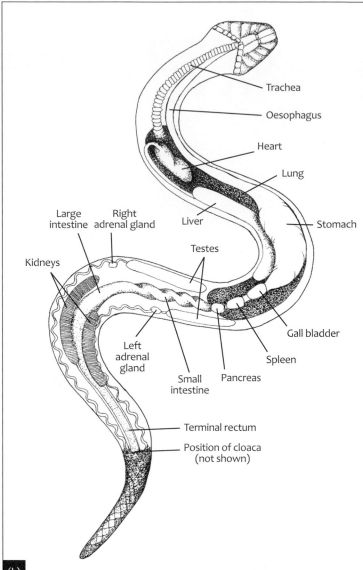

Trachea

Oesophagus

Heart

Lung

Large intestine

Right adrenal gland

Liver

Stomach

Kidneys

Testes

Left adrenal gland

Small intestine

Pancreas

Gall bladder

Spleen

Terminal rectum

Position of cloaca (not shown)

(b)

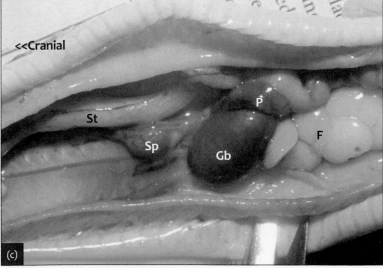

<<Cranial

St

P

Sp

Gb

F

(c)

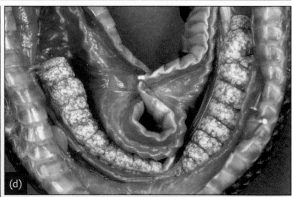

(d)

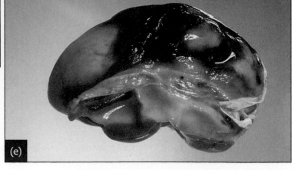

(e)

14.15 Snake necropsy. (a) View of a snake showing the position and length of the initial incision (one ramus has been cut and the jaw reflected). (b) Ventral view showing the main organs visible in the body cavity. (c) Prosected royal python: F = fat; Gb = gall bladder; P = pancreas; Sp = spleen; St = stomach. (d) Some macroscopic changes are very typical; the kidney of this Jamaican boa is white, indicative of urate deposition. (e) This heart, from a python, is ruptured – the cause of death.

(c, Courtesy of Paul Raiti)

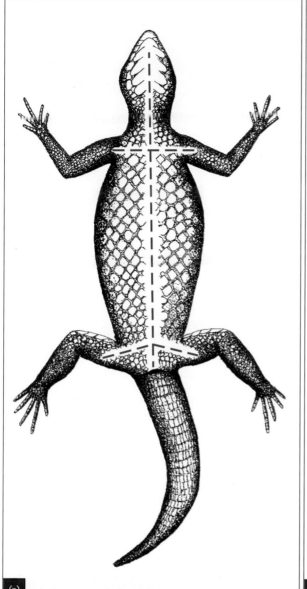

(a)

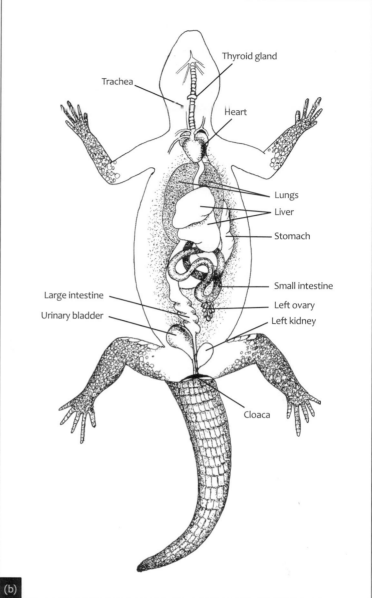

Thyroid gland

Trachea

Heart

Lungs

Liver

Stomach

Small intestine

Large intestine

Urinary bladder

Left ovary

Left kidney

Cloaca

(b)

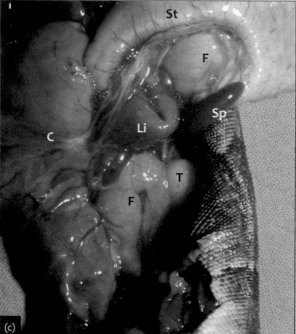

St

F

Sp

Li

C

T

F

(c)

14.16 Lizard necropsy. (a) Ventral view showing the position of the initial incision. (b) Ventral view showing the main organs visible in the body cavity. (c) Prosected juvenile green iguana: C = caecum; F = fat; Li = large intestine; Sp = spleen; St = stomach; T = testis.
(c, Courtesy of Paul Raiti)

Sample taking

Samples play an important part in the diagnosis of disease in reptiles and in the health monitoring of supposedly 'normal' animals. Those that may be taken from reptiles during or following post-mortem examination are listed in Figure 14.17. If no specific diagnosis has been made as a result of gross investigation, a whole range of tissues should be sampled. They may not all need to be processed (cost alone may preclude this) but it is better to have them available, in case they are needed, rather than regret the lack of them at a later date.

Correct sampling will help to yield reliable results and facilitate accurate interpretation and appropriate action. In legal ('forensic') cases such precision is even more important (Cooper and Cooper, 2007).

Mistakes can occur at various stages of sampling: selection; taking; packing; transportation; reception; processing.

The *purpose* for which samples are collected is all-important and will influence how they are collected, stored and transported. The investigations that are to be carried out often dictate how the sample is taken, presented and handled; for instance, hygienic ('sterile') precautions are essential when tissues are to be examined microbiologically but are less important than is careful handling with the correct (atraumatic) forceps when histopathological investigation is the aim. Likewise, techniques in the laboratory will depend upon the request received. Consistency in sampling methods is vital if results are to be reliable and different studies are to be comparable.

A summary of methods that can be used to preserve samples, to ensure flexibility in terms of laboratory testing, is given in Figure 14.18.

The time that elapses between taking a sample and processing it is also a fundamental consideration in assessing and interpreting results. Thus, for example, a delay in processing a set of swabs may result in the culture of fewer

Sample	Purpose	Comments
Faeces; stomach and intestinal contents	Parasitology; microbiology; chemical tests (e.g. for fat); toxicology	Samples can be removed during necropsy but examined later
Blood	Haematology; clinical chemistry; parasitology; serology; DNA technology	Even if insufficient blood is available for full haematological examination, smears can usually be made
Urine	Microbiology; clinical chemistry; cytology	Samples can often be obtained from the bladder or cloaca
Pus	Microbiology; cytology	Pus is usually caseous. Pus-like material from any species should be sampled and examined. Aerobic and anaerobic culture advisable
Tissues	Histology (histopathology and histochemistry); scanning/transmission electron microscopy; cytology; chemical analysis; toxicology; immunological tests (e.g. for detecting snake or scorpion venom); radiography; DNA technology	Samples should include not only internal soft tissues but also integument (scales) and skeleton. Some can be stored for later use

14.17 Post-mortem samples from reptiles.

Method of treatment	Advantages	Disadvantages	Comments
Chilled at +4°C	Good preservation for a few days	Autolysis continues to take place	The autolysis is slow and generally predictable
Frozen	Can be stored indefinitely and is necessary for samples required for toxicology	Causes artefacts in terms of both gross and histological changes. Pathogens generally not killed	Some allowance can be made for gross artefacts (e.g. corneal opacity) but confusion may arise
Fully fixed in formalin	As above. Pathogens are usually killed (not prions)	Permits histopathology but use of formalin makes DNA studies difficult. Affects appearance of organs – colour changes	Careful interpretation needed, as in embalmed cadavers
Fixed in ethanol or methanol	As above, but DNA extraction is little affected	Affects appearance of organs – colour changes	As above

14.18 Storage and treatment of carcases and tissues of reptiles. (Adapted from Cooper and Cooper, 2007)

bacteria, or perhaps an overgrowth of one species (such as *Proteus*), so that the findings cannot then reliably be compared with those from another set of swabs.

The taking and transportation of samples in the field, especially in relatively inaccessible or isolated areas, can present particular problems. Special equipment may be required and improvisation is often essential (Cooper and Samour, 1997; Cooper, 2013).

It is always wise to develop and to use protocols for sampling, whereby the method to be used is clearly defined and followed. It is also prudent to include details of the protocol in any published 'Materials and Methods' so that other investigators can employ the same techniques – or, at least, be aware of where discrepancies may have occurred that might have influenced the results.

Common abnormalities

The veterinary surgeon needs to be familiar with the normal post-mortem (or endoscopic) appearance of organs in order for significant lesions to be recognized accurately. While some changes associated with disease are common to all vertebrates, e.g. pale foci in the liver or kidney, distinct inflammatory changes (as seen in, for example, pericarditis, oophoritis or pneumonia), others may be specific to, or particularly significant in, the class Reptilia. The latter include the accumulation of urates in the kidney in nephropathies, nodules associated with helminths and a range of cloacal lesions. Some histological appearances in reptiles are shown in Figures 14.19–14.33. Certain of them are discussed in more detail below.

The *normal* appearance of organs in reptiles may lead an inexperienced investigator to suspect pathological change; for instance, many species store melanin in the liver (giving it a dark coloration) and some, e.g. certain chameleons and bearded dragons, have a heavily pigmented peritoneum. Glomerulogenesis is a normal feature of many reptiles (see Figure 14.28). Anatomical features, internal as well as external, may also prove confusing. For instance, snakes usually have only one functional lung, while in most chelonians the pericardial sac is continuous with the peritoneal (coelomic) membrane.

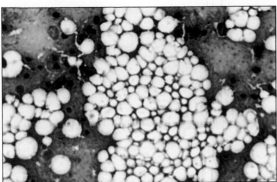

14.19 A cytological preparation from the liver of an obese reptile. Large numbers of adipocytes (fat cells) are present (quick stain).

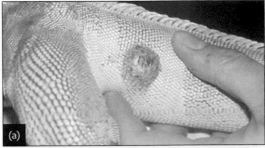

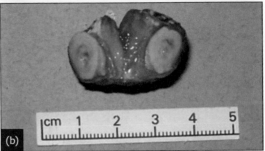

14.23 (a) A green iguana with a raised skin nodule, prior to surgical removal. (b) The lesion in (a), bisected. This is an abscess. Caseous material, composed of pus and fibrin, is visible in concentric layers.

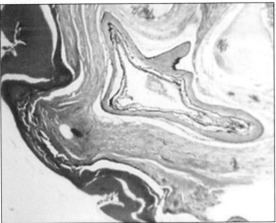

14.20 Marked hyperkeratinization over the eye of a lacertid lizard attributed to a chronic vitamin A deficiency (H&E).

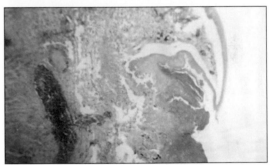

14.24 Necrotic dermatitis in a snake showing marked cellular infiltration. A scale is clearly visible (H&E).

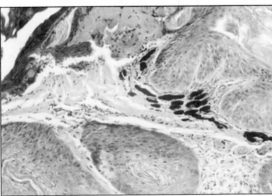

14.21 A papilloma of the skin of a lacertid lizard. Melanocytes (normal in this species) are present in the centre of the field (H&E).

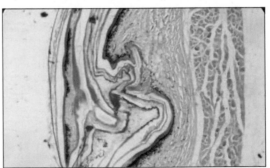

14.25 Retained slough and dysecdysis in a snake. There are several layers of keratin over the skin surface (H&E).

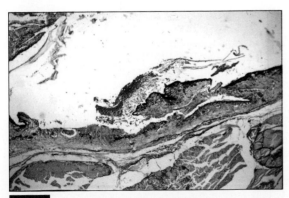

14.22 A fungal dermatitis in a snake (PAS).

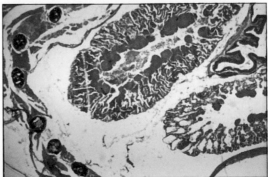

14.26 Pneumonia in a lacertid lizard. Note the thickened (inflamed) lung surface and inflammatory debris in the lumen (H&E).

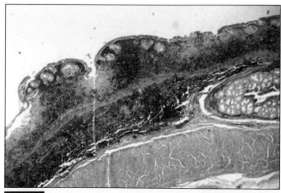

14.27   Haemorrhagic gastritis in a python (H&E).

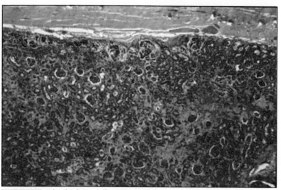

14.28   The kidney of a Mediterranean tortoise showing subcapsular glomerulogenesis (H&E). Continued development of glomeruli throughout life is a normal feature of many reptiles.

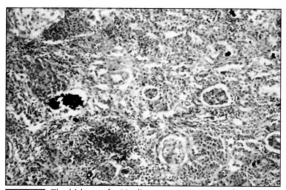

14.29   The kidney of a Mediterranean tortoise, showing interstitial nephritis and deposits of calcium (H&E). These were unexpected findings following post-mortem examination and suggested earlier infectious disease and a calcium:phosphorus imbalance.

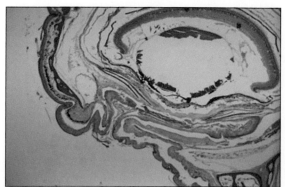

14.30   Sealed eyelids and mild conjunctivitis in a lacertid lizard, probably associated with a vitamin A deficiency (H&E).

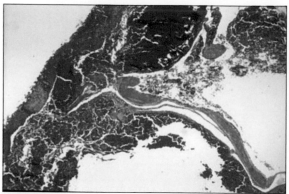

14.31   Haemorrhagic pneumonia in a Mediterranean tortoise (H&E).

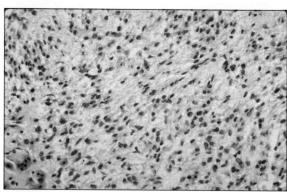

14.32   A neurilemmoma in a Hermann's tortoise (H&E). Histological examination of masses in reptiles is always wise; most are of infectious or traumatic origin but a few prove to be neoplasms, as in this case.

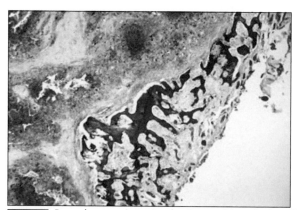

14.33   Bone abscesses in a ratsnake. Reasonably well mineralized osseous tissue is on the right; multiple pyogenic foci on the left (H&E).

Legal aspects

The collection, transportation and processing of samples (including carcases) are likely to be covered by legislation on postal and packaging regulations (UK), health and safety, and animal health, and the Convention on International Trade in Endangered Species of Wild Fauna and Flora (CITES) (Cooper, 1987). Even the smallest samples, assuming that they are 'recognizable derivatives', may require CITES permits if they originate from species of reptile that are listed in Appendix I or II of CITES, or (in the European Union) in the relevant annexes of the EU CITES regulations, or ('third'/non-EU countries) are subject to equivalent national CITES legislation. The international movement of samples – even histological sections of a lesion for a second opinion, to, say, North America – presents legal hurdles if the species from which they are taken is CITES-listed (Cooper, 1993, 2000a): CITES and, sometimes, animal health export and import permits are likely to be needed.

Zoonoses

There are potential health hazards when performing euthanasia on a live reptile, examining one post-mortem, or handling and processing samples. One of these is the risk of contracting a zoonosis – a disease or infection that is naturally transmitted between a vertebrate animal and a human (based on World Health Organization wording).

Reptiles are traditionally associated with certain bacteria – for example, *Salmonella* spp. and atypical *Mycobacterium* spp. – but many other organisms present in or on reptiles (such as *Pseudomonas* spp.) can potentially infect humans, especially if the latter are in some way immunocompromised (Palmer *et al.*, 1998).

So, what action should be taken to minimize the dangers to staff and clients? First and foremost, as in all work, a risk assessment is essential.

The five steps of a risk assessment are:

- Identify hazards
- Assess who might be harmed and how
- Evaluate risks and decide precautions
- Record findings
- Review assessment and update.

Laboratory investigations

A range of tests may be carried out, as emphasized earlier. Not all are necessary immediately, which is another good reason for retaining material after the post-mortem examination.

Environmental investigations, e.g. water and soil sampling, should be considered (in addition to tests on the animal's tissues), especially when a number of animals have died in a vivarium or enclosure.

Interpretation

This can present problems, especially if the practitioner has limited experience of reptiles or the species is one for which few or no reference data are available. Useful references to microorganisms include Cooper (1991 and 1999) and some information is given elsewhere in this manual (see Chapter 25). For interpretation of histological appearances, a particularly useful reference is Aughey and Frye (2001).

Laboratory results should be linked with clinical and post-mortem findings. For example, in hepatic lipidosis (not uncommon in reptiles) endoscopic observations (live animals), or the finding of a pale liver that is inclined to float in fixative (dead animals), will be associated on cytology or histology with an abnormal accumulation of lipid in hepatocytes (see Figure 14.19) (Divers and Cooper, 2000).

Artefactual changes can complicate histological interpretation; some of these are due to poor handling or processing of material. Guidelines for the examination of biopsy samples from reptiles are also relevant to post-mortem samples (Cooper, 1994). Distinguishing antemortem and post-mortem change can often present difficulties to the practitioner – see earlier.

Record keeping

Accurate record keeping is vital – particularly so in this litigious age – and the following points must be emphasized:

- Record all findings, even if some appear not to be significant or their relevance is unclear. During the examination itself, a tape recorder (preferably voice-activated and digital) is invaluable, especially if the person doing the necropsy is working alone; the recording can always be transcribed later. Photographs should be taken whenever possible; a 'clean' person should do the photography in order to minimize spread of pathogens
- Use a standard format for collation and storage of information and samples. For the former, a computerized system such as the Zoological Information Management System (ZIMS) may be appropriate, especially if working with a zoological collection. For samples follow published guidelines.

Forms

The use of standardized forms is recommended:

- Submission of material: Figures 14.3 and 14.4 show suggested forms for submission of dead reptiles and eggs
- Post-mortem examination: see Figure 14.8.

Retention of material

As mentioned earlier, retention of material after the necropsy is a wise precaution that is often overlooked, even by experienced pathologists. It means that one can return to the carcase later if, for example, histology suggests a fungal infection and samples need to be sent for culture. It can prove invaluable if litigation or a malpractice claim follows the examination (Cooper and Cooper, 2007, 2013).

Acknowledgements

I am grateful to my wife, Margaret E. Cooper, for reading and commenting on an early draft of this revised chapter. Sally Dowsett very kindly assisted with typing and formatting.

References and further reading

American Veterinary Medical Association (2001) 2000 Report of the AVMA Panel on Euthanasia. *Journal of the American Veterinary Medical Association* **218(5)**, 669–696

Aughey E and Frye FL (2001) *Comparative Veterinary Histology with Clinical Correlates.* Iowa State University Press, Ames, IA

British Veterinary Zoological Society (2003) *Guidelines for Acceptable Methods of Euthanasia for Zoo, Exotic Pet and Wildlife Species, No.1: Reptiles.* British Veterinary Zoological Society, London

Close B, Banister K, Baumans V *et al.* (1996) Recommendations for euthanasia of experimental animals: Part 1. *Laboratory Animals* **30(4)**, 293–316

Close B, Banister K, Baumans V *et al.* (1997) Recommendations for euthanasia of experimental animals: Part 2. *Laboratory Animals* **31(1)**, 1–32

Cooper JE (1986) The role of pathology in the investigation of diseases of reptiles. *Acta Zoologica et Pathologica Antverpiensia* **79**, 15–32

Cooper JE (1989a) Reptiles and amphibians. *Proceedings of the Second Symposium of the British Wildlife Rehabilitation Council*, pp. 76–77

Cooper JE (1989b) Health monitoring and quality control of reptiles and amphibians kept for biomedical research. *Proceedings of the Third International Colloquium on the Pathology of Reptiles and Amphibians*, pp. 4–7

Cooper JE (1991) Bacteriological studies on snakes. *Transactions of the Royal Society of Tropical Medicine and Hygiene* **85**, 847

Cooper JE (1994) Biopsy techniques. *Seminars in Avian and Exotic Pet Medicine* **3**, 161–165

Cooper JE (1999) Reptilian microbiology. In: *Laboratory Medicine: Avian and Exotic Pets*, ed. AM Fudge, pp. 223–227. WB Saunders, Philadelphia and London

Cooper JE (2000) Tumours (neoplasms) of reptiles: some significant cases from Jersey Zoo. *Dodo* **36**, 82–86

Cooper JE (2012) The estimation of *post-mortem* interval (PMI) in reptiles and amphibians: current knowledge and needs. *Herpetological Journal* **22**, 91–96

Cooper JE (ed.) (2013) Field Techniques in Exotic Animal Medicine. *Journal of Exotic Pet Medicine* **22(1)**

Cooper JE, Bloxam QMC and Tonge SJ (1998) Pathology of Round Island geckos *Phelsuma guentheri*: some unexpected findings. *Dodo* **34**, 153–158

Cooper JE and Cooper ME (1998) Forensic veterinary medicine. *Seminars in Avian and Exotic Pet Medicine* **7(4)**, 159–230

Cooper JE and Cooper ME (2007) *Introduction to Veterinary and Comparative Forensic Medicine*. Blackwell, Oxford

Cooper JE and Cooper ME (2013) *Wildlife Forensic Investigation: Principles and Practice*. CRC Press, Boca Raton, FL, USA

Cooper JE and Davies O (1997) Studies on morbidity and mortality in smooth snakes (*Coronella* spp.). *Herpetological Journal* **7**, 19–22

Cooper JE, Dutton CJ and Allchurch AF (1998) Reference collections: their importance and relevance to modern zoo management and conservation biology. *Dodo* **34**,159–166

Cooper JE, Ewbank R and Platt C (1989) *Euthanasia of Amphibians and Reptiles*. Universities Federation for Animal Welfare, Potters Bar, UK

Cooper JE, Ewbank R and Rosenberg ME (1984) Euthanasia of tortoises. *Veterinary Record* **114**, 635

Cooper JE and Jackson OF (1981) *Diseases of the Reptilia*. Academic Press, London

Cooper JE and Laurie A (1987) Investigation of deaths in marine iguanas (*Amblyrhynchus cristatus*) on Galapagos. *Journal of Comparative Pathology* **97**, 129–136

Cooper JE and Sainsbury AW (1994) Review: oral diseases of reptiles. *Herpetological Journal* **4**, 117–125

Cooper JE and Samour JH (1997) Portable and field equipment for avian veterinary work. *Proceedings of the 4th Conference of the European Committee of the Association of Avian Veterinarians*, pp. 50–60

Cooper JE and West CD (1988) Radiological studies on endangered Mascarene fauna. *Oryx* **22**, 18–24

Cooper JE and Williams DL (1995) Veterinary perspectives and techniques in husbandry and research. In: *Health and Welfare of Captive Reptiles*, ed. C Warwick *et al.*, pp. 98–112. Chapman and Hall, London

Cooper ME (1987) *An Introduction to Animal Law*. Academic Press, London and New York

Cooper ME (1993) Legal implications for the management of infectious disease in captive breeding and reintroduction programmes. *Journal of Zoo and Wildlife Medicine* **24**, 296–303

Cooper ME (2000a) Legal considerations in the international movement of diagnostic and research samples from raptors: conference resolution. In: *Raptor Biomedicine III*, ed. JT Lumeij *et al.*, pp. 337–343. Zoological Education Network, Lake Worth, FL, USA

Divers SJ and Cooper JE (2000) Reptile hepatic lipidosis. *Seminars in Avian and Exotic Pet Medicine* **9**, 153–164

Ewert J-P, Cooper JE, Langton T *et al.* (2004) *Background Information on the Species-Specific Proposals for Reptiles*, Presented by the Expert Group on Amphibians and Reptiles. Council of Europe, Strasbourg, GT 123 (2004) 15

Expert Panel (2013) *Analysis of Humane Killing Methods for Reptiles in the Skin Trade*, ed. Swiss Federal Veterinary Office (FVO). Swiss Confederation, Berne, Switzerland

Frye FL (1984) Euthanasia necropsy techniques and comparative histology of reptiles. In: *Diseases of Amphibians and Reptiles*, ed. GL Hoff *et al.*, pp. 703–755. Plenum Press, New York

Frye FL (1991) Euthanasia and necropsy. In: *Biomedical and Surgical Aspects of Captive Reptile Husbandry, 2nd edition*, pp. 513–525. Krieger, Melbourne, FL, USA

Kusuma A, Ten Donkelaar HJ and Nieuwenhuys R (1979) Chapter 2: Intrinsic organisation of the spinal cord. In: *Biology of the Reptilia, Volume 10*, pp. 59–11. Academic Press, London, New York, and San Francisco

Mader DR (2006) *Reptile Medicine and Surgery, 2nd edition*. Saunders Elsevier, St Louis, MO, USA

Mader DR and Divers SJ (2014). *Current Therapy in Reptile Medicine & Surgery*. Elsevier Saunders. St Louis, MO, USA.

Palmer SR, Lord Soulsby and Simpson DIH (1998) *Zoonoses: Biology, Clinical Practice, and Public Health Control*. Oxford University Press, Oxford

Rival F (1999) Euthanasie. *Le Pointe Vétérinaire* **30**, 237–238

Woodford MH (2001) *Quarantine and Health Screening Protocols for Wildlife Prior to Translocation and Release into the Wild*. OIE/Care for the Wild/IUCV/EAZWV, Paris

Zwart P (1996) *Post-mortem* examination of reptiles. *Proceedings of the British Veterinary Zoological Society/EARAV*, pp. 20–23

Chapter 15

Dermatology

Mary A. Fraser and Simon J. Girling

Skin disease is one of the commonest reasons that a reptile is presented in the veterinary clinic (Hellebuyck *et al.*, 2012). Reptilian skin is unique in its structure and physiology. Many of the problems encountered are related to poor husbandry and nutrition and will involve education of the owners in addition to treating the condition.

Anatomy and physiology

The skin is the largest organ of the body and has a large number of functions, including protection of internal organs, camouflage, water and electrolyte loss regulation, and hormone derivative synthesis (e.g. vitamin D precursor production).

Reptilian skin is similar in general construction to mammalian skin, in that it is composed of an outer epidermis and an inner dermis. In most reptiles the epidermis and dermis make up the scales and scutes of the skin. There is, however, much variation between reptile species at the cellular level, and variation in the skin over an individual reptile's body. For example, the skin may be thickened over the head and formed into accessory structures such as spines or horns.

More detailed information on the anatomy and physiology of reptilian skin is given in Chapter 1.

Ecdysis and dysecdysis

Ecdysis

Ecdysis is the process by which reptiles form a new skin and then shed the old overlying one. There is some variation between the species:

- Many lizards shed their skin in large patches
- Snakes shed the entire skin in one episode
- Chelonians shed scutes intermittently.

Four physiological stages have been described in ecdysis (Maas, 2013):

1. Resting stage.
2. Beginning of the growth cycle, where there is hypertrophy of the *stratum germinativum*.
3. Formation of new alpha-, beta- and Oberhautchen layers.
4. Separation of the layers through the actions of lymphatic fluids and proteolytic enzymes. This process takes an average of 2 weeks in lizards and snakes.

During the shedding process, the underlying newly formed outer layers are more permeable than at other times and this may lead to an increased risk of absorption of topical preparations and irritants.

A variety of physiological and environmental factors affect the success of ecdysis:

- **Age:** younger individuals often grow more quickly and shed more frequently than adults
- **Hydrational status:** dehydration will lead to dysecdysis
- **Local environment:** lack of abrasive substrate for snakes may prevent successful shedding; low humidity and low temperatures may retard shedding
- **Nutritional status:** hypoproteinaemia and hypovitaminosis A will lead to dysecdysis
- **Parasitism:** ectoparasites, such as *Ophionyssus natricis*, may cause repeated poor sheds
- **Seasonal influences:** e.g. daylight length, temperatures, rainfall/relative humidity
- **Systemic disease:** e.g. septicaemia, hormonal conditions
- **Wounds and scars:** may lead to retention of shed skin at the site of the wound, often for several cycles of shedding.

Dysecdysis

Dysecdysis is the term used to describe impaired shedding of the outer layers of the epidermis and is one of the most common conditions to affect reptile skin (Hellebuyck *et al.*, 2012). In snakes it may be taken that dysecdysis refers to any failure of the whole slough to come away in one attempt. In lizards and chelonians it is more difficult to evaluate, as these reptiles slough in a piecemeal fashion.

In lizards, however, extensive areas of sloughing, or evidence of multiple layers of keratin debris sloughing and the retention of slough over distal digits, tail tips and (if present) dorsal spines are indicative of dysecdysis. Indeed, the retention of sloughs around these small extremities commonly leads to gradual ischaemic necrosis as the dried slough contracts and the tissues swell. This is particularly common in leopard geckos and skinks. Eventually lizards so affected may lose these extremities permanently (Figure 15.1).

Skinks and geckos may have retained skin around the eyes, leading to conjunctivitis (see Chapter 16).

Frequent episodes of ecdysis may indicate a number of conditions, including hormonal problems such as hyperthyroidism, which has been reported in snakes (Frye, 1991), particularly older corn snakes.

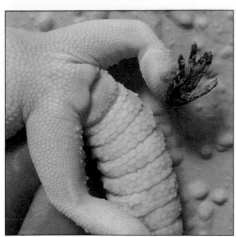

15.1 Dysecdysis with foot necrosis in a leopard gecko.

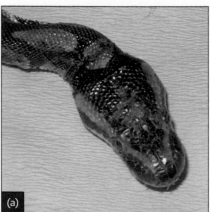

(a)

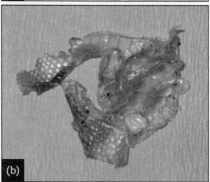

(b)

15.2 Dysecdysis in a royal python: (a) retained slough over the head and eyes; (b) slough following removal showing retained spectacles; (c) photomicrograph of a retained spectacle (arrowed) from a garter snake. (Haematoxylin and eosin stain; X10 objective)

Humidity

One of the many causes of dysecdysis is a low environmental relative humidity, leading to dehydration of the slough in the short term and dehydration of the reptile in the long term, particularly if it is coupled with inappropriate water provision (such as water bowls for drip feeders such as chameleons). Indeed, anything which may lead to dehydration can lead to a reduced lymphatic output during the process of ecdysis and so a reduction in the efficacy of the cleavage plane and dysecdysis. Therefore, one of the husbandry procedures that may be performed at the time of ecdysis is to raise the environmental humidity. This may be done by regular misting of the cage interior and the reptile (being aware of the difficulty in maintaining high relative humidity levels at higher environmental temperatures), provision of large-surface-area shallow trays of water for evaporative loss, and shallow warm-water bathing. In addition, the provision of a small enclosure (such as a plastic food container with a hole cut in the side) within the vivarium that can provide localized increased humidity, by means of a water-absorbent floor covering such as sphagnum moss or cotton wool, may also encourage shedding of retained sloughs. In the case of snakes with retained sloughs, encouraging the patient to move over a gently abrasive wet surface, such as a damp towel, can encourage shedding.

Retained spectacle

Retention of the ocular spectacle, commonly seen in snakes, can provide a challenge for the clinician (Figure 15.2). It is usually differentiated from the normal spectacle by its slightly wrinkled and more opaque appearance. Care should be taken, however, as previous ocular damage and dehydration may all leave a snake with a wrinkled non-retained spectacle.

A retained spectacle may be attached to the rest of a retained slough over the head of the snake and therefore may be removed after gently soaking the area in warm water, and peeling the slough with the spectacles away with moist cotton buds. Alternatively, if only the spectacles are retained, the author prefers using hypromellose (non-proprietary; a methyl-cellulose-containing tear replacer) eye drops to lubricate the spectacle, which may then be lifted gently from the lateral canthus with a moistened cotton bud or a blunt dental gingival probe. Extreme care should be taken not to damage the underlying normal spectacle.

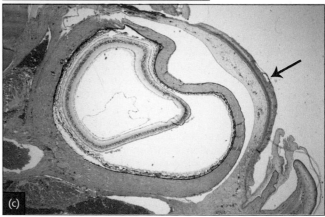

(c)

Clinical evaluation

Carrying out a skin work-up in a reptile is similar to that for a cat or dog. Obviously, specific conditions such as a retained slough are only found in reptiles, but the taking of a history and carrying out a clinical examination need to be logical so that important information is not missed. As home environment and nutrition are so important, owners must also be asked in detail about these aspects. In an ideal world a skin examination would be carried out as a work-up with appropriate time devoted to it; however, it is possible to ask owners questions while carrying out a basic work-up during a busy evening surgery.

History

Gaining a detailed history from the owner is extremely valuable. Questions about the origin (wild-caught *versus* captive-bred) of the reptile and its current environment (e.g. type of housing, substrate, heating source, relative humidity, diet) are vital to make a diagnosis. See Figure 15.3 for an example of a checklist that can be used.

Dermatology work-up

Date ....

Owner ....

Animal name/identity ....

Age ....

Species ....

Sex ....

Wild-caught/captive-bred ....

History:

Primary complaint...

Initial problem...

Areas affected:

Eyes ☐   Nose ☐   Mouth ☐   Abdomen ☐   Back ☐   Tail ☐   Digits ☐   Claws ☐

How long has the problem been present?...

Other animals kept and/or affected:..

Date of last normal and/or abnormal slough...

Any other health problems (e.g. weight loss, anorexia, etc.)..

Do owners have any skin lesions?..

Endoparasiticide/ectoparasiticide regime (if any):..

Housing and cleaning information:..

Products used:..

Is a UV light used? ....Type? ....Date last renewed?................................

Temperature range within the enclosure? ....

Is the heating ever turned off?...

Medications already prescribed:..

Reptile's regular diet?..

List type and frequency of any vitamins/supplements:...

Other comments ....

Clinical examination: Weight ....Body condition ....

Heart rate at preferred body temperature (PBT): ....Respiratory rate at PBT:..................

Primary lesions:

Macule ☐   Papule ☐   Fibriscess ☐   Patch ☐   Nodule ☐   Vesicle ☐   Plaque ☐

Bullae ☐   Wheal ☐   Tumour ☐   Cyst ☐   Stress bars on nails ☐

Secondary lesions:

Retained slough ☐   Scale ☐   Erosion ☐   Excoriation ☐   Sinus ☐   Crust ☐   Ulcer ☐   Fissure ☐

Reddening of skin ☐   Scar ☐   Callus ☐   Lichenification ☐   Hyperpigmentation ☐

Hyperkeratosis ☐   Hypopigmentation ☐   Necrosis ☐   Gangrene ☐

Skin changes:

Normal ☐   Thick ☐   Thin ☐   Fragile ☐

Configuration of lesions:

Linear ☐   Annular ☐   Follicular ☐   Grouped ☐   Other ☐

Other findings on examination:...

....

15.3   Reptile dermatology work-up checklist. (continued)   ▶

Laboratory:

Gross examination for parasites/use magnifying glass...

Tape – plain...

Tape – stained..

Impression smear...

Swab/scrape/culture...

Fine-needle aspirate of lump..

Faecal examination...

Biochemistry...

Haematology...

Blood culture...

Radiography..

Histopathology..

Viral work/PCR/ELISA/isolation..

Differential diagnosis..

....

....

Further investigation...

....

Treatment...

....

Review...

....

15.3 (continues) Reptile dermatology work-up checklist.

Examination

After a thorough physical examination (see Chapter 6), further investigation of any skin lesions may be performed. The dermatological examination of a reptile follows a similar protocol to that for cats and dogs.

The location and description of any lesions should be recorded accurately to allow monitoring of treatment. If possible, pictures should be taken to allow a comparison at review. A listing of the more commonly seen presenting signs, their possible aetiologies, diagnosis and treatment is given in Figure 15.4.

Ectoparasites such as leeches, ticks and mites may be observed with the naked eye. Mites in particular tend to accumulate in the folds of skin around the axillae and stifles in lizards, and around the rim of the eye or gular folds in snakes. Alternatively, mites may be seen floating in water bowls or baths. If in doubt, collection of surface debris may be attempted using adhesive tape strips pressed against the skin surface in multiple sites, before being adhered to a glass slide and examined microscopically.

Any moist lesions, such as ulcers, may be examined further using impression smears on glass slides. These may be stained with Gram's stain for bacterial evaluation, or a Giemsa-style stain (e.g. Diff-Quik®) to examine any cells present. In addition, samples of exudate may be collected for bacterial and fungal culture and sensitivity testing.

Skin biopsy may also be performed, and indeed is preferred for suspected fungal conditions and bacterial problems such as mycobacteriosis or dermatophilosis where culture of the causative organism may be difficult. Skin biopsy is possible under local anaesthetic with lidocaine, but it is preferable to sedate or anaesthetize the patient first. Wedge biopsies are easier to perform than punch biopsies, owing to the toughness of the scales and yet thin nature of the skin. Any biopsy material taken should be sufficient to allow one part to be placed in dilute formal saline for histopathological analysis, and the other to be sent for attempted fungal/bacterial culture and sensitivity testing.

In more complicated cases, and where budget and time allow, other analytical procedures such as radiography, ultrasonography, haematology and biochemical assessment are all helpful adjuncts to direct sampling.

Clinical sign	Possible causes	Diagnosis	Treatment options (depending on cause)
Blisters	Excessively damp environment; bacterial infections; parasites (e.g. cestodes and subcutaneous filarids); thermal burns	Aspirate sample aseptically for culture and sensitivity testing	Antibiosis – systemic and topical (e.g. silver sulfadiazine cream for burst blisters); anthelmintics; reduce environmental water content
Colour change	Trauma; injection-site reaction; systemic disease; ectoparasites; hypothermia; thermal burns; 'stress'	History; examination of vivarium; physical examination for mites (check water bowls)	No treatment for minor injection-site reactions; remove ectoparasites (treat with ivermectin for squamates); treat burns (topical silver sulfadiazine, fluid therapy, systemic antibiosis, dressings, surgical grafts)
Dysecdysis	Systemic disease; decreased relative humidity; ectoparasites; wounds	History; examination of vivarium; physical examination for mites (check water bowls) and wounds	Correct humidity; remove ectoparasites; correct systemic disease (e.g. fluid therapy for dehydration)
Epidermal/dermal separation	Iatrogenic hypervitaminosis A; renal disease; cachexia/hypoproteinaemia	History; species (boas and pythons re hypovitaminosis C); oedema, anuria, polyuria suggestive of renal disease	Treat as burns (fluid therapy, systemic antibiosis, topical silver sulfadiazine, analgesia, grafts/dressings); vitamin C injection 10–20 mg/kg q24h; renal disease see Chapter 20
Excessive sloughing	Iatrogenic hypervitaminosis A; hyperthyroidism	History; species (older corn snakes; green iguanas)	Methimazole 1–1.25 mg/kg orally q24h for 30 days (Frye, 1991) for hyperthyroidism, or surgical removal of adenoma
Nodule	Granuloma or abscess due to bacterial/fungal infection; subcutaneous parasite (e.g. filarial worm)	History; biopsy/fine-needle aspiration; radiography	Surgical removal of subcutaneous parasite; surgical removal of granuloma/abscess with systemic antibiosis based on culture/sensitivity; antibiotic-impregnated beads for deep/bone-associated infections (see Chapter 13)
Oedema	Vasculitis; septicaemia; renal disease; cardiovascular disease; bruising; infection	History; renal function tests; echocardiography	Systemic antibiosis, preferably based on culture/sensitivity, or using antibiotics effective against Gram-negative bacteria; diuretics for cardiovascular failure (see Chapter 19)
Patches	Burns; viral infection (grey patch disease in green turtles); avascular necrosis; injection-site reaction	History; examination of vivarium; species (green turtles)	No treatment for grey patch disease but separation of affected/unaffected individuals, reducing stocking density and improving environmental hygiene reduce severity of disease; treat large areas of skin necrosis as burns
Petechiation	Septicaemia; warfarin-derivative poisoning (snakes consuming poisoned prey); thrombocytopenia	History; blood sampling/culture and complete blood count; blood smear evaluation	Antimicrobial therapy based on blood culture/sensitivity or effective against Gram-negative bacteria in particular; vitamin K therapy; blood transfusion or use of haemoglobin products such as haemoglobin glutamer (Oxyglobin)
Swelling (discrete)	Abscess; granuloma; tumour; subcutaneous parasite	History; biopsy/fine-needle aspirate ± culture and sensitivity; radiography	Surgical excision of tumour/abscess; surgical removal of parasite; systemic antibiosis based on culture/sensitivity after removal of abscess/granuloma (focus on capsule for culture)
Ulceration	Trauma; bacterial disease ± septicaemia; parasite attachment site (e.g. leeches) Fungal disease (CANV)	History; physical examination for ectoparasites; microbial culture of abscess ± aseptically collected blood sample	Debridement with 0.05% chlorhexidine or 0.01% povidone iodine (latter effective against *Pseudomonas* spp.) under local/general anaesthesia; systemic antibiosis based on culture/sensitivity; manual removal of leeches/topical ivermectin; correct husbandry

15.4 A summary of the more commonly seen dermatological presentations.

Diseases

Viral infections

Viruses associated with skin disease include herpesvirus, papillomavirus, poxviruses, flavivirus and arenavirus (Jacobson, 2007; Maas, 2013).

Herpesvirus

A herpesvirus has been shown to be responsible for grey patch disease in green turtles (Rebell *et al.*, 1975). This condition is generally seen in individuals less than 3 months of age that are raised in pools. Clinically, papular lesions are seen anywhere on the body and gradually increase in size as the condition progresses. Owing to the epidemiology of the condition it has been suggested that it may be related to increased water temperature and overcrowding (Harkewicz, 2001). No cure has been demonstrated. Herpesviruses have also been isolated from oral lesions in tortoises (Cooper *et al.*, 1988).

Fibropapillomatous disease syndrome has been reported in loggerhead, hawksbill and olive ridley turtles (Jacobson and Origgi, 2002), caused by herpesvirus and not papillomavirus as previously believed. Multiple papillomas can affect the axillary and inguinal regions, the eyelids, conjunctiva and cornea, impairing vision and the ability to swim and feed. Since these lesions may lead to considerable fluid drag in the water, increased calorie usage and inevitable weight loss, individuals are often presented in poor body condition. Treatment includes nutritional support and fluid therapy, antimicrobial therapy and surgery, utilizing laser surgery if possible.

Papillomavirus

Viral particles similar to both Reoviridae and Papovaviridae have been found in papillomatous skin lesions (Hellebuyck *et al.*, 2012). Papovaviridae are now classified as Papillomaviridae and Polyomaviridae (Bernard *et al.*, 2010). Two main species of Papillomaviridae that are of interest are *Caretta caretta papillomavirus* 1, which is responsible for cutaneous papillomas in loggerhead sea turtles (*Caretta caretta*) and *Chelonia mydas papillomavirus* 1, which causes cutaneous fibropapillomas in green sea turtles (*Chelonia mydas*) (Herbst *et al.*, 1995; Herbst *et al.*, 2009; Rector and van Ranst, 2013).

Papillomaviruses have been isolated from European green lizards (Raynaud and Adrian, 1976) and side-necked turtles (Jacobson *et al.*, 1982), where they were associated with the development of papillomas, in the case of the lizards chiefly along the dorsal surface of the body.

A related virus, thought to be a papovavirus, has been associated with squamous papillomas in inland bearded dragons, presenting with firm crusty lesions over the body (Greek, 2001). This condition was noted to spread between in-contact reptiles.

Poxvirus

Poxviruses have been reported in a variety of species. Clinically poxviruses can cause necrotizing dermatitis; in some cases this has been reported to cause a chronic debilitating disease, whereas others regressed spontaneously. A Hermann's tortoise presented with papules on the eyelids and rostrum, associated with anorexia and weight loss (Orós *et al.*, 1998). It has been suggested that reptiles may carry the virus asymptomatically, and when stressed they can develop overt disease and shed the virus, or that arthropods may play a role in its transmission (Horner, 1988). Poxvirus lesions are generally self-limiting.

Flavivirus

Flaviviruses are transmitted by haematophagous arthropods and include the West Nile virus (WNV). American alligators infected with mosquito-transmitted WNV exhibit proliferative lymphohistiocytic cutaneous lesions.

Arenavirus

Arenaviruses (Bodewes *et al.*, 2013) are now thought to be the causal agent of inclusion body disease (IBD). They have been associated with dysecdysis in pythons, possibly due to the fact that the virus causes incoordination, which may prevent effective removal of the slough.

Bacterial infections

Bacterial skin conditions are commonly seen as secondary problems following traumatic wounds, or associated with poor/filthy husbandry conditions. They are exacerbated by excessive moisture, contamination of substrate, and the lowering of the reptile's immune system defences by inappropriate (usually too low) environmental temperatures and/or malnutrition. Many of the bacteria excreted from the digestive tract of reptiles may act as opportunistic pathogens (e.g. *Pseudomonas*, *Aeromonas*, *Salmonella*); therefore, regular and thorough cleansing of vivaria should be performed by owners to reduce the likelihood of wound contamination. Anaerobic bacteria such as *Clostridium*, *Bacteroides* and *Fusobacterium* spp. are part of the normal bacteria found on reptile skin, but they can also be involved in skin disease (Hellebuyck *et al.*, 2012).

Blister disease/vesicular dermatitis

This condition has been known by a variety of names, including blister disease, vesicular dermatitis, necrotizing dermatitis and scale rot. It is a condition of snakes, usually due to a high relative humidity, and has been associated with parasitism (both internal and external) and 'stress' (Branch *et al.*, 1998). Clinically affected snakes develop erythema and blistering of the scutes ventrally. These may burst and become secondarily infected, particularly in poor/filthy vivarium conditions, with resultant skin sloughing and even septicaemia (Figure 15.5). Diagnosis may be made based on careful history taking and clinical signs. Aseptic sampling of any unburst blisters and swabbing of any sores should be performed to attempt bacterial culture and sensitivity. Direct smears of aspirated vesicles should also be done to identify transcutaneous nematode penetration. Haematology and plasma biochemical analysis will rule out any concurrent disease conditions, which may affect the choice of a particular parenteral antibiotic.

Treatment is based on sensitivity testing and should be both topical and systemic in nature. Bathing in dilute chlorhexidine (0.05%) or povidone iodine (0.01%; more likely to be effective against *Pseudomonas* spp.) and provision of a paper substrate soaked in antiseptic may be useful for extensive sores. Initial debridement of wounds, with systemic antibiotics and creams such as silver sulfadiazine, is recommended.

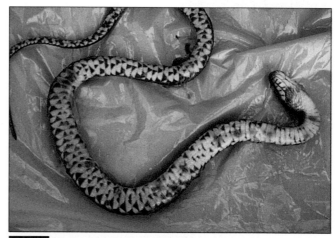

15.5 Blister disease in a garter snake.

Necrotic dermatitis/shell disease

This condition affects freshwater chelonians in particular and is caused by a variety of bacterial organisms, including *Aeromonas hydrophila*, *Citrobacter freundii* and *Serratia* spp.. These may gain access through abrasions to the skin and shell, caused by inappropriate substrates or due to continuous soaking of the shell and skin. The latter is often caused by a lack of a basking area for the turtle to haul itself out of the water. Feeding the turtle in its daytime tank may also lead to fouling of the water and an explosion in environmental bacteria, making this condition more likely. Clinically, the reptile presents with ulceration of the shell and skin; erythema of the scute suture lines may also be noticed, and some become lethargic and collapsed as septicaemia sets in. Other causes of shell ulceration that may lead to septicaemia include the ingestion of shellfish contaminated with the bacterium *Beneckea chitonovora* (Wallach, 1977). It has been suggested that trauma damages the blood supply of osteoscutes, resulting in tissue damage/death allowing secondary infection (Figure 15.6) (Maas, 2013). Terrestrial chelonians may suffer from shell necrosis due to haematogenous bacterial spread or by direct infection from untreated wounds (Figure 15.7).

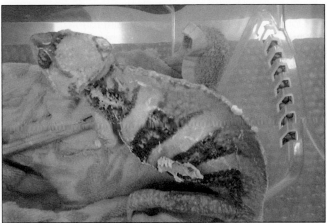

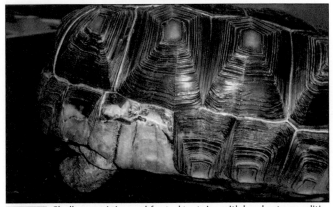

15.6 Casque osteomyelitis and dorsal spine necrosis in a panther chameleon with bacterial septicaemia and end arteriole disease.

15.7 Shell necrosis in a red-footed tortoise with local osteomyelitis as the result of shell trauma.

Treatment is based on systemic antibacterials chosen on the basis of sensitivity testing of samples from ulcers and, if septicaemia is suspected, an aseptically collected blood sample. Shell ulcers may be debrided under anaesthetic and packed with a waterproof paste (e.g. Orabase) mixed with an antibiotic such as amikacin or gentamicin (the author [SG] uses 2 g of antibiotic powder per 100 g of paste).

Abscessation

Infection of the skin will often result in abscessation. A variety of bacteria have been isolated from reptilian abs-cesses – mainly Gram-negative bacteria such as *Pseudomonas*, *Edwardsiella*, *Enterobacter*, *Escherichia coli*, *Klebsiella*, *Micrococcus* and *Salmonella* – but also some Gram-positive bacteria such as *Staphylococcus* and *Streptococcus*. Anaerobes such as *Bacteroides*, *Clostridium*, *Fusobacterium* and *Peptostreptococcus* have also been isolated.

The process by which reptiles deal with infection is different to that of mammals. In reptiles, the presence of infective material elicits an inflammatory response where fibrin exudes into the affected area, leading to the formation of granulomatous abscesses called 'fibriscesses' (Huchzemeyer and Cooper, 2001). Pathogens, however, can be trapped within this matrix of fibrin thus allowing a chronic infection to develop. This results in a solid appearance to reptile abscesses, instead of the liquid pus expected in mammals. Treatment of fibriscesses/abscesses is best performed by surgical excision (see Chapter 13) as their solid nature makes lancing impossible.

A common presentation of fibriscess/abscess formation is the aural abscess afflicting the middle ear of chelonians (Figure 15.8). This presents as a swelling of the tympanic membrane caudal to the eye, and may be associated with a suppressed immune system due to poor husbandry conditions (e.g. low environmental temperatures, poor nutrition). Treatment is best performed by surgical excision (see Chapter 13) coupled with systemic antibiotics.

A common condition reported in savannah monitor lizards is abscessation of the hindfeet with Gram-negative bacteria (Stahl, 2003). This has been associated with high humidity and an abrasive substrate. It often presents as dramatic swelling of the plantar surface, with cellulitis, and may quickly progress to osteomyelitis of the digits.

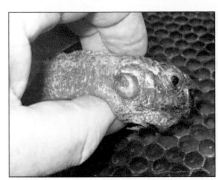

15.8 Aural abscess in a spur-thighed tortoise.

Dermatophilosis

Skin disease due to infection with *Dermatophilus congolensis* has been recorded in a variety of reptiles, including the inland bearded dragon, green iguana, collared lizard and common boa. *D. chelonae* has been isolated from captive chelonians (Masters *et al.*, 1995) and can be carried asymptomatically by the bearded dragon (Hellebuyck *et al.*, 2009). Typical lesions include hyperkeratosis, necrotic dermatitis and ulceration, although mortality has been recorded in agamids (Hellebuyck *et al.*, 2009). A recent outbreak associated with a Ranavirus was reported in a population of 100 inland bearded dragons resulting in the death of 15 reptiles with 50 affected with skin lesions (Tamukai *et al.*, 2016). The dermatophilus organism isolated in this case was *Austwickia chelonae*. It is rare for humans to be infected with dermatophilus organisms but they are considered zoonotic (Burd *et al.*, 2007).

Diagnosis by culture of the pathogen is difficult. Biopsy is the preferred tool for diagnosis, where the organism may be visualized using Gram's or periodic acid–Schiff (PAS) stains. Treatment based on culture and sensitivity is advised, although systemic enrofloxacin and topical diluted povidone iodine can be used (Origgi *et al.*, 1999).

Other bacteria-associated skin diseases

Other bacterial dermatological diseases include a necrotizing dermatitis and haemorrhagic lesions in captive turtles and crocodiles due to *Aeromonas hydrophila*, and swollen limbs and granuloma formation due to mycobacteria (Rossi, 1996; Griffin, 2000).

Mycobacterial skin conditions are uncommon in reptiles but have been reported in Egyptian spiny-tailed lizards, where *Mycobacterium marinum* produced a dermatitis and swelling of the joints, but the disease was not found systemically (Morales and Dunker, 2001). Joint swellings have also been reported in an inland bearded dragon found to be infected with *M. marinum* (Girling and Fraser, 2007). A variety of different species of reptile have been reported to carry *Mycobacterium* spp. (Ebani *et al.*, 2012).

Demonstration of mycobacterial infection is best performed by histological examination using acid-fast stains. *Salmonella* has been found to cause dermatitis in addition to fibriscess formation (Mader and DeRemer, 1993).

A filamentous Gram-positive bacterium referred to as *Devriesea agamarum* has also been associated with lip and skin-fold dermatitis and septicaemia in many uromastyx (Figure 15.9), causing chronic hyperkeratosis. It has also been shown to be carried and transmitted by healthy inland bearded dragons (Devloo *et al.*, 2011). Providing adequate basking temperatures (43–48.5°C) and systemic antibiosis with drugs such as ceftiofur, as well as keeping the vivarium dry and cleaning all crusts/debris, are required as the bacterium is resistant to fluoroquinolones and can survive for prolonged periods in the environment (Hellebuyck *et al.*, 2009; Hellebuyck *et al.*, 2011).

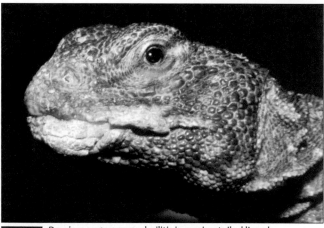

15.9 *Devriesea agamarum* cheilitis in a spiny-tailed lizard. (Courtesy of Paul Raiti)

Fungal infections

Fungal dermatitis is commonly observed in reptiles. Fungal spores are present in the environment and can continually contaminate healthy or damaged skin. Examination of the normal skin of 79 individual reptiles revealed 41 different fungal genera (Paré *et al.*, 2001). The most frequently isolated were *Aspergillus* spp., *Penicillium* spp. and *Paecilomyces lilacinus*. Fungi isolated from diseased tissue include *Aspergillus*, *Candida*, *Fusarium*, *Geotrichum*, *Oospora*, *Penicillium*, *Trichoderma*, *Trichophyton*, *Trichosporon*, *Alternaria* and *Sporothrix schenckii* (Cheatwood *et al.*, 1999; Nichols *et al.*, 1999; Rossi and Rossi, 2000). The primary fungal pathogen *Chrysosporium* anamorph of *Nannizziopsis vriesii* (CANV) which has now been reclassified will be discussed in more detail below.

Fungal dermatitis is often related to poor environmental conditions, such as excessively high humidity and inappropriate substrate of high organic content (e.g. damp hay/straw). Pre-existing wounds can also be a factor. Fungal dermatitis may be exacerbated by parasitism and malnutrition, confirming fungal pathogens as largely secondary opportunist pathogens.

Diagnosis

Visually, fungal dermatitis may resemble bacterial conditions, requiring the clinician to rely more on biopsy of affected areas. The skin surface should be wiped gently with dilute (0.05%) chlorhexidine to remove surface contaminants, and the biopsy performed under local or general anaesthetic. A minimum of two samples should be taken: one for histological examination in dilute formal saline, and the other for attempted culture and sensitivity. Histology should be performed using stains designed to highlight fungal elements, such as PAS.

Treatment

Treatment of fungal dermatitis includes correction of any underlying management problems such as humidity and substrate. Azoles such as ketoconazole, itraconazole and fluconazole (Mallo *et al.*, 2002) may be used systemically or topically, but it should be noted that ketoconazole has no effect against fungi such as *Aspergillus* spp. Itraconazole (1.5 mg/kg orally q36h) has been used successfully as an adjunct to surgical excision to treat a fungal granuloma in a corn snake (Girling, 2002). The use of metabolic scaling of itraconazole in reptiles has been described by Girling and Fraser (2009). Other topical medications include enilconazole, clotrimazole, dilute malachite green and acriflavine cream for treating superficial fungal infections. Topical application of dilute chlorhexidine can be useful and it may be applied to paper towels to cover the floor of a vivarium for species such as snakes and small lizards. A therapeutic challenge can be presented where patients such as turtles need to remain in water. The use of PC-7® epoxy paste applied over topical medication and a semi-occlusive dressing has been reported as successful (Neiffer *et al.*, 1998).

CANV

In recent years, *Chrysosporium* anamorph of *Nannizziopsis vriesii* (CANV) has been reported as a primary pathogen causing a severe or fatal dermatomycosis in a number of different species (Mitchell and Walden, 2013), including brown tree snakes (Nichols *et al.*, 1999), veiled chameleons, tentacle snakes, saltwater crocodiles, leopard geckos (Toplon *et al.*, 2012), inland bearded dragons (Bowman *et al.*, 2007), green iguanas (Abarca *et al.*, 2008) and a girdled lizard (Hellebuyck *et al.*, 2010). It has been shown that CANV is only rarely found on the skin of reptiles, but can affect terrestrial, semiaquatic and aquatic species (Paré *et al.*, 2003). Toplon *et al.* (2012) demonstrated that affected animals tend to be younger, recently wild-caught or crowded animals. CANV has been shown to be zoonotic to immunosuppressed individuals (Mitchell and Walden, 2013). Further molecular analyses revealed that the CANV pathogens belong in well-supported clades corresponding to three lineages within the family Onygenaceae of the order Onygenales (Sigler *et al.*, 2013). One lineage represents the genus *Nannizziopsis* and comprises *N. vriesii*, *N. guarroi*, and six additional species seen in skin disease of chameleons, geckos, crocodiles, agamid and iguanid lizards. Two other lineages comprise the genus *Ophidiomyces*, with the species *Ophidiomyces ophiodiicola* occurring only in snakes, and the genus *Paranannizziopsis* gen. nov., with species infecting squamates and tuataras. The newly described species seen in reptiles are *Nannizziopsis crocodili* (salt water crocodiles), *Nannizziopsis barbata* (coastal bearded dragon), *Nannizziopsis dermatitidis* (chameleons and geckos), *Nannizziopsis draconii* (inland bearded dragon), *Nannizziopsis chlamydospora* (inland bearded dragon), *Paranannizziopsis californiensis* (snakes), *Paranannizziopsis australasiensis* (tuatara and bearded dragons) and *Paranannizziopsis crustacea* (snakes). *Chrysosporium longisporum* has been reclassified as *Paranannizziopsis longispora* and has been reported in snakes. *N. guarroi* causes yellow fungus disease, a common infection in bearded dragons and green iguanas, and *O. ophiodiicola* is an emerging pathogen of captive and wild snakes (so called 'white nose disease') (Sigler *et al.*, 2013; Cabanes *et al.*, 2014).

Clinical signs of infection include dermatitis with ulceration, discoloration and nodule development, which can progress into a cellulitis (Figure 15.10). Diagnosis is based on histology, culture and polymerase chain reaction (PCR). Histologically, multifocal epidermal hyperplasia and hyperkeratosis are seen, along with epidermal degeneration, necrosis and intraepidermal vesicles. Hyphae may also be seen and can extend into the underlying tissue. Culture can be difficult owing to the presence of contaminant fungi; selective fungal culture media should be used.

Treatment with itraconazole or voriconazole has been described (Van Waeyenberghe *et al.*, 2010; Hellebuyck *et al.*, 2010).

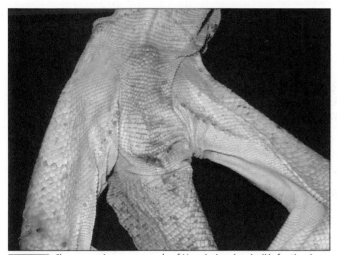

15.10 *Chrysosporium* anamorph of *Nannizziopsis vriesii* infection in a green iguana. Note yellow lesions on the ventral surface of the right hindlimb.

Algal infections

Algae can be found normally on the skin of reptiles such as aquatic turtles, but they may colonize wounds with resultant granuloma formation and shell necrosis. Superficial lesions may be removed manually, with a dilute solution of povidone iodine.

Parasites

A description of reptile parasites is included elsewhere in this text (see Chapter 24). The following section will examine those parasites that have a direct effect on the skin.

Ectoparasites

Mites: Snake and lizard mites are probably the most commonly observed ectoparasites on reptiles in general practice. The snake mite *Ophionyssus natricis* is ubiquitous and can often be found on lizards as well as snakes. Other species, such as *Hirstiella* spp., have also been reported in green iguanas (Stahl, 2003).

Mites are commonly uncovered around the spectacle and in the gular folds of snakes, and in the axillae and stifle skin folds of lizards. Physical damage to the skin as the mite feeds causes irritation, swelling, erythema and secondary bacterial infection. This may lead to dysecdysis,

and transmission of disease, for example *Aeromonas hydrophila* septicaemia (Rossi, 1996), haemoparasites and, hypothetically, IBD. Affected snakes may spend more time bathing in water bowls, as this gives temporary relief from the irritation.

Other mites that may be observed include harvest mites (*Neotrombicula autumnalis*) (Figure 15.11) and chigger mites (*Eutrombicula alfreddugesi* and *Trombicula irritans*), particularly in reptiles with access to the outdoors, but also in vivarium-housed reptiles that have hay, wood chips or straw as substrate. Johnson-Delaney (1996) reported dermatitis due to these mites in snakes, lizards and box turtles. The dermatitis is usually associated with the nymphal stages (often coloured red–orange), which attach to the reptile for dispersal reasons and coincidentally cause irritation, as on other domestic pets.

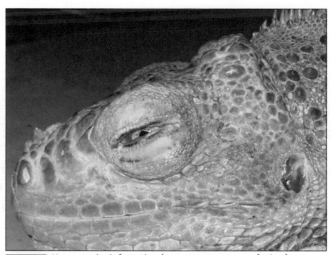

15.11 Harvest mite infestation (orange aggregates of mites) resulting in pruritus, self trauma and periocular oedema in a green iguana.

Treatment: Therapy for snake and lizard mites involves treating both the patient and the environment, as substantial portions of mite life cycles are spent off the host. Bathing the patient in warm water will remove some of the mites and should be followed by oral or subcutaneous ivermectin (DeNardo and Wozniak, 1997). The environment may also be sprayed with ivermectin diluted in water at 5 mg/l (it may first be diluted in a small volume of propylene glycol at a ratio of 1:2 to improve solubility). It should be noted that ivermectin is toxic to chelonians and should not be used for them (Teare and Bush, 1983; Szell *et al.*, 2001).

Topical pyrethroid and pyrethrin powders have also been used to treat mites in reptiles, but there have been reports of toxicity (principally due to poor ventilation post-application) (DeNardo and Wozniak, 1997).

Fipronil has also been used successfully by the authors and others to treat mites in snakes. Caution should be observed as the drug is in a strong alcohol carrier base and this may be irritant to delicate mucous and respiratory membranes. In addition, the drug has not been sufficiently tested to verify its safety margin in reptiles. The spray is applied to a gauze cloth and then wiped over the surface of the reptile, repeated at 2-week intervals on three or four occasions.

Ticks: Ticks are more commonly observed in wild-caught specimens and on animals that have regular access to the outside, and some species from the genera *Amblyomma*,

Aponomma and *Hyalomma* have been found on reptiles introduced into the USA (Burridge and Simmons, 2003). Some ticks (*Amblyomma marmoreum* and *A. sparsum*) transmit the rickettsial organism *Cowdria ruminantium*, the cause of heartwater disease (Burridge and Simmons, 2001). The relapsing fever tick (*Ornithodoros turicata*), Western black-legged tick (*Ixodes pacificus*) and *Ixodes ricinus* have all been found on reptiles (Johnson-Delaney, 1996). They are frequently found attached to loose skin around the base of the neck and in inguinal regions in chelonians, and around the head and neck in lizards. They cause local trauma, inflammation and secondary infection of the skin, which may result in abscess or granuloma formation.

Ticks may be removed by gentle manual removal, using a commercial tick remover or haemostat forceps and grasping the head close to the site of attachment, or by applying an acaricide such as fipronil directly on to the tick. Once dead, the tick is more easily removed.

Myiasis/fly strike: Maggots of flies such as *Phormia* spp., botflies and *Cistudinomyia cistudinis* can affect reptiles and chelonians in particular. Affected animals often suffer from faecal soiling or diarrhoea, which tends to attract flies to lay their eggs. Clinical signs include skin damage around the area of soiling, anorexia, presence of maggots and evidence of secondary septicaemia (such as reddening of scutes). Botflies often create discrete swellings with a central breathing hole. Treatment includes manual removal, cleaning and debridement of wounds. This may require sedation or light anaesthesia. Supportive therapy, including systemic broad-spectrum antibiosis and aggressive fluid therapy, is also advised.

Leeches: Leeches may also be seen on wild-caught reptiles, particularly aquatic/semiaquatic species. Clinical signs are similar to those for tick infestation, including secondary skin infections. There is also a risk of transmission of haemoparasites. Removal of the leech may be achieved manually after application of local anaesthetic, or topical ivermectin applied to the leech. Topical antibacterial creams such as silver sulfadiazine and systemic antibacterial medications effective against Gram-negative bacteria (e.g. fluoroquinolones, aminoglycosides) are recommended.

Endoparasites

Tapeworm larvae: The larval stages of cestodes (plerocercoids or spargana) of the family Diphyllobothriidae may be found in the subcutaneous and muscle layers of the skin, causing swellings resulting from bullae or cyst formation. They are found mainly in snakes imported from Australia, South America and East Asia. Treatment may be attempted with surgical removal of larvae and preferably treating with oral praziquantel (Rossi, 1996).

Tongue worms: Pentastomes are arthropod parasites of the respiratory tract of vertebrates (Paré, 2008), which can in some instances cause skin lesions when they burrow out of the animal. Pentastomes are also called tongue worms owing to the resemblance of one particular Genus of species (*Linguatula*) to the mammalian tongue, not because they affect the tongue. Larger carnivorous snakes, lizards and crocodilians are more likely to be affected, in particular wild-caught specimens. The infection is zoonotic (*Armillifer* and *Porocephalus* spp.); for this reason, and because the parasite is difficult to eradicate, serious thought should be given to whether the patient should be euthanased. However, in small numbers tongue

worms rarely seem to cause serious disease and, as they are spread via an intermediate prey host, spread within a collection is unlikely. Other options include oral or subcutaneous ivermectin, the use of other medications such as praziquantel, levamisole or tiabendazole and/or surgical removal under anaesthetic.

Flukes and filarial worms: Trematodes and filarial worms can cause skin disease due to the development of ischaemic necrosis following obstruction of an end arteriole by trematode eggs or by microfilariae released into the circulation. Clinically the condition is seen as swelling of the affected area followed by necrotizing dermatitis. Treatment may be difficult, due to the rapid development of ischaemic necrosis. Filarial infection may be treated by surgical removal of subcutaneous adults followed by ivermectin administration. Trematode infection may be treated with praziquantel. However, both these treatments may cause release of toxins and debris from dying worms and this, in itself, may lead to local and systemic damage.

Systemic diseases

Systemic disease may present as a dermatological problem, either directly related to the underlying problem or where there is a common predisposing factor.

- Any condition that causes protein loss (e.g. nephropathies, enteropathies or hepatic failure) may cause oedema with resultant swelling of the skin, particularly over the limbs.
- Oedema and skin swelling may also be seen with circulatory failure such as primary heart disease.
- Dehydration can be detected by a tightening of the skin and loss of elasticity.
- Cachexia and weight loss may also result in loss of skin elasticity, but is generally accompanied by an increase in the number of skin folds.

Septicaemia

Infection resulting in septicaemia can cause petechiation and ecchymosis (Figure 15.12). Initially these are seen ventrally in the interscalar or interscutal area, where the keratin layers are thinnest, but they can spread over the entire body. Jaundice may be detected as a yellowing of the interscalar area, although this is less common.

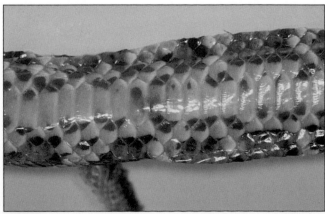

15.12 Petechiae and ecchymosis in an emaciated Burmese python with septicaemia.

Vascular obstruction

Parasites and bacteria may be associated with necrotizing dermatitis due to blockage of blood vessels and ischaemic necrosis (see above).

Hyperthyroidism

Hyperthyroidism has been associated with an increase in the rate of skin turnover and may present as an increased frequency of ecdysis, particularly in snakes. In a green iguana, hyperthyroidism was associated with a loss of the dorsal spines, as well as weight loss, increased aggression, tachycardia and polyphagia. The diagnosis was made based on clinical signs, a palpable thyroid and T4 levels of 30 nmol/l (normal reference range for *Calotes* and *Sceloporus* lizards 0.21–6.78 nmol/l) (Hernandez-Divers et al., 2001). Surgical removal of the adenoma resulted in regrowth of the dorsal spines, suggesting this was a hormonally induced condition.

Hypothyroidism

Hypothyroidism may lead to myxoedema, particularly in giant chelonians (Frye, 1991).

Husbandry-related problems

Husbandry-related skin problems are common (Hoppman, 2007); some common factors are listed in Figure 15.13. Nutrition-related problems are discussed separately, below.

Abrasions

These are commonly observed on the rostrum, starting off as traumatic injuries that rapidly become secondarily infected. They are more commonly found in highly active species (e.g. Asian water dragons) which are easily startled, and in many species of snake that seem to have an inability to perceive the solid nature of transparent glass or Perspex walls. Early lesions may be treated successfully using a combination of topical and systemic antibiotic therapy after initial debridement of the wound(s) under anaesthetic. If allowed to progress, however, the wounds may involve deeper structures, allowing osteomyelitis to occur, with a resultant worsening of the prognosis.

Bite wounds

Bites from live prey items may indicate an underlying pathology, or the reptile may be overfed and leave some prey alive. In the UK it is currently virtually illegal to feed live vertebrate prey, such as small mammals, to predators such as snakes, but instances and injuries do still occur. In addition, outdoor chelonians may be subject to dog and fox attacks. In small fine-skinned lizards, such as geckos, larger insect prey may also inflict wounds, particularly when the reptile is debilitated or anorexic, prompting the clinician to investigate further. A variety of bacterial and fungal contaminants may be isolated from any wounds. Treatment is based on systemic antibacterial therapy, debridement and wound closure, often in stages if there is heavy contamination of the wound, and the use of topical medications such as silver sulfadiazine, dilute chlorhexidine and acriflavine ointment.

Contact dermatitis

The use of substrates such as highly resinous cedar chips, or residues of cleaning fluids such as bleaches, may result in the formation of an irritant contact dermatitis. This will present as erythema between the scales, with fluid exuding from inflamed skin, petechial haemorrhage, blister formation and secondary infection. Treatment includes removal of the causal agent, copious flushing of any wounds with isotonic warmed fluids, and treating the wound(s) as for a thermal burn (see Burns, below).

Factor	Potential problems
Vivarium material	• Lack of water repellence • Excessively abrasive surfaces
Vivarium design	• Poor ventilation • Lack of visual barriers to prevent rostral trauma on vivarium walls • Sharp internal edges • Crevices/corners preventing adequate cleaning
Heat sources	• Unprotected focal heat sources • Lack of sufficient basking areas • Heat sources that also function as light provision
Mixing of species or sexes	• Intraspecific or interspecific fighting
Number of individuals housed	• Some species are aggressive and should be housed singly (e.g. kingsnakes)
Prey	• Feeding live vertebrate prey to snakes, which is virtually illegal in the UK, can lead to prey-induced injury • Small insectivorous lizards may be attacked by large insect prey
Substrate	• Soil/peat-based substrates may make it difficult to maintain hygiene levels and may carry a high microorganism load • Cedar wood chips are highly resinous, which may be irritant to delicate-skinned reptiles such as geckos
Vivarium plants	• Irritation • Toxicity
Humidity	• Excessively high humidity with poor hygiene may lead to blister disease • Excessively low humidity may lead to desiccation in semiaquatic species and dysecdysis even in desert species (e.g. leopard geckos require a focal area of raised humidity when sloughing)
Temperature	• Extremely high temperatures will lead to dysecdysis and sudden death through dehydration • Low temperatures lead to reduced metabolism, reduced sloughing and increased susceptibility to opportunistic infections

15.13 Husbandry factors associated with skin disease.

Overgrown claws or beak

These may be seen in cases where a juvenile reptile has been fed an excessively high calorie/protein-containing diet, leading to over-rapid growth. They may also be seen in chelonians kept and fed on smooth surfaces, where lack of abrasion prevents claw and beak wear. Trimming of claws, using proprietary cat claw clippers, is possible. Care should be taken not to trim certain species intended for breeding, such as male red-eared terrapins where the forelimb claws are used for mating display purposes. Beaks may be trimmed using commercial grinding tools, or dental drills.

Vascular injuries

Frostbite may be a problem in outdoor species, such as chelonians, that have been left outdoors overnight in late summer/early autumn. This leads to a number of problems, including central nervous system damage leading to blindness and vestibular disease, but may also result in damage to surface vessels, with resultant tissue necrosis of the extremities. Treatment is based on the use of analgesics and peripheral circulation stimulants, such as topical preparations containing yeast extracts, or oral medications such as isoxsuprine at 2–5 mg/kg q24h in an attempt to prevent vascular necrosis. Once necrosis has occurred, distal extremities may slough, and systemic antibiosis with topical dressings or even surgery may be required to encourage healing to occur.

Humidity

Excessively high humidity may result in blister disease and other conditions mentioned above. Excessively low humidity levels, particularly where access to free water is re-stricted, may also lead to desiccation and secondary dermatitis in species such as freshwater and soft-shelled turtles.

Fly strike/myiasis

Filthy conditions, and unobserved/untreated diarrhoea or excessive faecal soiling may all attract blowflies (see above). Owners should be instructed to perform regular careful examinations of captive reptiles; bathing soiled animals should be encouraged, as well as vivarium hygiene.

Lawnmower/strimmer injuries

Strimmers and rotary lawnmowers may induce severe lacerating injuries, particularly in outdoor chelonians. Treatment may involve extensive reconstructive shell surgery, with concomitant antibiosis, fluid therapy and analgesia. In addition, aquatic species may be subject to speedboat rotor damage in the wild.

Burns

Burns may occur under a variety of conditions:

- Close/direct contact with an unprotected focal heat or light source
- Chemical agents
- Faulty electrical equipment.

Heated simulated rocks with faulty thermostats have been associated with ventral burns in a number of reptiles. It has been suggested that reptiles do not have the same withdrawal reflex as mammals and do not recognize that the heat source is burning the skin (Mader, 1998). However, it may also indicate that a reptile is weak or lethargic and that there is something else clinically wrong. It is essential therefore to perform a full clinical examination of any patient that presents with burns, to determine if there is an underlying cause.

Clinically, burns can be classified according to the depth of damaged tissue.

First-degree burns:

- Superficial: damage confined to the epidermis
- Clinical signs: sloughing of damaged scales; erythema; colour change suggestive of bruising
- Damaged tissue heals in around 4 weeks
- Damaged tissue shed at next ecdysis.

Second-degree burns:

- Damage to underlying dermis as well as epidermis
- Clinical signs: as above plus blistering. Blisters may rupture, with loss of tissue fluid, and often become secondarily infected
- Healing is prolonged, taking 6–8 weeks
- Results in scab formation and scar development.

Third-degree burns:

- Destruction of epidermis, dermis and underlying adnexal structures. Destruction of associated nerves may lead to lack of pain sensation, which may lead to inadvertent self-trauma of the fragile wound
- Secondary bacterial and/or fungal infection is inevitable
- It can take >6 months for contraction and scar formation to occur (Figure 15.14)
- Overlying healed skin can take on a white or black appearance, due to the presence/absence of pigment cells moving in to the repairing wound.

Treatment: This is similar to that for mammals. Acute rapid cooling of burning skin is required, with the application of a cold compress for 15–20 minutes to reduce further burning and limit tissue swelling.

Where blisters form, every effort should be made to minimize trauma and resultant rupture so as to limit tissue fluid loss and prevent secondary infection. Topical therapy, such as dilute chlorhexidine (0.05%) and silver sulfadiazine cream, along with the use of non-adherent sterile dressings, is advised to limit secondary infection. Silver sulfadiazine is particularly useful owing to its broad-spectrum activity and its efficacy against *Pseudomonas* – common contaminants of serious burns in reptiles – as well as its ability to reduce

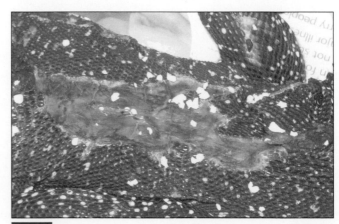

15.14 Third-degree burn in a monitor lizard.

further fluid loss by evaporation. Patients should also be kept on non-adherent substrates and so removed from bark chips etc. to minimize further wound trauma and infection; an empty glass enclosure is the simplest to keep clean. Parenteral fluid therapy, preferably intraosseous or intravenous, is required for second- and third-degree burns.

For extensive wounds, a semipermeable hydroactive wound dressing (e.g. Granuflex®) may be used to cover defects. For snakes, where dressings are difficult to apply, this may be sutured directly to healthy skin surrounding the wound; in other reptiles it can be bandaged in place. Such dressings prevent maceration of the wound by drawing fluids away from the wound surface. The fluid is held in a stable hydrocolloid gel within the dressing, so maintaining humidity levels and encouraging re-epithelialization. Other products that have been used widely in reptile medicine and surgery include the porcine xenograft dressing Vet BioSISt®, a sterile non-allergenic dressing that may be sutured over extensive wounds to provide a semipermeable membrane, protecting the granulation bed and encouraging rapid epithelialization. Analgesia, antibiotics and treatment for shock may also be required. Treatment can take anything from weeks to months, so owners need to be prepared for this.

Wounds

Wounds will arise for a number of reasons, in association with other disease or due to trauma. Stages of wound healing in reptiles are similar to those in mammals. The temperature at which reptiles are kept will obviously influence the rate at which healing takes place and the efficiency of the immune system in fighting any infection. Animals should also be kept at the correct level of humidity for their species. Basic husbandry and cleanliness apply. Consideration should be given to the location of the wound and the effect that this will have on future sheds.

Any foreign material that is present should be removed either consciously or under anaesthesia, depending on the species and temperament of the individual. Wounds can be flushed in a manner similar to that used in cats and dogs, utilizing 0.05% chlorhexidine, 0.1% iodine or sterile saline. Care should be taken not to force any foreign material further into the wound. Once cleaned, fresh lacerations can be sutured using an everting suture pattern and non-absorbable suture material. Drains are not often used in reptiles as they are not found to work well (Wellehan, 2005). Antibiotic therapy should also be implemented. Adhesive dressings can be used to protect the wound from environmental contamination if required.

Honey or sugar bandages have been used to slough dead tissue and promote healing in reptiles (Rudloff, 2005). Topical medications can be used; OpSite Spray can be used to protect wounds and is useful as it can be left in place until the next shed takes place. Ointments should be avoided as they have been associated with granuloma formation (Smith et al., 1988).

In the event of carapacial fractures radiographs should be made and carefully explored to identify any deeper trauma that may have occurred to the lungs.

Nutrition-related skin disease

Hypovitaminosis A

This is seen more commonly in aquatic or semiaquatic carnivorous chelonians, such as the red-eared terrapin and box turtle, as their captive diets are often suboptimal, frequently comprising unsupplemented meat and little

else. The condition affects dermal structure resulting in circumoral and occasionally body hyperkeratosis, palpebral oedema, xerophthalmia, conjunctivitis, ulcerative cheilitis, lethargy and anorexia (see Chapter 16). Treatment for chelonians is with vitamin A at 2000 IU/kg orally. Care should be taken not to overdose vitamin A. The best form of treatment is to correct the diet.

Chameleons have also been recorded with hypovitaminosis A, presenting with periocular dysecdysis. These were treated successfully with parenteral vitamin A (200 IU/30 g) on two occasions, 7 days apart (Harkewicz, 2001).

Iatrogenic hypervitaminosis A

This results from overdosage of parenteral vitamin A (doses recorded >10,000 IU/kg). Clinically, the condition presents with patches of dry skin and dysecdysis over the neck and limbs in chelonians. This may result in full-thickness sloughing of the skin with weeping wounds resembling second- and third-degree burns. Treatment should be along the lines of that for serious burns, with dressings, fluid therapy and covering antibiosis (see Burns above).

Hypovitaminosis C

This has been reported in anorexic/cachectic pythons and boas (Frye, 1991) and may be associated with a collagen defect. The condition presents with full-skin-thickness spontaneous ruptures, particularly over the dorsum. Treatment of the wounds by suturing/gluing and administration of 10–20 mg/kg vitamin C per day is advised.

Hypovitaminosis E

This is commonly seen with diets high in polyunsaturated fats, such as in piscivorous reptiles fed fish with a high oil content, particularly where rancidity may be present. Affected individuals show signs of steatitis, with sloughing of the skin, necrosis, granulation of subcutaneous fat deposits and opportunistic secondary infections. Treatment may be attempted with dietary change alongside vitamin E supplementation at doses of 1 IU/kg (Donoghue and McKeown, 1999).

Biotin deficiency

This may be found in species, such as monitor lizards, that consume large amounts of unfertilized eggs containing the anti-biotin hormone avidin. Although the main clinical signs are associated with neurological disease, there is often weakening and fracturing of keratin structures such as nails and abnormal sloughing. Treatment is by correction of the diet and biotin supplementation.

Hypocalcaemia/hypovitaminosis D

Feeding diets low in calcium and/or vitamin D, but with high energy content (see Excessive calorie or protein intake, below), can result in rapid growth and the development of shell deformities and soft shells, and rapid shedding of skin and scutes. Prevention is geared to ensuring correct calcium and energy contents in the diet, particularly in growing reptiles, and sufficient exposure to short-wavelength ultraviolet (UVB) light for vitamin D synthesis (see Chapters 4 and 22). However, once changes in the structure of dermal bone and scutes have occurred, they are extremely difficult to reverse, and abnormalities may be lifelong.

Excessive calorie or protein intake

Too high a calorie or protein content in the diet will result in rapid growth of beaks, shells and claws in chelonians (see Hypocalcaemia/hypovitaminosis D, above). Restriction of protein levels and calorie intake is necessary. Low relative humidity has also been shown to interact with high protein/calorie levels in this condition (see Chapters 4 and 22).

Neoplasia

Papillomas, fibropapillomas and squamous papillomas are discussed above (Herpesvirus and Papillomavirus sections).

Mast cell tumours are rare in reptiles but have been recorded in an iguana (Reavill *et al.*, 2000). Another rare condition is a cutaneous liposarcoma, which has been recorded in a boa and a chameleon (Reavill *et al.*, 2002). Multiple subcutaneous masses were found over the entire body. Reptiles have also been seen to develop squamous cell carcinomas, sometimes preceded by the development of a mass resembling a cutaneous horn, as described in humans (see Chapter 23). Bearded dragons have been specifically reported with squamous cell carcinomas with a predilection for the mucocutaneous junction of the periocular area (Hannon, 2011). Other reported skin neoplasms include fibromas (Figure 15.15), cutaneous melanomas (which appear to be often malignant, particularly in snakes) and epitheliomas.

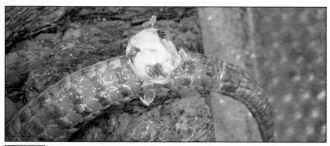

15.15 Benign slow-growing fibroma on the tail of a Berber skink.

Congenital and inherited conditions

Congenital cutaneous abnormalities may occur due to genetic aberrations, such as albinism and amelanism, which are frequently specifically bred.

Improper incubation conditions can also result in abnormalities. Eggs incubated at high environmental temperatures resulted in scale or scute abnormalities (Millichamp, 1989) such as clefting of scutes or abnormal colour patterns (Hammack, 1991). Incubation of eggs at low environmental humidity may be linked with pyramiding of the shell. Indeed, chelonian hatchlings placed on heat mats often show faster growth rates of the plastron than of the carapace.

An autosomal recessive scale agenesis has been reported (Rossi, 1996), as has amelanism in a Hermann's tortoise (Silvestre and Soler, 2001). An ichthyosis-like dermatopathy has been recorded in a California desert tortoise, although histology was not carried out to confirm this clinical diagnosis (Frye, 1991).

Miscellaneous

Impaction of the temporal gland in chameleons

The temporal gland in some species of chameleon is located at the lateral commissures of the mouth; it is a holocrine gland of dermal origin. The functions of this gland are variable; secretions can be used in defence, to mark territory and to attract insects. Impaction of the glands results in abscess formation, which may affect the orbit of the eye owing to its proximity (Klaphake, 2001). Possible causes of impaction include poor husbandry and diet, including hypovitaminosis A. Treatment involves manual removal of impacted material. The area is very vascular and profuse haemorrhage is common.

Leucoderma

This is the presence of abnormal white skin or scales following trauma such as severe infections, bites and burns. It is important to acknowledge that injections such as ketamine and enrofloxacin may cause chemical burns or irritation that can lead to the development of leucoderma.

Cutaneous dyskeratosis in tortoises

This has been reported in wild-caught desert tortoises (Jacobson *et al.*, 1994). Clinically, the shell developed a white/grey discoloration with a roughened flaky appearance. It was suggested that these lesions were due to a deficiency of vitamin A or zinc, or possibly an unknown toxicity.

Mineralized skin lesions

The presentation of mineralization within the skin may be classified according to the clinical findings:

- Calcinosis cutis describes the deposition of inorganic calcium and phosphate ions, and possibly other mineral salts, in the dermis, epidermis or subcutis (Reavill and Schmidt, 2002)
- Calcinosis circumscripta describes the formation of nodules of calcium deposition subcutaneously.

Calcinosis cutis and circumscripta have been described in various species of lizard (e.g. chameleons) (Reavill and Schmidt, 2002). The cases presented with multifocal crusting and thickened skin that, when it sloughed, left areas of ulceration and petechial haemorrhage. Discrete masses filled with white liquid crystalline material have also been reported.

The pathology behind calcium and mineral deposition in the skin is complicated. Dystrophic calcification can occur in damaged or necrotic tissue. Metastatic calcification may occur due to an abnormality in calcium metabolism, such as renal secondary hyperparathyroidism; hypervitaminosis D; or any condition leading to excessively high calcium to phosphorus ratios, including excessive dietary supplementation.

Fluoroquinolone toxicity

Administration of fluoroquinolones (e.g. enrofloxacin, marbofloxacin) to hatchling or juvenile chelonians can result in shell abnormalities. In chelonians and other reptiles, skeletal abnormalities may arise due to the ability of fluoroquinolone to cause cartilage growth derangement (see data sheets). Care should therefore be taken in using fluoroquinolones in juvenile reptiles.

Immune reactions

Experimentally induced skin reactions have been demonstrated in anoles (Cope, 2000). Topical application of a hapten of low molecular weight resulted in an Arthus (Type III) immune-mediated reaction, with swelling 4 hours after application. This suggests that immune-mediated conditions are a possibility in reptile species, but the clinical applications of these findings remain to be identified.

References and further reading

Abarca ML, Martorell J, Castella G, Ramis A and Cabanes FJ (2008) Cutaneous hyalohyphomycosis caused by a *Chrysosporium* species related to *Nannizziopsis vriesii* in two green iguanas (*Iguana iguana*). *Medical Mycology* **46**, 349–354

Bernard HA, Burk RD, Chen Z et al. (2010) Classification of papillomaviruses (PVs) based on 189 PV types and proposal of taxonomic amendments. *Virology* **401**, 70–79

Bodewes R, Kik MJ, Raj VS et al. (2015) Detection of novel divergent arenaviruses in boid snakes with inclusion body disease in the Netherlands. *Journal of General Virology* **96(6)**, 1206–1210

Bowman MR, Paré JA, Sigler L et al. (2007) Deep fungal dermatitis in three inland bearded dragons (*Pogona vitticeps*) caused by the *Chrysosporium* anamorph of *Nannizziopsis vriesii*. *Medical Mycology* **45**, 371–376

Branch S, Hall L, Blackshear P and Chernoff N (1998) Infectious dermatitis in a ball python (*Python regius*). *Journal of Zoo and Wildlife Medicine* **29**, 461–464

Brown DR, Lackovich JK and Klein PA (1999) Further evidence for the absence of papillomaviruses from sea turtle fibropapillomas. *Veterinary Record* **145**, 616–617

Burd EM, Juzych LA, Rudrik JT et al. (2007) Pustular dermatitis caused by *Dermatophilus congolensis*. *Journal of Clinical Microbiology* **45**, 1655–1658.

Burridge MJ and Simmons LA (2001) Control and eradication of exotic tick infestations on reptiles. *Proceedings of the Association of Reptilian and Amphibian Veterinarians Annual Conference*, pp. 21–23

Burridge MJ and Simmons LA (2003) Exotic ticks introduced into the United States on imported reptiles from 1962 to 2001 and their potential roles in international dissemination of diseases. *Veterinary Parasitology* **113**, 289–320

Cabanes, FJ, Sutton DA, Guarro J (2014) *Chrysosporium*–related fungi and reptiles: A fatal attraction. *PLOS Pathogens* **10**, e1004367

Cheatwood JL, Jacobson ER, May PG and Farrell TM (1999) An outbreak of fungal dermatitis and stomatitis in a wild population of pigmy rattlesnakes *Sistrurus miliaris barbouri*, in Volusia County, Florida. *Proceedings of the Association of Reptilian and Amphibian Veterinarians Annual Conference*, pp. 19–20

Cooper JE, Geschmeissner S and Bone RD (1988) Herpes-like virus particle in necrotic stomatitis of tortoises. *Veterinary Record* **123**, 544

Cope RB (2000) Sensitisation-dependent skin swelling responses to topical 2,4-dinitro-1-fluorobenzene in the Carolina (green) anole, *Anolis carolinensis*. *Journal of Herpetological Medicine and Surgery* **10(3/4)**, 11–14

DeNardo D and Wozniak EJ (1997) Understanding the snake mite and current therapies for control. *Proceedings of the Association of Reptilian and Amphibian Veterinarians Annual Conference*, pp. 137–148

Devloo R, Martel A, Hellebuyck T et al. (2011) Bearded dragons (*Pogona vitticeps*) asymptomatically infected with *Devriesea agamarum* are source of persistent clinical infection in captive colonies of dab lizards (*Uromastyx* sp.). *Veterinary Microbiology* **150(3/4)**, 297–301

Donoghue S and McKeown S (1999) Nutrition of captive reptiles. *Veterinary Clinics of North America: Exotic Animal Practice* **2**, 69–91

Ebani VV, Fratini F, Bertelloni F, Cerri D and Tortoli E (2012) Isolation and identification of mycobacteria from captive reptiles. *Research in Veterinary Science* **93**, 1136–1138

Frye F (1991) *Biomedical and Surgical Aspects of Captive Reptile Husbandry*, 2nd edition, Volumes 1 and 2. Krieger, Malabar, FL, USA

Girling SJ (2002) A fungal granuloma in a corn snake *Elaphe guttata guttata* due to *Aspergillus fumigatus* associated with a previously treated abscess. *ZooMed Bulletin of the British Veterinary Zoological Society* **2(1)**, 27–35

Girling SJ and Fraser MA (2007) Systemic mycobacteriosis in an inland bearded dragon (*Pogona vitticeps*). *Veterinary Record* **160**, 526–528

Girling SJ and Fraser MA (2009) Successful treatment of *Aspergillus* spp. infection in reptiles with itraconazole at metabolically scaled dosages. *Veterinary Record* **165**, 52–54

Greek TJ (2001) Squamous papillomas in a colony of bearded dragons, *Pogona vitticeps*. *Proceedings of the Association of Reptilian and Amphibian Veterinarians Annual Conference*, pp. 161–162

Griffin C (2000) Subcutaneous atypical mycobacteriosis in a ball python, *Python regius*. *Proceedings of the Association of Reptilian and Amphibian Veterinarians Annual Conference*, pp. 39–41

Hammack SH (1991) New concepts in colubrid egg incubation: preliminary report. *Proceedings of the 15th International Symposium on Captive Propagation and Husbandry*, pp. 103–108

Hannon D (2011) Squamous cell carcinomas in inland bearded dragons (*Pogona vitticeps*). *Proceedings of the Association of Reptilian and Amphibian Veterinarians Annual Conference*, p. 131

Harkewicz KA (2001) Dermatology of reptiles: a clinical approach to diagnosis and treatment. *Veterinary Clinics of North America: Exotic Animal Practice* **4**, 441–461

Hellebuyck T, Pasmans F Haesebrouck F and Martel A (2009) Designing a successful antimicrobial treatment against *Devriesea agamarum* infections in lizards. *Veterinary Microbiology* **139**, 189–192

Hellebuyck T, Baert K, Pasmans F et al. (2010) Cutaneous hyalohyphomycosis in a girdled lizard (*Cordylus giganteus*) caused by the *Chrysosporium* anamorph of *Nannizziopsis vriesii* and successful treatment with voriconazole. *Veterinary Dermatology* **21**, 429–433

Hellebuyck T, Pasmans F, Blooi M, Haesebrouck F and Martel A (2011). Prolonged environmental persistence requires efficient disinfection procedures to control *Devriesea agamarum* associated disease in lizards. *Letters in Applied Microbiology* **52**, 28–32

Hellebuyck T, Pasmans F, Haesebrouk F and Martel A (2012) Dermatological diseases in lizards. *Veterinary Journal* **193**, 38–45

Herbst LH, Jacobson ER and Klein PA (1995) Green turtle fibropapillomatosis: evidence for a viral etiology. *Proceedings of the Joint Conference of the American Association of Zoo Veterinarians, Wildlife Disease Association, and American Association of Wildlife Veterinarians*, Houston, p. 224

Herbst LH, Lenz J, van Doorslaer K et al. (2009) Genomic characterisation of two novel reptilian papillomaviruses *Chelonia mydas* papillomavirus 1 and *Caretta caretta* papillomavirus 1. *Virology* **383**, 131–135

Hernandez-Divers SJ, Knott CD and MacDonald J (2001) Diagnosis and surgical treatment of thyroid adenoma-induced hyperthyroidism in a green iguana (*Iguana iguana*). *Journal of Zoo and Wildlife Medicine* **32**, 465–475

Hoppman E (2007) Dermatology in reptiles. *Journal of Exotic Pet Medicine* **16**, 210–224

Horner RF (1988) Poxvirus in farmed Nile crocodiles. *Veterinary Record* **122**, 459–462

Huchzemeyer FW and Cooper JE (2001) Fibriscess, not abscess, resulting from localised inflammatory response to infection in reptiles and birds. *Veterinary Record* **147**, 515–516

Jacobson ER (2007) Viruses and viral diseases of reptiles. In: *Infectious Diseases and Pathology of Reptiles: Color Atlas and Text*, ed. ER Jacobson, pp. 395–460. CRC Press, Boca Raton, FL, USA

Jacobson ER, Cheatwood JL and Maxwell LK (2000) Mycotic diseases of reptiles. *Seminars in Avian and Exotic Pet Medicine* **9(2)**, 94–101

Jacobson ER, Gaskin JM, Clubb S and Calderwood M (1982) Papilloma-like virus infection in Bolivian side-necked turtles. *Journal of the American Veterinary Medical Association* **181**, 1325–1328

Jacobson ER and Origgi F (2002) Use of serology in reptile medicine. *Seminars in Avian and Exotic Pet Medicine* **11(1)**, 33–45

Jacobson ER, Popp JA, Shields RP and Gaskin JM (1979) Pox-like skin lesions in captive caimans. *Journal of the American Veterinary Medical Association* **175**, 937–940

Jacobson ER, Wronski TJ, Schumacher J, Reggiardo C and Berry KH (1994) Cutaneous dyskeratosis in free-ranging desert tortoises, *Gopherus agassizii*, in the Colorado Desert of southern California. *Journal of Zoo and Wildlife Medicine* **25**, 68–81

Johnson-Delaney CA (1996) Zoonotic parasites of selected exotic animals. *Seminars in Avian and Exotic Pet Medicine* **5(2)**, 115–124

Klaphake E (2001) Temporal glands of chameleons: medical problems and suggested treatments. *Proceedings of the Association of Reptilian and Amphibian Veterinarians Annual Conference*, pp. 223–225

Koplos P, Garner M, Besser T, Nordhausen R and Monaco R (2000) Cheilitis in lizards of the genus *Uromastyx* associated with filamentous Gram positive bacterium. *Proceedings of the Association of Reptilian and Amphibian Veterinarians Annual Conference*, pp. 73–75

Lilywhite HB and Maderson PFA (1982) Skin structure and permeability. In: *Biology of the Reptilia, Volume 12: Physiology*, ed. C Gans and FH Pough, pp. 397–442. Academic Press, London

Maas AK (2013) Vesicular, ulcerative and necrotic dermatitis of reptiles. *Veterinary Clinics of North America: Exotic Animal Practice* **16**, 737–755

Mader DR (1998) Understanding thermal burns in reptile patients. *Proceedings of the Association of Reptilian and Amphibian Veterinarians Annual Conference*, pp. 143–149

Mader DR and DeRemer K (1993) Salmonellosis in reptiles. *Vivarium* **4**, 12–13, 22

Mallo KM, Craig AH, Lewbart GA and Papich MG (2002) Pharmacokinetics of fluconazole in loggerhead sea turtles (*Caretta caretta*) after single intravenous and subcutaneous injections, and multiple subcutaneous injections. *Journal of Zoo and Wildlife Medicine* **33**, 29–35

Masters AM, Ellis TM, Carson JM, Sutherland SS and Gregory AR (1995) *Dermatophilus chelonae* sp. nov. isolated from chelonids in Australia. *International Journal of Systematic Bacteriology* **45**, 50–56

Millichamp NJ (1989) Congenital defects in captive-bred Indian pythons (*Python molurus molurus*). *Proceedings of the Third International Colloquium on Pathology of Reptiles and Amphibians*, p. 103

Mitchell MA and Walden MR (2013) *Chrysosporium* anamorph *Nannizziopsis vriesii*: an emerging fungal pathogen of captive and wild reptiles. *Veterinary Clinics of North America: Exotic Animal* **16**, 659–668

Morales P and Dunker F (2001) Fish tuberculosis, *Mycobacterium marinum*, in a group of Egyptian spiny-tailed lizards, *Uromastyx aegyptius*. *Journal of Herpetological Medicine and Surgery* **11(3)**, 27–30

Neiffer DL, Marks SK, Klein EC and Brady NJ (1998) Shell lesion management in two loggerhead sea turtles, *Caretta caretta*, with employment of PC-7 epoxy paste. *Bulletin of the Association of Reptilian and Amphibian Veterinarians* **8(4)**, 12–17

Nichols DK, Weyant RS, Lamairande EW, Sigler L and Mason RT (1999) Fatal myotic dermatitis in captive brown tree snakes (*Boiga irregularis*). *Journal of Zoo and Wildlife Medicine* **30**, 111–118

Origgi F, Roccabianca P and Gelmetti D (1999) Dermatophilosis in *Furcifer (Chameleo) pardalis*. *Bulletin of the Association of Reptilian and Amphibian Veterinarians* **9(3)**, 9–11

Orós J, Rodriguez L, Déniz S, Fernández L and Fernández A (1998) Cutaneous poxvirus-like infection in a captive Hermann's tortoise (*Testudo hermanni*). *Veterinary Record* **143**, 508–509

Paré JA (2008) An overview of pentastomiasis in reptiles and other vertebrates. *Journal of Exotic Pet Medicine* **17**, 285–294

Paré JA, Coyle KA, Sigler L, Maas AK and Mitchell RL (2006) Pathogenicity of the *Chrysosporium* anamorph of *Nannizziopsis vriesii* for veiled chameleons (*Chamaeleo calyptratus*). *Medical Mycology* **44(1)**, 25–31

Paré JA, Sigler L, Rypien K, Fe Gibas C and Hoffman TL (2001) Cutaneous microflora of healthy squamate reptiles and prevalence of the *Chrysosporium* anamorph of *Nanizziopsis vriesii*. *Proceedings of the Association of Reptilian and Amphibian Veterinarians Annual Conference*, pp. 43–44

Paré JA, Sigler L, Rypien KL *et al.* (2003) Survey for the *Chrysosporium* anamorph of *Nannizziopsis vriesii* on the skin of healthy captive squamate reptiles and notes on their cutaneous fungal mycobiota. *Journal of Herpetological Medicine and Surgery* **13(4)**, 10–15

Raynaud A and Adrian M (1976) Lésions cutanée à structure pilomateuse associées a des virus chez lézard vert (*Lacerta viridis Laur*). *Comptes Rendus de l'Académie de Sciences (Paris)* **283(Series D)**, 845

Reavill DR, Dahlhausen B, Zaffarano B and Schmidt R (2002) Multiple cutaneous liposarcomas in a red-tailed boa, boa constrictor and a chameleon. *Proceedings of the Association of Reptilian and Amphibian Veterinarians Annual Conference*, pp. 5–6

Reavill DR, Fassier AS and Schmidt RE (2000) Mast cell tumor in a common green iguana, *Iguana iguana*. *Proceedings of the Association of Reptilian and Amphibian Veterinarians Annual Conference*, p. 45

Reavill DR and Schmidt R (2002) Mineralised skin lesions in lizards. *Proceedings of the Association of Reptilian and Amphibian Veterinarians Annual Conference*, pp. 77–78

Rebell H, Rywlin A and Haines H (1975) A herpesvirus agent associated with skin lesions of green sea turtles in aquaculture. *American Journal of Veterinary Research* **36**, 1221–1224

Rector A and van Ranst M (2013) Animal papillomaviruses. *Virology* **445**, 213–223

Rossi J and Rossi R (2000) Fungal dermatitis in a large collection of Brazos water snakes, *Nerodia harteri harteri*, housed in an outdoor enclosure and a possible association with slugs. *Proceedings of the Association of Reptilian and Amphibian Veterinarians Annual Conference*, pp. 81–83

Rossi JV (1996) Dermatology. In: *Reptile Medicine and Surgery*, ed. DR Mader, pp. 104–117. WB Saunders, Philadelphia

Rudloff E (2005) How to use honey/sugar bandages in reptiles. *Proceedings of the North American Veterinary Conference, Volume 19*, Orlando, Florida, USA, p. 1307

Sigler L, Hambleton S and Paré JA (2013) Molecular characterization of reptile pathogens currently known as members of the *Chrysosporium* Anamorph of *Nannizziopsis vriesii* complex and relationship with some human-associated isolates. *Journal of Clinical Microbiology* **51**, 3338–3357

Silvestre AM and Soler J (2001) An amelanistic Hermann's tortoise (*Testudo hermanni hermanni*) from the Balearic Islands (Spain). *Testudo* **5(3)**, 35–36

Smith DA, Barker IK and Allen OB (1988) The effect of certain topical medications on healing of cutaneous wounds in the common garter snake (*Thamnophis sirtalis*). *Canadian Journal of Veterinary Research* **52**, 129–133

Stahl SJ (2003) Pet lizard conditions and syndromes. *Seminars in Avian and Exotic Pet Medicine* **12(3)**, 162–182

Szell Z, Sreter T and Varga I (2001) Ivermectin toxicosis in a chameleon (*Chamaeleo senegalensis*) infected with *Foleyella furcata*. *Journal of Zoo and Wildlife Medicine* **32**, 115–117

Tamukai K, Tokiwa T, Kobayashi H *et al.* (2016) Ranavirus in an outbreak of dermatophilosis in captive inland bearded dragons (*Pogona vitticeps*). *Veterinary Dermatology* **27**, 99–105

Teare JA and Bush M (1983) Toxicity and efficacy of ivermectin in chelonians. *Journal of the American Veterinary Medical Association* **183**, 1195–1197

Toplon DE, Terrell SP, Sigler L and Jacobson ER (2012) Dermatitis and cellulitis in leopard geckos (*Eublepharis macularius*) caused by the *Chrysosporium* anamorph of *Nannizziopsis vriesii*. *Veterinary Pathology* **50**, 585–589

Van Waeyenberghe L, Baert K, Pasmans F *et al.* (2010) Voriconazole, a safe alternative for treating infections caused by the *Chrysosporium* anamorph of *Nannizziopsis vriesii* in bearded dragons (*Pogona vitticeps*). *Medical Mycology* **48**, 880–885

Wallach JD (1977) Ulcerative shell disease in turtles: identification, prophylaxis and treatment. *International Zoo Yearbook* **17**, 170

Wellehan J (2005) Reptile medicine for the emergency clinician: things that slither in the night. *Proceedings of the North American Veterinary Conference, Volume 19*, Orlando, Florida, USA, pp. 1310–1311

Chapter 16

The reptile eye

David Williams

We like to think of reptiles as one group of animals: snakes, lizards, crocodiles, tortoises all classified together. They are all ectothermic and scaly after all. But evolutionary taxonomists tell us that phylogenetic analysis paints a very different picture (Shine, 2013). The dinosaurs and crocodiles are much more closely related to birds than are the snakes, lizards and chelonians, with the squamates (lizards and snakes) diverging from the crocodiles and turtles 200 million years ago. This inner diversity even in the face of apparent outward homogeneity accounts for differences between the eyes of different reptile species.

Anatomy and physiology

The irony of comparative ophthalmology is that all vertebrate eyes have the same basic morphology with the cornea, lens and retina providing the visual foundation, yet between species even as apparently closely related as different genera of reptiles, there can be substantial differences in the detail of the ocular structures. The eyes of lizards, snakes, crocodilians and chelonians are surprisingly different, these variations giving considerable insight into both the diversity of their evolutionary origins and their current residence in different ecological niches. Underwood's masterful chapter on the reptile eye in the second volume of Gans and Parsons' *Biology of the Reptilia* (Underwood, 1970) shows these variations. Different species have modified their basic ocular equipment to adapt to current conditions and evolutionary opportunities. Study of the eye may contribute to reconstruction of a group's phylogeny (Ott, 2006).

In the majority of reptile species, whether diurnal or nocturnal, vision is important and so the eye is relatively large. The lizard eye (Figure 16.1) can be divided into an anterior corneal and a posterior orbital segment. The cornea has a thin stroma but a relatively thick Bowman's layer devoid of cells and covered by a thin corneal epithelium. The iridocorneal angle is poorly developed compared with that of higher vertebrates. Overlapping scleral ossicles, around 10–14 in lizards, are found in the sclera immediately behind the limbus, overlying the ciliary body which surrounds the equator of the lens. The lens is fairly soft with epithelium that thickens markedly at the lens equator, forming the Ringwulst, bringing the lens into contact with the ciliary body. The ciliary muscle, as in birds, is divided into an anterior part (Crampton's muscle) and a posterior part (Brucke's muscle), inserting between the cornea and the

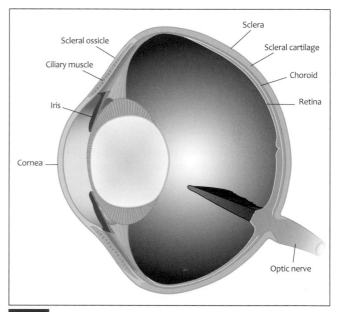

16.1 Cross-section of a lizard eye.

ciliary body and having both radial and circumferential fibres. This is a significantly different arrangement from that in the mammalian eye, which allows not only changes in spherical shape of the lens but also enhancement of the curvature of the cornea. Nocturnal lizards have a very large cornea, an almost spherical lens and a pupil that is hexagonal when dilated, allowing a much larger pupil diameter than that of a circular pupil, and closes to a slit on miosis. Diurnal lizards generally have a simple round pupil and a retina containing many cones with oil droplets, giving them specific responses to particular light wavelengths. Nocturnal lizards have cones that have the morphological features of rods, but still use cone photo-pigments in their visual transduction pathway.

The eyes of all snakes are covered by a spectacle formed from fused transparent eyelids (Underwood, 1970). The ophidian orbit has only the Harderian gland, which secretes a seromucous fluid between the spectacle and the cornea (Minucci *et al.*, 1981), while all other reptiles also have a lacrimal gland. Snakes accommodate changes in lens deformation but, more importantly, with forward movement of the lens (Ott, 2006). Snakes do not have scleral ossicles but rather an entirely fibrous sclera with a cartilaginous cup posteriorly. The cornea, not needing to have a protective function given that this is provided by the spectacle, is thin with an epithelium of only a very few cell layers. It is for this reason that if one accidentally removes the spectacle while attempting to dislodge a retained eye-cap, loss of the whole globe often results.

The chelonian eye varies markedly between species, depending on the different ecological niches they inhabit. The amphibious terrapin *Emys* species, for instance, has a relatively convex cornea and a thick lens with a thin annular pad (Pchelyakov, 1982) and uses the iris to squeeze the anterior face of the lens, dramatically increasing its curvature and refractive power. The terrestrial *Testudo* species have a lens which is less spherical, since the cornea plays an active part in light refraction. The small size of the eye in many of these species means that the lens cannot be as ovoid as that of larger mammals.

The lacrimal and Harderian orbital glands are large in most chelonians compared with other reptiles. In marine species these are important as they play a critical role in salt excretion (Abel and Ellis, 1966). Chelonians have a predominantly cone population of photoreceptors in which oil droplets accentuate colour vision as they do in birds (Walls, 1942). This may be important in detecting fruit, a key part of their diet.

What do reptiles see?

Nobody would attempt to answer as broad a question as 'what do mammals see?' in a single paragraph, yet somehow we expect to be able to cover what reptiles see in a few sentences. Reptiles range from crocodilians with dorsally placed eyes to boa constrictors and pythons with lateralized eyes, and from nocturnal species such as many of the geckos to diurnal animals like the iguanas, with obvious differences in vision. Nocturnal geckos have a rodless retina with nocturnal colour vision, since they have evolved from cone-dominated diurnal lizards (Roth and Kleber, 2004). Diurnal snakes such as the garter snake have a cone-rich retina (Silman *et al.*, 1997), while those that hunt nocturnally are more rod-dominated (Silman *et al.*, 2001). Such variations in activity at different light levels has an effect not just on the retina but on other areas of ocular anatomy. Diurnal snakes have round pupils, while those with nocturnal habits have slit pupils allowing a wider range of light entry (Malmström and Kroger, 2006).

Differences are also seen in the field of vision. Many snakes have laterally placed eyes giving an almost panoramic field of vision, while diurnal geckos have forward facing eyes with predominantly binocular vision. Studies of unilaterally anophthalmic snakes have shown that they need to use both eyes to assess movement of prey, even if this does not involve a truly stereo binocular field (Grace *et al.*, 2001). Unusual adaptations for optimizing prey location include multiple pupils seen in reptiles such as the Tokay gecko (Figure 16.2), whereby objects at the focal distance of the lens appear as one in-focus image on the retina, accurately determining the distance of a prey item prior to capture (Murphy and Howland, 1986).

Many reptiles do not rely on ocular vision alone as they also have a parietal eye, a structure homologous with the pineal gland of higher vertebrates and histologically similar to conventional eyes (Figure 16.3). This is an axial mid-brain structure, overlain by a dorsal foramen in the skull and translucent skin, allowing the parietal eye to play a central role in seasonal physiological and behavioural cycles through light detection.

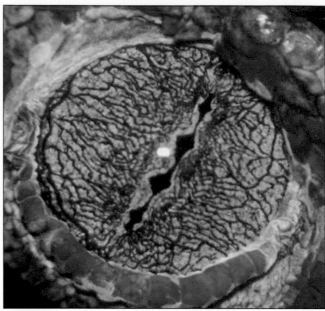

16.2 Eye of the Tokay gecko with its multiple pupils.
(© David Williams)

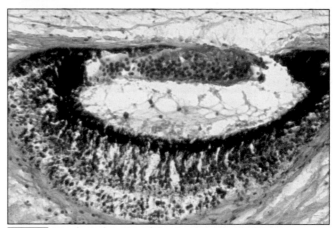

16.3 Histological section of the pineal gland or parietal eye.
(© David Williams)

In addition to ocular vision, boid snakes use infrared detection in predation with nerves from the infrared end organs located deep within invaginations between labial scales. This infrared system projects to the lateral descending nucleus of the trigeminal tract (LTTD). In crotaline pit vipers, the pit organ contains an infrared sensitive membrane from whence the nerves proceed to the LTTD. Deprivation of either sight or infrared detection did not alter rattlesnakes' strike behaviour or ability to catch prey in one study (Grace and Woodward, 2001), while obliteration of both systems led to poorer strike accuracy (Grace *et al.*, 2001).

Ophthalmic examination

Examination of the reptilian eye requires the same techniques as for any other species, with direct and indirect ophthalmoscopy as well as slit-lamp biomicroscopy all valuable in investigating conditions of the globe and adnexa. As many of the animals' eyes are very small, a slit-lamp can be useful in providing sufficient magnification to allow evaluation; if this is not available, then a set of magnifying loupes can be invaluable.

Ancillary tests used in companion mammals, such as those used to evaluate tear production and intraocular pressure, can also provide important data regarding ocular health in reptiles. The small size of many reptilian eyes renders the Schirmer tear test difficult, if not impossible, to perform; whereas, the phenol red thread test (PRTT) can be much more readily undertaken. Normal data for these tests are shown in Figure 16.4, but it should be borne in mind that different species have varying values of test wetting, even among animals of a similar size (e.g. the European pond turtle has a PRTT twice that of the red-eared terrapin).

Similarly, the small size of many reptilian eyes means that the rebound Tonovet tonometer is much preferred to the Tonopen applanation tonometer to measure intraocular pressure. Tonometric values from normal reptiles are given in Figure 16.5. As with tear production, reptile species similar in size and ecology can have quite varied values of intraocular pressure. This shows the value of comparing a diseased eye with a normal eye, either in the patient itself or in another individual of the same species.

Species	Method	Value	Reference
European pond turtle	PRTT PPTT EAPPT	4.8 ± 1.6 mm/15 sec 4.5 ± 1.2 mm/min 8.3 ± 0.6 mm/min	Rajaei et al., 2014
Red-eared slider	mSTT	2.55 ± 3.4 mm/min	Somma et al., 2015
Red-footed tortoise	STT EAPTT-1 EAPTT-2	12.0 ± 3.5 mm/min 15.9 ± 0.7 mm/15 sec 16.6 ± 0.4 mm/min	Oria et al., 2015a
Green Iguana	PRTT EAPPT STT	3.9 ± 1.7 mm/15 sec 8.5 ± 2.4 mm/min 1.0 ± 0.5 mm/min	Araujo et al., 2017
Andros island iguana	PRTT	11.4 ± 6.0 mm/15 sec	Woiick et al., 2013
Broad-snouted caiman	STT EAPTT	3.4 ± 3.6 mm/min 17.1 ± 2.5 mm/min	Oria et al., 2015b

16.4 Tear production in various reptile species. EAPPT = endodontic absorbent paper point test; mSTT = modified Schirmer tear test; PPTT = paper point tear test; PRTT = phenol red thread test; STT = Schirmer tear test.

Species	Method	Value	Reference
Red-footed tortoise	Applanation tonometry (Tonopen)	11.5 ± 2.8 mmHg male 14.0 ± 3.5 mmHg female	Oria et al., 2015a
Yellow-footed tortoise	Applanation tonometry (Tonopen)	14.2 ± 1.2 mmHg	Semi et al., 2003
Hermann's tortoise	Rebound tonometry (Tonovet)	15.74 ± 0.20 mmHg	Selleri et al., 2012
Red-eared slider	Rebound tonometry (Tonovet)	5.4 ± 1.7 mmHg	Somma et al., 2015
Broad-snouted caiman	Applanation tonometry (Tonopen)	12.9 ± 6.2 mmHg	Oria et al., 2015b
Green iguana	Rebound tonometry (Tonovet)	18.0 ± 1.7 mmHg	De Araujo et al., 2017
Andros Island iguana	Rebound tonometry (Tonovet)	4.9 ± 2.1 mmHg	Wojick et al., 2013
American alligator	Applanation tonometry (Tonopen)	23.7 ± 2.1 mmHg (>50 cm) 11.6 ± 0.5 cm (<50 cm)	Whittaker et al., 1995

16.5 Tonometry values from different reptile species measured with applanation and rebound tonometers.

Ocular diseases

Hypovitaminosis A in chelonians

The signs of hypovitaminosis A range from mild eyelid oedema to more severe eyelid swelling with chemotic conjunctival enlargement to the extent that no globe is visible and the animal rendered blind (Figure 16.6). The globe is exophthalmic as the orbital glands are enlarged through epithelial dyskeratosis; consequently, they cease to function as tear glands, which leads to dry eye and a build-up of necrotic debris. Dyskeratosis of the digestive epithelium renders absorption of dietary vitamin A poor. Given that chelonians feed by sight, these blinding ocular changes preclude natural feeding, further exacerbating the nutritional deficiency at the centre of the disease (Frye, 1991).

Hypovitaminosis A is particularly obvious in terrapins because the lacrimal and Harderian glands take up such a large proportion of the orbit and also, since being carnivorous they are more likely to have subnormal vitamin A intake than herbivorous chelonia. Geckos, chameleons and snakes have a well-developed Harderian gland, but even this does not rival the size of the chelonian orbital glands. Desquamated hyperkeratinized epithelium swells the conjunctiva and fills the orbit.

The pathognomonic appearance of vitamin A deficiency often renders biopsy unnecessary, but cytology can show numerous heterophils or bacteria, in which case topical or systemic antibiosis with a fluoroquinolone such as enrofloxacin is required. Additionally, excessive caseous debris located between the cornea and lids commonly has to be removed by flushing with sterile saline. Topical tear replacement therapy may also be valuable.

The most important part of managing the condition is restoration of the correct level of vitamin A, either by oral supplementation or, possibly, by weekly intramuscular injections of water-soluble vitamin A if oral dosing appears ineffective. This may occur if the intestinal epithelium is similarly dystrophic, rendering absorption of dietary vitamin A difficult, if not impossible. Having said that, it is important to be aware of the signs of hypervitaminosis A, which can be a side effect of overdose of injectable retinol.

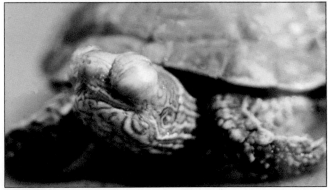

16.6 Terrapin with hypovitaminosis A. (Courtesy of Dr Edward Elkan Reference Collection)

Periocular lesions

Periocular adnexal lesions in reptiles may involve lid swelling, ocular discharge and conjunctival hyperaemia. Periocular lesions need to be differentiated from hypovitaminosis A and normal anatomy encountered in some species. For example, some varanid monitor lizards have a vivid red episclera, which is quite within normal limits, but in other species this would be a sign of ocular inflammation.

Caiman pox and herpesvirus infection have been reportedly associated with proliferative and often ulcerative skin lesions in sea turtles, as well as with tracheitis, conjunctivitis and periocular neoplasia. The most common cause of conjunctivitis in reptiles, where vitamin A deficiency has been excluded, is bacterial blepharitis. Clinical signs include blepharoedema and sometimes chemosis, occasionally with a mucoid discharge, but often with the eyelids being sealed shut with a dry caseous discharge (Figure 16.7). Often in such cases septicaemia may be a predisposing factor, although the lesions may be localized to the eye alone. Periocular *Aeromonas* spp. infection, for example, was noted to cause conjunctivitis and blepharitis in a colony of lacertid lizards (Cooper *et al.*, 1980), while *Pseudomonas* sp. was isolated from a group of anoles with conjunctivitis and blepharitis (Millichamp *et al.*, 1983). In the lacertid lizards, treatment with oral oxytetracycline and topical ocular bathing using a solution of the same drug was successful while the anoles responded well to topical gentamicin. Vivarium hygiene was improved and ventilation increased with some effect. The mealworms which comprised the majority of the animals' diet were thought to be a potential source of infection.

Chlamydia is generally considered a pathogen of birds rather than reptiles, but exudative conjunctivitis has been reported in association with *Chlamydia* sp. in hatchling and juvenile crocodiles, the problem being introduced by the non-quarantine addition of wild-caught animals into a farm (Huchzermeyer *et al.*, 1983). Such a report confirms the importance of ensuring strict biosecurity when introducing new individuals into any group of captive animals.

Other causes of conjunctivitis include irritation from physical causes, such as small pieces of vermiculite used as a substrate, and chemical agents, such as organochlorine pesticides reported to be associated with conjunctivitis and blepharitis in Eastern box turtles (Tandfredi and Evans, 1997).

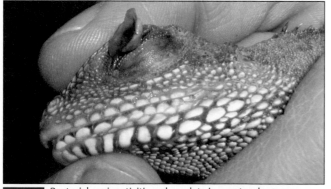

16.7 Bacterial conjunctivitis and exudate in a water dragon.
(Courtesy of Paul Raiti)

Periocular masses

Periocular masses present as firm swellings gradually increasing in size (Figure 16.8) with signs of secondary trauma caused by their growing bulk and blindness as a result of physical interference with vision. Most are inflammatory lesions resulting from Gram-negative bacterial or fungal infection. These inflammatory lesions are, for the most part, granulomatous in nature as the heterophils which populate them do not have the coagulative enzymes seen in mammalian neutrophils and a large amount of fibrin is secreted into the abscess. These lesions can be very difficult to differentiate from neoplasms, thus biopsy is indicated.

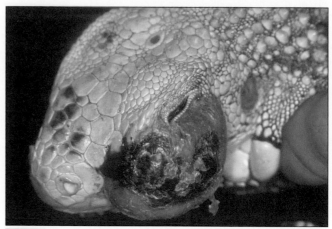

16.8 Iguana with a periocular inflammatory mass. In this case it was determined to be a fibriscess/granuloma.
(© David Williams)

Adnexal mass lesions may be inflammatory, infectious and neoplastic concurrently, as reported in a veiled chameleon with a squamous cell carcinoma that was diagnosed concurrently with abscessation caused by *Pseudomonas aeruginosa* (Abou-Madi and Kern, 2002). Other lesions are purely infectious, for example, the periorbital abscess reported by Schumacher *et al.* (1996) in a chameleon. Management of such a mass must clearly be dictated by the specific diagnosis reached, but in most cases surgical exploration and excisional biopsy will be important in both reaching a diagnosis and dealing with the lesion itself. The relatively thin skin of the ocular adnexa in reptiles means, however, that a mass in this area readily distorts the eyelid margins, potentially rendering vision problematic in many cases. Reconstructive surgery to bring the palpebral aperture into apposition with the globe can be difficult to undertake successfully.

Exophthalmos

Other causes of adnexal pathology include parasitic infestations, such as a filaroid worm causing exophthalmos in a chameleon (Abou-Madi and Kern, 1983; Reavill and Schmidt, 2012). Other causes of exophthalmos include dacryops, acquired lacrimal cysts (reported in a terrapin, resulting in periocular swelling together with exophthalmos; Allgoewer *et al.*, 2002), orbital neoplasms and abscesses (Mayer *et al.*, 2010), as well as orbital varices (rare), which cause both exophthalmos and periocular swelling.

Dacryocystitis

Inflammation of the nasolacrimal duct can be seen in different reptiles, even those in which, according to the anatomy books, no nasolacrimal duct exists! Thus, while some textbooks report that chelonians do not have a nasolacrimal duct, dacryocystitis has been reported in these species, with discharge and bubble formation at the medial canthus as signs of the condition. Animals with tear overflow or a purulent ocular discharge, particularly from the medial canthus, should be investigated for dacryocystitis with slit lamp biomicroscopy and placement of a drop of fluorescein dye in the eye to assess appearance of the dye at the external nares. Nasolacrimal flushing, while theoretically possible, is likely to be difficult in such a small eye.

Retained spectacles

All snakes and a number of lizards have a transparent layer over the cornea, acting as a protective cover. This is the spectacle or, as it used to be termed by the biologists who first investigated it, the 'brille'. The spectacle, derived from fusion of the eyelids, forms a closed space in which tears form, circulate and are drained through the nasolacrimal duct. This is clearly a marked difference from the open ocular surface of all other animals and has a substantial influence on the disease states experienced by the eye when the spectacle is present. The spectacle has characteristics of the skin scales from which it was formed, including blood vessels (Mead, 1976) (Figure 16.9). The spectacle is shed with the rest of the skin and during this period of ecdysis it becomes oedematous and opaque in the same way that the rest of the skin becomes dull, with fluid separating the old skin from the newly regenerating tissue underneath as a normal phase in the growth of the animal (Figure 16.10).

Retention of previously unshed spectacles manifests as a raised plaque of retained tissue, often opaque, in the ocular area (Figure 16.11). In many cases the animal is not presented until the condition has occurred several times, when such retained 'eye-caps' are multiple. Differential diagnoses include opacity of the spectacle as a result of infection or trauma, bullous spectaculopathy and subspectacular abscess. Another, but much less common, differential diagnosis would be a neoplastic process such as a keratocanthoma. The multiple nature of these retained layers of skin is normally obvious on close examination. Spectacle retention is often seen as part of a more generalized dysecdysis, where skin shedding is not complete. The underlying problem is a husbandry deficit, particularly too low humidity. Another aetiopathogenic factor may be infestation with the snake mite *Ophionyssus natricius* (Figure 16.12). The parasite undergoes several moults until it reaches adulthood and during each of these it takes a blood meal to increase its body size. The space between the spectacle and the first periocular skin scale is an ideal place to take such a blood meal. Multiple punctures here cause inflammation and lead to spectacle retention. The dark deposits around the spectacles in Figure 16.13 are the mites and the haemorrhagic remains of their multiple blood meals.

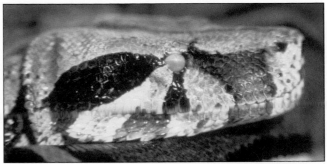

16.10 Oedematous spectacle in a snake about to shed its skin.
(Courtesy of Professor Elliott Jacobson)

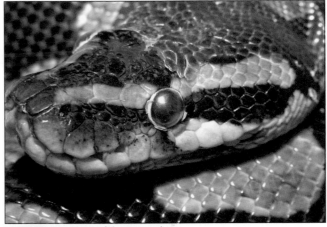

16.11 Retention of the spectacle.
(Courtesy of Dr Stephen Barten)

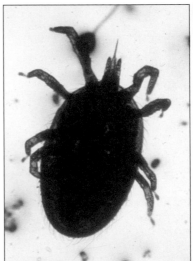

16.12 The snake mite *Ophinyssus natricius*.
(Courtesy of Dr Stephen Barten)

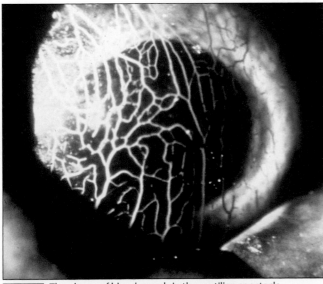

16.9 The plexus of blood vessels in the reptilian spectacle.
(Courtesy of Dr A Mead)

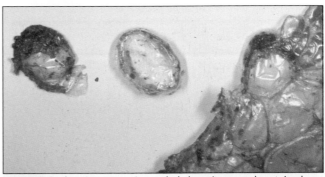

16.13 Snake mites appearing as dark deposits around a retained spectacle.
(Courtesy of Dr Stephen Barten)

Management

The key point to note in managing a case of retained spectacles is that no attempt should be made to remove the retained tissue by force using a pair of forceps. This can often result in removal of the entire spectacle, leading to severe keratitis (Figure 16.14). Given that low humidity is critical in many cases of retained spectacles, increasing the humidity at the time of the next ecdysis may be sufficient to promote a full shed with removal of the retained spectacles. If this is not the case, use of damp cotton paper in the vivarium against which the snake can rub itself or soaked cotton wool abraded against the retained spectacles can affect removal of the abnormal tissue. A recalcitrant mass of spectacles can on occasion be removed with forceps if no other less severe technique has a beneficial effect, but such a technique is best performed with the snake under general anaesthesia and using an operating microscope to ensure that the true spectacle and underlying eye are not damaged.

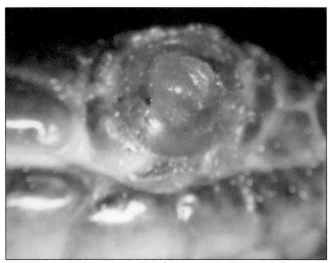

16.14 Severe keratitis resulting from attempted removal of a retained spectacle in a snake.

Prophylaxis

Keeping the snake in an appropriate humidity, especially around the time of shedding, is vitally important if dysecdysis and spectacle retention is to be avoided. The correct level of humidity differs depending on the species involved; a desert dwelling snake will require a lower humidity than one residing in a rainforest, although even desert dwelling species will often hide in rock crevices during the day, which can have a higher relative humidity than one would associate with a desert habitat. Providing a damp area within the vivarium is worthwhile and wetted paper added to the vivarium at the time of moulting is valuable, especially for an animal that has previously been affected by spectacle retention. Owners of affected snakes should be encouraged to check at each shed that the exuvium (the shed skin) includes both spectacles (Figure 16.15) to ensure that sets of retained spectacles do not build up and that preventative measures can be taken if dysecdysis occurs.

Bullous spectaculopathy

Obstruction of the nasolacrimal ducts in snakes leads to a build-up of tear fluid underneath the spectacle with resultant marked enlargement of the spectacle. The resulting

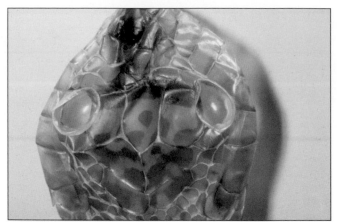

16.15 The spectacle shed with the rest of the exuvium in a normal ecdysis.
(Courtesy of Dr Stephen Barten)

appearance of the eye can be one of a protruberant opaque mass (Figure 16.16) or one where, while the spectacle is clearly distended, it remains transparent (Figure 16.17). The difficulty in snakes is differentiating bullous spectaculopathy from glaucoma, which in a non-spectacled animal would present in a similar manner but with globe enlargement, resulting in the clinical signs noted above. Indeed, in what is apparently the first mention of the condition in the literature, the term pseudobuphthalmos was used to indicate that it was not the globe that was enlarged but the spectacle alone (Boniuk and Lusquette, 1963). The authors noted 'this apparent buphthalmos has often been misinterpreted as the result of an underlying glaucoma'.

The nasolacrimal obstruction may be congenital, with developmental atresia of the duct being reported in a blood python (Millichamp et al., 1986). More commonly, it is caused by an acquired physical obstruction to the duct. In some cases, there is an infectious aetiology at its origin, in which case the condition should probably be termed a subspectacular abscess (see later). Interestingly, there are snakes which develop this condition just prior to ecdysis, when presumably the shed epithelium (which includes the

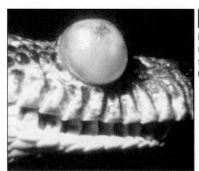

16.16 Exceptional spectacle swelling in a snake with an obstructed nasolacrimal duct and bullous spectaculopathy.
(Courtesy of Dr Frederic Frye)

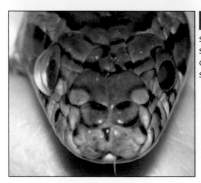

16.17 Less obvious distention of the spectacle of the right eye of a snake with nasolacrimal duct obstruction and mild bullous spectaculopathy.

nasolacrimal duct as well as the dermal epidermis) impedes tear drainage for a few days.

Simple aspiration of the lacrimal fluid with a needle under sedation or general anaesthesia is possible but will only provide temporary amelioration of the signs. Such a technique can also be useful if the sample obtained is submitted for bacteriological culture and cytology. However, the fluid produced by the lacrimal and Harderian glands can be viscous, precluding aspiration with a narrow-gauge needle. The standard treatment under general anaesthesia is to excise a ventral triangle of the spectacle, allowing continual drainage of tears until the next shed (Figure 16.18). This requires a microsurgical approach and should be performed by a specialist, ideally using an operating microscope. Such cases are thus best referred to a veterinary ophthalmologist with experience in exotic animal ophthalmology.

Often the initial problem causing the condition is an inflammatory obstruction, even when a clear abscess is not visible. Cytology and bacteriology of the aspirated fluid should be undertaken and a detailed examination performed of the buccal cavity. It is important to treat any underlying pathology to prevent recurrence.

A more profound infection of the ocular surface in snakes is seen as an abscess manifesting in the space between the cornea and spectacle. This is termed a subspectacular abscess. Such a condition should be relatively easy to diagnose, as a yellow mass is seen in the ventral subspectacular space or, in severe cases, occupying the entire ocular surface (Figure 16.19). However, it should be noted that it can be difficult to differentiate bullous spectaculopathy with opacity of the spectacle from a subspectacular abscess.

The optimal treatment for a subspectacular abscess is to create a 30-degree window in the ventral aspect of the spectacle, through which the infected and inflammatory debris can be removed by irrigation. The purulent material can be caseous in nature and not fluid, so it may be difficult to remove from the narrow space between the cornea and the spectacle. Persistence with saline or Hartmann's solution will eventually allow all the inflammatory debris to be removed. Samples obtained from flushing the subspectacular space should be submitted for bacteriological culture and cytology, together with samples from the oral

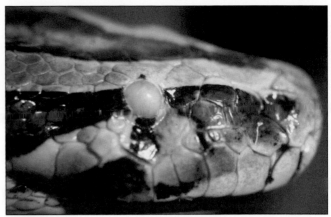

16.19 Subspectacular abscess in a python with necrotic stomatitis and an ascending infection up the nasolacrimal duct to the subspectacular space.

cavity, to assess the likelihood that necrotic stomatitis is the underlying cause of the ascending infection resulting in the ocular signs.

Corneal disease

Corneal disease in reptiles may be due to keratitis with or without attendant infection and possibly resulting from an excessive UV light provision (Gardiner *et al.*, 2009; Musgrave *et al.*, 2016), traumatic ulceration or lipid deposition. Each of these differential diagnoses display different clinical signs. The diagnostic work-up in cases of post-traumatic corneal ulcers in reptiles (other than snakes, where the spectacle protects the cornea from such trauma) is an area where we can extrapolate from existing knowledge of mammals more frequently seen in veterinary practice. Use of fluorescein dye in exactly the same way as might be employed in an ulcerated canine or feline cornea will demarcate the extent of the ulcer and its depth (Figure 16.20). Other tests to complete the diagnostic work-up should include bacteriology and cytology, the sample for the latter obtained with a cytobrush and smeared on to a clean slide, air-dried and stained with a modified Wright–Giemsa stain (e.g. Diff-Quik®).

The three questions which should be addressed for any ulcer are:

1. What is the cause of the ulcer?
2. How deep is the ulcer?
3. Is the ulcer healing?

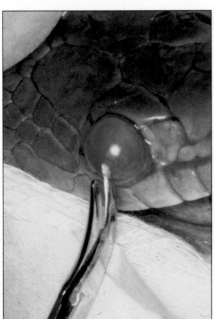

16.18 Incision to relieve distension of the spectacle in a snake with bullous spectaculopathy.
(Courtesy of Dr Daniel Priehs)

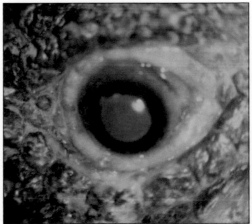

16.20 Central corneal ulcer in an aged tortoise following trauma.
(© David Williams)

Most ulcers in reptiles have a history of a traumatic incident, although some can be complicated by secondary infection. Many of these erosions are superficial, but care must be taken given the thickness of the cornea in many reptiles kept in captivity (for example, the total corneal thickness in Ridley's sea turtles is 288 ± 23 μm compared with 0.6–0.7 mm in dogs). Even a superficial ulcer in an iguana or a box turtle can involve a considerable proportion of the corneal thickness and so should be treated as an emergency.

Corneal ulcers usually heal rapidly, within 1 week, except where healing is delayed because of either an abnormality in the epithelial basement membrane (as seen in recidivistic epithelial erosions in Boxers) or due to age (see Figure 16.20 where a traumatic ulcer has failed to heal in a 38-year-old tortoise). In such cases, debridement of the redundant devitalized epithelium at the edge of the ulcer is important, followed by topical antibiotics to prevent secondary infection, although preservatives and stabilizers such as benzalkonium chloride have been shown to retard ulcer healing *in vitro* (Ayaki *et al.*, 2008).

Third eyelid flaps can be used to protect eyes with ulcers, but conjunctival pedicle flaps are difficult to fashion in small eyes such as those of the reptiles normally encountered in practice. Tear replacement drops such as those with a carbomer gel or sodium hyaluronate base can be useful to ensure rapid healing.

Corneal opacification

While a long-standing corneal ulcer could cause corneal opacification, predominantly through pigmentation, lack of transparency is more commonly related to a white discoloration of the cornea caused by either lipid, calcium or proteinaceous deposits. Chelonians with systemic circulating lipidaemia, either as a result of inherited dyslipoproteinaemia or dietary hyperlipidaemia, have corneal lipidosis that is not dissimilar to that seen in the dog. In these cases, the lesion appears as a diffuse milky white colour (Figure 16.21), but at higher magnification individual lipid crystals may be evident.

A denser and much more homogeneous white corneal lesion may be seen in reptiles, particularly following hibernation (Figure 16.22). Frye (1991) reported that these could be dissolved using Kymar ointment (a preparation of alpha-chymotrypsin), suggesting that the lesion is proteinaceous in nature, but unfortunately such treatment is not now widely available.

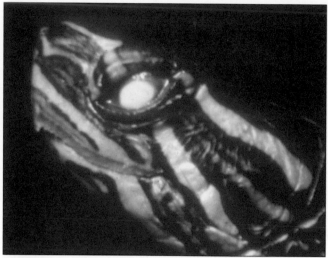

16.22 Post-hibernational corneal deposit in a terrapin.
(Courtesy of Dr Frederic Frye)

Amelioration of lipid-related corneal pathology is difficult in companion mammals, even if circulating lipid levels can be reduced. In the same way in reptiles, these opacities, once formed, can be very taxing to resolve. The key feature in dealing with lesions in reptiles (as with other species) is identifying the underlying cause and correcting it, with the hope that the corneal lipid deposition will gradually resolve in time. Assessing the diet of the individual is essential.

Uveitis

Inflammation of the uveal tract, normally manifesting as iritis, is rarely seen in reptiles but where it is encountered it can be a sign of systemic infection. The main clinical signs of anterior uveitis are the presence of inflammatory cells in the anterior chamber of the eye with either flare in mild cases giving a hazy appearance to the iris or more overt purulent deposits resulting in hypopyon (Booney *et al.*, 1978) (Figure 16.23).

The majority of cases in reptiles are associated with systemic infection by Gram-negative bacteria (Booney *et al.*, 1978; Millichamp *et al.*, 1983). It is unclear whether this association between septicaemia and intraocular inflammation represents the presence of infectious organisms in the eye. Circulating lipopolysaccharide (as would be seen with septicaemia) can lead to a breakdown of the blood–aqueous barrier with resultant flare; however, further research would be needed to determine if this is the case in reptiles.

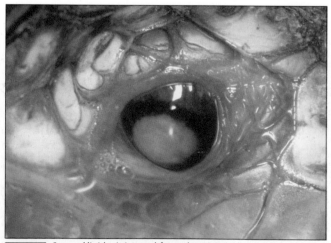

16.21 Corneal lipidosis in a red-footed tortoise.
(Courtesy of Dr Stephen Barten)

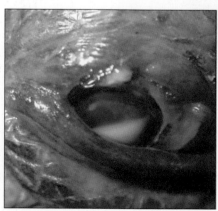

16.23 Uveitis in a tortoise with profound hypopyon.

Close examination with a slit lamp biomicroscope reveals early signs of inflammatory cell circulation and fibrin deposition in uveitis with aqueous flare. Due to the likelihood of association with systemic infection, blood samples for culture should be obtained as well as for routine haematological and biochemical assessment. From a therapeutic perspective, parenteral antibiosis should be provided, ideally based on bacteriological culture and sensitivity testing; however, even before bacteriology results are available, a broad-spectrum agent such as enrofloxacin should be administered orally or by injection.

Topical steroids or non-steroidal agents are worthwhile even in the face of infection, as reducing the inflammatory processes in the eye is essential. Attempts at surgical removal of the purulent debris has been reported in a case of fungal hypopyon, but without long-term success, with enucleation eventually being required (Zwart *et al.*, 1973). The striated muscle of the reptilian iris renders atropine ineffective, and the use of depolarizing or non-depolarizing muscle relaxants, while effective to provide mydriasis for fundoscopy, have yet to be reported in reptilian uveitis. While the author feels that using general anaesthesia to produce mydriasis is somewhat extreme, there is some evidence that suggests variable mydriasis may be achieved fairly consistently under general anaesthesia. (Montiani-Ferreira, 2008). This information source also states that the use of general anaesthesia to induce mydriasis for routine fundus examination in birds and reptiles is a reliable and safer method for achieving mydriasis rather than the use of curariform drugs.

Cataracts

Mature blinding cataracts are readily visible as a white opacity through the pupil of the eyes (Figures 16.24 and 16.25). Immature cataracts are more difficult to visualize without the use of ophthalmic equipment such as a direct ophthalmoscope or slit lamp biomicroscope. Incipient opacities in the lens are more difficult still to evaluate and the most useful technique is retro-illumination, viewing against the red reflex, using a direct ophthalmoscope at +10D.

As with any species, there are several factors involved in the generation of any lens opacity. Nutritional deficiency, particularly of antioxidants, may be a factor in causing lens opacification. Ultraviolet (UV) illumination, as widely used to prevent metabolic bone disease, may be a more likely aetiopathogenic agent in the development of cataracts. However, there is currently no direct evidence of UV light causing cataract development in reptiles.

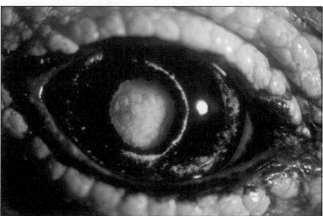

16.24 Mature cataract in a tree monitor lizard.
(© David Williams)

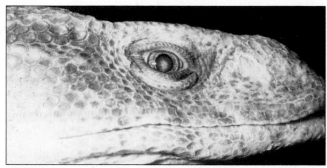

16.25 Cataract formation in a monitor lizard that was housed in close proximity to a UV light source. Although suggestive, there is currently no direct evidence of UV light causing cataracts in reptiles.
(© David Williams)

The author has recently examined the eyes of a number of inland bearded dragons and Chinese water dragons kept under the same UV irradiation (350–450 uW/cm²). The former species is exposed to considerable levels of UV irradiation in its natural environment, while the latter species (which resides under a leaf canopy) is adapted for a substantially lower UV light level. (It should be noted that two different species from similar environments have been shown to have significantly different degrees of skin absorption of UV light, and the same might be expected in relation to lens absorption.) The forest-dwelling lizards were found to have a significantly higher prevalence of nuclear cataract compared with the inland bearded dragons, the lens of which may be presumed to be adapted to high levels of UV light.

Freeze artefacts during hibernation have also been suggested as a cause of cataracts in tortoises (Lawton and Stokes, 1989), and the author's study investigating lens opacification in older *Testudo* species revealed that beyond 35 years of age, most if not all tortoises in this genus have some lens opacification (Williams, 2012), but without reported hibernational freezing in any of the animals examined. Cataract surgery using phacoemulsification has been reported in a monitor lizard (Colitz *et al.*, 2002) and a green sea turtle (Kelly *et al.*, 2005).

Glaucoma

Increased intraocular pressure has not been reported in reptiles, but several studies have reported the normal intraocular pressure in tortoise species and alligators (see Figure 16.5). The spectacle precludes the measurement of intraocular pressure in snakes by tonometry, as well as the assessment of globe size other than by ultrasonography. Tripathi's (1970) comprehensive account of aqueous outflow across the species gives a valuable insight into the drainage pathways of each reptile group. The differences between species of reptile occur because of the variation in anterior chamber depth and anatomy of the iridociliary cleft and ciliary musculature, which varies with the different mechanisms of accommodation (see above).

Microphthalmos and anophthalmos

As with any species, congenital abnormalities may be encountered in reptiles. Microphthalmos and, less commonly, anophthalmos are not infrequently seen (Millichamp and Jacobson, 1990; Da Silva *et al.*, 2015). Visual dysfunction occurs in many cases, ranging from total blindness in anophthalmic animals to mild visual impairment in microphthalmic animals (Figure 16.26). Blind reptiles experience

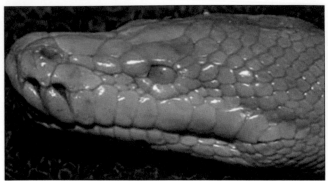

16.26 Microphthalmos and corneal oedema in a snake hatched from an egg incubated at too high a temperature.

(© David Williams)

great difficulty in eating since they are high visually motivated feeders. A common concurrent problem seen in moderate to severe cases is orbital infection; this is due to the conjunctival sac being increased in size as a result of the reduced globe diameter. These congenital defects may be associated with incubating eggs at too high a temperature. The pathogenesis is likely to involve increased metabolism with a relative hypoxia, which results in abnormalities of globe development.

Posterior segment lesions

While the reptile retina has been the subject of a number of studies, reports of retinal disease are vanishingly rare in the literature. Three exceptions to this paucity of data exist: the first is a report of post-hibernational freeze damage in *Testudo* species retinas leading to blindness (Lawton and Stoakes, 1989), although the relative contribution of retinal and central lesions to visual loss is difficult to assess with certainty. The second is the retinal toxicity of mercury in alligators in the Florida Everglades (Heaton-Jones, 1990). Changes in the electroretinogram were seen in mercury-intoxicated animals, reflecting the high concentrations of the metal toxin in the retinas, optic nerves and optic tracts of affected individuals. The third is a reported case of disseminated phaeohyphomycosis due to an *Exophiala* species in a Galapagos tortoise (Manharth *et al.*, 2005).

References and further reading

Abel JH and Ellis RA (1966) Histochemical and electron microscopic observations on the salt-secreting lachrymal glands of marine turtles. *American Journal of Anatomy* **118**, 337–358

Abou-Madi N and Kern TJ (2002) Squamous cell carcinoma associated with a periorbital mass in a veiled chameleon (*Chamaeleo calyptratus*). *Veterinary Ophthalmology* **5**, 217–220

Allgoewer I, Göbel T, Stockhaus C and Schaeffer EH (2002) Dacryops in a red-eared slider (*Chrysemys scripta elegans*): case report. *Veterinary Ophthalmology* **5**, 231–234

Boniuk M and Luquette GF (1963) Leukocoria and pseudobuphthalmos in snakes. *Investigative Ophthalmology* **2**, 283

Bonney CH, Hartfiel DA and Schmidt RE (1978) *Klebsiella pseumoniae* infection with secondary hypopyon in Tokay gecko lizards. *Journal of the American Veterinary Medical Association* **173**, 1115–1116

Colitz CM, Lewbart G and Davidson MG (2002) Phacoemulsification in an adult Savannah monitor lizard. *Veterinary Ophthalmology* **5**, 207–209

Cooper JE (1975) Exophthalmia in a Rhinoceros viper (*Bitis nasicornis*). *Veterinary Record* **97**, 130–131

Cooper JE, McClelland MH and Needham JR (1980) An eye infection in laboratory lizards associated with an *Aeromonas* species. *Laboratory Animals* **14**, 149–151

Cullen CL, Wheler C and Grahn BH (2000) Diagnostic ophthalmology: bullous spectaculopathy in a king snake. *Canadian Veterinary Journal* **41**, 327–328

Da Silva MAO, Bertelsen M, Wang T, Pedersen M, Lauridsen H and Heegaard S (2015) Unilateral microphthalmia or anophthalmia in eight pythons (*Pythonidae*). *Veterinary Ophthalmology* **18(S1)**, 23–29

Elkan E and Zwart P (1967) The ocular disease of young terrapins caused by vitamin A deficiency. *Pathology Veterinaria* **4**, 201–222

Frye FL (1981) *Biomedical and Surgical Aspects of Captive Reptile Husbandry.* Krieger Publishing, Malabar, Florida

Gardiner DW, Baines FM and Pandher K (2009) Photodermatitis and photokeratoconjunctivitis in a ball python (*Python regius*) and a blue-tongued skink (*Tiliqua* spp.). *Journal of Zoo and Wildlife Medicine* **40(4)**, 757–766

Grace MS and Woodward OM (2001) Altered visual experience and acute visual deprivation affect predatory targeting by infrared-imaging Boid snakes. *Brain Research* **919(2)**, 250–258

Grace MS, Woodward OM, Church DR and Catlisch G (2001) Prey targeting by the infrared-imaging snake Python: effects of experimental and congenital visual deprivation. *Behavioural Brain Research* **119**, 23–31

Hardon T, Fledelius B and Heegaard S (2007) Keratoacanthoma of the spectacle in a Boa constrictor. *Veterinary Ophthalmology* **10**, 320–322

Haverly JE and Kardong KV (1996) Sensory deprivation effects on the predatory behaviour of the rattlesnake *Crotalus viridis oreganus*. *Copeia* 419–428

Huchzermeyer FW, Langlet E and Putterill JP (2008) An outbreak of chlamydiosis in farmed Indopacific crocodiles (*Crocodylus porosus*). *Journal of the South African Veterinary Association* **79**, 99–100

Kelly TR, Walton W, Nadelstein B and Lewbart GA (2005) Phacoemulsification of bilateral cataracts in a loggerhead sea turtle (*Caretta caretta*). *Veterinary Record* **156**, 774–777

Lawton MPC and Stokes LC (1989) Post-hibernational blindness in tortoises (*Testudo* spp.) *Proceedings of the Third International Colloquium on Pathology of Reptiles and Amphibians, Orlando, Florida*, ed. ER Jacobson, pp. 56–58

Malmström T and Kröger RH (2006) Pupil shapes and lens optics in the eyes of terrestrial vertebrates. *Journal of Experimental Biology* **209**, 18–25

Manharth A, Lemberger K, Mylniczenko N *et al.* (2005) Disseminated phaeohyphomycosis due to an *Exophiala* species in a Galapagos tortoise, *Geochelone nigra*. *Journal of Herpetological Medicine and Surgery* **15(2)**, pp. 20–26

Martin GR (2009) What is binocular vision for? A birds' eye view. *Journal of Vision* **9(11)**, 14

Mayer J, Pizzirani S and DeSena R (2010) Bilateral exophthalmos in an adult iguana (*Iguana iguana*) caused by an orbital abscess. *Journal of Herpetological Medicine and Surgery* **20**, 5–10

Mead AW (1976) Vascularity in the reptilian spectacle. *Investigative Ophthalmology* **15**, 587

Montali RJ (1988) Comparative pathology of inflammation in the higher vertebrates (reptiles, birds and mammals). *Journal of Comparative Pathology* **99**, 1–26

Montiani-Ferreira F (2008) Ophthalmology. In: *Biology, Medicine and Surgery of South American Wild Animals*, ed. ME Fowler and ZS Cubas, p 443. Iowa State University Press, Ames, Iowa

Millichamp NJ, Jacobson ER and Dziezyc J (1986) Conjunctivoralostomy for treatment of an occluded lacrimal duct in a blood python. *Journal of the American Veterinary Medical Association* **189**, 1136–1138

Millichamp NJ, Jacobson ER and Wolf ED (1983) Diseases of the eye and ocular adnexae in reptiles. *Journal of the American Veterinary Medical Association* **183**, 1205–1212

Minucci S, Chieffi Baccari G and di Matteo L (1981) Histology, histochemistry and ultrastructure of the Harderian gland of the snake *Coluber viridiflavus*. *Journal of Morphology* **211**, 207–212

Murphy CJ and Howland HC (1986) On the gecko pupil and Scheiner's disc. *Vision Research* **26(5)**, 815–817

Musgrave KE, Diehl K and Mans C (2016) Aeromonas hydrophila keratitis in freshwater turtles. *Journal of Exotic Pet Medicine* **25(1)**, 26–29

Ott M (2006) Visual accommodation in vertebrates: mechanisms, physiological response and stimuli. *Journal of Comparative Physiology A: Neuroethology, Sensory, Neural and Behavioural Physiology* **192(2)**, 97–111

Pchelyakov VF (1981) Structural peculiarities of the cornea of the reptilian eye. *Neuroscience Behaviour and Physiology* **11**, 367–370

Reavil D and Schmidt RE (2012) Pathology of the reptile eye and ocular adnexia. *Proceedings of the Association of Reptilian and Amphibian Veterinarians*, pp. 87–97

Roth LS and Kelber A (2004) Nocturnal colour vision in geckos. *Proceedings of Biological Science* **271(Suppl. 6)**, S485–S487

Schumacher J, Pellicane CP, Heard DJ and Voges A (1996) Periorbital abscess in a chameleon (*Chameleon jacksonii*). *Veterinary and Comparative Ophthalmology* **6**, 30–33

Selmi AL, Mendes GM and MacManus C (2003) Tonometry in adult yellow-footed tortoises (*Geochelone denticulata*). *Veterinary Ophthalmology* **6**, 305–307

Shine R (2013) Reptiles. *Current Biology* **23(6)**, R227–R231

Silman AJ, Govardovskii VI, Röhlich P, Southard JA and Loew ER (1997) The photoreceptors and visual pigments of the garter snake (*Thamnophis sirtalis*): a microspectrophotometric, scanning electron microscopic and immunocyto-chemical study. *Journal of Comparative Physiology A* **181(2)**, 89–101

Silman AJ, Johnson JL and Loew ER (2001) Retinal photoreceptors and visual pigments in Boa constrictor imperator. *Journal of Experimental Zoology* **290(4)**, 359–365

Tangredi BP and Evans RH (1997) Organochlorine pesticides associated with ocular, nasal or otic infection in the eastern box turtle (*Terrapene carolina carolina*). *Journal of Zoo and Wildlife Medicine* **28(1)**, 97–100

Tomson FN, McDonnell SE and Wolf ED (1976) Hypopyonin a tortoise. *Journal of the American Veterinary Medical Association* **173**, 1115

Tripathi RC (1974) Comparative physiology and anatomy of the aqueous outflow pathway. In: *The Eye*, ed. H Davson and LT Graham, pp. 163–197. Academic Press, London and New York

Underwood G (1970) The eye. In: *Biology of the Reptilia Volume 2B*, ed. C Gans and TS Parsons, pp. 1–97. Academic Press, London and New York

Walls GL (1942) *The Vertebrate Eye and Its Adaptive Radiation*. Hafner Publishing Company, New York and London

Whittaker CJ, Heaton-Jones TG, Kubilis PS *et al.* (1995) Intraocular pressure variation associated with body length in young American alligators (*Alligator mississippiensis*). *American Journal of Veterinary Research* **56**, 1380–1383

Whittaker CJ, Schumacher J, Bennett AR *et al.* (1997) Orbital varix in a green iguana (*Iguana iguana*). *Veterinary and Comparative Ophthalmology* **7**, 101–104

Williams DL (2012) *Ophthamology of Exotic Pets*. Wiley-Blackwell, Oxford

Zwart P, Verwer MAJ, DeVries GA *et al.* (1973) Fungal infection of the eyes of the snake *Epicrates chendra maurus*: enucleation under halothane narcosis. *Journal of Small Animal Practice* **14(12)**, 773–779

Chapter 17

Gastrointestinal system

Sarah J.L. Brown, Adam D. Naylor, Ross A. Machin and Sarah Pellett

Diagnosis and treatment of gastrointestinal disease in reptiles can be challenging due to the huge anatomical and physiological diversity between species. A thorough and systematic approach to cases is essential.

Clinical approach

History and clinical examination

The case history and clinical examination may be suggestive of gastrointestinal disease, such as reports or evidence of regurgitation, vomiting, or changes in faecal quality or output. In many cases, however, gastrointestinal disease may present as non-specific signs including weight loss, lethargy and anorexia, and a comprehensive work-up is required in order to establish the underlying aetiology.

Diagnostic procedures

Faecal examination

Faecal examination is crucial to the reptile health assessment. Samples should be fresh so that parasites, especially motile protozoa, are not missed. If a fresh void cannot be obtained, warm bathing, gentle coelomic massage or a cloacal flush may yield a diagnostic sample.

Performing a cloacal flush:

1. Suitably restrain the animal.
2. Insert a lubricated smooth-ended urinary catheter just beyond the vent opening.
3. Infuse 1–2 ml of sterile saline per 100 g bodyweight.
4. Gently massage the caudal coelom.
5. Aspirate the sample and withdraw the catheter.

(NB: concentrating techniques, such as sedimentation, may improve diagnostic value).

Identification of a faecal parasite is important, but careful interpretation is required to determine its clinical relevance (see Chapter 24). Amplification of parasite burdens occurs when environmental hygiene is poor. This is commonly seen with oxyurid and protozoal infections (Figure 17.1). Serial faecal examinations will check the efficacy of anti-parasitic treatments.

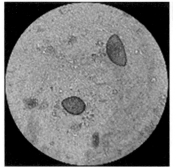

17.1 Oxyurid ovum (top) and *Nyctotherus* cyst (bottom) on a wet preparation from a Mediterranean spur-thighed tortoise; X400.

Faecal examination techniques:
Direct wet preparation: Qualitative technique for identifying helminth eggs and larvae, and protozoal trophozoites, oocysts and cysts. Sensitivity may be low and dependent on the level of parasite burden. This technique provides a valuable initial assessment; the presence of excessive amounts of undigested food or high numbers of a single organism may indicate abnormality.

Flotation: Uses a solution (sugar or salt) with a higher specific gravity than that of the eggs, cysts or oocysts of interest. Large eggs (e.g. spirurid nematodes, cestodes and trematodes) require higher density solutions for flotation. McMaster and Stoll techniques enable quantitative egg counts (expressed in eggs per gram).

Sedimentation: Filtration with centrifugation and sediment examination allows improved detection sensitivity for scarce parasites and large eggs not readily detected by flotation techniques.

Stained smears: Lugol's iodine or formalin immobilizes and allows identification of motile trophozoites and amoebic cysts. Acid-fast stains (e.g. modified Ziehl–Neelsen) are useful for *Cryptosporidium* identification (see also Chapter 24).

Haematology and plasma biochemistry

Characteristic changes in absolute white cell counts as well as shifts in the cell differential may help distinguish between acute and chronic gastrointestinal diseases and assist with alluding to the underlying aetiology. Interpretation must be made in conjunction with clinical signs and other diagnostic tests as leucogram changes in gastrointestinal disease are often non-specific (see also Chapter 8).

Biochemistry changes must also be interpreted with care. Enzyme activities in intestinal tissue are low and of poor diagnostic value. Low blood albumin levels are associated with gastrointestinal disease due to decreased uptake (e.g. anorexia or malabsorption), decreased production (e.g. liver disease) or increased loss (e.g. protein-losing enteropathies), but diseases of other systems must also be considered (e.g. protein-losing nephropathies). Hepatocellular damage can lead to elevations in numerous intracellular enzymes; however, wide distribution of these enzymes in other tissues, including muscle and kidney, limits their diagnostic value (Eatwell *et al.*, 2014).

Imaging

For further information, see Chapters 9 and 10.

Radiography: Plain radiography may be useful for identifying excessive gas or radio-dense foreign material within the gastrointestinal tract. Contrast radiography provides significant diagnostic advantages for the investigation of obstruction, motility issues, tract integrity and tract size, as well as allowing differentiation from other coelomic organs. Barium sulphate (Figure 17.2) and iodinated contrast agents have been evaluated in reptiles. Selection should be based on species and presentation (see below). Volumes in the range 5–25 ml/kg are appropriate.

Barium sulphate suspensions (25–70%) provide superior mucosal detail but have prolonged large intestinal clearance (due to water absorption reducing barium viscosity). They are not appropriate where tract integrity is compromised. The use of barium-impregnated polyethylene spheres (BIPS) may avoid some potential complications associated with liquid formulations, but will not provide mucosal detail or show filling defects; they are primarily used to evaluate motility disorders of the gastrointestinal tract.

Water-soluble iodides carry reduced risk of solidification in the large intestine and so may be more appropriate for herbivorous species with prolonged gut transit times. They are not recommended in dehydrated patients owing to their hyperosmolar properties, and progressive reduction of radiographic opacity during gut transit has been reported.

Gut transit times vary with different contrast agents, and with many physiological and environmental factors, so following a published study protocol when investigating hypomotility issues is advised. In particular, the type, concentration and volume of contrast agent; fasting time; and the environmental temperature should be taken into consideration. Transit contrast studies in a range of species are summarized by Mans (2013).

Ultrasonography: 7.5 MHz transducers are appropriate for the assessment of most pet species. The addition of a stand-off can be beneficial when evaluating very small patients. Visualization is good where the tract is fluid filled or empty but can be challenging when large amounts of gas are present (e.g. herbivorous species) or if access is limited (e.g. chelonians).

Assessment of the size and homogeneity of the liver and gall bladder is straightforward in most reptile species. Comparing hepatic echogenicity with the hyperechoic coelomic fat bodies in lizards and snakes allows objective interpretation and monitoring. Ultrasound-guided fine-needle aspirate sampling can be performed.

Endoscopy: For intraluminal diseases of the digestive tract, endoscopy provides a means of visual assessment, biopsy sample collection and foreign body retrieval. The

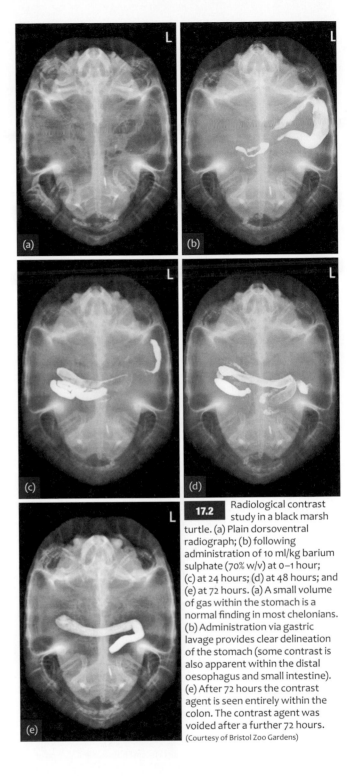

17.2 Radiological contrast study in a black marsh turtle. (a) Plain dorsoventral radiograph; (b) following administration of 10 ml/kg barium sulphate (70% w/v) at 0–1 hour; (c) at 24 hours; (d) at 48 hours; and (e) at 72 hours. (a) A small volume of gas within the stomach is a normal finding in most chelonians. (b) Administration via gastric lavage provides clear delineation of the stomach (some contrast is also apparent within the distal oesophagus and small intestine). (e) After 72 hours the contrast agent is seen entirely within the colon. The contrast agent was voided after a further 72 hours. (Courtesy of Bristol Zoo Gardens)

buccal cavity, oesophagus and stomach may be assessed via an oral approach, and the outflow of the large intestine (the coprodeum) may be visualized via a cloacal approach.

For visual assessment and diagnostic sample collection from the liver, pancreas and serosal surfaces of the digestive tract, a coelioscopic technique is required. In lizards and chelonians, this approach is extremely valuable owing to the small entry sites needed and excellent visualization achieved. In snakes, insufflation is difficult and multiple entry sites are required in order to make a full assessment. This may make other imaging modalities or coeliotomy more appropriate.

Advanced imaging modalities: Computed tomography evaluation is increasingly inexpensive and quick to perform. The close proximity and similar tissue opacities of the liver and digestive tract can make differentiation challenging, and so prior administration of oral contrast agents is recommended. The presence of gas within the digestive tract is easily recognized, making this modality useful for evaluation of herbivorous species where tract ultrasonography is more difficult. Evaluation of liver size and density may be particularly valuable; in Hermann's tortoises, low hepatic parenchyma densities have been strongly correlated with hepatic lipidosis (Gumpernberger, 2011).

Magnetic resonance imaging is superior to computed tomography for assessment of the liver and digestive system owing to its excellent soft tissue detail and intrinsic high tissue contrast. Currently the high cost has limited its use in pet reptiles.

Coeliotomy: While endoscopy is less invasive than coeliotomy, assessment of the entire digestive tract is not feasible using endoscopy alone and so exploratory coeliotomy has a valuable role to play in the assessment of gastrointestinal disease. Coeliotomy allows inspection of intestines and viscera as well as biopsy sample collection. If an obstructive or penetrating foreign body is suggested by imaging, exploratory coeliotomy is justified (see also Chapter 13).

Histopathology: Tissue samples for histopathological examination may be harvested endoscopically or via coeliotomy,

and from fatalities or sacrificed animals within a diseased group. Histopathology may offer significantly more reliable or detailed assessment than non-invasive diagnostic testing alone.

Molecular tests/viral isolation: A variety of viral diagnostic tests are available commercially including polymerase chain reaction (PCR) assays and virus isolation kits. Tests more commonly used in the investigation of gastrointestinal disease in pet reptiles include PCRs for herpes and ranaviruses in chelonians and for *Atadenovirus* in bearded dragons.

Diseases by region

See Figure 17.3 for clinical signs associated with specific regions of the gastrointestinal tract.

Beak abnormalities

Abnormalities or damage to the chelonian beak can result in anorexia due to impaired food prehension. Keratin sheaths cover the maxillary and mandibular crests. In tortoises, the rhinotheca (maxillary keratin sheath) is often seen overgrown to a rostral point (Figure 17.4), while overgrowth of the gnathotheca (mandibular keratin sheath) causes lateral protrusion (Figure 17.5).

Region	Common clinical signs		Non-specific signs
Oropharynx	• Dysphagia • Facial/gular swelling • Regurgitation • Hypersalivation • Oral discharge • Discoloration of oral mucosa Extension from or to respiratory disease (see Chapter 18; Respiratory system) Extension from or to ocular disease (see Chapter 16; Ophthalmology)		• Anorexia • Weight loss • Lethargy • Vomiting/regurgitation
Oesophagus	• Dysphagia • Regurgitation • Hypersalivation Extension from or to disease of the oropharynx and stomach		
Stomach	• Vomiting/regurgitation • Melaena/haematemesis (gastric ulceration) • Coelomic distension (coelomitis secondary to perforation, gastric distension and gastric hypertrophy (*Cryptosporidium* infection of snakes))		
Liver	• Non-specific (see right) • Biliverdinuria/jaundice (advanced disease) • Diarrhoea (acute hepatitis) • Coelomic distension (hepatomegaly and ascites secondary to hypoproteinaemia)		
Pancreas	• Non-specific (see right) • Hyperglycaemia (rare)		
Small intestine	• Melaena • Steatorrhoea	• Constipation/obstipation • Vomiting • Diarrhoea • Tenesmus • Cloacal organ prolapse	
Large intestine	• Haematochezia • Mucoid faeces	• Coelomic distension (ascites secondary to protein-losing enteropathies, coelomitis secondary to perforation, and intestinal distension) • Borborygmi/flatus	
Cloaca	• Cloacal organ prolapse • Diarrhoea • Tenesmus		

17.3 Clinical signs associated with specific regions of the gastrointestinal tract.

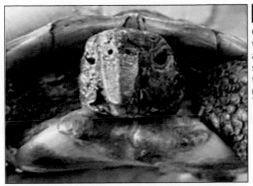

17.4

Overgrowth of the rhinotheca in a Mediterranean spur-thighed tortoise.
(Courtesy of Norfolk Tortoise Club)

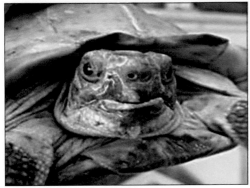

17.5

Overgrowth of the gnathotheca in a Horsfield's tortoise.
(Courtesy of Norfolk Tortoise Club)

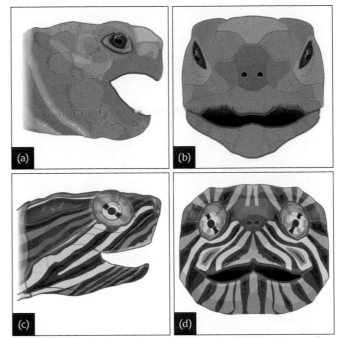

17.6 Lateral and rostral views of (a–b) a spur-thighed tortoise and (c–d) a red-eared terrapin, showing normal beak anatomy. Note that marked differences in normal beak anatomy occur between chelonian species, so literature review before corrective trimming is advised.

Aetiology

Beak overgrowth has been associated with nutritional secondary hyperparathyroidism, hypovitaminosis A, accelerated growth, congenital abnormalities, infection and trauma. Symmetrical overgrowth is often associated with nutritional aetiologies, while asymmetrical abnormalities can suggest localized infection or trauma.

Treatment

The beak can be easily trimmed to restore functional (and ideally natural) anatomy using a high-speed burr. Serial treatments are usually necessary. Concurrent osteomyelitis should be ruled out and underlying factors such as nutritional and husbandry deficiencies addressed.

Aquatic chelonians that normally consume shellfish and crustaceans (e.g. diamondback terrapins) have broad maxillary and mandibular dental plates which are used to crush food items. These may also become overgrown.

Performing corrective beak trimming:

1. Review normal species beak anatomy (Figure 17.6).
2. Suitably restrain the patient; for large/aggressive species, sedation or anaesthesia may be necessary.
3. Place an oral gag (e.g. syringe case or tongue depressor):
   - For correction of rhinothecal overgrowth, the flat surface of a circular cutting disc or a parallel-sided bar burr on a high-speed woodwork tool (e.g. Dremel multi drill) is used to gradually reduce the rostral beak length. A conical burr or small dental burr is then used to shape the lateral rhinothecal walls
   - For correction of gnathothecal overgrowth, a conical burr or small dental burr is used to reduce the lateral edges. Full return to natural anatomy is often not achieved.

Periodontal disease

Periodontal disease is a significant cause of morbidity in lizards with acrodont dentition, particularly the chameleons and agamids (e.g. water dragons and bearded dragons). Acrodont teeth are not continuously replaced and are ankylosed directly to the exposed crests of the mandibular and maxillary bones. The teeth of most snakes and other lizards are regularly replaced (pleurodont) so dental disease is uncommon in these species.

Early stages of disease are frequently not detected by owners. More advanced cases may be presented with anorexia or systemic illness. Examination findings include facial swelling over the mandibles or maxillae, gingival erythema, gingival swelling, formation of calculus, gingival recession or hyperplasia, osteomyelitis of the facial bones, and loosening or loss of teeth.

Aetiology

An inappropriately soft diet (predominantly fruit or soft-bodied insects) may predispose to bacterial colonization and development of periodontal disease (McCracken and Birch, 1994). Other factors which may lead to bacterial colonization or loosening and damage of the teeth include nutritional secondary hyperparathyroidism, extension of infection from rostral abrasions, mouthing inappropriate cage furniture and immunosuppression resulting from underlying systemic disease.

Initially, plaque and calculus build-up leads to an inflammatory response in the marginal gingiva causing gingivitis and gingival recession (Figure 17.7). As disease progresses, osteomyelitis is common owing to bone exposure. Gram-negative bacteria often predominate and culture of anaerobic bacteria, spirochaetes and fungal agents is common. Ultimately, infection leads to tooth loss and facial bone disintegration (Figure 17.8). Spread of infection by thromboses to other organs, such as the liver, has been reported (Redrobe and Frye, 2001).

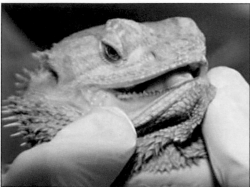

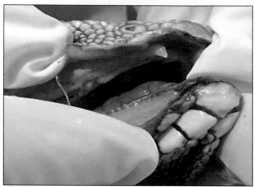

17.7 A bearded dragon displaying discoloration of the mandibular teeth, calculus build-up and gingival recession.

17.8 An Asian water dragon displaying advanced periodontal disease; marked gingival recession, loss of teeth, and missing sections of the maxillary and mandibular bone are noted.

Treatment

General anaesthesia is required to investigate periodontal disease lesions and remove calculus by ultrasonic or instrumental descaling. Radiographic assessment is useful initially and throughout treatment; pathological fractures, sequestrum formation, periosteal proliferation and bone lysis are reported. Aggressive debridement of necrotic bone and curettage of abscess lesions may be necessary; lizards often cope well with extensive loss of bone (deficits eventually fill with fibrous tissue). Regular irrigation of the mouth with 0.05% chlorhexidine solution is useful in mild cases and as a long-term adjunct to treatment in more severe disease. Systemic antibiotic therapy should be based on culture and sensitivity. Local application of antibiotic-impregnated polymethyl methacrylate beads can also be considered (Mans, 2013). Fungal periodontal osteomyelitis has been reported (Heatley *et al.*, 2001), emphasizing the need for diagnostic testing (culture, cytology and/or histopathology) in order to avoid treatment failures. Analgesia is recommended and supportive feeding (ideally via oesophagostomy tube) may be necessary. Environmental and dietary issues must be addressed. Providing harder, more chitinous invertebrates such as cockroaches and beetles may help prevent recurrence.

Rostral abrasions

Snout and rostral maxilla damage can occur from repeated contact with glass or plastic vivarium walls. Sequelae include stomatitis, gingivitis, and osteomyelitis of the mandible and maxilla. Rostral trauma is common in nervous lizards such as Asian water dragons, which may run into the walls of their enclosure when startled (Figure 17.9). It is also commonly seen in snakes repeatedly

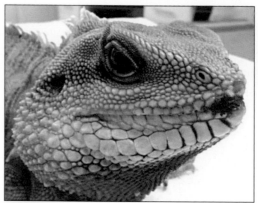

17.9 Mild rostral abrasions in an Asian water dragon affecting the rostral maxilla and mandible. At this stage, management changes alone may be sufficient in preventing further progression.

attempting to escape from inappropriately small enclosures (e.g. large boas and pythons), in breeding males attempting to reach receptive females, and in nervous or aggressive species striking at movement outside the enclosure (e.g. arboreal boas and pythons) (Figure 17.10). Other causes of facial trauma include bites from live prey and burns from unshielded heat sources.

Treatment

Systemic antibiotics, ideally based on culture and sensitivity results, and medicated barrier ointments can be helpful in managing secondary infections, while severe cases (with osteomyelitis of facial bones) can be managed similarly to periodontal disease. Environmental factors must be addressed, with the addition of visual barriers at the animal's eye level and shelter from external stressors. Tape strips or one-way glass can be used in addition to increasing cage furniture and shade, and reducing human disturbance. Moving the enclosure to a low-traffic area may help.

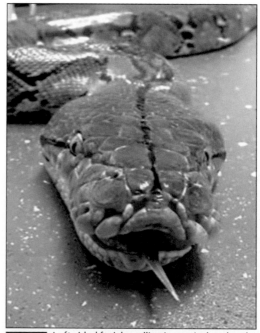

17.10 Left-sided facial swelling in a reticulated python. Inflammation and secondary infection resulted from repeated trauma on the vivarium glass wall.

Jaw fractures

Fractures of the mandibular symphysis or ramus are relatively common, particularly in individuals with poor bone health due to metabolic bone disease (see Chapter 22) or advanced periodontal infections. Care should be taken to avoid iatrogenic jaw fractures when examining reptiles' mouths and when using solid stomach tubes. Snakes may injure their jaws when attempting to strike prey items.

Treatment involves internal fixation (e.g. pins, tension band wires or external fixators) or external coaptation, depending on the species, fracture site and individual's bone quality (see Chapter 13). Owing to the prevalence of metabolic bone disease, caution is advised before considering internal fixation. Alternatively, if the fracture is well aligned, the jaw may be taped shut and an oesophagostomy tube placed for feeding while healing takes place. All affected individuals will require nutritional support, usually with oesophagostomy tube placement.

Stomatitis

Stomatitis, or 'mouth rot', involves mucosal inflammation and necrosis of the oral cavity. It can occur in any reptile species where husbandry is deficient, but in chelonians a strong primary viral association has been made. Left untreated, infection may spread to the facial bones resulting in osteomyelitis, ascend the nasolacrimal ducts to involve the eyes, or descend the trachea resulting in pneumonia. Without intervention death is not uncommon. A comprehensive work-up and aggressive treatment is recommended.

Clinical signs include anorexia, dysphagia, hypersalivation, perioral swelling, and inflammation of the oral mucosa and tongue. Diphtheritic/caseous plaques and haemorrhagic, mucoid or purulent oral discharge may be apparent. Stomatitis in chelonians is often referred to as stomatitis–rhinitis–conjunctivitis complex, as these clinical signs commonly appear together. However, respiratory or ocular signs in any species also warrant oral examination for stomatitis. Concurrent clinical signs depend on the underlying causative agent.

Aetiology

The aetiology is often multifactorial, commonly related to underlying husbandry factors and causes of immunosuppression such as poor enclosure hygiene, low environmental temperatures, overcrowding, excessively long or poorly controlled hibernation, and nutritional deficiencies. Hypovitaminosis A has been implicated as a primary cause of stomatitis in numerous reptile species (Stahl, 2013). Ulcerative stomatitis secondary to renal disease (uraemic ulceration) is uncommon in reptiles; however, deposition of uric acid crystals in the soft tissues of the gastrointestinal tract (visceral gout) may occur and is an important non-infectious differential for stomatitis (Figure 17.11).

Chelonians: The most common cause of chelonian stomatitis is viral infection, specifically with chelonian herpesviruses and ranaviruses (of the Iridoviridae family). Currently four chelonian herpesviruses are recognized. Exposure results in permanent infection with cycles of latency and recrudescence, often associated with immune status. Infections spread rapidly through colonies and consequently the virus is common in Mediterranean tortoises farmed for the pet trade. Ranaviruses have recently emerged as a significant cause of mortality in wild chelonian populations. Disease in pet species is usually associated with exposure to other infected reptiles or

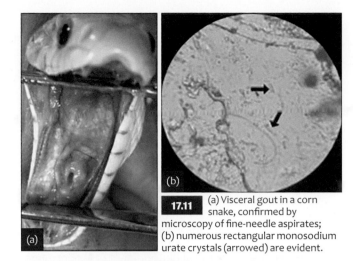

17.11 (a) Visceral gout in a corn snake, confirmed by microscopy of fine-needle aspirates; (b) numerous rectangular monosodium urate crystals (arrowed) are evident.

amphibians. Infection with either virus is typified by ulcerative to diphtheroid necrotizing stomatitis, with rhinitis and conjunctivitis. Damage to other organs such as the liver is reported with both viruses, and central nervous system signs have been seen with chronic herpesvirus infection. Bacterial infections including *Mycoplasma* are a rare primary cause of stomatitis; however, infection may result in immunosuppression and secondary stomatitis or recrudescence of concurrent herpesvirus infection. Irritation and ulceration of the oral mucosa may also be seen with ingestion of highly abrasive or caustic plants.

Squamates: Extension of infection from periodontal disease in lizards and rostral abrasions in all squamates frequently results in stomatitis (see above). Trauma to the mouth caused by prey items and iatrogenic damage from assisted feeding are also commonly implicated. Adenoviruses should be considered as a possible infectious differential for stomatitis, and in boid snakes stomatitis is frequently seen in association with inclusion body disease infection, probably secondary to immunosuppression.

Diagnosis

Cases require a comprehensive work-up and critical review of captive husbandry. Clinical examination, haematology and plasma biochemistry are recommended. Culture of oral lesions may help guide treatment; common secondary bacterial agents include *Pseudomonas*, *Klebsiella*, *Aeromonas* and *Salmonella* spp., and opportunistic fungal agents are not uncommon (e.g. *Candida albicans*). Cytology may be useful as, for example, oral lymphosarcoma may mimic infectious aetiologies. Radiography may identify underlying osteomyelitis.

An underlying viral aetiology may be suggested by clinical history, cytology or histopathology. For confirmation, PCR testing is generally preferred. A tortoise herpesvirus PCR detecting all four viruses is now widely available in the UK, in addition to PCRs targeting individual viruses. A ranavirus PCR has also been developed.

Treatment

Treatment and stabilization of affected individuals may be prolonged and is focused on optimizing immune function and treating underlying infections. Treatment should include:

- **Providing optimal environmental conditions:** e.g. UVB lighting, heat provision and humidity appropriate to the species. Vivarium design should aim to reduce stress levels (see rostral abrasions)

- **Treating active infections:**
  - **Systemic** – systemic antibacterial and antifungal treatments should be based on culture and sensitivity. Acyclovir (30–80 mg/kg orally q8h) has shown positive clinical response against herpesvirus infection (McArthur *et al.*, 2004), but may not eliminate it, and continued shedding after treatment is possible (Gibbons, 2013). Valacyclovir (40 mg/kg orally q24h) has also been proposed for herpesvirus treatment, and is rapidly converted to acyclovir after oral administration (Allender *et al.*, 2013)
  - **Topical** – cleaning lesions with 0.01% povidone iodine solution or 0.05% chlorhexidine solution is appropriate and topical antimicrobials such as silver sulfadiazine creams can be considered (Mehler and Avery Bennett, 2006). Topical acyclovir cream has been used with some success for viral lesions. In severe cases, surgical debridement of lesions under anaesthesia and continued conscious cleaning (daily) with reapplication of topical agents is recommended. Analgesia should be provided.
- **Providing nutritional support/fluid therapy:** nutritional support should be provided for anorexic, debilitated or cachectic patients. Oesophagostomy tube placement is recommended. Fluids may be provided orally, parenterally or via bathing (see management of anorexia and nutritional support)
- **Reduce spread of infection:** strict biosecurity with barrier nursing should be applied, treating all animals as potentially infectious. Optimizing immune status may reduce viral shedding but clearance is unlikely, so maintaining closed collections is recommended in these cases.

Prognosis will depend on the underlying cause of the stomatitis, the presence of concurrent disease and the individual's immune status. Cases involving osteomyelitis tend to carry more guarded prognoses.

Tongue prolapse

Prolapse and damage to the tongue are seen most frequently in species with long extendable tongues, such as chameleons, and snakes. Animals with generalized stomatitis may suffer infection of the tongue or tongue sheath resulting in prolapse. In chameleons, weakening of retractor muscles leading to permanent extension of the tongue is often the result of hypocalcaemia in animals suffering from nutritional secondary hyperparathyroidism (Figure 17.12). Iatrogenic prolapse and subsequent desiccation can also occur during anaesthesia, particularly in snakes.

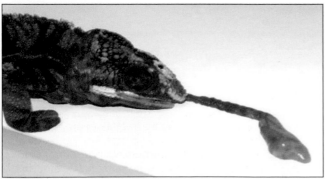

17.12 Tongue paresis in a panther chameleon due to nutritional secondary hyperparathyroidism.

The exposed tongue should be protected from desiccation using water-based lubricants, while underlying factors such as hypocalcaemia and stomatitis are addressed. Assisted feeding should be performed with care to prevent further trauma. Owing to contamination with substrate, desiccation and trauma, restoration of normal tongue function may be impossible. Euthanasia or amputation must be considered in these cases. With tongue amputation, long-term assisted feeding is required and quality of life must be considered carefully.

Oesophagitis and oesophageal ulceration

Oesophagitis in reptiles is commonly associated with extension of stomatitis or gastritis, the presence of foreign bodies – such as hooks embedded in the upper gastro-intestinal tract of aquatic turtles (Figure 17.13) – or iatrogenic injury sustained during assisted feeding. Oesophagitis is reported in association with stomatitis-causing viruses of chelonians, and also with adenovirus infection in several species of reptile across the order. Suggestive clinical signs of oesophagitis include dysphagia, regurgitation, hypersalivation and anorexia.

Diagnosis

A presumptive diagnosis may be made based on clinical signs, oral examination and history; however, endoscopic examination of the oesophageal mucosa, with or without biopsy, is preferred (see Chapters 9 and 10) (Figure 17.14). Specific viral testing may be warranted and oesophageal contrast studies may be useful.

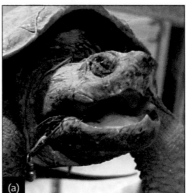

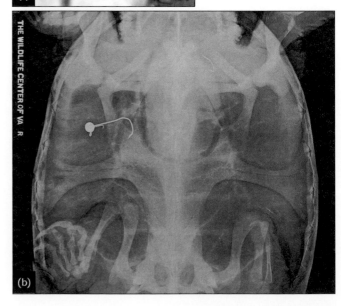

17.13 (a) A wild common snapping turtle presented with fishing tackle protruding from the mouth. (b) Dorsoventral radiography confirms the presence of two fishing hooks; one in the cranial and one in the caudal oesophagus. Both were removed using oral endoscopy under anaesthesia.
(Courtesy of Wildlife Center of Virginia)

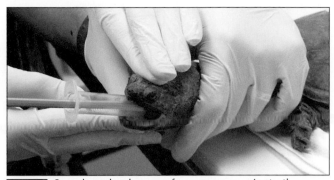

17.14 Oesophageal endoscopy of a common snapping turtle performed under sedation; a plastic syringe case is used as an oral gag to prevent damage to the scope.
(Courtesy of Wildlife Center of Virginia)

Treatment

In addition to treatment of underlying conditions, administration of sucralfate (500–1000 mg/kg orally q6–8h) and histamine receptor antagonists such as cimetidine (4 mg/kg i.m., orally q8h) may be beneficial. To avoid iatrogenic causes, round-ended gavage tubes should be used and careful attention paid to correct technique. Where repeated oral medication or feeding is required, oesophagostomy tube placement is recommended.

Gastric disease and gastric ulceration

Acute aetiologies of gastritis include thermal burns following feeding of inappropriately hot food items (e.g. snakes fed with microwave-defrosted rodents), toxic plant ingestion, gastric foreign bodies, and the effects of non-steroidal anti-inflammatory drugs or corticosteroids. Gastritis has also been associated with chronic poor husbandry (specifically inappropriate environmental temperatures and inappropriate diet), neoplasia (e.g. neuroendocrine carcinomas in bearded dragons) and a number of infectious agents (e.g. cryptosporidium, adenoviruses). An association between gastritis/gastric ulceration and stress is unproven in reptiles but should be considered.

Initial clinical signs may be subtle, including anorexia, lethargy and weight loss. Vomiting and regurgitation are possible but can be difficult to differentiate in reptiles as ejected food is often simply found within the enclosure. Regurgitation is common in snakes owing to a lack of distinct division between the oesophagus and stomach. In lizards and chelonians, regurgitation is unusual and vomiting is frequently associated with advanced gastric disease. With gastric ulceration, vomiting of haemorrhagic stomach contents and melaena are reported. Perforation may result in peritonitis and ascites. Mid-body swellings may be apparent in snakes with gastric hypertrophy caused by cryptosporidiosis.

Diagnosis

Thorough anamnesis is often beneficial to help distinguish between acute and chronic causes of gastric disease. Gastroscopy and gastric mucosal biopsy are recommended. Gastric lavage sampling, plain and contrast radiography, coelomic endoscopy (see Chapter 10), faecal analysis (see Chapter 8), and exploratory coeliotomy may all be warranted. Blood analysis may suggest protein loss, and anaemia was reported as a consistent clinical finding in a case series of green iguanas with gastric ulcers (Kubisch *et al.*, 2006).

Treatment

Specific treatment depends on the underlying cause. Husbandry correction, fluid therapy (with correction of electrolyte imbalances) and nutritional support are warranted. Administration of sucralfate (500–1000 mg/kg orally q6–8h) and histamine receptor antagonists such as cimetidine (4 mg/kg i.m., orally q8h) will be beneficial in most cases. Blood transfusion should be considered for severe anaemia associated with gastric ulceration (see Chapter 7), and perforating ulcers require aggressive therapy including coeliotomy for coelomic lavage. Partial and complete gastrectomies have been performed with success in several species (Figure 17.15) (see Chapter 13).

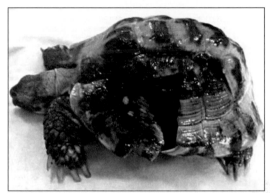

17.15 A Mediterranean spur-thighed tortoise with severe external and internal trauma, having been hit by a car. Gastric rupture was identified and partial gastrectomy (30%) was required prior to repair of the carapace. An oesophagostomy tube was placed to facilitate fluid and nutritional support. The tortoise went on to make a full recovery.

Enterocolitis and dysbiosis

Enterocolitis and dysbiosis are common in pet reptiles. Primary types of enterocolitis include those caused by infectious agents (primarily viruses, such as adenovirus; protozoa, such as *Cryptosporidium*; and helminths) and drug induced (e.g. following non-steroidal anti-inflammatory and corticosteroid administration). Enterocolitis also occurs secondary to dysbiosis (i.e. bacterial, fungal and/or protozoal overgrowth). This is frequently associated with underlying husbandry issues; feeding diets high in sugars (e.g. fruit) to Mediterranean tortoises or providing inappropriate temperatures to all species may result in fermentation and putrefaction of food within the gut. Prolonged antimicrobial use may lead to fungal dysbiosis.

Anorexia, lethargy, weight loss, excessive gas production resulting in tympany, and diarrhoea are all commonly reported. The differences between small and large intestinal disease observed in canine and feline medicine are less common in reptiles. In some reports, steatorrhoea and melaena have been associated with small intestinal disease, and haematochezia and increased mucus production with diseases of the large intestine, but this differentiation is often unclear. Septicaemia may result if the condition is not treated.

Diagnosis

The underlying cause should be identified. Faecal parasitology is valuable, in addition to ultrasonography, endoscopy (± biopsy), and plain and contrast radiography. Blood work may suggest protein-losing enteropathy and dehydration. Thorough anamnesis to rule out husbandry problems is recommended and testing for specific infectious agents may be indicated.

Faecal bacteriology may be misleading as normal reptilian gut flora is not well documented. Pure bacterial cultures, particularly of Gram-negative organisms, have been isolated in both sick and healthy reptiles. Fungal overgrowth is indicative of underlying husbandry problems or immunosuppression.

Treatment

Underlying husbandry issues should be addressed. Where dysbiosis (bacterial, fungal or protozoal) is suspected, husbandry and dietary correction frequently leads to resolution without the need for medical therapy.

Most cases will benefit from fluid therapy and appropriate nutritional support. Transfaunation (feeding of faeces from a clinically 'normal' reptile) has been advocated, but risks possible disease transmission. Probiotics have been used with mixed response in reptiles. Pectin-containing products have been used anecdotally for the management of diarrhoea.

Targeted use of antimicrobials can be considered; nystatin may be used for fungal overgrowth and metronidazole used to reduce anaerobic bacterial populations. Treatment is, however, controversial as it may potentiate ongoing dysbiosis.

Cloacal organ prolapse (including colon prolapse)

Organs which may prolapse through the cloaca (and out through the vent) are the cloacal wall, colon, urinary bladder (if present), phallus (chelonians and crocodilians) or hemipenes (all other reptiles) in males, or oviduct in females. It is important to note that gastrointestinal diseases do not only cause colonic prolapses, and indeed prolapse of the colon is frequently associated with diseases of other body systems. A multisystemic approach is therefore required.

Aetiology

Any condition resulting in tenesmus, increased coelomic pressure or muscle/sphincter weakness may be associated with abnormal prolapse of tissue through the vent (see Figure 17.16). Temporary prolapse of the phallus/hemipenes may be normal, associated with sexual behaviour, but may also be associated with diseases of other systems. Common underlying aetiologies are summarized in Figure 17.16.

In a recent retrospective study of 56 cases, cloacal prolapses were most commonly seen in chelonians and lizards (Hedley and Eatwell, 2014). Colonic prolapses were only seen in lizards (despite being reported commonly in all reptiles) and were significantly more common in females, with a variety of underlying aetiologies including metabolic bone disease, enteritis and spondylosis.

Diagnosis

The prolapsed organ should first be identified:

- **Cloaca:** shiny, pink, may or may not have a lumen depending on the extent of tissue prolapsed
- **Colon:** shiny, pink, with a lumen (faeces can frequently be obtained from the lumen) (Figure 17.17)
- **Bladder** (not present in snakes and some lizards): thin, diaphanous wall, no lumen, may appear fluid filled despite being everted owing to filling with coelomic fluid
- **Oviduct:** thin walled, flabby, plicated (accordion-like), with a lumen

Conditions resulting in tenesmus	
Gastrointestinal system: • Obstipation • Dehydration (more common in species requiring high humidities, e.g. green tree pythons) • Overfeeding • Suboptimal environmental temperature • Hypocalcaemia/metabolic bone disease • Space-occupying lesions • Foreign body • Stricture • Gastrointestinal parasitism • Enteritis/colitis • Neoplasia	Reproductive system: • Dystocia • Salpingitis • Neoplasia Urinary system: • Urolithiasis • Cystitis • Neoplasia Other: • Cloacitis

Conditions resulting in increased coelomic pressure	
Space-occupying lesions: • Organomegaly • Intracoelomic neoplasm • Intracoelomic abscess • Constipation/obstipation • Urolithiasis • Follicular stasis • Preovulatory (follicles) • Postovulatory (eggs)	• Obesity • Trauma • Crushing injuries to the coelomic cavity • Pneumocoelom • Dyspnoea

Conditions resulting in muscle/sphincter weakness
• Hypocalcaemia/metabolic bone disease • Spinal disease

17.16 Underlying aetiologies of cloacal organ prolapse.

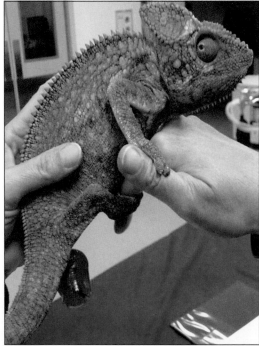

17.17 Cloacal prolapse in an Oustalet's chameleon secondary to hepatomegaly; the prolapsed structure is shiny, pink and has a lumen containing faecal material, consistent with prolapse of the colon. (Courtesy of A. Barratclough, Lowry Park Zoo)

- **Phallus** (chelonians): fleshy, extends from ventral floor of the cloaca, distal end pointed, groove running down dorsal midline, no lumen
- **Hemipenes** (lizards and snakes): paired, often barbed surface, extend from the caudal–lateral corners of the vent (often only one is prolapsed).

Investigations should then aim to identify the underlying cause of the prolapse. Radiography (plain or contrast), ultrasonography, cloacal palpation, blood haematology and biochemistry, and faecal/cloacal wash examination may be indicated.

Treatment

Avoidance of further trauma and desiccation of prolapsed tissues is crucial. Pet owners calling to report a prolapse should be directed to apply a non-adhesive covering to protect the tissue (a cling film 'nappy' or sling is useful) and present the animal as quickly as possible.

On presentation, prolapsed tissues should be cleaned by flushing with sterile saline. Water-soluble lubricants may be applied to help prevent desiccation. Application of hyperosmolar solutions such as glycerine, mannitol, or concentrated sugar or salt solutions (not granules) can help to reduce oedema if the tissue is significantly engorged. Fluid therapy, antibiosis and analgesia should all be considered. Unless the prolapsed tissue is small, healthy, and easily replaced using gentle pressure with a digit or moistened cotton bud, the authors advocate reapplication of a cling film dressing at this stage, while underlying causes are investigated.

It is essential that underlying causes are addressed; Hedley and Eatwell (2014) found that all cases of recurrent prolapse occurred where underlying causes had not been investigated or resolved prior to prolapse replacement. For management of gastrointestinal aetiologies see appropriate sections (Enterocolitis and dysbiosis, Hypomotility/constipation/obstipation, Gastrointestinal foreign bodies, Neoplasia, and Infectious diseases affecting the gastrointestinal tract). For management of non-gastrointestinal causes, see Chapters 19–21. Treatment of prolapsed tissues other than the colon, are discussed elsewhere (see Chapters 13 and 20).

Treatment of colon prolapse: Once underlying causes have been addressed, viable tissues are replaced under general anaesthesia. For small prolapses of the colon, gentle manipulation may be used to replace it through the vent (Figure 17.18). Enlarging the opening, by incising the vent laterally on each side, may be necessary to allow swollen tissues to be replaced. Once replaced, it should be ensured that the colon is completely inverted; water enemas may be useful.

Some authors advocate methods to stop re-prolapse while supportive structures are healing and underlying causes are being resolved. Use of a vent purse-string suture or two simple interrupted sutures (one at each of the lateral margins of the vent) are appropriate. They should be placed so that urination and defecation are still possible and are usually left in place for 7–10 days. It should be noted that this technique will not stop re-eversion of the colon into the cloaca, where it may go undetected. For non-surgical colopexy of the colon in lizards and snakes, a cotton bud may be passed into the inverted colon and angled out against the ventrolateral body wall. A monofilament simple interrupted suture is placed by passing the needle through the skin and colon into the cotton bud tip. The cotton bud is withdrawn (to confirm presence of suture material in the colon) and the suture material teased from the tip. The suture is then tightened and tied, fixing the colon against the body wall.

For large prolapses of the colon, coeliotomy may be necessary for replacement. Some underlying causes, including intestinal foreign bodies, uroliths and abnormal

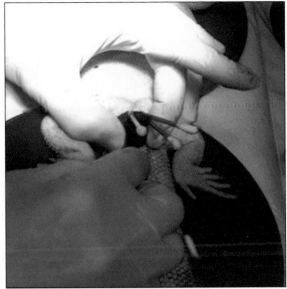

17.18 Prolapse of the colon secondary to heavy oxyurid burden in a bearded dragon; prolapsed tissues were replaced through the cloaca without coeliotomy.

eggs, may require coeliotomy for correction, so prolapsed tissues can be replaced at the same time (Figure 17.19). If coeliotomy is required, a surgical colopexy of the colon can be performed – either by suturing to the dorsal ribcage on the right-hand side (removal of the gonad on this side is recommended) or by inclusion of the distal colon into the body wall closure (see Chapter 13).

Non-viable tissues should never be replaced and require resection (Figure 17.20). Resection and anastomosis of de-vitalized colon has been reported with and without coeliotomy (Bennet and Mader, 2006).

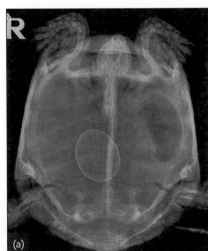

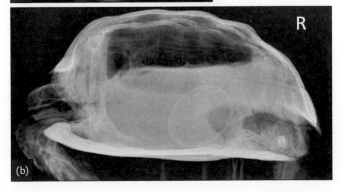

17.19 (a) Dorsoventral and (b) lateral radiographs of a Mediterranean spur-thighed tortoise with extensive cloacal prolapse. A single oversized egg causing obstructive dystocia is evident and required coeliotomy for removal. Prolapsed tissues were replaced during the same procedure.

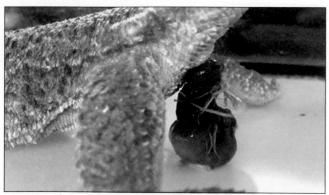

17.20 A bearded dragon with colon prolapse; tissues appear discoloured, oedematous and contaminated with substrate material. Owing to concerns regarding tissue viability, coeliotomy for partial enterectomy with end-to-end anastomosis was performed.

Hypomotility/constipation/obstipation

Gastrointestinal motility is affected by a number of intrinsic and extrinsic factors, with food ingestion instigating contractions. The rate of food passage through the gastrointestinal tract will vary with volume, type and composition of food; environmental temperature; the type and length of the gastrointestinal tract; and the reptile's general health status. Normal gut transit time may be as little as 2–4 days in small carnivorous lizards, and as long as 3–5 weeks in larger snakes and herbivorous chelonians and lizards (Mitchell, 2005).

There are numerous causes of reduced gastrointestinal motility (Figure 17.21).

Clinical signs

Clinical signs may be non-specific, such as lethargy. History may suggest infrequent or no faecal output, although keepers may be unaware of this. Tenesmus and

Primary husbandry causes

- Chronic dehydration due to inappropriate or insufficient water sources or low humidity levels (Wright, 2008)
- Inappropriate environmental temperature, lack of a temperature gradient or lack of a day/night temperature difference
- Insufficient space/opportunity for exercise
- Ingestion of substrate material
- Dietary:
  - Lack of fibre
  - Long-haired prey
  - Hard-shelled insect prey
  - Overfeeding (too frequent/large meals) (Griffin, 2006)

Other causes (often secondarily associated with husbandry factors)

- Endoparasitism (Hnizdo and Pantchev, 2011)
- Chronic systemic disease
- Hypocalcaemia (e.g. associated with metabolic bone disease)
- Narrowing of the pelvic canal (secondary to metabolic bone disease and/or fractures)
- Neuropathies and spinal cord damage
- Gastrointestinal strictures
- Space-occupying lesions causing obstruction:
  - Renomegaly
  - Uroliths
  - Cloacoliths
  - Neoplasia
  - Abscesses
  - Eggs (see Figure 17.19) or fetuses
- Brumation-associated constipation – described in a red diamond rattlesnake resulting from dehydration and reduced gastrointestinal motility during brumation (Corbit et al., 2014)

17.21 Causes of reduced gastrointestinal motility.

haematochezia are possible and secondary intussusception and/or cloacal prolapse can occur. Some reptiles present with coelomic distension and pain due to build-up of faeces or gas (tympany). Distended loops of bowel impinging on the lungs may cause dyspnoea. Vomiting or regurgitation may occur. Faecal impactions may be palpable in lizards and snakes. Clinical signs of concurrent or associated disease such as metabolic bone disease may also be present.

Diagnosis

A full history may identify diet and husbandry issues. Faecal examination will rule out endoparasitism. Radiography is useful to confirm constipation (Figure 17.22) and assess for other pathology (contrast radiography may rule out obstruction). Blood work can be used to assess for dehydration and underlying conditions such as hypocalcaemia or renal disease. Endoscopy or coelioscopy may be valuable depending on the underlying aetiology and region of tract affected. Ultrasonography can be valuable in the diagnosis of obstruction but is challenging where excess gas build-up is present. Diagnosis of ileus should be made with caution as extrapolation from domestic mammals may be misleading owing to the normal slow tract motility of most reptiles. *Atadenovirus* PCR testing should be considered, particularly in bearded dragons with recurrent gastrointestinal motility issues where husbandry causes have been ruled out.

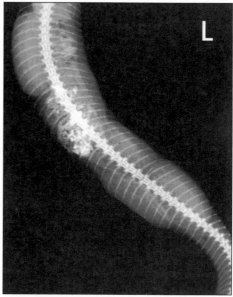

17.22 Dorsoventral radiograph of a kingsnake showing constipation secondary to gravidity.

Treatment

Underlying causes should be addressed and husbandry issues corrected, particularly with respect to temperature and water provision. Fluid therapy is paramount, with the route dependent on the patient's clinical condition. Endoparasites should be treated.

Cloacal washes or enemas can be useful. Warmed water is instilled via a lubricated catheter or ball-tipped crop tube. In species with a functional bladder, there is a risk of entering the urinary bladder instead of the rectum; the tube should be inserted in a dorsal direction to try to avoid this. Bearded dragons, which commonly present with constipation (Wright, 2008), do not have a urinary bladder, so this is not an issue. Daily or twice daily soaking in warm water may encourage defecation (and rehydration). Gentle massage of the colon may also aid defecation.

If cloacal washes, bathing, enteral fluid therapy and correction of environmental issues do not resolve the constipation, medical treatment may be considered. Lactulose (0.5 ml/kg orally q24h) and psyllium laxatives can be used (Mans, 2013). The use of prokinetics such as cisapride (0.5–2 mg/kg orally q24h) or metoclopramide (0.05–1 mg/kg orally, i.m. q24h) remains controversial (and contraindicated in cases of obstruction). There are anecdotal reports indicating good responses (Hnizdo and Pantchev, 2011), while one study showed minimal effectiveness in the desert tortoise, where higher doses may be required (Tothill *et al.*, 2000).

Surgery may be indicated in refractory cases (i.e. faecolith removal via enterotomy), or where indicated by other pathology (e.g. intussusception or presence of a urolith) (see Chapter 13).

Gastrointestinal foreign bodies

Foreign bodies within the gastrointestinal system are generally ingested, but it is possible for uroliths to move into the cloaca and cause acute obstruction. Ingested foreign bodies are relatively common in reptiles and may be accidental (e.g. substrate entering the mouth with food items) or deliberate. Pica, or geophagy, is common in some species (Diaz-Figueroa and Mitchell, 2006), although the reason for the behaviour is unknown (speculated reasons include aiding mechanical digestion of food, detoxification of plant toxins, endoparasite control or maintenance of beak shape). Some reptiles have been observed to seek out white material, such as bone or white stones, if calcium is deficient or during periods of increased calcium demand (McArthur *et al.*, 2004).

Ingestion of substrate material such as woodchips and 'digestible' calcium carbonate sands by insectivorous lizards (e.g. bearded dragons and leopard geckos) and woody plant material or stones by tortoises appears to be overrepresented (Mitchell, 2005) (Figure 17.23). Bearded dragons in particular appear predisposed to ingest inappropriate objects; in addition to substrate material, the authors have removed marbles and paper clips, amongst other gastrointestinal foreign bodies. Snakes present more rarely (Figure 17.24) and usually after ingestion of substrate when taking prey items. In addition to causing obstruction, trauma to the intestinal tract from ingestion of foreign bodies (or sharp food items) may also result in bacterial

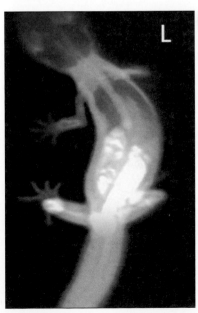

17.23 Dorsoventral radiograph of a leopard gecko showing radiodense (mineral opacity) material within the mid to caudal coelom, consistent with a sand substrate impaction.

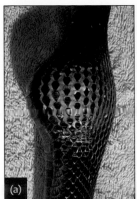

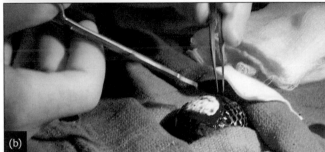

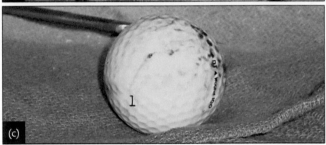

17.24 (a) A wild black ratsnake presented with a mid-body focal swelling. Radiography confirmed a spherical mineral opacity within the intestinal tract. (b) Coeliotomy for enterotomy was performed, and (c) a golf ball removed. While foreign body ingestion is uncommon in captive snakes this case is not isolated in wild snakes which presumably perceive these objects to be eggs, which form part of their natural diet.
(Courtesy of Wildlife Center of Virginia)

granuloma and stricture formation leading to signs of partial or full obstruction despite the inciting cause no longer being present.

Clinical signs

Gastrointestinal foreign bodies may cause clinical disease due to obstruction. Many, however, will be asymptomatic incidental findings on radiography. Clinical signs (if present) are usually non-specific, for example anorexia, dehydration and lethargy. Chronically affected reptiles may show weight loss and cachexia. Regurgitation or vomiting may occur, but are relatively uncommon (except in snakes). There may be coelomic distension visible in snakes and lizards, and the foreign body (or proximally impacted faeces) may be palpable.

Diagnosis

There may be a history of foreign-body ingestion or reduced faecal output, although many keepers will be unaware. Radiography may show radiodense foreign material within the gut (see Figure 17.23). Materials such as plastic or wood will be less obvious and radiographic contrast studies, ultrasonography or computed tomography may be useful (see Chapter 9).

Treatment

It is important to differentiate between obstructive foreign bodies (which will require surgical treatment) and non-obstructive material that is likely to pass. The latter tends to be asymptomatic or mildly affecting and cases can be treated as for constipation (see Hypomotility/constipation/obstipation).

Removal of obstructive foreign bodies is usually via enterotomy during exploratory coeliotomy. Plastronotomy is usually required in chelonians, although an endoscope-assisted enterotomy performed through the prefemoral fossa has been described (Kik and Nickel, 2001). Oral endoscopic removal of oesophageal or gastric foreign bodies may be possible. Care should be taken to inspect the entire gastrointestinal tract for tissue viability, perforation or further foreign bodies. Intussusception (Figure 17.25) and volvulus secondary to the presence of a foreign body are considered rare (Diaz-Figueroa and Mitchell, 2006; Mans, 2013).

Access to further potential foreign bodies should be prevented and inappropriate substrate issues addressed. Feeding animals on solid surfaces (e.g. a bowl) can avoid accidental substrate ingestion.

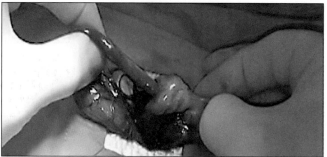

17.25 Intussusception in a bearded dragon secondary to obstruction caused by a gastrointestinal foreign body.

Hepatic disease

Liver disease in itself is not a diagnosis as there are numerous possible aetiologies (both primary and secondary). Onset may be acute or chronic and disease may be inflammatory (hepatitis) or degenerative (hepatosis) (Divers, 2013b). Diseases of other organ systems may also affect the liver, for example, visceral gout.

Acute hepatitis often occurs owing to an infectious cause:

- **Bacterial:** bacterial hepatitis commonly results from systemic bacterial infection (e.g. septicaemia) and can lead to hepatomegaly, diffuse microabscesses, focal abscessation and infarcts. Common isolates from bacterial hepatitis cases include members of the Enterobacteriaceae (e.g. *Aeromonas* and *Salmonella* spp.). *Chlamydia* and *Mycobacterium* spp. have been less commonly identified (Hnizdo and Pantchev, 2011)
- **Viral:** hepatitis and hepatic necrosis have been associated with many viruses in numerous reptile species. In squamates, ranaviruses, herpesviruses and adenoviruses have been implicated (Latney and Wellehan, 2013; Marschang, 2014). *Atadenovirus* in particular is a major cause of mortality in agamids, such as bearded dragons. In chelonians, herpesviruses and ranaviruses have been implicated. Adenovirus is newly recognized in chelonians, which can present with signs of hepatitis, necrotizing enterocolitis, oesophagitis, splenitis and encephalopathy. Prognosis is poor (Gibbons and Steffes, 2013)
- **Fungal:** fungal hepatitis has been reported, caused by a number of agents, including *Aspergillus* and *Candida* spp. (Hnizdo and Pantchev, 2011)

- **Parasitic:** *Entamoeba invadens* is a major cause of necrotic hepatitis and hepatic abscessation in snakes and carnivorous lizards. It has a direct life cycle, with the organism invading the intestinal wall. Amoebae can also penetrate the bloodstream and travel to the liver, causing necrotizing hepatitis. Coccidians may also travel from the small intestine to the liver and gall bladder, and in chelonians, *Hexamita parva* has been associated with cases of hepatic, intestinal and renal disease. Hepatic necrosis has been described in a case of systemic microsporidiosis in a bearded dragon (Jacobsen *et al.*, 1998).

Hepatic lipidosis

Hepatic lipidosis (fatty liver disease) is common in reptiles, especially chelonians, bearded dragons and large carnivorous lizards such as monitors and tegus. It is not a single isolated clinical disease, but more a metabolic derangement (Hernandez-Divers and Cooper, 2006; Divers, 2013a) implicated in many chronic disease states. It is a pathological increase in the amount of fat deposition within the liver that negatively affects hepatic function. This must be differentiated from normal physiological increases in intrahepatic fat deposition, which occur during specific processes such as hibernation and vitellogenesis (McArthur, 2004; Mans, 2013). This differentiation can be challenging, and illustrates the importance of thorough history taking and considering the individual's signalment and breeding history.

In the pathological state, hepatic lipidosis can be seen with a number of disease states or predispositions (Figure 17.26) (McArthur, 2004; McArthur *et al.*, 2004; Hernandez-Divers and Cooper, 2006; Divers, 2013a; Chitty and Raftery, 2013a). Most cases of hepatic lipidosis are chronic in nature, although acute toxic hepatic lipidosis is an exception.

Causal factors	Condition
Dietary	• Starvation (or anorexia due to other disease problem) • Chronic malnutrition (e.g. amino acid and protein deficiencies) • Inappropriate diets, high in fats and simple carbohydrates, causing obesity • Ad-lib feeding year-round in species that would naturally fast during periods of hibernation or brumation
Inappropriate husbandry	• Lack of exercise, leading to obesity • Incorrect environmental temperatures and/or photoperiods, stimulating inappropriate lipid deposition • Inappropriate hibernation (incorrect temperature and/or duration)
Endocrinopathies	• Chronic hyperparathyroidism (nutritional or renal in origin); high parathyroid hormone levels may be a natural cue for prehibernation fat deposition • Chronic hyperoestrogenism (e.g. preovulatory follicular stasis) • Hypothyroidism
Toxins	• Bacterial toxins and mycotoxins (may disturb lipid metabolism) • Ivermectin administration in chelonians is associated with iatrogenic hepatic lipidosis (causal relationship unclear) (Teare and Bush, 1983)
Species/sex/age factors	• Common in females without breeding opportunity (Divers, 2013a) • Chelonians and savannah monitors appear predisposed (Divers, 2013a) • Uncommon in juveniles

17.26 Predispositions or disease states associated with hepatic lipidosis.

Clinical signs

Clinical signs of liver disease are often non-specific (e.g. anorexia, depression, regurgitation, reduced fertility, weight loss) or absent. Clinical signs will depend on the underlying cause and whether disease is acute or chronic. Diarrhoea is relatively common in acute hepatitis cases (Divers, 2013b). Regurgitation is considered to be a poor prognostic sign in chelonians and lizards. Biliverdinuria and jaundice may occur in severe hepatic disease; however, it is important to note that a yellowish tinge to oral mucous membranes may be normal in some species (e.g. some colour-morph bearded dragons). Polydipsia and polyuria are unusual. Hepatomegaly or liver masses may be palpable in lizards and snakes; in small lizards such as geckos, transillumination is useful for hepatic silhouette assessment (Figure 17.27). Hypoalbuminaemia, due to reduced hepatic synthesis, can lead to the development of ascites (transudates).

Liver disease may only become clinically apparent during times of increased physiological demand, such as during hibernation or breeding. Cases often present relatively late in disease development as keepers may miss early signs.

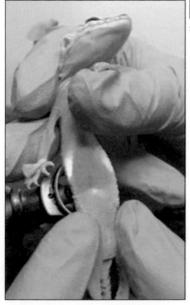

17.27 Transillumination to visualize the hepatic silhouette in a leopard gecko.

Diagnosis

Elucidating the underlying cause of hepatic disease in reptiles is a diagnostic challenge. Careful consideration of the history and signalment may guide diagnostic procedures.

Hepatic biopsy: Liver tissue sampling is likely to give the best chance of diagnosis. Endoscopy (see Chapter 10) allows visualization of the liver and biopsy (this can also be carried out surgically or via ultrasonographic guidance). Care should be taken as the liver tissue may be friable and at risk of haemorrhage. Samples should be submitted for histopathology and culture, and for viral testing where indicated (Mans, 2013).

Plasma biochemistry: Hepatocellular damage can lead to elevations of several enzymes, including aspartate aminotransferase (AST), gamma glutamyltransferase (GGT), alkaline phosphatase (ALP), alanine aminotransferase (ALT) and lactate dehydrogenase (LDH); however, none are organ specific. Wide tissue distribution of these enzymes in reptiles complicates interpretation. Assessment of creatinine phosphokinase (CPK) levels can help distinguish between muscle and non-muscle sources of enzyme elevations, but differentiation from increases caused by disease in other tissues is more challenging. Furthermore, in chronic hepatopathies, enzyme levels may remain within normal limits (Divers, 2000, 2013b; Wilkinson, 2004; Campbell, 2014). Hypoalbuminaemia may be present as a result of reduced hepatic production.

Bile acids measured in reptiles are 3 alpha hydroxy bile acids, rather than those routinely measured in mammals. Bile acid levels have only been evaluated in green iguanas (McBride *et al.*, 2007), where mean baseline values (following 48 hours fasting) were 7.5 μmol/l, rising to 33 μmol/l for at least 8 hours post-feeding. Divers (2013b) describes levels >60 μmol/l as suggestive of hepatic dysfunction (further work is needed). Most reptiles produce biliverdin, not bilirubin, as the major bile pigment; currently, no commercial assays for biliverdin are available. Cholesterol is an unreliable marker of hepatic disease (Campbell, 2014). Glucose elevations can be associated with hepatic disease (see Pancreatic disease) and beta-hydroxybutyrate elevations have been associated with hepatic lipidosis (Chitty and Raftery, 2013a) (see Chapter 8).

Haematology: Anaemia may be present in chronic liver disease (sometimes masked by dehydration). Heterophilia and monocytosis may occur with acute hepatitis or hepatic necrosis, whereas chronic bacterial hepatitis cases may show minimal white cell count elevation (Divers, 2013a). Eosinophilia may occur with parasitic disease. Red and white cell counts tend to be reduced in hepatic lipidosis.

Imaging: The hepatic shadow is often visible on horizontal beam radiographs of lizards, but less so in snakes and rarely in chelonians (see Chapter 9). Ultrasonography can be useful to assess hepatic size and echotexture. Changes may be focal, multifocal or diffuse, depending on the underlying process. Hepatic enlargement and homogeneous hyperechogenicity on ultrasonography are suggestive of hepatic lipidosis (Hochleithner and Holland, 2014).

Adjunctive tests: Faecal examination is useful to assess for parasitic causes of hepatic disease, particularly *Entamoeba invadens* (see Chapter 24). Ascitic fluid aspirates can be submitted for cytology and culture and sensitivity. Specific viral infections may be tested for by molecular means, e.g. *Atadenovirus* PCR (see Infectious diseases affecting the gastrointestinal tract).

Diagnosis of hepatic lipidosis is difficult and subjective with no discrete boundary from physiological to pathological processes. Diagnosis should be made on the basis of histopathological changes, taking into account clinical signs and individual patient signalment and circumstances (McArthur, 2004; Chitty and Raftery, 2013a). Grossly, lipidotic livers tend to look tan or yellow in colour, with rounded edges (Figure 17.28).

Treatment

Treatment will depend on the underlying cause. Husbandry and dietary issues should be corrected and concurrent disease addressed. If infectious disease is implicated, barrier nursing should be employed and biosecurity measures taken for collections.

Regardless of disease aetiology, supportive care is paramount. Patients will often be anorexic and nutritional support is essential, especially in cases of hepatic lipidosis, to avoid further mobilization of stored body fat (Mans, 2013)

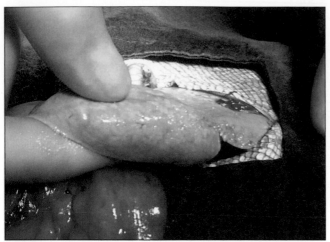

17.28 The liver of a female bearded dragon with preovulatory follicular stasis, showing the typical appearance of hepatic lipidosis.

(see Management of anorexia and nutritional support). Fluid therapy is also essential; with severe liver disease, lactate-containing fluids should be avoided (see Chapters 7 and 11). As long-term nursing care is likely to be required, placement of an oesophagostomy tube is recommended (particularly in chelonians) (see Management of anorexia and nutritional support).

Methionine (40–50 mg/kg orally q24h), carnitine (250 mg/kg orally q24h) and choline may promote hepatic function (Hernandez-Divers and Cooper, 2006; Divers, 2013a,b). Other empirical treatments include lactulose (0.5 ml/kg orally q24h) if hepatic encephalopathy is suspected, or silymarin (milk thistle) (50–100 mg/kg orally q24h) (Hernandez-Divers and Cooper, 2006; Divers, 2013b). Anabolic steroids (nandrolone, 0.5–1 mg/kg orally q7–28d) and thyroxine (levothyroxine, 20 µg/kg orally q2d) may improve hepatic fat metabolism, reduce catabolism and improve appetite in hepatic lipidosis cases (McArthur, 2004; Hernandez-Divers and Cooper, 2006; Divers, 2013a).

Changes in weight, body condition, appetite and demeanour should be closely monitored. Repeated liver enzymes and fasting bile acid levels may be useful to monitor trends. Serial ultrasound examinations and endoscopic biopsies for repeat histopathology are likely to improve prognostic advice, and contribute to further knowledge of hepatic disease (Hernandez-Divers and Cooper, 2006).

Prevention of hepatic disease is difficult, but regular health checks, including faecal and blood work, may pick up early signs. Client education regarding appropriate husbandry and diet is extremely important, as is the provision of species-appropriate hibernation or fasting periods. Overfeeding should be avoided and sufficient room for exercise provided. Reproductive management (e.g. elective ovariectomy) may prevent reproductive disease and hepatic lipidosis in non-breeding females. Consideration of collection hygiene and biosecurity is essential to try to prevent infectious hepatic disease outbreaks.

Pancreatic disease

Pancreatic disease appears rare in reptiles, with antemortem diagnosis extremely uncommon. Clinical signs are usually non-specific, such as anorexia, lethargy and depression; reptiles are often in poor clinical condition at presentation. Polydipsia and polyuria are uncommon. Coelomic pain may be noted in cases of acute necrotizing pancreatitis (Stahl, 2003).

Pancreatitis is rare. Cases have occurred secondary to bacterial, viral or protozoal infections (due to migration of nematodes, trematodes and coccidians) and to immunosuppression resulting from suboptimal husbandry (Stahl, 2003; McArthur et al., 2004; Hidalgo-Vila et al., 2011). One case of spontaneous autoimmune pancreatitis and diabetes mellitus was reported in a western pond turtle (Frye, 1999). Diabetes mellitus appears to be extremely rare and previously published cases may have had hyperglycaemia due to other causes. Other reported pancreatic diseases include ductal calculosis and neoplasia – generally carcinomas or adenocarcinomas (Mauldin and Done, 1996; Stern et al., 2010), although a functional pancreatic glucagonoma in a rhinoceros iguana (Frye et al., 1999) and a functional islet cell tumour in a savannah monitor (Naples et al., 2009) have been reported.

Diagnosis

Diagnosis is challenging, with most cases identified at postmortem; the entire pancreas and spleen and sometimes even portions of the gastrointestinal tract should be submitted for histopathology, owing to widespread and variable distribution of islet tissue outside the pancreas (Stahl, 2003, 2006). Pancreatic biopsy may prove helpful, but is rarely attempted owing to the poor clinical condition of cases and the difficulty in achieving representative samples.

Blood work and imaging (particularly endoscopy and ultrasonography) may be helpful. Elevated white blood cell counts may be associated with inflammatory or infectious conditions – e.g. acute necrotizing pancreatitis (Stahl, 2003). Reptile blood glucose levels appear to be regulated by insulin in the same way as in mammals, and so damage to the pancreas (e.g. due to trauma, autoimmune or other disease) would be expected to cause hyperglycaemia. There is, however, much variation in blood glucose levels, with physiological, environmental and metabolic factors playing a large part. Other disease processes may also cause hyperglycaemia, such as neoplasia (see later information on neuroendocrine gastric carcinomas in bearded dragons) and renal and hepatic disease. For this reason, clinicians should not rush to make a diagnosis of diabetes mellitus on finding hyperglycaemia. Stahl (2006) summarizes numerous reports of persistent blood glucose levels >11.1 mmol/l or >16.7 mmol/l as being potential candidates for diabetes mellitus, but this diagnosis must be made with caution. Blood insulin levels may prove useful, but further work is required to establish normal values and validate the use of mammalian assays in reptiles.

Treatment

Treatment options are limited – see Stahl (2006) for an overview – and the prognosis is often grave. Environmental, fluid and nutritional support should be provided, along with specific therapies as indicated – e.g. antibiosis in bacterial pancreatitis.

If the patient is a strong candidate for diabetes mellitus, empirical treatment with mammalian insulin may be considered at the following starting doses (Stahl, 2006): lizards and crocodilians 5–10 IU/kg q24–48h; snakes and chelonians 1–5 IU/kg q24–48h. These can be adjusted based on clinical response and serial blood glucose measurements. Insulin types used have not been reported and more research and documentation of cases are required in order to improve treatment protocols.

Toxicoses

A brief overview has been included in this chapter as most intoxicants will be ingested and treatment will usually be directed towards gastrointestinal decontamination. Some toxins may also directly affect the gastrointestinal system; Rotstein et al. (2003) reported a fatal case of suspected oak (Quercus spp.) poisoning in an African spurred tortoise where extensive necrosis was found within the oral cavity, stomach and intestine (as well as the kidneys). For a thorough overview of toxicoses, readers are directed to Fitzgerald and Vera (2006) and Fitzgerald and Newquist (2008). In the UK, the Veterinary Poisons Information Service (VPIS) holds a database of toxicoses, including those affecting reptiles, with a 24-hour emergency line available to members.

A variety of intoxicants have been described affecting reptiles, including heavy metals such as lead and zinc, toxic plants, and iatrogenic poisonings whereby a toxic drug or drug overdose has been administered. Tortoises kept in gardens commonly ingest poisonous plants such as rhododendrons, oleander and daffodils. Client education regarding the risks of exposure to toxins is important, as is clinician education regarding the safe administration of drugs at correct doses.

Clinical signs of toxicoses in reptiles are varied and non-specific; some species may vomit after ingesting poisonous plants (Chitty and Raftery, 2013c; Mans, 2013). Diagnosis is usually achieved via a thorough history and clinical examination. Contaminant analysis of blood, stomach contents or tissue may be carried out and radiography may be useful, particularly in cases of suspected heavy metal ingestion.

Treatment is often symptomatic and supportive, including fluid therapy, nutritional support and appropriate temperature provision. Oxygen may be required via ventilation if there is respiratory collapse (Chitty and Raftery, 2013c). More specific therapies include activated charcoal or psyllium to reduce gastrointestinal absorption of ingested toxins, calcium-EDTA (10–40 mg/kg i.m. q12h) for lead intoxication, midazolam (0.5–2 mg/kg i.m., i.v.) or diazepam (0.5 mg/kg i.m., i.v.) for seizures, and atropine (0.1–0.2 mg/kg i.m.) for organophosphate intoxication (Wellehan and Gunkel, 2004; Norton, 2005). Gastric lavage and endoscopic removal of ingested toxic material from the stomach may help to reduce exposure in acute cases.

Neoplasia

A full review of reptilian gastrointestinal neoplasia is beyond the scope of this chapter – see Chapter 23 and Hernandez-Divers and Garner (2003), Garner et al. (2004) and Mauldin and Done (2006).

Gastrointestinal neoplasia should be included in the differential diagnosis of oral, bodily or cloacal masses and swellings, and for non-specific clinical signs including anorexia, regurgitation or vomiting, weight loss, or obstipation.

- **Carcinomas and adenocarcinomas:** commonly documented in the gastrointestinal tract, liver and pancreas, particularly in snakes (rarely in chelonians and lizards). Clinical signs depend on the tumour site and can include constipation, regurgitation and progressive coelomic swelling (a major differential diagnosis for cryptosporidiosis in snakes). Cases are often presented late in tumour development, making treatment challenging.

- **Squamous cell carcinomas:** can occur within the oral cavity, especially in snakes. These tend to have poorly defined borders with haemorrhage and necrosis of adjacent tissues. Associated clinical signs include stomatitis, anorexia and oral discharge. Treatment involves surgery and/or radiation therapy (Reavill, 2004).

- **Gastric carcinomas:** an emerging issue in bearded dragons (Ritter et al., 2009; Kadoltaru, 2010, Lyons et al., 2010; Mans, 2013). Presenting signs include anorexia, lethargy, vomiting, melaena and weight loss, often with marked anaemia and hyperglycaemia. Most of the described cases were diagnosed as highly malignant neuroendocrine gastric carcinomas, immunohistochemically positive for somatostatin, suggesting that they may be somatostatinomas (Ritter et al., 2009; Lyons et al., 2010). They originate from the gastric mucosa, penetrate the gastric serosa, and metastasize primarily to the liver and kidneys. Diagnosis is often at post-mortem, but ante-mortem diagnosis can be attempted by gastroscopy or coeliotomy and biopsy (Raiti, 2012).

Definitive diagnosis of neoplasia will only be made by histopathological examination (or possibly cytological examination of an aspirated sample). It is important to submit samples to pathologists familiar with examining reptilian tissue. Blood work is usually non-specific but hyperglycaemia and anaemia in bearded dragons may increase the suspicion of gastric neuroendocrine carcinoma. Imaging (plain and contrast radiography, ultrasonography, endoscopy and advanced imaging modalities) may help to evaluate the degree of organ involvement, any metastases and adjacent tissue integrity.

Treatment options will be dictated by the size, location and type of neoplasm. Surgical excision, if possible, is usually the treatment of choice. Radiation therapy, chemotherapy (parenteral and intralesional) and photodynamic therapy have shown varying degrees of success in treating some reptile neoplasms (Mauldin and Done, 2006), but such techniques are still in their infancy in the treatment of reptiles.

Infectious diseases affecting the gastrointestinal tract

Viral diseases

Figure 17.29 lists viruses that can affect the gastrointestinal tract in reptiles (for further information, see Chapter 25).

Fungal diseases

True gastrointestinal mycoses are rare despite the high prevalence of fungal spores in the reptile gut. Fungal infection can be promoted by high humidity, inappropriate diet, overcrowding and inadequate environmental hygiene. Antibiotic use may also promote fungal overgrowth.

The presence of fungal organisms in faecal or gastric lavage samples should be interpreted with caution as many organisms may be normal commensals, e.g. Candida albicans. The clinician should address any dietary or husbandry issues before careful consideration as to whether anti-fungal therapy is necessary. Histopathology of biopsy samples showing fungal involvement in gastrointestinal lesions will give more support for drug therapy.

Nystatin (100,000 IU/kg q24h) may be used to treat fungal infections localized to the gastrointestinal system as it is not absorbed systemically. Ketoconazole (15–30 mg/kg orally q24h), itraconazole (5 mg/kg orally q24h) or

Viruses	Affected groups	Gastrointestinal signs	Diagnosis	Treatment
Herpesviruses e.g. testudinid herpesvirus 1–4	**Chelonians** Tortoises **Squamates** Uncommon (many unclassified viruses)	**Chelonians** Diphtheroid necrotizing stomatitis and hepatitis. Also respiratory, ocular and neurological signs **Lizards** Stomatitis and hepatitis **Snakes** Stomatitis and venom gland cell necrosis with reduced venom production	**Current preferred testing** PCR (TeHV PCR can be used for squamate herpesvirus detection). Histopathology useful **Samples** Ante-mortem – oral/choanal swabs Post-mortem – tongue, oesophagus, stomach, trachea, liver and brain tissue samples	Supportive care and management of secondary infections will often lead to resolution of signs Acyclovir may reduce viral replication but will not eradicate the infection Lifelong carrier status expected so consider culling in captive groups or managing as a closed group
Iridoviruses e.g. ranaviruses	**Chelonians** Numerous species **Squamates** Rarely reported	**Chelonians** Diphtheroid necrotizing stomatitis with subcutaneous cervical oedema, enteritis and hepatitis. Also respiratory and ocular signs, and peracute deaths **Lizards** Granulomatous liver lesions reported in a leaf-tailed gecko and mountain lizard **Snakes** Hepatic necrosis and necrotizing inflammation of the pharyngeal submucosa reported in tree pythons	**Current preferred testing** PCR or virus isolation **Samples** Ante-mortem – oral/cloacal swabs or whole blood Post-mortem – liver or gastrointestinal tract tissue samples	Supportive care Valacyclovir may have effect; further research required (Allender *et al.*, 2013)
Arenavirus (postulated cause of inclusion body disease)	**Snakes** Boas and pythons	Signs vary from subclinical carriers to severe neurological disease and death. Gastrointestinal signs include chronic regurgitation, diarrhoea and stomatitis	**Current preferred testing** Identification of eosinophilic intracytoplasmic inclusions on cytology and histopathology. Arenavirus PCR now available **Samples** Ante-mortem – EDTA blood and a fresh blood smear, an oesophageal swab, or surgical biopsy of the tonsils, liver or kidney Post-mortem – brain, oesophageal tonsils, liver, kidney, pancreas, gastrointestinal tract and respiratory tract	Supportive care. Chronic disease progression with long-term survival is possible No known effective treatment Consider culling in captive groups or managing as closed groups
Adenovirus e.g. agamid adenovirus (AdV), eublepharid AdV, chamaeleonid AdV	**Chelonians** Uncommon **Squamates** Numerous species	Gastrointestinal signs include anorexia, stomatitis, oesophagitis, enteritis, hepatitis and pancreatitis. Hepatic necrosis reported. Neurological, respiratory and dermatological signs also possible. Asymptomatic animals have also been identified. Concurrent infection with *Isospora amphiboluri* is common in bearded dragons	**Current preferred testing** PCR. Histopathology also useful **Samples** Ante-mortem – cloacal swabs in squamates, oral/choanal swabs and plasma in chelonians Post-mortem – liver and intestinal tissue	Supportive care Quarantine and screening important in captive groups. Consider culling or managing as closed groups
Paramyxovirus e.g. ferlaviruses	**Chelonians/lizards** Uncommon **Snakes** Numerous species	**Chelonians/lizards** Usually associated with respiratory signs **Snakes** May present with non-specific signs, e.g. anorexia, regurgitation, mucoid diarrhoea and malodorous stools. Respiratory and neurological signs predominate	**Current preferred testing** PCR and virus isolation. Histopathology also useful **Samples** Ante-mortem – oral and cloacal swabs Post-mortem – kidney, small intestine, lung, trachea, liver and heart tissue samples	Supportive care. Infection predisposed by poor husbandry and immune suppression. Quarantine and screening important in captive groups Consider culling of snakes in captive groups or managing as closed groups
Reoviruses	**Chelonians** Uncommon **Squamates** More common in snakes	**Chelonians** Stomatitis and rhinitis **Snakes** Usually respiratory or neurological signs **Lizards** Enteritis and skin lesions	**Current preferred testing** PCR and virus isolation **Samples** Ante-mortem – oral and cloacal swabs. Biopsies of skin lesions Post-mortem – lung, brain, skin and/or intestine	Supportive care
Nidovirus	Ball pythons (and other pythons and possibly boas)	Respiratory disease, often with severe stomatitis	**Current preferred testing** PCR and virus isolation **Samples** Oral swabs and tracheal washes	Supportive care

17.29 Viruses affecting the reptilian gastrointestinal tract.

fluconazole (5 mg/kg orally q24h) can be used for systemic mycoses. Care should be taken with amphotericin B (0.5 mg/kg i.v. q48–72h) owing to its potential nephrotoxicity. Stomatitis cases (see previous section) with fungal involvement may be treated topically with drugs such as povidone iodine, chlorhexidine, nystatin, miconazole or silver sulfadiazine.

Bacterial diseases

The presence of bacteria in samples from the reptilian gastrointestinal tract should be interpreted with care as some may be normal commensals, some opportunistic invaders, while others may be primary pathogens. Examples of bacteria which may cause opportunistic infections include *Salmonella*, *Clostridium*, *Bacteroides*, *Pseudomonas* and *Aeromonas* spp. The role of diet and husbandry deficiencies in causing immunosuppression and secondary bacterial invasion should not be underestimated. The significance of finding bacteria associated with lesions of the gastrointestinal system will depend on the reptile species, signalment, diet and husbandry history. For example, *Devriesea agamarum* may be considered part of the normal oral microflora in bearded dragons, which are generally asymptomatic, whereas *Uromastyx* lizards may show perioral lesions (Figure 17.30) (Devloo *et al.*, 2011).

The decision to use antibiotic therapy should be made on a case-by-case basis after a full work-up and after addressing any dietary or husbandry issues which may be causing immunosuppression. Antibiotic treatment should be based on culture and sensitivity results where possible, and care taken not to cause iatrogenic dysbiosis through inappropriate antimicrobial use.

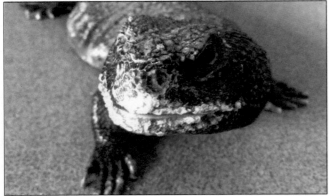

17.30 Cheilitis caused by *Devriesea agamarum* infection in a Saharan spiny-tailed lizard.

Parasitic diseases

Common parasites found within the reptile gastrointestinal tract are listed in Figure 17.31 (see also Chapter 24).

Management of anorexia and nutritional support

An essential part of the treatment of gastrointestinal disease in reptiles, nutritional support should be carefully planned, monitored and reassessed throughout the treatment period. Nutritional support is indicated when:

- 10% of bodyweight is lost acutely
- 20% of bodyweight is lost chronically
- Anorexia or injury prevents sufficient calorie intake to meet 85% of nutritional needs (Donoghue, 2006).

This can be difficult to ascertain in practice and so body condition evaluation, dietary history, blood results (e.g. albumin, triglyceride, glucose and electrolyte levels) and imaging (e.g. ultrasonography to assess intracoelomic fat bodies), can be useful guides (Donoghue, 2006; Pollock, 2012a,b,c). True anorexia can be difficult to differentiate from periods of physiological fasting (e.g. brumation or gravidity) and so full history, examination and clinical investigations are invaluable. Healthy brumating reptiles will not show an appreciable weight loss (<5% bodyweight).

In cases of prolonged anorexia, dehydration and electrolyte imbalances should be corrected prior to initiating nutritional support in order to prevent refeeding syndrome (see below). For most patients, fluids are administered at a rate of 4% bodyweight daily. This is continued until urination is achieved (indicating hydration) (see Chapter 11).

Refeeding syndrome

Refeeding syndrome is an electrolyte imbalance caused by sudden reintroduction of food after prolonged anorexia. In mammals, the onset of feeding results in complex metabolic and hormonal changes which result in shifts in electrolyte levels between intracellular and extracellular spaces. The hallmark of the syndrome is hypophosphataemia but levels of other plasma electrolytes, such as potassium and sodium, may also be abnormal. The syndrome has not yet been truly defined in reptiles, but in humans can lead to muscle weakness and tetany, seizures, myocardial dysfunction, haemolytic anaemia, water retention and death. After rehydration, nutritional support following prolonged anorexia should start with small volumes of food (no more than 50% of calculated metabolic energy requirements in the first 2–4 feeds), which should be gradually increased over 2–4 days. Monitoring phosphorus, potassium and glucose levels is suggested (Donoghue, 2006; Nevarez, 2009).

Techniques for nutritional support

Enteral feeding is usually via syringe feeding, stomach tubing or oesophagostomy tube (naso-oesophageal, gastrostomy and jejunostomy tubes are generally not suitable for reptiles). The technique(s) chosen for assisted feeding will depend on the species, temperament and clinical condition of the animal. Use of appetite stimulants, such as metronidazole in snakes, is generally not recommended as these usually do not result in adequate nutritional intake and do not address any underlying cause of anorexia.

Food presentation: Changing food presentation is a valuable first approach (particularly in snakes) but it is important to set limits on how long to persist with non-invasive techniques if they are unsuccessful.

- **Odour:** smell is an important appetite stimulant for reptiles, especially if vision is compromised:
  - 'Braining' vertebrate prey by opening the cranial vault to allow the reptile to smell and taste the brain
  - 'Scenting' prey by rubbing with other food items such as reptile skin or fish (depending on the species' dietary preferences); scenting commercially produced rats and mice with bedding from a gerbil enclosure often appears successful in snakes
  - Crushing fragrant leaves/other foods and placing under the nose may encourage feeding in herbivorous species (particularly tortoises).

Parasite	Species affected	Clinical features	Diagnosis	Life cycle and transmission	Control and treatment
Protozoa					
Ciliates e.g. *Balantidium* and *Nyctotherus*; Flagellates e.g. *Trichomonas* and *Hexamita*	Most species (common in herbivorous species such as chelonians)	Most are nonpathogenic commensals. Heavy burdens may cause disease; usually associated with underlying diet/husbandry problems and other causes of immune suppression. Clinical signs: • Weight loss, diarrhoea and anorexia. *Hexamita parva* – can cause fatal renal disease. Clinical signs include: • Anorexia, weight loss and polydipsia. *Giardia intestinalis* – not thought to cause primary disease in reptiles but is considered a potential zoonosis	• Fresh faecal sample (± formalin or Lugol iodine stain) for identification of motile parasites (see Figures 17.1 and 17.32). *Hexamita parva* – urine microscopy (distinctive morphology and 'torpedo-like' movement) and/or renal biopsy for histopathology. *Giardia* SNAP tests for cats/dogs are not validated for reptiles	Most have direct life cycle with faecal–oral transmission. *Hexamita parva* – transmitted in urine	Optimize diet/husbandry; overgrowth of commensal species may resolve without medical treatment. Metronidazole 50–100 mg/kg orally, repeated after 14 days. • Lower doses preferred – seizures and death reported with overdose • Indigo snake, tricolour kingsnake, Uracoan rattlesnake and milk snakes should receive a maximum of 40 mg/kg (Carpenter et al., 2001) • *Hexamita parva* may require high doses (250 mg/kg orally)
Amoebae e.g. *Entamoeba invadens* (most significant pathogen)	Snakes and carnivorous reptiles generally most susceptible. Disease increasingly recognized in omnivorous and herbivorous chelonians. Variable susceptibility seen between species	Clinical signs: • High morbidity and mortality in squamates, with anorexia, dehydration and wasting • Dysentery due to ulcerative gastritis and colitis • Can result in renal and hepatic focal necrosis or abscesses from haematogenous spread. Septicaemia possible	• Fresh faecal sample (± Lugol iodine stain) for identification of cysts or trophozoites (difficult to differentiate from non-pathogenic amoebae) • Histopathology of the gastro-intestinal tract and liver. Current commercial ELISA (enzyme-linked immunosorbent assay) tests for *E. histolytica* are not reliable for *E. invadens* detection	Direct life cycle with faecal–oral transmission. Spreads rapidly through collections. Can become endemic in large collections with resistant species acting as reservoirs	Metronidazole 50–100 mg/kg orally, repeated after 14 days or 20 mg/kg orally q48h for >2 weeks (Kolmstetter et al., 1997) • Lower doses preferred – seizures and death reported with overdose • Indigo snake, tricolour kingsnake, Uracoan rattlesnake and milk snakes should receive a maximum of 40 mg/kg (Carpenter et al., 2001) • Combination with iodoquinol (50 mg/kg orally q24h for 21 days) may improve efficacy against cyst stage (McArthur 2004; Hedley, 2012). Other treatments reported with variable success include tetracyclines, paromomycin (35–100 mg/kg orally q24h), and quinoline derivatives. Collection control: • New animals – quarantine, health check and pooled faecal screening • Strict hygiene and biosecurity essential • Repeat testing after treatment to ensure eradication
Coccidians e.g. *Isospora*, *Eimeria* and *Caryospora*	*Isospora* spp. common in bearded dragons, leopard geckos and chameleons. Numerous coccidians reported in lizards and snakes. *Eimeria* and *Caryospora* reported in chelonians	Healthy animals may shed coccidia asymptomatically. Heavy burdens may cause clinical disease; usually associated with poor environmental hygiene and causes of immune suppression such as co-infection with Atadenovirus. Clinical signs: Signs vary from mild diarrhoea and anorexia to severe haemorrhagic diarrhoea, emaciation, regurgitation and death	• Fresh faecal sample for identification of parasites. *Isospora* oocysts have two sporocysts (Figure 17.33) (unsporulated *Isospora* may also be seen in faeces). *Eimeria* oocysts have four sporocysts. *Caryospora* has one sporocyst	Direct life cycle with faecal–oral transmission. Oocysts show prolonged environmental survival so amplification common with poor environmental hygiene	Treatment of severely debilitated reptiles can be challenging owing to concurrent disease, malnutrition and chronic gastrointestinal tract damage. Supportive care is essential in addition to fastidious daily environmental cleaning. Medical treatment of asymptomatic animals is controversial – e.g. asymptomatic *Isospora amphiboluri* infections in bearded dragons. Complete elimination is often not possible (aim to reduce load): 'sulfa' drugs (ensure well hydrated and avoid in renal dysfunction): • Sulfadimethoxine 50 mg/kg orally q24h for 3–5 days, then q48h • Trimethoprim/sulphonamide 15–30 mg/kg orally, i.m. q24–48h for 5–21 days • Trimethoprim (16 mg/ml)/sulfamethoxazole (80 mg/ml), for treating coccidiosis in bearded dragons, 15–20 mg/kg orally, q24 for 7–14 days. Toltrazuril may be useful but more research is needed (Modry and Sloboda, 2007) • 5–15 mg/kg orally q24h for 3 days reported in bearded dragons (Doneley, 2006). Ponazuril 30 mg/kg orally q48h x 2 treatments in bearded dragons (Mitchell, 2008)

17.31 Parasites of the reptile gastrointestinal tract. SNAP = enzyme immunoassay for the detection of *Giardia* antigen. (continues)

Parasite	Species affected	Clinical features	Diagnosis	Life cycle and transmission	Control and treatment
Protozoa continued					

Cryptosporidium	Snakes, lizards and occasionally chelonians. Common in leopard geckos (Figure 17.34)	Clinical signs:
		• Weight loss, regurgitation and death are common
		• In snakes, hypertrophic gastritis can result in a firm mid-body swelling but enteritis without gastric hypertrophy is also possible (presenting with diarrhoea)
		• In lizards and chelonians, enteritis (without gastritis) is more common but gastritis and pancreatitis may occur
		• Asymptomatic carrier state with intermittent shedding is common
			• Gastric/intestinal biopsy for histopathology is gold standard
			• Fresh faecal sample, mucus from regurgitated food items, gastric lavage samples for:
			  • Microscopy using a modified acid-fast stain
			  • Immunofluorescent antibody test
			  • Intermittent shedding may give false negative results
				Direct life cycle with presumed faecal–oral transmission. Two types of oocysts can be formed; thin-walled oocysts immediately reinfect the host, while thick-walled oocysts are excreted in faeces allowing environmental persistence and transmission (Scullion and Scullion, 2009)	Numerous treatments have been suggested but none have shown consistent effect. Intensive supportive care and medical therapy may reduce shedding and prolong life but elimination is unlikely. Paromomycin has shown promise in some cases but numerous reports of recurrence also exist:
					• 300–360 mg/kg orally q48h for 14 days led to cessation of oocyst shedding for at least a year in two Gila monsters (Paré, 1997)
					• 360 mg/kg q48h for 10 days led to histological clearance in five hatchling bearded dragons (Grosset et al., 2011)
					Hyperimmune bovine colostrum dosed at 1% bodyweight led to histological clearance in 50% of snakes; treatment in leopard geckos was less efficacious (Graczyk et al., 1999)
					Collection control:
					• Euthanasia is reasonable in confirmed cases
					• New animals – quarantine, health check and pooled faecal screening
					• Strict biosecurity is essential
					• For decontamination, ammonia (5%) and formalin (10%) with 18 hours contact time at 4°C appears effective (Campbell and Tzipori, 1982). Steam cleaning, freezing and desiccation may also be used (Cranfield and Graczyk, 1996)

Helminths					
Trematodes e.g. digenetic flukes	Most species (especially aquatic species). Common in snakes – e.g. indigo, hognose, water, garter, Asian ratsnakes and kingsnakes	Clinical signs: • Non-pathogenic adult flukes may be seen in the oral cavity • Migration can result in granulomatous inflammatory lesions in the gastrointestinal, urinary and respiratory systems	• Observation of adult flukes in the mouth or cloaca • Fresh faecal sample for identification of adult flukes or ova (large, yellow-brown with a single operculum) • Identification of ova from lung washes	Indirect life cycle; snails are common intermediate hosts, along with fish and frogs. Infection by ingestion of intermediate hosts	Manually remove oral flukes. Freeze amphibian/fish food items for 3 days prior to feeding. Praziquantel 5–8 mg/kg orally, i.m., s.c. once, repeated after 2 weeks (Stewart, 1990). Topical treatment with spot-on emodepside–praziquantel has been reported; 1 ml/kg (corresponding to 21.5 mg emodepside and 85.5 mg praziquantel) (Mehlhorn et al., 2005; Brames, 2008; 2010). Further research is needed
Cestodes	Most species	Clinical signs: • Usually asymptomatic. Large burdens can cause malnutrition, enteritis and obstruction	• Fresh faecal sample for identification of eggs, proglottids or adult worms	Indirect life cycle; reptiles may be intermediate or definitive hosts. Invertebrate or mammalian intermediate hosts are common	Praziquantel 5–8 mg/kg orally, i.m., s.c. once, repeated after 2 weeks (Stewart, 1990). Consider topical emodepside–praziquantel (see above)
Ascarids	Most species	Clinical signs: • Usually asymptomatic. Large burdens can cause malnutrition, enteritis, obstruction and gastrointestinal perforation with subsequent coelomitis and death • Larval migration can result in ulceration and abscessation in other systems (e.g. lungs)	• Fresh faecal sample for identification of thick-walled ova or adult nematodes	Indirect and direct life cycles. Many snake ascarids use a rodent or amphibian intermediate host. Enclosures may become heavily contaminated with eggs leading to high rates of reinfection	Strict environmental hygiene to reduce reinfection. Removal of infected intermediate hosts will halt reinfection. Fenbendazole 50–100 mg/kg orally once, repeated after 2–4 weeks (Holt, 1982) or 50 mg/kg orally q24h for 3–5 days (Funk, 2000). Oxfendazole 66 mg/kg orally once, repeated 2 weeks later. Benzimidazole-associated morbidity and mortality have been increasingly reported (Alvarado et al., 2001; Neiffer et al., 2005). Consider topical emodepside–praziquantel (see above)

17.31 (continued) Parasites of the reptile gastrointestinal tract. SNAP = enzyme immunoassay for the detection of *Giardia* antigen. (continues)

Parasite	Species affected	Clinical features	Diagnosis	Life cycle and transmission	Control and treatment
Helminths continued					
Rhabdiasids e.g. *Strongyloides* Strongylids e.g. *Kalicephalus*	Snakes predominantly. Reported in lizards and aquatic chelonians	Clinical signs: • May include lethargy, regurgitation, diarrhoea and anorexia. • Granulomatous reactions may occur owing to adult nematodes embedding in the intestinal wall. • Respiratory disease can occur with larval migration	• Fresh faecal sample for identification of thin-shelled embryonated ova – difficult to differentiate from larvated *Rhabdia* spp. (lungworm)	Direct life cycle. Infection can occur via percutaneous route as well as by ingestion. Enclosures may become heavily contaminated with eggs leading to high rates of reinfection	Strict environmental hygiene to reduce reinfection. Fenbendazole 50–100 mg/kg orally once, repeated after 2–4 weeks (Holt, 1982) or 50 mg/kg orally q24h for 3–5 days (Funk, 2000). Oxfendazole 66 mg/kg orally once, repeated 2 weeks later. Benzimidazole-associated morbidity and mortality have been increasingly reported (Alvarado *et al.*, 2001; Neiffer *et al.*, 2005). Ivermectin 0.2 mg/kg s.c., i.m. once. Repeat every 2 weeks until faeces clear (Wilson and Carpenter, 1996). DO NOT GIVE AVERMECTINS TO CHELONIANS
Oxyurids	Common in chelonians and lizards. Reported in some snake species. Not recorded in crocodilians	Clinical signs: • Often asymptomatic and moderate burdens suggested to be beneficial to digestion • High numbers may lead to debilitation or obstruction and can be associated with enteritis and cloacal prolapse	• Fresh faecal sample for identification of adults, larvae or 'D'-shaped ova (see Figure 17.1)	Direct life cycle. Enclosures may become heavily contaminated with eggs leading to high rates of reinfection	Strict environmental hygiene with regular removal of faecal material to reduce reinfection. Medical treatment of asymptomatic animals is controversial. Various protocols cited, including: • Fenbendazole 50–100 mg/kg orally once, repeated 14–28 days later (Holt, 1982), or for 3 consecutive days (Girling, 2004). Innis (2008) has reported intracolonic administration per cloaca • Benzimidazole-associated morbidity and mortality have been increasingly reported (Alvarado *et al.*, 2001; Neiffer *et al.*, 2005)
Pentastomids					
Tongue worms	Snakes predominantly. Reported in other reptiles, e.g. leopard geckos	Found adhered to pharynx, or within lungs or subcutaneous tissue. Clinical signs: • Mostly associated with respiratory disease • Inflammatory reactions and secondary infections may affect the gastrointestinal tract	• Identification of large ova, with claw-like appendages in faeces or sputum • Adult pentastomids occasionally seen during surgeries or observed ultrasonographically	Indirect life cycle; mammalian intermediate hosts are probably rodents. Humans are possible intermediate hosts (i.e. zoonotic potential)	Endoscopic or surgical removal of adult parasites. Control access to intermediate hosts; often self-limiting in captivity owing to an absence of wild rodent hosts. Ivermectin has been reported to temporarily decrease ovum production but is not effective in eliminating mature pentastomids: • 0.2 mg/kg q48h in monitor lizards (Flach *et al.*, 2000) • Risk of antigenic/inflammatory damage due to death of large parasites DO NOT GIVE AVERMECTINS TO CHELONIANS

17.31 (continued) Parasites of the reptile gastrointestinal tract. SNAP = enzyme immunoassay for the detection of *Giardia* antigen.

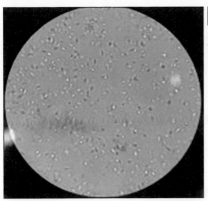

17.32 *Trichomonas* sp. on a wet preparation from a green tree python; X400.

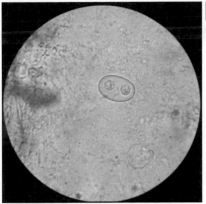

17.33 Sporulated coccidian (*Isospora* sp.) on a direct wet preparation from a veiled chameleon; X400.

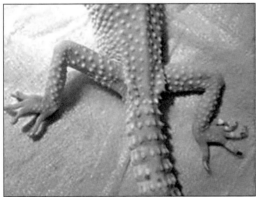

17.34 A leopard gecko with cachexia due to cryptosporidiosis; note loss of epaxial musculature and tail fat stores.

- **Temperature:** warming prey items will help enhance odour and activate thermoception senses used by some snake species, e.g. boas. Do not use a microwave for heating prey items.
- **Size:** offer differently sized food items or cut up prey items.
- **Colour:** most chelonians and lizards have good colour vision. Offering brightly coloured food items such as flowers (e.g. dandelions) to tortoises (especially testudinids) can be effective (Figure 17.35).
- **Location:** offer food within an appropriate area of the enclosure – e.g. in sheltered areas for shy species or in water for aquatic or semiaquatic species such as red-eared terrapins.
- **Circadian preferences:** offer food at appropriate times of day – e.g. nocturnal reptiles should be presented with food during evening hours.

- **Ontogenic preferences:** consider changes in diet preference as a reptile physically matures; e.g. some snake species may seek insects or small lizards when young but will switch to mammalian prey as they mature.
- **Reduce hunting challenge:** offering slow-moving invertebrate prey or putting prey into a smooth-sided dish (to prevent escape) may assist feeding in debilitated insectivores.

Hand-feeding: Hand-feeding with forceps or tongs is useful when patients are relatively bright and alert. Movement of food with tongs and placement under the animal's nose may encourage striking/prehending (see Figure 17.35). There are risks to attempting this in large and aggressive species and success is unlikely in shy species.

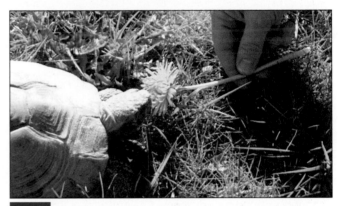

17.35 Hand-feeding anorexic tortoises may encourage appetite.

Force-feeding: Force-feeding guarantees food intake but can be highly stressful for the animal and risks oral cavity trauma. It should therefore be limited to short-term situations. Small pieces of food or small skinned and lubricated whole prey can be placed directly into the mouth or pushed down the oesophagus using atraumatic forceps.

Syringe feeding: Syringe feeding can be a viable option for home treatment by owners, particularly for the smaller lizard species. It can be stressful and aspiration pneumonia is possible if large volumes are given too quickly or if the animal has a poor swallowing reflex. Liquid formulations are trickled into the front or side of the mouth (small amounts frequently).

Stomach gavage: Gavage is a useful short-term option, provided the animal can be appropriately restrained. It is a stressful procedure and should therefore not be used long term. The risk of aspiration is reduced compared with force-feeding and it provides a useful option if coagulopathies or anaesthetic risks preclude oesophagostomy tube placement. Metal crop tubes, feeding tubes or canine urinary catheters are appropriate; using a gag will prevent perforation of thin-walled tubes (see Chapter 11).

Oesophagostomy tube placement: Oesophagostomy tube placement is the method of choice for longer-term (>3 weeks) nutritional support, fluid and oral medication administration, or in cases of severe upper gastrointestinal tract disease involving the head (e.g. mandibular fractures). It is useful in stressed, recalcitrant and aggressive individuals. Tubes are generally well tolerated and can be left in place for months at a time (Figure 17.36). Placement allows home nursing and animals will frequently start eating with the tube still in place. Anaesthesia or sedation is usually required for placement (see Chapter 13 for methodology).

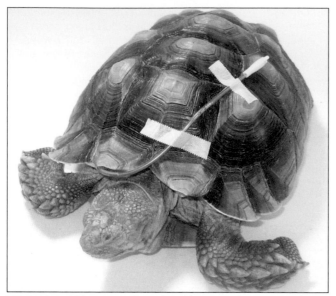

17.36 An African spurred tortoise with an oesophagostomy tube; the tube is taped along the ventral rim of the cranial carapace and then over the dorsum so as to prevent removal with the forelimbs.

Commercial enteral feeding products

Reptile critical care nutrition is still in relative infancy, with many extrapolations made from mammalian medicine, although with recent advances, newer commercial enteral feeding products more suitable for reptilian patients are being made available. These are usually in the form of a liquid or powder to be mixed with water and fall roughly into three categories (Chitty and Raftery, 2013b):

- **Simple nutritional mixes:** usually simple protein and carbohydrate mixes useful for short-term support (i.e. not a complete diet) and valuable in an acute critical care situation – e.g. Critical Care Formula (Vetark)
- **Elemental diets:** more complex nutritional mixes, providing nutrients in an easily assimilated form. For example, Emeraid (Lafeber) produces four different formulations (Herbivore, Carnivore, Omnivore and Piscivore), which can be mixed in different proportions to give the correct nutritional balance for a particular species. These can be fed for longer periods in cases of malabsorption or maldigestion, but herbivorous patients in particular should be moved on to recovery diets on signs of clinical improvement, as elemental diets may not provide enough fibre for normal gastrointestinal tract function
- **Recovery diets:** complete diets in liquid form, these require normal gastrointestinal tract function for digestion and so are suitable for long-term nutritional support – e.g. Carnivore Care and Critical Care (Oxbow).

The manufacturer's recommendations for quantity and dilution factors should be followed and ideally the food warmed before administration. For calculation of maintenance energy requirements, see Chapter 22. The volume given at each feed will be dependent on the species, age and clinical condition, and must not exceed the animal's stomach capacity; in lizards and chelonians 2–5% bodyweight is appropriate, and in snakes 5–10% bodyweight can be administered (Pollock, 2012a,b,c). Starting with small volumes and gradually increasing is advised (reduce if regurgitation is observed). One or two feeds a day appears suitable for most lizards and chelonians, while tube feeding in snakes is usually performed on a weekly or 'every-other-week' basis.

As the animal's condition improves, they will probably start to show interest in food and start eating voluntarily. Reduction or cessation of nutritional support should be based on an assessment of recovery and should ideally be tapered off within the reptile's own environment at home to avoid relapse when the animal is discharged.

Gastrointestinal zoonoses

Salmonella

Most reptiles are considered to harbour *Salmonella* spp. as normal inhabitants of the gut. Routine faecal screening for *Salmonella* is not advised, particularly as the organism may only be shed intermittently. Numerous efforts have been made to prevent *Salmonella* shedding in reptiles without success and with increased risk of antibiotic resistance.

The risk of contracting salmonellosis from eating contaminated food seems greater than from contact with reptiles (Gray, 2011). However, client and staff education is extremely important in preventing zoonotic infection. The Centers for Disease Control and Prevention (CDC) has developed guidelines for the prevention of salmonellosis in reptile owners (CDC, 2014). This advice will also apply to other zoonotic infections spread via the faecal–oral route.

Other zoonotic pathogens

Many bacteria present in the reptilian gastrointestinal tract pose a potential zoonotic risk, particularly in immunocompromised individuals, including *Escherichia coli*, *Campylobacter* and *Mycobacteria*, amongst many others.

Parasitic zoonoses include *Entamoeba invadens* and pentastomes (*Armillifer*). *Cryptosporidium* and *Giardia* spp. should also be considered as potential zoonoses, as although *Cryptosporidium serpentis* and *C. varanii* are now only considered to affect reptiles, there have been reports of *C. parvum* found in leopard geckos (Pedraza-Diaz *et al.*, 2009) and tortoises (Traversa *et al.*, 2008).

Acknowledgements

Thanks to Stuart McArthur for his assistance in the preparation of this chapter.

References and further reading

Allender MC, Mitchell MA, Yarborough J *et al.* (2013) Pharmacokinetics of a single oral dose of acyclovir and valacyclovir in North American box turtles (*Terrapene* sp.). *Journal of Veterinary Pharmacology and Therapeutics* **36(2)**, 205–208

Alvarado TP, Garner MM, Gamble K *et al.* (2001) Fenbendazole overdose in four Fea's vipers (*Azemiops feae*). *Proceedings of the Association of Reptilian and Amphibian Veterinarians Annual Conference*, Orlando, pp. 35–36

Bennet A and Mader D (2006) Cloacal prolapse. In: *Reptile Medicine and Surgery, 2nd edition*, ed. D Mader, pp. 751–755. Elsevier, St Louis, Missouri

Brames H (2008) Efficacy and tolerability of profender in reptiles: spot-on treatment against nematodes. *Exotic DVM* **10(3)**, 29–34

Brames H (2010) Risks, benefits and limitations of spot-on endo and ectoparasite treatment in reptiles. *Proceedings of the 1st International Conference on Reptile and Amphibian Medicine*, Munich, pp. 39–40

Campbell I and Tzipori S (1982) Effect of disinfectants on survival of *Cryptosporidium* oocysts. *Veterinary Record* **111**, 414–415

Campbell TW (2014) Clinical pathology. In: *Current Therapy in Reptile Medicine and Surgery*, ed. DM Mader and SJ Divers, pp. 70–92. Elsevier Saunders, Missouri

Carpenter JW, Mashima TY and Rupiper DJ (2001) Miscellaneous agents used in reptiles. In: *Exotic Animal Formulary, 2nd edition*, ed. JW Carpenter, pp. 76–78. WB Saunders, Philadelphia

CDC (2014) Reptiles, Amphibians, and Salmonella. CDC, Atlanta, GA. Available online at: http://www.cdc.gov/Features/SalmonellaFrogTurtle/

Chitty J and Raftery A (2013a) Hepatic lipidosis. In: *Essentials of Tortoise Medicine and Surgery*, pp. 222–224. Wiley Blackwell, Chichester, UK

Chitty J and Raftery A (2013b) Stomach tubing. In: *Essentials of Tortoise Medicine and Surgery*, pp. 93–96. Wiley Blackwell, Chichester, UK

Chitty J and Raftery A (2013c) Toxicoses. In: *Essentials of Tortoise Medicine and Surgery*, pp. 320–325. Wiley Blackwell, Chichester, UK

Corbit AG, Person C and Hayes WK (2014) Constipation associated with brumation? Intestinal obstruction caused by a fecalith in a wild red diamond rattlesnake (*Crotalus ruber*). *Journal of Animal Physiology and Animal Nutrition* **98(1)**, 96–99

Cranfield MR and Graczyk TK (1996) Cryptosporidiosis. In: *Reptile Medicine and Surgery, 2nd edition*, ed. D Mader, pp. 359–363. WB Saunders, Philadelphia

Devloo R, Martel A, Hellebuyck T *et al.* (2011) Bearded dragons (*Pogona vitticeps*) asymptomatically infected with *Devriesea agamarum* are a source of persistent clinical infection in captive colonies of Dab lizards (*Uromastyx* sp.). *Veterinary Microbiology* **150(3–4)**, 297–301

Diaz-Figueroa O and Mitchell MA (2006) Gastrointestinal anatomy and physiology. In: *Reptile Medicine and Surgery, 2nd edition*, ed. DR Mader, pp. 145–162. WB Saunders, Philadelphia

Divers SJ (2000) Reptilian liver and gastrointestinal testing. In: *Laboratory Medicine: Avian and Exotic Pets*, ed. AM Fudge, pp. 205–209. WB Saunders, Pennsylvania

Divers SJ (2013a) Hepatic lipidosis (reptiles). In: *Clinical Veterinary Advisor: Birds and Exotic Pets*, ed. J Mayer and TM Donnelly, pp. 103–105. Elsevier, MO

Divers SJ (2013b) Liver disease (reptiles). In: *Clinical Veterinary Advisor: Birds and Exotic Pets*, ed. J Mayer and TM Donnelly, pp. 115–117. Elsevier, MO

Doneley B (2006) Caring for the bearded dragon. *Proceedings of the North American Veterinary Conference*, pp. 1607–1611

Donoghue S (2006) Nutrition. In: *Reptile Medicine and Surgery, 2nd edition*, ed. DR Mader, pp.251–298. WB Saunders, Philadelphia

Eatwell K, Hedley J and Barron R (2014) Reptile haematology and biochemistry. *In Practice* **36(1)**, 34–42

Fitzgerald KT and Newquist KL (2008) Poisonings in reptiles. *Veterinary Clinics of North America: Exotic Animal Practice* **11(2)**, 327–357

Fitzgerald KT and Vera R (2006) Reported toxicities in reptiles. In: *Reptile Medicine and Surgery, 2nd edition*, ed. DR Mader, pp. 1068–1080. WB Saunders, Philadelphia

Flach EJ, Riley J, Mutlow AG *et al.* (2000) Pentastomiasis in Bosc's monitor lizards (*Varanus exanthematicus*) caused by an undescribed *Sambonia* species. *Journal of Zoo and Wildlife Medicine* **31**, 91–95

Frye FL (1999) Spontaneous autoimmune pancreatitis and diabetes mellitus in a western pond turtle, *Clemmys m. marmorata*. *Proceedings of the Association of Reptilian and Amphibian Veterinarians Annual Conference*, pp. 103–106

Frye FL, McNeely HE and Corcoran JH (1999) Functional pancreatic glucagonoma in the rhinoceros iguana *Cyclura c. figgensi*, characterized by immunocytochemistry. In: *Proceedings of the Association of Reptilian and Amphibian Veterinarians Annual Conference*, Columbus, OH, p. 315

Funk RS (2000) A formulary for lizards, snakes and crocodilians. *Veterinary Clinics of North America: Exotic Animal Practice* **3(1)**, 333–358

Garner MM, Hernandez-Divers SM and Raymond JT (2004) Reptile neoplasia: a retrospective study of case submissions to a specialty diagnostic service. *Veterinary Clinics of North America: Exotic Animal Practice* **7**, 653–671

Gibbons PM (2013) Advances in reptile clinical therapeutics. *Journal of Exotic Pet Medicine* **23(1)**, 21–38

Gibbons PM and Steffes ZJ (2013) Emerging infectious diseases of chelonians. *Veterinary Clinics of North America: Exotic Animal Practice* **16**, 303–317

Girling SJ (2004) Formulary. In *BSAVA Manual of Reptiles, 2nd edition*, ed. SJ Girling and P Raiti, pp. 352–356. British Small Animal Veterinary Association, Gloucester, UK

Graczyk TK, Cranfield MR and Bostwick EF (1999) Therapeutic efficacy of hyperimmune bovine colostrum treatment against *Cryptosporidium* infections in reptiles. *Proceedings of the Annual Meeting of the American Association of Zoo Veterinarians*, pp. 6–10

Gray TZ (2011) Update: reptiles and salmonella. *Journal of Exotic Pet Medicine* **20**, 14–17

Griffin C (2006) Severe obstipation as a result of power feeding in a red tail boa (*Boa constrictor*). In: *Proceedings of the Association of Reptilian and Amphibian Veterinarians Annual Conference*, Baltimore, MD, pp. 112–113

Grosset C, Villeneuve A, Brieger A *et al.* (2011) Cryptosporidiosis in juvenile bearded dragons (*Pogona vitticeps*): effects of treatment with paromomycin. *Journal of Herpetological Medicine and Surgery* **21(1)**, 10–15

Gumpernberger M (2011) Use of computed tomography to diagnose hepatic lipidosis in reptiles. *Proceedings of the Association of Reptilian and Amphibian Veterinarians Annual Conference*, Seattle, WA, pp. 173–174

Heatley JJ, Mitchell MA, Williams J *et al.* (2001) Fungal periodontal osteomyelitis in a chameleon (*Furcifer pardalis*). *Journal of Herpetological Medicine and Surgery* **11(4)**, 7–12

Hedley J (2012) Survey of Gastrointestinal parasites in tortoises in the United Kingdom. *RCVS Diploma*, Royal College of Veterinary Surgeons Library, London

Hedley J and Eatwell K (2014) Cloacal prolapses in reptiles: a retrospective study of 56 cases. *Journal of Small Animal Practice* **55(5)**, 265–268

Hernandez-Divers SJ and Cooper JE (2006) Hepatic lipidosis In: *Reptile Medicine and Surgery, 2nd edition*, ed. DR Mader, pp. 806–813. WB Saunders, Philadelphia

Hernandez-Divers SM and Garner MM (2003) Neoplasia of reptiles with an emphasis on lizards. *Veterinary Clinics of North America: Exotic Animal Practice* **6**, 251–273

Hidalgo-Vila J, Martínez-Silvestre A, Ribas A *et al.* (2011) Pancreatitis associated with the helminth *Serpinema microcephalus* (Nematoda: Camallanidae) in exotic red-eared slider turtles (*Trachemys scripta elegans*). *Journal of Wildlife Diseases* **47(1)**, 201–205

Hnizdo J and Pantchev N (2011) Diseases of the digestive system. In: *Medical Care of Turtles and Tortoises*, ed. J Hnizdo and N Pantchev, pp. 337–368. Chimaira Buchhandels, Frankfurt am Main

Hochleithner C and Holland M (2014) Ultrasonography. In: *Current Therapy in Reptile Medicine and Surgery*, ed. DM Mader and SJ Divers, pp. 107–127. Elsevier Saunders, MO

Holt PE (1982) Efficacy of fenbendazole against nematodes of reptiles. *Veterinary Record* **110**, 302–304

Innis C (2002) Clinical parasitology of the chelonia. *Proceedings of the North American Veterinary Conference*, Orlando, pp. 1783–1785

Jacobson ER (1999) Use of antimicrobial drugs in reptiles. In: *Zoo and Wild Animal Medicine: Current Therapy, 4th edition*, ed. E Fowler and RE Miller, pp. 190–200. WB Saunders, Philadelphia

Jacobsen ER, Green DE, Undeen AH, Cranfield M and Vaughn KL (1998) Systemic microsporidiosis in inland bearded dragons (*Pogona vitticeps*) *Journal of Zoo and Wildlife Medicine* **29**, 315–323

Kadekaru S, Suzuki T and Une Y (2010) Gastric carcinoid in three bearded dragons. *Journal of the Japan Veterinary Medical Association* **63(12)**, 945–949

Kik MJL and Nickel RF (2001) Removal of a foreign body from the intestine of a leopard tortoise (*Geochelone pardalis*) via laparoscopy. *Praktische Tierarzt* **82(3)**, 174–179

Kolmstetter CM, Frazier D, Cox S and Ramsay EC (1997). Metronidazole pharmacokinetics in yellow ratsnakes (*Elaphe obsolete quadrivitatta*). *Proceedings of the American Association of Zoo Veterinarians*, p. 26

Kubisch U, Fischer I and Hatt J (2006) Gastric ulcer in green iguanas (*Iguana iguana*). *Tieraerztliche Praxis Ausgabe Kleintiere Heimtiere* **34(1)**, 50–53

Lane TJ and Mader DR (1996) Parasitology. In: *Reptile Medicine and Surgery, 2nd edition*, ed. DR Mader, pp. 186–203. WB Saunders, Philadelphia

Latney LV and Wellehan J (2013) Selected emerging infectious diseases of Squamata. *Veterinary Clinics of North America: Exotic Animal Practice* **16(2)**, 319–338

Lyons JA, Newman SJ, Greenacre CB *et al.* (2010) A gastric neuroendocrine carcinoma expressing somatostatin in a bearded dragon (*Pogona vitticeps*). *Journal of Veterinary Diagnostic Investigation* **22**, 316–320

McArthur S (2004) Problem-solving approach to common diseases. In: *Medicine and Surgery of Tortoises and Turtles*, ed. S McArthur, R Wilkinson and J Meyer, pp. 333–349. Blackwell Publishing, Oxford

McArthur S, McLellan L and Brown S (2004) Gastrointestinal system. In: *BSAVA Manual of Reptiles, 2nd edition*, ed. SJ Girling and P Raiti, pp. 210–229. British Small Animal Veterinary Association, Gloucester, UK

McBride M, Hernandez-Divers SJ, Koch T *et al.* (2007) Preliminary evaluation of resting and post-prandial bile acid levels in the green iguana (*Iguana iguana*). *Journal of Herpetological Medicine and Surgery* **16**, 129–134

McCracken HE and Birch CA (1994) Periodontal disease in lizards: a review of numerous cases. *Proceedings of the American Association of Zoo Veterinarians*, pp. 108–115

Mans C (2013) Clinical update on diagnosis and management of disorders of the digestive system of reptiles. *Journal of Exotic Pet Medicine* **22**, 141–162

Marschang RE (2014) Clinical virology. In: *Current Therapy in Reptile Medicine and Surgery*, ed. DR Mader and SJ Divers, pp. 32–52. WB Saunders, MO

Marschang RE (2016) Viral diseases of reptiles. *In Practice* **38(6)**, 275–285

Marschang RE and Divers SJ (2014) Reptile viruses. In: *Current Therapy in Reptile Medicine and Surgery*, ed. DR Mader and SJ Divers, pp. 368–381. WB Saunders, MO

Mauldin GN and Done LB (1996) Oncology. In: *Reptile Medicine and Surgery, 2nd edition*, ed. DE Mader, pp. 299–322. WB Saunders, Philadelphia

Mehler SJ and Avery Bennett R (2006) Upper alimentary tract disease. In: *Reptile Medicine and Surgery, 2nd edition*, ed. DR Mader, pp. 924–930. WB Saunders, Philadelphia.

Mehlhorn H, Schmahl G, Frese M *et al.* (2005) Effects of a combination of emodepside and praziquantel on parasites of reptiles and rodents. *Parasitology Research* **97**, S64–S69

Mitchell MA (2005) Clinical reptile gastroenterology. *Veterinary Clinics of North America: Exotic Animal Practice* **8**, 277–298

Mitchell MA (2008) Ponazuril. *Journal of Exotic Pet Medicine* **17**, 228–229

Modry D and Sloboda M (2007) Control of coccidiosis in chameleons using toltrazuril: results of an experimental trial. In: *Proceedings of the 7th International Symposium on Pathology and Medicine in Reptiles and Amphibians*, 2004, Berlin, ed. J Seybold and F Mutschmann, pp. 93–97

Naples LM, Langan JN, Mylniczenko ND, Kagan R and Colegrove K (2009) Islet cell tumor in a savannah monitor (*Varanus exanthematicus*). *Journal of Herpetological Medicine and Surgery* **19**, 97–105

Neiffer D, Lydick R, Burks K *et al.* (2005) Haematological and plasma biochemical changes associated with fenbendazole administration in Hermann's tortoises (*Testudo hermanni*). *Journal of Zoo and Wildlife Medicine* **36(4)**, 661–672

Nevarez J (2009) Lizards. In: *Manual of Exotic Pet Practice*, ed. MA Mitchell and TN Tully, pp. 164–206. Saunders Elsevier, MO

Norton TM (2005) Chelonian emergency and critical care. *Seminars in Avian and Exotic Pet Medicine* **14(2)**, 106–130

Paré J (1997) Treatment of cryptosporidiosis in Gila monsters (*Heloderma suspectum*) with paromomycin. *Proceedings of the Association of Reptilian and Amphibian Veterinarians Annual Conference*, pp. 23–24

Pedraza-Díaz S, Ortega-Mora LM, Carrión BA, Navarro V and Gómez-Bautista M (2009) Molecular characterisation of *Cryptosporidium* isolates from pet reptiles. *Veterinary Parasitology* **160**, 204–210

Pollock C (2012a) Feeding the Hospitalized Lizard. Available online at http://www.lafebervet.com/vet/feeding-the-hospitalized-lizard/. LafeberVet

Pollock C (2012b) Feeding the Hospitalized Snake. Available online at http://www.lafebervet.com/vet/feeding-the-hospitalized-snake/. LafeberVet

Pollock C (2012c) Feeding the Hospitalized Turtle or Tortoise. Available online at http://www.lafebervet.com/vet/feeding-the-hospitalized-turtle-or-tortoise/. LafeberVet

Raiti P (2012) Husbandry, diseases, and veterinary care of the bearded dragon (*Pogona vitticeps*). *Journal of Herpetological Medicine and Surgery* **22(3–4)**, 117–131

Reavill DR (2004) Neoplasia. In: *BSAVA Manual of Reptiles, 2nd edition*, ed. SJ Girling and P Raiti, pp. 309–318. British Small Animal Veterinary Association, Gloucester, UK

Redrobe S and Frye FL (2001) Hepatic thrombosis and other pathology associated with severe periodontal disease in the bearded dragon, *Pogona vitticeps*. *Proceedings of the Association of Reptilian and Amphibian Veterinarians Annual Conference,* pp. 217–219

Ritter JM, Garner MM, Chilton JA *et al.* (2009) Gastric neuro-endocrine carcinomas in bearded dragons (*Pogona vitticeps*). *Veterinary Pathology* **46**, 1109–1116

Rotstein DS, Lewbart GA, Hobbie K *et al.* (2003) Suspected oak, *Quercus*, toxicity in an African spurred tortoise, *Geochelone sulcata*. *Journal of Herpetological Medicine and Surgery* **13(3)**, 20–21

Scullion F and Scullion M (2009) Gastrointestinal protozoal diseases in reptiles. *Journal of Exotic Pet Medicine* **18(4)**, 266–278

Stahl SJ (2003) Diseases of the reptile pancreas. *Veterinary Clinics of North America: Exotic Animal Practice* **6**, 191–212

Stahl SJ (2006) Hyperglycemia in reptiles. In: *Reptile Medicine and Surgery, 2nd edition*, ed. DR Mader, pp. 822–830. WB Saunders, Philadelphia

Stahl SJ (2013) Hypovitaminosis A. In: *Clinical Veterinary Advisor: Birds and Exotic Pets*, ed. J Mayer and TM Donnelly, pp. 110–112. Elsevier Saunders, St Louis, MO

Stenglein M, Sanders C, Kistler A *et al.* (2012) Identification, characterization, and *in vitro* culture of highly divergent arenaviruses from boa constrictors and annulated tree boas: candidate etiological agents for snake inclusion body disease. *mBio* **3(4)**, e00180–12

Stern AW, Velguth KE and D'Agostino J (2010) Metastatic ductal adeno-carcinoma in a western hognose snake (*Heterodon nasicus*). *Journal of Zoo and Wildlife Medicine* **41(2)**, 320–324

Stewart JS (1990) Anaerobic bacterial infections in reptiles. *Journal of Zoo and Wildlife Medicine* **21**, 180

Teare JA and Bush M (1983) Toxicity and efficacy of ivermectin in chelonians. *Journal of the American Veterinary Medical Association* **183(11)**, 1195–1197

Tothill A, Johnson J, Winsatt J and Mangone B (2000) Effect of cisapride, erythromycin, and metoclopramide on gastrointestinal transit time in the desert tortoise, *Gopherus agassizii*. *Journal of Herpetological Medicine and Surgery* **10**, 16–20

Traversa D, Iorio R, Otranto D, Modryc D and Slapeta J (2008) Cryptosporidium from tortoises: genetic characterisation, phylogeny and zoonotic implications. *Molecular and Cellular Probes* **22**, 122–128

Wellehan CFX and Gunkel CI (2004) Emergent diseases in reptiles. *Seminars in Avian and Exotic Pet Medicine* **13(3)**, 160–174

Wilkinson R (2004) Clinical pathology. In: *Medicine and Surgery of Tortoises and Turtles*, ed. S McArthur, R Wilkinson and J Meyer, pp. 141–186. Blackwell Publishing, Oxford

Wilson SC and Carpenter JW (1996) Endoparasitic diseases of reptiles. *Seminars in Avian and Exotic Pet Medicine* **5**, 64–74

Wright K (2008) Two common disorders of captive bearded dragons (*Pogona vitticeps*): nutritional secondary hyperparathyroidism and constipation. *Journal of Exotic Pet Medicine* **17(4)**, 267–272

Chapter 18

Respiratory system

John Chitty

Respiratory disease is common in reptiles, especially in snakes and chelonians. A large part of this is due to inappropriate husbandry practices and certain anatomical features of the reptile respiratory system, which include:

- Lack of a muscular diaphragm (in all except crocodilians) means that discharges cannot be coughed up
- A poorly developed mucociliary escalator in the airways also reduces the ability of the reptile to clear discharges
- The ability to withstand long periods of hypoxia means that respiratory diseases are often well advanced before clinical signs are seen.

Anatomy and physiology

An overview can be found in Chapter 1 of this volume, as well as Wyneken (2001), Gans and Gaunt (1998), and Wood and Lenfant (1976).

Anatomy

The respiratory system of reptiles is fundamentally different from that of mammals. Reptiles lack a bronchial tree leading to terminal alveolar sacs; air-exchange surfaces (ediculae and faveolae) are formed by small crypts in the lung parenchyma. Comparatively, reptiles have a much greater lung volume than a similar-sized mammal, although the simpler structure results in an absorptive surface approximately one-hundredth that of mammals. This mirrors the comparative differences in oxygen demand in reptiles and mammals.

The basic system is similar in all reptiles, with air entering via the nares to the nasal cavity, then passing through internal choanae to the glottis (situated at the base of the tongue in all species; see Chapter 1), trachea and bronchi and thence to the lungs. However, certain features are unique to each class (Figure 18.1).

Respiration

The differences in anatomy account for the differences seen in respiratory movements.

- In chelonians, antagonistic movements of the limbs stretch the *septum horizontale* (in the case of terrestrial species, via the pectoral girdle cranially and *transversus abdominis* muscle caudally) and pull it downwards. The negative pressure induced within the lungs facilitates inspiration.
- In lizards, expansion and contraction of the ribs result in movement of air through the lungs; unlike in mammals, both expiration and inspiration are active processes.

Structure/area	Chelonians	Lizards	Snakes	Crocodilians
Upper respiratory tract	Paired nares open to keratinized vestibule lined dorsally with olfactory epithelium and ventrally with mucous membrane. Vestibule divided by septum into left and right chambers. These open into single passage dorsal to hard palate, which opens into pharynx at choana	Similar to chelonians. Some (including green iguana) have salt glands that discharge via nares. Nasal septum continuous, so paired choanae open into pharynx	Similar to lizards but lacking salt glands*. Glottis very mobile, fitting into choanae during normal respiration but can be repositioned to allow breathing during swallowing *Sea snakes possess salt glands	Basic structure similar to lizards. Modifications allow breathing while mouth is open underwater: complete secondary palate; gular fold that closes off choanae and glottis from mouth (Figure 18.2)
Trachea/bronchi	Very short trachea in all except side-necked turtles and some terrapins. Trachea often bifurcates to paired bronchi just distal to glottis. Bronchi extremely flexible, allowing breathing while head withdrawn. Airways supported by complete cartilaginous rings	Long trachea supported by cartilaginous rings (complete or incomplete). In most species bronchi are short and open into lungs at cranial pole. In monitors, bronchi are longer and traverse length of lung	Long trachea supported by incomplete cartilaginous rings. Except for boids, trachea opens directly to lung	Similar to lizards but with much more complex system of bronchi (reflecting lung complexity)

18.1 Comparative anatomy of the reptilian respiratory system. (continues) ▶

Structure/area	Chelonians	Lizards	Snakes	Crocodilians
Lungs (Figures 18.3–18.5)	Paired (right larger than left in some Mediterranean species), separated by strong vertical septum. Fixed dorsally to coelomic membrane; ventrally to *septum horizontale* or pseudodiaphragm. Cranially, lungs consist of spongy 'alveolar' tissue where bronchi branch repeatedly. More distal to bronchial exits lungs become more sac-like	Variable structure: *Iguanids:* transitional lungs with single chamber divided by septa; intrapulmonary bronchus *Chameleons:* many hollow tubular diverticula extend from ventrocaudal surfaces *Geckos:* simple unlobed lungs *Monitors and helodermids:* more complex multichambered lungs reflecting more active lifestyle	Variable number: *Boids:* large right lung; left vestigial but functional *Others:* right lung only. Cranial part vascular, functions as respiratory lung; in many extends cranially into dorsal trachea forming 'tracheal lung'. Caudal part of the lung avascular, non-respiratory, acts as air sac. Elephant trunk snakes have tracheal air sacs	Highly vascularized, complex lungs. Breath can be held for long periods by means of glottic valve
Diaphragm	Non-muscular pseudodiaphragm	None, except for monitors/helodermids, which have incomplete postpulmonary septum	None	Complete muscular postpulmonary septum acts as diaphragm

18.1 (continued) Comparative anatomy of the reptilian respiratory system.

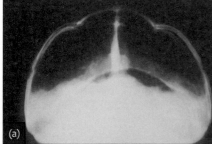

18.2 The paired choanae and glottis can be seen caudal to the gular fold in a young American alligator.

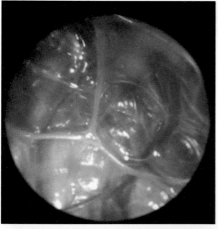

18.3 Endoscopic view of normal lung in a spur-thighed tortoise.

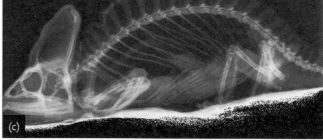

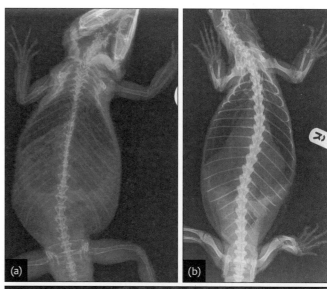

18.5 Extent of normal lungs and air sacs in lizards: (a) dorsoventral (DV) view of a bearded dragon showing the lungs and air sacs; (b) DV view of Bosc monitor showing the lungs and air sacs; (c) horizontal beam lateral view of a chameleon showing the air sacs.

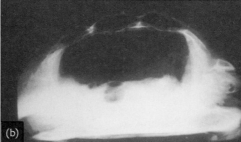

18.4 Normal lungs in tortoises: (a) craniocaudal radiograph of a leopard tortoise; (b) lateral radiograph of a leopard tortoise; (c) craniocaudal radiograph of a spur-thighed tortoise; note the normal asymmetry.

- In snakes, inspiration is achieved by expansion of the ribs (with a passive component where relaxation of expiratory muscles allows repositioning of the liver and other abdominal organs). Expiration is both passive (through relaxation of the muscles and natural recoil of the lungs) and active (via dorsolateral and ventrolateral muscle sheets) – i.e. respiration in snakes is a triphasic process: active expiration; inspiration; passive expiration.
- In crocodilians, respiratory movements are achieved by means of the intercostal muscles and the muscular diaphragm.

In both chelonians and lizards, gulping movements of the throat may be seen (gular pumping). It is thought that these are not linked to inspiration or expiration but are used to move air over the olfactory membranes in the oropharynx of lizards and nasal chambers of chelonians (except in freshwater turtles/terrapins and soft-shelled turtles, where some degree of oxygen exchange may occur in the pharynx). Additionally, the cloacal bursa and skin may be involved in respiration in aquatic chelonians.

The respiratory drive (in terms of rate: this is via alteration of the apnoea phase of the respiratory cycle) is principally by means of detection of low partial pressures of oxygen, rather than raised carbon dioxide levels as in mammals. This has implications for anaesthesia (see Chapter 12). It should also be noted that reptiles can withstand very low oxygen levels for extended periods. This may be due to their ability to switch from aerobic to anaerobic respiration (even the brain is able to utilize anaerobic respiration). Breathing cycles are discussed in Chapter 12. Markedly high carbon dioxide levels may also affect respiratory patterns in some species and situations, principally via alteration in tidal volume.

Other functions

In some species the respiratory system may have other functions:

- In aquatic species the dorsally placed lungs may act as a buoyancy aid
- In lizards the process of gular pumping is used to expand the lungs greatly, especially in chameleons where the tubular diverticula aid this process. This body size increase may be used in displays or for assisting crevice-dwelling lizards to resist capture. Some chameleons (e.g. Jackson's chameleon) have an accessory lung lobe in the ventral neck. This arises from the trachea just cranial to the forelimbs. Again, this is mainly used in gular pumping to increase body size. If infected, this lobe may fill with secretions and present as a ventral cervical swelling. Stored air may also be forcibly expelled in vocalizations.

Clinical evaluation

In all cases it is essential to perform a full clinical examination and take a detailed clinical history.

History

This should include a history of the current and previous disease problems, plus any preventive procedures such as parasite control and environmental disinfection. It is important to consider the species kept, whether there has been mixing of species and whether the owner has had contact with other reptiles (particularly important when considering viral spread in chelonians). Some problems may occur after addition of new animals, owing to contact with novel disease agents and/or stress effects.

The environment should be thoroughly assessed. The following may have a major role in promoting respiratory disease:

- Temperature – too high may cause chronic dehydration and drying of mucous membranes; too low may result in lowered immunity and resistance to infection
- Humidity – too high may promote excessive load of environmental microorganisms; too low will lead to mucous membrane drying
- Sanitation – poorly sanitized vivaria have been associated with an increased incidence of respiratory disease, especially in large snakes
- Vivarium size – this is especially relevant for large snakes, where inability to stretch out facilitates the build-up of discharges in the lungs. Arboreal or semi-arboreal species may also fail to clear discharges if they are unable to climb, as they may need to hang downwards to facilitate clearance
- Vivarium type – anecdotally it has been described by tortoise keepers that 'closed' vivaria, rather than 'open' type vivaria (or tortoise tables), are associated with respiratory disease in Mediterranean species. Clinically this appears untrue, especially as lower environmental temperatures appear more important and closed vivaria are better at maintaining these. Instead, it is more likely that the move to keep tortoises in vivaria rather than gardens coincided with the arrival in the UK of 'farmed' tortoises and increased prevalence of pathogen carriage.

The diet should also be assessed. Although malnutrition is rarely a primary cause of respiratory disease, it may be a contributory factor in stress and immunosuppression. Specifically, hypovitaminosis A has been described as an underlying cause of lower respiratory tract disease (LRTD) and upper respiratory tract disease (URTD) in reptiles, especially chelonians.

Clinical signs

The following may be indicative of respiratory disease:

- Open-mouth breathing
- Dyspnoea or tachypnoea (dyspnoea may take the form of an obviously exaggerated respiratory effort, increased gulping motions in the throat or an extended neck)
- Repeated yawning in snakes
- Tracheal discharges in snakes and lizards
- Respiratory noise
- Cyanosis or pallor of mucous membranes
- Nasal/ocular discharge – take care to distinguish from normal salt-gland secretions in some lizards
- Facial swellings in lizards where the nasolacrimal duct is involved; involvement of this duct (by erosion of surrounding bones, or direct entry of discharges into the duct) in snakes may result in bullous spectaculopathy
- Altered buoyancy in aquatic species (Figure 18.6) and/or obvious body hyperinflation.

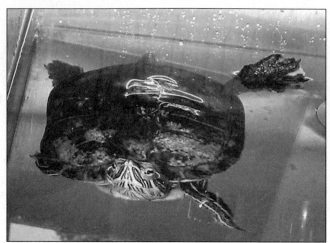

18.6 Red-eared terrapin with a right-lung pneumonia, showing altered buoyancy.

There may also be more generalized signs:

- Weight loss, lethargy, dehydration
- Altered behaviour
  - Large snakes may adopt a strange posture with the head and cranial part of the body raised vertically (Figure 18.7)
  - All species may seek cooler areas and become less active. This is designed to lower metabolic rate to enable the animal to cope better with hypoxia from respiratory disease
- Stomatitis: a careful examination should be made of the mouth as stomatitis and respiratory disease often occur together
  - Poor environmental conditions can be a part of the cause of either condition
  - Large snakes may inhale mucus containing large numbers of microorganisms, resulting in infection or even physical obstruction of the glottis
  - In chelonians apparent URTD and nasal discharge may be an extension of stomatitis because of the incomplete palate, meaning saliva may exit via the nasal cavity.

It is important to distinguish URTD from LRTD (Figure 18.8).

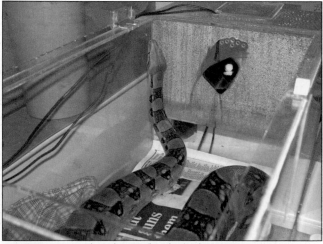

18.7 Common boa showing head-raised position with lower respiratory tract disease (LRTD).

Clinical sign	Upper respiratory tract disease (URTD)	Lower respiratory tract disease (LRTD)
Nasal discharge	Yes	No
Choanal discharge	Yes	No
Ocular discharge	Sometimes	No
Glottal discharge	No	Sometimes
Respiratory noise	Sometimes	Usually
Lung noises on auscultation	Rarely referred noise	Sometimes
Unwell/systemic signs	Often not	Usually
Open-mouth breathing/dyspnoea	Often	Often
Yawning	No	Sometimes in snakes
Attempts to 'cough'	No	Sometimes in snakes/lizards
Cyanosis	No	Sometimes
Behavioural changes	Rarely, unless secondary to systemic disease	Often
Tachypnoea	Rarely	Often
Altered buoyancy	No	Yes

18.8 Clinical signs of upper and lower respiratory tract disease.

Clinical examination

Before handling the patient, the character and rate of breathing should be observed. Cloacal temperature may be recorded, as this will give an indication of the reptile's environmental temperature and allow interpretation of the respiratory rate (as this will generally rise with increasing temperature).

The mouth should be examined closely, paying particular attention to evidence of cyanosis, inflammation and the presence of discharges from the internal choanae and the glottis.

Where there is respiratory noise, listen to the breathing with the mouth open and with the mouth closed. Absence of noise with the mouth open indicates upper respiratory noise.

The nares and eyes should be checked for discharges. It is very important in lizards to distinguish true respiratory discharges from salt emission from the salt glands (see Clinical signs, above). The nares should be checked for occlusion by pieces of retained skin or inflammatory reactions to ectoparasites. Discharges should be examined grossly for clarity, colour (Figure 18.9) and viscosity. Samples of discharges should be retained for cytology and microbiology.

Appearance	Significance
Clear	• Possible viral infection, irritation • Bacteria *unlikely* to be involved
Cloudy or yellow-green	• Bacterial, yeast, mycoplasmal or viral infection involved • Also may be seen with foreign bodies
Sanguineous	• More invasive process • May be related to infection or foreign body • More rarely seen with granulomas and tumours

18.9 Respiratory discharges: appearance and significance.

Auscultation

This is hard to achieve in reptiles as movement of the scales across the diaphragm of the stethoscope makes it difficult to pick up respiratory noises. Placing a damp cloth between the stethoscope and the skin decreases scale noise but also muffles respiratory noises. An electronic stethoscope, using ultrasound coupling gel between the stethoscope and the skin, allows auscultation of reasonable quality. An 8-MHz Doppler probe will not detect respiratory noise but is useful in detecting harsh cardiac murmurs typical of endocarditis, which is a frequent complication of septic conditions and carries a poor prognosis. Compared to mammalian medicine, auscultation of reptiles is a relatively insensitive method of diagnosing respiratory disease.

Diagnosis

Imaging

Radiography

This is one of the most useful diagnostic tools in LRTD. Techniques are discussed in Chapter 9. It is recommended that minimal sedation is used for performing radiography in dyspnoeic reptiles.

In URTD, radiography is less useful because of the many fine structures in this region and the lack of a well-developed sinus system. However, it may be useful in snakes and lizards where there is suspicion that there is deep infection and osteomyelitis. Lateral and dorsoventral (DV) views of the skull, as well as open-mouth oblique views of the nasal areas, should be taken.

Chelonians: DV, lateral and craniocaudal (CC) views are useful. Lateral and CC views must be performed using horizontal beam radiography, so that the coelomic organs do not fall into the lung space. Organomegaly, including distension of hollow viscera, and ascites may be causes of dyspnoea in the absence of respiratory disease through compression of lung space (Figure 18.10).

Lizards: DV, with limbs extended, and lateral (horizontal-beam) views are useful.

Snakes: DV (snake in extended position, not coiled) and lateral (horizontal beam) views are useful. It should be remembered that the lungs and air sacs may occupy a huge length in snakes and that lesions may be focal; therefore, multiple plates may be required.

Computed tomography and magnetic resonance imaging

Where funds allow and where there is access, these facilities may be useful, especially in chelonians (Murray, 2006; Chitty and Raftery, 2013).

Endoscopy

Use of rigid (or flexible in large snakes) endoscopy is extremely useful for visualizing lesions, sample taking and removal of foreign bodies or parasites (see Figure 18.11 and Chapter 10).

In dyspnoeic animals, tracheoscopy is recommended as foreign bodies, although unusual, are occasionally found (Figure 18.12).

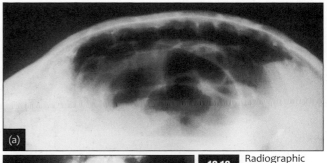

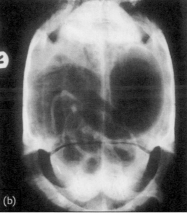

(a)

(b)

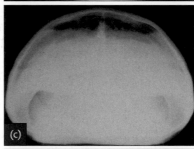

(c)

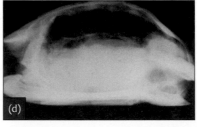

(d)

18.10 Radiographic changes seen in extra-respiratory disease of tortoises. (a) Lateral and (b) dorsoventral radiographs of a Turkish tortoise with gastric stasis. The initial presentation suggested lower respiratory tract disease (LRTD) but clinical signs resulted from compression of lung fields. (c) Lung compression in a case of egg-related peritonitis. The tortoise presented with dyspnoea: open-mouth breathing and gasping. (d) After abdominal drainage; respiratory signs improved markedly.

Route	Species	Comments
Tracheal	All	May also allow assessment of the cranial lungs, including the tracheal lung where present
Intrapulmonic: mid-lateral intra-rib approach	Lizards and snakes	Take care to avoid the heart (Divers, 1998)
Prefemoral	Chelonians	See Divers (2000) and Chapter 10. Take care when opening the septum; in the author's experience this may be accompanied by haemorrhage
Transcarapacial	Chelonians	See Divers (2000). This is the author's method of choice in chelonians. Radiography is essential for selecting the side and site for approach over a focal lesion. This approach allows placement of a catheter for localized therapy (Lewis, 2001)

18.11 Endoscopy of the lower respiratory tract.

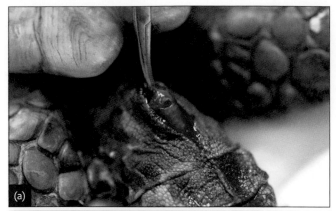

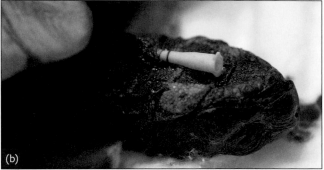

18.12 Marginated tortoise that presented severely dyspnoeic with respiratory noise. Tracheoscopy indicated an abscess at the bifurcation of the trachea, possibly associated with inhalation of tomato seed. (a) Tracheotomy was performed to remove the abscess. (b) Tracheotomy tube (modified catheter) placed into one bronchus and maintained during treatment and healing.

Laboratory tests

Haematology and biochemistry

Although unlikely to provide additional information about the respiratory disease, blood should be taken in all cases to gain information about the presence of underlying disease, degrees of immunosuppression and the scale of the systemic white-cell response to infection. The latter is very important in URTD as in many of these cases the infection appears localized without a systemic response and so systemic therapies are not always necessary. Also, serum may be submitted for serological examination for various infectious agents (see below).

Faecal examination

Lung parasites are not uncommon, especially in snakes, and so faecal examination can be of great value. It may also be useful in the overall assessment of underlying disease.

Nasal flush

Small samples can be obtained by placing a collecting vessel in the mouth under the choana and flushing small volumes of sterile saline (0.5 ml/kg chelonians and lizards; 1 ml/kg snakes) via the nostrils. This can be used for culture, cytology or polymerase chain reaction (PCR) investigations.

Tracheal wash

A sterile catheter may be inserted via the glottis and a small volume of saline syringed into the trachea and then re-collected (see Chapter 8). The sample may be submitted for bacteriology, mycology, cytology, parasitology and virology. However, it should be noted that where there are focal lung lesions this technique is unlikely to isolate significant organisms. In chelonians, an alternative approach is to perform a lung wash by inserting a needle via the prefemoral fossa. This is particularly appropriate in cases of unilateral diffuse pneumonia.

Microbiology

Swabs may be inserted into the nares or internal choanae (URTD) or through the glottis (LRTD) to obtain bacterial samples. As with tracheal washing, this is comparatively insensitive in isolating lung pathogens. In URTD it should be remembered that many of the organisms isolated in these non-sterile sites will be of secondary importance.

Tissue biopsy samples and tracheal washes or swabs may also be submitted for virological examination/culture. Similarly, PCR swabs may be taken from the pharynx (chelonians – *Chlamydia*/*Mycoplasma*/herpesvirus) or oesophagus (snakes – arenavirus; thought now to be the aetiological agent of inclusion body disease (IBD)). In all cases it is essential to rub the swab vigorously against the mucosa as these species can be poorly exfoliative. Serology may be appropriate where these infections are suspected (see below).

Cytology

Cytology is a very useful tool. Tracheal washes, swab samples from any region and endoscopically obtained lung biopsy samples may be submitted for cytology (see Chapter 10). This may give an idea of the type of organism present (e.g. yeast or bacteria) and so give an idea of appropriate therapy, while waiting for culture and sensitivity results. Cytology may also reveal the presence of parasitic ova or larvae.

Upper respiratory tract disease

Chelonians

URTD is extremely common in chelonians, especially tortoises (Figure 18.13). In some cases foreign bodies may be involved, such as pieces of hay or grass entering the nares; this results in a unilateral, rather than a bilateral, discharge (although dust irritation may be bilateral). More typical is an infectious disease often referred to as 'runny nose syndrome'. This generally involves inflammatory lesions of the nares, nasal cavity and, especially, the mouth and pharynx.

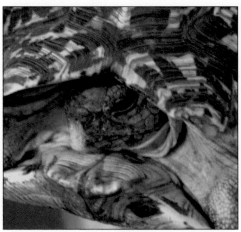

18.13 Upper respiratory tract disease in a leopard tortoise. Note the nasal discharge.

Topical antimicrobials are very useful. Where trans-carapacial endoscopy has been used, the resultant hole can be utilized to apply therapy to any focal lesions (Figure 18.24). Where endoscopy is not available, the site of a focal lesion can be determined radiographically and a hole drilled over this site under sedation or anaesthesia. A catheter may be inserted or the hole left intact but covered by moist chlorhexidine-soaked swabs. Therapy can then be applied daily to the affected lung. Typically, the author uses marbofloxacin (10 mg/kg using 1% injection) for bacterial infections, and amphotericin B (approximately 5 mg/kg of injectable solution made up to 10 mg/ml) in fungal disease. Alternatively, a solution of 1:250 dilution F10 may be introduced at 1 ml/kg. When the animal is recovered, the stoma may be sealed using epoxy resin or fibreglass.

Nebulization is another effective means of introducing topical therapy and for breaking up exudates. An advantage of the transcarapacial method of applying topical therapy is that the hole can be left open (or the catheter unplugged) while the tortoise is being nebulized, allowing drugs to penetrate via both trachea and stoma. As in URTD, it is vital to barrier nurse all cases.

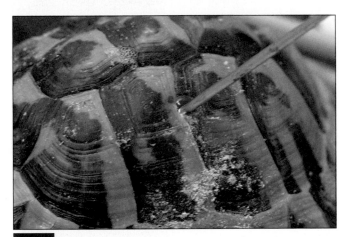

18.24 Transcarapacial endoscopy in a Hermann's tortoise.

Lizards

Foreign bodies are unusual but green iguanas in particular have been associated with a syndrome where human hair becomes tangled around the glottis, causing occlusion of the airway and respiratory distress. Masses (abscesses or, much more rarely, tumours) may impinge on the airway and cause problems. Similarly, trauma to the body in this region may result in dyspnoea. Infection (pneumonia) may be seen with a variety of aetiologies (Figure 18.25).

Clinical evaluation

In addition to basic history taking and examination, the following investigations should be performed:

- Radiography (Figures 18.26 and 18.27)
- Tracheal wash – for cytology (parasitic examination and stains for bacteria) and culture/sensitivity tests
- Endoscopy – where focal lesions are located in the lungs, percutaneous endoscopy (see Chapter 10) should be performed to collect samples of the lesion for cytology, culture/sensitivity and histopathology. This technique may also be used to deliver drugs to the site of infection
- Faecal examination – for parasites
- Haematology/biochemistry – to check for underlying disease.

Cause	Observation
Parasitic infection	Seen principally in wild-caught animals. Both nematodes (*Rhabdias* lungworms, *Entomelas* and *Strongyloides*) and pentastomids may provoke an inflammatory response, with a secondary bacterial pneumonia. It is important to remember that pentastomiasis may be zoonotic
Fungal infection	Very rare but may occur secondary to long-term antibiosis
Viral infection	Extremely rare. Paramyxovirus has been reported in Caiman lizards (Jacobson *et al.*, 2001) and antibodies to paramyxovirus have been found in various species in UK zoological collections, but disease has not yet been reported. Invertebrate-like and erythrocytic iridovirus infections are also reported in lizards, with the former being an important cause of disease possibly being derived from invertebrate livefoods (see Chapter 25)
Bacterial infection	Most common pneumonias. Generally secondary to husbandry problems or parasitic disease. There appear to be no primary bacterial pathogens, but infections typically involve overgrowth of commensals, e.g. *Pseudomonas*, *Aeromonas*, *Salmonella*

18.25 Causes of pneumonia in lizards.

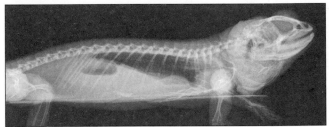

18.26 Horizontal beam lateral view of a diffuse pneumonia in a bearded dragon. Note the lack of air-sac inflation and the presence of air in the stomach (aerophagia).

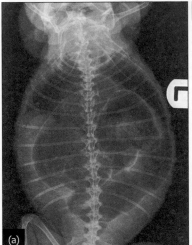

18.27 As in other species, respiratory signs may be induced by extra-respiratory causes. In this bearded dragon, gut ileus impinges on the air sacs and lungs, causing dyspnoea: (a) dorsoventral view; (b) horizontal beam lateral view.

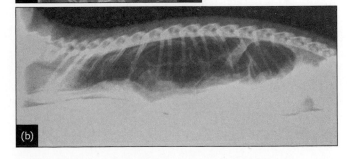

Treatment

Initial therapy may consist of full biological support. Underlying husbandry problems should be corrected. Typically, lizards should be hospitalized at the upper end of their Preferred Optimal Temperature Zone (POTZ) and in a slightly humidified atmosphere.

Antibiosis will be required. Broad-spectrum systemic antibiotics should be used while awaiting culture/sensitivity results. Suitable choices include ceftazidime, fluoroquinolones or amikacin. Nebulization may be of use.

Antiparasitic therapy is indicated where parasitic disease is diagnosed. Oxfendazole or ivermectin are appropriate for nematodes. Where pentastomids are identified, the only reliable therapy is surgery to remove them. This carries a poor prognosis owing to the invasive nature of the procedure; in some cases endoscopic removal may be possible. Occasional successes have been reported with use of ivermectin. It is important to stress the likely zoonotic risks when attempting therapy.

Snakes

Foreign bodies are rare, although asphyxiation due to inhalation of mucus or pus may occur in stomatitis cases. In severely dehydrated snakes, plugs of thick mucus may occlude the airway. Compression of the airway due to external masses is unusual but is possible (especially in cases of cardiomegaly). The snake's respiratory system is uniquely designed to function during compression to cope with the stresses placed on it while large prey items are being swallowed. Trauma to the body, especially the upper third, may result in respiratory signs. Infections (pneumonia) may occur due to a variety of aetiologies (Figure 18.28).

Husbandry is very important. The effect of small enclosures on large snakes cannot be overstressed. They cannot cough and therefore they have no active means of removing airway mucus on a large scale. Small amounts are removed via the mucociliary escalator, as in mammals. A small enclosure does not enable the snake to stretch out; the resulting compression of the lungs compounds and encourages the build-up of fluids and mucus in the lungs. Failure to allow arboreal species the ability to climb affects their ability to clear material, as they cannot use gravity. Underheating also appears to be very important in the aetiology of pneumonia as this may be linked to reduced movement (and therefore reduced clearing of discharges) and immunodeficiency.

In terms of infectious disease, paramyxovirus/ferlavirus and arenavirus (IBD) may be important. Parasitic disease, including pentastomids, may be possible in recently imported animals (or those mixed with imported animals).

Clinical evaluation

Investigation of LRTD in snakes should include a thorough history. It is important to evaluate the environment. The history of the collection is also important, as addition of new snakes (within the last 6–12 months) or the owner handling snakes in other collections or in pet shops may enable entry of IBD into the collection.

The following investigations should be performed:

- Tracheal wash – for cytology (parasites, bacteria, fungi), culture/sensitivity in cases of diffuse pneumonia; PCR – oesophageal swab for arenavirus (IBD)
- Radiography – of use in determining whether lesions are focal or diffuse

Cause	Observation
Parasitic infection	Both pentastomids and *Rhabdias* nematodes can be found in the lungs and may provoke an inflammatory response with secondary bacterial infection
Fungal infection	Very uncommon except in severely immunocompromised animals or following prolonged antibiosis
Viral infection	**Ophidian paramyxovirus (oPMV) also known as ferlavirus:** Mainly in viperid snakes but also in other species, including boids. Epidemiology and diagnosis are discussed in Chapter 25. Clinical signs vary from mild and non-specific to dyspnoea with tracheal haemorrhage. On post-mortem examination, infection is characterized by suppurative pneumonia with haemorrhage and pulmonary oedema. May also be associated secondary bacterial infection. Some reports suggest clinical signs may be associated with immunocompromised individuals (from e.g. poor husbandry, ageing) **Inclusion body disease (IBD):** Arenavirus infection: epidemiology and diagnostics are discussed in Chapter 25. IBD is seen in boids and causes a variety of signs, especially neurological and gastrointestinal; respiratory disease is seen in some cases. This may be a primary effect of the virus or may be due to a secondary bacterial infection. Arenavirus is an important differential diagnosis in boids with pneumonia
Bacterial infection	Extremely common, but generally secondary disease. Typical isolates are *Pseudomonas*, *Aeromonas* and *Escherichia coli*. Some important primary pathogens have been identified, e.g. *Mycoplasma* and *Mycobacterium*. Important predisposing factors are husbandry, viral infection, parasitism and stomatitis (due to inhalation of plugs of mucus)

18.28 Causes of pneumonia in snakes.

- Endoscopy
  - Tracheoscopy enables identification and sampling/clearing of mucous plugs and sampling of the tracheal lung, or for directed washing/flushing. This author finds flexible 2–4 mm endoscopes of value in most snakes, with 2 mm endoscopes allowing deep access in smaller individuals (e.g. corn snakes)
  - Percutaneous endoscopy enables accurate sampling of focal lesions and, even in diffuse pneumonia, collection of biopsy material for histopathology, bacterial or fungal culture/sensitivity, and virology
  - May be used to deliver drugs to the site of infection where there is a focal lesion
- Faecal examination – for parasites
- Haematology/biochemistry – for underlying disease and evaluation of the immune response
- Serology – for oPMV (paramyxovirus/ferlavirus) in recurrent/persistent cases or where there is an 'outbreak'.

Where there are deaths in a collection, post-mortem examination is essential as it enables early detection of the important viral diseases.

Treatment

Initial therapy should consist of biological support. As with lizards, snakes should be housed at the upper end of their POTZ and in a humidified atmosphere (Figure 18.29). A large enclosure should be provided. Death in these cases is often a result of asphyxiation on plugs of mucus. It is

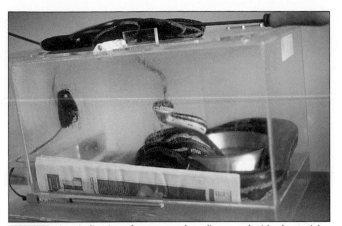

18.29 Hospitalization of a common boa diagnosed with a bacterial pneumonia. Use of an 'Aquabrooder' enables provision of a warm humid atmosphere.

therefore very important to clear the trachea each day. This can be done by suction, where a tube is placed into the trachea via the glottis in the conscious snake, or by coupage. The latter is especially useful in large snakes where the animal can be hung over a stepladder and the lungs and airways massaged to clear discharges via the glottis.

Identification and treatment of underlying disease should be achieved as soon as possible. Where viral disease is diagnosed, euthanasia is the logical choice, especially in collections. Where the animal is kept as an individual or where it is a particularly valuable specimen then supportive care (biological support, rehydration, nutritional support, etc.) may be used. As viral disease is relatively common (especially IBD in boids), any suspect case should be barrier nursed.

Where parasitic infection is suspected, relevant drugs should be given. Drug choices are similar to those used in lizards.

The choice between antibacterial and antifungal agents should be made on the basis of cytology results. When in doubt, it should be remembered that bacterial infections are much more common. Antibiotic choices are similar to those in lizards. However, it should be noted that in large snakes fluoroquinolones are often a poor choice as large injection volumes may be required and these can result in muscle and skin necrosis. Itraconazole (at 5–10 mg/kg by stomach tube q24h) or voriconazole is a good choice in fungal infections.

Nebulization may also be of use as it can allow penetration of antimicrobial drugs into the lungs and may also have an effect as an expectorant, although its use in snakes should be combined with coupage to remove discharges from the trachea and reduce the chance of obstruction.

Summary of management and therapeutics of respiratory disease

As in all reptilian medicine, it is vital to identify and correct underlying husbandry problems. It is also important to hospitalize respiratory cases at the upper end of their POTZ and in a humidified atmosphere.

In the author's clinic, humidification is typically achieved using a solution of 1:500 dilution F10. This prevents build-up of bacteria and fungi that could complicate disease in these patients. Except for large snakes and tortoises,

reptiles with respiratory disease are hospitalized in 'Aqua-brooders' (see Figure 18.29), where units can be easily disinfected between cases and it is easy to humidify the atmosphere from the heated water sleeve.

It is also vital to treat underlying disease and to provide fluid and nutritional support. For these reasons, most cases of respiratory disease seen in the author's practice are hospitalized for the duration of their therapy. While this may increase the cost of therapy, treating these cases on an outpatient basis is less successful, as underlying management or husbandry causes may not be corrected and supportive care may not be as intensive.

Drug therapy for respiratory disease varies little from that in other disease syndromes. However, it should be emphasized that antimicrobial agents given by the oral route may be more useful in URTD cases, as there is a considerable benefit from local therapy via the open internal choanae.

The following treatment modalities may be of specific benefit in respiratory disease.

Nebulization

This may be utilized in both URTD and LRTD. A standard asthmatic's nebulizer is used in the author's practice. A 1:250 dilution of F10 is very effective, as it has antiviral, antifungal and antibacterial action. It is also non-irritant and apparently safe for users and patients. This is provided for 30–45 minutes twice daily. If F10 is not available, the following may be used: amikacin (50 mg per 10 ml saline); piperacillin (100 mg per 10 ml saline). These have been used for 30 minutes two to four times daily (Murray, 2006).

Murray (2006) suggests that droplets >3 μm will not penetrate the lung but will be deposited in the trachea. However, in the author's experience nebulizers producing droplets larger than this still have a beneficial effect (in some mild LRTD cases, nebulization alone has resulted in cure). This may be as a result of the drugs still entering the lungs from the trachea, or due to the other beneficial supportive effects of nebulization, namely: hydration of mucous membranes; action as an expectorant, breaking down discharges and making them easier to clear; and encouragement of what mucociliary escalator the reptile possesses. Where a carapacial stoma is being used in chelonians, it is likely that droplet size is unimportant.

Raiti (2002) voiced concern that nebulization may be inappropriate in certain cases where areas of the lung may be excessively consolidated and aerosolized drugs may not penetrate. In these cases, intrapneumonic therapy may be more appropriate (see Intrapneumonic therapy, below). It is also possible that drugs may be absorbed from the lungs. It is therefore wise to use different antimicrobials to those used systemically in order to avoid overdosage.

Nasal flushing

In URTD, nasal flushing with a 1:250 dilution of F10 is of great benefit, not only in applying drugs directly to the affected area but also in mechanically flushing away debris and discharges.

Intrapneumonic therapy

Drugs may be delivered directly via an endoscope to focal lesions in snakes and lizards or via the carapace (with or without an indwelling catheter) in chelonians. This allows large amounts of drug to be delivered to the diseased area while lessening the risks of systemic toxicity, assuming that absorption is reduced in these areas; on this basis it is certainly wise to use different antimicrobials to those being used systemically in order to avoid inadvertent overdosage.

Oxygen therapy

In mammalian medicine it is common to administer 100% oxygen to animals in respiratory distress. However, in reptiles this may result in inhibition of respiratory drive, a lowered respiratory rate and, therefore, even lower rates of clearance of respiratory discharges. Also, administration of 100% oxygen may result in cooling and drying of the mucous membranes. It is therefore recommended that, if oxygen therapy is required, it should be administered at concentrations no greater than 30–40% in air, and this should be warmed and humidified (Murray, 2006). In collapsed reptiles, 100% oxygen may be given by ventilation (mechanical or manual) following tracheal intubation. It should be noted that few animals presented in this state survive.

References and further reading

Bennett T (2011) The chelonian respiratory system. *Veterinary Clinics of North America: Exotic Animal Practice* **14(2)**, 225–240

Chitty JR (2002) Use of a new disinfectant agent in the management of upper respiratory tract disease in Chelonia. *Scientific Proceedings, BSAVA Congress*, p. 634

Chitty JR and Raftery AP (2013) *Essentials of Tortoise Medicine and Surgery.* Wiley Blackwell, Oxford

Divers SJ (1998) An introduction to reptile endoscopy. *Proceedings of the Association of Reptilian and Amphibian Veterinarians Annual Conference*, pp. 41–45

Divers SJ (2000) Two techniques for endoscopic evaluation of the chelonian lung. *Proceedings of the Association of Reptilian and Amphibian Veterinarians Annual Conference*, pp. 123–126

Gans C and Gaunt AS (1998) *Biology of the Reptilia, Volume 19: Visceral Organs.* Society for the Study of Amphibians and Reptiles, University of Chicago Press, Chicago

Jacobson ER (2007) Bacterial diseases of reptiles. In: *Infectious Diseases and Pathology of Reptiles*, ed. ER Jacobson. CRC Press, Boca Raton, FL, USA

Jacobson ER, Origgi F, Pessier AP *et al.* (2001) Paramyxovirus infection in Caiman lizards (*Draecena guianensis*). *Journal of Veterinary Diagnostic Investigation* **13**, 143–151

Lewis W (2001) How to place intrapneumonic catheters in chelonians. *Exotic DVM* **3(5)**, 16–17

Murray MJ (2006) Pneumonia and lower respiratory disease. In: *Reptile Medicine and Surgery, 2nd edition*, ed. D Mader, pp. 865–877. WB Saunders, Philadelphia

Pericard JM and Blahak S (2013) Occurrence of *Mycoplasma*, *Chlamydia* and herpesvirus in land tortoises with respiratory or ocular diseases in the south of France. *Proceedings of the 1st International Conference on Avian, Herpetological and Exotic Mammal Medicine*, Wiesbaden Germany, p. 140

Raiti P (2002) Administration of aerosolised antibiotics to reptiles. *Proceedings of the Association of Reptilian and Amphibian Veterinarians Annual Conference*, pp. 119–123

Schumacher J (2011) Respiratory medicine of reptiles. *Veterinary Clinics of North America: Exotic Animal Practice* **14(2)**, 207–224

Soares JF, Chalker VJ, Erles K *et al.* (2003) Prevalence of *Mycoplasma agassizzi* and chelonian herpesvirus in captive tortoises (*Testudo* spp.) in the United Kingdom. *Proceedings of the Association of Reptilian and Amphibian Veterinarians Annual Conference*, p. 91

Stahl SJ (2013) Respiratory (lower) tract disease/pneumonia. In: *Clinical Veterinary Advisor: Birds and Exotic Pets*, ed. J Mayer and TM Donnelly. Elsevier, St Louis

Wood SC and Lenfant CJM (1976) Respiration: mechanics, control and gas exchange. In: *Biology of the Reptilia, Volume 5*, ed. C Gans and WR Dawson. Academic Press, London

Wyneken J (2001) Respiratory anatomy: form and function in reptiles. *Exotic DVM* **3(2)**, 17–22

Chapter 19

Cardiovascular and haemopoietic systems

Ben Hynes and Simon J. Girling

Reptiles are ectothermic and spend a lifetime expending far less energy (less than one-tenth) than a similarly sized endotherm. Their cardiovascular system does not have to perform with the perpetual high efficiency of a 'hot-blooded' mammal or bird. So, relatively, and more similar to amphibians, the reptile heart is small and works far less hard (Jensen *et al.*, 2014).

This ecological strategy is clearly reflected in their behaviour, with long periods of inactivity interspersed with only short energetic bursts to hunt, eat and reproduce. These long periods of inactivity coupled with a physiological tolerance of low oxygen levels and very low metabolic rate make recognizing illness caused by cardiovascular disease an uncommon challenge. Indeed, often it is not recognized until it is too late for a successful treatment outcome.

Nevertheless, heart disease does occur and familiarity with the anatomy and physiology of the reptile cardiovascular system is the key to its diagnosis. Since echocardiography has established itself as a non-invasive tool for cardiac examination in most veterinary clinics, its availability offers us the most useful opportunity to identify reptile cardiac disease. If we are going to progress from diagnoses made post-mortem and the paucity of published case studies, we should start by combining the skills of clinicians with an interest in exotic medicine with those who have expertise in echocardiology.

Lastly, the study of cardiovascular systems in comparative and evolutionary biology provides an excellent resource from which to start to investigate clinical cases. Research on reptiles has recently focused on the evolutionary position of reptiles as a step in how both birds and mammals, via separate pathways, arrived at a fully separated systemic and pulmonary circulation using a four-chambered heart. The techniques used are familiar to veterinary medicine and have included echocardiology, magnetic resonance imaging (MRI) and angioscopy. These studies should be the starting point in order to understand the anatomy and physiology of these fascinating animals (Jensen *et al.*, 2013a).

Specific relevant cardiovascular anatomy

This chapter will discuss cardiac disease in members of the Orders Testudinata (turtles and tortoises), Rhynchocephalia (tuatara), and Squamata (lizards and snakes). Crocodiles, with their unique four-chambered anatomy, will not be discussed, although reptiles in this chapter will be described as possessing a 'non-crocodilian' heart.

Three, four or six chambers?

The non-crocodilian heart in this group of reptiles has been consistently described throughout scientific literature as three-chambered: the basic heart plan being two atria emptying into a single ventricle. More accurately, from its gross external morphology, it is four-chambered due to the presence of the sinus venosus. Moreover, internally the ventricle is subdivided by muscular ridges, to a varying degree between species, into three relatively distinct subchambers. Hence, the heart of reptiles has even been described as functioning with six chambers (Pereira and Pizzi, 2012). Figure 19.1 shows an example of a snake heart and major vessels.

This reptile heart plan can usefully be seen as a step in evolution that started with the serial arrangement in fish and led to the high-performance version found in mammals and birds. In fact the reptile system is very similar to the early embryological heart of mammals and birds, before ventricular septation (Jensen *et al.*, 2013b). Starting

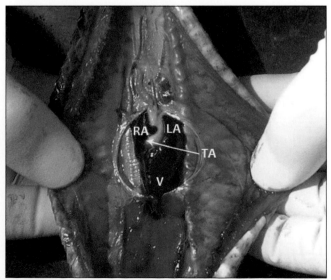

19.1 Post-mortem image of the heart and major blood vessels of a common boa, viewed from the ventral aspect. The pericardium has been opened to reveal the right (RA) and left atria (LA) and single ventricle (V). The truncus arteriosus (TA) corkscrews from the right of the ventricle.

from a pump within a serial tubular arrangement, the system can now be considered as folded back up on itself: the entrance adjacent to the exit. Consequently, when blood flows into the heart it is on its left side via the atria into a folded ventricle. To exit, the ventricle must eject the blood volume, onwards and upwards, to the right through three vessels that variously supply the lungs and body. This view, although simplistic, explains the unfamiliar anatomical position of the atrioventricular (AV) canal as an 'entrance' to the left of the midline and the truncus arteriosus as an 'exit' on the right, and the passage of blood between them, down and back out of the ventricle with its incomplete septal 'fold' (Figure 19.2).

Heart position

Diagrams of the placement of internal organs in chelonians, lizards and snakes are provided in Chapter 1.

- **Chelonians:** the heart typically lies in the ventral midline bordered dorsally by the lungs, laterally by the lobes of the liver, and ventrally by the acromion and coracoid processes. Flattening of the body plan in the soft-shelled turtles of the family Trionychidae has led to the heart being positioned to the right of the midline (Girgis, 1961).
- **Lizards:** in most species the heart lies in the midline within the pectoral girdle. However, in varanid lizards the heart lies caudal to the sternum.
- **Snakes:** the heart is positioned at 15–45% along the total body length. Its position is more cranial in arboreal and more caudal in aquatic species (Gabriel *et al.*, 2010).

Pericardium

The heart is located within the pericardium and is bathed with clear colourless to yellow pericardial fluid. In some snakes, lizards (except varanids) and tortoises/turtles, the ventricular apex and caudal pericardial sac share a fibrous attachment to the peritoneum termed the gubernaculum cordis (GC).

Chamber morphology and blood flow through the heart

The heart of lizards, snakes and chelonians consists of a sinus venosus upstream of the right atrium, a paired but smaller left atrium and a single ventricle (see Figure 19.2).

Systemic blood flow returns to the sinus venosus within the pericardial cavity positioned over the dorsum of the heart. The sinus venosus contracts to empty the poorly oxygenated blood from the systemic circulation into the right atrium via myocardial flap-like (sino-atrial) valves. Spontaneous contractile tissue is present within the wall of the sinus venosus and is believed to function as the dominant cardiac pacemaker.

The right atrium is larger than the left atrium. The size difference can be double in some cases, and should not be mistaken for pathological enlargement. The atrial walls are very thin and trabeculate.

The left atrium receives oxygenated blood from the lung or lungs via the paired pulmonary veins; conflicting reports dispute the presence or absence of valves at this orifice.

Both atria empty through the atrioventricular (AV) canal, a funnel-like entrance into the ventricle, past the AV valve complex. The AV canal is positioned to the left of the cardiac midline. The valve is bell-shaped and composed entirely of connective tissue; the concave side faces towards the ventricle.

The ventricle has a cortex of thin compact myocardial tissue surrounding a thicker inner medulla of spongy myocardium. Its internal structure is complex and although it is described as a single ventricle, it is internally divided to varying degrees by three septa in all the non-crocodilian reptiles. These septa divide the ventricle into three subchambers: the cavum arteriosum (CA), cavum venosum (CV) and cavum pulmonale (CP).

Analogous to the left ventricle, the CA is partially divided from the CV by the vertical septum (VS). The VS is composed of trabeculate sheets of myocardium; these span the ventricle but stop short of the AV base. This incomplete division creates a structure with a crest over, and septa through which blood can pass.

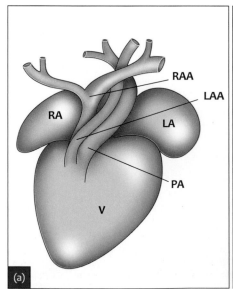
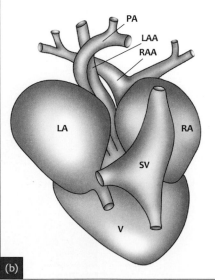
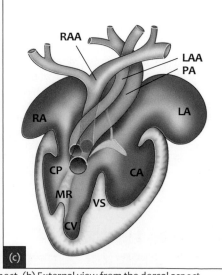

19.2 The heart and main vessels of a non-crocodilian heart. (a) External view from the ventral aspect. (b) External view from the dorsal aspect. (c) Internal structure, with ventricular and atrial walls removed. CA = cavum cavernosum; CP = cavum pulmonale; CV = cavum venosum; LA = left atrium; LAA = left aortic arch; MR = muscular ridge; PA = main pulmonary artery; RA = right atrium; RAA = right aortic arch; SV = sinus venosus; V = ventricle; VS = vertical septum.

A spiral shelf termed the muscular ridge (MR) divides the CV from the part of the heart analogous to a right ventricle, the CP. The MR has a finger-like projection visible in the transverse and sagittal planes within the ventricular lumen. The MR faces, and may abut, the third identifiable anatomical septum, the bulbus lamella (BL) on the right wall of the ventricle.

On the horizontal sections, the AV valve can be seen to be tethered centrally to the mobile interatrial septum (see Figure 19.2). The AV valve has an important role in directing blood into the ventricle. During the rapid diastolic filling it is forced or sucked on to the MR and VS, which also stretches the interatrial septum. Mesh-like strands of connective tissue below the AV valve in tortoises and varanid lizards appear to interact with the AV valve and perform a similar role (see Figure 19.2).

Ultrastructurally, the atrial and ventricular walls are composed of a mixture of thick inner spongy and compact outer myocardium. The spongy cardiomyocytes receive nutrition by diffusion from luminal blood via intramural flow; a coronary circulation supplies the compact myocardium of the ventricles (Jensen *et al.*, 2010a).

Exceptions to the rule: non-crocodilian reptiles, pythons and varanid lizards

In the heart of a healthy adult mammal or bird, the volume of blood ejected from the right and left ventricles is equal. In the majority of non-crocodilian reptiles this is not the case. This is because their blood mixes in a single ventricle, and it is the outflow resistance of the arteries that determines in which direction and at what volume the blood flows.

The exceptions to the general rule within the non-crocodilian reptiles of a ventricle acting as a single pressure pump are the pythons and varanid lizards. In pythons, the CV is reduced to such an extent the CA and CP are adjacent chambers throughout most of the ventricle and the CV is reduced to a crossing point for blood entering and leaving separated ventricle rather than a chamber in its own right (see Figure 19.3c). The three large internal septa – MR, BL and VS – contain specialized compact layers of myocardium that act as pressure-tight seals. This creates differential pressure between the systemic and pulmonary circulations, at levels similar to mammals, throughout the cardiac cycle. Interestingly, it is not understood why pythons have evolved this specialism when other similar-sized snakes with similar lifestyles (i.e. sit-and-wait predators) have not (Jensen *et al.*, 2010c).

Varanid lizards are behaviourally active and have larger hearts with a distinct ventricular anatomy that in function is similar to pythons, in that it creates pressure-tight separation of the systemic and pulmonary circulation. In contrast, they have a mesh of trabecular tissue that interacts with the AV valve complex in the ventricle.

Cardiac conduction

In order for contraction to occur in any heart, an electrical impulse must travel in an ordered sequence through the heart chambers in order to regulate effective contraction of the cardiomyocytes. Reptiles lack the insulated conducting system seen in mammals and birds, and despite extensive searches no specialized pathway has been found. However, in order to time the atrial and ventricular contractions, various areas of cardiomyocytes slow conduction between the compartments and function to create marked delays. These are clearly visible on any reptile's electrocardiogram (ECG), characteristically creating a rapid systolic phase and far slower diastolic one (see Electrocardiography section). Therefore, in function, the spongy myocardium of the ventricle serves the dual purpose of conduction and contraction (Jensen *et al.*, 2012).

Veterinary significance of cardiovascular anatomy and physiology

Cardiac blood flow and mechanisms of shunting

The existence of the single ventricle has always led to speculation over its functional significance in shunting blood in reptiles. The presence of a single ventricular chamber means oxygenated and deoxygenated blood might be expected to mix (or shunt) together. This is in direct contrast to the divided circulatory system existing in mammals and birds. The significance of a divided ventricle is that it allows the separated pulmonary and systemic circulations to work at lower and higher pressures respectively. This led to the evolution of highly efficient yet delicate alveoli for gas exchange, which would otherwise be damaged by higher pressures, and the capability to supply large oxygen- and nutrient-hungry capillary beds in organs distant from the heart. The expectation was that reptiles derived their own evolutionary benefit from a single ventricle that could control shunting blood away from or towards the lungs during behaviours such as breath holding or diving.

It is now believed that instead of being an adapted trait, the presence of mixed oxygen-rich and poor blood in most species of reptile is not significant enough in its impact on the reptile's survival to be selected against. See Figure 19.3 for blood-flow patterns through the heart in various species of reptiles.

Postprandial cardiac hypertrophy

After a large meal, oxygen consumption increases in carnivorous reptiles to meet a dramatically increased metabolic demand. In response, Burmese pythons have been shown to exhibit a remarkable hypertrophy that may increase cardiac muscle mass by up to 40% (Andersen *et al.*, 2005) (Figure 19.4). The hypertrophy is facultative and not obligatory, and triggered by an oxygen supply–demand mismatch (Slay *et al.*, 2014).

Breath holding

Many reptiles are intermittent lung breathers, reliant on pulmonary oxygen storage during periods of so-called 'quiet breathing'. In these animals, ventilation can be interspersed with apnoea of variable duration. In tortoises, apnoea is associated with vagally induced bradycardia and a pulmonary bypass shunt (right to left). In contrast, apnoea of monitor lizards is associated with tachycardia. The conscious examination, sedation and general anaesthesia of normal and diseased animals must take into consideration these specializations. Even the seemingly simple pronouncement of death must be carefully considered;

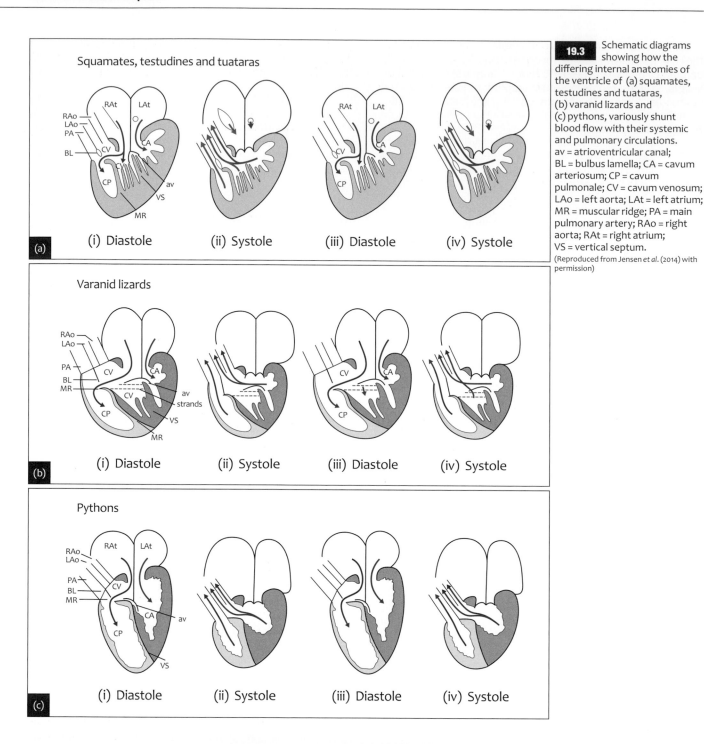

19.3 Schematic diagrams showing how the differing internal anatomies of the ventricle of (a) squamates, testudines and tuataras, (b) varanid lizards and (c) pythons, variously shunt blood flow with their systemic and pulmonary circulations. av = atrioventricular canal; BL = bulbus lamella; CA = cavum arteriosum; CP = cavum pulmonale; CV = cavum venosum; LAo = left aorta; LAt = left atrium; MR = muscular ridge; PA = main pulmonary artery; RAo = right aorta; RAt = right atrium; VS = vertical septum. (Reproduced from Jensen et al. (2014) with permission)

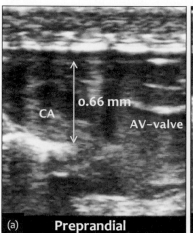

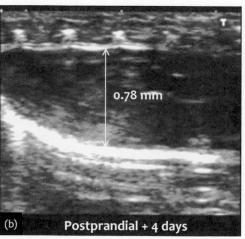

19.4 Echocardiographic long-axis images of a small (approximately 500 g) rock python that attempt to show physiological cardiac hypertrophy: (a) after a 2-week fast; (b) 4 days postprandially. An ECG trace (not shown) was used to synchronize ventricular measurements within the cardiac cycle.

Doppler blood-flow measurement and echocardiography are recommended in such cases, but due to reptiles' ability to withstand extended periods of apnoea, the cessation of a heart beat and blood flow does not result in instantaneous death.

Congestive failure

In varanid lizards and pythons, the functional separation of the systemic from the pulmonary circulation coincides with the development of a mean arterial pressure difference between them. When a disease process affects them, because of this separation it is the more delicate pulmonary tissues that will be affected. Exposure to higher circulating pressure results in congestive failure. Congenital and acquired heart diseases in these species are characterized by the development of respiratory signs: dyspnoea; cyanosis; and oedema fluid bubbling from the mouth or nose (Jensen and Wang, 2009; Pizzi et al., 2009; Schilliger et al., 2010b).

The renal portal system

The presence of a renal portal system (RPS) means that an injection given in an area drained by the caudal, hypogastric or iliac veins may be excreted by the kidneys before it enters the rest of the circulation. There is also concern with respect to potentially nephrotoxic drugs administered at these sites (such as the aminoglycoside family), as it is theoretically possible for the drug to be channelled into the kidney parenchyma very rapidly and at high concentrations, leading to enhanced toxic effects. The reality is that the RPS shunting mechanism is not as straightforward as this, and many facets of the shunting process have not been fully elucidated. Common practice has been to avoid giving potentially nephrotoxic medications in the caudal half of the reptile patient.

Diagnostic techniques

History and clinical examination

Cardiac disease should be considered in any reptile that is lethargic, inappetent and in poor body condition. Oedema and signs of congestive heart failure are frequently associated with heart failure (Figure 19.5). Snakes will demonstrate overt cardiomegaly that can distend the body outline (Figure 19.6).

Heart rate

Reptiles with cardiac disease appear to exhibit tachycardia in relation to clinically normal similar species in identical temperature and environmental conditions. However, reptiles' heart rate also varies with body temperature, body size, metabolic rate, season, respiratory rate, physiological conditions and sensory stimuli (Wyneken, 2009). Relevant to veterinary physical examination is that even normal reptiles demonstrate a marked tachycardia when handled.

Within the Preferred Optimal Temperature Zone (POTZ), allometric scaling may be used for the prediction of heart rate (Sedgwick, 1991); however, this can overestimate heart rate in some species, e.g. bearded dragons (Hunt, 2013):

Heart rate (beats/min) = 33.4 x [bodyweight (kg)]$^{-0.25}$

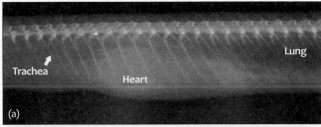

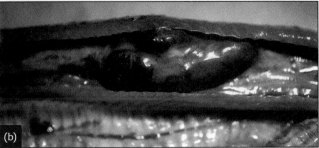

19.5 (a) Plain lateral radiograph of a corn snake demonstrating cardiomegaly secondary to pulmonary hypertension. (b) Post-mortem photograph of the above demonstrating cardiomegaly. Note the asymmetrical atria; this is normal in several species of snake and should not be misinterpreted as chamber enlargement.

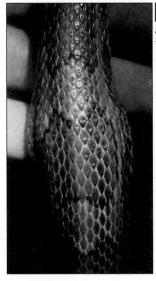

19.6 Dorsal view of the corn snake whose radiograph and post-mortem are shown in Figure 19.5. Note the coelomic distension.

Auscultation

External cardiac and pulmonary auscultation is generally unrewarding. A wet or gel-soaked swab or towel between the stethoscope and the body wall improves sound conduction, but even under ideal conditions for auscultation it is difficult to eliminate contact noise. An audible murmur has also been described in cases of AV valve disease (Clippinger, 1993; Rishniw and Carmel, 1999; Schilliger et al., 2010a). However, it may be only pythons and varanid lizards that can produce the flow velocity required to create an audible murmur. Pulmonary auscultation may indicate the presence of oedema by increased lung sounds. Under anaesthesia, the heart can be auscultated using an oesophageal stethoscope (see Chapter 12).

Breathing rate

Intermittent breathing makes accurate determination of respiratory rate difficult. A range between one and six respiratory cycles per minute appears normal in snakes (Valentinuzzi, 1969).

Pulse oximetry

Pulse oximeters non-invasively assess functional oxygen saturation (SpO_2) of haemoglobin and pulsatile blood flow. Most pulse oximeters in practice will have been optimized for mammalian use; reptile haemoglobin is significantly different so caution should be taken when assessing the SpO_2 of a reptile patient. For consistent results, and best contact between mucosa containing capillary bed and probe, the probe is placed into the proximal oesophagus or cloaca of the anaesthetized reptile for anaesthesia monitoring. Changes of SpO_2 as trends during anaesthesia may then be assessed.

Doppler ultrasonic blood-flow monitoring

Doppler blood-flow ultrasound devices give an acoustic qualitative assessment of the intensity and speed of blood flow through the vessel being monitored (Figure 19.7). Used during the course of an anaesthetic, this form of monitoring is an extremely sensitive means of detecting pulse quality and its alteration. Indeed, probes emitting frequencies of 5–8 MHz may measure blood flow in creatures as small as a leopard gecko weighing 50 g. Care should be taken to ensure a good coupling between probe and skin, which is enhanced with standard aqueous ultrasonic gel. Movement of the reptile, or weakening of the coupling, may create the false impression of a weakened pulse.

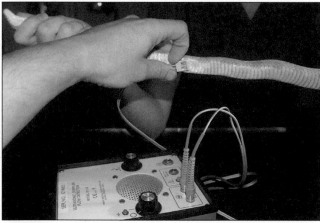

19.7 Heart rate using pulsatile blood flow can be obtained in this case using a Parks Medical 8-MHz Doppler ultrasound flow detector placed directly over the heart. The snake was only turned briefly to show the sensor position. In this healthy individual, handling alone markedly affected heart rate.

Blood pressure monitoring

Indirect blood pressure measurement has not been proven but is easily performed. A paediatric cuff on the hindlimb or tail gives a reproducible systolic reading; however, the results have been found unreliable when compared to direct arterial measurement. Direct measurement is well described in laboratory studies in comparative physiology and blood pressures for many reptile species have been published (Jensen *et al.*, 2014).

Radiography

Radiography is beneficial in the investigation of the vascular and pulmonary systems, but is of limited usefulness with suspected cardiac disease. High-detail screen film and good radiographic technique (collimation, restraint and positioning) are essential to gain most benefit from the images obtained (see Chapter 9).

Chelonians

The cardiac outline is indiscernible from the heterogeneous soft-tissue appearance of the viscera filling the ventral coelom. MRI is an alternative but expensive option.

Lizards

The radiographic anatomy of lizards varies between those species with an intrapectoral heart, where it lies in the midline at the base of the neck – e.g. green iguanas and bearded dragons (Figure 19.8) – and those where the heart is positioned much further back behind the sternum, such as the varanid lizards. Cardiomegaly is identifiable with severe cardiac disease, and in one case (Pizzi *et al.*, 2009) a sibling was used for comparison to confirm this.

The great vessels are visible: the aortae on the lateral view arise from the heart base in the truncus then separate cranially and caudally within the coelom; the pulmonary vessels can be followed through the lung. Metastatic calcification of the great vessels may occur with metabolic vascular disease (Figure 19.9).

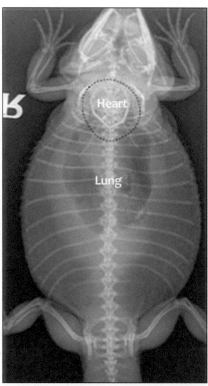

19.8 Plain dorsoventral radiograph of an inland bearded dragon, demonstrating the position of the heart within the pectoral girdle (yellow line), that is obscured by the sternum (dotted line).

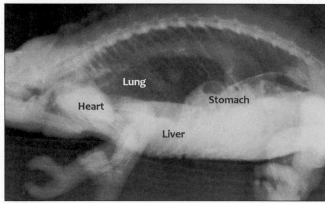

19.9 Plain lateral radiograph of a Meller's chameleon. Metastatic calcification of the blood vessels is apparent in the great vessels within the coelom.

Snakes

The trachea courses from the glottis to its termination above the cardiac outline roughly parallel to the spine. The heart has uniform soft-tissue density and an ellipsoid shape.

Cardiomegaly is indicated by displacement of the trachea and visible change of the body outline (see Figure 19.5). Remember, these species undergo dramatic cardiac postprandial hypertrophy, so cardiac size will also depend on the metabolic status of the animal. The authors would consider body-wall distension to be only associated with pathological, not physiological, hypertrophy.

Angiography has been described to outline the cardiovascular system in a Burmese python with a septic thrombus affecting the right atrium and sinus venosus (Jacobson *et al.*, 1991).

Electrocardiography

Electrocardiography records the electrical events associated with cardiac contraction via electrodes on the surface of the body. In reptiles, an ECG trace will show electrical activity of the heart and can be used to determine the timing of the cardiac cycle when performing echocardiography. It will also provide a heart rate if Doppler blood-flow or ultrasound equipment is unavailable. Without an internal conduction system (see Specific relevant cardiovascular anatomy) the only point in assessing different limb leads is to provide the clearest trace; only one lead above and one below the heart with a neutral are needed.

Electromechanical dissociation, or the equivalent in reptiles, where cardiac activity is dissociated from cerebral function, is well recognized, so do not rely on an ECG as a sole indicator of life.

Leads can be attached using human surface-adhering electrodes, but they may have to be cut to fit into available windows on the body (Figure 19.10). They can be held in place with small strips of cohesive tape if required. Blunted crocodile clips and needles may be used as electrodes.

- **Chelonians:** the cranial lead is placed on the cervical or axillary skin folds and caudal lead and neutral on the skin folds caudal to the hindlimb.

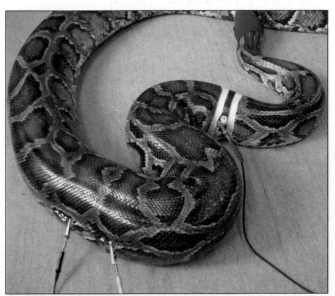

19.10 Electrocardiography lead position and placement on a Burmese python, demonstrating different attachment methods. The cranial lead uses a human skin-surface electrode; the caudal leads are placed with crocodile clips.

- **Lizards:** cranial leads are placed on the skin of the axilla, forelimb in varanids, or in species with an intrapectoral heart, on the neck; caudal leads are placed on the crural or popliteal fold (Hunt, 2013).
- **Snakes:** a base–apex reading is taken with electrodes placed two heart lengths cranial and caudal to the heart on the lateral aspect.

Interpretation

Reptile electrocardiograms demonstrate P wave, QRS complex and T wave deflections familiar to cardiologists. An additional SV waveform preceding the P wave, representing depolarization of the sinus venosus, may be seen. Note that the vector creating the ECG deflection is not proportional to the size of the animal, so bigger traces do not reflect larger body size (Figure 19.11).

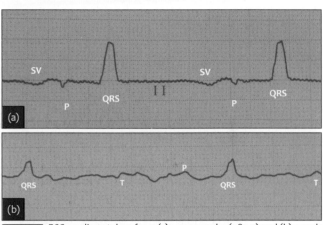

19.11 ECG readings taken from (a) a corn snake (385 g) and (b) a rock python (536 g) demonstrating the familiar sinus venosus (SV)–P–QRS–T waveform deflections from the baseline. These can be used for cardiac rate and rhythm measurements, and during echocardiography aid interpretation of the cardiac cycle.

Normal ECG findings include:

- Pleomorphism of the P wave – single, peaked or biphasic
- Q and S deflections absent so ventricular activity represented by a single R wave
- Long ventricular repolarization phase (QT interval).

These deflections describe the rapid diastolic but long systolic phase that reptiles exhibit.

Abnormal findings include:

- Tachycardia
- Increased amplitudes of P and QRS waves compared with similar-sized conspecifics (Figure 19.12).

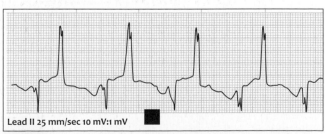

Lead II 25 mm/sec 10 mV:1 mV

19.12 Base–apex ECG from the corn snake in Figures 19.5 and 19.6, demonstrating notched P and QRS complexes. Increased amplitudes are suggestive of generalized cardiomegaly. Tachycardia is also seen: heart rate is approximately 50 beats/min (calculated normal heart rate should be 33.4 x (kg$^{0.25}$) = 26 beats/min).

Echocardiography

Ultrasonography has become the most useful modality for the assessment of cardiac structure and function in conscious reptiles. Two-dimensional cross-sectional views of the heart allow rapid assessment of cardiac morphology and an indication, at least subjectively in reptiles, of systolic and diastolic function.

Two-dimensional, colour, power and spectral (pulsed-wave and continuous-wave Doppler) echocardiography can all be used to investigate cases with suspected cardiac disease in lizards, snakes and chelonians.

Ultrasonography of the heart is straightforward in snakes; using a ventral midline acoustic window the majority of the standard views can be obtained (Schilliger et al., 2006). The shell of chelonians and pectoral girdle or sternum in lizards prevent access to the orthogonal views that echocardiologists usually prefer for standardizing views. Smaller patients with small hearts are difficult to image well, especially without a specialist high-frequency (>10 MHz) phased array probe, if only because of the small footprint. However, in larger patients an image with decent resolution can be obtained with most probes with a high enough frequency range.

> **PRACTICAL TIP**
>
> Do not restrict yourself to cardiac presets – use abdominal, musculoskeletal, vascular and/or fetal cardiac settings, and use harmonics, speckle reduction or compound imaging, if your machine has them, to optimize the image

Chelonians

The cervical window (between the base of the neck and proximal forelimb) is preferred in most species, but the ventral positioning of the heart means orientation of the probe is limited by the shell. The right and left cervical windows allow visualization of the structures within the heart and major vessels (Figure 19.13).

In species where it is difficult to extend the head manually (e.g. sulcata and leopard tortoises), it is difficult to maintain the cervical window. An improved view may be achieved by inserting the probe between the forelimbs and using the dorsal nuchal window to scan the cardiac structures elevated by the contraction of the forelimb musculature (Figure 19.14).

Cardiac structures are seen in an oblique sagittal long-axis craniocaudal direction (see Figure 19.14), although lateral movement allows a degree of image manipulation towards the horizontal plane.

The cranially positioned right and left atria can be seen as homogeneous distensible structures. Atrial fractional shortening (the contraction of the atrial walls as a percentage of the total atrial diameter) has been reported as 30–50% (Redrobe and Wilkinson, 2002). On the dorsal surface and emptying into the right atrium, the sinus venosus is visible, with two echogenic valve leaflets. The pulmonary artery and caudal vena cava on the dorsal cardiac surface may be visible.

Colour Doppler is useful to identify and confirm laminar blood flow and to distinguish the great vessels. The ventricle has a poorly defined endocardium owing to spongy myocardium. Orientation of the probe across the cardiac base provides a linear view of the main pulmonary artery and right and left aortae.

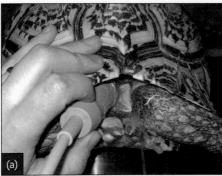
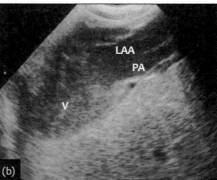
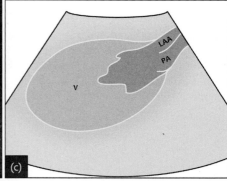

19.13 (a) This Horsfield tortoise habituated to handling allows a lateral cervical window to be used to provide an oblique long-axis view of the heart and great vessels. (b) Two-dimensional echocardiographic oblique long-axis view and (c) line drawing that highlights the left aortic arch (LAA) ventral to the pulmonary artery (PA) as they exit the ventricle (V). Note the homogeneity of the ventricle wall and blood within due to spongy myocardium.

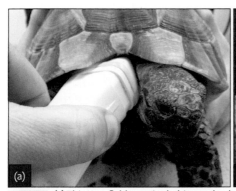
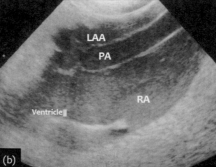
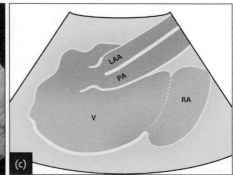

19.14 (a) Performing echocardiography on a leopard tortoise using a dorsal nuchal window. (b) The right atrium (RA) sits dorsal to the pulmonary artery (PA) and left aortic arch (LAA). (c) The line drawing again highlights the lack of contrast within the chambers between blood and spongy myocardium found in tortoises.

Lizards

The heart can be examined with ultrasonography using an axillary window (cranial to the shoulder joint) in species with an intrapectoral heart, providing long- and short-axis views of the cardiac structures (Figures 19.15 and 19.16). The size of the animal determines whether the entire heart can be placed in the acoustic window. In species with a caudally placed heart (e.g. monitor lizards, Komodo dragon), scan from the sub-xiphoid region, from where you can obtain sagittal and transverse views.

Snakes

The two-dimensional echocardiographic anatomy of the heart of the Burmese python has been well described and even standardized (Snyder *et al.*, 1999, Schilliger *et al.*,

2006, Jensen *et al.*, 2010c). Standard views are essential to create reproducible images and objective measurements using M-mode and spectral Doppler flow. Admittedly, these will only be useful for future comparison with the same animal during treatment or, if available, with healthy conspecifics. The same standard approach obviously applies to all species of snake, although the internal ventricular anatomy varies quite considerably (Figure 19.17).

Conscious examination of small snakes (<1 kg) is relatively straightforward; however, sedation, anaesthesia and a water bath have been used to produce optimal conditions for echocardiography. The ribs are unfused at the level of the heart, so the majority of views can be obtained from a ventral midline position. Linear probes that are usually avoided due to acoustic shadowing from ribs in domestic pets are well suited to snakes (Figure 19.18).

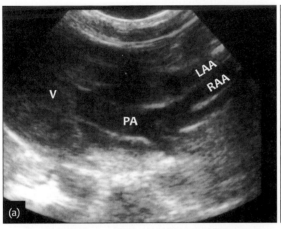
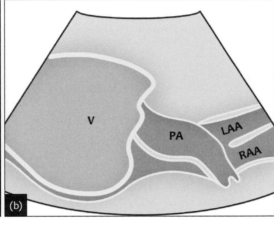

19.15 (a) Two-dimensional echocardiographic long-axis view from the right side of a green iguana. (b) The line drawing clarifies the relationship of the great vessels as these exit the heart and corkscrew dextrally to the right of the image. LAA = left aortic arch; PA= pulmonary artery; RAA= right aortic arch; V= ventricle.

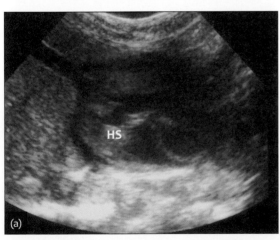
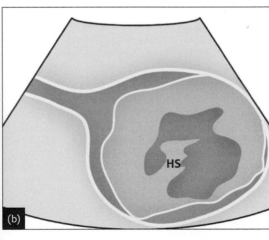

19.16 (a) Two-dimensional short-axis echocardiographic view of the ventricle of a green iguana. (b) The line drawing shows the horizontal septum (HS), a finger-like projection from the muscular ridge into the ventricle that subdivides the chamber internally.

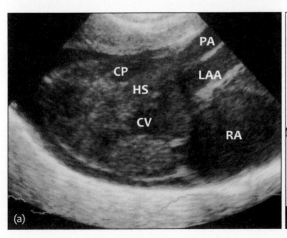
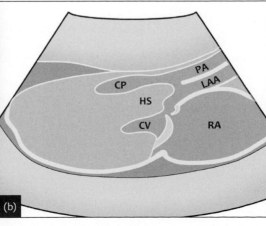

19.17 (a) Two-dimensional midline long-axis echocardiographic view of a Burmese python. (b) The line drawing demonstrates how the prominent horizontal septum (HS) on the muscular ridge effectively divides the ventricle into distinct subchambers, the cavum pulmonate (CP) and reduced cavum venous (CV). The right atrium (RA) is separated far more clearly by the AV valves (unlabelled). LAA = left aortic arch; PA = pulmonary artery.

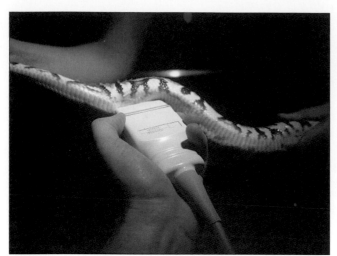

19.18 Echocardiography of a rock python that was undergoing ecdysis (NB: dead skin may interfere with ultrasound wave transmission) using the ventral window, and in the long axis provides a rapid assessment of cardiac morphology and subjective impression of systolic and diastolic function.

The snake heart lies parallel with the sagittal plane; the apex points to the tail and base cranially. Orienting the transducer with the beating heart in the sagittal plane produces images described as long-axis views, with a 90-degree rotation to the transverse plane providing the short-axis views. Horizontal (intercostal) views are obtained moving laterally up the body wall (from the 6 o'clock to a 3 or 9 o'clock position). Convention places the cranial aspect of the heart to the right side of the screen in echocardiology (Figure 19.19).

The heart is best identified using the screen image to find the contracting structures. Concurrent base–apex electrocardiogram leads will provide detail of the cardiac cycle if your scanner is equipped with this feature. Copious amounts of coupling gel are required to minimize air trapping between the scutes. It is important to allow time for the gel to penetrate the keratin skin layer; this will improve the images obtained.

Rotating the transducer through 90 degrees provides short-axis/transverse views, allowing identification of the VS, MR and BL within the ventricle, and a characteristic 'Mickey Mouse' appearance of the three major vessels that

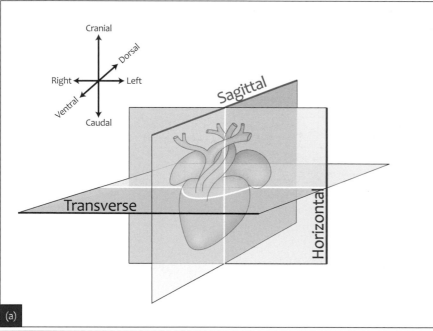

19.19 These diagrams show how the standard echocardiographic views are obtained. (a) The standard image planes with the probe positioned under the reptile can provide (b) the ventral short-axis view (probe in transverse plane) and (c) the long-axis view (probe in sagittal plane). Moving to the lateral aspect of the patient will allow (d) the intercostal view to be obtained (probe in horizontal plane).

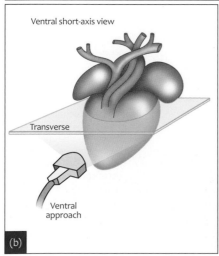

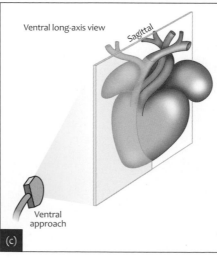

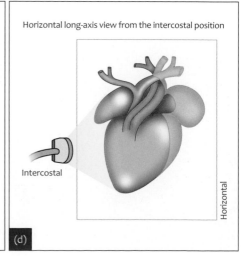

exit the ventricle, combining to make the truncus arteriosus. The laterally positioned aortic arches form the 'ears' and the pulmonary artery the 'face' (Figure 19.20). This is an easily recognizable reference point during the echocardiographic investigation. The presence of pericardial fluid is normal and allows a degree of axial rotation of the ventricle during the cardiac cycle due to the pattern of myocardial contraction. The spongy myocardium can make interpretation of the internal structures difficult. The atria are easier to identify as rapidly distensible ovoid structures in the craniodorsal position above the single ventricle with its incomplete internal septa.

Orientating the transducer to the right of the midline reveals the distensible sinus venosus with the bicuspid valve, caudal vena cava and pulmonary artery overlying the heart.

Scanning ventrally in the long axis permits identification of the truncus arteriosus; four chambers; internal ventricular cavae of the ventricle, including apposition of the MR and BL; and the AV canal (Figure 19.21).

In the ventral midline the CV may be identifiable in the ventricle, using the pulmonary artery exiting the ventricle in a cranial direction as an anatomical guide. At this level, the MR and BL separate the blood flow entering the pulmonary artery and CP from the left aortic arch and CV (Figure 19.22). The bicuspid pulmonary artery and left leaflet of the aortic valve complex are visible and define the origin of these vessels. It is not possible to view all three major vessels on the same long-axis sagittal view as they exit the ventricle. The right aortic arch is visualized immediately to the right of the AV canal, and adjacent and dorsal to the left aortic arch.

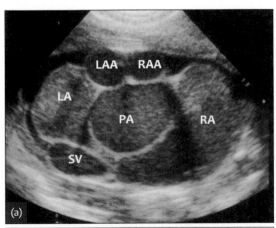

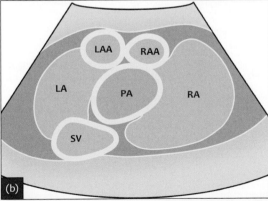

19.20 (a) Two-dimensional ventral short-axis echocardiographic ('Mickey Mouse') view, demonstrating the normal anatomy of a Burmese python. (b) The line diagram shows the three dorsal heart chambers, the sinus venosus (SV) and the right atrium (RA) and left atrium (LA), with the easily identifiable 'Mickey Mouse' face of the pulmonary artery (PA) and left aortic arch (LAA) and right aortic arch (RAA).

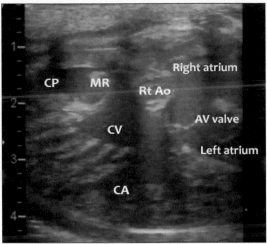

19.21 Long-axis horizontal view annotated echocardiographic image from a video of a yellow anaconda. Note the anaconda's internal ventricular septation characterized by sheets instead of a single vertical septum. AV = atrioventricular; CA = cavum arteriosum; CP = cavum pulmonale; CV = cavum venosum; MR = muscular ridge; Rt Ao = right aortic arch.
(Reproduced from Jensen et al. (2014) with permissio)

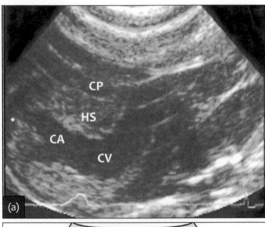

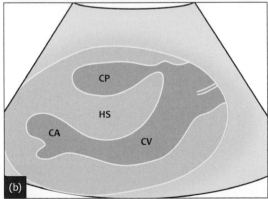

19.22 (a) Two-dimensional, non-standard view and (b) line diagram of a Burmese python that shows the almost complete separation of the cavum pulmonale (CP) by the muscular ridge and its horizontal septum (HS) from the cavum venosum (CV) and cavum arteriosum (CA).

Colour wave Doppler may be used to follow the direction of blood flow through the heart. In the normal animal, flow through the heart is laminar except for small areas of turbulence at the AV canal. Colour Doppler echocardiography has identified turbulent blood flow resulting from suspected congenital AV valvular dysplasia in a juvenile carpet python diagnosed with chronic heart failure (Rishniw and Carmel, 1999).

Laboratory investigations

Routine haematological, biochemical (electrolytes) and faecal analyses should be performed in the clinical investigation of cardiovascular disease. In addition, fresh haematological and faecal smears should be prepared at the time of sample collection and examined for evidence of any haemoparasites or endoparasites (see Chapters 8 and 24).

Biochemical analysis may reveal evidence of multiple organ dysfunction in cases of cardiac failure, with elevations in plasma uric acid levels suggesting renal compromise, and elevations in aspartate aminotransferase (AST) suggesting hepatocellular leakage. In cases of intravascular haemolytic anaemia, such as is seen with some haemoparasitic and autoimmune diseases, the plasma may become obviously icteric. It should be noted that the predominant bile pigment in reptiles is biliverdin; therefore, plasma bilirubin levels may not be elevated significantly.

With weight loss, elevations in creatinine kinase and AST may be seen as catabolism of muscle, and tissue anoxia occurs. Very little is known about specific cardiac enzymes or isoenzymes in reptiles.

Blood sampling by sterile technique for culture of bacteria in suspected cases of septicaemia/bacteraemia may be performed via routine venepuncture sites (see Chapter 8).

Cardiocentesis is commonly used to collect blood samples in snakes. Although generally safe in healthy reptiles, in a suspected case of heart disease this technique has proven fatal (Selleri and Di Girolamo, 2012). Remember to ensure needle placement is directed into the most caudal aspect at the apex of the ventricle, as the delicate structures such as the truncus arteriosus and atria are positioned cranially.

Cardiac disease

Congenital and acquired cardiac diseases are rarely reported in reptiles; a literature review revealed fewer than 40 reported cases of cardiac-associated disease in non-crocodilian reptiles (Figure 19.23).

Behavioural inactivity, low metabolic rates and tolerance to low oxygen levels appear to make primary cardiac disease rare in reptiles. In general, the signs of cardiac failure can be usefully separated into those of backward and forward failure (Figure 19.24). There may be a pattern appearing where pythons and varanids are more susceptible to lung oedema due to their separated systemic and pulmonary circulations.

- **Backward failure** implies increased cardiac filling pressures and failure to empty the venous circulation, resulting in congestion and oedema.
- Signs of **forward failure** result from an inability of the heart to supply blood commensurate with the metabolic needs of the body tissues. In reptiles, predominant signs of forward failure are rare, due to the inactivity of reptiles and their low metabolic requirements (approximately one-tenth that of a similar-sized mammal). Several cases report a clinical deterioration coinciding with the increased metabolic demands of ecdysis or prey capture (Jacobson et al., 1979; Rush et al., 2001).

Species	Clinical signs/diagnosis	Reference
Various	Nutritional vitamin E deficiency Atherosclerosis	Frye (1991b) Williams (1992)
All reptiles	Microfilaria from filarial nematodes	Murray (2006)
Chelonians		
Barbour's map turtle	*Flavobacterium meningosepticum* infection; multisystemic involvement (including myocardium); subcutaneous oedema and lethargy	Jacobson et al. (1989a)
Green turtle	Spirorchid fluke granulomas causing arteritis, thrombus, aneurysm, endocarditis Chlamydiosis; multisystemic disease, including necrotizing myocarditis resulting in lethargy, anorexia and inability to dive	Gordon et al. (1998); Greiner et al. (1980) Homer et al. (1994)
Leatherback turtle	*Vibrio damsela* septicaemia causing valvular endocarditis; route of infection thought to be via the gastrointestinal tract	Obendorf et al. (1987)
Loggerhead turtle	Metastatic neoplasia; multicentric lymphoblastic lymphoma	Oros et al. (2001)
Spur-thighed tortoise	Pericardial effusion and atrial dilation in association with oedema and liver disease	Redrobe and Scudamore (2000)
Lizards		
Central bearded dragon	Atherosclerosis/pericardial effusion	Shilliger et al. (2010a)
Frilled lizard	Granulomatous myocarditis (*Mycobacterium* spp.)	Murray (1996)
Green iguana	Aortic stenosis and secondary atrioventricular dilation Myocardial abscess and haemopericardium Atherosclerosis	Clippinger (1993) Innis (2000) Schuchman and Taylor (1970)
Komodo dragon	Atrial septal defect	Pizzi et al. (2009)
Savannah monitor	Myocardial and hepatic suspected adenovirus; sudden death	Jacobson and Kollias (1986)
Snakes		
Ball python	Congenital septal defect (to the muscular ridge)	Jensen and Wang (2009)
Black kingsnake	Cardiomyopathy Rhabdomyosarcoma (cardiac)	Wagner (1989) Catão-Dias and Nichols (1999)

19.23 Cases of cardiac disease in reptiles. (continues) ▶

Species	Clinical signs/diagnosis	Reference
Snakes (continued)		
Boa constrictor imperator	Granulomatous myocarditis	Selleri and Di Girolamo (2012)
Burmese python	Valvular insufficiency; pneumonia	Shilliger *et al.* (2010b)
	Aortic aneurysm and subsequent cardiopulmonary arrest while swallowing prey item	Rush *et al.* (1999)
	Bacterial endocarditis (*Salmonella* and *Corynebacterium*)	Jacobson *et al.* (1991)
Carpet python	Congenital valvular disease; right atrioventricular valvular insufficiency and congestive heart failure	Rishniw and Carmel (1999)
Copperhead	Haemangiosarcoma	Catão-Dias and Nichols (1999)
Corn snake	Cardiac haemangioma	Stumpel *et al.* (2012)
	Metastatic chondrosarcoma	Schmidt and Reavill (2010)
	Metastatic oviductal adenocarcinoma	Pereira and Viner (2008)
Deckert's ratsnake	Congestive heart failure; hepatic inclusions also found	Jacobson *et al.* (1979)
Madagascan Dumeril's boa	Granulomatous myocarditis and coelomic effusion due to *Salmonella enterica arizonae*	Schilliger *et al.* (2003)
Mole kingsnake	Cardiomyopathy	Barten (1980)
Puff adder	*Chlamydia* infection	Jacobson *et al.* (1989a)
Rattlesnakes	Obesity resulting in hyperlipidaemia and cardiovascular disease	Bauer and Jacobson (1989)
Rosy boa	Viral myocarditis (associated lesion with an adenovirus-like infection)	Schumacher *et al.* (1994)

19.23 (continued) Cases of cardiac disease in reptiles.

Clinical sign	Failure of cardiac output	Congestive failure (backward cardiac failure)
Anorexia	+++	+++
Inactivity	+++	+++
Poor body condition and weight loss	+++	++
Pericardial effusion	+	+++
Tissue oedema – cutaneous and visceral oedema (hepatomegaly, renal and intestinal)	–	+++
Pulmonary crackles	–	++
Cardiomegaly	++	++
Tachycardia	+++	++
Mucosal pallor	+++	+
Sudden death (e.g. during more strenuous activity)	+	+
Cardiac murmur	+	+

19.24 Clinical signs of heart disease in reptiles. +++ = almost always present; ++ = sometimes present; + = rarely present; – = never present.

Vascular and haemopoietic diseases

Haemoparasites

Haemoparasites are relatively common in reptiles, particularly in wild-caught and imported species. A list of the more commonly seen parasites is given in Figure 19.25 and some haemoparasites are illustrated in Chapter 8. The majority of parasites are non-pathogenic. The most serious pathogens are malarial parasites (*Plasmodium*), which may produce significant haemolytic anaemias and clinical disease in chelonians.

Other parasites

Any parasite that adds sufficiently to the general debility of a sick reptile may enhance the likelihood of a chronic anaemia developing. Some parasites may cause anaemia more directly:

- The snake mite *Ophionyssus natricis* may cause anaemia due to its blood-sucking nature (see Chapters 15 and 24). The mites *Hirstiella* and *Ophionyssus* may transmit the haemoparasite *Karyolysus* spp., but this has not been reported as causing anaemia
- The intestinal hookworm *Kalicephalus* may also be associated with anaemia and malnutrition, particularly in snakes (see Chapters 17 and 24)
- Leeches may cause anaemia in juvenile aquatic species if attached in sufficient quantities. They may also act as vectors for haemoparasites such as haemogregarines and trypanosomes, which may lead to haemolytic anaemia.

Metabolic vascular disease

Metastatic mineralization can be caused by hypervitaminosis D3 or by abnormalities in the calcium to phosphorus ratio, which may be caused by renal disease. Garner (2001) discusses the occurrence of pulmonary vessel metastatic calcification, associated with an erythroid response (although no anaemia had occurred) in green iguanas and a plumed basilisk. The latter also showed evidence of aortic mineralization. The majority of reptiles examined in this study were suffering from chronic renal disease and renal gout, hyperphosphataemia, or an inverted Ca:P ratio.

Frye (1991c) and Shilliger *et al.* (2010b) discuss vascular dystrophic mineralization as being associated with atherosclerosis related to stress, an unbalanced diet, hypercholesterolaemia, hepatic lipidosis and lack of exercise.

Haemoparasite	Reptiles commonly affected	Intermediate hosts/vectors	Description in blood	Pathogenicity reported
Protozoa – phylum Apicomplexa, subclass Coccidiasina				
Order Eucoccidiorida, Suborder Adeleorina family Haemogregarinidae				
Haemogregarina (sporogeny occurs in invertebrate intermediate host; may also accumulate in liver, spleen and lung)	Aquatic species – mainly freshwater turtles (e.g. *H. stepanovi* in the European pond turtle), tortoises of genera *Geoemyda* and *Testudo*, the tuatara, most snakes, and some crocodilians	Leeches	Erythrocytic inclusions, micro- and macrogametocytes rarely refractile	Rare, but pathogenic *H. crocodilinorum* reported in wild American alligators
Haemolivia	Tortoises as intermediate host (e.g. *H. mauritanica* in spur-thighed and marginated tortoises)	The reptile is the intermediate host – the chelonian tick *Hyalomma aegyptium* is thought to be the final host	Erythrocytic inclusions, micro- and macrogametocytes rarely refractile	Rarely pathogenic
Hepatozoon (sporogeny in invertebrate intermediate host; may also accumulate in liver, spleen and lung)	Terrestrial snakes	Arthropods, e.g. mites (no development occurs in vector)	Erythrocytic inclusions, micro- and macrogametocytes rarely refractile	Rarely pathogenic
Karyolysus (sporogeny in invertebrate intermediate host; may also accumulate in liver, spleen and lung)	Old World lizards and tree snakes (Frye, 1991a; Campbell, 1996)	Arthropods, e.g. lizard mite; transmitted through faeces of intermediate host	Erythrocytic inclusions, micro- and macrogametocytes rarely refractile	Rarely pathogenic
Order Haemosporida				
Plasmodium	Common in chelonians, occasionally in snakes	Mosquitoes, dipteran biting insects	Depends on host; may see schizonts, micro- and macrogametocytes in cytoplasm of erythrocytes (Telford, 1984) as well as in mononuclear cells and endothelium of blood vessels	Can cause severe haemolytic anaemia. May see extra-medullary haemopoiesis as well as vascular occlusive disease in brain, heart, etc. due to swelling of endothelium of vessels. *P. mexicanum* reportedly fatal in juvenile lizards
Haemoproteus	Mainly lizards, some turtles, occasionally snakes	Dipteran biting flies and mosquitoes, possibly mites	Gametocytes seen in erythrocytes, refractile	Rarely pathogenic
Saurocytozoon	Lizards	Mosquitoes	Resembles *Leucocytozoon* in birds, with gametocytes in leucocytes and immature erythrocytes. Lacks pigmentation	Rarely pathogenic
Order Achromatorida, Suborder Piroplasmorina				
Sauroplasma	Lizards	Ticks and biting flies	Vacuoles with inclusions in thrombocytes and erythroid cells	Rarely pathogenic
Serpentoplasma	Snakes	Ticks and biting flies	Vacuoles with inclusions in thrombocytes and erythroid cells	Rarely pathogenic
Order Eucoccidiorida, Suborder Eimeriorina				
Lainsonia (sporogeny occurs in reptile)	Lizards	Thought to be mites of dipteran biting insects	Unpigmented inclusions in leucocytes and thrombocytes	Enters reticuloendothelial system but no pathogenicity reported
Schellackia (sporogeny occurs in reptile)	New World reptiles	Thought to be mites of dipteran biting insects	Found in leucocytes. Commonest in erythrocytes. Ovoid unpigmented inclusions deforming host nucleus	Also parasitizes gut of lizards as schizont. Sporozoites released into bloodstream. May cause anaemia
Order Trypanosomatidae				
Trypanosoma	All forms of reptile affected	Dipteran and phlebotomine flies; leeches for aquatic species	Parasite seen free in plasma – trypanomastigote – classical undulating cellular membrane	Rarely pathogenic
Leishmania	Common in wild-caught lizards	Phlebotomine sandflies	Amastigote form in erythrocytes; promastigote form free in plasma	Rarely pathogenic

19.25 Reptile haemoparasites (see also Chapters 8 and 24). (continues) ▶

Haemoparasite	Reptiles commonly affected	Intermediate hosts/vectors	Description in blood	Pathogenicity reported
Helminths – subfamily Dirofilariinae				
Microfilaria (e.g. *Foleyella*, *Oswaldofilaria*)	Lizards commonly seen – but may affect any reptile	Ticks, mites, mosquitoes	Filaroid worm-like organisms free in plasma	May cause blockage of terminal vessels
Trematodes – family Spirorchiidae				
Digenetic spirorchiid flukes (e.g. *Spirorchis*, *Henotosoma*, *Vasotrema*)	Chelonians, particularly marine turtles	Aquatic snails, e.g. *Lornea* spp.	Trematode eggs rarely seen in peripheral blood smears. Pulmonary tissue biopsy and squash preparation often required	Adult flukes rarely cause disease; occasionally endothelial hyperplasia in main vessels exiting heart. Main pathology associated with blockage of end arterioles with fluke eggs

19.25 (continued) Reptile haemoparasites (see also Chapters 8 and 24).

Neoplasia

Neoplastic disease of lymphoid or haemopoietic origin has been reported variously as comprising between 0% and 30.8% of cancers in reptile species (Ramsey *et al.*, 1996; Catão-Dias and Nichols, 1999). Hernandez-Divers and Garner (2003) describe the haemopoietic system as the most commonly reported body system to be affected, with Garner *et al.* (2004) suggesting that snakes (particularly vipers such as cobras and urutus) and lizards (particularly monitors such as the savannah monitor and bearded dragons) are the most commonly affected.

Cancers involving lymphoid cells frequently involve lymphosarcomatous infiltration of parenchymal organs, and so may or may not involve the bloodstream (see Chapter 23). Lymphoblast cells are rarely seen normally in the bloodstream of reptiles and so their presence in moderate to large numbers indicates a lymphocytic leukaemia. Figure 19.26 details reported cases of neoplasia of lymphoid or haemopoietic origin.

Thromboembolic disease

Salmonella embolic septicaemia has been reported as a cause of atrial thromboembolism in a green iguana (Innis, 2000). This may seed micro-thrombi into the bloodstream to affect other organs. Hepatic artery thromboembolism has been reported in inland bearded dragons (Redrobe and Frye, 2001) associated with severe periodontal disease and *Pseudomonas* bacteria. Periodontal disease may be a common under-diagnosed source of septic embolic disease in reptiles.

Tumour type	Species	Reference
Chelonians		
Myeloblastic leukaemia	Red-eared terrapin	Frye and Carney (1972)
Myelogenous leukaemia	Helmeted turtle	Harshbarger (1976)
Multicentric lymphoblastic lymphoma (lymphoma nodules throughout body including heart and aortae)	Loggerhead turtle	Oros *et al.* (2001)
Lizards		
Chronic monocytic leukaemia	Bearded dragon	Gregory *et al.* (2004)
Immunoblastic leukaemia	Green iguana	Miller *et al.* (2000)
Lymphoma (disseminated)	Green iguana	Hernandez-Divers and Garner (2003)
Lymphoma (pharyngeal)	Green iguana	Folland *et al.* (2011)
Lymphoma/lymphosarcoma	East Indian water lizard Asian water monitor	Zwart and Harshbarger (1972)
Lymphosarcoma with leukaemic blood profile	Savannah monitor	Schultze *et al.* (1999)
Multicentric lymphoma	Egyptian spiny-tailed lizards	Gyimesi *et al.* (2005)
Myelogenous leukaemia	Inland bearded dragon	Tocidlowski *et al.* (2001)
Plasma cell tumour	Nile monitor	Harshbarger (1974)
Plasma cell tumour (disseminated to lung, liver and stomach)	East Indian water lizard	Schmidt (1977)
Undifferentiated leukaemia	Desert spiny lizard	Goldberg and Holshuh (1991)
Snakes		
Lymphocytic leukaemia	Indian python Common boa Broad-banded copperhead	Finnie (1972) Frye and Carney (1972) Hruban *et al.* (1992)
Lymphocytic leukaemia with multicentric T-cell lymphoma	Diamond python	Raiti (2002)
Lymphosarcoma with lymphoid leukaemia	Aruba island rattlesnake	Lock *et al.* (2001)
Myelogenous leukaemia	Russell's viper and Honduran milk snake	Hruban *et al.* (1992)
Lymphoblastic lymphoma	Red-tailed boa	Schilliger *et al.* (2011)

19.26 Neoplasia of haemopoietic/lymphoid origin affecting reptiles.

Congenital and developmental vascular disease

Congenital aortic stenosis with secondary ventricular dilatation has been recorded in a green iguana that was presented with a history of inappetence, lethargy, an increased respiratory cycle and a change in skin coloration (Clippinger, 1993).

Jensen and Wang (2009) report two cases of congenital malformation of the MR of ball pythons leading to inability to maintain ventricular pressure separation; interestingly they both grew normally as juveniles. This case contradicts (in young animals at least) the theory that pythons would be expected to develop pulmonary oedema when exposed to the high systolic blood pressure usually maintained only in their systemic circulation. A Komodo dragon was diagnosed post-mortem with an atrial septal defect that had signs of ill thrift, cardiomegaly and anaemia (Pizzi et al., 2009).

Aneurysms

These have been reported in bearded dragons (Barten et al., 2006; Sweet et al., 2009) and Burmese pythons (Rush et al., 1999). They have been reported arising from the internal carotid artery or directly from the aorta. A firm but fluctuant swelling is often seen on the dorsolateral neck, but aneurysms have also been reported within the cranial coelomic cavity. The aetiology is unknown, postulated to be due to trauma as a result of the superficial position of the carotid arteries in the dorsolateral pharyngeal area. The author [SG] and Barten et al. (2006) have successfully removed such aneurysms, with patients surviving months to years afterwards (Figure 19.27).

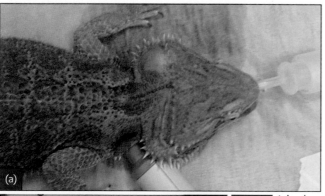
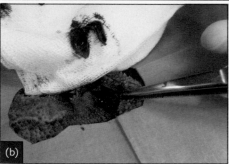

19.27 Inland bearded dragon with an aneurysm: (a) prior to surgery, demonstrating a swelling caudodorsal to the angle of the jaw on the left side, and (b) during removal.

Anaemia

Haemolytic

Pirhaemocyton was for many years classified as a protozoal haemoparasite, but the erythrocytic metachromatically staining inclusions have more recently been associated with viral assembly factories, consistent with viruses of the family Iridoviridae. Infection is known to cause haemolytic anaemia, although morbidity is only occasionally reported. There has been reported spontaneous resolution of the viraemia in a chameleon (Telford and Jacobson, 1993).

McCraken et al. (1994) described an erythrocytic virus in a diamond python causing an anaemia with a packed cell volume (PCV) of 7%. A total of 95% of the erythrocytes showed acidophilic intracytoplasmic inclusion bodies (0.5–3 μm diameter).

Immune-mediated haemolytic anaemia – of unknown aetiology – has been reported in a Parson's chameleon (Boyer, 2002) based on anaemia (PCV 7–8%), autoagglutination of erythrocytes, haemolytic serum with marked anisocytosis, and signs of lethargy and weakness. Treatment with prednisolone (see Appendix 2, Formulary) and a blood transfusion from sibling chameleons via the intraosseous route produced dramatic results. Side effects included osteomyelitis, which responded to antibiotic therapy.

Nutritional

A so-called 'nutritional anaemia' in a subadult coastal bearded dragon with a PCV of 14% and a total blood protein level of 34 g/l, presenting as profoundly cachexic, was reported by McCraken et al. (1994). A blood transfusion and the use of anabolic steroids resulted in a regenerative response. No pathogens were ever isolated from this patient, leading to the conclusion that profound malnutrition led to the original anaemia.

Toxic

Heavy-metal (lead and zinc particularly) poisoning has been reported as causing a non-regenerative anaemia in reptiles. It has been reported that the treatment, i.e. sodium calcium edetate, has resulted in haemolysis in chelonians (Saggese, 2009).

Haemoparasites

Most haemoparasites mentioned in Figure 19.25 rarely cause disease in reptiles, and so many are incidental findings and are not treated. However, for the more pathogenic parasites, such as *Plasmodium* in chelonians, treatment is often necessary (see Appendix 2, Formulary, for drug dosages) (Figure 19.28).

Other parasites

Mites and hookworms may be treated with ivermectin at 0.2 mg/kg s.c. given once. **Ivermectin should be avoided in chelonians owing to reported toxicity.** Doses should be repeated every 2 weeks until negative faecal or clinical examination have been reported. Environmental decontamination may be required, which involves removal of substrate and furniture (see Chapter 24 for further information).

Leeches may be removed manually after application of local anaesthetic directly to the parasite.

Excessive tick numbers may lead to anaemia and may be treated with ivermectin as detailed above, by manual removal or by careful application of fipronil – although the latter should be used with care as some toxicities have been reported.

Haemopoietic neoplasia

Chemotherapy is still very much in its infancy in reptile medicine. A summary of some case studies is given in Figure 19.29; see also Chapter 23.

Haemoparasite	Treatment	Reference
Protozoan haemoparasites of chelonians (e.g. *Plasmodium* spp.)	Chloroquine 125 mg/kg orally q48h on three occasions	Stein (1996)
Protozoan haemoparasites of snakes	Quinacrine 20–100 mg/kg orally q48h for 2 weeks	Raiti (2002)
Microfilaria	Maintaining the affected reptile at environmental temperatures of 35°–37°C for 24–48 hours to kill adult worms	Jacobson (1986)
Trematodes	Praziquantel 8 mg/kg orally once (may not be effective). Prevention is via control of aquatic snail intermediate host	Murray (1996)

19.28 Treatment of selected haemoparasite infections.

Case report	Treatment regimen	Problems encountered
Lymphoma in a green iguana (Folland *et al.*, 2011)	Initial 10 Gy fraction of radiation focused on cervical lesion plus regimen of vincristine, cyclophosphamide and prednisolone, and latterly doxorubicin (0.75 mg/kg i.v. q3w) and prednisolone (2 mg/kg q24h)	Initial regimen seemed to indicate cyclophosphamide was more effective than doxorubicin and vincristine; therefore, the latter two were ceased, but a relapse at 315 days meant a change back to stop cyclophosphamide and restart on doxorubicin at a dose of 0.75 mg/kg i.v. q3w, which reduced leucocyte count. Appeared to be in remission by day 1008
Lymphoma in king cobra (Willette *et al.*, 2001)	**Week 1:** Prednisolone 40 mg/m² orally q48h L-asparagine aminohydrolase 10,000 IU/m² s.c. once **Week 2:** Prednisolone 40 mg/m² orally q48h Vincristine 0.5 mg/m² i.v. once **Week 3:** Prednisolone 40 mg/m² orally q48h L-asparagine aminohydrolase 10,000 IU/m² s.c. once Initial treatment was successful, but regrowth occurred: new regimen started: Chlorambucil 2 mg/m² s.c. q24h for 30 days Prednisolone 40 mg/m² orally q48h	Poor skin sloughing Anorexia Reduced leucocyte count (immunosuppression in addition to desired effect) Hyperglycaemia Hypoalbuminaemia
Sarcomas (possible lymphoma) in a corn snake (Rosenthal, 1994)	Doxorubicin 1 mg/kg i.v.: q1w for two treatments, then q2w for two treatments, then q3w for two treatments	Anorexia Need for intravenous port problematic for course of treatment

19.29 Chemotherapy/radiotherapy of haemopoietic neoplasia.

Treatment of cardiovascular disease

Cardiac disease and failure

Initial therapy should be aimed towards reducing any additional metabolic demand and, depending on species, dosage with an appropriate parasiticide, antibiotic, fluid and nutritional support (Figure 19.30). Husbandry problems, as in all reptile diseases, should be identified if present, and then corrected.

A minimum database should be established with laboratory testing and echocardiography. Ultrasonography provides a rapid assessment of heart-chamber morphology and confirms suspected cardiomegaly. In a lizard, mineralization of great vessels on a radiograph may give you additional information so a dorsoventral view is warranted, but in a snake or chelonian probably provides no further information other than that gleaned from the physical examination.

Doppler blood flow will provide a heart rate and is an objective measure repeatable by the nursing team. Rhythm disturbances have not been described, so an ECG is not pertinent at this stage as the only information it will supply is duplicating that from the Doppler flow. Indirect blood pressure monitoring is as yet unproven, and direct arterial measurement beyond most general practitioners. Although fashionable and expensive, MRI is likely to provide far less information than can be obtained from a good echocardiologist.

- Maintain at lowest extent of POTZ to decrease metabolic demand
- Enrich local environment with oxygen
- Reduce stress with minimal handling
- Withhold food (for the short term, to decrease metabolic demand)
- Attempt short-term diuresis when signs of congestive heart failure are present:
  - Furosemide 2–5 mg/kg i.v. or i.m. q8–12h
  - Or hydrochlorothiazide 1 mg/kg q24h
  - Or spironolactone 2–4 mg/kg q24h
  - Enalapril has been used experimentally in alligators to ablate angiotensin I (Silldorff and Stephens, 1992) and in a spiny-tailed monitor to briefly manage/improve congestive heart failure at 0.5–0.7 mg/kg q24h (combined with spironolactone and furosemide) (Clayton *et al.*, 2007)
  - Monitor clinical response
- Blood culture + broad-spectrum antimicrobial (e.g. enrofloxacin and metronidazole or enrofloxacin and third-generation cephalosporin)
- Parasiticides (if suspect haemoparasites/microfilaria, or blood-sucking ecto/endoparasites, see Figure 19.29

19.30 Treatment protocol for suspected heart disease in a reptile.

When the patient is stable, more time can be spent handling and performing more specific diagnostic tests for any abnormalities detected in the blood tests and preliminary echo findings. If the heart is morphologically abnormal, e.g. a mass or segmental wall thickening, then a biopsy may be considered. Myocardial biopsy, although a risk, is most likely to differentiate the potential causes of acquired heart disease. Congenital disease may not always display obvious clinical signs in the juvenile, so should be considered, even in adults (Jensen and Wang, 2009).

If the patient is oedematous, then it is tempting to attempt diuresis as you would in a mammal. Reptile species have evolved in marine, freshwater or terrestrial environments with their variable challenges to osmoregulation. However, the reptile kidney lacks a loop of Henle (the target of loop diuretics like furosemide), and do not rely on the kidney for ion and water regulation. In turtles, furosemide has been shown to promote diuresis (Stephens and Robertson, 1985). Some evidence has been put forward to suggest that furosemide can work on sodium and chloride pumps found in the urinary bladder lining in those species possessing a urinary bladder, or in the terminal rectum where water may be reabsorbed after reflux from the cloaca (Ehrenspeck and Voner, 1985; Badia et al., 1987) Methylated xanthines (aminophylline 10 mg/kg i.m. per required need (prn); theophylline 5 mg/kg i.m. prn) can often be used successfully in reptiles for diuresis. Their diuretic effect may be partly due to their stimulatory effect on cardiac function, increased renal blood flow and increased glomerular filtration rate. The major diuretic effect of these compounds is apparently due to increased rates of excretion of sodium and chloride ions by renal tubules.

The prognosis in any case with heart failure will be poor, and treatment should only be started following a discussion with the owner to give a realistic expectation of success. However, recording and reporting outcomes is vital, and only by sharing knowledge about these cases will we progress from the current situation where a postmortem is the most likely diagnostic outcome.

Acknowledgements

Thanks to Dr Bjarke Jensen, Department of Bioscience and Zoophysiology, Aarhus University, Denmark, for his comments and permission to use images in Figures 19.3 and 19.21.

References and further reading

Andersen JB, Rourke BC, Caiozzo VJ, Bennett AF and Hicks JW (2005) Postprandial cardiac hypertrophy in pythons. *Nature* **434**, 37–38

Badia P, Gomez T, Diaz M and Lorenzo A (1987) Mechanisms of transport of Na$^+$ and Cl$^-$ in the lizard colon. *Comparative Biochemistry and Physiology. A, Comparative Physiology* **87(4)**, 883–887

Barten S (1980) Cardiomyopathy in a king snake (*Lampropeltis calligaster rhombomaculata*) *Veterinary Medicine Small Animal Clinics* **75**, 125–129

Barten S, Wyneken J, Mader D and Garner M (2006) Aneurysm in the dorsolateral neck of two bearded dragons (*Pogona vitticeps*). *Proceedings of the Association of Reptilian and Amphibian Veterinarians Annual Conference*, pp. 43–44

Bauer J and Jacobson ER (1989) Hyperlipidaemia and cardiovascular disease in obese rattlesnakes. *Colloquium on Pathology of Reptiles and Amphibians*, p. 11 [abstract]

Boyer T (2002) Autoimmune hemolytic anemia in a Parson's chameleon, *Calumma parsonii parsonii*. *Proceedings of the Association of Reptilian and Amphibian Veterinarians Annual Conference*, pp. 81–84

Campbell TW (1996) Hemoparasites. In: *Reptile Medicine and Surgery*, ed. D Mader, pp. 379–381. WB Saunders, Philadelphia

Catão-Dias JL and Nichols DK (1999) Neoplasia in snakes at the national zoological park, Washington, DC (1978–1997). *Journal of Comparative Pathology* **120**, 89–95

Clayton LA, Hadfield CA, Gore SR and Brazil AM (2007) Management of presumptive congestive heart failure in a spiny tailed monitor lizard (*Varanus acanthurus*). *Proceedings of the Association of Reptilian and Amphibian Veterinarians Annual Conference*, pp. 60–61

Clippinger TL (1993) Aortic stenosis and atrioventricular dilatation in a green iguana (*Iguana iguana*). *Proceedings of the American Association of Zoo Veterinarians*, pp. 390–393

Ehrenspeck G and Voner C (1985) Effect of furosemide on ion transport in the turtle bladder: evidence for direct inhibition of active acid base transport. *Biochimica et Biophysica Acta* **817(2)**, 318–326

Finnie EP (1972) Lymphoid leucosis in an Indian python (*Python molurus*). *Journal of Pathology* **107**, 295

Folland DW, Johnston MS, Thramm DH and Reavill D (2011) Diagnosis and management of lymphoma in a green iguana (*Iguana iguana*). *Journal of the American Veterinary Medical Association* **239**, 985–991

Frye F (1991a) Hemoparasites. In: *Biomedical and Surgical Aspects of Captive Reptile Husbandry, 2nd edition*, pp. 259–261. Krieger, Malabar, FL, USA

Frye F (1991b) Comparative histology. In: *Biomedical and surgical aspects of captive reptile husbandry, 2nd edition*, pp. 473–512. Krieger, Malabar, FL, USA

Frye F (1991c) Arteriosclerosis with medial mineralisation. In: *Biomedical and surgical aspects of captive reptile husbandry, 2nd edition*, p. 533. Krieger, Malabar, FL, USA

Frye F and Carney J (1972) Myeloproliferative disease in a turtle. *Journal of the American Veterinary Medical Association* **161**, 595

Gabriel EA, Gartner GE, Hicks JW et al. (2010) Phylogeny, ecology and heart position in snakes. *Physiological and Biochemical Zoology* **83(1)**, 43–54

Garner M (2001) Regenerative erythroid response without anemia in Iguanidae associated with soft tissue mineralization. *Proceedings of the Association of Reptilian and Amphibian Veterinarians Annual Conference*, pp. 213–216

Garner MM, Hernandez-Divers SM and Raymond JT (2004) Reptile neoplasia: a retrospective study of case submissions to a specialty diagnostic service. *Veterinary Clinics of North America: Exotic Animal Practice* **7**, 653–671

Girgis S (1961) Observations on the heart in the family Trionychidae. *Bulletin of the British Museum (Natural History) Zoology* **8**, 73–107

Goldberg SR and Holshuh HJ (1991) A case of leukaemia in the desert spiny lizard (*Scelporus magister*). *Journal of Wildlife Diseases* **27**, 521–525

Gordon AN, Kelly WR and Cribb TH (1998) Lesions caused by cardiovascular flukes (*Digenea: Spirorchidae*) in stranded green turtles (*Chelonia mydas*). *Veterinary Pathology* **35**, 21

Gregory C, Latimer K, Fontenot D et al. (2004) Chronic monocytic leukemia in an inland bearded dragon, *Pogona vitticeps*. *Journal of Herpetological Medicine and Surgery* **14(2)**, 12–16

Greiner EC, Forrester DJ and Jacobson ET (1980) Helminths of macri-culture reared green turtles (Chelonia mydas mydas) from Grand Cayman B.W.I. *Proceedings of the Helminthological Society of Washington* **47**, 142–144

Gyimesi ZS, Garner MM, Burns RB et al. (2005) High incidence of lymphoid neoplasia in a colony of Egyptian spiny-tailed lizards (*Uromastyx aegyptius*). *Journal of Zoo and Wildlife Medicine* **36**, 103–110

Harshbarger JC (1974) *Activities Report Registry of Tumors in Lower Animals, 1965–1973*. Smithsonian Institution, Washington, DC

Harshbarger JC (1976) *Activities Report Registry of Tumors in Lower Animals, 1975 supplement*. Smithsonian Institution, Washington, DC

Hernandez-Divers SM and Garner M (2003) Neoplasia of reptiles with an emphasis on lizards. *Veterinary Clinics of North America: Exotic Animal Practice* **6(1)**, 251–273

Homer BL, Jacobson ER, Schumacher J and Scherba G (1994) Chlamydiosis in macri-culture reared green turtles (*Chelonia mydas mydas*). *Veterinary Pathology* **31**, 1–7

Hruban Z, Vardiman E, Meehan T, Frye FL and Carter WE (1992) Hematopoietic neoplasms in zoo animals. *Journal of Comparative Pathology* **106**, 15–24

Hunt C (2013) Electrocardiography of the normal inland bearded dragon (*Pogona vitticeps*). *Royal College of Veterinary Surgeons Diploma in Zoological Medicine*, DZM-13-2, 23 September

Innis C (2000) Myocardial abscess and hemopericardium in a green iguana, *Iguana iguana*. *Proceedings of the Association of Reptilian and Amphibian Veterinarians Annual Conference*, pp. 43–44

Jacobson, ER (1986) Parasitic diseases of reptiles. In: *Zoo and Wild Animal Medicine, Current Therapy 2*, ed. ME Fowler, pp. 162–181. WB Saunders, Philadelphia

Jacobson ER, Gardiner CH, Barten SL, Burn DH and Bourgeois AI (1989a) Flavobacterium meningosepticum infection of a Barbour's map turtle (*Graptemys barbouri*). *Journal of Zoo and Wildlife Medicine* **20**, 474–477

Jacobson ER, Gaskin JM and Mansell J (1989b) Chlamydial infection in puff adders (*Bitis arietans*). *Journal of Zoo and Wildlife Medicine* **20**, 364–369

Jacobson ER, Homer B and Adams W (1991) Endocarditis and congestive heart failure in a Burmese python (*Python molurus bivittatus*). *Journal of Zoo and Wildlife Medicine* **22**, 245–248

Jacobson ER and Kollias GV (1986) Adenovirus like infection in a savannah monitor. *Journal of Zoo Animal Medicine* **17**, 149–151

Jacobson ER, Seely JC, Novilla MN and Davidson JP (1979) Heart failure associated with unusual hepatic inclusions in a Deckert's ratsnake. *Journal of Wildlife Diseases* **15**, 75–81

Jensen B, Abe AS, Andrade DV, Nyengaard JR and Wang T (2010a) The heart of the South American rattlesnake, *Crotalus durissus*. *Journal of Morphology* **271**, 1066–1077

Jensen B, Boukens BJD, Postma AV et al. (2012) Identifying the evolutionary building blocks of the cardiac conduction system. *PLoS One* **7**, e44231

Jensen B, Moorman AFM and Wang T (2014) Structure and function of the hearts of lizards and snakes. *Biological Reviews of the Cambridge Philosophical Society* **89(2)**, 302–336

Jensen B, Nielsen JM, Axelsson,M, Löfman C and Wang T (2010b) How the python heart separates pulmonary and systemic blood pressures and blood flows. *Journal of Experimental Biology* **213**, 1611–1617

Jensen B, Nyengaard JR, Pedersen M and Wang T (2010c). Anatomy of the python heart. *Anatomical Science International* **85(4)**, 194–203

Jensen B, van den Berg G, van den Deol R *et al.* (2013a). Development of the hearts of lizards and snakes and perspectives to cardiac evolution. *PLoS One* **8(6)**, e63651

Jensen B and Wang T (2009) Hemodynamic consequences of cardiac malformations in two juvenile ball pythons (*Python regius*). *Journal of Zoo and Wildlife Medicine* **40**, 752–756

Jensen B, Wang T, Christoffels VM and Moorman AFM (2013b) Evolution and development of the building plan of the vertebrate heart. *Biochimica et Biophysica Acta* **1833**, 783–794

Lock B, Heard D, Dunmore D and Ramaiah S (2001) Lymphosarcoma with lymphoid leukaemia in an Aruba island rattlesnake, *Crotalus unicolor. Journal of Herpetological Medicine and Surgery* **11(4)**, 19–23

McCraken H, Hyatt AD and Slocombe RF (1994) Two cases of anemia in reptiles treated with blood transfusions: (1) haemolytic anemia in a diamond python caused by erythrocytic virus (2) nutritional anemia in a bearded dragon. *Proceedings of the Association of Reptilian and Amphibian Veterinarians Annual Conference*, pp. 47–51

Miller DL, Bossart G, Randle K, Decker S and Zorgniotii F (2000) Immunoblastic leukemia in an iguana (*Iguana iguana*). *Proceedings of the American Association of Zoo Veterinarians*, p. 528

Murray MJ (1996) Cardiology and circulation. In: *Reptile Medicine and Surgery, 1st edition*, ed. DR Mader, pp. 95–104. Saunders Elsevier, St Louis, USA

Murray MJ (2006) Cardiopulmonary anatomy and physiology. In: *Reptile Medicine and Surgery, 2nd edition*, ed. DR Mader, pp. 124–134. Saunders Elsevier, St Louis, USA

Obendorf DL, Carson J and McManus TJ (1987) *Vibrio damsela* infection in a stranded leatherback turtle. *Journal of Wildlife Diseases* **23**, 666–668

Oros J, Torrent A, Espinose de los Monteros A *et al.* (2001) Multicentric lymphoblastic lymphoma in a loggerhead sea turtle. *Veterinary Pathology* **38**, 464–467

Pereira ME and Viner TC (2008) Oviduct adenocarcinoma in some species of captive snakes. *Veterinary Pathology* **45**, 693–697

Pereira Y and Pizzi R (2012) Echocardiography of the weird and wonderful: tarantulas, turtles and tigers. *Ultrasound* **20**, 113–116

Pizzi R, Martinez Pereira YM, Rambaud YF *et al.* (2009) Secundum atrial septal defect in a Komodo dragon (*Varanus komodoensis*). *Veterinary Record* **164**, 472–473

Raiti P (2002) Snakes. In: *BSAVA Manual of Exotic Pets, 4th edition*, ed. A Meredith and S Redrobe, pp. 241–256. BSAVA Publications, Gloucester, UK

Ramsay EC, Munson L, Lowenstine L and Fowler ME (1996) A retrospective study of neoplasia in a collection of captive snakes. *Journal of Zoo and Wildlife Medicine* **27(1)**, 28–34

Redrobe SP and Frye FL (2001) Hepatic thrombosis and other pathology associated with severe periodontal disease in the bearded dragon *Pogona vitticeps. Proceedings of the Association of Reptilian and Amphibian Veterinarians Annual Conference*, pp. 217–219

Redrobe SP and Scudamore CL (2000) Ultrasonographic diagnosis of pericardial effusion and atrial dilatation in a spur-thighed tortoise (*Testudo graeca*). *Veterinary Record* **146**, 183–185

Redrobe SP and Wilkinson RJ (2002) Reptile and amphibian anatomy and imaging. In: *BSAVA Manual of Exotic Pets, 4th edn*, ed. A Meredith and S Redrobe, pp. 193–207. BSAVA Publications, Gloucester, UK

Rishniw M and Carmel BP (1999) Atrioventricular valvular insufficiency and congestive heart failure in a carpet python. *Australian Veterinary Journal* **77**, 580–583

Rosenthal K (1994) Chemotherapeutic treatment of a sarcoma in a corn snake. *Proceedings of the Joint Conference of the American Association of Zoo Veterinarians and the Association of Reptile and Amphibian Veterinarians*, p. 46

Rush EM, Donnelly TM and Walberg J (1999) Aneurysm and subsequent cardiopulmonary arrest in a Burmese python (*Python molurus bivittatus*). *Proceedings of the American Association of Zoo Veterinarians*, p. 134–138

Rush EM, Donnelly TM and Walberg J (2001) What's your diagnosis? Cardiopulmonary arrest in a Burmese python: aortic aneurysm. *Laboratory Animals* **30**, 24–27

Saggese MD (2009) Clinical approach to the anemic reptile. *Journal of Exotic Pet Medicine* **18**, 98–111

Schilliger L, Lemberger K, Chai N, Bourgeois A and Charpentier M (2010a) Atherosclerosis associated with pericardial effusion in a central bearded dragon (*Pogona vitticeps*, Ahl. 1926). *Journal of Veterinary Diagnostic Investigation* **22(5)**, 789–792

Schilliger L, Selleri P and Frye FL (2011) Lymphoreticular neoplasm and leukemia in a red-tail boa (*Boa constrictor constrictor*) associated with concurrent inclusion body disease. *Journal of Veterinary Diagnostic Investigation* **23**, 159–162

Schilliger L, Tessier D, Pouchelon JL and Chetboul V (2006) Proposed standardization of the two-dimensional echocardiographic examination in snakes. *Journal of Herpetological Medicine and Surgery* **16**, 90–102

Schilliger L, Trehiou-Sechi E, Petit A *et al.* (2010b) Double valvular insufficiency in a Burmese python (*Python molurus bivittatus*, Linnaeus, 1758) suffering from concomitant bacterial pneumonia. *Journal of Zoo and Wildlife Medicine* **41(4)**, 742–744

Schilliger L, Vanderstylen D, Pietrain J and Chetboul V (2003) Granulomatous myocarditis and coelomic effusion due to *Salmonella enterica arizonae* in a Madagascarian Dumeril's boa (*Acrantophis dumerili*, Jan. 1860). *Journal of Veterinary Cardiology* **5**, 43–45

Schmidt RE (1977) Plasma cell tumour in an East Indian water lizard (*Hydrasaurus amboinensis*). *Journal of Wildlife Diseases* **13**, 47–48

Schmidt RE and Reavill DR (2010) Metastatic chondrosarcoma in a corn snake (*Elaphe guttata*). *Proceedings of the 1st International Conference on Reptile and Amphibian Medicine, Munich, Germany*, p. 147

Schuchman SM and Taylor DO (1970) Arteriosclerosis in an iguana (*Iguana iguana*). *Journal of the American Veterinary Medical Association* **157**, 614–616

Schultze AE, Mason GL and Clyde VL (1999) Lymphosarcoma with leukemic blood profile in a savannah monitor lizard (*Varanus exanthematicus*). *Journal of Zoo and Wildlife Medicine* **30**, 158–164

Schumacher J, Jacobson ER, Burns R and Tramontin RR (1994) Adenovirus-like infection in two rosy boas (*Lichanura trivirgata*). *Journal of Zoo and Wildlife Medicine* **25**, 461–465

Sedgwick CJ (1991) Allometrically scaling the data base for vital sign assessment used in general anaesthesia of zoological species. *Proceedings of the American Association of Zoo Veterinarians*, pp. 360–369

Selleri P and Di Girolamo N (2012) Cardiac tamponade following cardiocentesis in a cardiopathic boa constrictor imperator (*Boa constrictor imperator*). *Journal of Small Animal Practice* **53(8)**, 487

Silldorff EP and Stephens GA (1992) Effects of converting enzyme inhibition and alpha receptor blockade on the angiotensin pressor response in the American alligator. *General and Comparative Endocrinology* **87(1)**, 134–140

Slay C, Enok S, Hicks J and Wang T (2014) Reduction of blood oxygen levels enhances postprandial cardiac hypertrophy in Burmese python (*Python bivittatus*). *Journal of Experimental Biology* **217(10)**, 1784–1789

Snyder PS, Shaw NG and Heard DJ (1999) Two-dimensional echocardiographic anatomy of the snake heart (*Python molurus bivittatus*). *Veterinary Radiology and Ultrasound* **40**, 66–72

Stein G (1996) Reptile and amphibian formulary. In: *Reptile Medicine and Surgery*, ed. DR Mader, pp. 465–472. WB Saunders, Philadelphia, USA

Stephens CA and Robertson FM (1985) Renal responses to diuretics in the turtle. *Journal of Comparative Physiology* **155**, 387–393

Stumpel JB, Del-Pozo J, French A and Eatwell K (2012) Cardiac hemangioma in a corn snake (*Pantherophis guttatus*). *Journal of Zoo and Wildlife Medicine* **43**, 360–366

Sweet C, Linnetz E, Golden E and Mayer J (2009) What is your diagnosis? *Journal of the American Veterinary Medical Association* **234(10)**, 1259–1260

Telford SR (1984) Hemoparasites of reptiles In: *Diseases of Reptiles and Amphibians*, ed. GL Hoff, FL Frye and ER Jacobson, pp. 385–517. Plenum Press, NY, USA

Telford SR and Jacobson ER (1993) Lizard erythrocytic virus in East African chameleons. *Journal of Wildlife Diseases* **29**, 57–63

Tocidlowski ME, McNamara PL and Wojcieszyn JW (2001) Myelogenous leukaemia in a bearded dragon (*Acanthodraco vitticeps*). *Journal of Zoo and Wildlife Medicine* **32**, 90–95

Valentinuzzi ME (1969) Electrophysiology and mechanics of the snake heartbeat. PhD Dissertation: Bayler College of Medicine, Houston, Texas

Wagner A (1989) Clinical challenge case number one. *Journal of Zoo and Wildlife Medicine* **20**, 238–239

Willette MM, Garner MM and Drew M (2001) Chemotherapeutic treatment of lymphoma in a king cobra (*Ophiophagus hannah*). *Proceedings of the Joint Conference of the American Association of Zoo Veterinarians and the Association of Reptile and Amphibian Veterinarians*, pp. 20–24

Williams DL (1992) Cardiovascular system. In: *BSAVA Manual of Reptiles*, ed. PH Beynon, MPC Lawton and JE Cooper, pp. 80–87. BSAVA, Cheltenham, UK

Wyneken J (2009) Normal reptile heart morphology and function. *Veterinary Clinics of North America: Exotic Animal Practice* **12**, 51–63

Zwart P and Harshbarger JC (1972) Hematopoietic neoplasms in lizards: report of a typical case in *Hydrasaurus ambinensis* and of a probable case in *Varanus salvator. International Journal of Cancer* **9**, 548

Chapter 20

Urogenital system

Jay D. Johnson

The urogenital system of reptiles performs similar functions to that of other vertebrates, but there are significant anatomical and physiological differences. Understanding these differences and the abnormalities that can occur is essential for proper management of reptilian patients with urogenital disorders.

Renal system

Reptiles have paired metanephric kidneys. Their retroperitoneal location varies in different groups:

- In chelonians the kidneys are adherent to the inner carapace, craniodorsal to the pelvis
- In monitors and crocodilians the kidneys are located in the dorsocaudal coelomic cavity. The left kidney is larger than the right in crocodilians
- In most lizards the kidneys are in the dorsal aspect of the pelvic canal posterior to the iliac crest
- In snakes the kidneys occur in the caudal third of the coelomic cavity, with the right kidney slightly cranial to the left.

Anatomy and physiology

Most reptilian nephrons consist of a glomerulus, glomerular tuft of coiled capillaries, short neck piece, proximal convoluted tubule and distal collecting tubule that empties into the ureter-like mesonephric duct. The kidneys are often lobulated, with separate mesonephric ducts draining each lobule. Reptiles lack a urine-concentrating loop of Henle. In some males a sexual segment is present in the distal tubule where seminal fluids are produced and stored.

Urine passes from the mesonephric ducts into the urodeum and is then passed into the bladder, if present, or cranially into the colon. Water reabsorption and changes in electrolyte composition occur in the bladder or colon. Much less water is required for the renal excretion of uric acid in comparison to urea, thus decreasing water loss through the kidneys.

Reptiles are primarily uricotelic, with uric acid being the predominant nitrogenous waste product produced by the liver from the catabolism of proteins. Uric acid may comprise 80–90% of the total nitrogen excretion in terrestrial reptiles. Exceptions to this are in marine, aquatic and many semiaquatic species, where urea or ammonia is the primary end product formed.

Uric acid is secreted into the renal tubules and does not reflect glomerular filtration. Therefore, the clinician must realize that significant glomerular disease can be present without elevation in blood uric acid levels. Uric acid levels are lower in fasting reptiles and rise postprandially. Elevations in uric acid can occur with dehydration. Hyperuricaemia is also associated with gout and renal tubular disease. Uric acid levels of greater than 1190 μmol/l (20 mg/dl) are often seen with these two conditions. It is likely that significant functional kidney tissue must be damaged for blood uric acid levels to rise, thus, it is not sensitive for early diagnosis.

The lack of a loop of Henle in the nephron means that reptiles are unable to produce hypertonic urine and results in the inability to excrete excess electrolytes from the blood without further water loss. Many reptiles have evolved nasal salt glands that are used to excrete excess electrolyte loads. Reptiles with salt glands include many desert species (e.g. chuckwalla, desert iguana, Galapagos land iguana), arboreal tropical forest species (e.g. green iguana) and other arid-adapted iguanids. The only chelonians that have evolved with salt glands are those in marine environments, including loggerhead and other marine turtles, and diamondback terrapins.

Blood supply

Blood arrives from renal arteries and afferent renal portal veins. After passing through the capillary beds of the kidneys, blood leaves via the efferent renal veins, which then empty into the ascending vena cava. Blood may also be shunted from the afferent renal vein to mesenteric veins.

The renal portal system: The renal portal system (RPS) has been described differently by several authors. Holtz (1999) provides a good anatomical review of the RPS and discussion of its significance to the clinician. Simplistically, some blood from the caudal body has the potential to enter the kidneys directly, prior to circulating back to the heart. The blood that enters the kidneys via the RPS is used to perfuse the tubules and does not undergo glomerular filtration. Since reptiles cannot produce hypertonic urine, glomerular filtration must decrease to reduce water loss. When blood flow through the glomerulus decreases or ceases, the RPS continues to provide blood supply to the tubules, preventing ischaemic necrosis.

Drug effects and excretion

Some veterinary surgeons (veterinarians) have expressed concerns over administration of injectable medications in the caudal half of the body and the potential for nephro-toxicity or increased excretion owing to the RPS. Drugs excreted by glomerular filtration (i.e. aminoglycosides and sulphonamides) are likely *not* to have greater toxic effects on the kidney or increased excretion if injected in the caudal half of the body. Drugs with potential tubular toxic effects (i.e. quinolones, cephalosporins and penicillins) should be injected into the caudal half of the body with caution in the dehydrated patient. It is unlikely that the RPS has any significant effect on drug kinetics (Beck *et al.*, 1995; Holtz *et al.*, 1997, 2003).

Diseases

Inflammation of the nephron and/or surrounding tissues can occur owing to a variety of conditions in the reptilian patient. Infectious, parasitic, inflammatory, neoplastic and toxic damaging conditions can all occur. Glomerulonephritis, interstitial nephritis and tubulonephritis can occur as primary or secondary processes. Nephritis can occur secondary to abscesses, sepsis or chronic inflammatory diseases. The location of the damage to the nephrons can lead to differences in diagnostic abnormalities encountered.

Chronic clinical or subclinical dehydration may lead directly to renal damage or may exacerbate other causes of renal disease. Damage from nephrotoxic drugs, such as aminoglycosides and sulphur-containing antibiotics, can occur, especially if used while the patient is dehydrated. Dehydrated lethargic patients with infected lesions or abscesses should be managed for probable secondary glomerulonephritis. Vascular abnormalities decreasing perfusion or thromboemboli may cause damage to nephrons and lead to later renal failure.

Myolytic diseases and other toxins may also cause renal disease. Renal amyloidosis is relatively common. Amyloidosis occurring in reptiles is most likely a second-ary process due to chronic infection or inflammation.

Severe renal disease may occur in chelonians due to *Hexamita* spp. infections. *Entamoeba invadens*, coccidia and other protozoans can infect the kidneys. Trematodes also may be found in the kidneys. Identification of parasites that are known to infect the kidneys in faeces or urine may be useful in diagnosis. Renal biopsies are the only way to confirm the underlying pathology of the renal disease.

Diagnosis

Diagnosis of renal disease based solely on physical exam-ination is often not possible.

History and clinical signs: Abnormalities warranting evaluation of the kidneys as a cause for illness include:

- Excessive dietary protein for the species
- Lack of, or excessive, supplementation with vitamins and minerals
- Husbandry practices allowing for chronic subclinical or clinical dehydration
- Concurrent abscesses, infections and inflammatory conditions
- Geriatric patients
- Ingestion of toxic plants or other items
- Exposure to excessive heat (tortoises flipped on their backs for prolonged periods in the sun or under heat lamps).

Common presenting signs include:

- Lethargy and weakness
- Hyporexia or anorexia

- Weight loss
- Dehydration (sunken eyes, thickened saliva, increased skin turgor in some) (Figure 20.1).

In some lizards, enlargement of the kidneys can be palpated in the caudal coelomic cavity or via digital cloacal palpation (Figure 20.2). Dyschezia may occur if significant enlargement of the kidneys occurs within the pelvis. Observable polydipsia and polyuria are usually lacking in reptiles with renal disease. This is to be expected, since the kidneys do not concentrate urine. Polyuria is likely only a secondary process to polydipsia. Ascites and oedema are the most common presenting problems in aquatic reptiles with renal disease. Muscle tremors of the limbs may be seen in lizards. Uraemic encephalopathy may also occur.

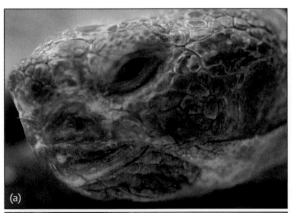
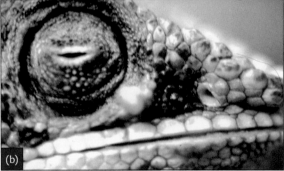

20.1 Sunken eyes in (a) a desert tortoise and (b) a chameleon, due to dehydration associated with renal disease.

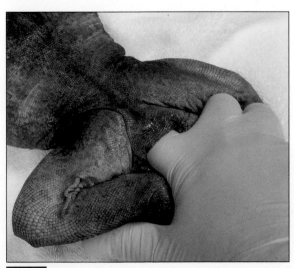

20.2 Cloacal palpation of the kidneys of a rhinoceros iguana.

Laboratory tests: A complete blood count and plasma biochemical profile should be performed as part of the work-up of the ill reptile patient (Figure 20.3). It should be noted that red and white blood cell counts, plasma blood urea nitrogen (BUN), creatinine, potassium and uric acid levels are not consistently altered with renal diseases in reptiles.

The most frequently observed abnormality is the elevation of plasma phosphorus. When phosphorus levels are elevated above those of calcium or are greater than 3.2 mmol/l (10 mg/dl), and the diet does not contain excess phosphorus, renal disease and renal secondary hyperparathyroidism should be considered. Mild hyperuricaemia can occur with dehydration, seasonal anorexia and catabolism, and seasonal foraging on higher-protein new growth of plants (up to 892 μmol/l, or 15 mg/dl; 1190 μmol/l or 20 mg/dl in some cases). Renal disease (or gout) should be suspected when significant hyperuricaemia (>1190 μmol/l, or 20 mg/dl) is present in the anorexic patient. Calcium is often normal or elevated in acute renal disease and more often decreased with chronic renal disease. Elevations in potassium occur most frequently with acute renal disease.

If leucocytosis is present, infectious conditions should be pursued. The presence of a non-regenerative anaemia is often associated with a chronic disease process. BUN is usually low owing to the uricotelic physiology of most reptiles. BUN may become elevated in some reptiles, especially those from desert environments, as a method of elevating plasma osmolality and thereby decreasing water loss (Jacobsen *et al.*, 1990). BUN does not appear to be elevated with renal disease in aquatic and semi-aquatic species.

Plasma uric acid values >2974 μmol/l (50 mg/dl) and phosphorus values >5.2 mmol/l (16 mg/dl) are often associated with end-stage renal failure and indicate a poor prognosis.

Parameter	Significance of results
Phosphorus	Most commonly elevated test with renal disease. Plasma levels higher than those of calcium and greater than 8–10 mg/dl are suggestive of renal disease
Uric acid	Mild hyperuricaemia can occur with dehydration (usually up to 15 mg/dl and in severe cases 20 mg/dl). Elevations occur postprandially (up to 20 mg/dl in some species), with renal tubular damage and with gout (20 mg/dl and higher)
Blood urea nitrogen (BUN)	Not sensitive for renal disease in species that produce uric acid. May be elevated, especially in desert reptiles, as a method of elevating plasma osmolality and decreasing water loss. Does not appear to be elevated with renal disease in aquatic and semiaquatic species. May increase with dehydration or anorexia
Creatinine	Not sensitive for renal disease
Calcium	May be increased or normal with acute renal disease. Often decreased in chronic renal disease
Potassium	May be elevated with renal disease and decreased with anorexia
Sodium and chloride	May be elevated owing to dehydration
Packed cell volume (PCV)	A non-regenerative anaemia may be associated with a chronic disease process
White blood cell count (WBC)	Leucocytosis may occur with infection or inflammation

20.3 Haematology and biochemistry results associated with renal diseases.

Urinalysis: The urine of reptiles is usually clear to pale yellow. Darker amber colours can result from diet and dehydration. Green discoloration may be indicative of biliverdin pigments in the urine secondary to liver disease or haemolysis.

Urine specific gravity (SG) can be affected by postrenal reabsorption of water in the bladder, colon or cloaca. Increases in urine SG may be seen with dehydration and anorexia. In herbivorous reptiles, as in most other herbivores, urine is normally alkaline. Shifts towards acidic urine production occur with anorexia, brumation/hibernation, improper diet and illness. Proteinuria, glycosuria and changes in urine pH may be seen with renal disease.

Uric acid crystals are normally present in the urine. Increased numbers of red blood cells and leucocytes are indicative of renal disease or cystitis. Casts may be found in the sediment when there is renal disease. Protozoan or other parasites present in the urine may be because of contamination from the faeces or may be indicative of renal parasitic infections. Urinary and faecal examination should be performed to look for parasites that can cause renal disease. Since urine is either stored in the cloaca or passed from the cloaca into the bladder, bacterial contamination from faeces is normal. However, heavy growth of a singular bacterial isolate from a urine culture may be indicative of disease. Figure 20.4 outlines urine parameters and interpretation of results.

Parameter	Normal values	Significance of results
Colour	Clear to yellow or amber	Green colour may indicate biliverdin from liver disease or haemolysis
Specific gravity	1.003–1.014	May be slightly elevated with dehydration and anorexia
pH	Alkaline in herbivores; usually acidic in others	Becomes acidic in herbivores with anorexia, brumation/ hibernation, illness or improper diet
Protein	Trace	Increased in renal disease
Glucose	Variable	More consistently present in renal disease
Renal epithelial cells	Few	Increased in renal disease
Renal casts	Absent	Indicative of renal disease
Red and white blood cells	Few	Increase indicates renal disease or cystitis. May get false positive results with commercial test strips. Confirm results with presence in sediment
Parasites	Absent	May be due to contamination from faeces or may indicate renal parasitism. Some parasites cause severe renal disease: *Hexamita* organisms are identified microscopically – they are small, oval and move rapidly in one direction, often in a straight or curved line
Crystals	Urates normal	Other crystals may form when disease is present
Bacteria	Bacterial contamination from faeces is normal	A heavy growth of a single bacterial isolate from a urine culture may be indicative of disease

20.4 Urinalysis results and their significance.

It is very important that the practitioner be able to differentiate *Hexamita* spp. from other flagellated protozoan parasites commonly present. *Hexamita* spp. are relatively small oblong flagellated protozoans with all the flagella at one end, causing rapid unidirectional motion.

Ultrasonography. Ultrasound examination of the kidneys may be beneficial in assessing size, shape and changes in echogenicity associated with renal abnormalities (see Chapter 9).

Biopsy: Renal biopsy is often needed for definitive diagnosis of the cause of the renal disease. Biopsies can be performed surgically, with the aid of ultrasonography or endoscopic techniques, or via percutaneous routes in some species (see Chapters 10 and 13). Biopsy samples should be submitted for both histopathology and microbiology.

Treatment

It is important, where possible, to determine whether the disease is acute or chronic. Most owners do not recognize the signs of chronic renal disease and patients are often presented for an acute failure emergency secondary to chronic disease. Treatment of acute and chronic renal disease is summarized in Figures 20.5 and 20.6.

- Identify and eliminate underlying cause when able
- Provide aggressive parenteral fluid therapy (20–40 ml/kg/day)
- Initiate broad-spectrum antibiotic therapy if bacterial disease suspected
- Provide proper species-specific thermal environment for recovery
- Provide nutritional support
- Consider allopurinol therapy if hyperuricaemia present

20.5 Treatment of acute renal disease.

- Identify and eliminate underlying cause when able
- Ensure ongoing good hydration with frequent soaking, misting, and increased cage or hiding-area humidity
- Administer oral phosphate binders (aluminium hydroxide) if hyperphosphataemia present
- Feed reduced amounts of high-quality protein foods
- Feed food items low in phosphorous
- Provide proper species-specific husbandry and thermoregulation ability
- Consider allopurinol therapy if hyperuricaemia is present

20.6 Treatment of chronic renal disease.

Fluid therapy: Appropriate fluid therapy should be initiated based on the patient's hydration and electrolyte status (Case 1). Plasma potassium and protein levels should ideally be determined prior to initiating fluid therapy. Reptile body-water distribution differs from that of mammals, and reptiles' plasma has been shown to vary in isotonicity between species (Dallwig *et al.*, 2010; Guzman *et al.*, 2011; Naverez *et al.*, 2012). Some have theorized which fluids would be beneficial, for a variety of reasons (Prezant and Jarchow, 1997; Rudloff, 2005). Fluids containing potassium should be used cautiously in anorexic patients and those with hyperkalemia or hypoproteinemia to prevent catabolism. No research so far has been performed to show which fluids or combinations of fluids are best for reptiles.

Reptiles are not as sensitive to electrolyte and pH disturbances as mammals. Short-term use of most buffered mixed-electrolyte and 0.9% saline replacement solutions to correct hypovolaemia are safe and effective. Routes of administration initially should include intravenous, intraosseous, intracoelomic (i.c.) or epicoelomic (e.c.) until the patient is stabilized. Initial fluid therapy rates should be 20–40 ml/kg/day. Close attention should be paid to the patient's plasma protein/albumin levels prior to initiation of infusion of large amounts of fluids. Weight and packed cell volume (PCV) should be monitored closely to assess patient hydration. Over-hydration should be avoided.

Soaking in shallow water baths can provide oral and cloacal intake, often sufficient for non-critical patients.

Drug treatment: Empirical broad-spectrum antibiotic therapy (e.g. ceftazidime 20–30 mg/kg i.m. q24–72h, depending on species) should be initiated if septic causes are suspected. Continuing antibiotic therapy should be based on culture and sensitivity of biopsied renal tissue, blood cultures or wounds thought to be the source of secondary bacterial nephritis (when possible). Antibiotics that are potentially nephrotoxic should be avoided.

If uric acid levels are significantly elevated, the use of allopurinol (25–50 mg/kg orally q24–72h) may be beneficial in decreasing production of uric acid by the liver. Nutritional support should be initiated gradually, using reduced high-quality protein and phosphorus diets.

Oedema associated with renal failure in aquatic reptiles can sometimes be managed by bathing in hypertonic solutions. Diuretics that work in the loop of Henle (e.g. furosemide) may not have any effect on reptiles unless working in other areas of the body. Some evidence has been put forward to suggest that they can work on sodium and chloride pumps found in the urinary bladder lining in those species possessing a urinary bladder, or in the terminal rectum where water may be reabsorbed after reflux from the cloaca (Ehrenspeck and Voner, 1985; Badia *et al.*, 1987). Methylated xanthines (aminophylline 10 mg/kg i.m. per required need (prn); theophylline 5 mg/kg i.m. prn) can often be used successfully in reptiles for diuresis. Their diuretic effect may be partly due to their stimulatory effect on cardiac function, increased renal blood flow and increased glomerular filtration rate. The major diuretic effect of these compounds is apparently due to increased rates of excretion of sodium and chloride ions by renal tubules.

If *Hexamita* spp. are found in urine or faeces of ill chelonians, treatment for both renal disease and the parasite should be given. Metronidazole (100 mg/kg orally q10d until samples are negative), a combination of metronidazole and fenbendazole (50 mg/kg orally q10d), or ronidazole (10 mg/kg orally q24h x 10 days) should be initiated. Treatment should be continued until faecal samples are negative for the parasite.

Thorough cleaning of the ventral plastron and vent area, in addition to disinfection of the enclosure with dilute sodium hypochlorite or other solutions that destroy protozoal cysts, should be performed routinely during treatment to prevent reinfection from cysts in the environment. Recovered chelonians should be kept in quarantine for 6–12 months and several faecal samples evaluated for the presence of the organism prior to exposure to other chelonians. At least two negative samples should be obtained prior to exposure to other chelonians.

Supportive care: If supportive care is provided for long enough for the kidneys to heal and resume function, complete recoveries can occur. Nutritional support should be initiated gradually for patients that have been anorexic. Anorexic or hyporexic patients my need assisted feeding depending on the duration of anorexia/hyporexia and the species. Oesophagostomy tube placement may facilitate better management in some chelonians. Moderately reduced amounts of increased-quality protein food items should be fed. Vitamin B supplementation may be helpful for appetite stimulation.

Oral phosphorus binders (e.g. aluminium hydroxide 1.0 ml/kg orally q24h) may be administered with nutritional support or voluntary diet to help reduce phosphorus absorption. This is likely to be more effective in treating hyperphosphataemia associated with diet, but may help to lessen the load associated with lack of renal excretion. High-quality protein food items low in phosphorus should be used. Treatment of hypocalcaemia should be initiated (e.g. calcium glubionate 23 mg/kg orally q24h) after hyperphosphataemia has been corrected. Supplementation of calcium and vitamin D3 in the face of hyperphosphataemia may lead to metastatic mineralization and worsening of the renal disease.

If chronic renal disease occurs, either in its own right or secondary to an acute renal disease episode, long-term therapy is likely to be needed. Management at home with frequent soaking in water baths should be continued for several weeks after acute disease, and long term if chronic disease is present.

Proper husbandry, including the ability for thermoregulation and improved humidity for the species, needs to be provided.

Follow-up: Critically ill patients hospitalized and treated with intravenous or intraosseous fluids should have follow-up plasma biochemistry performed after 48–72 hours to assess for improvement or progression of previously abnormal results.

Euthanasia should be considered if there is no improvement in clinical signs or biochemical abnormalities. Patients treated on an outpatient basis should have follow-up testing on a 2–3-week basis until normal. It may take 4–6 weeks, or longer, for problems to completely resolve in some cases. It is important to recheck phosphorus values regularly so as to prevent iatrogenic hypophosphataemia.

If chronic renal failure persists, lifelong treatment will be necessary.

Renal secondary hyperparathyroidism

Parathyroid hormone (PTH) is produced by the parathyroid glands in response to low blood calcium concentrations. In mammals, PTH maintains blood calcium levels by increasing calcium mobilization from the bone, increasing renal tubular reabsorption and stimulating hydroxylation of vitamin D3 to its active form (1,25-dihydroxycholecalciferol). Rising active vitamin D3 levels have an inhibitory effect on PTH production. Chronic renal disease frequently leads to decreased elimination of phosphorus via glomerular filtration. The hyperphosphataemia that occurs has a negative effect on hydroxylase activity. Decreased active vitamin D3 production causes decreased intestinal calcium absorption. Decreased calcium absorption leads to lower blood calcium levels which, in turn, stimulate PTH production. Decreased active vitamin D3 also decreases the inhibitory feedback on PTH production. Both of these add to an ongoing overproduction of PTH.

The chronic effects of hyperparathyroidism lead to continued osteoclastic activity in the bone. As the osteomalacia progresses, previously calcified bone is replaced by fibrous connective tissue (fibrous osteodystrophy). Clinically this appears as swollen bones, with the extremities and mandible being most noticeable in lizards. In chelonians, softening of the carapace and plastron may occur. In cases where the plasma levels of calcium and phosphorus become high enough for precipitation to occur and soft-tissue mineralization inhibitors fail, metastatic mineralization of tissues occurs. These tissues include the kidneys, major arteries, heart, pulmonary vasculature and gastric mucosa. Large amounts deposited in the kidneys add to further renal damage. This disease is very similar to nutritional secondary hyperparathyroidism, and differentiation between the two diseases can be difficult when diet and husbandry are inappropriate. Treatment is as for chronic renal disease.

Case 1

History
A 2–3-year-old male Saharan uromastyx presented for acute onset anorexia, lethargy, and weakness (Figure 20.7).

Physical examination
The patient was underweight, had slightly sunken eyes and thickened saliva.

Diagnostic testing
There was a leucocytosis of 12,000 white blood cells with 8600 heterophils, the rest of the complete blood count was normal. Phosphorus was 12.6 mg/dl. Calcium was 11.8 mg/dl. Sodium and chloride may have been slightly elevated depending on normal ranges used. The rest of the chemistry was normal.

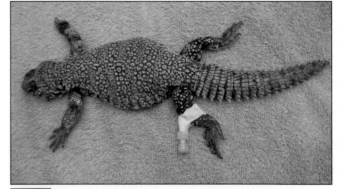

20.7 Uromastyx with an intraosseous catheter fitted.

Assessment
A presumptive diagnosis of pyelonephritis or infection with secondary nephritis was made.

Treatment
The patient was initially treated with intraosseous fluids and parenteral antibiotics. After 3 days, fluid therapy was changed to daily soaking. Judicious nutritional support was initiated with Oxbow Critical Care fine grind 5–10 ml/kg orally q72 (in the author's experience, more than this will cause problems for most uromastyx).

Follow-up
The patient was gaining weight, more alert and active, and starting to eat some food on its own after 2 weeks. Recheck labwork showed a normal white blood cell count and phosphorus of 8.6 mg/dl. At 4 weeks labwork was normal and the patient was back to normal.

Gout

Gout, although not a primary renal disease, may be exacerbated by improper functioning of the kidneys or may cause renal damage when uric acid crystals are deposited into the renal tissues.

The end product of protein metabolism by the liver of most reptiles is uric acid. Uric acid is cleared from the blood through renal tubular excretion. When uric acid levels become elevated in the blood or other bodily fluids, the uric acid may crystallize to form insoluble precipitates that are deposited in tissues of the body (Figure 20.8). Crystallization most frequently occurs in or around the joints, but can also occur in the viscera and in subcutaneous tissues. White nodular aggregates of crystals, called tophi, are often grossly visible. Swelling and inflammation often surrounds the tophi. Renal disease, dehydration and excessive protein in the diet may contribute to the disease.

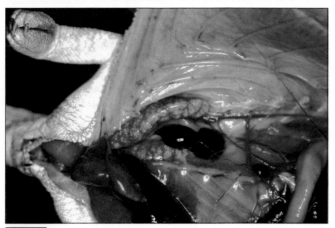

20.8 Visceral gout with tophi in the kidneys of a chameleon.

Diagnosis: This is based on clinical examination and history, and is further supported by plasma uric acid levels, cytology, radiography and endoscopy. Diet and hydration status need to be closely evaluated to rule out as causes for hyperuricaemia. Plasma uric acid is not always elevated in patients with gout. Cytology of affected joints often reveals uric acid crystals in the synovial fluid. Radiographs may reveal lesions in or around the joint. Definitive diagnosis is based on the histological finding of uric acid crystals or tophi within the affected tissue. Differentiation of gout should be made from the similar gross white calcified tissue appearance of dystrophic and metastatic mineralization.

Treatment: Allopurinol (25–50 mg/kg orally q24–72h) is often effective for managing the condition. Allopurinol inhibits the enzyme xanthine oxidase, decreasing degradation of xanthine to uric acid. Instead of uric acid, xanthine and hypoxanthine are eliminated via the kidneys. More water is lost in the elimination of these products in comparison to uric acid. Therefore, if allopurinol therapy is given, fluid therapy or frequent soaking should be initiated to prevent dehydration. In cases where joints are severely affected, surgery to remove tophi and flush the joint may provide some benefit. The use of corticosteroids (e.g. methylprednisolone 2.0 mg/kg i.m. q4–6wk prn) or non-steroidal anti-inflammatory drugs (NSAIDs) may provide some relief from inflammation and pain. Diets of high quality protein, with appropriate levels for the species, should be fed.

Urinary bladder

A urinary bladder exists in chelonians and in some lizards. Ureters empty into the urodeum of the cloaca; thus, urine is passed first into the urodeum and then into the bladder.

Anatomy and physiology

The urinary bladder arises from the ventral aspect of the cloaca and is connected to the urodeum via a short urethra. There is a main body to the bladder and, in some species, paired accessory bladders. In chelonians the bladder is often large and bilobed. Fluid retained in the bladder predominantly originates from the cloaca and is therefore not sterile. For urinalysis parameters and their interpretation, see Figure 20.4.

The urinary bladder mucosa is composed of smooth muscle and connective tissue and is supplied with many capillaries and lymphatics. It is likely that the vascular mucosa allows for significant water and electrolyte resorption to occur.

The desert tortoise and possibly other species cope with potassium, sodium and ammonium loads by precipitating them with uric acid. When tortoises ingest high levels of potassium without increasing protein intake, both the amounts of urate precipitated in the bladder and the concentration of potassium in these precipitates increase (Oftedal *et al.*, 1994). By storing these precipitates in the bladder and voiding them infrequently, tortoises are able to excrete potassium with minimal water loss. Desert tortoises have also been shown selectively to avoid diets high in potassium and low in protein when given the option (Oftedal *et al.*, 1995). Urea is produced in tortoises during periods of fasting and dehydration and contributes to increasing blood osmolarity. This increase in osmolarity helps to offset the rising osmolarity of urine in the bladder, preventing net flux of water from the blood into the bladder.

Medical conditions

Cystic calculi

Concretions of urates may occur in the bladders of chelonians and lizards. Small accumulations are normal and passed frequently. Larger more dense calculi may develop with time that cannot be passed through the urethra or anus/vent. Cystic calculi may form owing to dehydration, excess protein or potassium in the diet, decreased bladder emptying, or other conditions. Occasionally, eggs can pass through the urethra from the cloaca into the bladder of chelonians. These eggs often serve as a nidus where urates are deposited, and eventually grow into larger calculi. Over time calculi can grow to very large sizes, sometimes filling the entire bladder.

Clinical signs: Most reptiles with smaller calculi show no associated clinical signs. As 'stones' grow larger, haematuria; hindlimb dysfunction; tenesmus; audible 'grunting' noises; penile prolapse; and problems with passing eggs, urine or faeces may occur. In severe cases left untreated, bladder necrosis and death may occur. Some calculi may be passed through the urethra into the cloaca. Smaller calculi are usually voided, but large calculi can obstruct the vent.

Diagnosis: This is based on coelomic palpation of calculi and on radiography (Figure 20.9). In chelonians, coelomic palpation can be performed through the prefemoral fossae while tilting them from side to side.

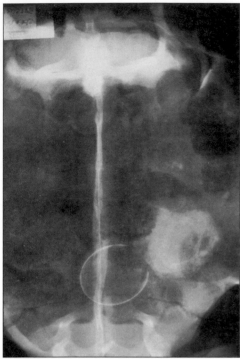

20.9 Radiograph of a cystic calculus causing eggshell fracture and dystocia in a desert tortoise.
(Courtesy of Dr Jim Jarchow)

Treatment: Coeliotomy and cystotomy are required to remove stones. In chelonians, cystotomy via marsupialization of the bladder through the prefemoral fossa can be used to remove most, if not all, calculi. Large calculi that do not fit through the marsupialization can usually be fragmented and removed in smaller pieces. The calculi should be grasped with sponge forceps and positioned in the opening of the marsupialization. A drill can be used to create multiple holes in the calculi. Carmalts or other heavy-duty forceps can then be used to fragment the calculi. Plastron osteotomy may be required for cystotomy access to remove larger stones that cannot be fragmented, or if bladder laceration occurs during surgery in chelonians. Calculi present in the cloaca can usually be removed with sedation and the use of forceps to fragment the calculi.

Male reproductive tract

Anatomy and physiology

Male reptiles, excluding tuataras, have paired testes and either a single penis or paired hemipenes. The testes are made up of interstitial cells, seminiferous tubules and blood vessels, encapsulated in connective tissue.

- In chelonians the testes are round to oval, smooth, variable in colour and located in the dorsal medial coelomic cavity.
- In snakes and lizards the testes are located cranial to the kidney(s).
- In crocodilians and chelonians the testes are attached to the coelomic membrane overlying the kidneys.

Sperm pass from the testes via efferent ductules into the epididymis. No epididymides are present in snakes. Sperm pass from the epididymis (if present) into the ductus deferens, which empties into the cloaca at the base of the copulatory organ.

- Chelonians and crocodilians have a single penis (phallus), which arises from the cranial ventral aspect of the cloaca.
- Snakes and lizards have paired hemipenes, which are inverted caudally into the base of the tail. Each hemipenis is held in an inverted resting position by a retractor muscle.

The penis/hemipenis is composed of a pair of corpora cavernosa, which fill with blood to cause erection. When erect, a dorsal groove, the sulcus spermaticus, forms a passage for sperm and fluids. The reptilian penis or hemipenis functions only as a copulatory organ. The ureters and urethra empty into the cloaca.

Medical conditions
Penile prolapse (paraphimosis)

The penis/hemipenis is everted and exteriorized for copulation. It may become prolapsed outside of its normal inverted position in the tail of snakes and lizards, or not retracted back inside the cloaca of chelonians (Figure 20.10). When the penis/hemipenis experiences prolonged periods outside of its normal position, the mucous membranes begin to desiccate and physical trauma usually occurs. Eventually the penis/hemipenis becomes necrotic.

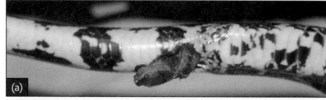

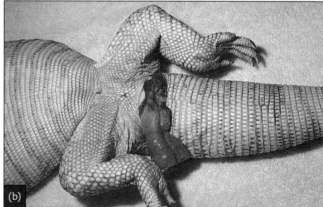

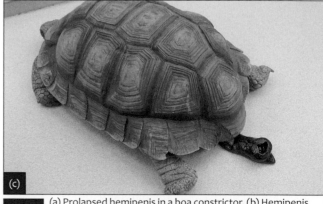

20.10 (a) Prolapsed hemipenis in a boa constrictor. (b) Hemipenis prolapse in a monitor lizard. (c) Prolapsed penis in a Chaco tortoise.
(a, Courtesy of Paul Raiti; b, Courtesy of Dr Fredric L Frye)

Treatment: Male copulatory organs with superficial necrosis, inflammation, trauma and penile retractor muscle fatigue can often be replaced under anaesthesia or sedation into their normal position and allowed to heal. Swelling of penile tissue can be reduced with hypertonic dextrose or saline solutions. The phallus/hemipenis should then be lubricated with an antibiotic plus steroid ointment and manipulated back into its normal position. Tacking sutures may be placed on either side of the cloaca in chelonians or directly over the hemipenis opening in snakes and lizards to retain the organ in its normal position. Sutures should be removed after 14 days in chelonians and after 14–21 days in snakes and lizards. Systemic antibiotic therapy should be initiated if superficial necrosis or traumatic lesions are present. If the penis re-prolapses after suture removal, it can be reduced and sutures replaced and left in longer, or amputated.

Necrotic phallus/hemipenes and complete paresis of the retractor muscles warrant amputation (Case 2). Hemipenis/phallus amputation is performed in most cases with the use of local anaesthetic only. A clamp is placed across the base of the organ. One to two transfixing ligatures with absorbable suture material are placed and the organ is transected distal to the ligation.

Hemipenal plugs

The sulci created by the inverted hemipenes of lizards and snakes can sometimes fill with firm caseous or waxy-appearing plugs. The aetiology of the plug formation is unknown, but it is likely that they are accumulations of desquamated epithelial cells along with other debris or exudates that enter into the sulcus. The plugs prevent the ability of the penis to evaginate and become erect. The plugs can also become large and appear to cause discomfort in some reptiles. On rare occasions abscessation can occur.

Plugs can be visualized by viewing the openings of the hemipenes in the caudal vent. Plugs can often be grasped with forceps and removed with gentle traction. Additional external pressure and manipulation at the caudal aspect of the hemipenal bulge may be required in some cases to remove the plug. If penile tissue bleeds, appears inflamed or becomes traumatized, infusion of the sulci with antibiotic cream or ointment may be beneficial.

Female reproductive tract

Anatomy and physiology

The female reproductive tract has paired ovaries and oviducts. Most reptiles lay eggs (oviparous) but some are live-bearing (viviparous and ovoviviparous) (see Chapter 5).

- The ovaries of chelonians, lizards and crocodilians are attached to the coelomic membrane at the level of, or cranial to, the kidneys.
- In snakes, the ovaries lie in the caudal half of the coelomic cavity, between the gall bladder and kidneys.

The ovaries comprise germinal cells, epithelial cells, connective tissue, nerves and blood vessels, encased in an elastic tunic. The gross appearance of ovaries varies depending on the stage of oogenesis. Inactive ovaries appear as a sheet of connective tissue with small granular nodules. Active ovaries appear as large clusters of vitellogenic follicles. Mature follicles tend to cluster along the cranial aspect, especially in chelonian ovaries. Corpora lutea and corpora albicans occur as in other vertebrates.

The mesotubarium connects the ovary to the oviduct. The oviduct lies lateral to the ovary and extends cranially around it, with the funnel-like ostium opening on the craniomedial aspect. The ostium receives the ovulated follicles. The oviducts of reptiles have five regions: the ostium, aglandular segment, magnum, shell gland (oviparous reptiles) and vagina. The caudal vaginal end of each oviduct empties into the urodeum of the cloaca. The oviducts become much more muscular and mobile in mature females.

During ovulation the ostium moves over the surface of the ovary, collecting ovulated follicles. The follicles pass through the aglandular segment into the magnum where albumen is added. The follicles then pass to the shell gland of oviparous species, where the protein and carbohydrate shell membranes and the shell matrix are secreted. Eggs then pass into the vaginal region, where they are held until deposition. At the time of deposition, eggs are passed into the cloaca and out of the vent into the nest.

In viviparous lizards and snakes, embryos may develop using yolk (lecithotrophy) or varying degrees of a placenta may be present to provide gas exchange and nourishment (matrotrophy).

Case 2

History
A male desert tortoise of approximately 50 years of age presented for a 1-week history of tissue dragging around behind him following aggressive courtship behaviours.

Physcial examination
The penis was prolapsed. The distal penis was necrotic. There was no strength in the penile retractor muscle.

Assessment
Amputation was elected due to both necrotic tissue and an inability to retract the penis.

Surgery
The penis was infused at its base with a mix of lidocaine and bupivacaine. A carmalt clamp was placed at the base of the penis to crush the tissue (Figure 20.11). A transfixing absorbable suture ligature was placed through the crushed tissue. The penis was transected distal to the suture and remaining stump placed back in the cloaca. Broad-spectrum antibiotics and analgesics were administered postoperatively.

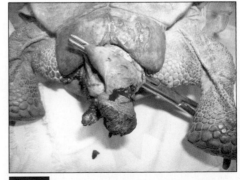

20.11 Desert tortoise with a necrotic phallus.

Medical conditions

Follicular stasis

Ovarian follicular disease is a relatively common problem in reptiles whose aetiology is not fully understood. Inappropriate diet and husbandry, lack of brumation/ hibernation for some species, stress, or other medical conditions probably lead to hormonal disturbances in the female reproductive cycle. Some species may be 'induced ovulators', i.e. only ovulate when a male is present. Hormonal disturbances may allow follicles to form without progression to ovulation.

Follicles may become atretic and be resorbed without illness. If resorption of follicles does not occur, over time inflammation of the follicles and ovary frequently occurs (Case 3). In snakes, and probably in many species of reptile, commensal *Salmonella* spp. exhibit a bacteraemia during vitellogenesis, effectively inoculating yolked follicles with potential (opportunistic) pathogens (Chiodini, 1982). Gram-negative bacteria are frequently cultured from septic follicles of snakes and lizards. This inflammatory or septic condition is likely to cause rupture or leakage of vitellin out of the follicle into the surrounding tissues. Vitellin is highly irritating and may cause severe coelomitis. The vitellin leakage may be a primary problem associated with follicular stasis and septic follicles, or secondary to trauma from activity or palpation.

Diagnosis: Presumptive diagnosis is based on history and physical examination. Anorexia, lethargy and sometimes coelomic distension are the most common complaints made by the owner. In some snakes and lizards, palpation of large clusters of follicles within the coelomic cavity is possible. For larger snakes, lizards and chelonians, ultrasonography or radiography can be helpful in identifying the follicles. Plasma chemistry results initially may show elevated triglycerides, calcium, phosphorus and albumin associated with vitellogenesis. With chronicity, hypoalbuminaemia from anorexia and hepatic lipidosis is common. Haematology of chronic cases often indicates anaemia of chronic disease and leucocytosis associated with inflammation and/or infection.

Ovarian disease should be considered when persistent elevations in plasma calcium occur in the female reptile patient outside of normal reproductive periods.

Treatment: Improvement of diet and husbandry (including proper photoperiod and the ability to thermoregulate properly), ability to have social interaction with a male, and providing suitable nesting areas for oviposition for non-ill patients with follicular stasis may be sufficient in resolving the problem. For patients that present for illness, ovariectomy or ovariosalpingectomy is indicated (see Chapter 13). Without surgical correction and aggressive medical care when coelomitis is present, prognosis is poor.

Dystocia

Given the wide variety of gestation periods among different species of reptiles (see Chapter 5) and even variation within a given species, diagnosis of dystocia can be difficult. If a female initiates delivery of eggs or fetuses and does not complete the process within 48–72 hours, dystocia should be investigated.

Many conditions can lead to dystocia in reptiles. These problems may be caused by obstructive anatomical or non-obstructive physiological abnormalities.

Obstructive dystocia: Anatomical abnormalities leading to dystocia include:

- Oversized fetuses or eggs
- Abnormally shaped eggs
- Abnormal maternal pelvic structure or size
- Oviductal stricture
- Neoplasia
- Other coelomic masses such as cystic calculi.

Diagnosis of obstructive dystocia is based on physical examination and radiography.

Non-obstructive dystocia: Non-obstructive conditions leading to dystocia may result from:

- Inappropriate husbandry; inability to thermoregulate properly, dehydration
- Lack of nesting site; reptiles may choose not to lay eggs when suitable nesting sites are not available
- Poor nutrition; may lead to hypocalcaemia and muscle atony
- Obesity and poor skeletal muscle tone
- Infection of the oviduct.

Non-obstructive conditions are usually identified with thorough discussion of diet and husbandry, physical examination findings and plasma biochemistry results.

Treatment: Non-obstructive dystocia associated with improper husbandry or lack of a nesting site, where the reptile does not appear ill, may be corrected simply by improving husbandry and providing an appropriate nesting area.

If illness is present, medical intervention should be initiated. Proper hydration should be ensured prior to initiating therapy. If hypocalcaemia is diagnosed or suspected based on clinical signs and history, treatment with calcium gluconate (100 mg/kg i.m., s.c. or i.c. q48–72h prn) should be initiated. Low doses of ketamine (10 mg/kg i.m.) are sometimes beneficial in reducing stress, relaxing vent musculature and allowing eggs to pass. In chelonians the use of oxytocin (1.0–10.0 IU/kg i.m.) is usually effective in initiating oviduct contractions and removal of eggs. Oxytocin (5.0–20.0 IU/kg i.m.) is rarely effective in lizards but ineffective in snakes. Oxytocin can be repeated again in 1 hour and then after 4–6 hours if eggs are not completely passed with initial treatment.

The efficacy of medical management varies depending on how long eggs have been in the oviducts. Eggs often become adherent to the walls of the oviducts if they are not passed at the appropriate time. The use of oxytocin in the presence of obstructive dystocia can cause oviductal rupture and allow passage of eggs into the coelomic cavity.

Gentle manipulation of eggs caudally via coelomic and cloacal palpation may be effective in removing retained eggs from snakes and lizards – sedation or anaesthesia may be required to perform this. In some lizards and snakes, percutaneous aspiration of yolk and egg contents (ovocentesis) may cause the egg to collapse, allowing for easier passage or removal (Case 4). Rehydration should always be performed before attempting to manipulate egg position. Some snakes will pass eggs after a combination of soaking and swimming activity. When manipulating eggs down the oviducts, care must be taken not to apply too much pressure, or oviductal rupture can occur and eggs pass into the coelomic cavity. Surgical intervention is usually required for obstructive causes of dystocia and dystocia unresponsive to medical management (see Chapter 13).

Prolapse

Prolapsed tissue protruding from the vent of female reptiles may include cloaca, intestine, oviduct or urinary bladder. Differentiation of prolapsed tissue should be attempted, using palpation or visualization with an otoscope or endoscope. Prolapsed oviducts may have a plicated appearance. Prolapses of the oviducts or bladder may occur owing to any condition causing straining or decreased muscular tone. Radiography is indicated to look for cystic calculi, eggs in the bladder, or abnormal eggs/fetuses in the oviducts. Blood tests should be performed to assess calcium levels and overall health.

Prolapsed tissues, irrespective of origin, are often inflamed, swollen and traumatized (Figure 20.14). Superficial or deep necrosis may be present, depending on how long the tissue has been prolapsed. Severely traumatized or necrotic prolapsed oviducts, bladder or intestine often require surgical intervention via coeliotomy (see Chapter 13). If underlying conditions such as cystic calculi or abnormal eggs are present, they should be addressed and corrected concurrently (see above).

Non-gastrointestinal prolapses of undetermined aetiology can often be managed medically. Hypertonic saline or dextrose solutions can be applied to reduce swelling.

Case 3

History
An 18-month-old female chameleon presented for a 2-week duration of anorexia, abdominal swelling, and progressive weakness (Figure 20.12a).

Physical examination
The chameleon was found to have sunken eyes, thickened saliva, a distended lobulated caudal coelomic cavity, poor skin coloration, and generalized weakness.

Diagnostic testing
Radiographs and blood tests were declined by the owner.

Assessment
A presumptive diagnosis of dystocia or ovarian disease was made. The owner declined surgery and elected instead for medical care.

Treatment
The patient received parenteral fluids, calcium gluconate, and broad-spectrum antibiotics along with appropriate husbandry. The patient showed no improvement with treatments and was euthanased 1 week later.

Necropsy
Generalized coelomitis with large ovarian follicles present. Many follicles were darker orange-red in colour (Figure 20.12b). The liver was also a pale orange suggestive of concurrent liver pathology.

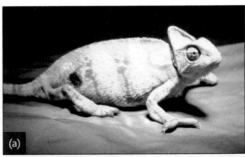
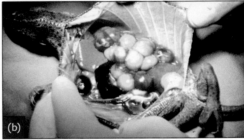

20.12 (a) A dehydrated chameleon with (b) follicular stasis.

CASE 4

History
A 6-year-old female grey-banded kingsnake presented for a caudal coelomic cavity swelling and anorexia persisting for several weeks after laying eggs.

Physical examination
A 2 x 4 cm oval semi-firm mass was present in the caudal coelomic cavity.

Assessment
A presumptive diagnosis of dystocia and retained egg was made.

Treatment
The snake was soaked for 30 minutes in a shallow warm-water bath. The egg could not be manipulated distally through the oviduct. Cloacoscopy using an otoscope showed no obvious problems. The egg was then aspirated percutaneously to remove its contents (Figure 20.13a). After being collapsed, the egg was able to be manipulated down the oviduct and out of the cloaca (Figure 20.13b). The patient was treated with broad-spectrum antibiotics, was doing well, and ate 2 weeks later.

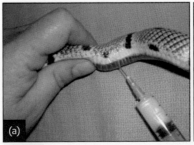
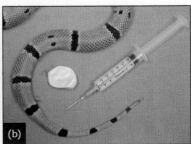

20.13 (a–b) Egg aspiration in a 6-year-old female grey-banded kingsnake.

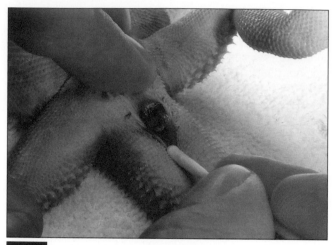

20.14 Oviduct prolapse in a bearded dragon.

The tissue should then be lubricated with an antibiotic plus steroid cream or silver sulfadiazine cream and manipulated back through the vent. Lateral tacking sutures should be placed on either side of the vent to hold tissues in, but allowing for some urination and defecation (similar to the procedure for replacement of chelonian penile prolapse). Sutures can be left in place for 14 days. Systemic antibiotic therapy should be initiated. Cloacopexy may be needed for recurring prolapses (see Chapter 13).

Neoplasia

Neoplasia has been reported throughout the urogenital tract of many species of reptile. Neoplastic conditions of the urogenital tract can be the underlying causes of renal diseases, dystocia, prolapses, cachexia and other problems. Whenever possible, histopathology should be performed when abnormal masses or abnormal tissues are identified.

Sterilization

Ovariectomy and ovariosalpingectomy should be considered for many female reptiles kept as pets, to reduce pet overpopulation and the risk of medical problems in species where it is of concern. Orchiectomy in males has not been shown to have any behavioural benefits as seen in many mammals. Phallectomy and penile amputations can be performed to prevent successful copulation.

References and further reading

Badia P, Gomez T, Diaz M and Lorenzo A (1987) Mechanisms of transport of Na[+] and Cl[-] in the lizard colon. *Comparative Biochemistry and Physiology A, Comparative Physiology* **87(4)**, 883–887

Beck K, Loomis M, Lewbart G, Spelman L and Papich M (1995) Preliminary comparison of plasma concentrations of gentamicin injected into the cranial and caudal limb musculature of the eastern box turtle, *Terrapene carolina carolina*. *Journal of Zoo and Wildlife Medicine* **26**, 265–268

Chiodini RJ (1982) Transovarian passage, visceral distribution, and pathogenicity of *Salmonella* in snakes. *Infection and Immunology* **35**, 710–713

Dallwig RK, Mitchell MA and Acierno MJ (2010) Determination of plasma osmolality and agreement between measured and calculated values in healthy adult bearded dragons (*Pogona vitticeps*). *Journal of Herpetological Medicine and Surgery* **20(2–3)**, 69–73

Ehrenspeck G and Voner C (1985) Effect of furosemide on ion transport in the turtle bladder: evidence for direct inhibition of active acid-base transport. *Biochimica et Biophysica Acta* **817(2)**, 318–326

Fox H (1977) *The Urogenital System of Reptiles. Biology of the Reptilia, Volume 6*, pp. 1–157 New York, NY. Academic Press

Guzman D, Mitchell MA and Acierno M (2011) Determination of plasma osmolality and agreement between measured and calculated values in captive male corn snakes (*Pantherophis [Elaphe] guttatus guttatus*). *Journal of Herpetological Medicine and Surgery* **21(1)**, 16–19

Holtz PH (1999) The reptilian renal-portal system: influence on therapy. In: *Zoo and Wild Animal Medicine: Current Therapy IV*, ed. ME Fowler and RE Miller, pp. 249–252. WB Saunders, Philadelphia

Holtz PH, Barker IK, Burger JP, Crawshaw GJ and Conlon PD (1997) The effects of the renal portal system on pharmacokinetic parameters in the red-eared slider, *Trachemys scripta elegans*. *Journal of Zoo and Wildlife Medicine* **28**, 386–393

Holtz PH, Burger JP, Pasloske K, Baker R and Young S (2003) Effects of injection site on carbenicillin pharmacokinetics in the carpet python, *Morelia spilota*. *Journal of Herpetological Medicine and Surgery* **12(4)**, 12–16

Naverez JG, Acierno MJ, Angel M and Beaufrere H (2012) Determination of agreement between measured and calculated plasma osmolality values in captive-reared American alligators (*Alligator mississippiensis*). *Journal of Herpetological Medicine and Surgery* **22(1–2)**, 36–41

Oftedal OT, Allen ME and Christopher TE (1995) Dietary potassium affects food choice, nitrogen retention, and growth of desert tortoises. *Proceedings of the Desert Tortoise Council*, pp. 58–61

Oftedal OT, Allen ME, Chung AL, Reed RC and Ullrey DE (1994) Nutrition, urates and desert survival: potassium and the desert tortoise (*Gopherus agassizii*). *Proceedings of the American Association of Zoo Veterinarians*, pp. 308–313

Prezant RM and Jarchow JL (1997) Lactated fluid use in reptiles: is there a better solution? *Proceedings of the Association of Reptilian and Amphibian Veterinarians Annual Conference*, pp. 83–87

Rudloff E (2005) Concepts in fluid therapy for the sick reptile. *Proceedings of the North American Veterinary Conference,* Orlando, Florida, pp. 1302–1304

Wyneken J (2013) Reptilian Renal Structure and Function. *Proceedings of the Annual Conference of Reptilian and Amphibian Veterinarians*, pp. 72–78

Chapter 21

Neurology

Simon J. Girling

The reptilian nervous system is similar to the mammalian and avian systems. There are some differences in reptiles which complicate the assessment of neurological function – one being the ectothermic nature of the class Reptilia as a whole. If a reptile is kept at suboptimal temperatures, neurological reflexes/responses will be reduced or may even be absent. Therefore, any attempt to assess neurological function in a reptile should be carried out when the reptile is at its preferred body temperature. Many disease processes, less common in mammals, may lead to neurological disease; for example, metabolic conditions, such as hypocalcaemia/hypovitaminosis D, are very common in reptiles, particularly lizards, and often present with neurological signs. Furthermore, some clinical signs of neurological disease in reptiles may appear in other body systems first – dysecdysis in snakes in particular is common where neurological disease is present. Finally, some species may 'play possum' and sham death/neurological disease, such as hognose snakes, which will invert themselves and become unresponsive in order to escape predation or attack.

Relevant anatomy and physiology

Anatomy and physiology of the central nervous system (CNS) are covered in more detail in Chapter 1. Some specific information relevant to neurological disease is given here as well:

- The spinal cord in chelonians enters the carapace after cervical vertebra 8 and exits at the sacral vertebra; therefore, injuries to the carapace in this region can lead to spinal cord and neurological damage
- There is no arachnoid mater or subarachnoid space. Cerebrospinal fluid (CSF) is instead found between the dura mater and inner leptomeninx. There is no CSF in the epidural space, but there are veins ventral and lateral to the cord itself which may be inadvertently entered when sampling for CSF
- CSF volumes are very small in reptiles, adding to the difficulty in sampling
- Reptiles appear able to regenerate nerve cells, both peripheral and central nervous system neurons, after injury, making prognoses for neurological damage better than comparable injuries in mammals or birds

- Cutaneous sense organs are present in many species of reptiles. These vary from heat-sensing pits around the head of snakes (the edge of the maxilla in boids and pythons and pits between the nares and eyes in pit vipers) to pressure-sensitive organs embedded within lateral scales in crocodilians, similar to the lateral line of fish, which alert the reptile to the presence of prey in the water
- Nociceptors are also found in reptiles, and both encapsulated nerve ending and non-encapsulated nerve ending nociceptors have been demonstrated throughout the dermis. It is therefore self-evident that reptiles can perceive pain and equally self-evident that analgesia is essential when a reptile is exposed to noxious stimuli/events
- A vago-vagal reflex exists in reptiles, as in mammals, but may be used to induce a reduction in heart and respiratory rate and immobility to allow radiography. It is elicited by gentle pressure on the eyes, but is rapidly ablated by stimuli such as noise or physical contact.

Clinical evaluation

History

A detailed history is always important when dealing with reptile disease. Recent introduction of new reptiles to a collection or disease in a recent acquisition may point towards an infectious agent. Clearly, the use of certain potentially toxic agents in the reptile's environment, such as chlorhexidine, permethrins, organophosphates, etc., is also likely to be significant in cases of neurological disease, as is the use of neurotoxic drugs such as ivermectin in chelonians. Trauma, access to poisonous plants or frost damage in outdoor chelonians are also significant, as are inappropriate environmental temperatures, leading to immunosuppression and potential septicaemia. Diet should also be evaluated as nutritional deficiencies can lead to neurological signs, such as diets deficient in calcium/vitamin D (often combined with a lack of ultraviolet light exposure in certain lizards and chelonians), biotin deficiencies in egg-eating species or thiamine deficiencies in captive reptiles fed previously frozen saltwater fish etc.

Clinical neurological examination

Signs of neurological disease are many and varied, but are similar to those seen in mammals and include: fitting;

paresis; paralysis; head tilts; opisthotonus/torticollis; circling and blindness. A standard neurological assessment focuses on an assessment of the reptile's behaviour, followed by a cranial nerve examination, an assessment of posture and spinal reflexes, and finally cutaneous sensation.

Reptile awareness

A four-point graded scale for assessing mentation and responsiveness from alert to obtunded (reduced responsiveness but can still be stimulated), stupor (will only respond to noxious stimuli) and finally coma, has been described by Mariani (2007). It should be noted, however, that there is a variation in alertness between species and some may feign death (e.g. hognose snakes), which may complicate assessment.

Posture assessment and reflexes

As with mammals, various postural reflexes may be affected, dependent on the level of peripheral/central nervous system damage.

Positional nystagmus and dull mentation suggest a central vestibular problem, as with mammalian species. Conversely, persistent horizontal nystagmus, head tilt, leaning and falling, and tight circling suggest a peripheral vestibular problem.

Cerebellar disease tends to produce intention head tremors as the reptile approaches food and will produce exaggerated limb movements.

Cerebral disease tends to produce loss of consciousness, or in less severe injuries may produce a lack of finely tuned movement.

The gait of the lizard or chelonian may be assessed in a similar way to that of a dog or cat. Hypermetria, hypometria, ataxia, paresis, paralysis and circling should all be noted. In snakes, the ability of the snake to propel itself using contraction of the ventral body wall muscles and the tone of these muscles may be assessed by running a finger down the ventrum of the snake. There should be a reflex contraction wave of the muscles (the Bauchstreich reflex) in snakes with normal neurological function.

Opisthotonus is common in many forms of central neurological disease of reptiles. Head bobbing may be seen in reptiles with respiratory disease as well as those suffering from neurological disease.

Positional reflexes of the feet in lizards may be possible to assess via knuckling and placing. This is, however, difficult to assess in chelonians and impossible, of course, in snakes.

A righting reflex is a basic postural reflex. Chelonians and lizards use their necks and forelimbs to help right themselves. Snakes turn their heads upright first and the rest of the body follows in a reflex muscle contraction. Snakes with a completely damaged spinal cord will not be able to turn over the body caudal to the lesion.

A cloacal reflex may also be assessed by examining the cloacal sphincter, which should hold the cloaca closed even at rest. Flaccidity or lack of contraction when inserting a blunt probe into the cloaca may indicate denervation.

Spinal reflex assessment

The level of damage to the spinal cord may be assessed by its effects on various segments of the body. It is important to remember that upper motor neuron damage will result in hyper-responses of the area affected. Lower motor neuron damage will result in hypo-response or no response of the area affected. For example:

- Damage to the cervical segment of the spinal cord will result in upper motor neuron deficit to the fore- and hindlimbs and vent, but with no interference, of course, with the cranial nerves
- Damage to the spinal cord that forms the brachial plexus will result in lower motor neuron deficit to the forelimbs, but upper motor neuron effects to the hindlimbs and vent. The head will be completely unaffected, as will the cranial nerves
- Damage to the thoracic section of the spinal cord will result in no head or forelimb lesions but upper motor neuron deficits to the hindlimbs and vent
- Damage to the lumbar and sacral elements of the lumbosacral plexus will result in no head or forelimb lesions but lower motor neuron deficits to the hindlimbs and vent
- Damage to the pudendal element of the lumbosacral plexus will result in no head, forelimb or hindlimb signs but lower motor neuron deficit to the vent
- In snakes, the level of the deficit may be noted by the point at which the Bauchstreich reflex ceases
- Pinch withdrawal reflexes can be used in limbed reptiles to assess the level of any injury
- Crossed extensor reflexes, as in birds and mammals, indicate upper motor neuron damage – but some authors argue that this reflex is never seen in reptiles (Mariani, 2007).

Cutaneous reflexes

A panniculus reflex is seen in reptiles, with the obvious exception of chelonians, and may help to identify the level of any spinal deficit. The skin of squamates may be gently pricked with a sterile hypodermic needle while watching for the muscular twitch elicited.

Cranial nerve assessment

For cranial nerve clinical assessment, see Figure 21.1.

Cranial nerve	Clinical assessment
I	This is difficult to assess – a history of loss of appetite has been reported
II and V	These may be assessed by performing a menace test (not useful in snakes and some geckos owing to fused eyelids)
II and III	These may be assessed by performing a pupillary light reflex test (although reptiles do have skeletal muscle in the iris which is under partial voluntary control)
III, IV and VI	Damage to these cranial nerves may be deduced by the presence of strabismus
V and VII	These may be assessed by the palpebral reflex (not in snakes and some geckos); may also be assessed by the degree of jaw tone
VIII (vestibulocochlear) and 3, 4 and 6	Damage may be deduced if oculocephalic or physiological nystagmus is seen
IX and X	Loss of function will result in a loss of the gag reflex
XI	Loss of function leads to poor neck movement (nerve not present in snakes and some lizards)
XII	Their loss of function leads to hypomotility of the tongue, which may be assessed by grasping the tongue to observe the withdrawal reflex response

21.1 Clinical assessment of cranial nerve function in reptiles.

Noxious stimuli response

Reptiles may respond to mild pain by muscular twitching, as with the panniculus reflex (Figure 21.2), or by head movement to-wards the stimulus. Deep pain sensation may be assessed by squeezing firmly over any extremity such as a digit or tail tip using forceps, digital pressure or haemostats (Figure 21.3). A normal response would typically include head movement towards the stimulus or an attempt to escape or attack the instigator of the stimulus. Lack of such a response, as with mammalian patients, indicates a severe injury with a guarded prognosis, although reptile patients do have the ability to regenerate neurons even in the CNS (Cruce, 1979; Srivastava, 1992).

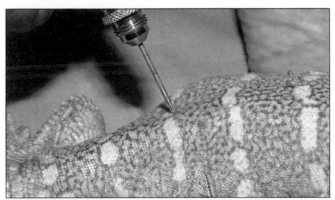

21.2 Evaluation of the panniculus reflex in a lizard.
(Courtesy of Paul Raiti)

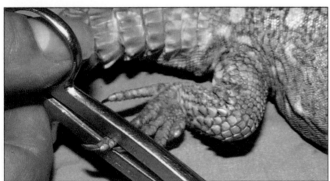

21.3 Elicitation of the limb withdrawal reflex is used to assess spinal cord segments in the lower back. The reflex was absent in this spiny-tailed lizard with hindlimb paralysis. A more vigorous noxious stimulus applied to the toes revealed an absence of deep pain, indicating serious damage to the spinal cord.
(Courtesy of Paul Raiti)

Differentiating central from peripheral neurological disease

Central neurological disease may present with vague clinical signs. These can include a reduced appetite and general dullness in mentation and can be difficult to diagnose in mild cases. In severe cases they can involve seizure, collapse and paralysis, opisthotonus, loss of the righting reflex, circling and torticollis.

Spinal and peripheral neurological disease clearly can affect one part of the body severely and yet leave other parts unaffected. Obvious examples include hemiparesis/paralysis, paresis/paralysis of one limb, segmental loss of pain response, loss of cloacal reflex and loss of panniculus reflex at a set point. However, peripheral vestibular disease may also result in head tilt and circling, as in mammals.

An attempt to locate the level of a neurological lesion is given in Figure 21.4.

Level of neurological lesion	Potential clinical signs	Common differentials
Forebrain	Seizures, opisthotonus, central blindness, dull mentation, behavioural changes, limb paresis and postural deficits, potentially cranial nerve involvement	Encephalitis (e.g. inclusion body disease (IBD), ferlavirus, adenovirus, reovirus, fungal, parasitic, bacterial meningoencephalitis), drug toxicity (e.g. metronidazole), plant toxicity (e.g. cannabis), pesticide toxicity (e.g. organophosphates/permethrins), head trauma, frost damage, thiamine deficiency, CNS neoplasia, cerebral xanthomatosis
Cerebellum	Ataxia, intention tremors, torticollis, nystagmus, hyper/hypometria	Trauma, encephalitis (as above), neoplasia
Spinal cord proximal to brachial plexus	Quadriplegia/paralysis, maintains spinal reflexes	Trauma, bacterial or fungal spinal lesion, parasitic migration
Spinal cord at brachial plexus	Quadriparesis, ataxia all four limbs, reduced/absent pain withdrawal reflex pectoral limbs	Trauma, bacterial or fungal spinal lesion, parasitic migration
Spinal cord distal to brachial plexus but proximal to pelvic plexus	Paraplegia, ataxia in pelvic limbs, panniculus reflex present cranial and absent caudal to lesion, righting reflex in snakes absent caudal to lesion and present proximal, local segmental spinal reflexes present	Trauma, bacterial or fungal spinal lesion, parasitic migration
Spinal cord at pelvic plexus	Paraplegia, ataxia in pelvic limbs, reduced/absent pelvic withdrawal reflexes, reduced/absent cloacal reflex	Trauma, bacterial or fungal spinal lesion, parasitic migration
Spinal cord distal to pelvic plexus	Paresis/paralysis of the tail	Trauma, bacterial or fungal spinal lesion, parasitic migration

21.4 Location of central nervous system (CNS) neurological damage. NB: for snakes, assume similar trunk neurological deficits caudal to the spinal lesion. Assume pain at the site of any spinal lesion on palpation.

Diagnostic imaging

This is essential where a history of spinal lesions is suspected. Common areas for reptiles to injure themselves are around the mid-spine in chelonians with carapacial wounds, the cervical region in snakes being held by the head and the lumbar area in lizards with metabolic bone disease. Radiography may help identify obvious spinal deformities associated with developmental disease such as poor calcium/vitamin D3 levels in the diet (Figures 21.5 and 21.6).

Myelography has been used in reptiles but, as with CSF collection, it is a difficult technique. The atlanto-occipital site is preferred but intrathecal injections in chelonians have been performed for local analgesia/anaesthesia in the coccygeal vertebrae, and may be used for contrast techniques to assess for spinal cord damage/compression.

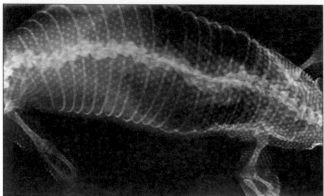

21.5 Beaded lizard with hindlimb paresis and kyphosis and scoliosis of the spine (dorsoventral view).

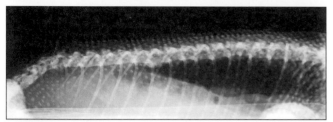

21.6 Beaded lizard with hindlimb paresis and kyphosis and scoliosis of the spine (lateral view). The head is to the right.

Computed tomography (CT) and magnetic resonance imaging (MRI) have been used in reptiles to aid diagnosis of neurological disease. CT is most useful in assessing bony changes to the spinal column and skull, and has been shown to be useful in chelonians in particular (Abou-Madi *et al.*, 2004). MRI is more useful for assessing soft tissue tumours in the spinal cord and brain and the presence of encephalocoeles/hydrocephalus. See Chapter 9 for more information.

Blood biochemistry, haematology and serology

Blood biochemistry and haematology should be carried out to determine a full cell count and liver/renal function as well as calcium levels and glucose. Organ failure such as liver or kidney failure can result in neurological signs such as seizures due to a build-up of toxins, and should be included in the list of extra CNS differential diagnoses. Hypoglycaemia has been reported as producing collapse in Crocodilia and hypocalcaemia has been reported causing flaccid paralysis in several species of lizard. Serological tests for diseases such as West Nile virus or paramyxovirus may also be helpful in diagnosing neurological disease.

Cerebrospinal fluid analysis

Cerebrospinal fluid (CSF) is produced by the choroid plexus within the ventricles of the brain. It then flows caudally in the subdural space. Due to its small volume and the narrow access site, collection can be a challenge. Two sites are possible for collection – the atlanto-occipital space and the lumbar region. The lumbar site (lumbosacral intervertebral space) is very difficult to access owing to the narrowness of the intervertebral space and minimal subdural space in this region (it is also very difficult to precisely locate in snakes) and so the atlanto-occipital site is preferred. The patient should be held still or preferably anaesthetized. The dorsum of the head is surgically prepared and then is ventroflexed. The landmarks used vary with the species, but the caudal edge of the skull should be identified and the body of the atlas behind, and the entry site is midline and halfway between the two. A spinal needle can be used in larger species, but in smaller patients a hypodermic needle may be used. Flow of CSF through the needle is slow or may not be obvious and volumes will be small – often only filling the needle. It is not advisable to aspirate as this can lead to blood contamination or, worse, CNS damage. Centrifugation should be carried out to assess cellularity and the fluid should be analysed for protein levels if sufficient volumes are collected. In the majority of cases, though, the sample is very small and so a smear should be made immediately after collection and analysed using Romanowsky stains.

In some species, such as chelonians, there is a venous sinus in this area and so a spinal needle with stylet should be used to prevent contamination while the needle traverses the sinus.

Normal values for CSF analysis in reptiles are sparse in the literature. One publication on American alligators suggests that the cellularity is similar to mammals, but there are normally higher protein levels (Bennett *et al.*, 2001). Clippinger *et al.* (2000) also described the isolation of *Mycoplasma* from the CSF of American alligators.

Electrophysiological testing

Techniques used in mammals may be applied to reptiles but there are some specific differences, as outlined below.

Electromyography assesses the health of the muscle cell and the integrity of the lower motor neuron (LMN) and can be used to help differentiate disease associated with the LMN and that associated with muscle tissue. General anaesthesia is needed in reptiles to carry out this procedure. The responses are similar to those seen in birds and mammals, but normal values are not readily available in the literature. The technique involves inserting the probe above the suspected injury close to the nerve and an electrical stimulus is then created. The response potential is measured in the associated muscle tissue. Nerve damage will obviously result in no, or reduced, potential in the muscle. Further complications can occur if the reptile is not kept at its preferred body temperature as low environmental temperatures can lead to a reduced body temperature and slowing of nerve conduction velocities. Interpretation otherwise is similar to that for mammals.

A nerve locator has been used in American alligators, Yacare caimans and dwarf crocodiles to determine the success of mandibular nerve blocks, and so may theoretically be used in other reptile species to assess nerve function (Wellehan *et al.*, 2006).

Conduction velocity may also be measured using mammalian techniques, but identification of the motor nerve can be difficult in small patients. However, if combined with electromyography, it can be used to distinguish between neurological and myological disease, as with mammals. Demyelination results in reduced velocities, whereas myopathies or axonal damage can produce a reduction in the potential produced (compound muscle action potential or CMAP).

F waves may also be measured as with mammalian patients and so may be used to assess the health of the ventral nerve root. Repetitive nerve stimulation can also be performed and is useful for assessing diseases of the neuromuscular junction, where the CMAP will decrease with progressive stimulation. Very little information on healthy or diseased reptile patients is available.

Other tests

Performing biopsy of nerves and associated muscles may also help in determining the cause of suspected neurological disease. It is particularly helpful in distinguishing between inflammatory muscle disease and primary neurological disease. Fresh tissue sampling is advisable as well as dilute formalin storage of collected samples to allow immunohistochemical tests to be performed if required.

Electroencephalography may be difficult to perform in reptiles owing to the lack of subcutaneous space over the skull in many species, the fact that it is affected by the environmental temperature/preferred body temperature and the small size of the patient's head. Surface electrodes have been used but, again, the lack of 'normal' readings from healthy reptiles can hamper interpretation.

However, waveforms have been reported in reptiles and suggest that their alert waveforms are similar to mammalian sleep patterns, as well as spikes and waves that would suggest epilepsy in mammals but which appear normal in reptiles (Flanigan, 1973; Gaztelu et al., 1991).

Nuclear scintigraphy has been used to diagnose brain tumours in reptiles although it is not so useful for inflammatory CNS lesions (Schumacher and Toal, 2001).

Diseases

A summary of published work on a selection of diseases resulting in neurological disease is provided in Figure 21.7.

Aetiological agent		Species of reptile	Reference	Presenting signs
Infectious agents				
Viral	Inclusion body disease	Pythons and boas principally but also palm vipers and eastern kingsnakes have been reported	Raymond et al., 2001; Vancraeynest et al., 2006; Jacobson, 2007	Predominantly neurological in pythons, with opisthotonus, disorientation, head tremors, loss of righting reflexes, paresis, paralysis and death. Boas may also show regurgitation and respiratory disease
	Ferlavirus (paramyxovirus)	Snakes from Boidae, Elapidae, Colubridae and Crotalidae	Folsch and Leloup, 1976; Jacobson et al., 1980, 1992; Kolesnikovas et al., 2006; Jacobson, 2007	Predominantly respiratory disease but neurological disease also reported causing head tremors but also regurgitation and sudden death
	Sunshine virus (paramyxovirus unrelated to Ferlavirus)	Australian pythons (spotted, diamond, etc.)	Hyndman et al., 2012	Lethargy, inappetence, head tremors, delayed righting reflex, respiratory disease including dyspnoea, opisthotonus, regurgitation
		Royal python	Marschang, 2013	
	West Nile virus	American alligator	Miller et al., 2003; Jacobson et al., 2005; Nevarez et al., 2005	Anorexia, tremors, swimming on side/spinning in water, opisthotonus. Also stomatitis, proliferative skin lesions and frequently hepatitis and death
	Reovirus	Prairie rattlesnake	Vieler et al., 1994	Opisthotonus, incoordination
	Chelonid herpesviruses	Mediterranean tortoises	Marschang, 2011	In addition to respiratory and oral signs may develop paresis, incoordination and paralysis of limbs
	Adenovirus	Bearded dragon	Jacobson et al. 1996; Kim et al., 2002	Head tilt, opisthotonus, circling, as well as liver disease, pneumonia, lethargy and wasting. Enteritis also reported
		Jackson's chameleon	Jacobson and Gardiner, 1990	
		Boa constrictor	Jacobson et al., 1986	
		Coastal mountain kingsnake	Raymond et al., 2003	
		Mountain kingsnakes	Wozniak et al., 2000	
Bacterial	Aeromonas spp.	Variety of species, particularly snakes	Jacobson, 2007	Stomatitis, septicaemia, seizures, opisthotonus and death
	Listeria monocytogenes	Bearded dragon	Girling and Fraser, 2004	Depression, seizures, septicaemia, collapse and death
	Mycobacterium marinum	Bearded dragon	Girling and Fraser, 2007	Collapse, paresis, reduction of righting reflex and withdrawal reflexes
	Providencia rettgeri	Saltwater crocodile hatchlings	Ladds et al., 1996	Seizures, meningitis and sudden death
	Clostridium botulinum	Green turtles	Jacobson, 1980	Paresis of all four limbs (so-called floppy flipper syndrome)
	Salmonella spp.	Green sea turtles	Raidal et al., 1998	Associated with cardiovascular trematode infections causing granulomatous meningoencephalitis, producing incoordination, paralysis and death
	Mycoplasma alligatoris	American alligators	Clippinger et al., 2000; Brown et al., 2001	Polyserositis, polyarthritis, dyspnoea, loss of righting reflex, incoordination, death

21.7 Selected aetiological agents reported in the literature as causing neurological disease in reptiles. (continues) ▶

Aetiological agent		Species of reptile	Reference	Presenting signs
Infectious agents continued				
Fungal	*Phycomyces* spp.	Massasauga rattlesnake	Williams *et al.*, 1979	Collapse, anorexia, skin ulceration, death
	Phaeohyphomycosis	Green iguana	Olias *et al.*, 2010	Paroxysmal paralysis
	Cryptococcus spp.	Anaconda	McNamara *et al.*, 1994	Loss of righting reflex, tremors of head, cachexia, lethargy
Parasitic	*Acanthamoeba* spp.	Variety of species including boa constrictor and Pacific coast rattlesnake	Frank, 1974	Spasmodic opisthotonus
	Entamoeba spp.	Green iguana	Frank, 1966	Fitting, collapse and meningoencephalitis
Non-infectious agents				
Neoplasia	Nerve sheath tumour	Bearded dragon	Lemberger *et al.*, 2005	Subcutaneous swellings
		Water moccasin	Ramis *et al.*, 1998	
	Pituitary cystadenoma	Everglades ratsnake	Dadone *et al.*, 2010	Hyperkeratosis, dysecdysis and inappetence but no neurological signs reported
	Spinal cord glioma	Ridge-nosed rattlesnake	Craig *et al.*, 2005	Egg retention and decreased motility of the caudal body
	Secondary metastasis of liposarcoma to spinal cord	Red coach-whip snake	Churgin *et al.*, 2013	Paralysis and death – associated with *Coccidioides* spp. intestinal disease
Nutritional	Hypoglycaemia	Crocodiles	Wallach, 1971	Collapse, muscle tremors, anorexia and lethargy
	Hypocalcaemia/ hypovitaminosis D	Herbivorous chelonians and lizards particularly susceptible	Bennett and Mehler, 2006	Muscle fasciculations, collapse, flaccidity or tetany, renal failure, metabolic bone disease, heart failure
	Hypovitaminosis E	Green iguana	Farnsworth *et al.*, 1986	Tremors of all four limbs, knuckling of the forelimbs, lethargy and anorexia
	Cerebral xanthomatosis	Water dragon	Kummrow *et al.*, 2010	Head bobbing, progressing to opisthotonus
		Geckos	Garner *et al.*, 1999	
		Great plated lizard	Gyimesi *et al.*, 2002	
	Hypovitaminosis B1	Water and garter snakes in particular but any reptile fed high levels of thiaminases	Girling, 2013	Opisthotonus, central blindness, dysphagia, loss of righting reflex and death
	Biotin	Egg-eating reptiles	Frye, 1984	Muscle tremors, generalized weakness
Toxins	Brevetoxicosis	Loggerhead sea turtles	Manire *et al.*, 2013	Head bobbing, nervous twitching and coma
	Ivermectin toxicity	Chameleon	Szell *et al.*, 2001	Paralysis, paresis, collapse and death
		Chelonians	Teare and Bush, 1983	Sudden death
		Common boa	Klingenberg, 1996	Sudden death (one case reported)
	Metronidazole toxicity	Indigo and kingsnakes (any species at doses >200 mg/kg)	Jacobson, 1988	Opisthotonus, seizures, death
	Chlorhexidine >2%	Various species but particularly chelonians	Bennett and Mehler, 2006	Flaccid paralysis, reduced withdrawal reflexes, loss of righting reflexes
	Levamisole toxicity	Most species	Rees-Davies and Klingenberg, 2004	Hepatotoxicity, head shaking, excitability, muscle tremors, salivation and death
	Permethrin/ organophosphate toxicity	Western fence lizard	Holem *et al.*, 2006	Seizures, collapse, tremors and death. 20% mortality and 70% clinical signs at 200 mg/kg malathion
	Lead	Western fence lizard	Holem *et al.*, 2006	30% mortality at 1000 mg/kg but only fine neurological signs, depression, etc., seen prior to this
	Cannabinoid toxicosis	Green iguana	Girling and Fraser, 2011	Seizures, tachycardia, tonic–clonic muscle contractions, loss of righting reflex, absence of pinch reflex, mydriasis, hyperaesthesia.
Miscellaneous	Compressive myelopathy	Komodo dragon	Zimmermann *et al.*, 2009	Quadriplegia, quadriparesis, dullness and anorexia
	Lymphocytic epaxial perineuritis	Boa constrictor	Fitzgerald *et al.*, 1990	Caudal coiling of the body, congenital

21.7 (continued) Selected aetiological agents reported in the literature as causing neurological disease in reptiles.

Viral infections

Paramyxovirus (*Ferlavirus*) infections

These have been reported in many species of snake and some lizards (Jacobson *et al.*, 1980). Various individual viruses have been isolated, predominantly within the *Ferlavirus* genus (Marschang *et al.*, 2009). However, a typed paramyxovirus unrelated to ferlaviruses has been isolated associated with neurological disease in Australian pythons and has been named sunshine virus (Hyndman *et al.*, 2012). *Ferlavirus* infection has been associated with pneumonia and neurological disease in snakes. Sunshine virus causes similar pathology in Australian boids and pythons but has also now been reported in Europe in a royal python (Marschang, 2013). Diagnosis of paramyxovirus infections has historically relied on serology (haemagglutination inhibition tests) due to the cross-reactivity of squamate antibodies with avian paramyxovirus 3 and 7. Problems exist though in acute infections as seroconversion takes 6–8 weeks. However, real-time polymerase chain reaction (PCR) has been developed which can be used to detect ferlaviruses and sunshine virus from swabs or washes of the trachea and lungs ante-mortem and multiple tissues post-mortem. See Chapter 25 for more information.

Inclusion body disease

An arenavirus has been isolated from cases of inclusion body disease (IBD) seen primarily in boas and pythons and is now thought to be the most likely aetiological agent (Stenglein *et al.*, 2012). However, historically IBD was thought to be due to a retrovirus and has also been reported in elapids and colubrids as well as boids and pythons. In pythons the disease is severe with infectious stomatitis, pneumonia and neurological signs such as loss of the righting reflex, disorientation and blindness, often followed rapidly by death (Figure 21.8). In boas, the disease is fatal in young individuals. In older patients, the disease produces more chronic neurological signs with chronic anorexia, vomiting and pneumonias. Neurological signs are milder with a loss of ability to chew and swallow prey, and a loss of the striking reflex. Transmission is thought to be via the snake mite *Ophionyssus natricis* and bodily secretions. Diagnosis is currently based on biopsy of affected organs, principally the liver, kidney, spleen and oesophageal tonsils, which will show classical eosinophilic intracytoplasmic inclusion bodies. Early in the course of the disease there may be a leucocytosis (white blood cell count >30 x 10^9/l). Real-time PCRs as well as electron microscopy and virus isolation have been reported in the diagnosis of the condition but there are no serological tests currently available – see Chapter 25 for more information.

Other viruses

Chelonian herpesviruses have been associated with neurological disease including paralysis and incoordination as well as the more typical respiratory signs. Real-time PCRs are available to diagnose the condition and classical eosinophilic inclusion bodies may be seen on cytology/histopathology.

Adenoviruses have been associated with opisthotonus and death in chameleons (Jacobson and Gardiner, 1990) and neurological signs in other lizards (Kim *et al.*, 2002). PCRs are available for diagnosis.

Reoviruses (Reoviridae) have been isolated from lizards and snakes and associated with respiratory and neurological disease. Real-time PCRs have been developed and may be used on lung, oral and cloacal swabs.

West Nile virus (Flaviviridae) has been isolated from American alligators, and associated with opisthotonus and fatalities, as well as skin lesions, pneumonia, myocarditis, etc. Real-time PCRs and virus isolation on blood samples and serological tests have been used to diagnose infection (Jacobson *et al.*, 2005; Marschang, 2011).

Bacterial infections

Bacterial abscesses/granulomas of the spinal cord or the brain may result in neurological disease. Most are Gram-negative in nature, but mycoplasmal and chlamydophilal organisms have also been reported, as have mycobacterial infections such as *Mycobacterium marinum* which have resulted in paresis and collapse (Girling and Fraser, 2007) (Figure 21.9). *Mycoplasma alligatoris* was reported in American alligators presenting with neurological signs, including lethargy, muscle weakness and paraparesis, as well as pneumonia, tissue oedema and fatalities (Clippinger *et al.*, 2000).

Middle ear infections in aquatic chelonians are common and may result in peripheral vestibular disease. There is often an underlying vitamin A deficiency problem, particularly in carnivorous chelonians; however, it may be seen in herbivorous chelonians with no obvious vitamin A deficiency (Figure 21.10).

Listeria monocytogenes has been reported as a cause of septicaemia and neurological signs in a bearded dragon fed previously frozen mouse pups which were demonstrated to be infected (Girling and Fraser, 2004).

Osteomyelitis of the spinal column is also common, particularly in snakes. It can result in a range of spinal lesions including osteolysis and vertebral collapse, osteoarthropathy, and hyperostosis producing physical distortion as

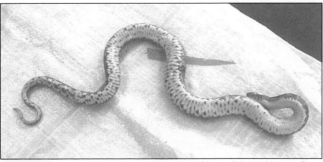

21.8 Boa constrictor showing ataxia and loss of the righting reflex with inclusion body disease infection.

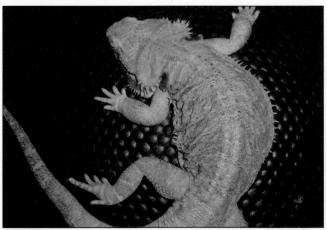

21.9 Bearded dragon with systemic *Mycobacterium marinum* infection with episodic collapse, weakness and tremors.

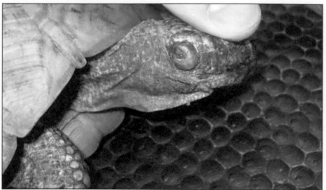

21.10 Aural abscess in a spur-thighed tortoise showing signs of peripheral vestibular disease.

well as neurological paresis or paralysis distal to the lesion. Again, Gram-negative bacteria such as *Aeromonas* and *Pseudomonas* spp. are commonly isolated. In addition, *Salmonella* spp. and *Streptococcus* spp. have also been isolated from blood cultures of snakes with these lesions. Blood cultures, collected in an aseptic manner, are advisable in these cases to identify the causal pathogen. *Mycobacterium* spp. have also been isolated occasionally, but are not easily cultured from a blood sample. See Chapter 9 for radiographic images.

Fungal infections

Migration of fungal disease from other body organs such as the lungs can involve the spinal column or disseminate into the central nervous system and cause neurological disease. Cerebral phaeohyphomycosis has been reported in a green iguana, resulting in a paroxysmal paralysis of all four limbs (Olias *et al.*, 2010). The fungus was only found in the left cerebrum and left ventricle of the brain, showing nervous system tropism. Phycomycosis has also been reported in a rattlesnake, affecting the CNS by extension from skin/sinuses (Williams *et al.*, 1979).

Cryptococcus neoformans has also been described in an anaconda, resulting in neurological disease, gaining access to the blood stream and CNS via the lungs (McNamara *et al.*, 1994).

Cases of respiratory aspergillosis have resulted in septicaemic migration of fungal elements to the CNS. Systemic disease associated with *Chrysosporium* anamorph of *Nannizziopsis vriesii* (CANV) infections that have resulted in neurological signs has also been reported, and seen by this author (Figure 21.11).

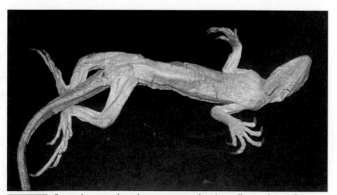

21.11 Green iguana showing severe cachexia, collapse, loss of righting reflex and tremors due to *Chrysosporium* anamorph of *Nannizziopsis vriesii* (CANV) infection and renal failure.

Parasites

Acanthamoebic meningoencephalitis

This is a condition seen primarily in snakes caused by the gut parasites of the *Acanthamoeba* genus. Fits and opisthotonic seizures are seen. Treatment is generally unsuccessful once the central nervous system is involved but may be attempted with metronidazole.

Other parasites

Toxoplasma and *Encephalitozoon* infections have also been reported as a cause of meningoencephalitis in reptiles, but the latter showed no neurological disease (Richter *et al.*, 2013). *Entamoeba invadens* has also been reported causing opisthotonus and seizures in snakes and green iguanas (Frank, 1966).

Cardiovascular trematode infections are common in aquatic chelonians and may result in blockage of vessels supplying nervous tissue, amongst others, and so may result in neurological signs. These are often associated with secondary Gram-negative bacterial infections and granulomata (Raidal *et al.*, 1998).

Systemic diseases

Septicaemia may result in a number of clinical signs including neurological signs such as seizures, tremors, paralysis and paresis. Septicaemic spread to the CNS has also been reported in bacterial and fungal disease and may result in neurological signs. Finally, viral septicaemia commonly affects the CNS and may produce neurological disease – see sections above.

Organopathies, as previously mentioned, may also result in neurological disease, with hypoglycaemia and renal and liver failure often being associated with neurological signs such as collapse, paresis, paralysis and seizures.

Husbandry-related problems

Inappropriate environmental temperatures may result in neurological signs. Low environmental temperatures, as previously mentioned, will lead to slower neurological responses or even ablation of response. Increased environmental temperatures may do the same. Severely low temperatures, those approaching or falling below freezing point, can lead to permanent neurological damage. Frost damage in *Testudo* spp. is not uncommon in the UK in outdoor-hibernated tortoises. Clinical signs can include blindness (both central due to CNS damage and peripheral due to cataract formation) and vestibular disease (often seen as circling with a head tilt). In addition, reduction of environmental temperature will lead to a reduction in the immunocompetence of the reptile and so may allow gastrointestinal or environmental bacteria and fungi to gain access to the bloodstream and result in septicaemia and concurrent neurological disease.

Treatment has been attempted with short-acting corticosteroids, supportive therapy and slow warming. However, if cellular necrosis has occurred, the prognosis is guarded, although neural cell regeneration is more likely in reptiles than in mammals or birds.

Metabolic-related neurological disease

Hypocalcaemic collapse

This is commonly seen in gravid lizards, such as green iguanas, where the blood calcium levels drop too low owing to egg production and insufficient dietary provision of calcium/vitamin D3. The female becomes flaccidly paralysed and unresponsive (Figures 21.12 and 21.13). Occasionally, fine-muscle tremors will be seen. See the section on musculoskeletal diseases for more information.

Treatment: This is by dietary correction of the deficiency in the long term, and by intravenous or intramuscular injection of 100 mg/kg calcium gluconate in the short term. Long-term correction of dietary calcium and vitamin D3 levels/ultraviolet light provision should also be carried out.

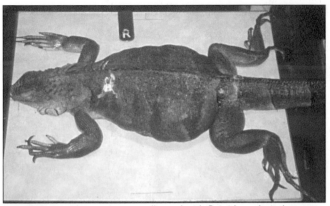

21.12 Gravid green iguana collapsed with flaccid paralysis due to hypocalcaemia.

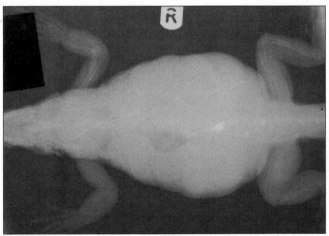

21.13 Gravid green iguana dorsoventral radiograph showing extensive demineralization of the skeleton and pathological fractures associated with nutritional hyperparathyroidism.

Hypovitaminosis B1

Hypovitaminosis B1 is common in aquatic snakes owing to the presence of thiaminases in the diet which cause the destruction of thiamine. A source of these thiaminases is thawed frozen saltwater fish, which may be fed to piscivorous reptiles such as garter snakes, red-eared terrapins and gharials. There are thiamine antagonists present in blackberries, beetroot, coffee, chocolate and tea, when considering the diet of herbivores. When a relative deficiency occurs neurological signs result, including opisthotonus, weakness and head tremors. In garter and water snakes, a classical inability of the animal to right itself occurs, with the snake continually flipping on to its back. In addition, fungal infections are reported as more likely after a vitamin B1 deficiency.

Treatment: Recommended minimum levels for reptiles are 20–35 mg/kg food offered. In addition, if marine fish such as smelt, which are high in thiaminases, are to be fed, cooking the fish for 5 minutes at 80°C has been recommended to deactivate the thiaminase. In a reptile with thiamine deficiency, doses of 50–100 mg/kg thiamine/kg bodyweight are recommended; because of this problem it is often advised feeding garter and water snakes on rodent prey. Scent transfer is done by wiping the rodent prey with the fish to cover the scent.

Biotin deficiency

This is seen in species fed mainly on unfertilized hens eggs, which contain large amounts of the anti-biotin vitamin, avidin. This produces a relative deficiency in biotin which leads to muscle tremors and general weakness. Monitor lizards and egg-eating snakes in captivity are commonly affected.

Treatment: This is long term by changing the diet. In the short term, a multi-B vitamin containing biotin should be administered.

Hypovitaminosis E/selenium deficiency

This has been reported in a green iguana presenting with tremors of all four limbs, knuckling of the forelimbs, lethargy and anorexia (Farnsworth *et al.*, 1986). The iguana responded to vitamin E/selenium injections although no muscle/nerve biopsy was performed to confirm the diagnosis.

Hypoglycaemia

This is a condition seen in farmed crocodiles exposed to excessive social stressors such as overcrowding or attacks by other crocodiles. Muscle tremors and weakness are seen.

Treatment: This involves oral administration of 3 g/kg glucose solution (Stein, 1996).

Cerebral xanthomatosis

This has been reported in green water dragons, geckos, great plated lizards, a Russian viper and a Cuban anole. Many showed progressive neurological signs, some with head bobbing and opisthotonus, and cases were thought to be associated with a high-cholesterol diet (Schmidt and Hubbard, 1987; Garner *et al.*, 1999; Gyimesi *et al.*, 2002; Kummrow *et al.*, 2010). Blood cholesterol levels, where measured, were elevated in all cases and diagnosis was suggested by MRI in some, but the majority were only confirmed at post-mortem with plaques in the forebrain in particular. Treatment once deposits have occurred is unlikely to be successful.

Neoplasia

Spinal cord glioma has been reported in a ridge-nosed rattlesnake associated with a prolonged history of egg retention and decreased motility of the caudal body (Craig *et al.*, 2005). This was diagnosed at post-mortem. Secondary metastasis of malignant neoplasms to the CNS has also been reported in a number of reptiles and may result in neurological disease (Churgin *et al.*, 2013).

Pituitary cystadenoma has been reported in an Everglades ratsnake resulting in hyperkeratosis, dysecdysis and inappetence. The dermatological signs were attributed to endocrine derangements associated with the pituitary neoplasm (Dadone *et al.*, 2010).

Multicentric benign peripheral nerve sheath tumours have been reported in related bearded dragons (Lemberger *et al.*, 2005). The tumours were restricted to the subcutaneous tissue and grossly resembled fat deposits. Malignant nerve sheath tumour has been reported in a water moccasin, again in a peripheral subcutaneous site, producing a white firm tumour which penetrated the coelomic cavity and compressed the liver (Ramis *et al.*, 1998).

Neurofibromas have been reported in many species of animal and may also occur in reptiles (Figure 21.14)

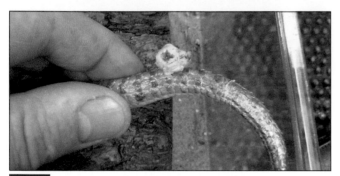

21.14 Neurofibroma on the tail of a Berber skink.

Congenital and inherited conditions

Hydrocephalus has been reported in snakes and may result in dullness, lethargy, seizures and loss of the righting reflex. Whether this is linked to hypovitaminosis A has never been definitively proven in reptiles, but it is one differential.

Congenital ataxia has been reported in snakes, as has so-called 'coiling syndrome', whereby kyphosis or scoliosis of the spine, usually in the caudal third of the body, can occur. This condition appears particularly in boa constrictors and radiographically the vertebrae often appear normal and the CNS does not seem to be affected; rather, there appears to be a mononuclear inflammatory infiltrate of the peripheral motor nerves, suggestive of a viral or other inflammatory disease (Fitzgerald *et al.*, 1990).

Toxins
Pyrethrin/organophosphate poisoning

These are most likely to be associated with mite treatments. Overdose will result in opisthotonus, head tilts, fits and death. Management with atropine in cases of organophosphate poisoning may be successful but is rarely so in pyrethrin cases. Supportive therapy in mildly affected animals may be sufficient to allow recovery.

Chlorhexidine

A 2% solution applied topically or as a soak has been associated with neurological signs such as flaccid paralysis leading to death, and has been reported as more likely in chelonians (Bennet and Mehler, 2006).

Heavy metal toxicosis

Lead poisoning has been reported in chelonians and experimental disease in western fence lizards. It usually results in gut stasis and liver/kidney damage, but may present as neurological disease in reptiles. Treatment with 10–40 mg/kg sodium calcium EDTA q12h has been used. Normal values have been published in green iguanas with whole-blood lead levels as averaging 0.06 µg/ml and zinc plasma levels as 2.68 µg/ml (Burns and Paul-Murphy, 2009).

Ivermectin

Ivermectin has been shown to cause neurological disease and result in fatalities in chelonians, even at therapeutic doses, and so should not be used. It is thought that their increased susceptibility to the paralytic effects of the drug is due to the large number of gamma-aminobutyric acid (GABA) receptors present within the CNS in chelonians. Ivermectin has also been associated with mortality in a chameleon with microfilarial disease. The cause of death, however, could not be proven to be due to ivermectin and could have been associated with a toxic reaction to the death of large numbers of microfilaria (Szell *et al.*, 2001).

Levamisole

This anti-parasitic has a narrow safety margin and neurological toxicity has been reported in reptiles (Rees-Davies and Klingenberg, 2004).

Metronidazole

This has been reported as toxic to indigo snakes and kingsnakes at above 40 mg/kg and in other reptiles periodically above 100 mg/kg (Jacobson, 1988). Hepatotoxicity is seen as well as seizures, opisthotonus and ataxia. Treatment is supportive.

Brevetoxicosis

This has been reported in marine turtles associated with algal blooms, resulting in head bobbing, nervous twitching, oedema and coma (Manire *et al.*, 2013). Dehydration, supportive therapy and antihistamine administration proved successful in some cases.

Plant toxins

Cannabis consumption and toxicity has been reported, resulting in seizures, muscle fasciculations, hyperaesthesia, jaw clamping, loss of toe-pinch reflexes and loss of the righting reflex to varying degrees in three green iguanas (Girling and Fraser, 2011). Symptomatic therapy to control seizures (diazepam and in one case full anaesthesia with propofol and isoflurane), support of the cardiovascular system with fluid therapy and removal of remaining cannabis plant material from the stomach resulted in full recovery.

Oxalate poisoning has resulted in renal damage and hypocalcaemia and has been seen in chelonians in particular consuming plants such as spinach and rhubarb leaves.

Andromedotoxin poisoning associated with rhododendron and azalea poisoning has also been reported in chelonians and iguanas, resulting in neurological signs including seizures and death (Barten, 1996).

Cedarwood and other highly resinous pine chips used as substrate may result in neurological (as well as localized dermatological) disease including loss of righting reflex, weakness, lethargy and seizures. If removed from the source of the problem quickly, most cases are self-resolving.

Miscellaneous
Trauma

Causes of trauma can be many and varied but examples include spinal trauma from lawnmower injuries, car accidents, owners stepping on/driving over their pets, etc. Many injuries can be severe and life-threatening. In most species, paresis or paralysis of the body and limbs caudal to the lesion are obvious (Figure 21.15), with loss of

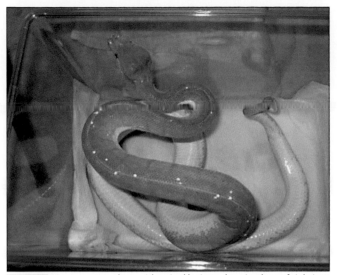

21.15 Green tree python with spinal lesions showing loss of righting reflex caudal to the lesion.

reflexes including righting and withdrawal. It may be necessary to assess spinal trauma, requiring radiography, myelography, and potentially CT and MRI to determine the extent of the problem in addition to electromyographic techniques. Reptiles do have an ability to regrow some damaged nerve cells, even within the CNS; therefore, their prognosis is not as guarded as for a mammal or bird with similar injuries.

Compressive myelopathy has been reported in Komodo dragons with instability in cervical vertebrae 1–4, resulting in quadriplegia, quadriparesis, dullness and anorexia (Zimmermann *et al.*, 2009). One of these cases was due to trauma, but for the other three cases the causal process was unknown.

References and further reading

Abou-Madi N, Scrivani PV, Kollias GV and Hernandez-Divers SM (2004) Diagnosis of skeletal injuries in chelonians using computed tomography. *Journal of Zoo and Wildlife Medicine* **35(2)**, 226–231

Barten S (1996) Lizards. In: *Reptile Medicine and Surgery, 1st edition*, ed. D Mader, pp. 141–148. WB Saunders, Philadelphia

Bennett RA, Hart SH, McSherry LJ *et al.* (2001) Analysis of cerebrospinal fluid in the American alligator. *BSAVA Congress Scientific Proceedings*, p. 554

Bennett RA and Mehler SJ (2006) Neurology. In: *Reptile Medicine and Surgery, 2nd edition*, ed. DR Mader, pp. 239–250. Saunders Elsevier, St Louis, MO, USA

Brown DR, Noguiera MF, Schoeb TR *et al.* (2001) Pathology of experimental mycoplasmosis in American alligators. *Journal of Wildlife Disease* **37(4)**, 671–679

Burns RP and Paul-Murphy J (2009) Determination of lead and zinc concentrations in the blood and liver of the captive common green iguana (*Iguana iguana*). *Journal of Zoo and Wildlife Medicine* **40(3)**, 495–500

Churgin SM, Garner MM, Swenson J *et al.* (2013) Intestinal coccidioidomycosis in a red coachwhip snake (*Masticophis flagellum piceus*). *Journal of Zoo and Wildlife Medicine* **44(4)**, 1094–1097

Clippinger TL, Bennett A, Johnson CM *et al.* (2000) Morbidity and mortality associated with a new *Mycoplasma* species from captive American alligators (*Alligator mississippiensis*). *Journal of Zoo and Wildlife Medicine* **31(3)**, 303–314

Craig LE, Wolf JC and Ramsay EC (2005) Spinal cord glioma in a ridge-nosed rattlesnake (*Crotalus willardi*). *Journal of Zoo and Wildlife Medicine* **36(2)**, 313–315

Cruce WL (1979) Spinal cord in lizards. In: *Biology of the Reptilia: Neurology B, volume 10*, ed. C Gans, RG Northcutt and P Ulinski, pp. 111–131. Academic Press, New York

Dadone LI, Klaphake E, Garner MM *et al.* (2010) Pituitary cystadenoma, enterolipidosis, and cutaneous mycosis in an Everglades ratsnake (*Elaphe obsoleta rossalleni*). *Journal of Zoo and Wildlife Medicine* **41(3)**, 538–541

Farnsworth RJ, Brannian RE, Fletcher KC and Klassen S (1986) A vitamin E-selenium responsive condition in a green iguana. *Journal of Zoo Animal Medicine* **17**, 42–45

Fitzgerald SD, Janovitz EB, Burnstein T and Axthelm MK (1990) A caudal coiling syndrome associated with lymphocytic epaxial perineuritis in newborn boa constrictors. *Journal of Zoo and Wildlife Medicine* **21(4)**, 485–489

Flanigan WF Jnr (1973) Sleep and wakefulness in iguanid lizards, *Ctenosaura pectinata* and *Iguana iguana*. *Brain Behavioural Evolution* **8**, 401–436

Folsch DW and Leloup P (1976) Fatale endemische Infektion in einem Serpentarium. *Tierärztliche Praxis* **4**, 527–536

Frank W (1966) Generalised amoebiasis without intestinal symptoms in an iguana (*Iguana iguana*) (Reptilia, Iguanidae) caused by *Entamoeba invadens* (Protozoa, Amoebozoa). *Zeitschrift für Tropenmedizin und Parasitologie* **17(3)**, 285–294

Frank W (1974) Limax – amoebae from cold-blooded vertebrates. *Annales de la Société Belge de Médecine Tropicale* **54(4,5)**, 343–349

Frye FL (1984) Nutritional disorders in reptiles. In: *Diseases of Amphibians and Reptiles*, ed. GL Hoff, FL Frye and ER Jacobson, pp. 633–660. Springer US

Garner MM, Lung NP and Murray S (1999) Xanthomatosis in geckos: five cases. *Journal of Zoo and Wildlife Medicine* **30**, 443–447

Gaztelu JM, Garcia-Austt E and Bullock TH (1991) Electrocorticograms of hippocampal and dorsal cortex of two reptiles: comparison with possible mammalian homologs. *Brain Behavioural Evolution* **37**, 144–160

Girling SJ (2013) Reptile and amphibian nutrition. In: *Veterinary Nursing of Exotic Pets, 2nd edition*, pp. 286–296. Wiley-Blackwell, Oxford

Girling SJ and Fraser MA (2004) Listeriosis in an inland bearded dragon, *Pogona vitticeps*. *Journal of Herpetological Medicine and Surgery* **14(3)**, 6–12

Girling SJ and Fraser MA (2007) Systemic mycobacteriosis in an inland bearded dragon (*Pogona vitticeps*). *Veterinary Record* **160(15)**, 526–528

Girling SJ and Fraser MA (2011) Cannabis intoxication in three green iguanas (*Iguana iguana*). *Journal of Small Animal Practice* **52(2)**, 113–116

Gyimesi ZS, Stedman NL and Crossett VR (2002) Cholesterol granulomas in a great plated lizard, *Gerrhosaurus major*. *Journal of Herpetological Medicine and Surgery* **12**, 36–39

Holem RR, Hopkins WA and Talent LG (2006) Effect of acute exposure of malathion and lead to sprint performance of the western fence lizard (*Sceloporus occidentalis*). *Archive of Environmental Contaminant Toxicology* **51(1)**, 111–116

Hyndman TH, Shilton CM, Doneley RJ and Nicholls PK (2012) Sunshine virus in Australian pythons. *Veterinary Microbiology* **161(1–2)**, 77–87

Jacobson E, Gaskin JM, Simpson CF and Terrell TG (1980) Paramyxo-like virus infection in a rock rattlesnake. *Journal of the American Veterinary Medical Association* **177(9)**, 796–799

Jacobson ER (1980) Infectious diseases of reptiles. In: *Current Veterinary Therapy VII*, ed. RW Kirk, pp. 625–633. Saunders, Philadelphia

Jacobson ER (1988) Use of chemotherapeutics in reptile medicine. In: *Exotic Animals*, ed. ER Jacobson and GV Kollias Jnr, pp. 35–48. Churchill Livingstone, New York

Jacobson ER (2007) Viruses and viral diseases of reptiles. In: *Infectious Diseases and Pathology of Reptiles*, ed. ER Jacobson, pp. 395–460. CRC Press, Boca Raton, FL, USA

Jacobson ER and Gardiner CH (1990) Adeno-like virus in oesophageal and tracheal mucosa of a Jackson's chameleon (*Chameleo jacksonii*). *Veterinary Pathology* **27**, 210–212

Jacobson ER, Gaskin JM and Gardiner CH (1986) An adenovirus-like infection in a boa constrictor. *Journal of the American Veterinary Medical Association* **187**, 1226–1227

Jacobson ER, Gaskin JM, Wells S, Bowler K and Schumacher J (1992) Epizootic of ophidian paramyxovirus in a zoological collection: pathological microbiological and serological findings. *Journal of Zoo and Wildlife Disease* **23**, 318–327

Jacobson ER, Johnson AJ, Hernandez JA *et al.* (2005) Validation of an enzyme-linked immunosorbent assay for the detection of antibodies to West Nile virus in American alligators (*Alligator mississippiensis*) in Florida. *Journal of Wildlife Diseases* **41(1)**, 107–114

Jacobson ER, Kopit W, Kennedy FA, and Funk RS (1996) Coinfection of a bearded dragon, *Pogona vitticeps*, with adenovirus- and dependovirus-like viruses. *Veterinary Pathology* **33(3)**, 343–346

Kim DY, Mitchell MA, Bauer RW, Poston R and Cho D-Y (2002) An outbreak of adenoviral infection in inland bearded dragons (*Pogona vitticeps*) coinfected with dependovirus and coccidial protozoa (*Isospora* sp.). *Journal of Veterinary Diagnostic Investigation* **14**, 332–334

Klingenberg RJ (1996) Therapeutics. In: *Reptile Medicine and Surgery, 1st edition*, ed. D Mader, pp. 299–321. Saunders, Philadelphia

Kolesnikovas CKM, Grego KF, Rameh de Albuquerque LC *et al.* (2006) Ophidian paramyxovirus in Brazilian vipers (*Bothrops alternatus*). *Veterinary Record* **159**, 390–392

Kummrow MS, Berkvens CN, Paré JA and Smith DA (2010) Cerebral xanthomatosis in three green water dragons (*Physignathus cocincinus*). *Journal of Zoo and Wildlife Medicine* **41(1)**, 128–132

Ladds PW, Bradley J and Hirst RG (1996) *Providenicia rettgeri* meningitis in hatchling saltwater crocodiles (*Crocodylus porosus*). *Australian Veterinary Journal* **74(5)**, 397–398

Lemberger KY, Manharth A and Pessier AP (2005) Multicentric benign peripheral nerve sheath tumors in two related bearded dragons (*Pogona vitticeps*). *Veterinary Pathology* **42(4)**, 507–510

Manire CA, Anderson ET, Byrd L and Fauquier DA (2013) Dehydration as an effective treatment for brevetoxicosis in loggerhead sea turtles (*Caretta caretta*). *Journal of Zoo and Wildlife Medicine* **44(2)**, 447–452

Mariani CL (2007) The neurologic examination and neurodiagnostic techniques for reptiles. *Veterinary Clinics of North America: Exotic Animal Practice* **10(3)**, 855–891

Marschang RE (2011) Viruses infecting reptiles. *Viruses* **3**, 2087–2126

Marschang RE (2013) First detection of sunshine virus in pythons (*Python regius*) in Europe. *Proceedings of the Association of Reptilian and Amphibian Veterinarians Annual Conference*, p.15

Marschang RE, Papp T and Frost JW (2009) Comparison of paramyxovirus isolates from snakes, lizards and a tortoise. *Virus Research* **144**, 272–279

McNamara TS, Cook RA, Behler JL, Ajello L and Padhye AA (1994) Cryptococcosis in a common anaconda (*Eunectes murinus*). *Journal of Zoo and Wildlife Medicine* **25**, 128–132

Miller DL, Mauel MJ, Baldwin C *et al*. (2003) West Nile Virus in farmed alligators. *Emerging Infectious Diseases* **9**, 794–799

Nevarez JG, Mitchell MA, Kim DY, Poston R and Lampinen HM (2005) West Nile Virus in alligator ranches from Louisiana. *Journal of Herpetological Medicine and Surgery* **15**, 4–9

Olias P, Hammer M and Kopfleisch R (2010) Cerebral phaeohyphomycosis in a green iguana (*Iguana iguana*). *Journal of Comparative Pathology* **143(1)**, 61–64

Raidal SR, Ohara M, Hobbs RP and Prince RI (1998) Gram-negative bacterial infections and cardiovascular parasitism in green sea turtle (*Chelonia mydas*). *Australian Veterinary Journal* **76(6)**, 415–417

Ramis A, Pumarola M, Fernandez-Moran J *et al*. (1998) Malignant peripheral nerve sheath tumor in a water moccasin (*Agkistrodon piscivorus*). *Journal of Veterinary Diagnostic Investigation* **10(2)**, 205–208

Raymond JT, Garnber MM, Nordhausen RW and Jacobson ER (2001) A disease resembling inclusion body disease of boid snakes and captive palm vipers (*Bothriechis marchi*). *Journal of Veterinary Diagnostic Investigation* **13**, 82–86

Raymond JT, Lamm M, Nordhausen R, Latimer K and Garner MM (2003) Degenerative encephalopathy in a coastal mountain kingsnake (*Lampropeltis zonata multifasciata*) due to adenoviral-like infection. *Journal of Wildlife Disease* **39**, 431–436

Rees-Davies R and Klingenberg RJ (2004) Therapeutics and medication. In: *BSAVA Manual of Reptiles, 2nd edition*, ed. SJ Girling and P Raiti, pp. 115–130. British Small Animal Veterinary Association, Gloucester, UK

Richter G, Csokai J, Graner I *et al*. (2013) Encephalitozoonosis in two inland bearded dragons (*Pogona vitticeps*). *Journal of Comparative Pathology* **148(2–3)**, 278–282

Schmidt RE and Hubbard GB (1987) Central nervous system. In: *Atlas of Zoo Animal Pathology, Volume 2*, pp. 117–124. CRC Press, Boca Raton, FL, USA

Schumacher J and Toal RL (2001) Advanced radiography and ultrasonography in reptiles. *Seminars in Avian and Exotic Pet Medicine* **10**, 162–168

Srivastava VK (1992) Functional recovery following reptilian (*Calotus calotus*) spinal cord transection. *Indian Journal of Physiology and Pharmacology* **36**, 193–196

Stein G (1996) Reptile and amphibian formulary. In: *Reptile Medicine and Surgery*, ed. DR Mader, pp. 465–472. WB Saunders, Philadelphia

Stenglein MD, Sanders C, Kistler AL *et al*. (2012) Identification, characterization, and *in vitro* culture of highly divergent arenaviruses from boa constrictors and annulated tree boas: candidate etiological agents for snake inclusion body disease. *mBio* **3**, doi:10.1128/mBio.00180-12

Szell Z, Sreter T and Varga I (2001) Ivermectin toxicosis in a chameleon (*Chamaeleo senegalensis*) infected with *Folyella furcata*. *Journal of Zoo and Wildlife Medicine* **32(1)**, 115–117

Teare JA and Bush M (1983) Toxicity and efficacy of ivermectin in chelonians. *Journal of the American Veterinary Association* **183**, 1195–1197

Vancraeynest D, Pasmans F, Martel A *et al*. (2006) Inclusion body disease in snakes: a review and description of three cases in boa constrictors in Belgium. *Veterinary Record* **158(22)**, 757–761

Vieler E, Baumgartner W, Herbst W and Kohler G (1994) Characterisation of a reovirus from a rattlesnake *Crotalus viridis* with neurological dysfunction. *Archives of Virology* **138**, 341–344

Wallach JD (1971) Environmental and nutritional diseases of captive reptiles. *Journal of the American Veterinary Medical Association* **159**, 1632–1643

Wellehan JFX, Gunkel CI, Kledzik D, Robertson SA and Heard DJ (2006) Use of a nerve locator to facilitate administration of mandibular nerve blocks in crocodilians. *Journal of Zoo and Wildlife Medicine* **37(3)**, 405–408

Williams LW, Jacobson E, Gelatt KN, Barrie KP and Shields RP (1979) Phycomycosis in a western massasauga rattlesnake (*Sistrurus catenatus*) with infection of the telencephalon, orbit and facial structures. *Veterinary Medicine Small Animal Clinics* **78(8)**, 1181–1184

Wozniak EJ, DeNardo DF, Brewer A, Wong V and Tarara RP (2000) Identification of adenovirus and dependovirus-like agents in an outbreak of fatal gastroenteritis in captive born California mountain kingsnakes, *Lampropeltis zonata multicincta*. *Journal of Herpetological Medicine and Surgery* **10**, 4–7

Zimmermann DM, Douglass M, Sutherland-Smith M *et al*. (2009) Compressive myelopathy of the cervical spine in Komodo dragons (*Varanus komodiensis*). *Journal of Zoo and Wildlife Medicine* **40(1)**, 207–210

Chapter 22

Nutritional problems

Matthew Rendle and Ian Calvert[†]

Nutritionally related problems are regularly seen in captive reptiles. Many are predominantly related to disorders of vitamin D and calcium metabolism. Inadequate ultraviolet B exposure leads to severe vitamin D deficiency in many reptiles, even those given oral supplementary vitamin D. Reptiles are adapted for very specific photomicrohabitats; many commonly kept reptiles come from regions where high UVB irradiance may be accessible for most of the year. Reproducing suitable levels of UVB exposure in indoor vivaria is often perceived as difficult to achieve and monitor satisfactorily, and can also seem an expensive option to some owners. To confound the problem, reptiles are also often fed diets which are calcium deficient or have inappropriate calcium-to-phosphorus ratios. Consequently, metabolic bone disorder (MBD) of nutritional origin is frequently encountered.

Problems resulting from deficiencies in other vitamins and minerals (such as vitamins A, B1, C, E, biotin and iodine) have also been described. In this chapter, clinical approaches to anorexia will also be considered.

Metabolic bone disorder

Metabolic bone disorder (MBD) is a term in widespread use which actually covers a range of disease entities with very different aetiologies. Nutritional secondary hyperparathyroidism (NSHP) is the commonest cause of MBD in reptiles, but this must be distinguished from renal secondary hyperparathyroidism, typical of chronic renal disease, since their treatments are very different.

Other bone disorders, including hypertrophic osteopathy, osteopetrosis and Paget's disease, have also been recorded in reptiles (Mader, 2006b). Deficiencies in vitamins A or K may also be implicated in bone disorders in some cases.

Nutritional secondary hyperparathyroidism

Nutritional secondary hyperparathyroidism (NSHP) may result from:

- Vitamin D3 deficiency
- A deficiency of calcium in the diet
- Impaired calcium absorption from the diet; for example, from high dietary oxalates (e.g. spinach) or phytates (e.g. cereal products)

- An imbalance in the calcium-to-phosphorus ratio in the diet; for example, from feeding unsupplemented commercially reared insects
- A combination of several of these factors.

Hypervitaminosis A may inhibit calcium uptake by antagonizing calcitriol and increase the risk of MBD (Johansson and Melhus, 2001).

Vitamin D

Although knowledge of vitamin D metabolism in reptiles is fairly rudimentary, this steroid continues to be the subject of extensive research in human medicine. In mammals vitamin D and its hormonal metabolites are known to play a pivotal role in a large number of physiological processes. Appreciating the complexity of this hormonal system is essential when trying to determine why problems have arisen under a particular reptile husbandry regime, and deciding how to correct them.

Vitamin D3 (cholecalciferol) is a precursor to the hormone 1,25-dihydroxy vitamin D3 (1,25(OH)2D3), more usually referred to as calcitriol, which has a vital endocrine function: the maintenance of calcium and phosphorus homeostasis. However, calcitriol also has multiple autocrine and paracrine functions, currently being elucidated. Calcitriol is an extremely potent hormone with widespread actions. Intracellular vitamin D receptors (VDRs) have now been found in almost every organ in the vertebrate body. Calcitriol binds to VDRs and this complex, in turn, binds to DNA sequences on target genes as a heterodimer with a retinoid-X receptor. Transcription factors attach to this complex to complete the process of up-regulating or down-regulating the gene's activity.

Photobiosynthesis of vitamin D

In most vertebrates, the primary source of vitamin D is through the action of ultraviolet light on skin, although many can also absorb pre-synthesized vitamin D from their diet. The crucial wavelengths for natural cutaneous vitamin D synthesis in sunlight are 295–315 nm, within the UVB section of the electromagnetic spectrum.

UVB converts 7-dehydrocholesterol (7-DHC) in the epidermal layers of the skin into previtamin D3 while attached to the keratinocyte plasma membrane; this then undergoes a temperature-sensitive isomerization to produce vitamin D3, which is released from the membrane. This is taken up by a vitamin D binding protein (VDP) and transported from the epidermis into the circulation. Any excess previtamin D3 and vitamin D3 building up in the epidermis are, however, further converted by solar UVB and short-wavelength UVA into apparently inert photo-isomer derivatives (principally lumisterol, tachysterol and suprasterols). Prolonged exposure to natural sunlight does not therefore produce toxic levels of vitamin D3. Production of vitamin D3 is, however, extremely slow at sub-optimal temperatures, as demonstrated in green iguana skin samples incubated at 25°C and 5°C by Holick *et al.* (1995). Therefore both UVB and an adequate skin temperature are crucial for vitamin D biosynthesis.

Once in the circulation, vitamin D3 is transported to the liver where it is enzymatically converted into photostable 25-hydroxy vitamin D3 (25(OH)D3), also sometimes known as calcidiol or calcifediol, which re-enters the circulation, again bound to VDP. This is the circulating storage form of the vitamin. Serum 25(OH)D3 levels are considered a reliable indicator of vitamin D status.

25(OH)D3 has low biological activity when in normal concentrations, and has a long half-life in the circulation, which varies with species and the body's current rate of usage, but which has been estimated at weeks or months for most species. In man, estimates from isotope-labelling studies range from around 15–25 days in apparently healthy individuals (for example, Lips, 2007; Jones, 2008), although serum levels may fall very sharply, presumably owing to increased bodily requirements, in illness or trauma, including surgery (Heaney, 2011). Only a few basic measurements of the fall in serum 25(OH)D3 with UVB and/or dietary vitamin D deprivation have been conducted in reptiles. The results suggest a longer half-life in some species; for example, 128–139 days in black-throated monitor lizards (Ferguson *et al.*, 2009).

In humans, liver disease can result in vitamin D deficiency as a result of a reduced ability to hydroxylate vitamin D3 into 25(OH)D3. To date, this does not appear to have been studied in reptiles.

Calcitriol production

Circulating 25(OH)D3 is the substrate for the active hormone, calcitriol. Calcitriol synthesized within renal cells is released into the circulation, once again bound to VDP, and has vital endocrine functions that have been well known for many years.

However, many other types of cells, including cells in the brain and vascular smooth muscle and macrophages, have recently been discovered to possess not only VDRs but also the enzymatic ability to produce intracellular calcitriol, which has a purely autocrine and paracrine function within these cells.

Endocrine functions of calcitriol

Calcitriol produced by the kidneys has a very short half-life in the bloodstream. Estimates range from 7–20 hours in humans (Lips, 2007; Jones, 2008). Serum calcitriol levels are normally about 1000 times lower than those of 25(OH)D3 (and thus only in the picomole range) and held within narrow physiological limits. Renal calcitriol production is closely regulated, increasing in response to raised parathyroid hormone (PTH) levels and low serum calcium or phosphorus. Conversely, hyperphosphataemia will inhibit calcitriol synthesis, and elevated serum calcium will depress PTH release and thereby also reduce the synthesis of calcitriol. Excess serum calcitriol will also inhibit its own production by the kidney, and increase metabolic clearance of both itself and its substrate, 25(OH)D3.

Because of the tight physiological control of serum levels and very rapid turnover, serum calcitriol levels do not indicate vitamin D status; their measurement is unhelpful in this respect. Moreover, in NSHP, calcitriol levels may be normal or even elevated despite vitamin D insufficiency, since high serum PTH will stimulate increased production of calcitriol.

Circulating calcitriol acts upon intestinal epithelial cells by up-regulating expression of genes encoding an epithelial calcium channel and a calcium-binding protein. These enable increased active transport of calcium ions from the intestine into the circulation. Phosphate ions follow the calcium, and so both calcium and phosphorus uptake is increased. Passive uptake of calcium between enterocytes across a diffusion gradient is not affected by calcitriol, and in some species, given high enough enteral calcium concentrations, it is sufficient in itself to maintain calcium homeostasis. This appears to be the case with, for example, leopard geckos. Other species, such as day geckos, appear to rely far more upon active transport and hence upon adequate vitamin D status; with these, merely increasing dietary calcium is ineffective in preventing NSHP (Allen *et al.*, 1996).

In most species, low levels of calcitriol are adequate to maintain calcium homeostasis via control of enteral uptake. However, if serum calcium levels fall despite increased intestinal absorption, raised PTH concentrations stimulate further actions (DeLuca, 2004). In the kidneys, when PTH is elevated, calcitriol up-regulates calcium reabsorption from the glomerular filtrate, raising serum calcium by preventing its loss. Calcitriol from the bloodstream also acts to release calcium from bone cells. Calcitriol binds to VDRs in osteoblasts, which in conjunction with PTH causes them to release a specific cytokine, RANKL, which stimulates the maturation of osteoclasts. These release calcium and phosphate ions from bone into the bloodstream, thereby raising serum calcium and phosphorus levels and restoring homeostasis.

Rising serum calcium exerts a negative feedback on the production of PTH from the parathyroid gland, thus 'turning off' the mechanism. Should serum calcium continue to rise, however, the hormone calcitonin is released from the ultimobranchial gland. This inhibits osteoclast activity in bones, inhibits calcium absorption by the gut, and inhibits renal reabsorption of calcium and phosphorus, thereby increasing their excretion.

Figure 22.1 is a simplified diagram of the hormonal regulation of serum calcium in mammals. The system is likely to be very similar in reptiles; PTH, calcitriol and calcitonin are found in all reptiles, and the effect of parathyroidectomy in some reptile species is similar to that in mammals. Some turtles, however, appear to be able to maintain normal blood calcium levels without PTH, possibly utilizing the large stores of calcium and phosphate in their carapace bone (Clark, 1983), while in a number of species there are seasonal changes in the structure of the parathyroid glands.

Paracrine and autocrine functions of calcitriol

Calcitriol is thought to regulate the expression of as many as 2000 genes, controlling, in addition to calcium metabolism, a wide range of biological processes including cellular proliferation and differentiation during growth and healing, hormonal responses to seasonal changes, and the production of insulin and renin. It also has a major influence upon the effectiveness of the immune system. In lower vertebrates the innate immune system is of particular

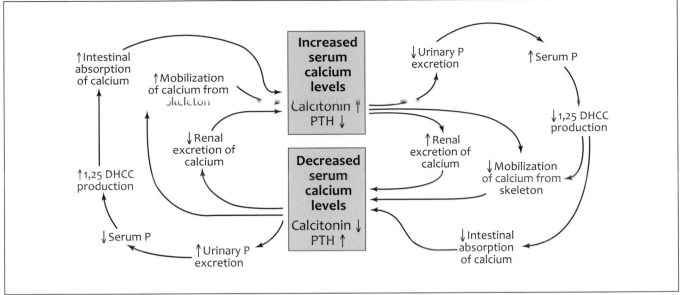

22.1 Some factors affecting blood calcium levels in mammals. Current information suggests the system is similar in reptiles. The two prime controls are PTH and calcitonin. 1,25 DHCC = 1,25-dihydroxycholecalciferol; P = phosphorus; PTH = parathyroid hormone.
(Courtesy of Dermod Malley and Peter Scott)

importance; vitamin D has important effects on toll-like receptors and upon the differentiation of monocytes to macrophages and their activation, as well as on the adaptive immune system through modification of T cell differentiation. It promotes synthesis of anti-inflammatory cytokines and stimulates the production of antimicrobial peptides. (For a detailed review, see Hossein-nezhad and Holick, 2013.)

Reptiles suffering from even moderate vitamin D deficiency may therefore display a higher incidence of problems as diverse as reduced immunocompetence, disturbed glucose metabolism and cardiovascular disease, in addition to increased risk of conditions related to calcium deficiency, such as smooth- and striated-muscle weakness, tetany, reproductive failure and NSHP.

Photobiosynthetic ability

Evidence continues to accumulate regarding the ability of many reptiles to synthesize vitamin D3 endogenously; however, there appear to be marked differences between species. For example, studies have demonstrated vitamin D3 synthesis, as indicated by increases in 25(OH)D3, following exposure to UVB in species as diverse as corn snakes (Acierno *et al.*, 2008), red-eared slider turtles (Acierno *et al.*, 2006), Hermann's tortoises (Selleri and Di Girolamo, 2012), chuckwallas (Aucone *et al.*, 2003), veiled chameleons (Hoby *et al.*, 2010) and black-throated monitors (Ferguson *et al.*, 2009), but no significant elevation in 25(OH)D3 levels were measured following exposure of a small group of ball pythons to UVB lighting (Hedley and Eatwell, 2013).

Differences in the amount of UVB exposure required for optimal vitamin D production have been found between lizard species. The Texas spiny lizard and the Mediterranean house gecko have similar quantities of 7-DHC per unit area of skin. However, when exposed to equal amounts of UVB the gecko produced larger quantities of previtamin D3 per unit time than the spiny lizard (Carman *et al.*, 2000) (Figure 22.2). It has long been assumed that nocturnal reptiles

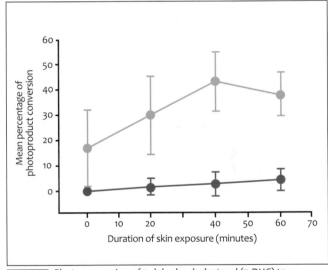

22.2 Photoconversion of 7-dehydrocholesterol (7-DHC) to previtamin D in the skin of the nocturnal house gecko (green) and the diurnal Texas spiny lizard (red).
(Reproduced from Carman *et al.* (2000) with the permission of the American Society of Ichthyologists and Herpetologists)

obtain vitamin D solely from their food; however, these results suggest that geckos have a sensitive response to UVB, and may synthesize sufficient vitamin D3 by exposing themselves to even small amounts of UVB, possibly from daylight reaching their diurnal retreats, or during brief periods of exposure to weak sunlight at dawn or dusk. This is likely to be a crucial behaviour since their invertebrate diet contains virtually no vitamin D. Similarly, a shade-dwelling species of anole lizard has skin with greater photobiosynthetic ability than that possessed by a more heliophilic anole species (Ferguson *et al.*, 2005).

It is likely that the skin of species which occupy microhabitats with more intense solar radiation has evolved a more protective function, with a balance achieved between damage prevention and vitamin D synthesis. The corollary of this is that such species will require greater UVB exposure in captivity, than shade-dwelling species, to achieve normal levels of vitamin D3 synthesis.

Dietary vitamin D

Vitamin D3 is a fat-soluble molecule which can be absorbed from the intestinal tract of many species, especially carnivores, enabling them to utilize the vitamin D3 initially synthesized and stored by their prey. From the gut, it is primarily transported to the liver in chylomicrons and lipoproteins, as opposed to VDPs; in humans, at least, this results in more rapid but less well sustained rises in serum 25(OH)D3 levels (Haddad *et al.*, 1993), and some vitamin D3 may remain unhydroxylated and become sequestered in fat stores.

Plants produce a related analogue, vitamin D2 (ergocalciferol), which can be metabolized in a similar manner to vitamin D3. However, the biological activity of vitamin D2 and its metabolites is much lower than vitamin D3 in most vertebrates (Hay and Watson, 1977; Armas *et al.*, 2004). Thus, when using vitamin supplements as the sole source of vitamin D for reptiles it is important to know what form of vitamin D is being used; vitamin D3 (cholecalciferol) is always preferable.

Appropriate vitamin D sources for different reptiles

As in mammals, a range of species-specific strategies seem to be used to obtain adequate amounts of vitamin D. Many rely entirely on photobiosynthesis, others use dietary sources, others use a combination, and some may require hardly any. Failure to recognize this spectrum has led to much confusion in the reptilian literature.

Chelonians: Vitamin D3 and calcium metabolism in chelonians is not yet well understood. Apparently, healthy captive desert tortoises housed outdoors in the Mojave Desert had serum 25(OH)D3 levels ranging from less than 12.5 nmol/l (5 ng/ml) to 41.3 nmol/l (16.5 ng/ml) (Eatwell 2008b). Juvenile desert and African spurred tortoises kept indoors with no UVB exposure and fed 2000 IU vitamin D3 daily remained apparently healthy despite similarly low 25(OH)D3 levels; moreover, single doses of 20,000 IU/kg dry matter (DM) of diet or 8.5 IU/g bodyweight, respectively, had no measurable effect on these levels (Ullrey and Bernard, 1999). This suggests that these species rely upon cutaneous synthesis for their vitamin D3, but do not maintain high circulating levels despite ample basking opportunities with high UV irradiance.

Much higher 25(OH)D3 levels may be normal for other chelonian species. A group of Hermann's tortoises kept outdoors exposed to Mediterranean sunlight maintained serum 25(OH)D3 levels from an initial mean value of 356 nmol/l (142 ng/ml), whereas in a group moved indoors for only 35 days, housed under weak sources of UVB (branded mercury vapour and fluorescent UVB reptile lamps), levels fell to means of 156 and 134 nmol/l respectively (62 and 54 ng/ml) (Selleri and Di Girolamo, 2012). In captivity in higher latitudes, however, Mediterranean species may not be able to maintain high vitamin D levels even with free access to sunlight. Eatwell (2008b) took samples from apparently healthy captive Mediterranean tortoises housed outdoors in the UK and determined a mean 25(OH)D3 serum value of only 28.4 nmol/l (11.4 ng/ml). This is not merely a result of reduced hours of sunshine in the cloudy British climate. Solar UVB is attenuated by the atmosphere, and solar

altitude is a major determinant of the thickness of atmosphere through which the sunlight must pass. At higher latitudes, the sun remains lower in the sky, even at midday, and photobiosynthetic opportunity is thereby greatly reduced.

Disorders of calcium metabolism and vitamin D deficiency may also play a role in the development of pyramiding in tortoises (see later).

Based on current research it seems sensible to assume that oral supplements of vitamin D3 alone may be inadequate for many species of lizards and tortoises until experimental evidence proves otherwise. However, artificial sources of UVB light vary widely in their spectrum and output, and some of these may also prove inadequate to enable sufficient vitamin D3 synthesis.

Lizards: Carnivorous species might be expected to obtain most of their vitamin D3 requirement from their natural diet, but this may not always be the case. Gillespie *et al.* (2000) measured normal serum 25(OH)D3 levels in wild Komodo dragons within the range of 117–324 nmol/l (46.8–130 ng/ml), with median 183 nmol/l (73 ng/ml). However, two juvenile Komodo dragons in captivity at Louisville Zoo, Kentucky, were unable to maintain normal 25(OH)D3 levels without exposure to UVB from natural sunlight. Despite being fed diets containing 1600–3000 IU vitamin D3 per kg DM, one animal lost over 50% of circulating 25(OH)D3 after being moved indoors for about 8 months (Gyimesi and Burns, 2002).

Vitamin D3 is not synthesized by plants or insects, so it is not normal for obligate herbivores and insectivores to obtain vitamin D3 from the diet. Some species, such as green iguanas and Madagascar day geckos, appear unable to utilize dietary vitamin D3 effectively (Allen *et al.*, 1996). Normal circulating 25(OH)D3 levels do not seem to have been measured from wild green iguanas, but in his investigations Allen reported levels of up to 1000 nmol/l (400 ng/ml) in captive green iguanas housed outdoors and fed diets containing 5000 IU vitamin D3 per kg DM. Green iguanas kept indoors, despite being fed a diet containing 2000 IU vitamin D3 per kg DM, had serum concentrations of 25(OH)D3 <12.5 nmol/l (5 ng/ml). The indoor iguanas, perhaps not surprisingly, developed skeletal abnormalities.

Madagascar day geckos fed crickets containing either 319 IU or 720 IU vitamin D3 per kg DM, without UVB exposure, grew poorly; all but one died, and all had pliable bones at necropsy. In contrast, leopard geckos fed the same diets without UVB exposure but with high dietary calcium developed normally, and only those on a low-calcium diet developed MBD (Allen, 1989ab).

Perhaps more surprisingly, field-caught juveniles of the heliophilic insectivorous western fence lizard, kept without access to UVB light and fed diets deficient in vitamin D3 (but not calcium) for 10 weeks, had almost identical concentrations of calcium and phosphorus in their serum and bones to those in a group of animals reared in the wild, and grew at a similar rate (Gehrmann *et al.*, 1991). This seems to confirm that some species are able to take in sufficient calcium from their diet via passive absorption.

Studies aiming to compare the effectiveness of oral supplementation *versus* provision of UVB have added to the confusion, largely because of wide variation in estimates for appropriate amounts of dietary vitamin D3 and in the measurement of UVB exposure. The species studied to date include veiled chameleons (Hoby *et al.*, 2010), green iguanas (Allen *et al.*, 1996; Hibma, 2004), bearded dragons (Oonincx *et al.*, 2010; Kroenlein *et al.*, 2011) and black-throated monitor lizards (Ferguson *et al.*, 2009).

Some researchers have included measurements of the total UVB available within the basking area, but no studies have explored the effect of spectral differences between lamps and sunlight, which can have profound implications for the resulting photoproducts (MacLaughlin et al., 1982). Some results suggest that abnormally short wavelength (less than 290 nm) UVB may disrupt natural mechanisms preventing overproduction of vitamin D. For example, the green iguanas in the Allen et al. (1996) study were subjected to low levels of UVB from a phototherapy lamp emitting very short wavelength UVB, and some developed extraordinarily high 25(OH)D3 blood levels, up to 1280 nmol/l (513 ng/ml).

Other researchers have described conflicting and even bizarre results, which may be related to differences in irradiance and/or spectrum between lamp brands. Kroenlein et al. (2011) raised groups of bearded dragons, all given diets containing some vitamin D3, under different lamps. Inexplicably, the serum 25(OH)D3 levels in a group housed for 11 weeks under a household compact fluorescent lamp emitting apparently insignificant UVB were reported to be around 350 nmol/l (140 ng/ml), significantly higher than from groups housed with a branded reptile UVB fluorescent tube and a mercury vapour lamp, both of which emitted approximately eight times more UVB than the household bulb, and from a control group housed outdoors in natural sunlight where even higher irradiances could be obtained. 25(OH)D3 in these groups ranged from around 50–200 nmol/l (20–80 ng/ml). Conversely, Oonincx et al. (2010) reported 18 times greater 25(OH)D3 levels in young bearded dragons reared with a reptile UVB compact fluorescent lamp (178.4 nmol/l; 71.4 ng/ml) than in a group reared with no UVB lamp but given vitamin D3 orally (18.6 nmol/l; 7.4 ng/ml).

The Hoby et al. (2010) study demonstrated that 25(OH)D3 serum concentrations above 250 nmol/l (100 ng/ml) and healthy bone growth were achieved with juvenile veiled chameleons when both dietary vitamin D3 and UVB from a branded reptile UVB compact lamp were supplied. Dietary vitamin D3 or UVB in isolation raised serum values above 100 nmol/l (40 ng/ml), indicating that veiled chameleons can utilize vitamin D3 from either source, but skeletal deformities consistent with NSHP were seen in the group without dietary supplementation. The UVB provided was apparently insufficient, on its own, to prevent vitamin D deficiency. Whether a lamp with greater UVB irradiance would have proven sufficient, of course, remains unknown.

Basking, although primarily thermoregulatory in function, may in some species include behavioural regulation of UV exposure. Panther chameleons fed diets low in vitamin D3 spent more time basking at locations where UVB levels were high, than did individuals fed diets with high levels of vitamin D3 (Ferguson et al., 2003; Karsten et al., 2009). Similar results were obtained with the heliophilic brown anole, but not with the sympatric shade-dwelling grey anole in Jamaica (Ferguson et al., 2013). It therefore appears that some species which can obtain vitamin D3 both from the diet and via photobiosynthesis will voluntarily increase their UVB exposure if vitamin D deficient. The presence of VDRs in the reptile brain suggests that a physiological mechanism may exist for such behavioural regulation (Bidmon and Stumpf, 1996).

Snakes: Most snakes consume diets containing high levels of calcium and adequate amounts of vitamin D, and rarely display evidence of NSHP. However, snakes fed entirely on all-meat diets or those with little bone, such as neonatal (pinkie) mice may risk calcium and/or vitamin D deficiency, particularly if the pinkie mice had not suckled, or if the dams of the mice were themselves deficient. Some species of snake, as described above, can demonstrably obtain vitamin D3 by photobiosynthesis; many diurnal snakes naturally bask in sunlight, which would make cutaneous synthesis a likely resource for them. Nevertheless, the provision of UVB lighting for captive snakes remains a rarity, except in some naturalistic terraria as seen in some zoos.

Vitamin D supplementation and its problems

Vitamin D3 is commercially produced by the irradiation of sheep's lanolin, which contains 7-DHC. It is available as a supplement either in powdered form or dissolved in edible oil. However, mixing vitamin D with fats and oils may reduce its shelf life because it is prone to oxidation by unsaturated fatty acids. Vitamin D can also be damaged by iron and copper in foodstuffs, and is photolabile. Products containing vitamin D should be marked with an expiry date. Vitamin D3 in powdered form mixed with calcium carbonate, with or without an additional mineral and vitamin supplement, is widely sold 'over the counter' as a dusting powder for use with feeder insects or sprinkled on the food. However, the amount of vitamin D3 varies widely between brands, and even if the labelling accurately reflects the content and it is stored properly, accurate daily 'dosing' with 'pinches' of dusting powder is virtually impossible.

The amount actually consumed by the reptile may also bear little relationship to the amount added to the food. Donoghue (2006) cites a case study in which veiled chameleons were treated successfully for NSHP with exposure to UVB light and natural sunlight, and feeding of crickets dusted with a supplement containing 32,000 IU/kg. It was estimated that only 7% of the supplement applied to the crickets actually stuck to them long enough to be ingested. It was therefore calculated that its use resulted in a diet containing 2000–5500 IU/kg DM. Following treatment, the chameleons were maintained apparently successfully, with UVB light and sun exposure, on a supplement containing 19,000 IU/kg, which, applied in the same way to the crickets, was estimated to result in a diet containing 2000–3000 IU/kg DM.

Veterinary and human medicinal vitamin D3 products with guaranteed analysis are suitable resources for controlled supplementation during treatment. A serious problem facing both owners and veterinary surgeons (veterinarians) is that suitable dosages for supplementation are still unknown for any species. Published 'general recommendations' cover a wide range; for example, calcium 0.6–1.5% DM, phosphorus 0.5–0.8% DM, vitamin D3 200–2000 IU/kg DM, with a maximum tolerance of 5000 IU/kg DM (Donoghue, 2006). However, green iguanas fed diets containing 1.5% calcium, 0.7% phosphate and 2000 IU vitamin D3 per kg DM still developed NSHP (Ullrey and Bernard, 1999).

Hypervitaminosis D and hypercalcaemia

Fortunately, contrary to popular belief, it is quite difficult to over-supplement reptiles to the point of toxicity with oral vitamin D preparations. Some species, as previously described, seem unable to absorb vitamin D from the gut. In species which can absorb it, one might expect excessive doses to cause toxicity from hypercalcaemia, as it does in mammals. However, this has not been observed, and even parenteral administration of high doses may not always cause harm.

If massive overdoses of parenteral vitamin D preparations are given, hypercalcaemia may be encountered. Daily injections of 1000 IU/kg bodyweight vitamin D or 100 IU/kg calcitriol to an Asian water snake for 15 days caused significant hypercalcaemia and hyperphosphataemia (Srivastav *et al.*, 1995). Similarly, injecting yellow monitors with vitamin D3 (20,000 IU/kg) produced hypercalcaemia within 3 days (Swarup *et al.*, 1987), but neither research group noted adverse effects.

Green iguanas given a massive oral dose of 8500 IU/kg bodyweight vitamin D3 (equivalent to 1,200,000 IU vitamin D3 per kg of dietary DM) showed no ill effects (Allen *et al.*, 1996). Likewise, Ferguson *et al.* (2009) dosed groups of black-throated monitors with either 5000, 10,000 or 15,000 IU/kg bodyweight parentally weekly for 13 weeks, and observed a 600% rise in 25(OH)D3 levels above an initial mean value of 185 ng/ml (461.7 nmol/l); however, no toxicity was seen.

In humans, chronic elevation of serum calcium and phosphorus levels can lead to metastatic calcification of a wide range of soft tissues, particularly blood vessels and especially the aorta and pulmonary arteries. Metastatic calcification occurs when serum levels exceed the calcium x phosphate solubility product (i.e. serum phosphate (mg/100 ml) x serum calcium (mg/100 ml) >50).

Cases of metastatic calcification have occasionally been reported in reptiles and ascribed to hypervitaminosis D; however, no controlled studies have been performed to identify toxic doses of vitamin D in reptiles. Zwart (1980) reported calcification in young iguanas fed a diet containing only 100 IU vitamin D3 per kg DM, but this is unlikely to have been due to hypervitaminosis D. In a study where serum levels of vitamin D were actually measured, the levels were extremely low compared with wild iguanas, confirming that vitamin D toxicity was not the cause of the tissue calcification (Rickman *et al.*, 1995). Calcitriol production in reptiles inhibits the further secretion of PTH; reptiles with chronic renal disease (or failure) are deficient in calcitriol and so PTH continues to be secreted, which leads to metastatic mineralization.

Metastatic calcification, which occurs in otherwise normal tissues, must also be distinguished from dystrophic calcification, which occurs in damaged or necrotic tissues and may be completely unrelated to elevated serum calcium or phosphate.

Normal serum calcium levels in most reptiles are within 8–11 mg/dl. Ionized calcium, however, is the active form with clinical significance and this is held within a very narrow physiological range in all vertebrates; hence, elevated ionized calcium levels have greater clinical significance.

Hypercalcaemia due to hypervitaminosis D is rare, though, as are other possible causes such as primary hyperparathyroidism or tumours stimulating vitamin D production (e.g. sarcoidosis). A far more common finding is hypercalcaemia in female reptiles early in the breeding season. Hypercalcaemia is a normal response to follicular development, in response to oestrogens. The calcium in this case is protein bound, destined primarily for vitellogenesis. Total serum calcium may rise fourfold, with no adverse effects since ionized calcium levels remain within normal limits.

Hypercalcaemia due to abnormally elevated calcitriol can be treated with fluid therapy (Divers, 1999) and cortisol, which inhibits the conversion of 25(OH)D3 to calcitriol.

Disorders of the vitamin D system

In addition to primary vitamin D deficiency, in mammals abnormal bone mineralization may be caused by a range of genetic disorders that cause malfunctions in the metabolism of vitamin D (Haussler *et al.*, 1998). Similar disorders have been seen in reptiles (Mader, 2001), although many can go undetected unless calcifediol levels are measured. Reptiles with genetic disorders are unlikely to respond to improvements in nutrition and UVB exposure.

It is also known that there is considerable polymorphic variation in VDR proteins in humans; this ultimately affects vitamin D and calcium requirements and manifests itself as differences in bone strength and density in individuals on comparable diets (Morrison *et al.*, 1994; Uitterlinden *et al.*, 2002). The vitamin D system is evolutionarily very old and similar VDR protein variants are likely to occur in reptiles; thus, some individuals may be affected more severely by lack of UVB light and/or calcium deficiency than others.

Ultraviolet lighting for reptiles

Benefits of UV light

Reptiles are quite literally 'solar powered'; every aspect of their lives is governed by their daily experience of solar light and heat – or the artificial equivalent, when they are housed indoors. They require all wavelengths from infrared to ultraviolet, in amounts which depend upon their microhabitat and normal basking behaviour (or lack thereof). Each part of the spectrum has specific effects (Figure 22.3). Careful provision of lighting is essential for a healthy reptile in captivity.

When discussing lighting, most reptile owners assume that the light is only necessary for vision. However, non-visual perception of light is equally vital to reptiles. The length of day and night, the sun's position in the sky, the intensity and the amount of short-wavelength light in the sunlight all give precise information about the time of day and season of the year; in response, the reptile adjusts its activity levels and its daily and seasonal behaviour. The eyes, and the parietal eye (third eye) in those species which have one, transmit information to the neuroendocrine system mediated via the pineal body and suprachiasmatic nuclei. There are even deep brain photoreceptors in the base of the lateral ventricles of the reptile brain that respond directly to the glow of sunlight which penetrates the skull. Light alters production of melatonin, serotonin and pituitary hormones and adjusts body clocks controlling functions as diverse as thermoregulation 'set points', the immune system and reproductive cycles (Ralph *et al.*, 1979; Vigh *et al.*, 2002).

Some reptiles appear to select a basking site based upon the intensity of its illumination. If heat and light sources are separated, reptiles may not choose what would appear to be the optimal 'hot spot' nor UVB zone; presumably a bright patch of sunlight is attractive to heliotherms because they evolved to receive heat, light and UV from the same location (Dickinson and Fa, 1997).

It would therefore seem important to position high-intensity visible light, UVB and heat sources close together in the vivarium, to create a well-defined basking zone. This is the ideal way to create a good thermal gradient, vital for thermoregulation. It also makes it easy to provide shade and shelter in other parts of the vivarium.

Even nocturnal species govern their behaviour by monitoring day and night from their hiding places during daylight hours (Sievert and Hutchison, 1988). It follows that even nocturnal reptiles may benefit from the provision of patches of artificial 'sunlight' in the daytime, even if they do not bask in them. Many also sleep in places reached by daylight, if not direct sunlight, thus enabling cutaneous vitamin D synthesis throughout the day.

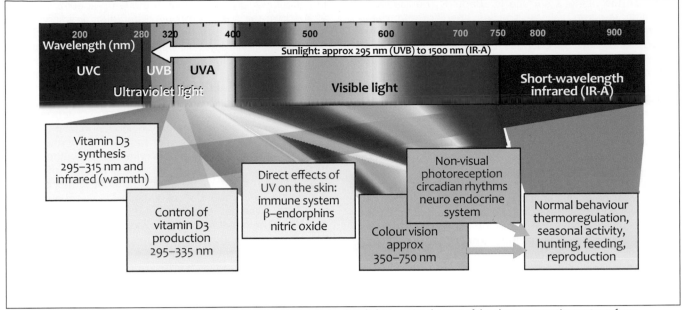

22.3 The utilization of all parts of the solar spectrum by reptiles. Natural sunlight contains the part of the electromagnetic spectrum from medium-wavelength UVB around 290–295 nm (depending upon solar altitude) to short-wavelength infrared. Earth's atmosphere blocks solar radiation with wavelengths shorter than 290 nm.
(Courtesy of Frances M. Baines)

Ultraviolet is a normal component of sunlight. Most reptiles see UVA-wavelength light as a 'colour in their rainbow', and utilize it in recognizing conspecifics and food items; its provision within the spectrum is therefore very important (Moehn, 1974; Fleishman *et al.*, 1993; Honkavaara *et al.*, 2002).

As well as its role in enabling and regulating cutaneous vitamin D synthesis, as described above, ultraviolet light has direct effects upon skin which include the destruction of bacteria, fungi and viruses; the induction of pigment formation; and the modulation of the cutaneous immune system. It also stimulates production of beta endorphins (giving sunlight its 'feel-good' factor), improves skin barrier functions and induces nitric oxide production, which has localized protective effects (Juzeniene and Moan, 2012).

Provision of UV light
Natural unfiltered sunlight

This is ideal wherever the climate makes it possible. Outdoor enclosures for temperate reptiles such as Mediterranean tortoises are highly beneficial. As far as UVA and visible light are concerned, useful levels are available worldwide at any time of the year. However, because of stronger atmospheric absorption, levels of UVB in sunlight are much attenuated when the sun is low in the sky. In high latitudes, such as in the UK, low solar altitudes and increased cloud cover result in much lower UVB levels year-round, but especially in winter. In humans, levels drop to below those necessary for adequate cutaneous D3 synthesis for up to 5 months of the year at approximate latitude 50°N (Holick, 2004). For reptiles evolved to live in tropical sunlight, even full outdoor access in summer in the UK may not provide sufficient UVB to maintain adequate vitamin D3 levels.

Sunlight passing through specialized UV-transmitting glass or acrylic

Provided that the undesirable build-up of heat caused by sunlight is prevented, the admission of natural daylight and even sunlight to large enclosures through skylights or roofing for 'greenhouse' enclosures can be very beneficial. However, ordinary glass blocks 98–99% of all UVB and a high percentage of short-wavelength UVA. Polycarbonates and most other plastics used for glazing panels also block UVB and, in some cases, all the UVA. Pure acrylic permits high UV transmission; however, most acrylics used for glazing are deliberately treated with UV-blocking substances. UV-transmitting acrylic sheeting ('sunbed acrylic') has been used in zoos and private collections and appears very effective (Baines and Davis, 2005). Brands such as Lucite Perspex XT0X02 and Irpen Policril, providing 84–86% UVB transmission, are currently available from a few specialist UK suppliers. A high-quality German twin-wall acrylic product actually designed for glazing commercial greenhouses, Plexiglas Alltop SDP16, transmits approximately 78% UVB; breeding success in tuataras at a New Zealand collection housed indoors has been obtained following its installation in skylights (Price, 2011). Low-iron high-light-transmission architectural glass sold under the brand names Pilkington Optiwhite and AGC Planibel Clearvision allowed 50–56% transmission in tests.

Recently, UV-transmitting flexible plastic polytunnel sheeting has also become available, under brand names such as Lumisol Clear by Bpi.Visqueen, with 66% transmission at 300 nm, and Sunmaster Clear by XL Horticulture Ltd, with 58% transmission at 300 nm. Partial covering of outdoor enclosures with UVT materials can create sheltered microclimates while maintaining adequate solar exposure for vitamin D synthesis (Highfield, 2015).

Artificial lighting

General aspects: A wide range of lighting products are sold for reptiles. Tungsten and halogen incandescent bulbs and LEDs do not emit UVB. Some metal halide and mercury vapour lamps, fluorescent tubes and 'compact' fluorescent lamps do; however, types and brands vary widely. The suitability of any lamp is governed by two features: its quality (the spectrum) and quantity (the intensity of the light and the shape of the beam).

The template for the ideal spectral power distribution is the solar spectrum, under which life evolved and to which all life on the planet's surface is adapted. The irradiance (intensity) required will be species specific, and determined by the animals' microhabitat, as will the photoperiod. The natural changes in both spectrum and intensity which occur in nature owing to the changing position of the sun in the sky, the seasons and the weather are far more difficult to imitate, but creative solutions with timers, dimmers and use of lamps with different spectral power distributions at different times of day can be very effective, for example, simulating 'dawn' and 'dusk'.

Lighting the vivarium is not simply a matter of choosing a bulb. Each type of lamp has a characteristic spectrum, level of intensity and beam spread, with a mixture of optimal and suboptimal features when comparing the light source with solar illumination. It is unlikely that just one bulb will ever provide a full solution. Lamps must be selected and combined to create the specific environment required by that species, taking into account the ambient light levels required, the provision of heating and the presence or absence of a distinct basking spot with a higher level of illumination.

All lamps should also be directly above the animals, so that the light source is never in their direct line of sight, shining straight into their eyes. UVB-emitting lamps should always be positioned in close proximity to non-UVB lamps emitting bright visible light and infrared, enabling instinctive responses to sunlight, which is a continuous spectrum of radiant heat, light and UV. Such combinations also create a much more complete simulation of a solar spectrum, i.e. a much better quality light. In addition, if the animal looks up at the light, the intensely bright visible light will be aversive, protecting the animal's eyes from prolonged UV exposure.

The desired level of UVB will, of course, govern the choice of lamps and determine the distance at which they will need to be placed above the animal. The Ferguson Zones (see below) may provide 'ballpark' estimates of suitable target ultraviolet index (UVI) values.

No ordinary plastic or glass must be placed between the lamp and the reptile as this selectively blocks UVB (as described above). Wire mesh allows the passage of all wavelengths of light including UV light; its effect is to physically block a percentage of this light. Mesh screen commonly used for terrarium lids typically blocks 30–35%. This must be taken into account when planning lamp placement.

All lamps lose their UVB output slowly as they age and their outer glass solarizes, blocking the shortest wavelengths first. For this reason, checks on the UV output of all lamp units should be made regularly. Monthly checks with a UV meter (such as the Solarmeter 6.5 UV Index meter, Solartech Inc., Harrison Township, MI) are likely to be sufficient unless a problem is suspected or a lamp appears to be coming to the end of its useful life. Most products undergo a fairly rapid initial decay as the lamp chemistry settles down. After several weeks the rate of decay in high-quality lamps becomes very slow; most fluorescent tubes, for example, will maintain a good output for at least 12 months.

Spectral analysis (quality): Vitamin D3 synthesis is a process in which a fine balance of photoproducts (7-DHC, previtamin D3, lumisterol and tachysterol) forms in the skin. The precise spectral power distribution between about 295 and 335 nm determines the percentage of each photoproduct, and hence controls vitamin D3 production. Ideally, the lamp's UV spectrum should therefore resemble that of natural sunlight as closely as possible. In addition, UVA wavelengths longer than 350 nm are visible to reptiles; these

too should ideally be present in the lamp spectrum. Figure 22.4 shows the spectral power distribution (irradiances not to scale) of samples of typical lamp types compared with a subtropical midday solar spectrum (solar altitude 85.4 degrees, San Bartolomé, Gran Canaria).

The spectrum of most high-quality UVB fluorescent tubes follows the solar spectral power distribution fairly closely in the relevant UVB region; however, a deficit in the longer-wavelength UVA is common. The spectrum of a mercury vapour arc is extremely discontinuous; it consists primarily of powerful 'spikes' of radiation in narrow bands of wavelengths. These enable vitamin D synthesis but this very different spectrum alters the balance of photoproducts; it may therefore affect the control mechanisms preventing overproduction of vitamin D3 (MacLaughlin *et al.*, 1982). Whether this has any clinical significance is unknown. The metal halide has a much more sun-like spectral power distribution than the mercury vapour, including a high UVA component in the reptile-visible range.

Irradiance and beam shape (quantity): Research on the UV output of a range of lamps has been published by Gehrmann and his colleagues from 1993 onwards (for a more recent review see Gehrmann, 2006) and Lindgren (2004); however, most of the lamps tested in those studies are no longer on sale. Moreover, they have analysed the output of the lamps as measured at a standard distance from the lamp, regardless of the lamp type and the shape of the beam. These features are extremely important. A fluorescent tube which irradiates a diffuse, relatively low level of UVB from its entire surface will produce a very different UVB gradient and basking opportunity than a mercury vapour spot lamp which emits a very narrow beam of intense UVB light, maybe only a few centimetres across.

A broadband UVB meter is a practical instrument, both for measuring the irradiance from a lamp at specific distances, and for plotting the shape of the beam, as an iso-irradiance chart. The Solarmeter 6.5 UV Index meter has proven its worth in this respect. Unlike most broadband UVB meters, which respond to the entire range of UVB wavelengths, the Solarmeter 6.5 has a response curve that follows the action spectrum for vitamin D synthesis, making it ideal for estimating the vitamin D synthesizing potential of both sunlight and artificial sources. The readings are displayed in the unitless UV Index, which is beneficial for interpretation as it is a well-known measurement of 'sun strength' as determined by human erythema, which has a similar action spectrum (Figure 22.5).

One of the most important features determining the usefulness of a UVB lamp is the shape of the beam – the UV gradient, or the UV 'footprint' in the basking area. Ideally, the whole reptile should receive warmth, light and UVB while basking. Figure 22.6 gives examples of the four main types of UVB lamp currently available, with typical iso-irradiance charts from each group.

Artificial sunshine is not ideal but there are now many combinations of lamps, bulbs and tubes that will, used with care and sensitivity, go a long way towards meeting the needs of all reptiles in captivity.

Ordinary tungsten or halogen 'household' flood lamps: These provide excellent heat and light, which can be thermostatically controlled, at a basking spot. Their light is predominantly red and yellow, is very deficient in blue and UVA, and has no UVB. These complement UVB reptile lamps, which have little red or yellow light, extremely well. A simple golden dawn and dusk effect can be produced by using timers to switch them on just before, and off just after, the UVB lamps.

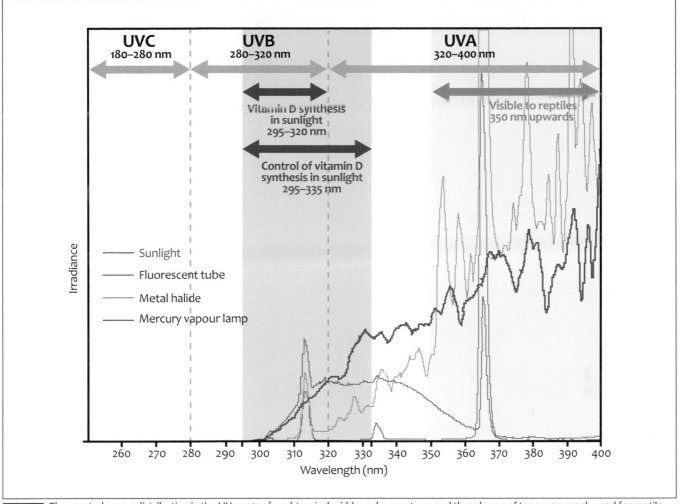

22.4 The spectral power distribution in the UV range of a subtropical midday solar spectrum and three lamps of types commonly used for reptile lighting. Solar spectrum was recorded under clear-sky conditions, solar altitude 85.4 degrees, San Bartolomé, Gran Canaria (27° 55' N, 15° 31' W), 21 June 2011, local time 14:00. Fluorescent tube: ZooMed 5.0 T5-HO 24 W fluorescent tube. Metal halide: ExoTerra SunRay 70 W metal halide lamp. Mercury vapour lamp: ReptileUV MegaRay 100 W PAR38 lamp.

(Courtesy of Frances M. Baines)

There is no need to purchase special 'reptile' basking lamps, since they are virtually identical to their household equivalents. It is very important to use flood lamps with wide diffused beams, mounted at safe distances (ideally >30 cm above the animal) to create sufficiently large basking areas and minimize hot spots. These lamps should be used with dimming thermostats which should be set to maintain safe temperatures in the cool end of the vivarium.

Lamps coated with neodymium produce light with a slightly more blue colour, but not because they emit more blue light – the neodymium merely filters out some of the red and orange wavelengths.

'Daylight' fluorescent tubes: These are sometimes called 'full spectrum' but they either produce no UVB, or insufficient for vitamin D3 synthesis at distances greater than a few centimetres. They can be very useful for improving general light levels in cooler areas of a vivarium. They are of historical interest. In the late 1960s, NSHP was a serious problem in zoo animals. Trials with two household brands of fluorescent tubes, DuroTest VitaLite and Optima, were first carried out with reptiles by one Jozsef Laszlo, in Houston Zoo, Texas. His short description of their successful use (Laszlo, 1969) led to their widespread recommendation.

UV Index colour code		
	Typically occurs in:	*World Health Organization category*
11+	Full tropical midday sun	Extreme
10	Full tropical late morning sun; full summer sun in subtropical areas	Very high
9		
8		
7	Full tropical mid-morning sun or under light cloud at midday	High
6		
5	Full tropical early morning sun; light shade or overcast weather at midday	Moderate
4		
3		
2	Very early morning sun; shade at midday	Low
1		
0		

22.5 The UV Index as defined by the World Health Organization (WHO) and the international colour coding system. Since the solar altitude is a major determinant of the UV Index, it is possible to predict the likely range of UV Index readings which might be expected in the tropics at different times of day in fully exposed sunlit positions. Reptiles are rarely seen in full tropical sunlight between mid-morning and mid- to late afternoon.

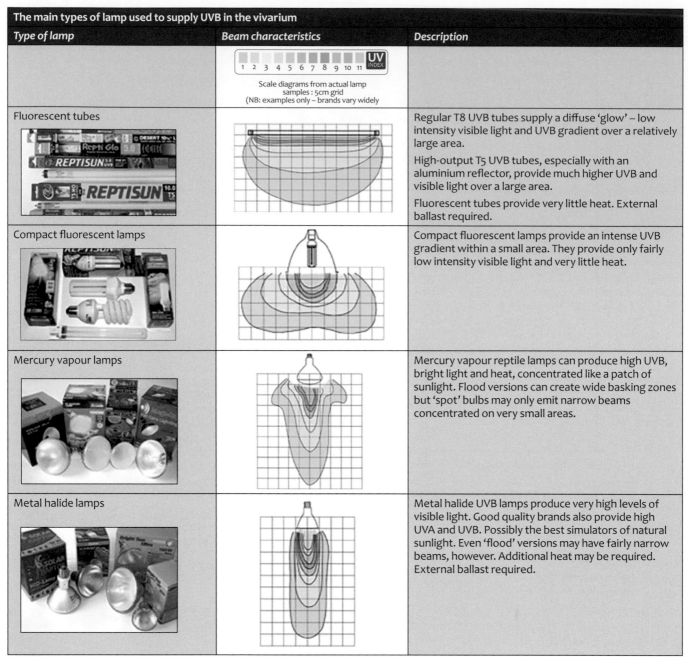

Type of lamp	Beam characteristics	Description
	Scale diagrams from actual lamp samples : 5cm grid (NB: examples only – brands vary widely)	
Fluorescent tubes		Regular T8 UVB tubes supply a diffuse 'glow' – low intensity visible light and UVB gradient over a relatively large area. High-output T5 UVB tubes, especially with an aluminium reflector, provide much higher UVB and visible light over a large area. Fluorescent tubes provide very little heat. External ballast required.
Compact fluorescent lamps		Compact fluorescent lamps provide an intense UVB gradient within a small area. They provide only fairly low intensity visible light and very little heat.
Mercury vapour lamps		Mercury vapour reptile lamps can produce high UVB, bright light and heat, concentrated like a patch of sunlight. Flood versions can create wide basking zones but 'spot' bulbs may only emit narrow beams concentrated on very small areas.
Metal halide lamps		Metal halide UVB lamps produce very high levels of visible light. Good quality brands also provide high UVA and UVB. Possibly the best simulators of natural sunlight. Even 'flood' versions may have fairly narrow beams, however. Additional heat may be required. External ballast required.

22.6 Characteristics of the four main types of UVB lamp often used in vivaria.
(Courtesy of Frances M. Baines)

These and other similar misleadingly called 'full-spectrum' lamps (some of which are still sold for human lighting) only emit traces of UVB around 313 nm, barely within the wavelengths necessary for vitamin D synthesis, along with small amounts of UVA. 'Blacklights' also found favour for a while; however, these also only emit traces of UVB; their output is almost entirely UVA.

At the close of the twentieth century, the development of a lamp containing a blend of phosphors emitting visible light and UVB marked a turning point in reptile husbandry (Ullrey and Bernard, 1999). This might be considered a prototype of some of the best fluorescent UVB lamps available today.

UVB fluorescent tubes: Modern high-quality UVB fluorescent lamps are made with improved phosphor blends and high-transmission borosilicate glass which blocks all undesirable short-wavelength UVB and UVC. Inferior brands do not always contain phosphors producing similar spectra, however, and some are still manufactured in quartz glass, which permits transmission of very short wavelength UVB and even UVC if there are defects in the inner phosphor coating. Such products have caused photokeratoconjunctivitis and photodermatitis in reptiles (Gardiner et al., 2009).

Standard 26 mm diameter (designated 'T8') UVB-emitting fluorescent tubes are available in a variety of lengths. They can be operated with regular magnetic or electronic ballasts. Most brands offer different 'strengths' with names such as 'tropical' and 'desert', or state the UVB as a percentage of the total light output (5%, 10%, etc.). However, the output from different 'strengths' from different brands can vary widely, both in spectral quality and in quantity (i.e. total irradiance), both of which are determinants of the effectiveness of vitamin D3 synthesis.

Typical T8 tubes produce diffuse, low levels of UVB resembling outdoor shade on a sunny day at practical distances (i.e. >20–25 cm), but very little visible light. They should always be combined with a higher-quality visible-light source.

UVB-emitting T5 (16 mm diameter) 'high-output' (HO) fluorescent tubes were first sold for use with reptiles in 2010. The output of visible light and UV is greatly increased compared with standard T8 tubes. Large effective UVB gradients can be produced at distances of 30–60 cm or more from some T5-HO tubes fitted with efficient aluminium reflectors. Indeed, at close range, UVB irradiance can be very high, requiring a minimum safe distance to be observed. T5-HO tubes require dedicated electronic ballasts. These operate at a frequency of 20,000 Hz or higher, creating a flicker-free light. Matching ballast controllers with end caps and clip-on reflectors are available, as are attractive all-in-one 'luminaires' which can be fixed inside vivaria or placed over mesh-screen tops.

UVB, just like visible light, is additive; if two lamps are placed over a surface, the irradiance is doubled at that point. Therefore, mounting an array of T5-HO fluorescent tubes together will provide effective UVB over a much larger area and at a much greater distance from the lamps. To provide high-intensity UVB lighting over a basking area for very large reptiles housed in zoo enclosures, an aluminium unit housing six 120 cm T5-HO tubes has been developed by the UK company Arcadia. One unit can provide a UV index of 3.4 at 1.5 m distance, and create a UVB zone 2 m wide. At ZSL London Zoo, four of these units suspended, with ceramic heater panels, 2.5 m above a group of Galapagos tortoises has created a giant brightly lit basking zone which the animals find attractive (Figure 22.7).

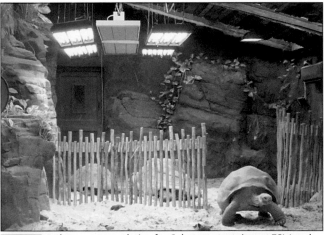

22.7 Indoor accommodation for Galapagos tortoises at ZSL London Zoo. UVB, UVA and visible light are provided by four Arcadia SuperZoo T5-HO fixtures, each holding six 1150 mm, 54 W Arcadia T5 D3+ 12% UVB Reptile Lamp fluorescent tubes. Infrared radiation is provided by two ceramic heater panels suspended between the lighting units. (Courtesy of Frances M. Baines)

Compact fluorescent lamps: The 'energy-saving' compact fluorescent lamp is basically a small fluorescent tube coiled into a spiral or bar shape, controlled by a miniature electronic ballast built into the lamp base. UVB-emitting versions of these, designed for use with reptiles, were first introduced in the early 2000s. They produce diffuse, low levels of UVB at practical distances, but they typically produce a very steep UVB and visible-light gradient over a relatively small area, making good positioning difficult. If not placed inside a dome fixture, horizontal mounting above the basking zone is recommended, to prevent the unshielded lamp from hanging in the reptile's direct line of sight.

These decay more rapidly than tubes, owing to a higher operating temperature, and may need replacement after 6 months' use.

Mercury vapour lamps: These vary widely in quality and UVB output. A good-quality lamp will have a wide, well diffused beam, evenly illuminating a zone at least as large as the entire body of the reptile, with adequate UVB at a minimum distance of at least 30 cm. Some brands, however, have a low UVB output, only effective at close range, or a higher output that is restricted to a narrow beam. Some cheap imports, typically large reflector bulbs with clear glass faces, may emit extremely tightly focused beams with dangerous intensity at the centre of the beam.

Even the best quality mercury vapour lamps are not ideal as sole light sources for animals. The spectrum of a mercury vapour arc is extremely discontinuous with many wavelengths absent from the light. The lamps thus have very poor colour rendering, even to a human eye. The lamps are also difficult to use in a small vivarium because their heat output cannot be thermostatically controlled.

Metal halide lamps: These are externally ballasted arc lamps, similar in principle to mercury vapour lamps but producing a far brighter white light, which can approach the intensity of natural sunlight at basking distances. Unshielded, uncoated metal halide arc tubes emit all wavelengths from hazardous UVC to infrared, but suitable glass outer bulbs render them safe. Some of the best quality metal halide bulbs designed for human lighting, with colour temperatures between 5000 and 6500 K, are capable of producing wide beams with true 'full-spectrum' solar simulation in the UVA and visible wavelengths – but no UVB.

However, by modifying the glass and inner coatings, metal halide bulbs emitting suitable UVB have now been developed. Dedicated ballasts are required; lamp-holder sets are available. Their visible light has not yet reached the high standard of the best 'human' metal halides. Nevertheless, their light is far brighter and their spectrum is much more sun-like than a mercury vapour lamp. Unfortunately, the beams of these lamps are relatively narrow and create small effective UVB zones, although the miniature 35 W version from several brands, curiously, produces a very high output at close range which makes it unsuitable for use in very small enclosures.

The effective UVB output of metal halide lamps appears to be short-lived, around 6 months of normal use. However, the technology appears to be in its infancy and these lamps look promising for the future.

LED lighting: LEDs are also being considered for lighting animal enclosures, although none emitting UV for vitamin D3 synthesis have yet been developed. There are still major disadvantages to be overcome with LEDs, owing to their wavelength specificity; it is very difficult to produce a full-spectrum output across the human visible range, even by using arrays with many different individually coloured units. At present, although UVA- and UVB-emitting LEDs can be created, their output is extremely low and, of course, wavelength specific, whereas a very broad spectrum of UVB and UVA wavelengths is required to enable natural vitamin D synthesis, and for natural colour vision in those species with UV perception.

Many reptile owners lack accurate knowledge about the proper provision of UVB. During any consultation, owners should always be questioned about their use of UVB lighting, as this will often reveal some of the common mistakes listed in Figure 22.8.

- Inappropriate lamp choice for species (considering heat and visible light, as well as UVB)
- Lamp placed too far away from animal (insufficient UVB for vitamin D3 synthesis)
- Lamp placed too close to animal (risk of damage to eyes and skin)
- Failure to provide areas for sheltering from light
- Lamp with beam too narrow to cover whole body of animal when basking
- Lamp placed at animal level or in its line of sight, rather than above basking zone
- Lamp placed behind a sheet of glass or plastic cover (blocking UVB)
- Lamp placed some distance away from basking zone, so reptile does not receive UVB while basking with warm skin
- Lamp not replaced often enough. Brands vary; usually UVB is maintained for 6–12 months
- UVB fluorescent lamp also used as sole heat source
- 'Full-spectrum' or 'daylight' lamp thought to be same as UVB-emitting lamp
- Aquarium UVA 'actinic' lamp (or even sterilizing UVC lamp) thought to be same as UVB lamp
- UVB regarded as a substitute for calcium
- Lamp switched on for too short a time period each day (lamps should be on timers)
- Attempted use of thermostat with UVB lamp
- Poor lamp installation and maintenance leading to premature lamp failure

22.8 Some common mistakes made when using UVB lamps.

How much UVB is needed?

The absorption of UV light by a reptile's body will vary depending upon not just the weather but also its microhabitat (e.g. on open ground, under light vegetation or in a burrow); its behaviour (e.g. periods of activity, basking preferences); and body characteristics, such as thick or thin skin, heavy or light pigmentation (Carman *et al.*, 2000; Ferguson *et al.*, 2005). With regard to vitamin D3, the reptile's body characteristics and behaviour will have evolved together to optimize the level of vitamin D3 it synthesizes. Some reptiles even specifically self-regulate their UVB exposure, which they increase if their vitamin D levels become suboptimal (Ferguson *et al.*, 2003, 2013; Karsten *et al.*, 2009).

At present there is very little scientific data upon which to base a recommendation of any particular level of UVB exposure for any species. Records of solar irradiance from meteorological stations in the species' country of origin are unhelpful because they indicate only maximum levels in completely exposed locations, which are vastly different from the irradiances recorded in the microhabitats where reptiles live. A small number of researchers have made, and are making, field recordings but so far data is deficient for all but a very few species.

Another problem in determining the UVB requirement for vitamin D3 synthesis is that there is only available knowledge of the normal serum 25(OH)D3 levels for a handful of free-living, wild reptile species (see Figure 22.16). There is wide variation between species in their synthetic ability (Carman *et al.*, 2000) and there may also be wide variation in the optimum serum levels between species. A small number of experiments measuring serum 25(OH)D3 levels under artificial sources suggest that this can be very successful in eliciting vitamin D3 synthesis (see Figure 22.16); however, most of these studies used different UVB sources (some of them very weak, some with the irradiance unrecorded) and different exposure times, so little can be deduced about optimum levels. Research on this topic is in its infancy, even with regard to human beings.

The British and Irish Association of Zoos and Aquaria's Reptile and Amphibian Working Group (BIAZA RAWG) have developed a working document for estimating suitable UVB levels for species held in captivity in zoos (BIAZA RAWG UV-Tool Focus Group, 2012; Baines *et al.*, 2016). This is based upon the few existing studies assessing UVB levels in different microhabitats. Their underlying premise is that optimal UV levels are likely to be the natural ones the reptile chooses to experience when environmental conditions (heat, light and UV) are favourable in its microhabitat, since it has evolved to thrive in that precise location. If heat, light and UV gradients similar to those created by sunlight in that microhabitat are provided, using suitable lighting combinations in captivity, the reptile should then be able to self-regulate its day-to-day exposure to all three of these parameters.

Ideally, measurements should be taken at the precise location of each species in the wild. In the absence of this data, however, knowledge of the species' natural behaviour in the wild and the range of UVB exposures typical of its microhabitat should be sufficient for an adequate estimate of the likely gradient needed. Gradients are vital as they allow animals room to manoeuvre.

The Ferguson Zone concept: The BIAZA UV-Tool estimates suitable UV gradients using a concept described by Dr Gary Ferguson and his team from Texas Christian University (Ferguson *et al.*, 2010). They recorded the daily UV exposure of 15 species of reptiles, in the field, as measured with the Solarmeter 6.5 UV Index meter. They allocated species into four sun-exposure groups or 'zones', which have since been designated 'UVB Zones' or 'Ferguson Zones' (Carmel and Johnson, 2014; Ferguson *et al.*, 2014; Baines *et al.*, 2016).

The Ferguson Zones are:

- Zone 1 = crepuscular or shade dweller, thermal conformer
- Zone 2 = partial sun/occasional basker, thermoregulator
- Zone 3 = open or partial sun basker, thermoregulator
- Zone 4 = midday sun basker, thermoregulator.

Ferguson *et al.* calculated 'Zone ranges' by averaging all the UVI readings for the microhabitats at the time and place the reptiles were found. This included readings when the animals were seen in shade as well as in sun, over the course of the day. They also noted the maximum UVI at which each species was seen during the study. The BIAZA UV-Tool interpreted the 'Zone ranges' as representing a suitable mid-background level of UVB for the species in question, neither in full sun nor full shade; and the maximum UVI as an indication of a rough guide to the upper acceptable limit for the UVB gradient to be provided in captivity.

Differences between the way UVB lamps produce such gradients (see Figure 22.6) suggest two ways of supplying UVB to reptiles kept indoors in captivity:

- The 'Shade method' provides low-level 'background' UV over a large proportion of the animal's enclosure, with a gradient to zero into full shelter. This would normally be the method of choice for shade-dwelling reptiles and occasional baskers, i.e. all those in zones 1 and some in zone 2. The 'Zone range' described by Ferguson *et al.* is used as a guide to the required level. Fluorescent T8 (26 mm diameter) UVB tubes are suitable for this
- The 'Sunbeam method' is designed to provide a higher level of UV for species known to bask in direct sunlight. The aim is to provide UV similar to that of an early- to mid-morning basking period – the time when most

reptiles bask. This higher level needs to be restricted to the basking zone ('like a sunbeam') with a gradient to zero into full shelter. This method would seem appropriate for reptiles in zones 3 and 4, and for some in zone 2, and uses the maximum UVI reported by Ferguson et al. as the upper acceptable limit at the closest point of access to the lamp. Mercury vapour lamps, metal halide UVB lamps and high-output T5 (T5-HO) UVB fluorescent tubes (16 mm diameter) tubes may be used in this way.

The BIAZA UV-Tool allocates each of the 254 species currently listed to a Ferguson Zone based upon their basking behaviour and known microhabitat. Figure 22.9 uses the current Ferguson Zone allocations to estimate suitable UV ranges for some reptiles commonly kept as pets. This is a very simplistic assessment, with very wide interpretations possible. This is intentional: the concept is designed to enable creation of wide, safe UV gradients alongside heat and light gradients in the vivarium. All guidelines to date are still very experimental and it is vital to watch the animals' responses and record results.

The following suggestions are therefore based on Ferguson's study results:

- Zone 1 – Shade method, gradient with UVI 0–0.7
- Zone 2 – Shade method, gradient with UVI 0.7–1.0 or in a larger vivarium; Sunbeam method, UVI with a maximum of 1.1–3.0 in basking zone
- Zone 3 – Sunbeam method, UVI with a maximum of 2.9–7.4 in basking zone
- Zone 4 – Sunbeam method, UVI with a maximum of 4.5–8.0 in basking zone.

Although some zone 3 and 4 reptiles have been observed basking above UVI 7.0–8.0, even these spend the majority of their basking time at far lower levels, in the early morning and late afternoon, when levels are around UVI 3.0–5.0. Since the UV spectrum from artificial lighting is not the same as from natural sunlight, the UV-Tool specifies that, for safety, UVI 7.0–8.0 should be considered the maximum UVI at reptile level for these reptiles.

A special situation exists when considering ultraviolet lighting for albino and hypopigmented morphs of any species. Reduced or absent pigmentation greatly increases sensitivity to UV. To avoid damage to their skin and eyes, lower levels of UV will be essential. Fortunately, it is likely that adequate vitamin D synthesis will still be possible, since reduced pigmentation allows more UVB to enter the epidermal cells.

Figure 22.10 illustrates possible configurations for three different UV lighting arrangements, using iso-irradiance charts from actual lamps to visualize typical UVB gradients which can be obtained for 'Shade' and 'Sunbeam' methods.

Choosing a UV meter: Ideally, reptile keepers should use their own UVI readings from a Solarmeter 6.5 or similar laboratory-grade UVI meter, to aid positioning of a UV lamp. Cheap so-called UVI meters, e.g. those sold as suntan aids, should never be used. Most of these rely on inexpensive sensors responding almost entirely to UVA. These are very inaccurate with most UVB lamps, which have spectra different from sunlight.

Before the development of the Solarmeter 6.5 UV Index meter, many keepers and veterinary surgeons obtained the original Solarmeter 6.2 UVB meter. This is a reliable and sensitive instrument which responds to the entire UVB spectrum, and gives a readout in microwatts per square centimetre (μW/cm^2). This is extremely useful for checking and monitoring the output of UV lamps. However, since the readout indicates the total UVB, not just the shorter wavelengths responsible for most of the vitamin D synthesis, the meter cannot be used to compare readings between different lamps and sunlight. Many UVB lamps have a greater percentage of their UVB output in the shorter wavelengths; total UVB readings may underestimate their potential.

A set of typical Solarmeter 6.5 readings for 30 different UVB lamps widely available in the UK at the time of publication are provided in Figure 22.11. The spectra from these lamps revealed no significant abnormally short wavelength UVB radiation. These figures must only be taken as rough guidelines, however, since no two lamps are ever identical, and individual lamps also vary in their UVB output depending upon many factors including their age, the precise voltage of the electrical supply and external temperature.

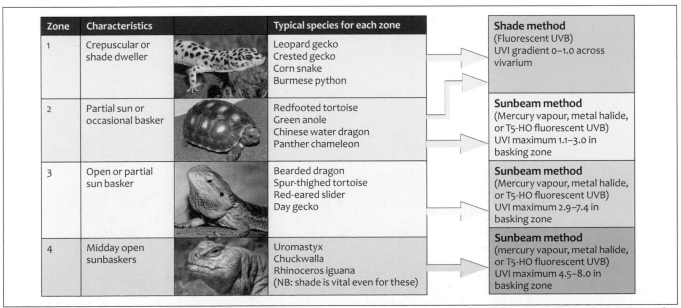

Zone	Characteristics		Typical species for each zone	
1	Crepuscular or shade dweller		Leopard gecko Crested gecko Corn snake Burmese python	**Shade method** (Fluorescent UVB) UVI gradient 0–1.0 across vivarium
2	Partial sun or occasional basker		Redfooted tortoise Green anole Chinese water dragon Panther chameleon	**Sunbeam method** (Mercury vapour, metal halide, or T5-HO fluorescent UVB) UVI maximum 1.1–3.0 in basking zone
3	Open or partial sun basker		Bearded dragon Spur-thighed tortoise Red-eared slider Day gecko	**Sunbeam method** (Mercury vapour, metal halide, or T5-HO fluorescent UVB) UVI maximum 2.9–7.4 in basking zone
4	Midday open sunbaskers		Uromastyx Chuckwalla Rhinoceros iguana (NB: shade is vital even for these)	**Sunbeam method** (mercury vapour, metal halide, or T5-HO fluorescent UVB) UVI maximum 4.5–8.0 in basking zone

22.9 The Ferguson Zones, as described by Ferguson et al. (2010). The 'zone ranges' and 'maximum UVI recorded' were for the original 15 species of reptiles in their natural habitat in Jamaica and the south and west of the USA. The examples of typical species are species commonly found in the pet trade, assigned to Ferguson Zones based upon their known basking behaviour. Arrows link animals from each zone to either 'Shade' or 'Sunbeam' methods of UV provision, as proposed by the BIAZA RAWG UV-Tool Focus Group (2012), and indicate typical lamp types used for each method.
(Courtesy of Frances M. Baines)

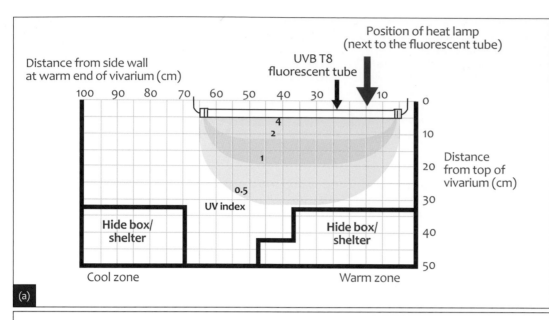

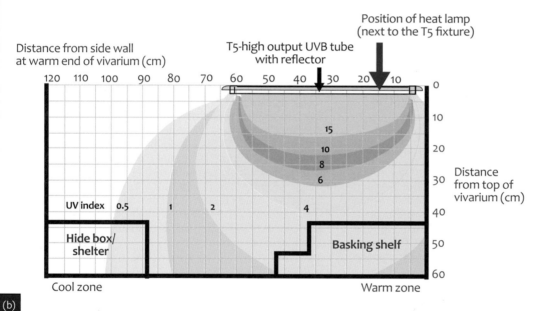

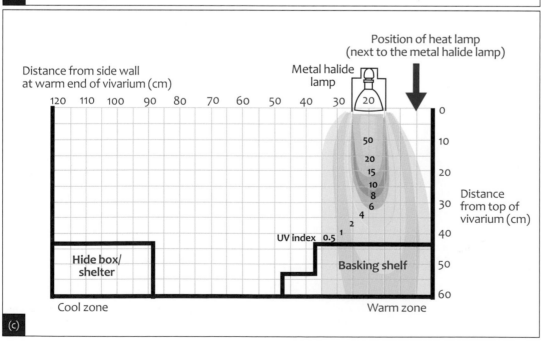

22.10 Examples of UVB lighting for vivaria.
(a) Shade method using typical T8 UVB fluorescent tube, suitable for Ferguson Zone 1 reptile. 100 × 50 cm vivarium. Iso-irradiance chart for Arcadia T8 D3 6% UVB Reptile Lamp T8 (18 W 610 mm tube).
(b) Sunbeam method using typical T5-HO UVB fluorescent tube with aluminium reflector, suitable for Ferguson Zone 3–4 reptile. 120 x 60 cm vivarium. Iso-irradiance chart for Arcadia T5 D3+ 12% UVB Reptile Lamp (24 W 550 mm tube) fitted with Arcadia T5 aluminium strip reflector.
(c) Sunbeam method using typical UVB metal halide lamp, suitable for Ferguson Zone 3–4 reptile. 120 x 60 cm vivarium. Iso-irradiance chart for ExoTerra SunRay 70 W metal halide lamp.
All methods may require the use of non-UVB-emitting lamps for warmth and additional visible light; these should be controlled by dimming thermostats. Hides, basking shelves and other fixtures should be added as appropriate for the species; shelter must always be provided.
(Courtesy of Frances M. Baines)

Brand name and type	Wattage (W)	Distance (cm)			
		20	30	40	50
T8 fluorescent tubes (610 mm length)					
ExoTerra Repti-Glo 2.0	20	0			
Arcadia Natural Sunlight 2% UVB T8	18	0.3	0.2	0.1	0.1
Arcadia D3 Reptile 6% UVB T8	18	0.7	0.4	0.2	0.2
ExoTerra ReptiGlo 5.0	20	1.5	0.9	0.6	0.4
ZooMed Reptisun 10.0 T8	18	1.5	0.9	0.6	0.4
Arcadia D3+ 12% Reptile UVB T8	18	1.5	0.9	0.6	0.4
Arcadia D3+ 12% Reptile UVB T8 with clip-on reflector	18	3.2	2.0	1.3	0.9
T5 high-output fluorescent tubes (550 mm length)					
ZooMed Reptisun T5-HO 5.0	24	0.7	0.5	0.3	0.2
ZooMed Reptisun T5-HO 5.0 in ZooMed Reptisun Terrarium Hood	24	2.1	1.2	0.8	0.6
Arcadia D3 Reptile 6% UVB T5	24	2.0	1.2	0.7	0.5
ZooMed Reptisun T5-HO 10.0	24	1.2	0.8	0.5	0.4
ZooMed Reptisun T5-HO 10.0 in ZooMed Reptisun Terrarium Hood	24	3.5	2.1	1.4	0.9
Arcadia D3+ Reptile 12% UVB T5	24	3.1	1.8	1.2	0.8
Arcadia D3+ Reptile 12% UVB T5 in Arcadia Slimline Luminaire	24	6.3	3.6	2.3	1.6
Arcadia D3+ Reptile 12% UVB T5 with clip-on reflector	24	(11.0)	6.4	4.2	2.9
Arcadia D3+ Dragon 14% UVB T5	24	4.6	2.7	1.8	1.2
Arcadia D3+ Dragon 14% UVB T5 with clip-on reflector	24	(13.1)	7.8	5.0	3.5
Compact fluorescent lamps					
ExoTerra Reptile UVB 100 (coil lamp)	25	1.6	0.8	0.4	0.3
ExoTerra Reptile UVB 200 (coil lamp)	25	1.8	0.9	0.5	0.3
Arcadia Natural Sunlight Compact Lamp (3-bar lamp)	20	0.5	0.2	0.1	0.1
Arcadia D3+ 10% UVB Compact Reptile Lamp (3-bar lamp)	23	1.4	0.6	0.4	0.2
ZooMed ReptiSun 5.0 Compact Lamp (3-bar lamp)	26	0.5	0.3	0.1	0.1
ZooMed ReptiSun 10.0 Compact Lamp (3-bar lamp)	26	1.8	0.9	0.4	0.3
Metal halides					
Lucky Reptile Bright Sun UV Desert 35 W PAR30	35	(27.9)	(15.1)	(9.6)	6.5
Lucky Reptile Bright Sun UV Desert 70 W PAR30	70	(14.8)	6.8	3.6	2.1
Lucky Reptile Bright Sun Flood Jungle 150 W PAR 38	150	(14.1)	6.3	3.5	2.1
ExoTerra SunRay 35 W PAR30	25	(26.2)	(10.3)	5.4	3.3
ExoTerra SunRay 50 W PAR30	50	(11.0)	5.0	2.8	1.7
ExoTerra SunRay 70 W PAR30	70	(17.3)	7.4	4.0	2.4
ZooMed Powersun HID PAR36	70	7.2	3.3	1.9	1.2
Mercury vapour lamps					
ExoTerra Solar Glo 125 W	125	5.3	2.9	1.8	1.2
ExoTerra Solar Glo 160 W	160	1.7	1.0	0.5	0.4
ZooMed Powersun 100 W	100	5.7	3.0	1.8	1.2
ZooMed Powersun 160W	160	(8.5)	4.7	2.9	2.0
Natural tropical sunlight: Kakadu, NT, Australia. Latitude 12°39′ S. October 4th 2006					
09:00h Solar altitude 40°	3.5				
10:00h Solar altitude 50°	7.6				
12:30h Solar altitude 80°	13.5				

22.11 Typical UVI meter readings from UVB lamps. Lamps were all tested after approximately 100 hours of use, to allow initial 'burning-in' to complete. Readings were taken with no mesh between lamp and meter, and with no reflector unless specified. Note the numbers in brackets: UV Index too high (>UVI 8.0) – lamp is unsuitable at this distance.
(Courtesy of Frances M. Baines)

Calcium requirements

Precise calcium requirements have not been determined for most reptiles. Nutritionists currently recommend 0.42–0.7 mg of calcium/kJ or about 1% of dietary DM, based on extrapolation from other animals (see Chapter 4). Many veterinary texts suggest that reptile diets should contain calcium and phosphate at a ratio of 1.5:1–2:1. This appears to be an extrapolation from data obtained in the poultry industry and it is possible that the figure may be inappropriate for some reptile species (Klaphake, 2001).

As with any animal, reptiles' calcium requirements vary considerably with life stage. Growth and reproduction place the highest demands, with requirements reducing considerably in adults with well formed bone stores.

Measuring calcium

In healthy mammals about 50% of total plasma calcium is in an unbound, ionized form (i.e. not complexed with albumin, globulins or anions). Ionized calcium is the physiologically active portion and so it is this fraction that needs to be monitored. Levels can be measured with ion-selective electrodes (Endres and Rude, 1996). The fraction of 'free' calcium varies with serum pH; it is always best to consult the laboratory with regard to requirements for storage and handling *en route* (Rosol and Capen, 1997).

Mean levels in 30 healthy green iguanas were reported as 1.47 ± 0.105 mmol/l (Dennis *et al.*, 2001) and 1.38 ± 0.1 mmol/l in another group of 23 (Hernandez-Divers *et al.*, 2005) but very little information is available for other species.

Variations in albumin concentrations will cause considerable changes to total calcium measurement but not to the concentration of free calcium. This phenomenon is particularly important in reproductively active reptiles and birds. During vitellogenesis, oestrogens stimulate the production of vitellogenins, which bind considerable amounts of calcium and are used to transport the mineral to the developing eggs. Consequently, elevated levels of total calcium and phosphate in female lizards are often indicative of folliculogenesis rather than hypercalcaemia. However, sequestration of calcium by these proteins may precipitate a hypocalcaemic crisis (low ionized calcium) in reptiles that previously had marginal NSHP, and the problem may not be obvious if only total plasma calcium is measured.

Dietary calcium supplementation

Various calcium compounds have been used to supplement diets in order to prevent hypocalcaemia (Figure 22.12), especially in cricket-fed insectivorous lizards. The cheapest is probably calcium carbonate, but this seems unpalatable to many animals.

Various mineral supplements containing calcium salts are sold commercially for dusting on to food items. In one study, crickets dusted with an 11% calcium product only contained 0.12% 3 hours later, so insects need to be eaten soon after dusting (Trusk and Crissey, 1987). An extension of this approach has been the development of a variety of calcium-rich gut-loading diets for enhancing the mineral content of prey insects (Klasing *et al.*, 2000). A study by Allen and Oftedal (1989) found that gut-loading diets need to contain at least 8% calcium in order to produce prey with a 1:1 Ca:P ratio. Unfortunately, diets containing this level of calcium are unpalatable and unbalanced for insects, and can lead to high mortality rates (Allen and

Calcium compound	Approximate calcium content (mg/g)	Comments
Calcium acetate (anhydrous)	253	
Calcium carbonate	400	
Calcium chloride (dehydrate)	273	
Calcium citrate (tetrahydrate)	211	Acidified
Calcium glubionate (monohydrate)	66	Best for oral use
Calcium lactate (anhydrous)	184	
Calcium lactate (trihydrate)	147	
Calcium lactate (pentahydrate)	130	
Calcium lactate gluconate (dehydrate)	129	Best for parenteral use
Calcium lactobionate (dihydrate)	51	
Calcium hydrogen phosphate (dihydrate)	233	Fairly inert; used more as an excipient and antacid
Calcium phosphate	388	Insoluble and fairly inert

22.12 Calcium compounds and their calcium content.

Oftedal, 1989). It is advisable to use such calcium-enriched diets no more than 24–48 hours before the insects are used as food (Allen, 1997). The best method of delivering vitamins A and E, calcium, and phosphorus seems to be a combination of dusting and gut-loading (Sabatini *et al.*, 1998; Finke, 2003).

A clinical approach to NSHP

Normal bone is not inert but is subject to continuous remodelling activity. Achieving and maintaining normal bone structure depends on a complex interplay between dietary vitamins and minerals, systemic hormones, local factors, and the mechanical loading (Banu *et al.*, 1999; Frost, 2000) produced by exercise. The latter is often overlooked but may be a significant factor in young active reptiles as these are often kept in vivaria that are too small to allow sustained exercise.

Developmental causes

The vitamin D, calcium and genetic statuses of the parents are key contributory factors to bone disorders in their offspring. In poultry, it is well known that the vitamin D and calcium status of a hen and the incubation temperature and humidity have a major influence on the hatchability of eggs and chick growth, including bone mineralization. Calcium and 25(OH)D3 are transported into the egg during its formation and are intimately involved in bone formation during the incubation period (Kubota *et al.*, 1981; Guinotte and Nys, 1991). Similar processes seem to occur in reptilian eggs (Stewart and Ecay, 2010)

Green iguana eggs kept at higher humidity produce heavier hatchlings with a higher calcium content (Packard *et al.*, 1992). Incubation temperature also influences skeletal development and post-hatching basking behaviour (Phillips *et al.*, 1990). A similar situation has also been observed in turtles. Hatchlings from most oviparous reptiles emerge with only a small reserve of calcium to support growth and skeletal development (Packard and Clark, 1996), and consequently require a good dietary source of calcium and access to UVB soon after birth.

Skeletal development during embryonic development may have a profound influence on bone quality in later life. Eggs produced from females with vitamin or mineral deficiencies which are then incubated under suboptimal conditions will give rise to offspring that are more prone to NSHP, especially if they are then kept under poor husbandry conditions. In such cases it may be difficult or impossible to reverse the damage already done to the developing bone.

Clinical signs of calcium and vitamin D deficiency and nutritional secondary hyperparathyroidism

History and diagnosis

Trying to distinguish the causality of NSHP is challenging as these cases are often multifactorial. Obtaining a detailed history should always be the first stage and will often highlight husbandry misconceptions. It should initially be directed towards identifying possible causes of calcium or vitamin D3 deficiency.

Before 25(OH)D3 assays were commercially available, the precise aetiology of bone disease was difficult to determine, so animals presenting with typical signs of calcium or vitamin D deficiency were often referred to as suffering from metabolic bone disorder (MBD). Where possible, a more specific diagnosis should be made.

Extreme care should be exercised when examining animals with NSHP as it is very easy to fracture weakened bones.

Reptiles with NSHP with any, or a combination, of the three causes usually present with:

- Anorexia
- Weight loss
- Muscular tremors are seen frequently in squamates, but do not occur in chelonians who tend to show general motor weakness
- Inability to maintain a normal stance – this usually starts with the pelvic limbs and progresses to the forelimbs (Figure 22.13)
- Lameness, often associated with folding fractures in juveniles or more conventional fractures in adults (Figure 22.14)
- Preovulatory ovostasis and dystocia may occur secondary to calcium deficiency
- Cloacal prolapse and intestinal stasis resulting from smooth muscle weakness
- Scoliosis and kyphosis have also been associated with MBD (Boyer, 1996), although no specific studies have been carried out to confirm the aetiology.

Classically, vitamin D deficiency during growth results in the following, but none of these should be considered pathognomonic:

- Poor calcification of the organic matrix of cartilage and bone
- Failure of cartilage cells to mature, leading to accumulation rather than destruction of the joints
- Compression of proliferating cartilage
- Enlargement and swelling of cartilaginous areas.

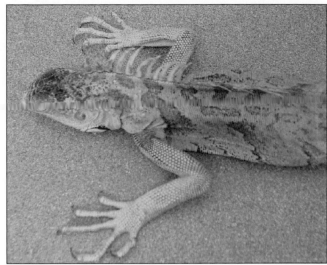

22.13 Lack of truncal lifting in a young green iguana with metabolic bone disorder (MBD).

The net effect is usually termed rickets. In adults, minerals are slowly lost from developed bone to cause osteomalacia, shown as unmineralized osteoid on the bone surface. Histologically, osteomalacia can be distinguished from other bone remodelling disorders by the presence of more than four birefringent lamellae in the osteoid seams (Recker, 1999). Prolonged exposure to PTH in green iguanas leads to excessive calcium loss from the bone with replacement by connective tissue. This produces the characteristic periosteal lesions of fibrous osteodystrophy (Rosol and Capen, 1997) (see Figure 22.15).

Juveniles affected during growth may have poorly mineralized and pliable mandibles – this is usually a sign of prolonged NSHP as mineralization of the jaw usually takes precedence over the long bones. In lizards, the soft jaw bones are often distorted by tension from the attached jaw muscles, leading to a characteristic facial 'smile'. The chelonian rhamphotheca (beak) develops a parrot-beak-like appearance (see Figure 6.6). Chameleons with NSHP often have difficulty protruding or retracting the tongue. In some chelonians, the scutes may be soft enough to deform with digital pressure.

Unless the NSHP is severe, calcium and phosphate levels may appear normal; blood mineral values will decrease only after skeletal sources have been exhausted. If a hypocalcaemia develops, there may be a progression from tremors to muscular fasciculations and finally paresis and death if it goes untreated.

Radiography

Husbandry details and dietary history often suggest a diagnosis, but this is best confirmed radiographically. Radiolucent transverse processes in the caudal (coccygeal) vertebrae are pathognomonic for this disease in lizards (Figure 22.14); in some reptiles almost all the bones may be radiolucent. The costo-chondral junctions may also enlarge and become distorted (rachitic rosettes). In some individuals there is a marked fibrous osteodystrophy in the long bones, with the femur commonly being affected. The uneven and gross thickening of the bone cortex that results, makes the hindlimbs look very muscular and is often mistaken for healthy tissue until the hard mass is revealed by palpation or radiography (Figure 22.15).

Blood samples can be used to check free (ionized) calcium and 25(OH)D3 status.

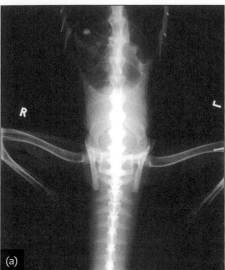

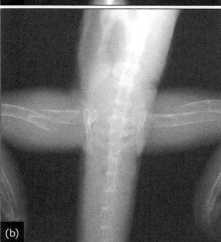

22.14
(a) Radiograph of a normal green iguana, showing distinct transverse processes in the tail. (b) In metabolic bone disorder the transverse processes are radiolucent and there are thin femoral cortices. Note the bilateral femoral fractures.

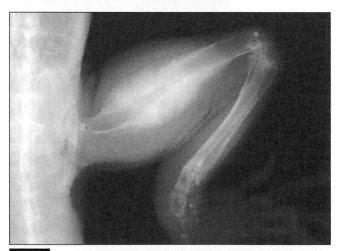

22.15 Fibrous osteodystrophy in a green iguana.

25(OH)D3 assay

Since 25(OH)D3 is the principal circulating metabolite of vitamin D, measuring its serum concentration is the best way of assessing an animal's vitamin D status.

The measurement of 25(OH)D3 can be performed by use of immunoassay. Enzyme-immunoassays (EIAs) and enzyme-linked immunosorbent assays (ELISAs) are now available for the measurement of serum 25(OH)D3 that require very small sample volumes of frozen serum (25 µl in EDTA or heparin).

Recently, however, 25(OH)D3 assays using liquid chromatography mass spectrometry have been developed which may be performed on single dried blood spots on test cards submitted to the laboratory. This makes it possible to obtain test results from very small reptiles. City Assays, Birmingham (www.vitamindtest.org.uk), are one such laboratory offering this test, with a turnaround time of 5 working days. However, at the present time very little documented information on normal 25(OH)D3 levels in reptiles is available, since ideally these values must come from wild, or at least free-living, animals in their native microhabitat. Figure 22.16 lists several reported values of 25(OH)D3 in reptiles.

There is no guarantee that apparently normal animals housed indoors or far from their country of origin will be vitamin D sufficient; thus, normal values can not be inferred from sampling these. In various studies worldwide, it has been estimated that 20–80% of European, American and Canadian humans are vitamin D deficient (Hossein-nezhad and Holick, 2013), presumably owing mainly to indoor lifestyles and sun avoidance. Given the prevalence of NSHP in captive reptiles, it seems reasonable to speculate that subclinical deficiency in these animals is equally widespread.

Calcitriol assay

As described previously, serum calcitriol (1,25(OH)2D3) levels are not a reliable indicator of vitamin D3 status. This potent steroid hormone is not stored, and has a half-life of a few hours. Owing to its up-regulation by PTH in response to hypocalcaemia, calcitriol levels in NSHP and vitamin D deficiency may be normal or even elevated, until its substrate, 25(OH)D3, is depleted, at which time calcitriol levels will fall.

Low calcitriol levels are, however, a marker for chronic kidney disease and secondary renal hyperparathyroidism, in which renal production of calcitriol has been compromised. It should be possible, however, to differentiate renal disease from vitamin D deficiency by investigating serum phosphate levels, elevated in chronic renal disease, in which serum 25(OH)D3 levels may be normal.

Parathyroid hormone assay

PTH levels are elevated in response to hypocalcaemia in vitamin D deficiency and/or calcium deficiency. PTH is also elevated in chronic renal disease when calcitriol production has failed, since calcitriol normally inhibits proliferation of the parathyroid gland. Unfortunately, at the current time no commercial PTH assay is available for reptiles.

Treatment

Initial treatment should address improving calcium intake and access to appropriate UVB light.

In an emergency, animals with clinical hypocalcaemia (free calcium <0.9 mmol/l) and hypocalcaemic tetany, where renal failure has been ruled out, can be treated with parenteral calcium injections. However, this is a dangerous procedure; reptiles given parenteral calcium should be monitored carefully (via a Doppler unit) in case the injection precipitates cardiac arrhythmia.

Calcium injections can be painful if given intramuscularly, and may cause tissue reactions if given subcutaneously or perivascularly. High dosages can also cause severe kidney damage.

Calcium gluconate is the preferred compound for injection and can be used at a maximum dose of 100 mg/kg i.v., s.c., i.m., i.o. or i.c. q6–12h, until the patient is stable enough

Reptile	Serum 25(OH)D3 (nmol/l)		Reference
Wild	**Mean**	**Range**	
Alligator snapping turtles – Florida	13.0	10–16	Chaffin et al. (2008)
Chuckwallas – Arizona	211	137–323	Aucone et al. (2003)
Green iguanas – Costa Rica	365		Laing et al. (2001)
Green sea turtles – North Carolina coast	36	16.1–72.1	Stringer et al. (2010)
Komodo dragons – Komodo, Indonesia	183	117–324	Gillespie et al. (2000)
Rhinoceros iguana – Dominican Republic	332	260–369	Ramer et al. (2005)
Ricord's iguana – Dominican Republic	554	250–1118	Ramer et al. (2005)
In captivity			
Agamids and iguanids – very low UVB indoors	44		Laing et al. (2001)
Agamids and iguanids outdoors in 3 Australian zoos	105		Laing et al. (2001)
Ball pythons – UVB indoors		78–203	Hedley and Eatwell (2013)
Bearded dragons – high UVB indoors	198.5	122–234	Oonincx et al. (2010)
Bearded dragons – high UVB indoors	181.4	48.0–267.5	Oonincx et al. (2013)
Bearded dragons – no UVB, oral D3 indoors	15.9		Oonincx et al. (2010)
Black-throated monitors – high UVB indoors		461.7–302.0	Ferguson et al. (2009)
Blandings turtles – low UVB indoors	36.1		Acierno et al. (2006)
Blandings turtles – no UVB	6.6		Acierno et al. (2006)
Chuckwallas – high UVB indoors	234	175–350	Aucone et al. (2003)
Chuckwallas – no UVB	103	85–112.5	Aucone et al. (2003)
Corn snakes – low UVB indoors	196	121–232	Acierno et al. (2008)
Corn snakes – no UVB	57.2	21–128	Acierno et al. (2008)
Crocodile and water monitors – no UVB	<100		Gillespie et al. (2000)
Crocodile and water monitors – UVB indoors	>100		Gillespie et al. (2000)
Day geckos – very low UVB indoors	40.0		Allen et al. (1996)
Desert and sulcata tortoises indoors	<12.5		Eatwell (2008b)
Desert tortoises outdoors in Nevada		12.5–41.3	Eatwell (2008b)
Fijian iguanas – partially outdoors, very low UVB indoors	78		Laing et al. (2001)
Grand Cayman iguana – no UVB indoors	283.75		Ramer et al. (2002)
Grand Cayman iguana – outdoors 4–6 weeks in summer in Indianapolis	475		Ramer et al. (2002)
Green iguanas – high UVB indoors	750		Allen et al. (1996)
Green iguanas – high UVB indoors		825–1437.5	Bernard et al. (1996)
Green iguanas – high UVB indoors	560		Oftedal et al. (1997)
Green iguanas – no UVB	<12.5		Allen et al. (1996)
Green iguanas – no UVB	<25		Oftedal et al. (1997)
Green iguanas – outdoors in El Salvador – females	233.8	74.8–392.8	Nevarez (2002)
Green iguanas – outdoors in El Salvador – gravid females	264.3	121.9–406.7	Nevarez (2002)
Green iguanas – outdoors in El Salvador – males	188.9	51.1–326.7	Nevarez (2002)
Green iguanas outdoors in Costa Rica	365		Allen et al. (1996)
Green iguanas outdoors in Honolulu	1000		Allen et al. (1996)
Green sea turtles – no UVB >75 days	27.5	17.2–64.6	Stringer et al. (2010)
Green sea turtles – no UVB, 6–8 years indoors		5–27	Purgley et al. (2009)
Green sea turtles – outdoors in Nevada		62.5–65.0	Purgley et al. (2009)
Hermann's tortoises – outdoors at native latitude, Italy	411.5		Selleri and DiGirolamo (2012)
Hermann's tortoises – UVB 5 weeks indoors		134.4–155.69	Selleri and DiGirolamo (2012)
Hermann's tortoises after hibernation	356	313.7–387.7	Selleri and DiGirolamo (2012)
Jamaican iguana – no UVB indoors	125		Ramer et al. (2002)
Jamaican iguana – outdoors 4–6 weeks in summer in Indianapolis	565		Ramer et al. (2002)
Komodo dragon indoors		4–32	Gyimesi and Burns (2002)
Komodo dragon outdoors		279–450	Gyimesi and Burns (2002)

22.16 Blood levels of 25(OH)D3 in reptiles. (continues) ▶

Reptile	Serum 25(OH)D3 (nmol/l)		Reference
In captivity continued			
Komodo dragons – low UVB indoors	29	4–97	Gillespie *et al.* (2000)
Komodo dragons – no UVB		18–31	Nijboer *et al.* (2007)
Komodo dragons – UVB indoors		195–291	Nijboer *et al.* (2007)
Komodo dragons outdoors in Indonesia and USA	168	83–260	Gillespie *et al.* (2000)
Leopard geckos – no UVB, high vitamin D diet	102.5		Allen *et al.* (1996)
Leopard geckos – no UVB, low vitamin D diet	11.8		Allen *et al.* (1996)
Mali uromastyx – outdoors in El Salvador		62·4–406·8	Mitchell *et al.* (2005)
Mediterranean tortoises outdoors in UK–females		21–30	Eatwell (2008b)
Mediterranean tortoises outdoors in UK–males		38–61	Eatwell (2008b)
Ornate and Egyptian uromastyx – no UVB		12.5–107.5	Raphael *et al.* (1999)
Panther chameleons – high UVB indoors – females	1315	225–2400	Ferguson *et al.* (2005)
Panther chameleons – low UVB indoors – females	91.8		Ferguson *et al.* (2003)
Panther chameleons – low UVB indoors – females	604		Ferguson *et al.* (2003)
Red-eared sliders – low UVB indoors	71.7	34.0–155.0	Acierno *et al.* (2006)
Red-eared sliders after outdoor hibernation	10.7	5.0–14.0	Acierno *et al.* (2006)
Rhinoceros iguana – no UVB indoors	118.75		Ramer *et al.* (2002)
Rhinoceros iguana – outdoors 4–6 weeks in summer in Indianapolis	406.25		Ramer *et al.* (2002)
Rhinoceros iguana – outdoors in Dominican Republic	317	220–519	Ramer *et al.* (2005)
Rhinoceros iguanas indoors in winter in Texas	32	16–49.5	Ferguson *et al.* (2015)
Rhinoceros iguanas outdoors in summer in Texas	239	157–312.5	Ferguson *et al.* (2015)
Tunisian tortoise – hypocalcaemic	63.0		Eatwell (2008a)
Veiled chameleons – no UVB, oral D3 indoors	102		Hoby *et al.* (2010)
Veiled chameleons – UVB and oral D3 indoors	>250		Hoby *et al.* (2010)
Veiled chameleons – UVB indoors	142		Hoby *et al.* (2010)

22.16 (continued) Blood levels of 25(OH)D3 in reptiles.

for oral preparations. Dilution with an equal volume of 0.9% NaCl and intracoelomic injection into the caudolateral ab-domen seems to cause the least problems.

Parenteral treatment should only be given until clinical signs, such as muscular fasciculations, cease.

It is usually only necessary to use injections for 12–24 hours, even in severe cases, if oral supplementation is also started at the same time. In some situations the easiest way to ensure that lizards and tortoises receive adequate amounts of calcium (Figure 22.17) is to syringe-feed calcium glubionate/lactobionate; this is sold as a sweet paediatric syrup and can be administered at the same dose as calcium injection. As calcium can cross the intestine via the paracellular route (see above), feeding poorly ionized calcium salts will elevate blood levels if luminal concentrations are higher. Response to calcium supplementation is easily monitored via blood samples and clinical response. If mineralized bone loss is severe, this form of calcium supplementation may be necessary for 1–3 months.

Vitamin D status is best addressed by exposure to appropriate UVB irradiation (see above) rather than by injection, provided liver and kidney functions are normal. If the reptile has liver disease or renal failure (recall the effect of prolonged exposure of kidneys to PTH) then exposure to UVB or vitamin D3 injection may have either a reduced or no effect on the production of calcitriol.

Calcium supplementation calculator for lizards						
Daily requirements						
	B	C	D	E	F	G
	Reptile weight (g)	Scaled weight	SMR (kJ/d)[a]	SMR x 1.5	mg calcium calculated as 0.7 mg/kJ SMR (equivalent to approximately 1% DM intake)	Calcium Sandoz 22 mg Ca/ml[b] (1 mmol = 1.85 ml) maintenance (ml/day)
Calculation[c]		(B/1000)^0.82	C*51.37	D*1.5	0.7*E	F/22
	1	0.00	0.18	0.27	0.19	0.01
	10	0.03	1.29	1.94	1.35	0.06
	20	0.04	2.25	3.37	2.36	0.11

22.17 Calcium supplementation spreadsheet calculator for a generalized lizard (SMR = 51.37 kg weight [0.82]) assuming daily energy requirements are 1.5 SMR. [a] A more accurate calculation can be obtained by substituting a specific SMR for the particular species if this is known (see Figure 4.2). Blood calcium levels should always be checked to avoid overdosing, especially in mature animals. [b] A mixture of 0.218 g/ml calcium glubionate and 0.145 g/ml calcium lactobionate. [c] Figures used in calculation cells in Excel to produce the spreadsheet. ^ = Excel symbol for 'to the power of'; SMR = standard metabolic rate. (continues)

Calcium supplementation calculator for lizards						
Daily requirements continued						
	B	C	D	E	F	G
	Reptile weight (g)	Scaled weight	SMR (kJ/d)[a]	SMR x 1.5	mg calcium calculated as 0.7 mg/kJ SMR (equivalent to approximately 1% DM intake)	Calcium Sandoz 22 mg Ca/ml[b] (1 mmol = 1.85 ml) maintenance (ml/day)
Calculation[c]		(B/1000)^0.82	C*51.37	D*1.5	0.7*E	F/22
	30	0.06	3.11	4.66	3.26	0.15
	40	0.08	3.91	5.87	4.11	0.19
	50	0.09	4.68	7.01	4.91	0.22
	60	0.11	5.41	8.12	5.68	0.26
	70	0.12	6.12	9.18	6.43	0.29
	80	0.13	6.81	10.22	7.15	0.33
	90	0.15	7.48	11.23	7.86	0.36
	100	0.16	8.14	12.21	8.55	0.39
	150	0.22	11.26	16.89	11.82	0.54
	175	0.25	12.74	19.11	13.38	0.61
	250	0.33	16.95	25.42	17.79	0.81
	300	0.38	19.61	29.41	20.59	0.94
	350	0.43	22.18	33.27	23.29	1.06
	400	0.48	24.68	37.02	25.91	1.18
	450	0.53	27.12	40.68	28.48	1.29
	500	0.57	29.50	44.26	30.98	1.41
	550	0.62	31.84	47.76	33.43	1.52
	600	0.66	34.14	51.21	35.84	1.63
	650	0.71	36.39	54.59	38.21	1.74
	700	0.75	38.62	57.93	40.55	1.84
	750	0.79	40.81	61.21	42.85	1.95
	800	0.84	42.97	64.46	45.12	2.05
	850	0.88	45.11	67.66	47.36	2.15
	900	0.92	47.22	70.83	49.58	2.25
	950	0.96	49.30	73.96	51.77	2.35
	1000	1.00	51.37	77.06	53.94	2.45

22.17 (continued) Calcium supplementation spreadsheet calculator for a generalized lizard (SMR = 51.37 kg weight [0.82]) assuming daily energy requirements are 1.5 SMR. [a] A more accurate calculation can be obtained by substituting a specific SMR for the particular species if this is known (see Figure 4.2). Blood calcium levels should always be checked to avoid overdosing, especially in mature animals. [b] A mixture of 0.218 g/ml calcium glubionate and 0.145 g/ml calcium lactobionate. [c] Figures used in calculation cells in Excel to produce the spreadsheet. ^ = Excel symbol for 'to the power of'; SMR = standard metabolic rate.

Vitamin A deficiency has marked effects on reptilian bone and this should be assessed and addressed (see Hypovitaminosis A).

Salmon calcitonin injections have been used (50 IU i.m. q7d for two treatments) as a method of increasing calcium uptake into depleted bones in green iguanas (Mader, 2006b). The treatment appeared, empirically, to speed up improvement in green iguanas with NSHP; controlled studies have not yet been done. Calcitonin has no effect on several other reptile species (Copp and Kline, 1989) and can cause life-threatening hypocalcaemia as it also enhances renal calcium and phosphorus clearance.

Animals with NSHP that have fractured bones should initially have these stabilized with external coaptation (see Chapter 13); however, once a positive calcium balance has been established a good repair can often be achieved with careful external fixation. In lizards weighing 1.5 kg or less, repair with intramedullary pins will often lead to further fracturing of the bone and should therefore be avoided; lightweight external fixation is often the most appropriate option.

Hypovitaminosis A

Hypovitaminosis A is relatively common in reptiles. Deficiency causes a multifocal squamous cell metaplasia and hyperkeratosis in a wide range of epithelial tissues, e.g. eyes, lungs and kidneys (Frye, 1984). In birds and mammals, normal growth and cartilage maturation are adversely affected; this also appears to be true for at least some reptiles.

Vitamin A levels have only occasionally been measured in reptiles and the different methodologies used have made comparisons difficult (0.3 μg retinol = 1 IU): pancake tortoises 3.2 μg/l (10.67 IU/l) for females and 6.2 μg/l (20.67 IU/l) for males (Raphael et al., 1994); wild anacondas 0.08 μg/l plasma (0.27 IU/l) (Calle et al., 1994); green iguanas 52 μg/l plasma (173 IU/l) (Raila et al., 2002). Reported levels for reptiles are quite low compared with those found in mammals (100–1000 μg/l) (Schweigert, 1995). Normal livers of monitor lizards and snakes contained >1000 IU/g

(Elkan and Zwart, 1967); the same researchers reported liver vitamin A levels in two map turtles with hypovitaminosis A as 9 and 19 IU/g, respectively.

Clinical signs

Panther chameleons raised on a diet with low levels of vitamin A (retinol) had a reduced growth rate, periocular oedema, excessive ocular secretion, swollen lips, loss of posture control, gular oedema, hemipenal impaction, vertebral kinking, tail-tip necrosis, and reduced reproduction and egg viability. This study also documented MBD with poorly formed irregular cement lines and bones with normal calcium but higher ash content (Ferguson et al., 1996).

Swollen eyes are a common clinical sign caused by expansion of the anteromedial Harderian gland and posterior lacrimal gland and the accumulation of desquamated debris (Elkan and Zwart, 1967) (see Chapter 15). This eventually causes eversion of the conjunctiva and gross swelling of the eye to such an extent that it may be difficult to open the eyelids. Although often seen in inappropriately fed terrapins, the condition is also relatively common in insectivorous lizards (Figure 22.18) where owners have failed to pre-feed (gut-load) prey insects. Secondary infections may develop in the necrotic epithelial tissue owing to reduced ocular immunity, and can lead to misdiagnosis of the underlying cause.

Chronically affected chelonians may often have hyperkeratosis of the beak and are prone to develop secondary respiratory infections, such as 'runny-nose syndrome' and pneumonia (Fowler, 1980).

In severe cases there may also be metaplasia of the cuboidal cells of the pancreas, kidneys, ureters and-bladder, and fatty degeneration of the liver. Inguinal and axillary swelling due to oedema caused by kidney failure (Lawton, 1989) can also occur.

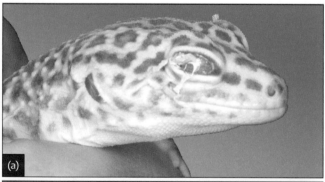

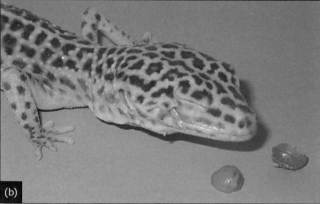

22.18 Hypovitaminosis A in a leopard gecko. (a) Appearance of the eyes before the removal of caseous deposits. (b) Caseous debris removed from the eyes. A round-ended earwax cleaner will usually remove the plug after moistening with saline.

Supplementation

Based on panther chameleon studies, the vitamin A dose recommended is 1000–2000 IU/kg per week (Abate et al., 2003). How far this can be extrapolated to other reptiles is difficult to say without appropriate research. This is reflected in the type and quantity of vitamin A in commonly sold reptile vitamin supplements; some only contain beta-carotene, some no vitamin A and some very large amounts >6000 IU/g.

Care should be taken when treating animals with injectable preparations. These are usually designed for large food animals and contain 100,000–500,000 IU/ml of vitamin A. The only way to measure out such concentrated solutions with any accuracy is by using a 0.3 ml insulin syringe; otherwise it is easy to produce iatrogenic hypervitaminosis A. This usually causes blistering and sloughing of the epidermis. NB: prior to treatment, always check that a reptile has not been given a vitamin injection within the recent past.

Lower-dose oral preparations for human paediatric use are a useful alternative. Most of these preparations also contain vitamin D; however, if the preparation is used primarily as a source of vitamin A and an appropriate dose is used it is unlikely that a vitamin D overdose will be given even if the reptile is exposed to UVB.

In humans, the ratio of vitamins A, D and E seems to be critical and these vitamins are usually supplied in a 100:10:1 ratio. Commercial reptile vitamin preparations sold in pet shops vary considerably in terms of their composition (see Chapter 4).

Hypovitaminosis B1 (thiamine deficiency)

In captivity, piscivorous garter and Eurasian water snakes and turtles can often become thiamine deficient.

Thiamine may be depleted if frozen fish is left to thaw for several hours prior to feeding, because thiaminases in some species (e.g. whitebait, mackerel, goldfish) are not destroyed by freezing. The loss can be reduced by defrosting the fish in hot water (80°C for 5 minutes) to denature the enzymes and then adding 20 mg of thiamine per kg of fish. Alternatively, a small quantity of brewer's yeast, or reptile supplement containing thiamine, can be inserted into the fish before feeding. Some leafy vegetables such as brackens and ferns contain phytothiaminases and can cause similar problems (Frye, 1991). This is usually encountered when owners make up and freeze batches of vegetable salads for herbivores such as iguanas.

Nervous tremors, incoordination, torticollis, opisthotonus, convulsions and apparent blindness are typical signs of thiamine deficiency, caused by cerebral cortical necrosis and peripheral neuritis (Zwart and van Ham, 1980).

Reptiles showing clinical signs can be treated parenterally or orally with thiamine preparations at 50–100 mg/kg q24h.

Biotin deficiency

Monitor lizards, Gila monsters and Mexican beaded lizards all relish raw eggs. In the wild these would only be part of a diet and would often be embryonated. If reptiles are fed almost exclusively on hens' eggs (which are infertile and so contain the anti-biotin vitamin avidin) they may show signs of biotin deficiency (Frye, 1991). This appears as muscular weakness and tremors.

Hypovitaminosis C (ascorbic acid deficiency)

Garter snakes are able to synthesize vitamin C, but how far this applies to other reptiles is unknown (Vosburgh et al., 1982). Although most bird species are able to synthesize vitamin C it has been found that dietary supplementation of this vitamin during periods of stress or infection has a beneficial effect (Peebles and Brake, 1985). In mammals and birds, biosynthesis of vitamin C is inhibited if vitamin A, E or biotin is deficient. Biosynthesis of vitamin C is poor in juvenile poultry, and dietary supplementation has been found to improve bone strength.

A study on juvenile Asian water dragons found that giving lizards 100 mg/kg vitamin C q24h did not affect bone calcium and phosphorus, but did have a positive effect on tibial bone-breaking strength and bone length (Oyarzun et al., 1995). Supplementing the diet of the Chinese soft-shelled turtle with vitamin C produced a significant effect on non-specific immune function, provided the amount was >2500 and <5000 mg/kg of diet (Zhou et al., 2002). Based on these limited data, there may be some merit in providing supplemental vitamin C to juveniles and stressed individuals that are not consuming fresh fruit, and to individuals with liver disease. The turtle study suggests that dose may be critical, but optimal doses have not been determined for other species.

Dose rates of 10–250 mg/kg i.m. have been suggested in the treatment of ulcerative stomatitis in snakes (Stein, 1996).

Hypovitaminosis E (tocopherol deficiency)

Whole fish are similar in nutrient composition to small mammal prey but fat content can vary widely with species and season. Many species have high levels of the fat-soluble vitamins A, D and E. However, the polyunsaturated fatty acids in fish undergo rapid oxidation after death, which quickly depletes the vitamin E content (Allen and Baer, 1989). Nutrient quality can also decline rapidly secondary to bacterial spoilage if the fish are not stored at low temperatures soon after being caught. Anorexia, steatitis and fat necrosis secondary to vitamin E deficiency have been recorded in alligators fed poor-quality fish (Larsen et al., 1983).

Hypovitaminosis E has been seen in crocodilians fed mackerel, in terrapins fed oily fish (e.g. whitebait) and in some snakes fed overweight laboratory rodents (Dierenfeld, 1989). Steatitis is seen as hard fatty nodules under the skin in the legs of chelonians, and linear ulcerations of the cloacae of crocodilians (Frye, 1991). Often the only presenting sign is anorexia, followed by death. High levels of polyunsaturated fats present in the diets of captive reptiles can cause depression of vitamin E levels and also lead to steatitis. Fat necrosis and steatitis are not seen in wild reptiles and therefore must be considered a disease of captivity due to inappropriate nutrition.

The suggested vitamin E supplementation dose for reptiles is approximately 1 IU/kg q24h (20–80 mg/kg of diet (DM)), based on extrapolation from mammals.

Selenium deficiency is a common problem in mammals and causes similar clinical signs to vitamin E deficiency. However, the role of this mineral has not been investigated in reptiles. In mammals the requirement is usually between 0.3 and 0.5 ppm, with higher levels being toxic.

Gout

Gout (see also Chapter 20) is a problem in uricotelic species when anything reduces the efficiency of renal excretion of uric acid. Diets high in protein and purines, with or without dehydration, are considered to be the major cause of gout in reptiles, although work on birds suggests other factors may be involved, such as starvation (Ekstrom and Degernes, 1989).

Gout is well recognized in commercially farmed American alligators, primarily due to overfeeding a high-protein diet when temperatures are below 20–25°C (when anabolism is less efficient) (Foggin, 1987).

In most reptiles, uric acid is the end product of the breakdown of purines, which results from degradation of nucleic acids in the diet or synthesized in the liver during protein metabolism. Uric acid and urate salts are relatively insoluble and easily crystallize out of solution. Collections of crystals (tophi) may be deposited in joints, lungs, spleen, kidney (see Figure 20.8), liver or the subcutaneous tissues (Mader, 2006a). Bennet (1996) has also reported neurological signs due to formation of tophi in the central nervous system. Often the primary deposition sites are the kidney tubules, possibly as a result of reduced filtration, treatment with nephrotoxic antibiotics or changes in the pH of the primary filtrate. This damages the tubules and the kidneys then cease to clear uric acid from the circulation.

For the treatment and management of visceral and renal gout, the reader is referred to Chapter 20.

Pyramidal growth syndrome in chelonians

Pyramidal-shaped scutes are considered normal in a few species (e.g. Indian star and African tent tortoises), but in others their development is pathological, and severe deformities can be debilitating and compromise the individual's welfare. Pyramidal growth syndrome, or 'pyramiding', is commonly seen in captive-reared tortoises. There is typically thickening and excessive growth of the scutes of the carapace, resulting in the centre of each scute being raised above the level of its margins, giving the appearance of pyramids. The underlying bone is also deformed, with thickened fibrous weakly structured bone in the areas of greatest stress at the centre of the vertebral scutes (Gerlach, 2004).

The aetiology of pyramiding has been much debated for many years. Overfeeding leading to too-rapid growth, excessive dietary protein (possibly leading to renal secondary hyperparathyroidism), calcium and phosphorus imbalances, and vitamin D deficiency leading to NSHP have all been proposed as the underlying cause. More recently, pyramiding as a result of low environmental humidity has become a popular theory, largely owing to a much-cited publication by Weisner and Iben (2003), despite significant methodological difficulties having been identified in their study by others. The true aetiology, however, is likely to be multifactorial. Highfield (2010) attributes pyramiding to a progression of events:

- Deficiencies in calcium in the diet and/or vitamin D3 from inadequate UVB or dietary supplementation leads to NSHP
- Overnutrition, arising from highly digestible, very low fibre diets which provide high energy levels (some also with high protein levels), leads to abnormally rapid growth

- The resulting poorly mineralized, rapidly growing and pliable bones are distorted by the pull of their muscle attachments, creating the typical bowing of the carapace, with bulging around the thorax and flattening above the pelvis
- Dehydration of the outer keratin layers of the carapace occurs, mainly due to the extreme drying effects of artificial heat sources (in particular, infrared radiation from overhead heat lamps)
- This causes the keratin to become very hard, inflexible and resistant to sideways expansion, and also stimulates its overproduction, thickening the scutes
- This produces a discrepancy between bone growth and scute growth, accentuated further if there is abnormally rapid bone growth due to overnutrition
- The hardened keratin then exerts a further, very significant, force upon the poorly mineralized skeleton beneath, which is remodelled to conform to the shape of the thickened inflexible scute – creating the typical pyramid-shaped distortions
- And in captivity, there is very little 'wear and tear' on the scutes, whereas in the wild, digging, burrowing, abrasion from rocks and foliage, and erosion by soil microorganisms naturally wear away old keratin from the surface of scutes, preventing thickening.

Highfield (2010) highlights the problems associated with the widespread use of small heat lamps with narrow beams at close range, which may heat only the top of the carapace (possibly to an unacceptable degree) while the rest of the tortoise remains poorly warmed, prolonging the period it spends under the lamp. He also acknowledges that increasing the humidity around the carapace will soften the keratin and reduce the stresses on the skeleton; however, he points out that this does not address any underlying bone pathology, and high humidity is not normal in the microhabitats of many desert tortoise species.

However, moderate humidity may be obtained in burrows, and evaporation from the surface of the body may be greatly reduced by self-burying in loose substrate, even if it is dry, as practised by many sheltering tortoises in the wild.

Recommendations to prevent pyramiding include providing a high-fibre low-calorie diet with adequate calcium and phosphorus. There must be access to natural sunlight or suitable UVB levels indoors; if this is not possible, oral supplementation of vitamin D3 could be considered as a last resort. A suitably large basking area with appropriate temperature gradient is necessary, to ensure whole-body warming to the preferred optimum temperature of the species without localized overheating and dehydration of the carapace. A moist hide, such as a box filled with damp moss, will provide shelter combined with localized high humidity. Tortoises should also have permanent access to water in a shallow container which they can drink from, and some authors recommend weekly soaking (e.g. Donoghue, 2006).

Once pyramiding has occurred the carapace deformity is permanent, but with treatment of any associated NSHP and improved diet and husbandry, further growth may be normal.

Secondary iodine deficiency

Secondary iodine deficiency has been reported in herbivorous lizards and chelonians (especially the larger species) due to the feeding of green forage that contains goitrogens (particularly brassicas such as kale, broccoli, Brussels sprouts and cabbage) and soybean-based products (Frye, 1991). Lethargy and swelling at the thoracic inlet are reported clinically. Treatment requires supplementation with thyroxine (T4) (Wilkinson, 2004) and dietary correction.

Dried kelp or dried kelp tablets can be added to these diets as a source of iodine. In excess, iodine is toxic, so it is important not to over-supplement diets.

Anorexia

All reptiles that present with anorexia should have their husbandry reviewed and investigated. Factors such as inappropriate thermal gradient, stress from overcrowding or lack of hides can quickly lead to not eating. Ingestion and impaction of substrate (Figure 22.19) is common, and can be due to poor nutrition and/or dehydration.

Some species will have natural periods of not eating, which may be in correlation with mating and courtship activity in males and gravidity in females, or may be due to a species, such as the Horsfield's tortoise, coming from an environment where food is not available all year round.

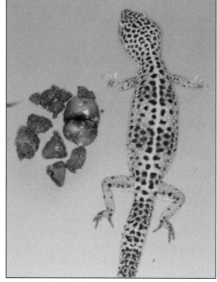

22.19 A large quantity of walnut-chip substrate removed from an anorexic leopard gecko.

Chelonians

Diagnosing anorexia in chelonians can be challenging; again, a review of husbandry is key, followed by an assessment to ensure it is not a normal seasonal occurrence. If these investigations are unrewarding, then faecal screening and blood samples are often good first stages to an investigation, as is radiography, but inappropriate husbandry must always be at the forefront of differential diagnosis.

Lizards

In the wild it is normal for many lizards to go for long periods without eating. If they have evolved to live in an environment where food is not available all year round or are 'sit-and-wait' predators, their metabolism copes with this lack of food very well, often with very little weight loss. In the wild, white-throated monitor lizards may fast for almost 7 months in the dry season (Secor and Phillips, 1997).

Reptiles have very active and flexible fat bodies that accumulate fat when surplus food is available. This fat is then used as an energy source when food is scarce or unavailable. Prior to hibernation, one-third of the body-weight of the common wall lizard is fat. At low temperatures this is more than adequate to fuel a fast of 6–7 months over the winter period (Avery, 1970).

Snakes

Male snakes often become anorexic during the breeding season, especially if a female is present or within olfactory distance. In contrast, females may eat voraciously at this time. In some species males may refuse to eat for many months. Male breeding-season anorexia has been observed in most reptiles, but especially North American snakes (Boyer and Boyer, 1993). The most extreme examples are male emerald tree boas, which undergo fasts of 5–9 months, and there are anecdotal accounts of African house snakes starving to death when not removed from females. It is therefore always worth checking the sex of an anorexic snake and determining whether a female is present in the collection, even if not in the same vivarium, and if it is the time of year this species normally breeds.

Weight loss can be dramatic. In the wild, male water pythons rapidly lose up to 17% of their bodyweight over 6 weeks during the breeding season and suffer no ill effects. In contrast, females that cease feeding for 3 months lose an average of 44% of their body mass over this period and experience increased mortality (Madsen and Shine, 2000).

Recent research has shown that boids and crotalids are adapted physiologically to undergoing long periods of anorexia as part of a sit-and-wait predatory lifestyle (Secor and Diamond, 2000). (For average feed intervals for different genera, based on feeding data of wild individuals, see Chapter 4.) During prolonged fasts, the intestines of these snakes are metabolically inactive, which enables their standard metabolic rate (SMR) to be lower than that of other snakes (Galvão et al., 1965). The small intestines have complexly folded pseudostratified mucosal epithelium that expands and increases in mass by up to three times within 48 hours of ingesting prey (Starck and Bleese, 2001). This size increase is energetically expensive and involves a 5–7-fold increase in metabolic rate (Secor and Diamond, 1998), termed the specific dynamic action. In pythons, 32% of a meal's energy yield is used to power this change in digestive capacity.

Enterocytes fill with large lipid droplets as they expand in size during digestion and appear to act as an energy source for a mitotic cycle 7–10 days post feeding (Starck and Bleese, 2001). In energetic terms it is more advantageous for these species to eat large infrequent meals than smaller more frequent ones.

Feeding a diet of high protein/fat content, which is easily digested, may be the way to stimulate digestive processes in these snake species (Secor et al., 2002). In practical terms, the main difficulty with snakes is determining when anorexia is part of normal physiology or when it is pathological and driven by underlying disease or poor management. From the limited information available it seems sensible to consider weight losses of >15% for males and >20% in females to be indicators for intervention in pythons and boas, and losses of 10% and 15% in other male and female snakes, outside the breeding season. However, weight loss should not be the sole criterion used to diagnose anorexia. Clinical assessment and changes in parameters such as intestinal parasites, total protein, uric acid levels, and red and white blood cell counts are all possible indicators for intervention.

Some temperate juvenile snakes born in autumn will hibernate after hatching and delay feeding until the following season; however, neonates that lose >30% of their body-weight usually die. Where intervention is warranted, enteral nutritional support is easily carried out in most snakes.

Post-brumation anorexia in tortoises

Brumating species in the wild will generally have a long period of warm weather to prepare for a short brumation period. During brumation in captivity, they may be exposed to a short period of warm weather to prepare for a notably long period of dormancy, inactivity and brumation. It may not be possible for their metabolism to adapt to these differences. Brumation in captivity should be restricted to a maximum of 3 months regardless of size. Juvenile animals may be hibernated for as little as a month.

In addition, leucopenia is common following long periods of brumation. This may be due to poor health prior to brumation, stress and seasonally related changes in reproductive hormones or to the fact that the life expectancy of white blood cells is limited and thus when hibernation is prolonged, cell numbers may decline to extremely low levels (NB: during normal brumation metabolic rest occurs, which aids the thyroid, bone marrow and gastro-intestinal tract).

Such leucopenic animals awake with compromised immune systems. When leucopenic tortoises are warmed (naturally or artificially), bacteria and fungal and viral agents within them appear to replicate quickly, often before the tortoise's immune system can recuperate. In such circumstances stomatitis, rhinitis and systemic infections are common.

This scenario appears to be exacerbated by failing to allow a tortoise to reach its preferred body temperature during hibernation recovery and allowing it to chill below its Preferred Optimal Temperature Zone (POTZ) at night, therefore compromising the immune system and favouring the pathogens. This is exacerbated by owner failure to observe that the individual is no longer hibernating. This results in dehydration, malnutrition and further debilitation. In addition, many chelonians may have experienced frost damage or rodent attacks during hibernation if not properly supervised (see Chapter 5 for additional information on brumation protocol).

Diagnosis

A detailed history of previous disease, prehibernation weight and health examinations is essential. Most chelonians urinate, defecate and eat within a week of hibernation recovery.

An initial pre-treatment biochemistry assessment is an essential part of evaluating the post-hibernation anorexia patient. A general tortoise profile would include:

- Haematology (including a differential white cell count)
- Examination for haemoparasites
- Blood biochemistry: total protein, potassium, urea, uric acid, albumin, alkaline phosphatase, aspartate aminotransferase, lactate dehydrogenase, glutamate dehydrogenase, calcium (ionized and total), alpha-hydroxybutyrate (an indicator of how chronic the non-feeding episode has been), phosphate, sodium, creatine kinase and glucose.

A baseline profile on admission allows sequential blood monitoring during hospitalization and recovery.

Following the results of a general profile, it is normal to monitor critical parameters such as packed cell volume, albumin, uric acid, urea and potassium throughout the stabilization period. Through these parameters the response to fluids, nutrition and medication, such as allopurinol, can be assessed.

Urine acidity, urine specific gravity and blood alpha-hydroxybutyrate (BHB) appear to be additional parameters worth monitoring when stabilizing a dehydrated terrestrial chelonian. In the immediate post-hibernation period of herbivorous chelonians it was found that urine pH was 5.0–6.0, but this rose to 8.0–8.5 after 1 month of normal feeding. Acidic urine (pH <7) is suggestive of catabolism and is a consistent feature of herbivorous chelonians suffering from prolonged anorexia.

BHB is thought to be a good indicator of ketogenesis in reptiles; in the desert tortoise, plasma levels of BHB ranged between 0.4 and 0.75 mmol/l in times of significant rainfall (and food availability), but increased to 2.0 mmol/l after 2 months of drought (Christopher et al., 1994). In contrast, ketogenesis did not appear to be important during brumation.

Treatment

Encouragement to urinate, defecate and eat is aided by soaking in warm shallow (2–3 cm deep) water. However, in post-hibernation Mediterranean tortoise species with hyperuricaemia, hyperkalaemia and hypoglycaemia, urgent fluid therapy (possibly in conjunction with drugs inhibiting further uric acid production, such as allopurinol) is essential to preserve life. Fluid therapy may involve the use of orogastric tubes, oesophagostomy tubes and intracoelomic, intraosseous, intravenous or epicoelomic routes (see Chapter 11).

In hyperuricaemic, hyperkalaemic cases it appears to be safe to give fluids by the intraosseous, oral or epicoelomic routes at up to 4 ml/100 g per day until urination is achieved. Following this, fluid levels are generally reduced to 2 ml/100 g per day, by pharyngostomy or stomach tube, as uric acid and blood potassium levels fall. Maintenance is continued for several weeks at least, at about 0.5–1 ml/100 g per day. Hospitalization and intensive treatment are advised for *Testudo* tortoises with the following signs or biochemical markers:

- Hyperuricaemia (uric acid >500 μmol/l (>11.76 mg/dl))
- Hyperkalaemia (K+ >5 mmol/l (>19.5 mg/dl))
- Anuria (no urine within the previous 10 days).

These animals are generally hospitalized on a fluid-therapy protocol until repeated urination, decreasing uric acid levels and decreasing potassium levels are achieved.

1. Allopurinol should be administered to all chronically ill chelonians with uric acid levels >1000 μmol/l (16.81 mg/dl). Generally, allopurinol is given at 20 mg/kg q24h by dissolving a 100 mg tablet in 5 ml of water and then offering 1 ml/kg q24h orally or by stomach/oesophagostomy tube. In most cases, treatment is continued for about 3 months, with further therapy dictated by regular blood biochemistry assessment.
2. Animals with uric acid levels >2000 μmol/l (33.61 mg/dl) and potassium levels >9 mmol/l (approximately 35 mg/dl) often demonstrate no urine output despite active fluid therapy. Treatment can be attempted with aggressive dialysis and the use of diuretics, but positive outcomes are rare; therefore, euthanasia

should be considered in these cases, as death in such animals is very likely to occur, due to cardiac failure associated with hyperkalaemic arrhythmias.
3. Following initial urination, nutritional support should be offered and initially should involve small but increasing levels of calories and nutrients in order to reduce the possibility of 'refeeding syndrome'. However, in hyperkalaemic patients it is advantageous to give glucose to drive potassium ions into the cells. Emeraid® herbivore (Lafeber), initially double diluted, may be used for this purpose. This means half the recommended feeding amount is given initially in order to counter refeeding syndrome (see paragraph below).

Nutritional support for sick reptiles

Nutritional support may be required for animals that have recently undergone surgery or have suffered malnutrition for prolonged periods. Food should be introduced slowly if malnutrition has occurred over an extended period, since life-threatening hypophosphataemia and hypokalaemia are potential problems (Bounos, 1972). This 'refeeding syndrome' is caused by the sudden insulin-stimulated cellular uptake of potassium and phosphate ions, which depletes already marginal plasma electrolyte reserves. This mammalian phenomenon has also been documented in malnourished Argentine side-necked turtles (DaSilva and Migliorini, 1990).

In mammals, nutritional support is calculated on the calorific requirement at the current weight of the animal, and phased in over several days. This can be achieved by providing half the required calories on day 1, three-quarters of the required calories on day 2 and the full calorific requirement on day 3. This method is extrapolated from cats and dogs but has been tried and tested in reptiles; however, it is imperative to consider the metabolic nature of the species and the individual reptile before drawing up such plans. For example, species with high metabolic rates and short gut-transit times such as day geckos may require feeding numerous times a day. However, they are also a small species and so need more calorie-concentrated foods.

Care should be taken with the use of hyperosmolar solutions initially because intravascular fluid will equilibrate with these across the small intestine resulting in an osmotic diarrhoea. This can cause an initial hypotension (Shils, 1988). Plasma osmolality in most healthy reptiles is about 300 mOsmol/l (slightly lower in crocodilians and freshwater turtles, and slightly higher in marine turtles and some desert lizards, but there is still a limited amount of data published) (Minnich, 1982).

In mammals, the intestinal mucosa only acts as a barrier to bacteria when there are nutrients present in the lumen (Alverdy, 1990), so some enteral feeding is likely to be useful even if the reptile is being supported parenterally, to avoid sepsis. In reptiles, enteral feeding is best done via a flexible silicon feeding tube (e.g. human nasogastric tube). If tube feeding is required for an extended period of time the placing of a pharyngostomy tube is indicated; this will require sedation and local anaesthesia or general anaesthesia (see Chapter 12). These are well tolerated and simplify feeding and medication, and if placed correctly (i.e. so the access to the tube end is well away from the head and out of direct sight of the patient) will massively reduce stress to the patient and often allow feeding to be carried out without restraint in the case of chelonians. A volume of 2–10% of bodyweight is usually fed, depending on the reptile's condition and the energy density of the mixture. The calculation of basal energy requirement (BER) in reptiles can be complicated, and difficulty in coming up with this figure should never be a cause of delay in starting a feeding plan; weighing the animal daily and looking for a steady weight gain is a good indication of the appropriateness of what is being given, which in most cases will be a reflection of rehydration initially.

BMR (basal metabolic rate) = K x (weight in kg)$^{0.75}$, where the factor K is assumed to be 10 for reptiles. The BER is usually 1.5 times the BMR for a healthy reptile. Therefore, for sick reptiles, the BER may be increased by 1.5–2 times for sepsis and trauma (as for mammals), or slightly reduced for reptiles that are long-term cachexic cases, to avoid refeeding syndrome (usually 0.75 times the BER).

Normally urates will be passed first and this is a good indication of improving hydration and kidney function. This is hopefully followed by faeces; however, the first faeces passed after an extended period of anorexia are often hard and desiccated, resulting in constipation. This may require enemas, which should always be given with caution in female reptiles as there are many anecdotal accounts of faecal material being flushed, retrogradely, into the reproductive tract, resulting in infection. Therefore, small volumes of sterile solutions such as lactated Ringer's solution are indicated in these cases, and ensuring the tube is correctly placed into the rectum rather than just the cloaca.

In addition to being of appropriate composition, an enteral food must also pass easily down a feeding tube. A solution such as Duphalyte (Pfizer), containing dextrose, amino acids and minerals, is a good simple starter solution that can be given enterally or parenterally. As it has a high potassium content, it should be used with care in herbivores.

There are many diets sold as dry pellets by manufacturers; these can be ground to a fine powder in a coffee grinder. The resulting powder can then be mixed with water or an enteral solution to form slurry, although these tend to be messy and often clog and block all but the wider-bore feeding tubes.

Several enteral solutions are sold for veterinary use (Figure 22.20) and there is also a plethora of human products with varying properties; these are subject to strict regulatory control and many are designed to be nutritionally complete (for humans). All the human products have guaranteed analysis and energy-density data.

Product	Comments	Composition	Energy content[a]
Critical Care Formula (Vetark Professional)	Protein concentrate, maltodextrins and amino acids Mix 1:2 with water	Protein: 14.4 g/100 g	1511 kJ/100 g (361 kcal/100 g) 5.86 kJ/ml (1.4 kcal/ml) made-up
Critical Care for Herbivores (Oxbow Pet Products)	Based on timothy grass, wheat and soybean meals Mix 1:1.5 with water NB: for herbivores only	Protein: 16% Fat: 3.2% Crude fibre: 21% Vitamin A: 214 IU/100 g Vitamin D: 71 IU/100 g Vitamin C: 28 mg/100 g	1045 kJ/100 g (250 kcal/100 g) 5.25 kJ/ml (1.25 kcal/ml) made-up
Science Recovery for Herbivores (Supreme Petfoods Ltd)	Alfalfa, oatfeed, wheat, wheatfeed, soybean meal, peas, milk powder, synthetic cellulose, sugar-beet pulp, probiotic, casein, anise, fenugreek Fed as 20 g concentrate mixed with 70 ml water NB: for herbivores only	Protein: 13–17% Fat: 2% Crude fibre: 20% Ash: 5% Calcium 1.3–1.8% Vitamin A: 1200 IU/100 g Vitamin D3: 150 IU/100 g Vitamin C: 1 mg/100 g Vitamin E: 8 mg/100 g Copper: 1.2 mg/100 g	1305 kJ/100 g (312 kcal/100 g) 2.9 kJ/ml (0.7 kcal/ml) made-up
Dry juvenile inland bearded dragon food (T-Rex)[b,c]	Mix 1:4 with water	Protein: 18% Fat: 6.5% Crude fibre: 5.0% Ash: 5% Moisture: 10%	1346 kJ/100 g (322 kcal/100 g) 2.69 kJ/ml (0.64 kcal/ml) made-up
Dry juvenile aquatic turtle food (T-Rex)[b,c]	Mix 1:4 with water	Protein: 34% Fat: 10% Crude fibre: 5% Ash: 5% Moisture: 10%	1420 kJ/100 g (339 kcal/100 g) 2.36 kJ/ml (0.56 kcal/ml) made-up
Dry juvenile iguana food (T-Rex)[b,c]	Mix 1:4 with water	Protein: 19% Fat: 5% Crude fibre: 6% Ash: 6.5% Moisture: 10%	1287 kJ/100 g (307 kcal/100 g) 2.57 kJ/ml (0.61 kcal/ml) made-up
Alfalfa powder (also sold as tablets; available from health-food shops)	Can be used to increase the protein content of an enteral solution for a herbivorous reptile	Protein: approximately 950 mg/g Vitamin A: approximately 345 IU/g Calcium: approximately 26 mg/g	Approximately 13.87 kJ/g (3.31 kcal/g)

22.20 Enteral products that can be tube fed to reptiles. Specific combinations can be tailored to the species and its individual requirements where known. [a] Values given are calculated energy content and based on composition and moisture content, which may vary between limits set by the manufacturer. Values assume 100% digestibility but this is more likely to be 70–85%. [b] Typical values of individual products will vary; always use the juvenile versions of these diets as they have a higher protein content. [c] Most dry products can, with the aid of a coffee grinder, be reduced to a fine powder suitable for tube feeding. Dilutions can be varied but it is difficult to pass solutions that are too concentrated through a syringe or small-bore pharyngostomy tube and solutions with high osmotic pressures may adversely affect fluid uptake in the gut. (continues) ▶

Product	Comments	Composition	Energy content[a]
Horse alfalfa pellets (Dengie)[c]	Can be used as above after grinding to a powder	Protein: 16% Crude fibre: 32% Ash: 6.5% Moisture: 10% Oil: 2.5%	9 kJ/g (2.15 kcal/g)
ZooMed Anole Diet (ZooMed)	Almost 100% dried fruit flies; can be easily powdered and mixed with another enteral product to provide a mix for insectivorous reptiles	Protein: 63.2% Fat: 15.3% Fibre: 14.5% Moisture: 9.8%	1588 kJ/100 g (379 kcal/100 g)
Isosource Fibre (Novartis Animal Health)	Nutritionally complete for humans; like Ensure but has added fibre	Protein: 3.8 g/100 ml Carbohydrate: 13.6 g/100 ml Fat: 3.4 g/100 ml Fibre: 1.4 g/100 ml	418.68 kJ/100 ml (100 kcal/100 ml)
Enlive (Abbott Nutrition)	Not nutritionally complete but fat free	Protein: 4 g/100 ml Carbohydrate: 27 g/100 ml	532 kJ/100 ml (125 kcal/100 ml)
Peptisorb (Nutricia)	Nutritionally complete but low fat	Protein: 4 g/100 ml Carbohydrate: 17.6 g/100 ml Fat: 1.7 g/100 ml	419 kJ/100 ml (100 kcal/100 ml)
Ensure (Abbott Nutrition)	Nutritionally complete for humans; comes in savoury as well as fruit flavours	Protein: 4 g/100 ml Carbohydrate: 13.6 g/100 ml Fat: 3.4 g/100 ml	419 kJ/100 ml (100 kcal/100 ml) Ensure Plus: 628 kJ/100 ml (150 kcal/100 ml)
Ensure mixes (homemade)	Various Ensure mixes have been used in the USA for herbivores	1: Ensure 4.2 g; alfalfa meal 1 g 2: Ensure 1.5 g; banana 1 g	Approximately 419 kJ/100 ml (100 kcal/100 ml) Approximately 544 kJ/100 ml (130 kcal/100 ml)
Elemental 028 Extra (SHS International)	Nutritionally complete; high density; available as unflavoured powder	Protein: 12.5 g/100 ml Carbohydrate: 55 g/100 ml Fat: 59 g/100 ml	1855 kJ/100 g (443 kcal/100 g)
Generaid (SHS International)	Not nutritionally complete Used for cases of chronic liver disease in humans	Protein: 81 g/100 ml Carbohydrate: <5 g/100 g Fat: 5 g/100 g	1629 kJ/100 g (389 kcal/100 g)
Caloreen (Nestlé)	Not nutritionally complete	Glucose polymer; low electrolytes	1633 kJ/100 g (390 kcal/100 g)
Protifar (Nutricia)	Not nutritionally complete	Protein: 88.5 g/100 g	1292 kJ/100 g (308 kcal/100 g)

22.20 (continued) Enteral products that can be tube fed to reptiles. Specific combinations can be tailored to the species and its individual requirements where known. [a] Values given are calculated energy content and based on composition and moisture content, which may vary between limits set by the manufacturer. Values assume 100% digestibility but this is more likely to be 70–85%. [b] Typical values of individual products will vary; always use the juvenile versions of these diets as they have a higher protein content. [c] Most dry products can, with the aid of a coffee grinder, be reduced to a fine powder suitable for tube feeding. Dilutions can be varied but it is difficult to pass solutions that are too concentrated through a syringe or small-bore pharyngostomy tube and solutions with high osmotic pressures may adversely affect fluid uptake in the gut.

Semi-elemental feeding mixtures have been used in humans for decades and are well proven. Ranges for reptiles from several commercial sources are now available (e.g. Emeraid (Lafeber); Critical Care Formula (Vetark)), which are easy to use and come with feeding-volume guides for most species. These diets tend not to be complete or balanced so should be used only for short periods of time, but as they are solutions, they easily pass through a narrow-bore tube.

Long-term anorexic snakes are often fed a whole prey item, and in the author's opinion this has a high risk of inducing refeeding syndrome, with potential mortalities. Anorexic snakes, like all anorexic reptiles, require careful rehydration and electrolyte support before any food is given in whatever form. Tube feeding with liquid semi-elemental diets works well, but has to be done correctly as snakes have evolved to be able to regurgitate food items with great ease and often as a response to a stressful situation. Therefore, if manually restrained and tube fed and put back immediately, they will regurgitate and in some cases inhale liquids and die acutely from asphyxiation, or more likely die days later from a pneumonic infection. The most effective method is to continue to hold the snake vertically with its head uppermost for 2–15 minutes (depending on size: larger snakes will require holding for a longer duration) after administration. This allows the food to drain well down into the gastrointestinal tract. During these feeding sessions the body must always be supported to avoid spinal damage, and in large constrictors this will take several people. If it is decided the best approach is to feed a whole prey item to a snake, the snake must be well hydrated and selection of what to feed is key (Barten, 1995). Several small items are easier to administer than one big one. They must be well lubricated with a water-based lubricant such as KY jelly, and any sharp parts removed, such as large incisor teeth in the case of rodents and spurs on birds such as quail (there are anecdotal accounts of sharp teeth or spurs lacerating the oesophagus and/or heart). They must always be introduced head first and slowly advanced down to as near to the stomach as possible using long feeding forceps or tongs. Sometimes it is possible to massage the food item down the oesophagus externally into the stomach; great care must be taken to not leave the food item in the oesophagus overlying the heart, as this can lead to a restriction of cardiac output and occasionally death.

Acknowledgements

We are grateful to Frances Baines for all her assistance with this chapter.

References and further reading

Abate A (1997) Nutrition part V: vitamin A and chameleons. *Chameleon Information Network Newsletter* **26**, 9–17

Abate AL, Coke R, Ferguson G and Reavill D (2003) Roundtable: chameleons and vitamin A. *Journal of Herpetological Medicine and Surgery* **13(2)**, 23–31

Acierno MJ, Mitchell MA, Roundtree MK and Zachariah TT (2006) Effects of ultraviolet radiation on 25-hydroxyvitamin D3 synthesis in red-eared slider turtles (*Trachemys scripta elegans*). *American Journal of Veterinary Research* **67**, 2046–2049

Acierno MJ, Mitchell MA, Zachariah TT *et al.* (2008) Effects of ultraviolet radiation on plasma 25-hydroxyvitamin D3 concentrations in corn snakes (*Elaphe guttata*). *American Journal of Veterinary Research* **69**, 294–297

Allen ME (1989a) Dietary induction and prevention of osteodystrophy in an insectivorous reptile *Eublepharis macularius*: characterization by radiography and histopathology. *Third International Colloquium on the Pathology of Reptiles and Amphibians Eastern States Veterinary Association,* Gainsville, Florida, pp. 83–89

Allen ME (1989b) Nutritional Aspects of Insectivory. PhD dissertation, Michigan State University

Allen ME (1997) From blackbirds to thrushes ... to the gut-loaded cricket: a new approach to zoo animal nutrition. *British Journal of Nutrition* **78**, S135–S143

Allen ME and Baer DJ (1989) Fat soluble vitamin concentrations in fish commonly fed to zoo animals. *Proceedings, Annual Meeting of the American Association of Zoo Veterinarians*, p. 104

Allen ME and Oftedal OT (1989) Dietary manipulation of the calcium content of feed crickets. *Journal of Zoo and Wildlife Medicine* **20**, 26–33

Allen ME, Oftedal OT and Horst RL (1996) Remarkable differences in the response to dietary vitamin D among species of reptiles and primates: is ultraviolet B light essential? In: *Biologic Effects of Light 1995*, ed. MF Holick and EG Jung, pp. 13–38. Walter de Gruyter, New York

Alverdy JC (1990) Effect of glutamine supplemented diets on immunology of the gut. *Journal of Parenteral and Enteral Nutrition* **14(4)**, 109S–113S

Anderson MP and Capen CC (1976a) Fine structural changes of bone cells in experimental nutritional osteodystrophy of green iguanas (*Iguana iguana*). *Virchows Archive B, Cell Pathology* **20**, 169–184

Anderson MP and Capen CC (1976b) Nutritional osteodystrophy in captive green iguanas (*Iguana iguana*). *Virchows Archive B, Cell Pathology* **21**, 229–247

Annis JM (1992) Hypervitaminosis A in chameleons; are we unknowingly overdosing our animals with vitamin A? *Chameleon Information Network Newsletter* **9**, 18–25

Annis JM (1993) Hypervitaminosis A in chameleons; vitamin A is not the whole story! *Chameleon Information Network Newsletter* **10**, 13–16

Armas LA, Hollis BW and Heaney RP (2004) Vitamin D2 is much less effective than vitamin D3 in humans. *Journal of Clinical Endocrinology and Metabolism* **89(11)**, 5387–5391

Arnaud CD and Sanchez SD (1990) Calcium and phosphorus. In: *Present Knowledge in Nutrition, 6th edn*, ed. ML Brown, pp. 212–223. Nutrition Foundation, Washington DC

Aucone BM, Gehrmann WH, Ferguson GW, Chen TC and Holick MF (2003) Comparison of two artificial light sources used for chuckwalla *Sauromalus obesus* husbandry. *Journal of Herpetological Medicine and Surgery* **13(2)**, 14–17

Avery RA (1970) Utilization of caudal fat by hibernating common lizards, *Lacerta vivipara*. *Comparative Biochemistry and Physiology* **37**, 119–121

Baines F, Chattell J, Dale J *et al.* (2016) How much UV-B does my reptile need? The UV-Tool, a guide to the selection of UV lighting for reptiles and amphibians in captivity. *Journal of Zoo and Aquarium Research* **4(1)**, 42–63

Baines F and Davis C (2005) Natural light in the vivarium. *Natterjack, Newsletter of the British Herpetological Society* **127**, 9–12

Banu MJ, Orhii PB, Mejia W *et al.* (1999) Analysis of the effects of growth hormone, voluntary exercise and food restriction on diaphyseal bone in female F344 rats. *Bone* **25**, 479–480

Barten SL (1995) Methods of tube-feeding, force-feeding and assist feeding reptiles. *Proceedings of the Association of Reptilian and Amphibian Veterinarians Annual Conference*, pp. 50–55

Bell NH, Shaw S and Turner RT (1984) Evidence that 1,25-dihydroxyvitamin D3 inhibits the hepatic production of 25-hydroxyvitamin D3 in man. *Journal of Clinical Investigation* **74**, 1540–1544

Bennett RA (1996) Neurology. In: *Reptile Medicine and Surgery*, ed. DR Mader, pp. 141–148. WB Saunders, Philadelphia

Bernard JB, Oftedal OT and Barbosa PS (1991) The response of vitamin D deficient green iguanas (*Iguana iguana*) to artificial ultraviolet light. *Proceedings of the American Association of Zoo Veterinarians*, pp. 147–150

Bernard JB, Oftedal OT and Ullrey DE (1996) Idiosyncrasies of vitamin D metabolism in the green iguana (*Iguana iguana*). *Proceedings of the Comparative Nutrition Society Symposium*, 11–14

BIAZA RAWG UV-Tool Focus Group (2012) *Reptile and Amphibian Working Group UV-Tool*. Available at: www.uvguide.co.uk/BIAZA-RAWG-UV-Tool.htm

Bidmon HJ and Stumpf WE (1996) Vitamin D target systems in the brain of the green lizard *Anolis carolinensis. Anatomy and Embryology* **193(2)**, 145–160

Bounos G (1972) Enteral hyperalimentation with elemental diet. *Canadian Medical Journal* **107**, 607–608

Boyer TH (1996) Metabolic bone disease. In: *Reptile Medicine and Surgery*, ed. DR Mader, pp. 385–392. WB Saunders, Philadelphia

Boyer TH and Boyer DM (1993) Breeding season anorexia in snakes. *Bulletin of the Association of Reptilian and Amphibian Veterinarians* **3**, 6

Calle P, Rivas J, Muñoz M *et al.* (1994) Health assessment of free-ranging anacondas (*Eunectes murinus*) in Venezuela. *Journal of Zoo and Wildlife Medicine* **25**, 53–62

Carman EN, Ferguson GW, Gehrmann WH, Chen TC and Holick MF (2000) Photobiosynthetic opportunity and ability for UVB generated vitamin D synthesis in free-living house geckos (*Hemidactylus turcicus*) and Texas spiny lizards (*Sceloporus olivaceous*). *Copeia* **2000(1)**, 245–250

Carmel B and Johnson R (2014) Lighting. In: *A Guide to Health and Disease in Reptiles and Amphibians*, pp. 55–61. Reptile Publications, Burleigh

Cassidy MJ, Owen JP, Ellis HA *et al.* (1985) Renal osteodystrophy and metastatic calcification in long-term continuous ambulatory dialysis. *Quarterly Journal of Medicine* **54**, 29–48

Chaffin K, Norton TM, Gilardi K *et al.* (2008) Health assessment of free-ranging alligator snapping turtles (*Macrochelys temminckii*) in Georgia and Florida. *Journal of Wildlife Diseases* **44(3)**, 670–686

Christopher MM, Brigman R and Jacobson ER (1994) Seasonal alterations in plasma beta-hydroxybutyrate and related biochemical parameters in the desert tortoise (*Gopherus agassizii*). *Comparative Biochemistry and Physiology A* **108**, 303–310

Clark NB (1983) Evolution of calcium regulation in lower vertebrates. *American Zoologist* **23**, 719–727

Clements MR, Johnson L and Fraser DR (1987) A new mechanism for induced vitamin D deficiency in calcium deprivation. *Nature* **325**, 62–65

Copp DH and Kline LW (1989) Calcitonin. In: *Vertebrate Endocrinology: Fundamentals and Biomedical Implications, Volume 3 – Regulation of Calcium and Phosphate*, ed. PKT Pang and MP Schreibman, pp. 79–103. Academic Press, San Diego, CA

Coulson RA and Hernandez T (1964) *Biochemistry of the Alligator*. Louisiana State Press, Baton Rouge, LA

DaSilva RS and Migliorini RH (1990) Effects of starvation and refeeding on energy-linked metabolic processes in the turtle. *Comparative Biochemistry and Physiology A* **96**, 415–419

DeLuca HF (2004) Overview of general physiologic features and functions of vitamin D. *American Journal of Clinical Nutrition* **80(6)**, 1689S–1696S

Dennis PM, Bennett RA, Harr KE and Lock BA (2001) Plasma concentration of ionized calcium in healthy iguanas. *Journal of the American Veterinary Medical Association* **219(3)**, 326–328

Dickinson HC and Fa JE (1997) Ultraviolet light and heat source selection in captive spiny-tailed iguanas *Oplurus cuvieri. Zoo Biology* **16(5)**, 391–401

Dierenfeld ES (1989) Vitamin E deficiency in zoo reptiles, birds and ungulates. *Journal of Zoo and Wildlife Medicine* **20**, 3–11

Divers SJ (1999) Administering fluid therapy to reptiles. *Exotic DVM* **1(2)**, 5–10

Donoghue S (2006) Nutrition. In: *Reptile Medicine and Surgery, 2nd edn*, ed. D Mader, pp. 287–288. Saunders Elsevier, St. Louis, MO

Eatwell K (2008a) Hypocalcemia in a Tunisian tortoise (*Furculachelys nabeulensis*). *Journal of Herpetological Medicine and Surgery* **18(3–4)**, 117–121

Eatwell K (2008b) Plasma concentrations of 25-hydroxycholecalciferol in 22 captive tortoises (*Testudo* species). *Veterinary Record* **162**, 342–345

Ekstrom DD and Degernes L (1989) Avian gout. *Proceedings of the Association of Avian Veterinarians*, pp. 130–138

Elkan E and Zwart P (1967) The ocular disease of young terrapins caused by vitamin A deficiency. *Pathologia Veterinaria* **4**, 201

Endres DB and Rude RK (1996) Mineral and bone metabolism. In: *Tiez' Fundamentals of Clinical Chemistry, 4th edn*, ed. CA Burtis and ER Ashwood, pp. 685–706. WB Saunders, Philadelphia

Ferguson GW, Brinker AM, Gehrmann WH *et al.* (2010) Voluntary exposure of some western-hemisphere snake and lizard species to ultraviolet-B radiation in the field: how much ultraviolet-B should a lizard or snake receive in captivity? *Zoo Biology* **29(3)**, 317–334

Ferguson GW, Gehrmann WH, Bradley KA *et al.* (2015) Summer and Winter Seasonal Changes in Vitamin D Status of Captive Rhinoceros Iguanas (*Cyclura cornuta*). *Journal of Herpetological Medicine and Surgery* **25(3–4)**, 128–136

Ferguson GW, Gehrmann WH, Brinker AM and Kroh GC (2014) Daily and seasonal patterns of natural ultraviolet light exposure of the western sagebrush lizard (*Sceloporus graciosus gracilis*) and the dunes sagebrush lizard (*Sceloporus arenicolus*). *Herpetologica* **70(1)**, 56–68

Ferguson GW, Gehrmann WH, Chen TC, Dierenfeld ES and Holick MF (2002) Effects of artificial ultraviolet light exposure on reproductive success in the female panther chameleon (*Furcifer pardalis*) in captivity. *Zoo Biology* **21**, 525–537

Ferguson GW, Gehrmann WH, Chen TC and Holick MF (2005) Vitamin D-content of the eggs of the panther chameleon *Furcifer pardalis*: its relationship to UVB exposure/vitamin D-conditions of mother, incubation and hatching success. *Journal of Herpetological Medicine and Surgery* **15**, 9–13

Ferguson GW, Gehrmann WH, Karsten KB *et al.* (2003) Do panther chameleons bask to regulate endogenous vitamin D3 production? *Physiological and Biochemical Zoology* **76(1)**, 52–59

Ferguson GW, Gehrmann WH, Karsten KB *et al.* (2005) Ultraviolet exposure and vitamin D synthesis in a sun-dwelling and a shade-dwelling species of *Anolis:* are there adaptations for lower ultraviolet B and dietary vitamin D3 availability in the shade? *Physiological and Biochemical Zoology* **78(2)**, 193–200

Ferguson GW, Gehrmann WH, Peavy B *et al.* (2009) Restoring vitamin D in monitor lizards: exploring the efficacy of dietary and UVB sources. *Journal of Herpetological Medicine and Surgery* **19(3)**, 81–88

Ferguson GW, Jones JR, Gehrmann WH *et al.* (1996) Indoor husbandry of the panther chameleon: effects of dietary vitamins A and D and ultraviolet radiation on pathology and life-history traits. *Zoo Biology* **15**, 279–299

Ferguson GW, Kingeter AJ and Gehrmann WH (2013) Ultraviolet light exposure and response to dietary vitamin D3 in two Jamaican anoles. *Journal of Herpetology* **47(4)**, 524–529

Finke MD (2003) Gut loading to enhance the nutrient content of insects as food for reptiles: a mathematical approach. *Zoo Biology* **22(2)**, 147–162

Fleishman LJ, Loew ER and Leal M (1993) Ultraviolet vision in lizards. *Nature* **365**, 397

Foggin CM (1987) Diseases and disease control on crocodile farms in Zimbabwe. In: *Wildlife Management: Crocodiles and Alligators*, ed. GJW Webb, SC Manolis and PJ Whitehead, pp. 351–362. Surrey Beatty, Chipping Norton, NSW

Fowler ME (1980) Comparison of respiratory infection and hypovitaminosis in desert tortoises. In: *Comparative Pathology of Zoo Animals*, ed. RJ Montali and G Migaki, pp. 93–97. Smithsonian Institution, Washington DC

Frost HM (2000) The Utah paradigm of skeletal physiology: an overview of its insights for bone cartilage and collagenous tissue organs. *Journal of Bone and Mineral Metabolism* **18**, 262–278

Frye FL (1984) Nutritional disorders in reptiles. In: *Diseases of Amphibians and Reptiles*, ed. GI Hoff, FL Fry and ER Jacobson, pp. 640–642. Plenum Press, New York

Frye FL (1991) *Biomedical and Surgical Aspects of Captive Reptile Husbandry*, 2nd edn. Kreiger, Malabar, FL

Galvão PE, Tarasantchi J and Guertzenstein P (1965) Heat production of tropical snakes in relation to body weight and body surface. *American Journal of Physiology* **209**, 501–506

Gardiner DW, Baines FM and Pandher K (2009) Photodermatitis and photokeratoconjunctivitis in a ball python (*Python regius*) and a blue-tongue skink (*Tiliqua* spp.). *Journal of Zoo and Wildlife Medicine* **40(4)**, 757–766

Gehrmann WH (1994) Spectral characteristics of lamps commonly used in herpetoculture. *Vivarium* **5(5)**, 16–29

Gehrmann WH (1998) Reptile lighting: a current perspective. *Vivarium* **8**, 44–46, 62

Gehrmann WH (2006) Artificial lighting. In: *Reptile Medicine and Surgery, 2nd edn*, ed DR Mader, pp. 1081–1084. WB Saunders, New York

Gehrmann WH, Ferguson GW, Odom TW, Roberts DT and Barcellona WJ (1991) Early growth and bone mineralization of the Iguanid lizard *Sceloporus occidentalis* in captivity: is vitamin D3 supplementation or ultraviolet B irradiation necessary? *Zoo Biology* **10**, 409–416

Gerlach J (2004) Effects of diet on the systematic utility of the tortoise carapace. *African Journal of Herpetology* **53(1)**, 77–85

Gillespie D, Frye FL, Stockham SL and Fredeking T (2000) Blood values in wild and captive Komodo dragons (*Varanus komodoensis*). *Zoo Biology* **19**, 495–509

Guinotte F and Nys Y (1991) The effects of a particulate calcium source in broiler breeder hens upon their egg quality, reproductive traits, bone reserves, chick weight and tibia strength characteristics. *Archiv für Geflugelkunde* **55**, 170–175

Gyimesi ZS and Burns RB (2002) Monitoring of 25-hydroxyvitamin D concentrations in two Komodo dragons *Varanus komodoensis*: a case study. *Journal of Herpetological Medicine and Surgery* **12(2)**, 4–9

Haddad JG, Matsuoka LY, Hollis BW, Hu YZ and Wortsman J (1993) Human plasma transport of vitamin D after its endogenous synthesis. *Journal of Clinical Investigation* **91(6)**, 2552–2555

Haussler MR, Whitfield GK, Haussler CA *et al.* (1998) The nuclear vitamin D receptor: biological and molecular regulatory properties revealed. *Journal of Bone and Mineral Research* **13(3)**, 325–349

Hay AW and Watson G (1977) Vitamin D2 in vertebrate evolution. *Comparative Biochemistry and Physiology B* **56(4)**, 375–380

Heaney RP (2011) Serum 25-hydroxyvitamin D is a reliable indicator of vitamin D status. *American Journal of Clinical Nutrition* **94(2)**, 619–620

Hedley J and Eatwell K (2013) The effects of UV light on calcium metabolism in ball pythons (*Python regius*). *Veterinary Record* **173(14)**, 345

Hernandez-Divers SJ, Stahl SJ, Stedman NL *et al.* (2005) Renal evaluation in the healthy green iguana (*Iguana iguana*): assessment of plasma biochemistry, glomerular filtration rate, and endoscopic biopsy. *Journal of Zoo and Wildlife Medicine* **36(2)**, 155–168

Hibma JC (2004) Dietary Vitamin D3 and UV-B Exposure Effects on Green Iguana Growth Rate: Is Full-Spectrum Lighting Necessary? *Bulletin of the Chicago Herpetological Society* **39**, 145–150

Highfield AC (2010) The causes of 'pyramiding' deformity in tortoises: a summary of a lecture given to the Sociedad Herpetologica Velenciana Congreso Tortugas on 30 October. Available at: www.tortoisetrust.org/articles/pyramiding.html

Highfield AC (2015) The 'Climate Frame' Outdoor Terrarium with Natural UV-B and WiR-A Available at: http://www.tortoisetrust.org/articles/climateframe.html

Hoby S, Wenker C, Robert N *et al.* (2010) Nutritional metabolic bone disease in juvenile veiled chameleons (*Chamaeleo calyptratus*) and its prevention. *Journal of Nutrition* **140(11)**, 1923–1931

Holick MF (1990) The use and interpretation of assays for vitamin D and its metabolites. *Journal of Nutrition* **120**, 144–164

Holick MF (1995) Vitamin D: new horizons for the 21st century. *American Journal of Clinical Nutrition* **60**, 619–630

Holick MF (2004) Vitamin D: importance in the prevention of cancers, type 1 diabetes, heart disease, and osteoporosis. *American Journal of Clinical Nutrition* **79(3)**, 362–371

Holick MF, Tian XQ and Allen M (1995) Evolutionary importance for the membranous enhancement of the production of vitamin D3 in the skin of poikilothermic animals. *Proceedings of the National Academy of Sciences of the United States of America* **92**, 3124–3126

Honkavaara J, Koivula M, Korpimaki E, Siitari H and Viitala J (2002) Ultraviolet vision and foraging in terrestrial vertebrates. *Oikos* **98**, 505–511

Hossein-nezhad A and Holick MF (2013) Vitamin D for health: a global perspective. *Mayo Clinic Proceedings* **88(7)**, 720–755

Johansson S and Melhus H (2001) Vitamin A antagonises calcium response to Vitamin D in man. *Journal of Bone and Mineral Research* **16**, 1899–1905

Jones G (2008) Pharmacokinetics of vitamin D toxicity. *American Journal of Clinical Nutrition* **88(2)**, 582S–586S

Juzeniene A and Moan J (2012) Beneficial effects of UV radiation other than via vitamin D production. *Dermatoendocrinology* **4**, 109–117

Karsten KB, Ferguson GW, Chen TC and Holick MF (2009) Panther chameleons, *Furcifer pardalis*, behaviorally regulate optimal exposure to UV depending on dietary vitamin D3 status. *Physiological and Biochemical Zoology* **82(3)**, 218–225

Kass RE, Ullrey DE and Trapp AL (1982) A study of calcium requirements of the red-eared slider turtle (*Pseudemys scripta elegans*). *Journal of Zoo Animal Medicine* **13**, 62–69

Klaphake E (2001) A review of phosphorus for the reptile practitioner. *Proceedings of the Association of Reptilian and Amphibian Veterinarians Annual Conference*, pp. 281–286

Klasing KC, Thacker P, Lopez MA and Calvert CC (2000) Increasing the calcium content of mealworms (*Tenebrio molitor*) to improve their nutritional value for bone mineralization of growing chicks. *Journal of Zoological and Wildlife Medicine* **31(4)**, 512–517

Kroenlein KR, Zimmerman KL, Saunders G and Holladay SD (2011) Serum vitamin D levels and skeletal and general development of young bearded dragon lizards (*Pogona vitticeps*), under different conditions of UV-B radiation exposure. *Journal of Animal and Veterinary Advances* **10**, 229–234

Kubota M, Abe E, Shinki T *et al.* (1981) Vitamin D metabolism and its possible role in the developing chick embryo. *Biochemistry Journal* **194**, 103–109

Laing CJ and Fraser DR (1999) The vitamin D system in Iguanian lizards. *Comparative Biochemistry and Physiology B* **123**, 373–379

Laing CJ, Trube A, Shea G. and Fraser DR (2001) The requirement for natural sunlight to prevent vitamin D deficiency in iguanian lizards. *Journal of Zoo and Wildlife Medicine* **32(3)**, 342–348

Larsen RE, Buergelt C, Cardeilhac PT and Jacobson ER (1983) Steatitis and fat necrosis in captive alligators. *Journal of the American Veterinary Medical Association* **183**, 1202–1204

Laszlo J (1969) Observations on two new artificial lights for reptile display. *International Zoo Yearbook* **9**, 12–13

Lawton MPC (1989) Health problems associated with feeding. *Testudo* **3(1)**, 75

Lindgren J (2004) UV-lamps for terrariums: their spectral characteristics and efficiency in promoting vitamin D3 synthesis by UVB irradiation. *Herpetomania* **13(3–4)**, 13–20

Lips P (2007) Relative value of 25(OH)D and 1,25(OH)2D measurements. *Journal of Bone and Mineral Research* **22(11)**, 1668–1671

MacLaughlin JA, Anderson RR and Holick MF (1982) Spectral character of sunlight modulates photosynthesis of previtamin D3 and its photoisomers in human skin. *Science* **216(4549)**, 1001–1003

Mader DR (1993) Use of calcitonin in green iguanas with metabolic bone disease. *Bulletin of the Association of Reptilian and Amphibian Veterinarians* **3(1)**, 5

Mader DR (2000) Nutritional secondary hyperparathyroidism. In: *Kirk's Current Veterinary Therapy XIII: Small Animal Practice*, ed. JD Bonagura and R Kersey, pp. 1179–1182. WB Saunders, Philadelphia

Mader DR (2001) Metabolic bone disease in reptiles. *Proceedings of the Association of Reptilian and Amphibian Veterinarians*, pp. 287–289

Mader DR (2006a) Gout. In: *Reptile Medicine and Surgery, 2nd edn*, ed. D Mader, pp. 793–800. Saunders Elsevier, St Louis, MO

Mader DR (2006b) Metabolic bone diseases. In: *Reptile Medicine and Surgery, 2nd edn*, ed. D Mader, pp. 841–851. Saunders Elsevier, St. Louis, MO

Madsen T and Shine R (2000) Energy versus risk: costs of reproduction in free-ranging pythons in tropical Australia. *Australian Journal of Ecology* **25(6)**, 670–677

Massfelder T, Parekh N, Endlich K *et al.* (1996) Effect of intrarenally infused parathyroid hormone-related protein on renal blood flow and glomerular filtration rate in the anaesthetized rat. *British Journal of Pharmacology* **118(8)**, 1995–2000

Menon J, Shah RV and Hiradhar PK (1981) Effect of thyroidectomy on carbohydrate metabolism during tail regeneration in the gekkonid lizard *Hemidactylus flaviviridis*. *Indian Journal of Experimental Biology* **9**, 1018–1026

Messonier SP (1995) Incorrect ultraviolet usage. *Bulletin of the Association of Reptilian and Amphibian Veterinarians* **5(3)**, 4

Meulemans CCE and Werner IM (1995) *Light Sources for Photobiology and Phototherapy*. Phillips, New York, USA

Milne ML and Baran DT (1985) End product inhibition of hepatic 25 hydroxy vitamin D3-hydroxy vitamin D production in the rat: specificity and kinetics. *Archives of Biochemistry and Biophysics* **242**, 488–492

Minnich JE (1982) The use of water. In: *Biology of the Reptilia, Volume 12 – Physiology, C – Physiological Ecology*, ed. C Gans and F Harvey Pough, p. 323. Academic Press, London and New York

Mitchell MA, Riggs S, Singleton CB, Hale-Mitchell L and Carboni D (2005) Characterizing hematologic and plasma biochemistry values for captive mali uromastyx (*Uromastyx maliensis, Agamidae*). *Proceedings of the 12th Annual Conference of the Association of Reptilian and Amphibian Veterinarians*, p. 52. Tuscon, USA

Moehn LD (1974) The effect of quality of light on agonistic behaviour of iguanid and agamid lizards. *Journal of Herpetology* **8(2)**, 175–183

Morrison NA, Qi JC, Tokita A et al. (1994) Prediction of bone density from vitamin D receptor alleles. *Nature* **367(6460)**, 284–287

Nevarez JG, Mitchell MA, Le Blanc C and Graham P (2002) Determination of plasma biochemistries, ionized calcium, vitamin D3 and hematocrit values in captive green iguanas (*Iguana iguana*) from El Salvador. *Proceedings of the Ninth Annual Conference of the Association of Reptilian and Amphibian Veterinarians*, pp. 87–93. Reno, USA

Nijboer J, van Brug H, Tryfonidou MA and van Leeuwen JPTM (2007) *UV-B and Vitamin D3 Metabolism in Juvenile Komodo Dragons (Varanus komodoensis)*. Filander Verlag, Furth, Germany

Oftedal OT, Chen TC, Schulkin J (1997) Preliminary observations on the relationship of calcium ingestion to vitamin D status in the green iguana (*Iguana iguana*). *Zoo Biology* **16**, 201–207

Ooninicx DGAB, Stevens Y, Van Den Borne JJGC, Van Leeuwen JPTM and Hendriks WH (2010) Effects of vitamin D3 supplementation and UVB exposure on the growth and plasma concentration of vitamin D3 metabolites in juvenile bearded dragons (*Pogona vitticeps*). *Comparative Biochemistry and Physiology B* **156(2)**, 122–128

Ooninicx DGAB, van de Wal MD, Bosch G et al. (2013) Blood vitamin D3 metabolite concentrations of adult female bearded dragons (*Pogona vitticeps*) remain stable after ceasing UVb exposure. *Comparative Biochemistry and Physiology Part B: Biochemistry and Molecular Biology* **165(3)**, 196–200

Oyarzun SE, Dufresne AL, Valdes EV, Crawshaw GJ and Leeson S (1995) Effect of vitamin D/ascorbic acid supplementation on growth and tibial characteristics of green water dragons (*Physignathus cocincinus*). *Proceedings of the First Annual Conference of the Nutritional Advisory Group (NAG) of the American Zoo and Aquarium Association*, pp. 87–89

Packard MJ and Clark NB (1996) Aspects of calcium regulation in embryonic lepidosaurians and chelonians and a review of calcium regulation in embryonic archosaurians. *Physiological Zoology* **69**, 435–466

Packard MJ, Phillips JA and Packard GC (1992) Sources of mineral for green iguanas (*Iguana iguana*) developing in eggs exposed to different hydric environments. *Copeia* **3**, 851–858

Peebles WD and Brake J (1985) Relationship of dietary ascorbic acid to broiler breeder performance. *Poultry Science* **64**, 2041–2048

Phillips JA, Garel A, Packard GC and Packard MJ (1990) Influence of moisture and temperature on eggs and embryos of green iguanas (*Iguana iguana*). *Herpetologica* **46**, 238–245

Price M (2011) Too many tuatara with nowhere to go. *Otago Daily Times*, 6 June. Available at: www.odt.co.nz/your-town/invercargill/163463/too-many-tuatara-nowhere-go

Purgley H, Jewell J, Deacon JE, Winokur RM and Tripoli VM (2009) Vitamin D3 in captive green sea turtles (*Chelonia mydas*). *Chelonian Conservation and Biology* **8(2)**, 161–167

Raila J, Schumacher A, Gropp J and Schweigert FJ (2002) Selective absorption of carotenoids in the common green iguana (*Iguana iguana*). *Comparative Biochemistry and Physiology A* **132**, 513–518

Ralph L, Firth BT and Turner JS (1979) The role of the pineal body in ectotherm thermoregulation. *American Zoologist* **19**, 273–293

Ramer J, Maria R, Reichard T and Tolson P (2002) Vitamin D status of free-ranging Ricord's iguanas (*Cyclura ricordi*) and captive and free-ranging rhinoceros iguanas (*Cyclura cornuta cornuta*) in the Dominican Republic. *Proceedings of the American Association of Zoo Veterinarians*, pp. 309–311. Milwaukee, USA

Ramer JC, Roberto M, Reichard T et al. (2005) Vitamin D status of wild Ricord's iguanas (*Cyclura ricordii*) and captive and wild rhinoceros iguanas (*Cyclura cornuta cornuta*) in the Dominican Republic. *Journal of Zoo and Wildlife Medicine* **36(2)**, 188–191

Raphael BL, James SB and Cook RA (1999) Evaluation of vitamin D concentrations in *Uromastyx* spp. with and without radiographic evidence of dystrophic mineralization. *Proceedings of the American Association of Zoo Veterinarians*, pp. 20–23

Raphael BL, Klemens MW, Moehlman P, Dierenfeld E and Karesh WB (1994) Blood values in free-ranging pancake tortoises (*Malacochersus tornieri*). *Journal of Zoo and Wildlife Diseases* **25(1)**, 63–67

Recker RR (1999) Bone biopsy and histomorphometry in clinical practice. In: *Primer on the Metabolic Bone Diseases and Disorders of Mineral Metabolism*, ed. MJ Flavus, pp. 169–174. Lippincott, Williams & Wilkins, Philadelphia

Reichel H, Koeffler HP and Norman AW (1989) The role of the vitamin D endocrine system in health and disease. *New England Journal of Medicine* **320(15)**, 980–991

Rickman LK, Montali RJ and Allen ME (1995) Paradoxical pathological changes in vitamin D deficient green iguanas (*Iguana iguana*). *Proceedings of the Joint Conference of the American Association of Zoo Veterinarians and American Association of Wildlife Veterinarians*, pp. 231–232

Rosol TJ and Capen CC (1997) Calcium-regulating hormones and diseases of abnormal mineral (calcium, phosphorus, magnesium) metabolism. In: *Clinical Biochemistry of Domestic Animals, 5th edn*, ed. JJ Kaneko, JW Harvey and ML Bruss, pp. 619–702. Academic Press, San Diego, CA

Sabatini JA, Dierenfeld ES, Fitzpatrick MP and Hashim L (1998) Effects of internal and external supplementation on the nutrient content of crickets. *Vivarium* **9(4)**, 23–24

Schweigert FJ (1995) Comparative aspects of vitamin A and carotenoid metabolism in exotic mammals. In: *Research in Captive Propagation*, ed. U Ganslosser, JK Hodges and Kaumanns, pp. 130–146. Filander Verlag, Fürth, Germany

Secor SM and Diamond J (1998) A vertebrate model of extreme physiological regulation. *Nature* **395**, 659–662

Secor SM and Diamond J (2000) Evolution of regulatory responses to feeding in snakes. *Physiological and Biochemical Zoology* **73(2)**, 123–141

Secor SM, Lane JS, Whang EE, Ashley SW and Diamond J (2002) Luminal nutrient signals for intestinal adaptation in pythons. *American Journal of Physiology: Gastrointestinal and Liver Physiology* **283(6)**, G1298–G1309

Secor SM and Phillips JA (1997) Specific dynamic action of a large carnivorous lizard *Varanus albigularis*. *Comparative Biochemistry and Physiology A* **117**, 515–522

Selleri P and Di Girolamo N (2012) Plasma 25-hydroxyvitamin D3 concentrations in Hermann's tortoises (*Testudo hermanni*) exposed to natural sunlight and two artificial ultraviolet radiation sources. *American Journal of Veterinary Research* **73(11)**, 1781–1786

Shadrix CA, Crotzer DR, McKinney SL and Stewart JR (1994) Embryonic growth and calcium mobilization in oviposited eggs of the scincid lizard (*Eumeces fasciatus*). *Copeia* **2**, 493–498

Shils ME (1988) Enteral (tube) and parenteral nutritional support. In: *Modern Nutrition in Health and Disease*, ed. ME Shils and VR Young, pp. 1023–1066. Lea and Febiger, Philadelphia

Sievert LM and Hutchison VH (1988) Light versus heat: thermoregulatory behavior in a nocturnal lizard (*Gekko gecko*). *Herpetologica* **44(3)**, 266–273

Srivastav AK, Srivastav SK, Singh S and Norman AW (1995) Effect of various vitamin D metabolites on serum calcium and inorganic phosphate in the freshwater snake *Natrix piscator*. *General and Comparative Endocrinology* **100(1)**, 49–52

Starck JM and Bleese K (2001) Structural flexibility of the intestine of Burmese python in response to feeding. *Journal of Experimental Biology* **204**, 325–335

Stein G (1996) Reptile and amphibian formulary. In: *Reptile Medicine and Surgery*, ed. DR Mader, p.469. WB Saunders, Philadelphia

Stewart JR and Ecay TW (2010). Patterns of maternal provision and embryonic mobilization of calcium in oviparous and viviparous squamate reptiles. *Herpetological Conservation and Biology* **5(341)**, 341–359

Stringer EM, Harms CA, Beasley JF and Anderson ET (2010) Comparison of ionized calcium, phosphorus, parathyroid hormone, and 25-hydroxyvitamin D in rehabilitating and healthy wild green sea turtles (*Chelonia mydas*). *Journal of Herpetological Medicine and Surgery* **20(4)**, 122–127

Swarup K, Pandey AK and Srivastav AK (1987) Calcaemic responses in the yellow monitor, *Varanus flavescens*, to vitamin D3 administration. *Acta Physiologica Hungarica* **70**, 375–377

Thorington L (1985) Spectral, irradiance, and temporal aspects of natural and artificial light. *Annals of the New York Academy of Sciences* **453**, 28–54

Trusk AM and Crissey S (1987) Comparison of calcium and phosphorus levels in crickets fed a high calcium diet versus those dusted with supplement. *Proceedings of the 7th Dr Scholl Conference on the Nutrition of Captive Wild Animals*, pp. 93–95

Uitterlinden AG, Fang Y, Bergink AP et al. (2002) The role of vitamin D receptor gene polymorphisms in bone biology. *Molecular and Cellular Endocrinology* **197**, 15–21

Ullrey DE and Bernard JB (1999) Vitamin D: metabolism, sources, unique problems in zoo animals, meeting needs. In: *Zoo and Wild Animal Medicine*, ed. ME Fowler and RE Miller, pp. 63–78. WB Saunders, Philadelphia

Vieth R, Milojevic S and Peltekova V (2000) Improved cholecalciferol nutrition in rats is noncalcemic, suppresses parathyroid hormone and increases responsiveness to 1,25-dihydroxycholecalciferol. *Journal of Nutrition* **130**, 578–584

Vigh B, Manzano MJ, Zádori A et al. (2002) Nonvisual photoreceptors of the deep brain, pineal organs and retina. *Histology and Histopathology* **17**, 555–590

Vosburgh KM, Brady PS and Ullrey DE (1982) Ascorbic acid requirements of garter snakes: plains (*Thamnophis radix*) and eastern (*T. sirtalis sirtalis*). *Journal of Zoo Animal Medicine* **13**, 38–42

Weissman C, Kemper M and Hyman AI (1989) Variation in the resting metabolic rate of mechanically ventilated critically ill patients. *Anaesthetics and Analgesics* **68**, 457–461

Wiesner CS and Iben C (2003) Influence of environmental humidity and dietary protein on pyramidal growth in the carapaces of African spurred tortoises (*Geochelone sulcata*). *Journal of Animal Physiology and Animal Nutrition* **87**, 66–74

Wilkinson R (2004) Formulary. In: *Medicine and Surgery of Tortoises and Turtles*, ed. R Wilkinson, S McArthur and J Meyer, p. 496. Blackwell Publishing Ltd, Oxford, UK

Wright K (1997) In my experience: two products useful for tubefeeding herbivorous reptiles. *Bulletin of the Association of Reptilian and Amphibian Veterinarians* **7(3)**, 5–6

Yokoyama K (1993) A study of vascular calcification in patients on continuous ambulatory dialysis: special reference to vitamin D treatment. *Japanese Journal of Nephrology* **35**, 1171–1180

Zhou X, Niu C, Sun R and Li Q (2002) The effect of vitamin C on the non-specific immune response of the juvenile soft-shelled turtle (*Trionyx sinensis*). *Comparative Biochemistry and Physiology A* **131**, 917–922

Zwart P (1980) Nutrition and nutritional disturbances in reptiles. *Proceedings of the European Herpetological Symposium*, pp. 75–80

Zwart P and van Ham B (1980) Keeping, breeding and raising garter snakes (*Thamnophis radix*). In: *The Care and Breeding of Captive Reptiles*, ed. S Townson, NJ Millichamp, DG Lucas and AJ Millwood, pp. 81–85. British Herpetological Society, London

Chapter 23

Neoplasia

Drury R. Reavill

Neoplastic diseases of reptiles are frequently documented and tabulated in the literature. Several large reviews have been published and the reader is directed to these extensive lists for further information (Schlumberger and Lucke, 1948; Harshbarger, 1976; Effron *et al.*, 1977; Frye, 1994; Ramsay *et al.*, 1996; Hernandez-Divers and Garner, 2003; Garner *et al.*, 2004; Mauldin and Done, 2006; Sykes and Trupkiewicz, 2006). This chapter will concentrate on common tumours as well as those in which more detailed clinical information has been collected.

General diagnostics

Cytology

Aspiration cytology is recommended if a mass lesion is discovered on examination. For most external masses this procedure can be done during an office visit and can provide rapid clinical information. Cytology may help to differentiate between neoplasms and other disease processes, such as granulomatous inflammation and discrete granulomas, which can closely mimic neoplasia (Figure 23.1). Collecting aspirates in conjunction with excisional biopsy is valuable for correlation since, to date, little has been described for reptilian oncology cytology.

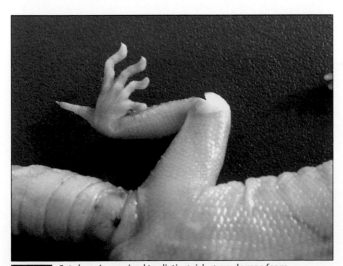

23.1 Cytology is required to distinguish granulomas from neoplasia. This white mass over the joint of a leopard gecko is articular gout (arrowed).

In general, the cell morphology of tissue hyperplasia is usually indistinguishable from that of benign neoplasia. The cells in both benign and hyperplastic lesions are immature, exhibit cytoplasmic basophilia, and have pale vesicular nuclei. There may be a high mitotic index with normal-appearing mitotic figures and a uniform nucleus-to-cytoplasm ratio. It is important to remember that fibrous or epithelial cell hyperplasia is common in inflammatory lesions, and these hyperplastic changes should not be confused with neoplasia. With malignant neoplasms, the sample may be highly cellular owing to the loss of normal cell-to-cell interactions. Neoplastic cells tend to be highly polymorphic with marked variations in nuclear size and nucleus-to-cytoplasm ratios. Some malignancies will have a high mitotic index and the cell nuclei may have irregular chromatin (coarse, hypochromatic, irregularly clumped). Another finding suggestive of neoplasia is the presence of chronic haemorrhage in an area without a history of trauma. For example, the presence of chronic haemorrhage in the coelomic cavity, coupled with radiographic evidence of a mass, suggests neoplasia even without evidence of neoplastic cells.

Carcinomas usually exfoliate well and the cells are in aggregates. The cells may be round to polyhedral with distinct cytoplasmic margins. Sarcomas provide poorly cellular samples because they are usually embedded within an extracellular matrix. For this reason, sarcomas require a traumatic exfoliation to obtain a reasonable sample. The cells of a sarcoma are generally spindle shaped with poorly defined cytoplasmic borders and usually exfoliate as individual cells or in small clusters. Discrete cell tumours or round cell tumours provide highly cellular samples and the cells exfoliate individually.

Biochemistry and haematology

In general, many tumours are associated with anaemia (regenerative or non-regenerative) and leucocytosis. Serum biochemical changes may occur depending on the extent of organ involvement and the specific system affected. Unfortunately, for many reptilian cases, serum biochemistry values are either not reported or poorly correlate to the tumour-induced changes.

Radiography

Radiographic studies with or without contrast are useful in evaluating the degree of organ involvement, identifying metastases and providing important information about the integrity of adjacent tissues. Computerized tomography and ultrasonography are additional tools. Each of these modalities can provide information about prognosis and may be used for guidance in obtaining excisional or aspiration biopsy samples.

Biopsy

The definitive diagnosis frequently relies on an appropriate biopsy. Performing an excisional biopsy may also be an important part of the treatment, allowing the tumour to be completely removed or at least debulked prior to exploring other forms of therapy.

Treatment

Treatment regimes for neoplasms for exotic animals, especially reptiles, are generally described as individual case reports. Surgical excision of cutaneous masses, along with supportive care, appears to be the most common treatment modality. Additional options include radiation therapy, cryotherapy, chemotherapy and photodynamic therapy. The lack of readily accessible peripheral vessels for intravenous administration of agents, the need to determine specific treatment protocols (dosages, time intervals, etc.) and difficulty in monitoring the systemic effects of treatment are some of the limitations associated with chemotherapy in reptiles. Inadequate follow-up has also limited the collection of important information such as occurrence of metastases and even the response to treatments. Figure 23.2 summarizes attempted therapy of malignant neoplasms in reptiles.

Tumours found in reptiles

There are exhaustive tabulations of reptile tumours, particularly in lizards and snakes, as well as numerous case reports listed in the references at the end of the chapter. The various tumours recognized both from the literature and from cases seen by the author in chelonians are listed in Figure 23.3.

Species	Tumour	Therapy given	Outcome	Reference
Chelonians				
Diamondback terrapin	Lymphoblastic leukaemia	Prednisone 2.5 mg orally q48h Cytosine arabinoside 5 mg s.c. q7d Chlorambucil 1 mg orally q7d	In progress at time of report	Silverstone et al. (2002)
Eastern box turtle	Squamous cell carcinoma of the leg	Strontium-90 requiring four different fields (7–8 mm each) to treat the affected area. Each field received 20,000 cGy to the surface, and second treatment with strontiium-90 (15,000 cGy surface dose per field) was given to two areas	Euthanased when recurred	Greenacre and Roberts (2000)
Red-eared slider	Malignant ovarian teratoma	Surgical removal	Died intraoperatively	Newman et al. (2003)
Lizards				
Bearded dragons	Squamous cell carcinoma	Surgical removal	No recurrence by 16-month recheck	Hannon et al. (2011)
Green iguana	Thyroid adenoma	Surgical removal	No recurrence 1 year and returned to euthyroid state	Hernandez-Divers et al. (2001)
Green iguana	Lymphoma	A single 10 Gy radiation fraction and, through a vascular access port, doxorubicin, vincristine, cyclophosphamide, and prednisone	Remission at 1008 days	Folland et al. (2011)
Green tree monitor	Chronic T-cell leukaemia	Prednisone and one treatment of chlorambucil	Clinical signs improved but death at 210 days post-presentation demonstrated tumour infiltrates	Georoff et al. (2009)
Snakes				
Boa constrictor	Squamous cell carcinoma of labial margin	Photodynamic treatment with a second-generation sensitizer, chloroaluminium sulphonated phthalocyanine (caspc) 1 mg of caspc per kg bodyweight 48 hours prior to irradiation with 675 nm light	Recurred but then in remission	Roberts et al. (1991)
Boa constrictor	Fibrosarcoma, subcutis of the body wall	A total dose of 48 Gy was delivered in 16 equivalent 3 Gy fractions by a cobalt radiation unit over a 21 day period. Additional chemotherapy consisting of 50 mg of intralesional carboplatin was administered following radiation	The mass enlarged over the course of radiation therapy and a post-radiation complete blood count revealed that the animal had developed a leucopenia (white blood cell count 2.7 x 10³ cells/µl) with severe lymphopenia (0 cells/µl). A severe granulomatous cellulitis with intralesional acid-fast bacilli was also present and the snake was euthanased	Langan et al. (2001)

23.2 Reported therapies for reptile tumours. (continues) ▶

Species	Tumour	Therapy given	Outcome	Reference
Snakes continued				
Burmese python	Fibrosarcoma of the mandible	Removed with three freeze–thaw cycles (cryosurgery)	Survived 23 months then died with disseminated metastases	Frye and Williams (2002)
Burmese python	Mixed sarcoma and carcinoma, under palatine bone	Photodynamic treatment with caspc 1 mg of caspc per kg bodyweight 48 hours prior to irradiation with 675 nm light	Recurred	Roberts *et al.* (1991)
Common death adder	Melanoma under scales of rostrum	Radiotherapy; lesion implanted with Au-198 for a dose of 40 Gy	Euthanased as tumour enlarged	Bryant *et al.* (1997)
Corn snake	Haemangiosarcoma, spleen	Surgical removal	Died 6 weeks postoperative	Tuttle *et al.* (2006)
Diamond python	Fibrosarcoma, oral	Cryosurgery. Three freeze–thaw cycles with liquid nitrogen	Euthanased as tumour continued to enlarge	Bryant *et al.* (1997)
Eastern kingsnake	Mast cell tumour	Implanted with 192-iridium	Died and there were metastases	Schumacher *et al.* (1998)
European viper	Adenocarcinoma of the cloaca and oviduct	Photodynamic treatment with caspc 1 mg of caspc per kg bodyweight 48 hours prior to irradiation with 675 nm light	Died	Roberts *et al.* (1991)
Madagascar ground boa	Squamous cell carcinoma, pharyngeal	Palliative radiation 10 Gy weekly for three weeks	The tumour was resistant	Steeil *et al.* (2013)
Rhinoceros viper	Lymphoma	Cytosine arabinoside	Died after chemotherapy with severe renal tubular necrosis	Jacobson and Ackerman (1981)
Spitting cobra	Angiosarcoma of hard palate	Radiation	Local regression but tumour metastasis	Leach *et al.* (1991)
Yellow ratsnake	Chromatophoroma, malignant	Radiation therapy; 6000 cGy delivered four equivalent fractions to the field on days 15, 23, 27 and 30. Scales in field became brownish and rough; resolved	After two surgeries and radiation, died 10 months later with a similar gross lesion found within coelom	Leach *et al.* (1991)

23.2 (continued) Reported therapies for reptile tumours.

Location	Tumour type	Chelonian	Comments	Reference
Carapace	Neurilemmal	Hermann's tortoise		Cooper *et al.* (1983)
Coelom	Malignant round cell tumour	Narrow-breasted snake-necked turtle	No metastases	Sykes and Trupkiewicz (2006)
Digestive	Haemangioma	Red-eared slider		Gal *et al.* (2009)
Heart	Rhabdomyoma	Black terrapin		Schlumberger and Lucke (1948)
Haemopoietic	Leukaemia	Diamondback terrapin		Silverstone *et al.* (2002)
Haemopoietic	Leukaemia	Helmeted turtle		Harshbarger (1976)
Haemopoietic	Leukaemia	Mobile terrapin		Frye and Carney (1972)
Haemopoietic	Leukaemia	Hermann's tortoise		Cooper *et al.* (1983)
Haemopoietic	Leukaemia	Chinese box turtle	Immunohistochemistry supports T-cell lymphoid leukaemia	Bezjian *et al.* (2013)
Haemopoietic	Leukaemia	Tortoise, species not provided		Rosskopf *et al.* (1981)
Haemopoietic	Lymphoma	Greek land tortoise	Multicentric	Machotka (1984)
Haemopoietic	Lymphoma	Sulcatta tortoise	Multicentric	ZEPS (2014)
Haemopoietic	Lymphoma	Burmese star tortoise	Multicentric	Frye (1994)
Haemopoietic	Lymphoma	Yellow-footed tortoise	Multicentric	ZEPS (2014)
Haemopoietic	Myeloproliferative disease	Burmese star tortoise		Frye (1994)
Haemopoietic	Myeloproliferative disease	Red-eared slider		Frye (1994)
Kidney	Adenocarcinoma	Box turtle	Liver metastasis	Machotka (1984)
Kidney	Renal tubular adenocarcinoma	African black mud turtle	No metastases	Sykes and Trupkiewicz (2006)
Kidney	Renal tubular adenoma	African black mud turtle	No metastases	Sykes and Trupkiewicz (2006)
Liver	Lipoma	Yellow-spotted Amazon river turtle		ZEPS (2014)
Liver	Biliary cystadenoma	Piedmont terrapin	No metastases	Sykes and Trupkiewicz (2006)

23.3 Tumours in tortoises. (continues)
(ZEPS (2014) indicates cases from the files of the Zoo/Exotic Pathology Service in California)

Location	Tumour type	Chelonian	Comments	Reference
Lung	Fibroadenoma	Horsfield's tortoise		Schlumberger and Lucke (1948)
Lung	Fibroadenoma	European pond turtle		Machotka (1984)
Oral cavity	Carcinoma	Tortoise, species not provided		ZEPS (2014)
Ovary	Benign ovarian teratoma	Red-eared slider		Hidalgo-Vila et al. (2006)
Ovary	Benign ovarian teratoma	Mediterranean tortoise		Martorell et al. (2009)
Ovary	Malignant teratoma	Red-eared slider	No metastases present at time of surgical removal	Newman et al. (2003)
Ovary	Ovarian dysgerminoma	Common snapping turtle		Machotka et al. (1992)
Oviduct	Oviductal leiomyoma	Desert tortoise		Frye (1994)
Parathyroid gland	Adenoma	South African red-footed tortoise	Lethargy, anorexia, demineralization of the skeleton and carapace, decreased blood calcium and increased phosphorus	Frye and Carney (1975)
Parathyroid gland	Adenoma	Desert tortoise	Multiple primary tumours developed in this chelonian (parathyroid adenoma)	Frye (1994)
Skin	Fibroma	Common snapping turtle	On plantar surface of forelimb	Gonzales-Viera et al. (2012)
Skin	Haemangiosarcoma	Common snapping turtle	On leg	ZEPS (2014)
Skin	Mast cell tumour	Desert tortoise		Frye (1994)
Skin	Mast cell tumour	Galapagos tortoise	No recurrence at 11-month recheck	Santoro et al. (2008)
Skin	Myxoma	Russian tortoise		ZEPS (2014)
Skin	Osteoma cutis	European pond turtle	Surgical removal was curative	Frye et al. (2009)
Skin	Papilloma	Musk turtle		Schlumberger and Lucke (1948)
Skin	Squamous cell carcinoma	European pond turtle	Metastasis to liver	Billips and Harshbarger (1976)
Skin	Squamous cell carcinoma	Red-eared slider	Large mass on the neck and involving the tympanic membrane	Ardente et al. (2011)
Skin	Squamous cell carcinoma	Ceylon terrapin		Cowen (1968)
Skin	Squamous cell carcinoma	Hermann's tortoise		Zwart (2002)
Skin	Squamous cell carcinoma	British Indian turtle	No metastases	Sykes and Trupkiewicz (2006)
Skin	Squamous cell carcinoma	Spiny softshell turtle	No metastases	Sykes and Trupkiewicz (2006)
Skin	Squamous cell carcinoma	Common snake-necked turtle	No metastases	Sykes and Trupkiewicz (2006)
Skin around beak	Squamous cell carcinoma	Turtle, species not provided		ZEPS (2014)
Skin on carapace	Squamous cell carcinoma	Soft-shelled turtle		ZEPS (2014)
Skin of leg	Squamous cell carcinoma	Eastern box turtle	Strontium-90 was ineffective, mass extended into coelomic cavity	Greenacre and Roberts (2000)
Skin of leg	Squamous cell carcinoma	California desert tortoise	Mass on forelimb	ZEPS (2014)
Skin on neck	Squamous cell carcinoma	Turtle, species not provided	Associated with dysphagia	ZEPS (2014)
Skin of eyelids	Squamous cell carcinoma	California desert tortoise	Swollen eyelid for many months, refractory to treatment	ZEPS (2014)
Stomach	Adenocarcinoma	Giant tortoise		Schlumberger and Lucke (1948)
Stomach	Carcinoma	Black side-necked turtle		Cowen (1968)
Stomach	Carcinoma	Red-eared slider		Frye (1994)
Testis	Interstitial cell tumour	Desert tortoise	Incidental finding	Frye et al. (1988)
Thymus	Thymoma	Desert tortoise		Frye (1994)
Thyroid gland	Adenoma	Desert tortoise		Frye (1994)
Thyroid gland	Adenoma	Brazilian freshwater turtle		Schlumberger and Lucke (1948)
Thyroid gland	Papillary adenoma	Greek tortoise	Mass cranial to heart	ZEPS (2014)
Thyroid gland	Carcinoma	Ceylon terrapin		Cowen (1968)
Thyroid gland	Papillary carcinoma	Red-eared slider		Gál et al. (2010)
Tongue	Papilloma	Box turtle		ZEPS (2014)
Tongue	Squamous cell carcinoma	Russian tortoise		ZEPS (2014)

23.3 (continued) Tumours in tortoises.
(ZEPS (2014) indicates cases from the files of the Zoo/Exotic Pathology Service in California)

Alimentary tract tumours

The majority of gastrointestinal tumours are reported in snakes, and they are reported uncommonly in lizards and chelonians (Schlumberger and Lucke, 1948; Jessup, 1980; Jacobson and Ackerman, 1981; Martin et al., 1994; Latimer and Rich, 1998; Hernandez-Divers and Garner, 2003; Garner et al., 2004; Sykes and Trupkiewicz, 2006) These tumours result in variable clinical signs referable to the digestive tract, including constipation, regurgitation and progressive enlargement of the coelom.

Gastric adenocarcinomas and carcinomas in snakes tend to be invasive and associated with scirrhous reaction resulting in thickening of the gastric sections. The differential for this gastric thickening should include gastric cryptosporidia infections. Metastases are uncommon. The author has identified metastases from a gastric carcinoma into the intestine and liver of a carpet python. Intestinal adenocarcinomas seem to be identified more commonly in colubrids (Garner et al., 2004). One intestinal tumour in a corn snake had metastases to the liver (Garner et al., 2004). Colonic and cloacal adenocarcinomas again seem more common in colubrids such as king- and ratsnakes, and are seen rarely in Boidae. No metastases from this location have been described.

The gastrointestinal adenocarcinomas/carcinomas are uncommon in lizards. Reports have included a cloacal carcinoma in a desert iguana (Krause et al., 2015) (Figure 23.4), an intestinal adenocarcinoma in an iguana and a cloacal tumour in a chuckwalla (Garner et al., 2004). There are rare reports of metastases in the literature, including a colonic adenocarcinoma in a Mexican beaded lizard, with foci in the liver and spleen (Sykes and Trupkiewicz, 2006).

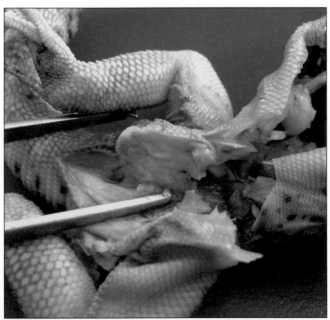

23.4 Cloacal carcinoma in a desert iguana. This is a formalin-fixed specimen.

In young bearded dragons, there is a highly malignant gastric neuroendocrine carcinoma that readily metastasizes (Ritter et al., 2009; Lyons et al., 2010). These dragons commonly present with anorexia, vomiting, hyperglycaemia, melaena and anaemia. The metastases commonly are found in the liver. Based on immunohistochemistry staining (positive somatostatin and negative gastrin and chromogranin AB) most tumours were identified as somatostatinomas (Ritter et al., 2009; Lyons et al., 2010). On transmission electron microscopy (TEM), neurosecretory granules in the neoplastic cells confirmed a neuroendocrine carcinoma (Lyons et al., 2010).

Therapy has rarely been attempted as many cases present in a terminal condition. A colonic adenocarcinoma in a corn snake was resected and this alleviated the intestinal obstruction for at least 4 months, after which the snake was lost to follow-up (Latimer and Rich, 1998) A Burmese python was euthanased because of complications following resection of a segmental colonic adenocarcinoma (Chandra et al., 2001). A European viper with a cloaca and oviduct adenocarcinoma died after photodynamic therapy with chloroaluminium sulphonated phthalocyanine (Roberts et al., 1991).

Hepatic tumours

Primary tumours of the liver, which can arise from the bile ducts or hepatocytes, are uncommonly reported in reptiles. Lizards seem to more frequently develop tumours of the biliary system (Frye, 1991; Wilson et al., 2004; Garner et al., 2004). Coelomic distension, coelomic fluid accumulation and a palpable mass approximately mid-coelom are common findings in both lizards and snakes. Biliary adenocarcinomas (cholangiocarcinomas) may appear as multiple masses in the liver and are rarely reported to metastasize (Garner et al., 2004; Sykes and Trupkiewicz, 2006). A metastasis to the pancreas was reported in a spiny-tailed iguana (Sykes and Trupkiewicz, 2006). Benign biliary adenomas are most frequently recognized as an incidental finding at post-mortem examination (Garner et al., 2004). A cystic variation on the benign tumour, a biliary cystadenoma, was reported in a Piedmont terrapin (Sykes and Trupkiewicz, 2006).

A wedge biopsy and histology are recommended for diagnosis of liver tumours. These tumours can easily be confused with severe chronic fibrosing liver disease and pseudocarcinomatous biliary hyperplasia if inadequate samples are collected (Wilson et al., 2004).

Hepatocellular hepatomas and carcinomas are recognized in both snakes and lizards (Sykes and Trupkiewicz, 2006). The benign hepatomas can be difficult to differentiate from hepatic nodular hyperplasia unless a sizeable section can be examined. The hepatoma will be associated with compression or alteration of adjacent parenchyma and lack portal tracts (Garner et al., 2004). One hepatocellular carcinoma in a snake had a metastasis to the lung.

Chondroid and osteoid tumours

Tracheal cartilaginous hyperplasia and/or chondroma

Tracheal cartilaginous nodules are described primarily in ball pythons. It is unknown if these are true chondromas or foci of cartilaginous hyperplasia that develop in response to damage. Whether they are benign cartilage tumours or cartilaginous hyperplasia, these proliferative growths expand into the lumen of the trachea and result in intermittent dyspnoea characterized by periods of open-mouth breathing, loud respirations, expiratory wheezing and vertical posturing (Figure 23.5). Radiodense space-occupying masses are visible in the trachea on radiographs. On sectioning, the masses are discrete and firm, and may be grey or grey-white. Histologically, the nodules are composed of a variably disorganized dense chondroid matrix and are populated by quiescent normal-appearing chondrocytes

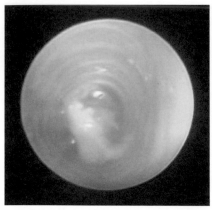

23.5 Endoscopic view of a tracheal chondroma in a ball python.
(Courtesy of Angela Lennox)

within lacunae. These lesions must be differentiated from abscesses or granulomas caused by infectious agents or migrating foreign bodies. Treatment is surgical resection with tracheal anastomosis (Diethelm *et al.*, 1996). Complications may include stenosis and there is a risk of suffocation owing to failure of the glottis to fully extend when swallowing prey.

A periosteal chondroma arising near the shoulder joint was described in a Mali uromastyx (Gal *et al.*, 2007). The slow-growing mass resulted in partial atrophy of the skeletal muscles and the lizard was euthanased owing to degradation in quality of life.

Chondrosarcoma

Chondrosarcomas are malignant tumours with tumour cells that produce a matrix of cartilage with no osteoid or bone-forming elements. They can arise in bone or periosteum, although the latter site is rare in animals. In a review of reptile tumours, one chondrosarcoma (site not provided) was listed in a corn snake (Mauldin and Done, 2006). Additional cases in corn snakes include vertebral chondrosarcomas (Garner *et al.*, 2004), most arising in the vertebral articulations and being locally invasive and sometimes associated with pathological fractures. One vertebral chondrosarcoma and one arising from the mandible developed multiple visceral metastases (Dawe *et al.*, 1980; Schmidt and Reavill, 2012) (Figure 23.6). A case of vertebral chondrosarcoma metastatic to the liver was reported in a grey ratsnake (Honour *et al.*, 1993). Chondrosarcomas have been reported in a snake of undetermined species (Gregory *et al.*, 1995), an Indian monitor (Schlumberger and Lucke, 1948) and unspecified saurians (Hernandez-Divers and Garner, 2003).

Chondrosarcomas are usually readily diagnosed with routine haematoxylin and eosin staining, and immuno-histochemical staining is not routinely indicated. S-100 and vimentin are usually positive in low- and intermediate-grade sarcomas, but can be focally negative in high-grade tumours.

Osteoma and osteosarcoma

Neoplasms originating from the mesenchymal precursors of bone or cartilage are rare in reptiles.

Osteomas are benign lesions that originate from bone, generally the mandible and long bones. Rarely these bone tumours arise from the integument (osteoma cutis). In a European pond turtle the removal of an osteoma returned normal neck movement (Frye *et al.*, 2009).

Osteosarcoma of the vertebra and proximal ribs was described in a California mountain kingsnake (Latimer *et al.*, 2000). An osteochondrosarcoma (compound osteosarcoma) has been reported in the cervical area of a Bengal (yellow tree) monitor (Frye, 1991). Chondroblastic osteosarcomas (osteoid chondrosarcomas) were identified in two young (5 and 6 months) and related spiny-tailed monitors (Needle *et al.*, 2013). The tumours were large firm multilobulated masses arising in the pelvic girdle. A similar tumour developed in a desert monitor mandible and had metastases to the tail, ribs and femur (Schonbauer *et al.*, 1982).

These tumours typically present as firm swellings associated with bone. The diagnosis of a bone or cartilage tumour is greatly enhanced by including both the clinical and radiographic findings with tissue sample submissions. The lesions of metabolic bone disease, osteomyelitis and reactive bone are more common and can mimic the cellular features and stromal patterns of neoplasia. Effective therapy for these tumours has not been described.

Cutaneous tumours

Squamous cell carcinoma

Squamous cell carcinoma (SCC) is a malignant tumour composed of nests and infiltrative cords of moderately undifferentiated to poorly differentiated squamous cells. The cells may form central cores of compressed laminated keratin ('keratin pearls') or individual cells may be keratinized (Figure 23.7). The primary tumour sites are the skin and oral cavity.

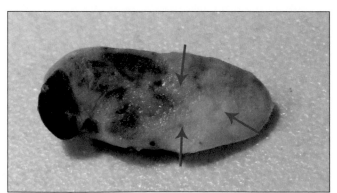

23.6 Longitudinal sections through the heart of a corn snake supporting metastatic foci (arrowed) of a chondrosarcoma. The foci are white and glisten.

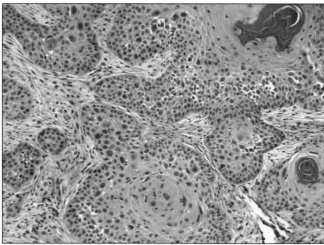

23.7 Histology of a cutaneous squamous cell carcinoma from a bearded dragon. (Haematoxylin and eosin stain; X10 objective)

Oral cavity SCCs (frequently involving the lips) are more commonly reported in snakes (Hill, 1977; Roberts *et al.*, 1991), and oral SCCs have been a cause of death in varanid species (Mendyk *et al.*, 2013). The tumours have poorly defined borders and are associated with haemorrhage and necrosis of the surrounding tissues. These lesions lead to a chronic stomatitis and may contain caseous material. Common clinical signs for tumours in these locations include stomatitis, anorexia, oral discharge and, if further caudal in the oral cavity, respiratory clinical signs such as wheezing and gurgling. Another common location is the cloacal region, arising from the scent glands, hemipenes or skin (Garner *et al.*, 2004)

On the skin, SCCs appear as proliferative irregular broad-based masses or wound-like ulcers. Reports in lizards include a periorbital mass in a veiled chameleon (Abou-Madi and Kern, 2002), an ulcerative lesion on the back of a leopard gecko associated with long-term dysecdysis, SCC in the ear canal in a leopard gecko (Sykes and Trupkiewicz, 2006; Duarte and Baines, 2009), and multiple sites in a series of tumours described in bearded dragons (Hannon *et al.*, 2011). A common location reported in bearded dragons is the periocular region, generally in proximity to a mucocutaneous junction (Hannon *et al.*, 2011).

There are rare reports of SCC in chelonians. An Eastern box turtle (Greenacre and Roberts, 2000) developed an SCC at the site of a forelimb amputation. Based on gross appearance, the differentials include chronic ulcerated dermatitis and abscesses; this illustrates the need to perform a biopsy on skin and oral lesions that are non-responsive to antimicrobial therapy. SCCs have also been reported in a British Indian turtle, a spiny softshell turtle and a common snake-necked turtle (Sykes and Trupkiewicz, 2006). A red-eared slider developed a large mass that effaced the right side of his face, preventing retraction of the head. The primary differential was of an aural abscess; however, on histology a well differentiated SCC was identified (Ardente *et al.*, 2011).

Reptilian SCCs are often associated with chronic inflammation and/or infection, and a link between chronic inflammation and tumour development has been speculated (Mendyk *et al.*, 2013). Neoplastic proliferation due to inflammation has been demonstrated experimentally in other species. The tumour formation in the oral cavity could be triggered by rostral trauma, abrasions and stomatitis secondary to abnormal captive behaviours, such as nose rubbing and trauma during prey strikes and escape attempts. This suggests that inflammatory lesions in reptiles should be treated aggressively and biopsy performed if they are non-responsive to appropriate therapy.

SCCs are locally aggressive but metastases are rarely reported in the few fully examined reptile cases. One tumour that started as a lesion on the tail of a diamondback rattlesnake invaded into adjacent blood vessels (Anderson *et al.*, 2010a). When SCC occurs in accessible areas, standard therapy includes surgical excision and/or radiation therapy. Photodynamic therapy in a boa has been described, with no tumour recurrence after therapy (Roberts *et al.*, 1991), while strontium-90 therapy in an eastern box turtle was unsuccessful (Greenacre and Roberts, 2000). Complete surgical removal obtained remission for greater than 16 months in two bearded dragons (Hannon *et al.*, 2011). Palliative radiation (10 Gy q7d for 3 weeks) was administered to a Madagascar ground boa with a caudal pharyngeal SCC (Steeil *et al.*, 2013).

Chromatophoroma

Chromatophoromas are common neoplasms of pigment-producing chromatophores. They have been described within the subcutis of snakes (Frye *et al.*, 1975; Ryan *et al.*, 1981; Leach *et al.*, 1991; Ramsay *et al.*, 1996; Bryant *et al.*, 1997; Gregory *et al.*, 1997; Kusewitt *et al.*, 1997), veiled chameleons (Reavill and Schmidt, 2004; Bronson *et al.*, 2006), a green iguana (Irizarry-Rovira *et al.*, 2006), a Mexican beaded lizard (Sykes and Trupkiewicz, 2006), bearded dragons and unspecified saurians (Hernandez-Divers and Garner, 2003). Tumours may arise from melanophores (melanin-pigment-producing cells), iridophores (cells with birefringent intracytoplasmic particles that refract and reflect light), erythrophores (red/orange-pigment-producing cells) and xanthophores (which produce yellow pigments) (Figure 23.8). Although most of these tumours involve only one type of pigment cell, multiple pigment cell types have been involved in some cases (Jacobson *et al.*, 1989). Generally, the morphological features described for chromatophoromas are similar to those of malignant melanomas in higher vertebrates. The differentiation between the chromatophoromas generally relies on electron microscopy (EM) and recognition of the pigment types. Melanophomas are immunoreactive for Melan-A and S100-antigen negative. The intracytoplasmic pigment granules on transmission electron microscopy were round to oval and had a single-layer membrane surrounding a markedly electron-dense melanin core (Irizarry-Rovira *et al.*, 2006).

Grossly, tumours are variable in size, multilobulated and may be partially encapsulated. They can vary from orange to red to black.

Of the several cases of chromatophoromas (or melanomas) reported in snakes, most have been malignant with local invasion, local recurrence and/or distant metastases (oesophagus, pericardium, coelom). A small number of cases have been described in lizards, and several of these describe metastasis (Mikaelian *et al.*, 2000; Hernandez-Divers and Garner, 2003; Reavill and Schmidt, 2004; Bronson *et al.*, 2006).

Therapy for chromatophoromas has been unsuccessful. Reports include using radioactive gold implants in a death adder (Bryant *et al.*, 1997) and radiation therapy in a yellow ratsnake (Leach *et al.*, 1991).

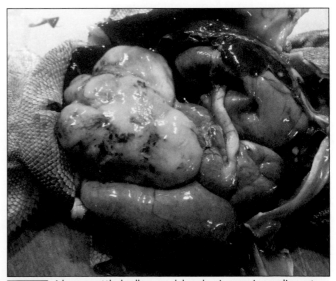

23.8 A large mottled yellow caudal coelomic mass is a malignant chromatophoroma in a bearded dragon. The coelomic fat pads have atrophied.

Lipomas and liposarcomas

Lipomas and infiltrative lipomas are benign connective tissue tumours composed of mature fat cells that are infrequently described in reptiles. The majority of reports have been of infiltrative lipomas in corn snakes and a black ratsnake. The tumours have generally been located in the caudal one-third of the body (Burkert *et al.*, 2002; Reavill and Schmidt, 2003; Haag *et al.*, 2008). The infiltrative lipoma has a locally aggressive behaviour and can be difficult to remove completely; however, it does not metastasize. A common complication is obstipation due to the mass effect resulting in mechanical interference at the level of the colon.

Lipomas have been described as masses in the subcutis of boa constrictors and there have been several cases involving the subcutis of monitors, and one in the liver of a Nile crocodile (Hernandez-Divers and Garner, 2003; Garner *et al.*, 2004). Although lipomas in chelonians have not been described in the literature, the author has seen a lipoma in the liver of a yellow-spotted Amazon river turtle. Grossly, lipomas are soft, pale yellow, encapsulated and lobulated. Histologically they are indistinguishable from normal adipose tissue. If cutaneous lipomas are traumatized, they may become inflamed and necrotic. Recommended therapy is early surgical removal. Gross inspection at the time of surgery is important in determining completeness of removal.

Liposarcomas, malignant tumours of lipocytes and lipoblasts, are rare. They have been described in a Burmese python, a shingleback skink, a boa and a veiled chameleon (Garner *et al.*, 1994; Reavill *et al.*, 2002) (Figure 23.9). They appear as yellow-to-grey poorly circumscribed masses of the subcutis, and differ from lipomas in that they are firmer and more infiltrative and vascular. Liposarcomas are expected to be aggressive, and in two reports they presented as multiple subcutaneous masses. Since cytological examination of an aspirate may not differentiate between a liposarcoma and a lipoma, surgical biopsy is recommended. Immunohistochemistry (IHC) and EM may be important contributing diagnostic tests. The additional tests may be necessary because features of cell morphology and architectural arrangement may not be sufficient to distinguish between the various soft-tissue sarcomas, particularly the poorly differentiated aggressive tumours often described in reptiles. An accurate histological classification will significantly contribute to establishing the prognosis, as liposarcomas are usually resistant to radiation and hyperthermia. The proposed therapy is wide and aggressive surgical excision.

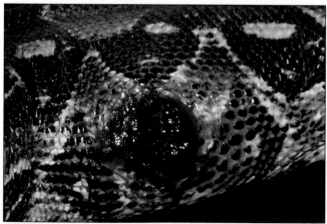

23.9 An ulcerated liposarcoma in a boa constrictor.
(Courtesy of Bob Dahlhausen)

Mast cell tumour

Although mast cell tumours are among the most common skin neoplasms of domestic dogs, cats and ferrets, they are rare in reptiles. A single case has been reported in an eastern kingsnake (Schumacher *et al.*, 1998). This snake presented with a poorly differentiated cutaneous tumour which was locally aggressive with neoplastic lymphatic emboli and multi-organ metastases. Treatment was attempted; however, the snake died after the start of radiation therapy. There are rare reports of well differentiated multicentric cutaneous and mucosal mast cell tumours with peripheral blood mastocytosis in green iguanas (Reavill *et al.*, 2000). The reported masses were subcutaneous, firm and white in colour (Figure 23.10). These must be differentiated from the more common bacterial or fungal granulomas and cutaneous lymphosarcomas. Effective therapy was not reported.

There are two reports in tortoises: a desert tortoise and a Galapagos tortoise (Frye, 1994; Santoro *et al.*, 2008). The Galapagos tortoise developed a skin mass on the ventral neck that was removed and identified as a cutaneous mast cell tumour. There was no regrowth at an 11-month recheck (Santoro *et al.*, 2008).

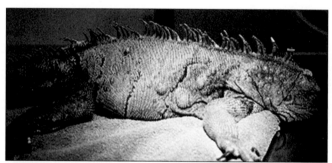

23.10 Subcutaneous mast cell tumours in a green iguana.
(Courtesy of Sarah Fassler)

Endocrine tumours

Tumours arising from the endocrine organs (pancreas, adrenal gland, thyroid gland and pituitary gland) are not commonly reported in reptiles.

Thyroid adenomatous hyperplasia and follicular adenomas have been reported in lizard, snake and turtle species (Frye, 1991; Hernandez-Divers *et al.*, 2001; Garner *et al.*, 2004; Hadfield *et al.*, 2012), whereas thyroid carcinomas in reptiles are rare. Thyroid carcinomas have been described in a Chinese crocodile lizard (Whiteside and Garner, 2001), a red-eared slider (Gál *et al.*, 2010), an Indian black turtle (Cowen, 1968), and a rough knob-tailed, a smooth knob-tailed and a marbled velvet gecko (Hadfield *et al.*, 2012). The clinical signs in the lizards included an intraoral mass, ventral neck swelling, oral haemorrhage and weight loss. The thyroid carcinoma metastasized to the liver and lungs in the rough knob-tailed gecko (Hadfield *et al.*, 2012). The functional aspects of these tumours are rarely described either by blood hormone levels or by clinical signs (Hadfield *et al.*, 2012). One iguana with a thyroid adenoma presented with polyphagia, aggression and tachycardia. The elevated total T4 (30.0 nmol/l) resolved to a euthyroid state after surgical removal (Hernandez-Divers *et al.*, 2001) (Figure 23.11).

Pancreatic islet cell tumours are uncommon but have been reported in a hognose snake, a Komodo dragon, a roughneck monitor and two green iguanas (Garner *et al.*, 2004; Sykes and Trupkiewicz, 2006). From the limited clinical information, there did not seem to be any evidence of these being functional tumours.

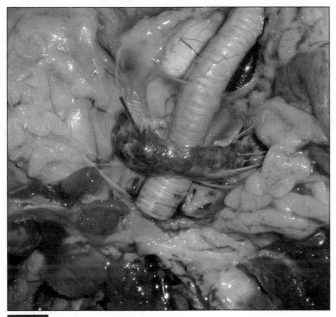

23.11 A thyroid adenoma in a green iguana (arrowed).

A C-cell carcinoma of the thyroid gland in a Chinese crocodile lizard metastasized to the liver and mesentery (Sykes and Trupkiewicz, 2006).

Only three cases of pituitary tumours have been described in snakes. A pituitary adenoma suspected to be arising from the pars distalis was associated with neurological clinical signs of poor muscle tone, fasciculations and abnormal righting reflex in a black-headed python (Linn et al., 1996). The 1-cm diameter round firm red-to-tan pituitary mass displaced the brain dorsolaterally. A Dumeril's ground boa also presented with poor muscle tone, dull mentation and postural abnormalities. The pituitary mass was 1.5 cm and compressed the brain. The histological features suggested this pituitary adenoma arose from the pars intermedia (Gyimesi and Garner, 2007). A pituitary cystadenoma was linked to diffuse hyperkeratosis in an Everglades ratsnake. The benign tumour arose from the pars intermedia, and the skin lesion was associated with bacteria and fungi (Dadone et al., 2010).

Haemopoietic and lymphatic organs

Lymphomas, histiocytic sarcomas, leukaemias and other myeloproliferative disorders are well documented in lizards, squamates and chelonians (Zwart and Harshbarger, 1972; Jacobson et al., 1980; Jacobson et al., 1981; Bodri, 1992; Rest et al., 1995; Romagnano et al., 1996; Tocidlowski et al., 2001; Raiti et al., 2002; Silverstone et al., 2002; Hernandez-Divers and Garner, 2003; Gyimesi et al., 2005; Chinnadurai et al., 2008; Bezjian et al., 2013; Mendyk et al., 2013). These are all round cell tumours arising from the haemopoietic cell lines. Leukaemias present as massive invasions of primitive haemopoietic cells within the vascular system, and sarcomas develop solid tumour masses in various organs. These two presentations can occur together (Schultze et al., 1999; Gyimesi et al., 2005; Chinnadurai et al., 2008; Georoff et al., 2009; Bezjian et al., 2013). Myeloproliferative disorders can be associated with proliferation of either myeloid or erythroid series cells, and these can be difficult to differentiate histologically. These disorders can also present as leukaemias or sarcomas (granulocytic sarcomas) (Rosskopf et al., 1981; Stanley, 1999; Sykes and Trupkiewicz, 2006).

Immunohistochemistry (IHC) which is routinely employed in mammals to determine the cell of origin, is rarely reported in reptiles and the accuracy of many markers for lymphocytes is poorly documented (Rest et al., 1995; Tocidlowski et al., 2001; Raiti et al., 2002; Silverstone et al., 2002; Hernandez-Divers and Garner, 2003; Gyimesi et al., 2005). Flow cytometric immunophenotyping and IHC were used to describe a chronic lymphocytic leukaemia of T-cell origin in a green tree monitor (Georoff et al., 2009). Cytochemical and IHC positive reaction for CD3 and alpha-naphthyl butyrate esterase confirmed a diagnosis of T-cell lymphoid leukaemia in a Chinese box turtle (Bezjian et al., 2013).

Transmissible viruses cause lymphomas and leukaemias in a wide variety of mammalian species, including humans, cattle, cats and, most recently, ferrets (Moulton, 1990; Erdman et al., 1995). In dogs and humans, chromosome abnormalities are associated with lymphoma (Hahn et al., 1994). Retroviral particles have been described in Burmese pythons with recurrent undifferentiated mesenchymal round cell tumour (lymphosarcoma) of the oral cavity, uterus and ovary, and there was diffuse involvement of the spleen. The relationship of the intraneoplastic viral particles to the aetiology of the tumours is uncertain (Chandra et al., 2001). Definitive viral inclusions have not been found in other reports (Jacobson et al., 1980; Chinnadurai et al., 2008; Bezjian et al., 2013). In one colony of Egyptian spiny-tailed lizards there was a high incidence of lymphoid tumours over 8 years. While IHC was not reliable for further characterization, by light and electron microscopy some tumours had plasmacytoid morphological features suggesting B-cell origin. Viruses were not detected through EM nor attempts at isolation, and no known toxic exposures were identified (Gyimesi et al., 2005).

Malignant lymphoma (lymphosarcoma) represents the majority of the documented cases in reptiles. These neoplasms can involve not only the spleen and bone marrow but also any organ or tissue. Many initially present as cutaneous or oral tissue masses that are found to be metastatic disease (Chinnadurai et al., 2008) (Figure 23.12). Grossly, they are grey-white or cream masses that are soft

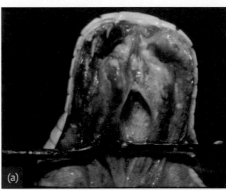

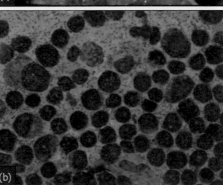

23.12

(a) Stomatitis in a diamond python with lymphoma.
(b) New methylene-blue staining of an oral swab demonstrating lymphoblasts.
(Courtesy of Paul Raiti)

to relatively firm. Necrosis and haemorrhage may be present. Therapy is uncommon but has included prednisone with a partial response in a savannah monitor (Hernandez-Divers et al., 2003). A green iguana, with a lymphoma identified in the cranial cervical area and a leukaemia, was treated with a single 10 Gy fraction radiation, and through a vascular access port given doxorubicin, vincristine, cyclophosphamide and prednisone. The iguana was still in remission at 1008 days from the start of the therapy (Folland et al., 2011).

Differentiation for tumour types is done by histology, with lymphomas being composed of small or large lymphoid cells forming diffuse sheets. Histiocytic sarcomas differ only in cell morphology. IHC for B- or T-cell lineage determination has been described in rare cases; however, the stains proved inconclusive (Hernandez-Divers and Garner, 2003). Granulocytic sarcomas, which are rare in reptiles but have been reported in a king cobra (Stanley, 1999) and a boa (Gregory et al., 2000), generally have poorly staining intracytoplasmic granules. Therapy has been unsuccessful in the rare reports (Jacobson et al., 1981).

With leukaemias, the animals are generally found dead or suffering non-specific clinical signs of weight loss and anorexia. Therapy is seldom reported. A combination of prednisolone, cytosine arabinoside and chlorambucil was used in a case of lymphoblastic leukaemia in a diamondback terrapin (Silverstone et al., 2002). Prednisone and chlorambucil resulted in clinical improvement in a green tree monitor with chronic T-cell leukaemia; however, the animal died with neoplastic infiltrations in multiple organs (Georoff et al., 2009).

Renal tumours

The primary renal tumours reported in reptiles include adenocarcinoma, adenoma and nephroblastoma (characterized by a metanephric blastema, and stromal and epithelial derivatives). These tumours have been described in lizards, snakes and chelonians (Burt et al., 1984; Jacobson et al., 1986; Barten et al., 1994; Gravendyck et al., 1997; Sykes and Trupkiewicz, 2006; Keck et al., 2011). From a survey, renal adenocarcinomas are most common in snakes, particularly kingsnakes (Garner et al., 2004). In snakes, swelling in the caudal third of the body cavity is typical, along with anorexia, regurgitation and constipation. Grossly, one or both kidneys may have irregular masses within the parenchyma (Figure 23.13).

A genetic and/or environmental factor is suspected in some cases. Three genetically related Cape coral snakes and two related red spitting cobras all developed renal

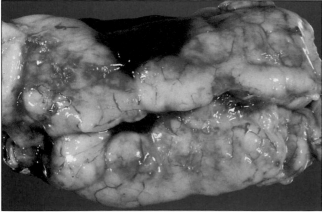

23.13 A renal carcinoma in a boa constrictor.
(Courtesy of Robert Schmidt)

adenocarcinomas, supporting a genetic component or a species predilection in some snake species (Keck et al., 2011; Belasco-Zeitz et al., 2013).

In lizards, renal tumours present as firm swellings in the caudal coelom and can occasionally be palpated extending cranially past the rim of the pelvis. Renal tubular adenomas are most common but are seldom associated with clinical signs of disease (Garner et al., 2004).

Differential diagnoses for renal tumours include acute and chronic renal disease in lizards and impacted eggs in snakes. Occasionally in snakes, renal tumours mistaken for impacted eggs have been massaged out of the body through the cloaca. Metastasis is unusual but has been reported. Sites include the liver, lung and perirenal abdominal wall. These tumours frequently have associated development of urate tophi and urate stasis. Early surgical removal of renal tumours is recommended.

Vascular tumours

These are tumours that arise from vascular endothelium. Haemangiomas, benign vascular tumours, have been reported sporadically. A cardiac haemangioma arising from the left atrial wall was associated with cranial oedema and swelling of the cardiac region in a corn snake. Attempts to remove it were unsuccessful (Stumpel et al., 2012). One tumour developed in the wall of the oesophagus of a red-eared slider (Gal et al., 2009). It mechanically interfered with swallowing. Additional cases (locations not provided) have been reported in unspecified lizards and a snake (Garner et al., 2004). The author has diagnosed haemangioma in the skin of turtles, a bearded dragon, blue-tongued skinks and red-tailed boas. The majority of the skin lesions had a history of raised pink masses which readily haemorrhaged. One blue-tongued skink had a haemangioma arise within the coelomic fat pad.

Haemangiosarcomas have been described in the liver of a pine snake and the spleen of a corn snake (Sykes and Trupkiewicz, 2006; Tuttle et al., 2006). The splenic tumour presented as a prominent mid-body swelling and it was surgically removed. Despite aggressive care, the snake died 6 weeks post-removal. The histological sections of this tumour were examined with IHC to confirm origin from the vascular system; however, factor VIII did not stain the tumour cells. A complete postmortem did not identify any metastases. Additional cases (locations not provided) have been reported in an unspecified lizard and snakes (Garner et al., 2004). The author has seen haemangiosarcomas in the leg tissues of a common snapping turtle, in the heart in a bearded dragon and a crocodile monitor, and in an unknown location in a rainbow boa and a leopard gecko. The animals with tumours in the heart both had a history of chronic fluid accumulation in the coelomic cavity.

Miscellaneous

Fibrosarcoma

Fibromas are benign mesenchymal tumours that are rarely reported in the literature. One tumour developed on the plantar surface of a forelimb on a common snapping turtle and appeared as a raised mass with a central ulceration (Gonzales-Viera et al., 2012). The tumour cells expressed vimentin, but not desmin.

Fibrosarcomas are locally aggressive tumours that originate from fibrous connective tissue. Myxosarcomas are variant fibrosarcomas which arise from primitive pleomorphic fibroblasts that produce excessive mucin. Diagnosis is generally made by examination of haematoxylin–eosin-stained tissue sections. However, these two tumour types are part of the family of soft-tissue spindle cell sarcomas including leiomyosarcoma, liposarcoma, peripheral nerve sheath tumours (see below), ganglioneuroma and ganglioneuroblastoma, and as they become less well differentiated they may have significant overlap of morphological features. More definitive determination of the tissue of origin may require IHC and EM. Fortunately, in many species, these tumours have similar biological behaviour.

In snakes, fibrosarcomas and myxosarcomas most commonly affect the subcutaneous intermandibular tissues, while they are more frequently recognized within the subcutis and muscle tissues in chelonians and saurians. Rare cases have been reported within internal organs such as the liver, lungs, heart and kidney. The tumour masses are firm with irregular and indistinct borders. Fibrosarcomas and myxosarcomas are locally invasive, do not commonly metastasize, and have a moderate to high potential for recurrence. In Burmese pythons, type-C-like retroviral particles have been found in an intermandibular fibrosarcoma (Chandra *et al.*, 2001). This can suggest a possible viral aetiology; however, retroviral-type particles have also been identified in other tumour types. In a Saharan horned viper a subcutaneous fibrosarcoma had metastatic foci in the vertebral bodies, ribs, lung, heart, ovaries and body wall. No virus particles were identified by TEM; however, this snake had high levels of hepatic cadmium (Oros *et al.*, 2009).

Radiation, intralesional chemotherapy (carboplatin) (Langan *et al.*, 2001) and cryosurgery (Bryant *et al.*, 1997; Frye and Williams, 2002) have been attempted in several snakes with fibrosarcomas. Only a partial response is reported. In general, most spindle cell tumours warrant a guarded prognosis.

Peripheral nerve sheath tumours

Peripheral nerve sheath tumours (PNSTs) are tumours that are reported to arise from the peripheral nerve sheath (Schwann cells, fibroblasts or perineural cells). They are classified under many names, including neurinomas, neurilemmomas, schwannomas, neurofibromas and neurofibrosarcomas, as histologically they are morphologically similar. The tumours should be evaluated by additional testing such as IHC and/or ultrastructural features for better understanding of their biological behaviour. The few cases in reptiles have included malignant as well as benign and multicentric tumours (Lemberger *et al.*, 2005; Diaz-Figueroa *et al.*, 2005) (Figure 23.14).

A mid-body subcutaneous swelling in a water moccasin was associated with flaccid paralysis distal to the lesion. The malignant PNST was removed; however, it regrew within 3 months. It invaded the coelomic cavity and the vertebral canal, compressing the spinal cord. Metastases were present in the liver. The tumour cells were IHC positive for S-100, moderate for vimentin, and negative for actin (Ramis *et al.*, 1998).

Multiple tumour masses were identified in three bearded dragons, two of which were related (Mikaelian *et al.*, 2001; Lemberger *et al.*, 2005). These well-demarcated masses were identified in the subcutis and resembled adipose tissue. After surgical removal and histological evaluation, additional IHC stains and transmission electron microscopic diagnostics were performed. The neoplastic cells were positive for neuron-specific enolase and negative for desmin and smooth muscle actin. Two were S-100 positive and one was vimentin positive. A continuous basal lamina separating intertwining cells was identified by TEM. Local recurrence occurred 1 year later in one incompletely excised mass. Numerous metastatic foci were identified in the lungs, liver and cardiac ventricle in the unrelated animal. A surgically removed firm encapsulated polycystic mass in the coelom from a savannah monitor was determined to be a benign PNST (schwannoma) based on IHC of positive staining with S-100a and vimentin and negative staining for desmin (Diaz-Figueroa *et al.*, 2005). It was speculated that this tumour arose from either paravertebral muscle or a peripheral nerve/ganglion around the intercostal space.

Teratoma

Teratomas are composed of tissues derived from at least two of the three embryonic germ layers (endoderm, mesoderm and ectoderm). Typically, they arise from the gonads and most are benign. The ovaries are common sites for teratoma development in the green iguana (Anderson *et al.*, 1996; Garner *et al.*, 2004; Levine, 2004) and other unspecified saurians (Hernandez-Divers and Garner, 2003) (Figure 23.15). Rare gonadal tumours have been described in chelonians, and only benign and malignant ovarian teratomas have been reported in red-eared sliders, with a benign ovarian teratoma in a Mediterranean tortoise (Machotka *et al.*, 1992; Newman *et al.*, 2003; Martorell *et al.*, 2009; Hidalgo-Vila, 2006).

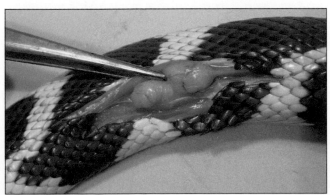

23.14 Multicentric and malignant peripheral nerve sheath tumour (PNST) in a kingsnake.

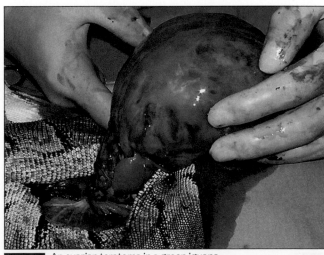

23.15 An ovarian teratoma in a green iguana.
(Courtesy of Chris Sanders)

Clinical signs are the result of a space-occupying mass and may include digestive and respiratory dysfunction as well as coelomic cavity distension. In the red-eared slider with a malignant teratoma there was subcutaneous swelling of all four limbs and severe respiratory distress (Newman et al., 2003). The Mediterranean tortoise with the benign ovarian teratoma presented with tetraparesis (Martorell et al., 2009).

Differential diagnoses for these masses in females include neoplasia or granuloma of the ovary or oviduct, cystic ovary, segmental pyosalpinx, and neoplasm or granuloma of the adrenal gland or spleen. In the few described cases the tumours in the lizards exhibited rapid growth, and in one iguana metastatic foci were identified 2.5 months after surgical removal of the original tumour (Levine, 2004). Intracoelomic carboplatin was attempted in this case with little response. Early surgical removal is recommended.

Xanthomas

Although xanthomas are not considered to be neoplasms they have many similar behaviours, with locally invasive growth and, in some animals, disseminated disease. The lesions, which are commonly found within the coelomic cavity or central nervous system, are composed of foamy macrophages, multinucleated giant cells and cholesterol clefts. Multiple xanthomas are not an unusual finding in female geckos, both in the coelom and in the central nervous system (Cooper et al., 1998; Garner et al., 1999). Central nervous system involvement has also been reported in other saurians, including water dragons, the Cuban anole and the great plated lizard (Schmidt and Hubbard, 1987; Gyimesi et al., 2002; Kummrow et al., 2010). The author has identified xanthomas in a black-lined plated lizard, green iguana, green crested basilisk (plumed basilisk) and blue-tongued skink. The clinical signs, as expected with a mass within the confines of the central nervous system, include opisthotonus, head bobbing and ataxia. Magnetic resonance imaging was performed on one water dragon with significant neurological clinical signs; however, no structural abnormalities were noted. Disease conditions that alter cholesterol metabolism may predispose animals to xanthoma formation. The multiple xanthomas which developed in the geckos, including lesions within the brain, were suspected to be due to dietary factors, folliculogenesis, follicular degeneration and yolk coelomitis. A serum cholesterol screening examination may be helpful in identifying female geckos at risk. Only one attempt at surgical removal resulted in resolution in a gecko (Reed et al., 2007).

The lesions are rarely described in snakes, but there are reports in a Russian viper, a long-nosed snake and a gopher snake (Ryan and Whitney, 1980; Schmidt and Hubbard, 1987; Anderson et al., 2010b). As with many of the saurians, there is a sex predilection for females.

References and further reading

Abou-Madi N and Kern TJ (2002) Squamous cell carcinoma associated with a periorbital mass in a veiled chameleon (Chamaeleo calyptratus). Veterinary Ophthalmology 5(3), 217–220

Anderson ET, Kennedy-Stoskopf S, Sandy JR et al. (2010a) Squamous cell carcinoma with vascular invasion in a diamondback rattlesnake (Crotalus adamanteus). Journal of Zoo and Wildlife Medicine 41(4), 745–748

Anderson ET, Troan BV, Stringer EM, Chinnadurai SK and DeVoe RS (2010b) Cerebral xanthoma in a long-nosed snake (Rhinocheilus lecontei). Journal of Herpetological Medicine and Surgery 20(2–3), 58–60

Anderson NL, Williams J, Sagartz JE and Barnewall R (1996) Ovarian teratoma in a green iguana (Iguana iguana). Journal of Zoo and Wildlife Medicine 27(1), 90–95

Ardente AJ, Christian LS, Borst LB and Lewbart GA (2011) Clinical challenge: squamous cell carcinoma. Journal of Zoo and Wildlife Medicine 42(4), 770–773

Barten SL, Davis K, Harris RK and Jacobson ER (1994) Renal cell carcinoma with metastases in a corn snake (Elaphe guttata). Journal of Zoo and Wildlife Medicine 25(1), 123–127

Barten SL and Frye FL (1981) Leiomyosarcoma and myxoma in a Texas indigo snake. Journal of the American Veterinary Medical Association 179(11), 1292–1295

Belasco-Zeitz M, Pye GW, Burns RE and Pessier AP (2013) Clinical challenge: renal adenocarcinoma in a spitting cobra. Journal of Zoo and Wildlife Medicine 44(3), 807–810

Bezjian M, Diep AN, de Matos R and Schaefer D (2013) Chinese box turtle (Cuora flavomarginata) with lymphoid leukemia characterized by immunohistochemical and cytochemical phenotyping. Veterinary Clinical Pathology 42(3), 368–376

Billips LH and Harshbarger JC (1976) Neoplasia: reptiles. In: Handbook of Laboratory Science, Volume III, ed. EC Melby and NH Altman, pp. 343–356. CRC Press, Cleveland, OH

Bodri MS (1992) Metastatic large granular cell lymphoma in a boa constrictor. Journal of Small Exotic Animal Medicine 1(3), 115–116

Bronson E, Pereira M, Sanchez C and Murray S (2006) Iridophoroma in a veiled chameleon, Chamaeleo calyptratus. Journal of Herpetological Medicine and Surgery 16(2), 58–60

Bryant BR, Vogelnest L and Hulst F (1997) The use of cryosurgery in a diamond python, Morelia spilota spilota, with fibrosarcoma and radiotherapy in a common death adder, Acanthophis antarcticus, with melanoma. Bulletin of the Association of Reptilian and Amphibian Veterinarians 7(3), 9–12

Burkert BA, Tully TN, Nevarez J, Mitchell MA and Camus AC (2002) Infiltrative lipoma in a corn snake, Elaphe guttata guttata. Journal of Herpetological Medicine and Surgery 12, 33–35

Burt DG, Crisp CE, Gillett CS and Rush HG (1984) Two cases of renal neoplasia in a colony of desert iguanas. Journal of the American Veterinary Medical Association 185(11), 1423–1425

Chandra AM, Jacobson ER and Munn RJ (2001) Retroviral particles in neoplasms of Burmese pythons (Python molurus bivittatus). Veterinary Pathology 38(5), 561–564

Chinnadurai SK, Brown DL, Van Wettere A et al. (2008) Mortalities associated with sepsis, parasitism, and disseminated round cell neoplasia in yellow-lipped sea kraits (Laticauda colubrina). Journal of Zoo and Wildlife Medicine 39(4), 626–630

Cooper JE, Bloxam QMC and Tonge (1998) Pathology of Round Island geckos Phelsuma guentheri: some unexpected findings. Dodo 34, 153–158

Cooper JE, Jackson OF and Harshbarger JC (1983) A neurilemmal sarcoma in a tortoise (Testudo hermanni). Journal of Comparative Pathology 93, 541–545

Cowen DF (1968) Diseases of captive reptiles. Journal of the American Veterinary Medical Association 153, 848–859

Dadone LI, Klaphake E, Garner MM et al. (2010) Pituitary cystadenoma, enterolipidosis, and cutaneous mycosis in an Everglades ratsnake (Elaphe obsoleta rossalleni). Journal of Zoo and Wildlife Medicine 41(3), 538–541

Dawe CJ, Small JD, Banfield WG and Woronecki DE (1980) Chondrosarcoma of a corn snake (Elaphe guttata) and nephroblastoma of a rainbow trout (Salmo gairdneri) in cell culture. In: The Comparative Pathology of Zoo Animals, ed. R Montali and G Migaki, pp. 603–612. Smithsonian Institution Press, Washington DC

Diaz-Figueroa O, Mitchell MA, Roberts ED and Kim D-Y (2005) Diagnostic challenge. Seminars in Avian and Exotic Pet Medicine 14(1), 65–70

Diethelm G, Stauber E, Tillson M and Ridgley S (1996) Tracheal resection and anastomosis for an intratracheal chondroma in a ball python. Journal of the American Veterinary Medical Association 209(4), 786–788

Duarte AR and Baines FM (2009) Squamous cell carcinoma in a leopard gecko. Exotic DVM 11(2), 19–22

Effron M, Griner L and Benirschke K (1977) Nature and Rate of Neoplasia Found in Captive Wild Mammals, Birds, and Reptiles at Necropsy. Journal of the National Cancer Institute 59(1), 185–198

Elkan E and Cooper JE (1976) Tumours and pseudotumours in some reptiles. Journal of Comparative Pathology 86(3), 337–348

Erdman SE, Reimann KA, Moore FM et al. (1995) Transmission of a chronic lymphoproliferative syndrome in ferrets. Laboratory Investigation 72(5), 539–546

Ewing PJ, Setser MD, Stair EL, Waurzyniak B and Cowell RL (1991) Myxosarcoma in a Sinaloan milksnake. Journal of the American Veterinary Medical Association 199(12), 1775–1776

Folland DW, Johnston MS, Thamm DH and Reavill D (2011) Diagnosis and management of lymphoma in a green iguana (Iguana iguana). Journal of the American Veterinary Medical Association 239(7), 985–991

Frye FL (1991) Common pathologic lesions and disease processes. In: Biomedical and Surgical Aspects of Captive Reptile Husbandry, pp. 529–619. Krieger Publishing Company, Malabar, FL

Frye FL (1994) Diagnosis and surgical treatment of reptilian neoplasms with a compilation of cases 1966–1993. In Vivo 8(5), 885–892

Frye FL and Carney J (1975) Parathyroid adenoma in a tortoise. Veterinary Medicine, Small Animal Clinician 70, 582–585

Frye FL and Carney JD (1972) Myeloproliferative disease in a turtle. Journal of the American Veterinary Medical Association 161(6), 595–599

Frye FL and Carney JD (1973) Acute lymphatic leukemia in a boa constrictor. *Journal of the American Veterinary Medical Association* **163(6)**, 653–654

Frye FL, Carney JD, Harshbarger JC and Zeigel RF (1975) Malignant chromatophoroma in a western terrestrial garter snake. *Journal of the American Veterinary Medical Association* **167(7)**, 557–558

Frye FL, Dybal NO and Harshbarger JC (1988) Testicular interstitial tumor in a desert tortoise (*Gopherus agassizi*). *Journal of Zoo and Wildlife Medicine* **19**, 55–58

Frye FL, Modry D and Siroky P (2009) Pathology in practice: primary osteoma cutis (benign). *Journal of the American Veterinary Medical Association* **235(5)**, 511–512

Frye FL and Williams DL (2002) Clinical snapshot #1. *Compendium of Continuing Education for the Practicing Veterinarian* **24(3)**, 200–219

Gál J, Csikó G, Pásztor I, Boleskey–Molnár A and *Mihály A* (2010) First description of a papillary carcinoma in the thyroid gland of a red-eared slider (*Trachemys scripta elegans*). *Acta Veterinaria Hungarica* **58(1)**, 69–73

Gal J, Jakab C, Balogh B, Toth T and Farkas B (2007) First occurrence of periosteal chondroma (juxtacortical chondroma) in *Uromastyx maliensis* (Reptilia: Sauria: Agamidae). *Acta Veterinaria Hungarica* **55(3)**, 327–331

Gál J, Jakab C, Szabo Z et al. (2009) Haemangioma in the oesophagus of a red–eared slider (*Trachemys scripta elegans*). *Acta Veterinaria Hungarica* **57(4)**, 477–484

Garner M, Johnson C and Funk R (1994) Liposarcoma in a shingleback skink (*Trachydosaurus rugosus*). *Journal of Zoo and Wildlife Medicine* **25(1)**, 150–153

Garner MM, Collins D and Joslin J (1995) Vertebral chondrosarcoma in a corn snake. *Proceedings of Joint Conference of the American Association of Zoo Veterinarians, Wildlife Disease Association, and American Association of Wildlife Veterinarians,* Houston, pp. 332–333

Garner MM, Hernandez–Divers SM and Raymond JT (2004) Reptile neoplasia: a retrospective study of case submissions to a specialty diagnostic service. *Veterinary Clinics of North America: Exotic Animal Practice* **7(3)**, 653–671

Garner MM, Lung NP and Murray S (1999) Xanthomatosis in geckos: five cases. *Journal of Zoo and Wildlife Medicine* **30(3)**, 443–447

Georoff TA, Stacey NI, Newton AN et al. (2009) Diagnosis and treatment of chronic T-lymphocytic leukemia in a green tree monitor (*Varanus prasinus*). *Journal of Herpetological Medicine and Surgery* **19(4)**, 106–114

Goldberg SR and Holshuh HJ (1991) A case of leukemia in the desert spiny lizard. *Journal of Wildlife Diseases* **27(3)**, 521–525

Gonzales-Viera O, Bauer G, Bauer A et al. (2012) Cutaneous fibroma in a captive common snapping turtle (*Chelydra serpentina*). *Journal of Comparative Pathology* **147(4)**, 574–576

Gravendyck M, Marschang RE, Schroder-Gravendyck AS and Kaleta EF (1997) Renal adenocarcinoma in a reticulated python (*Python reticulatus*). *Veterinary Record* **140(14)**, 374–375

Greenacre CB and Roberts R (2000) Effect of strontium–90 on squamous cell carcinoma in an eastern box turtle (*Terrapene carolina*): discussion of alternative treatment modalities. *Proceedings of the International Virtual Conference in Veterinary Medicine: Diseases of Reptiles and Amphibians, University of Georgia College of Veterinary Medicine*

Gregory CR, Harmon BG, Latimer KS et al. (1997) Malignant chromatophoroma in a canebrake rattlesnake (*Crotalus horridus atricaudatus*). *Journal of Zoo and Wildlife Medicine* **28(2)**, 198–203

Gregory CR, Latimer KS, Breckwoldt RA and Campagnoli RP (2000) Granulocytic sarcoma in a boa (*Boa constrictor*). *Proceedings of the International Virtual Conference in Veterinary Medicine: Diseases of Reptiles and Amphibians, University of Georgia College of Veterinary Medicine*

Gregory CR, Latimer KS, Howerth EW and Harmon BG (1995) A retrospective study of histologic lesions diagnosed in reptiles at the University of Georgia (January, 1989 to January, 1995). *Proceedings of Joint Conference of the American Association of Zoo Veterinarians, Wildlife Disease Association, and American Association of Wildlife Veterinarians,* Houston, pp. 463–484

Gyimesi ZS and Garner MM (2007) Pituitary adenoma in a Dumeril's ground boa, *Acrantophis dumerili*. *Journal of Herpetological Medicine and Surgery* **17(1)**, 16–18

Gyimesi ZS, Garner MM, Burns RB et al. (2005) High incidence of lymphoid neoplasia in a colony of Egyptian spiny-tailed lizards (*Uromastyx aegyptius*). *Journal of Zoo and Wildlife Medicine* **36(1)**, 103–110

Gyimesi ZS, Stedman NL and Crossett VR (2002) Cholesterol granulomas in a great plated lizard, *Gerrhosaurus major*. *Journal of Herpetological Medicine and Surgery* **12**, 36–39

Haag KM, Hernandez-Divers SM, Latimer KS and Hernandez-Divers SJ (2008) Infiltrative lipoma in a black rat snake, *Elaphe obsolete*. *Journal of Herpetological Medicine and Surgery* **17(4)**, 129–131

Hadfield CA, Clayton LA, Clancy MM et al. (2012) Proliferative thyroid lesions in three diplodactylid geckos: *Nephrurus amyae*, *Nephrurus levis*, and *Oedura marmorata*. *Journal of Zoo and Wildlife Medicine* **43(1)**, 131–140

Hahn KA, Richardson RC, Hahn EA and Chrisman CL (1994) Diagnostic and prognostic importance of chromosomal aberrations identified in dogs. *Veterinary Pathology* **31(5)**, 528–540

Hannon DE, Garner MM and Reavill DR (2011) Squamous cell carcinomas in inland bearded dragons (*Pogona vitticeps*). *Journal of Herpetological Medicine and Surgery* **21(4)**, 101–106

Harshbarger JC (1976) *Activities Report of the Registry of Tumors in Lower Animals, 1975 Supplement,* pp. 14–22. Smithsonian Institution Press, Washington, DC

Hernandez-Divers SJ, Knott CD and MacDonald J (2001) Diagnosis and surgical treatment of thyroid adenoma-induced hyperthyroidism in a green iguana (*Iguana iguana*). *Journal of Zoo and Wildlife Medicine* **32(4)**, 465–475

Hernandez-Divers SM and Garner MM (2003) Neoplasia of reptiles with an emphasis on lizards. *Veterinary Clinics of North America: Exotic Animal Practice* **6**, 251–273

Hernandez-Divers SM, Orcutt CJ, Stahl SJ et al. (2003) Lymphoma in lizards: three case reports. *Journal of Herpetological Medicine and Surgery* **13(1)**, 14–22

Hidalgo-Vila J, Martinez-Silvestre A and Diaz-Paniagua C (2006) Benign ovarian teratoma in a red-eared slider turtle (*Trachemys scripta elegans*). *Veterinary Record* **159(1)**, 122–123

Hill JR (1977) Oral squamous cell carcinoma in a California king snake. *Journal of the American Veterinary Medical Association* **171(9)**, 981–982

Honour SM, Ayroud M and Wheler C (1993) Metastatic chondrosarcoma and subcutaneous granulomas in a grey rat snake (*Elaphe obsoleta obsoleta*). *Canadian Veterinary Journal* **34(4)**, 238–240

Irizarry-Rovira AR, Wolf A and Ramos-Vara JA (2006) Cutaneous melanophoroma in a green iguana (*Iguana iguana*). *Veterinary Clinical Pathology* **35(1)**, 101–105

Jacobson E, Calderwood MB, French TW et al. (1981) Lymphosarcoma in an eastern king snake and a rhinoceros viper. *Journal of the American Veterinary Medical Association* **179(11)**, 1231–1235

Jacobson ER (1984) Chromomycosis and fibrosarcoma in a mangrove snake. *Journal of the American Veterinary Medical Association* **185(11)**, 1428–1430

Jacobson ER and Ackerman N (1981) What is your diagnosis? Snake swelling. *Journal of the American Veterinary Medical Association* **179(11)**, 1311–1312

Jacobson ER, Ferris W, Bagnara JT and Iverson WO (1989) Chromatophoromas in a pine snake. *Pigment Cell Research* **2**, 26–33

Jacobson ER, Long PH, Miller RE et al. (1986) Renal neoplasia of snakes. *Journal of the American Veterinary Medicinal Association* **189(9)**, 1134–1136

Jacobson ER, Seely JC and Novilla MN (1980) Lymphosarcoma associated with virus-like intranuclear inclusions in a California king snake (Colubridae: *Lampropeltis*). *Journal of the National Cancer Institute* **65(3)**, 577–583

Jessup DA (1980) Fibrosing adenocarcinoma of the intestine of a gopher snake (*Pituophis melanoleucus*). *Journal of Wildlife Diseases* **16(3)**, 419–421

Keck M, Zimmerman DM, Ramsay EC, Douglass M and Reavill DR (2011) Renal adenocarcinoma in Cape coral snakes (*Aspidelaps lubricus lubricus*). *Journal of Herpetological Medicine and Surgery* **21(1)**, 5–9

Krause K, Reavill DR and Weldy SH (2015) Cloacal Carcinoma in a Desert Iguana (*Dipsosaurus dorsalis*). *Proceedings ExoticsCon,* San Antonio, TX, pp. 655

Kummrow MS, Berkvens CN, Paré JA and Smith DA (2010) Cerebral xanthomatosis in three green water dragons (*Physignathus cocincinus*). *Journal of Zoo and Wildlife Medicine* **41(1)**, 128–132

Kusewitt DF, Reece RL and Miska KB (1997) S-100 immunoreactivity in melanomas of two marsupials, a bird, and a reptile. *Veterinary Pathology* **34(6)**, 615–618

Langan JN, Adams WH, Patton S, Lindermann K and Schumacher J (2001) Radiation and intralesional chemotherapy for a fibrosarcoma in a boa constrictor, *Boa constrictor ortoni*. *Journal of Herpetological Medicine and Surgery* **11**, 4–8

Latimer KS and Rich GA (1998) Colonic adenocarcinoma in a corn snake (*Elaphe guttata guttata*). *Journal of Zoo and Wildlife Medicine* **29(3)**, 344–346

Latimer KS, Rich GA and Gregory CR (2000) Osteosarcoma in a California mountain kingsnake (*Lampropeltis zonata*). *Proceedings of the International Virtual Conference in Veterinary Medicine: Diseases of Reptiles and Amphibians, University of Georgia College of Veterinary Medicine*

Leach MW, Nichols DK, Hartsell W and Torgerson RW (1991) Radiation therapy of a malignant chromatophoroma in a yellow rat snake (*Elaphe obsoleta quadrivittata*). *Journal of Zoo and Wildlife Medicine* **22**, 241–244

Lemberger KY, Manharth A and Pessier AP (2005) Multicentric benign peripheral nerve sheath tumors in two related bearded dragons, *Pogona vitticeps*. *Veterinary Pathology* **42(4)**, 507–510

Levine BS (2004) Treatment of a malignant ovarian teratoma in a green iguana. *Exotic DVM* **6(4)**, 12–14

Linn MJ, McNamara T, Steinberg JJ and Kress Y (1996) Pituitary adenoma in a black-headed python (*Aspidites melanocephalus*). *Proceedings of the American Association of Zoo Veterinarians,* Puerto Vallarta, Mexico, p. 449

Lyons JA, Newman SJ, Greenacre CB and Dunlap J (2010) A gastric neuroendocrine carcinoma expressing somatostatin in a bearded dragon (*Pogona vitticeps*). *Journal of Veterinary Diagnostic Investigation* **22**, 316–320

Machotka SV (1984) Neoplasia in reptiles. In: *Diseases of Amphibians and Reptiles,* ed. GL Hoff, FL Frye and ER Jacobson, pp. 519–580. Plenum Press, New York

Machotka SV, Wisser J, Ippen R and Nawab E (1992) Report of dysgerminoma in the ovaries of a snapping turtle (*Chelydra serpentina*) with discussion of ovarian neoplasms reported in reptilians and women. *In Vivo* **6(4)**, 349–354

Martin JC, Schelling SH and Pokras MA (1994) Gastric adenocarcinoma in a Florida indigo snake (*Drymarchon corais couperi*). *Journal of Zoo and Wildlife Medicine* **25(1)**, 133–137

Martorell J, Soto S, Barrera S and Ramis A (2009) Case report: ovarian teratoma in a Mediterranean tortoise. *Compendium of Continuing Education for the Practicing Veterinarian* **31(4)**, 193–196

Mauldin GN and Done LB (2006) Oncology. In: *Reptile Medicine and Surgery, 2nd edition*, ed. DR Mader, pp. 299–322. Saunders Elsevier, St Louis, MO

McNulty E and Hoffman R (1995) Fibrosarcoma in a corn snake, *Elaphe guttata*. *Bulletin of the Association of Reptilian and Amphibian Veterinarians* **5(3)**, 7–8

Mendyk RW, Newton AL and Baumer M (2013) A retrospective study of mortality in varanid lizards (Reptilia: Squamata: Varanidae) at the Bronx Zoo: implications for husbandry and reproductive management in zoos. *Zoo Biology* **32(2)**, 152–162

Mikaelian I, Levine BS, Smith SG, Harshbarger JC and Wong VJ (2001) Malignant peripheral nerve sheath tumor in a bearded dragon, *Pogona vitticeps*. *Journal of Herpetological Medicine and Surgery* **11(1)**, 9–12

Mikaelian I, Lynch S, Harshbarger JC and Reavill DR (2000) Malignant chromatophoroma in a day gecko (*Phelsuma madagarescencis grandis*). *Exotic Pet Practice* **5(10)**, 1–2

Moulton JE (1990) *Tumors in Domestic Animals*. University of California Press, Berkeley, CA

Needle D, McKnight CA and Kiupel M (2013) Chondroblastic osteosarcoma in two related spiny-tailed monitor lizards (*Varanus acanthurus*). *Journal of Exotic Pet Medicine* **22(3)**, 265–269

Newman SJ, Brown CJ and Patnaik AK (2003) Malignant ovarian teratoma in a red-eared slider (*Trachemys scripta elegans*). *Journal of Veterinary Diagnostic Investigation* **15(1)**, 77–81

Oros J, Monagas P, Andrada M, Calabuig P and Pether J (2009) Metastatic fibrosarcoma in a captive Saharan horned viper (*Cerastes cerastes*) with high hepatic levels of cadmium. *Veterinary Record* **164(22)**, 690–692

Patterson-Kane JC and Redrobe SP (2005) Colonic adenocarcinoma in a leopard gecko (*Eublepharis macularius*). *Veterinary Record* **157(10)**, 294–295

Raiti P, Garner MM and Wojcieszyn J (2002) Lymphocytic leukemia and multicentric T-cell lymphoma in a diamond python, *Morelia spilota spilota*. *Journal of Herpetological Medicine and Surgery* **12**, 26–29

Ramis A, Pumarola M, Fernandez-Mora'n J *et al.* (1998) Malignant peripheral nerve sheath tumor in a water moccasin (*Agkistrodon piscivorus*). *Journal of Veterinary Diagnostic Investigation* **10(2)**, 205–208

Ramsay EC, Munson L, Lowenstein L and Fowler ME (1996) A retrospective study of neoplasia in a collection of captive snakes. *Journal of Zoo and Wildlife Medicine* **27(1)**, 28–34

Reavill DR, Dahlhausen B, Zaffarano B and Schmidt R (2002) Multiple cutaneous liposarcomas in a red-tailed boa, Boa constrictor, and chameleon. *Proceedings of the Association of Reptile and Amphibian Veterinarians*, Reno, Nevada, pp. 5–6

Reavill DR, Fassler SA and Schmidt RE (2000) Mast cell tumor in a common green iguana (*Iguana Iguana*). *Proceedings of the Association of Reptile and Amphibian Veterinarians*, Reno, Nevada

Reavill DR and Schmidt RE (2003) Lipomas In cornsnakes (*Elaphe guttata guttata*): a series of four cases. *Proceedings of the Association of Reptile and Amphibian Veterinarians*, Reno, Nevada

Reavill DR and Schmidt RE (2004) Malignant chromatophoromas in three veiled chameleons, *Chamaeleo calyptratus*. *Proceedings of the Association of Reptile and Amphibian Veterinarians*, Naples, Florida, pp. 131–132

Reed SD, Reed FM and Castleman WL (2007) Successful surgical management of advanced xanthomatosis in a leopard gecko, *Eublepharis macularius*. *Journal of Herpetological Medicine and Surgery* **17(1)**, 19–21

Rest JP, Haire RN, Litman RT, Ross S and Litman G (1995) Identification and characterization of T-cell antigen receptor-related genes in phylogenetically diverse vertebrate species. *Immunogenetics* **42**, 204–212

Ritter JM, Garner MM, Chilton JA, Jacobson ER and Kiupel M (2009) Gastric neuroendocrine carcinomas in bearded dragons (*Pogona vitticeps*). *Veterinary Pathology* **46**, 1109–1116

Roberts WG, Klein MK, Loomis M, Weldy S and Berns MW (1991) Photodynamic therapy of spontaneous cancers in felines, canines, and snakes with chloro-aluminum sulfonated phthalocyanine. *Journal of the National Cancer Institute* **83(1)**, 18–23

Romagnano A, Jacobson ER, Boon GD *et al.* (1996) Lymphosarcoma in a green iguana (*Iguana iguana*). *Journal of Zoo and Wildlife Medicine* **27(1)**, 83–89

Rosskopf WJ, Howard EB and Gendron AP (1981) Granulocytic leukemia in a tortoise. *Modern Veterinary Practice* **62(9)**, 701–702

Ryan MJ, Hill DL and Whitney GD (1981) Malignant chromatophoroma in a gopher snake. *Veterinary Pathology* **18(6)**, 827–829

Ryan MJ and Whitney GD (1980) Xanthoma in a gopher snake. *Veterinary Medicine, Small Animal Clinician* **75(3)**, 503–507

Santoro M, Stacy BA, Morales JA *et al.* (2008) Mast cell tumour in a giant Galapagos tortoise (*Geochelone nigra vicina*). *Journal of Comparative Pathology* **138(2–3)**, 156–159

Schlumberger HG and Lucke B (1948) Tumors of fishes, amphibians, and reptiles. *Cancer Research* **8(12)**, 657–754

Schmidt RE and Hubbard GB (1987) Central nervous system. In: *Atlas of Zoo Animal Pathology, Volume 2*, pp. 117–124. CRC Press, Boca Raton, FL

Schmidt RE and Reavill DR (2012) Metastatic chondrosarcoma in a corn snake (*Pantherophis guttatus*). *Journal of Herpetological Medicine and Surgery* **22(3–4)**, 67–69

Schönbauer M, Loupal G and Schönbauer-Längle A (1982) Osteoid chondro-sarcoma in a desert monitor (*Varanus griseus*). *Berliner und Münchener Tierärztliche Wochenschrift* **95(10)**, 193–194

Schultze AE, Mason GL and Clyde VL (1999) Lymphosarcoma with leukemic blood profile in a savannah monitor lizard. *Journal of Zoo and Wildlife Medicine* **30(1)**, 158–164

Schumacher J, Bennett RA, Fox LE *et al.* (1998) Mast cell tumor in an eastern kingsnake (*Lampropeltis getulus getulus*). *Journal of Veterinary Diagnostic Investigation* **10(1)**, 101–104

Silverstone AM, Garner MM, Wojcieszyn JW and Couto CG (2002) Lymphoblastic leukemia in a diamondback terrapin (*Malaclemys terrapin*). *Proceedings of the Sixth International Symposium on the Pathology of Reptiles and Amphibians*, Saint Paul, MN, pp. 117–122

Stanley B (1999) Granulocytic sarcoma in a king cobra. *Twenty-Seventh Annual Southeastern Veterinary Pathology Conference*, Tifton, GA

Steeil JC, Schumacher J, Hecht S *et al.* (2013) Diagnosis and treatment of a pharyngeal squamous cell carcinoma in a Madagascar ground boa (*Boa madagascariensis*). *Journal of Zoo and Wildlife Medicine* **44(1)**, 144–151

Stumpel JBG, Del-Pozo J, French A and Eatwell K (2012) Cardiac hemangioma in a corn snake (*Pantherophis guttatus*). *Journal of Zoo and Wildlife Medicine* **43(2)**, 360–366

Suedmeyer WK and Turk JR (1996) Lymphoblastic leukemia in an inland bearded dragon, *Pogona vitticeps*. *Bulletin of the Association of Reptilian and Amphibian Veterinarians* **6(4)**, 10–12

Sykes JM and Trupkiewicz JG (2006) Reptile neoplasia at the Philadelphia Zoological Garden, 1901–2002. *Journal of Zoo and Wildlife Medicine* **37(1)**, 11–19

Tocidlowski ME, McNamara PL and Wojcieszyn JW (2001) Myelogenous leukemia in a bearded dragon (*Acanthodraco vitticeps*). *Journal of Zoo and Wildlife Medicine* **32**, 90–95

Tuttle AD, Harms CA, Grafinger MS, Lewbart GA and Van Wettere AJNJ (2006) Splenic hemangiosarcoma in a corn snake, *Elaphe guttata*. *Journal of Herpetological Medicine and Surgery* **16(4)**, 140–143

Whiteside DP and Garner MM (2001) Thyroid adenocarcinoma in a crocodile lizard, *Shinisaurus crocodilurus*. *Journal of Herpetological Medicine and Surgery* **11(1)**, 13–16

Wilson GH, Fontenot DK, Brown CA *et al.* (2004) Pseudocarcinomatous biliary hyperplasia in two green iguanas, *Iguana iguana*. *Journal of Herpetological Medicine and Surgery* **14(4)**, 12–18

Zwart P (2002) Pictorial guide to selected reptilian tumors. *Exotic DVM* **4(2)**, 20–21

Zwart P and Harshbarger JC (1972) Hematopoietic neoplasms in lizards: report of a typical case in *Hydrosaurus amboinensis* and of a probable case in *Varanus salvator*. *International Journal of Cancer* **15(9)**, 548–553

Chapter 24

Parasitology

Kevin Eatwell and Joanna Hedley

Parasitic infections are extremely common diseases seen in reptile medicine. Owners are often aware of the need for prophylactic control of parasites and many pharmaceutical products are available online or in pet shops without the need to consult a veterinary surgeon (veterinarian). However, there are side effects and contraindications to many of the potential medications that could be used, such as ivermectin, fenbendazole and metronidazole.

It is up to the veterinary surgeon to correctly diagnose the need for therapy. It is not just a question of identifying parasites in diagnostic samples, but determining if treatment is required. Parasites by definition are organisms that live on or in another (usually larger) host organism in order to obtain nutrients, while contributing nothing to the survival of the host. Parasites may not be detrimental to the host, but most clinicians consider them to be potential pathogens. Thus, diagnosing a parasitic infection in a sick reptile may not be related to the current illness, and eradication of the parasites may not yield the recovery of that animal. Both over- and under-treatment of parasites are therefore potential problems seen in veterinary medicine.

Parasites can have direct or indirect life cycles. Captive reptiles are rarely exposed to the intermediate hosts required for transmission of those species with indirect life cycles. Thus, recently imported animals may well have parasites with indirect life cycles not typically seen in the captive reptile population. These parasites are often short-lived and are only found in recently imported animals. The exceptions to this rule are the pentastomids, which can live for years (Riley and Self, 1980).

Parasites with direct life cycles do not require an intermediate host and are therefore commonly seen in captive reptiles. One of the problems in parasite control is environmental hygiene. Some parasites, such as *Cryptosporidium*, can have extremely resistant environmental stages which can be difficult to eradicate.

Specific genus identification of parasites may not be required in the clinical setting, provided the type of parasite is correctly identified and standard treatment employed with subsequent re-evaluation of samples to confirm successful treatment. However, should the clinician be unfamiliar with parasitology, then images can be taken and forwarded to more experienced parasitologists or references sought with photograph galleries of parasites for comparison, such as Foreyt (2001b). Many clinicians may prefer to send diagnostic samples directly to an external laboratory for evaluation.

This chapter covers methods for the diagnosis of parasite infection, followed by the common species identified, and ends with the treatment, prevention and control of parasitic infections.

Diagnosing a parasitic infection

Specimen collection

Generally, diagnostic samples are taken from the reptile directly or from its immediate environment. It is considered worthwhile performing parasite screening in healthy individuals as well, as part of a diagnostic work-up for a sick reptile. The most commonly analysed sample will be a faecal sample.

It is good practice to encourage owners to bring in a fresh sample of their pet reptile's faeces when presenting it for either a health check or illness. Many owners routinely screen their reptiles for endoparasites and faecal samples can often be posted to the clinic so that the results are available when the reptile arrives for its consultation. Samples are often taken from the enclosure of group-housed reptiles or can be pooled from multiple faecal deposits. In these cases, the concern is with the general parasite load and often all individuals in the group are treated based on the findings.

It is important that faecal samples are as uncontaminated as possible, as free-living organisms from soil or aged water can lead to confusion when analysing samples. Ideally, samples should be taken from the surface of the base of the enclosure, e.g. from the plastic or wooden base, from the sheet newspaper used as substrate, or from the surface of rocks or slates used. It is important that the sample is fresh and not desiccated (for example, it is best to avoid samples voided directly under a heat lamp). Owners should be advised on the suitable packaging of samples, both in terms of keeping the sample moist during transit (by wrapping a sample in cling film or using a screw-top container) and preventing leakage of the sample and contamination of the outer layers of the parcel. It is also important that owners are able to distinguish faecal material from solid urates. This is generally more of a problem with snakes, which only pass faeces intermittently. The owners should be instructed to wear disposable gloves when collecting the sample, and use a wooden spatula to scrape the faeces into the container. They should wash their hands afterwards. If there is a delay in sending the samples they should be refrigerated and double bagged.

Reptiles can often present because of anorexia, and this can cause problems as there can be limited faecal output. In these cases, providing assisted feeding and warmth may increase gastrointestinal motility, enabling a sample to be collected. Handling a reptile may promote faecal passage. Otherwise, bathing the reptile in clean, tepid water can encourage voiding and is an effective way of obtaining a sample; however, there is a risk of breakdown and dilution of the sample so any faeces passed should be removed immediately. This method of collection also risks bacterial contamination of the sample, which may compromise the reliability of culture results. Alternatively, a faecal sample can be collected directly from the reptile by performing a cloacal wash. The reptile is gently restrained with the cloaca facing the person collecting the sample. Initially, a gloved finger can be used to stimulate the cloaca and, in larger individuals, be inserted into the cloacal opening. This can encourage voiding of the cloacal contents, a technique that works very well in tortoises, and may yield a much better sample. If this fails, a catheter or solid crop needle can be inserted into the cloaca (Figure 24.1). Gentle manipulation may again encourage the reptile to void faeces, but if this is unsuccessful too, the tube should be directed dorsally (in order to try to avoid entering the bladder in those species that have one). Ideally, the end of the tube should be in the distal colon, but in practice it can be difficult to guarantee this placement unless the reptile is small (one can feel it pass through the rectum). An appropriate amount of either warmed water or physiological saline is infused according to the size of the animal, at 1–2 ml per 100 g bodyweight (McArthur *et al.*, 2004) (up to 1% of bodyweight). The reptile is gently manipulated and the sample aspirated.

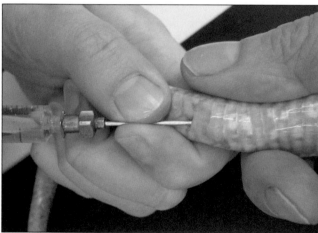

24.1 Cloacal flush being performed on a corn snake using an avian crop tube.

Faecal sample analysis

There are a number of techniques used to evaluate faecal samples. Initially, a simple gross examination of the submitted sample is appropriate. Firstly, it is important to confirm that faecal material is present and then to evaluate the volume. This will determine the suitability of differing tests. For example, an accurate McMaster egg count will require 3 g of faeces using standard laboratory techniques. Obtaining 3 g of faeces can be difficult in most of the species commonly seen in practice. Common gross abnormalities seen in faecal samples include:

- Changes in consistency: fresh normal faeces should be somewhat formed, depending on the species. Diarrhoea or constipation may be an indicator of parasitic infection
- Changes in coloration may be affected by food eaten or indicate malabsorption from the intestinal tract or parasites

- A reddish-brown/dark tarry discoloration may indicate the presence of digested blood and bright red streaks may be apparent if there is fresh blood loss. Blood of any description may indicate severe parasitic infection or a serious intestinal disease
- Mucus can be the result of parasitic infection or a digestive disorder
- Adult parasites or tapeworm segments may be found (Figure 24.2).

Faecal analysis can be easily performed in-house by both veterinary surgeons and veterinary nurses/technicians. If the practice lacks the facilities or experience of faecal analysis, the samples can be sent to an external laboratory. Generally, in-house testing is more economical and quicker than external laboratories. Quantitative techniques are less commonly used unless the clinician is testing the efficacy of a treatment protocol. The routine protocols in common use are detailed in Figures 24.3 and 24.4.

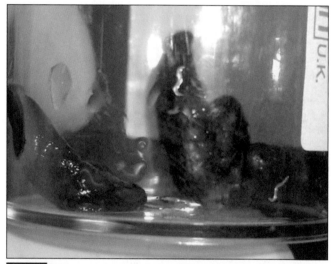

24.2 Oxyurids can be seen in this faecal sample pot from a tortoise.

Flotation	Usage
Salt flotation	These are used most commonly, but can severely distort parasite eggs. The maximum specific gravity obtainable is only 1:200, which allows heavier eggs to remain submerged. However, it is easy and economical to make up the solution from rock salt, which is added to water until no more dissolves and can be seen on the bottom of the container (usually 40 g per 100 ml). Heavy eggs (such as fluke eggs) will not float in this solution
Zinc sulphate flotation	Add approximately 371 g of zinc sulphate to 1 litre of water while stirring continuously (mild heating can be used to hasten the dissolution process). If possible, check the specific gravity and adjust as needed
Sodium nitrate flotation	Add approximately 400 g of sodium nitrate to 1 litre of water while stirring continuously (mild heating can be used to hasten the dissolution process)
Sugar flotation	Pour 355 ml of **warm** water into a beaker and place on a hot plate. Heat water on high but **do not boil**. Slowly add 454 g granulated sugar, stirring constantly until dissolved completely. Remove from heat and cool

24.3 Flotation solutions in common use.
(More detail can be found in Foreyt, 2001a)

Technique	Details	Notes
Wet preparation	Commonly used as a simple screen. A small amount of faecal material is suspended in a drop of warmed saline or water on a glass slide. This is mixed thoroughly with an applicator stick to form a homogeneous solution. Large pieces of faecal material should be removed. The smear should be thin enough to read print through. This can be examined under the X10 objective for eggs and larvae and then under X40 for motile protozoa and cysts. If the sample has been chilled it can be rested on a heated coin to encourage motility on the slide. A wet preparation is the first test performed on any faecal sample	This is used to get a general feel for parasite numbers and will readily allow for the identification of eggs and motile parasites. There will be increased amounts of particulate faecal matter, which can lead to problems with accurate identification of parasites
Faecal flotation	Up to 2 g of faeces are added to 10–20 ml of the flotation solution and gently mixed thoroughly. This is poured through a tea strainer (or alternative) and large particulate matter is discarded. The filtered liquid is titrated into a small container and topped up with flotation solution to form a meniscus. A coverslip is gently placed on top of the tube. The tube is allowed to rest for 20–30 minutes. This is necessary for eggs to float to the surface, but not long enough for the eggs to become waterlogged and sink again or become distorted. The coverslip is then removed by pulling it vertically off the top and is placed on to a glass slide. This is then examined under X10 and X40 objectives. A flotation can be performed easily in practice	This is a useful technique for small samples and is generally used alongside a wet preparation to reduce the risk of low levels of eggs being missed (Hedley *et al.*, 2013). There is usually less contamination of the sample with particulate matter, making it easier to identify the eggs present. This technique is of no use for the detection of motile parasites
McMaster technique	Mix 3 g of faeces with 42 ml of flotation solution (approximately 45 ml total volume) and strain through a tea strainer. Leave the solution to stand for 20–30 minutes. Remove the meniscus with a pipette and load the McMaster chamber on both sides. Count all eggs which lie within the lined 1 cm² of the counting chamber and repeat for the second side. The calculation is based on the fact that the depth of the chamber is 1.5 mm and the volume of fluid examined is 0.15 ml, which is 1/300 of the original volume of 45 ml. Therefore, each egg counted represents 300 per 3 g of faeces, which is equivalent to 100 eggs/g. When done in duplicate, the total count of the two chambers is multiplied by 100 and divided by 2	This is useful if the sample obtained is large enough and the volumes used are accurate. Owing to the small size of many faecal samples, a standard McMaster technique may be impossible; however, it is often used for larger reptiles
Modified McMaster technique	Weigh out 1 g of faeces and mix with 15 ml of flotation solution. Strain through a tea strainer and fill up both sides of the McMaster slide. Leave to stand for 20–30 minutes. Examine both grids, counting the number of worm eggs present in both. This can be performed with half the volume necessary for the McMaster technique, and the calculation is the same as above. A quantitative float can be performed on small sample sizes should quantitative egg counts be required	Useful down to 0.5 g of faeces. If the sample is smaller still, then use it all for a flotation technique
Sedimentation technique	Mix the faeces with water or saline. Strain the mixture through a tea strainer and pour into a centrifuge tube. Centrifuge the tube (with a balance) for 3 minutes at 1500 rpm. Slowly pour the liquid off the top without disturbing the sediment layer (including fine silty material) on the bottom. Using a Pasteur pipette, transfer a small amount of the sediment to the microscope slide – dilute with water if too thick	Useful if there is only a small volume of faeces, or if a cloacal wash has been performed
Formalin and ethyl acetate concentration	Place 6 ml of 10% buffered formalin into a centrifuge tube. Add faeces and emulsify thoroughly. Leave overnight on the bench; many parasites will form cysts and ova will be preserved by the formaldehyde. The following morning, mix gently and strain the sample through a tea strainer. Add 5 ml ethyl acetate and mix gently, leave for 10 minutes for the fat globules to dissolve and centrifuge at 1500 rpm for 30 seconds. Decant the supernatant off and resuspend the deposit by flicking the tube and, using a pipette, place a drop on the slide and dilute with water if too thick. Examine under the microscope. A formalin ethyl acetate concentrate can be stored overnight and used to detect very small numbers of faecal parasites	This method is ideal for tiny samples as all faeces received are concentrated. It is also useful for speed if you have no chance to look immediately. The risk of catching any zoonotic diseases is also reduced. However, this is not to be used for any motile parasites

24.4 Routine faecal analysis.
(More detail can be found in Zajac and Conboy, 2012)

Staining of faecal smears

Staining of faecal samples is often used for the detection of protozoa. Staining generally kills off protozoa and encourages them to encyst, and so these techniques are often used alongside a wet preparation for motile ciliates and flagellates.

Iodine staining can be used by adding a drop of Lugol's iodine to the saline mixture to fix and stain protozoa prior to smearing the sample on a glass slide. This, however, prevents motility and so is less commonly performed. However, one commonly used staining method is for *Cryptosporidium* detection. *Cryptosporidium* staining kits are commercially available (Pro-Lab *Cryptosporidium* Staining Kit, Pro-Lab Diagnostics) and are a modified cold Ziehl–Neelson stain (Figure 24.5). Using a swab, make a paper-thin smear of faeces or stomach contents on a slide. Smears can also be made from swabs taken from the outside of regurgitated matter. Smears should be almost transparent, and adding physiological saline to the sample can facilitate smearing. The slide is air dried and covered with a fixative (methanol) and left for approximately 10–15 minutes, until the fixative has evaporated. The slide is then flooded with strong carbol fuchsin and left for a further 10 minutes. It is then washed off with tap water and flooded with Differentiator 1 (hydrochloric acid), and left until no more pink colour appears to come out. This process is repeated a second time, again until no more pink colour appears to come out. The slide is given another rinse and flooded with malachite green and left for 30 seconds. The slide is given a final rinse and then examined under the X100 oil-immersion objective. Oocysts appear as bright red ovals approximately 4 μm in length, whereas bacteria and yeasts stain pale green (Figure 24.6). Casemore *et al.* (1985) describe the techniques for *Cryptosporidium* detection in more detail. *Cryptosporidium* can also be detected by immunofluorescent staining, which is 16 times more sensitive than acid-fast staining (Graczyk *et al.*, 1995, 1996a).

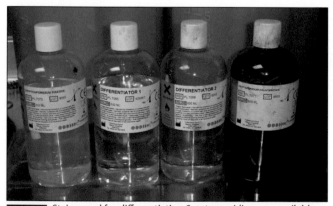

24.5 Stains used for differentiating *Cryptosporidium* are available commercially.

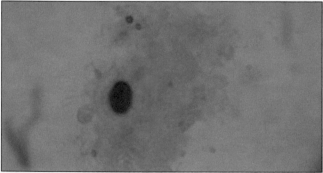

24.6 A faecal sample smear from a gecko, highlighting one red *Cryptosporidium* oocyst on a green background.

Detection of ectoparasites

Ectoparasites such as mites can be seen quite often on lizards and snakes. Typically, adhesive tape strips are used to remove parasites and these are examined directly under the microscope. Many ectoparasites have motile stages, and these may also be identified in the environment. Ectoparasites can also be identified on the shed skin of lizards and snakes. Ticks can be identified on recently imported specimens. These are often removed using commercially available tick removers. Cytological assessment of external lesions using skin scrapings or tape cytology may also yield ectoparasites. Cytology is covered in more detail in the diagnostic sampling and laboratory tests chapter (Chapter 8).

Haemoparasites

These can be intracellular or extracellular and are often detected on blood smears; they are covered in detail in Chapter 8.

Other methods of diagnosis

Histopathology can be used to identify parasites in tissues. Typically, specimens from gastric biopsies are used for the detection of *Cryptosporidium* in snakes, aiming to identify a host pathological response to the parasite to rule out misidentification with mammalian *Cryptosporidium* from the prey. Parasites are also often identified on post-mortem examination of tissue for histopathology.

Indeed, it is possible for parasites to be identified during imaging (for example, endoscopy) or to be found in tissue samples submitted for histopathology or cytology. It is important to have parasitism on your list of differentials and rule it out.

Pseudoparasites

It is important to ensure that any diagnosis of parasitism is accurate. Debris, pollen and other faecal material can mimic parasites, leading to a misdiagnosis. It is also important to realize that reptiles can shed parasites from prey items in their faeces, which have no effect on the reptile host. In snakes, one such example is the faecal shedding of mouse mites in the faeces, or the ingestion of ectoparasites such as snake mites (Figure 24.7). Of more concern is the shedding of *Cryptosporidium parvum*. In those species feeding on mammalian prey (such as

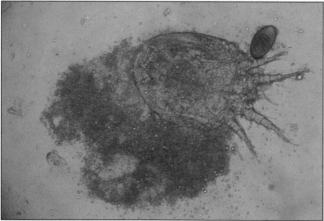

24.7 A snake mite and an oxyurid egg have been identified in this faecal sample from a water dragon. The mite must have been ingested by the lizard.

snakes), *Cryptosporidium* from the prey can be passed in the faeces of the reptile. This can be detected on faecal *Cryptosporidium* stains, which will not differentiate between mammalian and reptilian *Cryptosporidium*. This demonstrates the importance of confirming the pathogenicity of any parasite identified in a faecal sample. Reptiles may also ingest mites from their environment or from shed skin, with a typical example being *Ophionyssus*.

Types of parasites

Ectoparasites

Mites are the most common ectoparasite seen on pet reptiles, and of these *Ophionyssus natricis* is the most significant. Although it is generally known as the 'snake mite', lizards and even tortoises can also be susceptible (Wiechert, 2007). Animals are commonly presented after mites have been seen either on the reptiles themselves or in their environment. Scratching or rubbing behaviour may be observed, or alternatively other behavioural changes such as hyperactivity or increased bathing time because of irritation. Mites may cause physical skin damage, or lead to dysecdysis and even secondary bacterial or fungal skin infections. More serious consequences include dehydration and anaemia following heavy infestations or potentially the transmission of blood-borne infections. Humans may occasionally be infected too and dermatitis has been reported as a consequence of mite infection (Schultz, 1975).

On physical examination, mites may be found attached between scales, especially around the eyes (Figure 24.8), ears, corners of the mouth, axillae, inguinal folds and cloaca. Different species of mites have different morphology, and species may be confirmed by microscopic examination. *Ophionyssus* mites may be red, tan, grey or black depending on the stage in their life cycle and whether they have fed recently. Other mites which may be seen include pterygosomatid mites such as *Hirstiella*, a small red mite which can affect lizards (Figure 24.9). Trombiculid mites (harvest mites) may also be found on reptiles kept outdoors, but although the larvae (chiggers) may cause local skin irritation, adults are free-living in the environment and do not appear to feed on reptiles or cause disease.

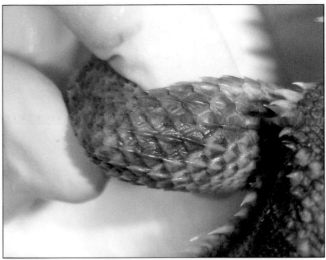

24.9 Pterygosomatid mites present between the scales of a bearded dragon.

Mite problems can escalate quickly and spread rapidly throughout reptile collections owing to their short life cycle of 7–16 days (Wozniak and DeNardo, 2000). Eggs are laid in the environment in warm humid crevices, such as cracks in wood, hide boxes or under the enclosure lid, where they hatch into larvae. Development to adult mite involves both feeding and non-feeding life stages and adults are able to persist for up to 40 days with or without feeding. Consequently, thorough prolonged treatment of both the reptile and the environment is required to target both phases of the life cycle and eliminate infection. Mite infestations are often associated with cramped conditions, poor hygiene or the introduction of new animals to a collection without a period of quarantine, so any underlying husbandry problems should also be corrected.

Ticks are an uncommon problem in captive-bred reptiles but may be seen in animals kept outside or those that have been recently imported. Low numbers may cause minor skin irritation and secondary infection but rarely result in significant problems. High numbers, however, usually indicate poor husbandry or underlying disease. Ticks are also vectors of various bacterial, viral and protozoal blood-borne infections, such as haemoparasites for example. These infections may not necessarily cause clinical disease in a reptile but could result in reptiles acting as reservoirs for infections. This was a significant concern in tortoises imported from Africa to Florida, which were found to harbour ticks infected with *Cowdria ruminantium* (heartwater) (Burridge *et al.*, 2000). All newly imported animals should be carefully examined for the presence of ticks, and reptiles kept outside should also be regularly checked and ticks manually removed if found. Fly strike (myiasis) can also be a problem in reptiles kept outside (Sales *et al.*, 2003). Blowflies such as *Calliphora* and *Lucilia* may deposit eggs on any area of broken skin or prolapsed tissue (Figure 24.10), and even around the eyes, nares and cloaca in debilitated animals. Eggs rapidly develop into larvae which burrow further into the tissue resulting in extensive damage, secondary infections and potentially fatal toxin release. Early detection of the larvae is vital and any deep infected wounds should be carefully examined for the presence of larvae or eggs. Larvae may be manually removed or the affected region may need to be surgically excised. Supportive treatment including analgesia, antibiotics and fluid therapy should be considered and in severe cases euthanasia may be necessary.

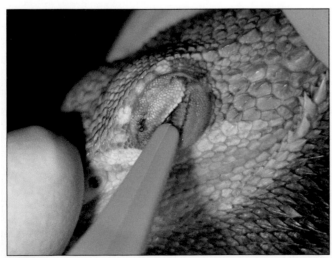

24.8 Snake mites around the eye of a bearded dragon.

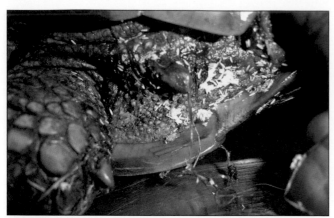

24.10 Fly eggs have been laid on this spur-thighed tortoise with a cloacal prolapse.

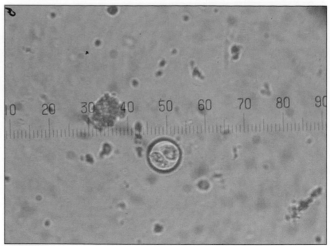

24.11 *Isospora amphiboluri* oocyst in a faecal flotation from a bearded dragon.

Leeches are rarely seen in pet reptiles although they can be found on wild-caught individuals from aquatic environments. In low numbers they rarely cause damage but in high numbers local trauma, inflammation, secondary infection and potentially anaemia may occur. Leeches have also been implicated as a mechanical vector for fibropapilloma-associated herpesvirus in marine turtles (Greenblatt *et al*., 2004). Manual removal is possible, but saltwater soaks for freshwater species (or freshwater for marine species) may be necessary to encourage detachment of the leeches' mouthparts without causing further tissue damage.

Gastrointestinal parasites

Protozoa

Flagellates: Flagellates, primarily trichomonads, are a common finding in faecal samples from both healthy and sick reptiles and are generally considered to be non-pathogenic in low numbers. High numbers, however, are often associated with anorexia, weight loss and diarrhoea, especially in carnivorous species, and treatment of animals with clinical signs is recommended. Tortoises may also be infected by a more significant flagellate, *Hexamita parva*, which can potentially result in fatal renal disease (Zwart and Truyens, 1975). Individuals affected by hexamitiasis may show non-specific signs of illness including lethargy, anorexia and weight loss and, more specifically, liquid mucogelatinous urine may be passed. Infection is thought to occur by ingestion of an infective cyst which passes through the gastrointestinal tract and via the cloaca up the ureters to the kidneys, where the parasite encysts resulting in renal damage. Although shed in the urine, *Hexamita* may be seen in faecal samples owing to mixing within the cloaca. It can, however, be easily missed owing to its small size and rapid movements and, as with other flagellates, will rapidly desiccate and die in small samples. Definitive diagnosis requires detection of the parasite on renal biopsy with associated inflammatory changes. Both specific parasite treatment such as metronidazole and supportive care for renal disease are recommended for these cases.

Coccidia: Coccidia are another common finding in faecal samples, especially in agamids, chameleons and geckos. Various coccidian species may be seen, and types of oocysts are generally differentiated by the number of sporocysts contained within an oocyst (Barnard and Upton, 1994). *Eimeria* species normally contain four sporocysts, *Isospora* (Figure 24.11) and *Sarcocystis* contain two, and *Caryospora* contains one. A low number of any of these coccidia can often live within the intestines without causing clinical disease. However, numbers may rapidly escalate in young animals, especially in association with poor hygiene, overcrowding or concurrent disease. *Isospora amphiboluri* is a common problem in young bearded dragons and may result in enteritis in high numbers. Concurrent infection with adenovirus is also possible, leading to a wide range of clinical signs. Animals are often presented for anorexia, lethargy, weight loss, diarrhoea, tenesmus or prolapses, and death may occur if untreated. Treatment of coccidia is therefore recommended for young animals or those with a moderate to high parasite burden.

Alternatively, some coccidia may colonize organs beyond the intestinal tract. For example, *Choleoeimeria* is a coccidia which develops in the gall bladder of lizards and can eventually result in bile duct obstruction, gallbladder dilatation and death. Reptiles may show clinical signs of lethargy, weight loss and jaundice, although in species with pigmented mucous membranes this may be hard to assess. Faeces should be examined for oocysts, but they may not always be detected especially if the bile duct has become obstructed (Schneller and Pantchev, 2008a). Intranuclear coccidiosis has also been described in a number of different chelonian species, with variable clinical signs including anorexia, lethargy, wasting and oculonasal discharges. Numerous organs may be affected, including the liver, kidneys and pancreas. Histopathology is required for diagnosis (Innis *et al*., 2007). Treatment with standard anticoccidials so far appears ineffective for non-intestinal coccidiosis.

Cryptosporidium is a small coccidian parasite frequently encountered in a wide variety of wild and captive reptiles worldwide. Unlike other coccidia, pathogenicity does not appear to depend on number of parasites, but instead reduced immunocompetence of the host or presence of other concurrent disease. In snakes it generally causes hypertrophic gastritis (Figure 24.12), with signs including gastric swelling, regurgitation, weight loss and eventual death (Brownstein *et al*., 1977). In lizards, enteritis is the more common form, with associated anorexia, diarrhoea, weight loss and again eventual death (Terrell *et al*., 2003). Less common presentations include aural polyps, cloacal prolapse and cystitis (Fitzgerald *et al*., 1998; Kik *et al*., 2011). Alternatively, an asymptomatic carrier state appears to be common (Deming *et al*., 2008). Disease is uncommonly diagnosed in chelonians (Hedley *et al*., 2013). Both gastric and intestinal forms may occur.

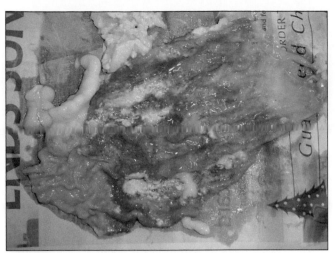

24.12 The stomach lining of a corn snake on post-mortem examination. Hypertrophy and excessive mucus are present. *Cryptosporidium* was identified on microscopy of the mucus.

Diagnosis is challenging owing to variable shedding of the oocysts in faeces. Repeat testing is therefore usually recommended to screen for the parasite (Deming *et al.*, 2008). Alternatively, samples may be obtained (depending on the species) from the mucus of regurgitated food items, by gastric lavage or cloacal washes, or from post-mortem cytology (Graczyk *et al.*, 1996). *Cryptosporidium serpentis* and *C. varanii* (= *C. saurophilum*) appear to be the main species involved in infection in pet reptiles (Fayer, 2010). Unlike mammalian strains, none of the reptile strains of *Cryptosporidium* have been reported to be zoonotic so far. However, *C. parvum* and *C. muris* have also been identified in faecal samples, and have been suggested to originate from mammalian prey and pass through the reptile gastrointestinal system without causing pathology in the reptile (Pedraza-Diaz *et al.*, 2009). A positive result from an asymptomatic snake should therefore be interpreted with caution, and ideally the species of *Cryptosporidium* determined by polymerase chain reaction (Xiao *et al.*, 2004). Alternatively, histopathology may be performed to confirm the presence of the parasite within a vacuole at the border of epithelial cells. Biopsies may be performed surgically or endoscopically, but the parasite can have a patchy distribution within the stomach, so false negative results are not uncommon. Immunofluorescent antibody testing can be used to confirm the species of *Cryptosporidium*.

Treatment of cryptosporidiosis is another challenge, with no completely successful treatment regime reported. Paromomycin treatment in Gila monsters reduced clinical signs and led to a cessation of oocyst shedding, but results appear inconsistent (Paré, 1997). Bovine hyperimmune colostrum has shown more promise, with small studies in snakes and monitors showing a significant reduction in oocyst shedding, in addition to histopathological resolution of disease after a course of treatment (Graczyk *et al.*, 1998, 2000). In geckos, however, in which intestinal cryptosporidiosis is more common, colostrum treatment appeared less efficacious, possibly owing to changes to the structure of colostrum immunoglobulins after passing through the stomach (Graczyk *et al.*, 1999). Supportive treatments, including the use of an immunomodulator consisting of inactivated virus and equine serum protein, have also been advocated, although mechanism of action and efficacy are not described (Schneller and Pantchev, 2008b). In view of the lack of successful treatment regimes, cryptosporidiosis within a collection is normally best controlled by good management, such as quarantine and multiple testing of new arrivals to reduce the risk of introduction to an existing collection, alongside routine monitoring of the collection by screening and post-mortem examination. Disinfection of the environment is important to limit the spread of disease, but oocysts can be difficult to totally eradicate. Iodophors, cresylic acid, sodium hypochlorite, benzalkonium chloride and sodium hydrochlorite have all been trialled and found to be ineffective. Ammonia (5%) and formalin (10%) appear effective, but with a contact time of 18 hours at 4°C these may not be the most practical solutions (Campbell and Tzipori, 1982). Currently, moist heat (45°–60°C for 5–9 minutes), freezing or desiccation appear to be the most effective ways to clear the environment (Cranfield and Graczyk, 1996).

Euthanasia should always be considered if *Cryptosporidium* is causing clinical disease within an individual, or being shed within a collection. Although diagnosis is difficult, repeated *Cryptosporidium* screens should always be included as part of quarantine procedures within a collection. Any animals found to be shedding should be isolated in a separate room with separate feeding and cleaning utensils, treated at the end of the day, and potentially euthanased. Eradication once infection is established within a collection could be attempted by identification of infected reptiles and their removal, but owing to the low sensitivity of readily available economical diagnostic tests and the difficulty in eradicating environmental oocysts, this approach would be difficult. Instead, preventing infection from entering the collection is of utmost importance.

Ciliates: Ciliates such as *Balantidium* and *Nyctotherus* (Figure 24.13) are common findings in faecal samples of herbivorous reptiles (particularly tortoises) and are generally considered non-pathogenic. The *Balantidium* trophozoite may be identified by its ciliate appearance and oval shape, and measures 60 x 40–45 µm, while cysts are round and a similar size. *Nyctotherus* trophozoites are larger, measuring 50–260 x 30–90 µm, and cysts are ovoid and operculated (Barnard and Upton, 1994). It has been suggested that ciliates may play a useful role in digestion of plant material. They are often seen in high numbers in association with intestinal disease, but it is unclear if the protozoa are the inciting factor or increased as a consequence of disease. Occasionally, *Balantidium* has been reported to penetrate the intestinal mucosa, resulting in extensive necrosis and liver abscessation. Treatment is therefore recommended if there are gastrointestinal signs, but otherwise unlikely to be necessary.

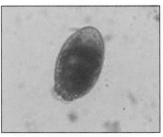

24.13 *Nyctotherus* identified on a wet preparation from a spur-thighed tortoise.

Amoebae: Various species of amoebae may be present within the gastrointestinal tract of herbivorous reptiles but are typically considered non-pathogenic. The main exception is *Entamoeba invadens*. Originally it was believed that this parasite was another commensal in the intestinal tract of herbivorous reptiles, with initial reports of disease described only in carnivorous species of snakes and lizards. Herbivorous chelonians were thought to be just carriers of this disease and never clinically affected. More recently, however, a variety of reports have described fatal amoebiasis in a variety of omnivorous and herbivorous tortoises (Hollamby *et al.*, 2000; Ozaki *et al.*, 2000; Philbey 2006). Juvenile tortoises have been suggested to be more susceptible, and both lack of food within the gastrointestinal tract and environmental temperature appear to play a role in parasite proliferation. A variety of clinical signs may occur but mucoid dysentery appears characteristic in most cases, with associated anorexia, wasting, dehydration and eventual death. Diagnosis of amoebiasis is possible by identification of amoebae, trophozoites (9–38.6 μm) or quadrinucleate cysts (9–24 μm) in a fresh faecal smear stained with iodine. Alternatively, on postmortem, intestinal ulceration, abscessation and areas of necrosis within many visceral organs, hepatitis, nephritis, and myonecrosis may be seen. Disease can spread rapidly owing to the parasite's direct life cycle, and is difficult to eradicate fully because of the resistance of both the trophozoite and the cysts, which can survive in the environment for over 14 days (McConnahie, 1955). Treatment targeting both trophozoites and cysts is therefore necessary in addition to thorough environmental decontamination. Agents such as paromomycin or iodoquinol are often combined with metronidazole in such cases.

Helminths

Nematodes: There are a wide variety of oxyurids (pinworms) found in reptiles, including *Oxyuris*, *Tachygonetria* and *Ozolaimus*. Tortoises and herbivorous or insectivorous lizards appear commonly affected. Eggs have a variable appearance but are generally thin walled, measuring ~130 x 40 μm, and may appear either oval or asymmetrical (D-shaped) (Figure 24.14) (Thapar, 1925). Adult worms are small-to-medium sized, measuring 1.5–7 mm in length, and live in the large intestine where they feed on intestinal contents and have a direct life cycle. They are generally considered to be commensals within the intestinal tract and have been suggested to have a beneficial effect in churning up faecal matter and so preventing constipation. However, intense infections of oxyurids have also been associated with anorexia, cloacal prolapse, stunted growth and even death, so treatment of high numbers should be considered (Martinez-Silvestre, 2011). Treatment is most commonly performed using benzimidazoles orally alongside environmental hygiene and is discussed later.

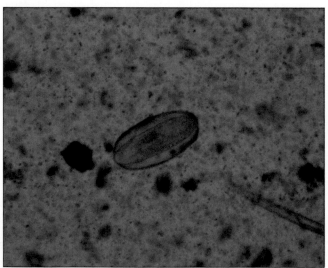

24.14 *Tachygonetria* ovum identified on a wet preparation from a Hermann's tortoise.

Ascarids: Ascarids are usually medium-to-large worms which live attached to intestinal mucosa and may affect a wide variety of reptile species. A variety of ascarids have been reported, including *Angusticaecum* and *Sulcascaris*. Adults are large and may be seen in faeces. Eggs are round with a thick shell and typically measure 80–100 x 60–80 μm (Jacobson, 2007) (Figure 24.15). In tortoises, ascarids appear to have a direct life cycle so may build up in captivity. In low numbers they may not cause any obvious problems, but in high numbers, weight loss, impaction, intussusception, gastrointestinal ulceration and coelomitis can all occur. Visceral migration of larvae may also result in pathology including pulmonary lesions and aural abscessation (Cutler, 2004). Treatment (typically with benzimidazoles) should therefore be considered. Ascarids of snakes and lizards, in contrast, usually have an indirect life cycle so are less likely to cause problems in captivity if there is no access to intermediate hosts, which are typically wild prey items such as rodents or amphibians.

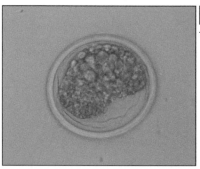

24.15 Ascarid ovum from a flotation from a Horsfield's tortoise.

Strongylids: Strongylids (hookworms) affect many species of reptiles but the most common is *Kalicephalus* infection in snakes. Eggs may be identified on faecal examination and measure ~70–100 x 40–50 μm. They appear thin walled with blunt ends, and the developing embryo fills most of the shell (Greiner and Mader, 2006). Adults are small worms ~1–1.5 cm in length and live in the gastrointestinal tract. At low levels they may cause no clinical signs, but significant damage to mucosa, weight loss and even anaemia can occur with heavier burdens. As they have a direct life cycle they can multiply rapidly in captivity and have been associated with gastrointestinal impaction and death, so treatment with benzimidazoles is generally recommended (Klaphake *et al.*, 2005).

Rhabditids: Rhabditids (threadworms) such as *Strongyloides* may affect both snakes and lizards. Infection occurs by oral or percutaneous penetration of larvae. These migrate to the lungs where they develop before passing up the trachea and back to the small intestine where they live as adults. Consequently, both respiratory and intestinal signs may be seen in an infected reptile. Thin-walled embryonated eggs may be detected on faecal examination and measure ~60 x 35 μm, but will appear similar to those of *Rhabdias* (Jacobson, 2007). *Rhabdias* has a similar life cycle except that adult worms live in the lungs, so respiratory signs are often more severe and pneumonia may result. Treatment with benzimidazoles for these parasites is recommended.

Cestodes: Cestodes (tapeworms) in reptiles require one or more intermediate hosts (i.e. molluscs, amphibians, fish, etc.) in order to replicate, so rarely build up to high numbers in reptiles in captivity. They may be found most commonly in aquatic or semiaquatic reptiles, although they have been identified in terrestrial species too, and are suggested to be non-pathogenic as long as they do not have access to an intermediate host in order to replicate. Adults live in the small intestine where they produce proglottids filled with eggs, which are shed in the faeces. Individual eggs may be distinguished by their variable number of refractile hooklets and should be distinguished from the tapeworm eggs of prey species (Frye, 1991). Sometimes whole adult worms may also be passed in the faeces. Problems can be seen in malnourished hosts or in animals where high numbers have led to intestinal damage. Signs include weight loss, regurgitation, constipation or diarrhoea. Treatment is therefore recommended to prevent potential problems. Parenteral praziquantel is often used as the agent of choice for these cases. Occasionally, reptiles can themselves become an intermediate host to some tapeworms. In these cases infective larvae may migrate throughout the body, potentially resulting in organ damage or subcutaneous swellings. Physical removal of larvae may be required.

Trematodes: Trematodes (flukes) are usually reported in wild-caught reptiles associated with an aquatic habitat as most require aquatic molluscs, fish or amphibians as their intermediate host. Consequently, they are rarely encountered in captivity as in most situations access to an intermediate host will be limited. They are generally thought to be relatively non-pathogenic except for the spirorchiids. These are a group of flukes which affect turtles and live within the heart and blood vessels. Consequently, they may potentially block small blood vessels causing ischaemia, necrosis and potentially organ failure (Johnson *et al.*, 1998). Trematode eggs are shed in faeces and are yellow–orange in colour, thin shelled and often operculated. Diagnosis generally requires specialized faecal sedimentation techniques (Wilkinson, 2004). Treatment with praziquantel is recommended to prevent potential problems.

Pentastomids: Pentastomids (tongue worms) are a significant problem owing to their zoonotic potential. They are generally found in imported reptiles as they require an intermediate host. They are not true 'worms' but actually primitive arthropods, and these parasites migrate through viscera causing significant damage. Clinical signs of disease are not always apparent in wild reptiles, although respiratory problems and excessive mucus in the mouth may be seen. Young animals may die of high parasite burdens. Eggs containing larvae with hooks may be detected in faeces, and will naturally then be ingested by an intermediate host such as a fish (Jacobson, 2007). Larvae will develop in this host, be eaten by the reptile and migrate to the lungs where they live as adults. Adult parasites appear superficially segmented and worm-like but have a hard cuticle and should be physically removed if possible. This can be achieved using coelioscopic techniques if they are in the lungs. Treatment with ivermectin is recommended.

Other parasites

Many different haemoparasites are reported in reptiles, including *Hepatozoon*, *Haemoproteus* and *Plasmodium*. Most require ectoparasite vectors such as ticks, flies or leeches, so do not appear to cause significant problems in captivity unless an aberrant host species is infected, where haemolytic anaemia can be a consequence (Wozniak and Telford, 1991). Diagnosis is usually made on examination of a blood smear (see Chapter 8). Treatments include the use of chloroquine or other antimalarial agents.

Microsporidian infections have been reported in bearded dragons, although the exact species has not been identified. Signs of systemic infection are variable, including anorexia, lethargy, weight loss and collapse. A variety of organs may be affected, including the liver, kidneys, ovaries (Figure 24.16), lungs and gastrointestinal tract, and diagnosis has so far only been made postmortem (Jacobson *et al.*, 1998). More recently, several cases of microsporidian conjunctivitis have been reported in bearded dragons, diagnosed on conjunctival biopsy. These appeared to resolve in response to treatment with fenbendazole, although it is unclear if they were genuinely localized infections or if these animals were actually systemically infected (Stidworthy *et al.*, 2008).

Filarial nematodes such as *Foleyella*, *Macdonaldius* and *Oswaldocruzia* are commonly seen in wild-caught reptiles, but less in captivity as they require a vector such as a mosquito for transmission (Mancianti *et al.*, 2001). Adult worms may live anywhere in the body but are often found in subcutaneous swellings and may cause irritation or physical damage to body organs. Alternatively, developing microfilaria may be found in blood vessels and can be detected on a blood smear. In large numbers they may potentially result in occlusion and ischaemic damage. Treatment with ivermectin has been attempted and appears to decrease the number of microfilaria but has not been found to be effective against adult worms (Bielli, 2007). Toxicity has been reported in some cases, so care should be taken with dosage of ivermectin used and supportive treatment may be necessary (Széll *et al.*, 2001). If possible, physical removal of all adult parasites is recommended.

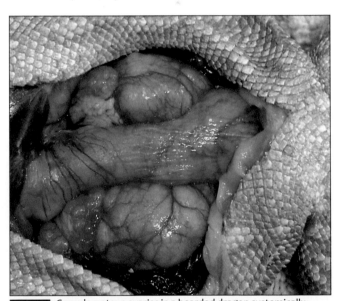

24.16 Granulomatous ovaries in a bearded dragon systemically infected with *Microsporidium*.

Prevention, treatment and control of parasitic infections

Prevention of parasitic disease starts with the routine screening of individuals for common parasites, indicating the need for treatment and control methods. It is generally considered that a quarantine period of 30–60 days is required to reduce the risk of parasites entering a collection, with routine testing and treatment being advocated during this period. Routine testing is typically recommended at the start of the quarantine period and would include evaluation for internal and external parasites. If any are identified, treatment can be provided alongside rigorous environmental hygiene. Subsequent testing is used to confirm that the treatment protocol has been effective. It is generally considered that it takes a longer time for faecal egg counts in reptiles to reduce to zero, up to 31 days in some species (such as terrestrial chelonians) (Giannetto et al., 2007). Subsequent testing of treated reptiles should be performed 14–28 days after the initial treatment course. A suggested quarantine protocol for the detection of parasites is outlined in Figure 24.17.

Days	Protocol
0	• Clinical examination for ectoparasites • Faecal wet preparation • Faecal flotation • *Cryptosporidium* testing
30	• Faecal wet preparation • Faecal flotation • *Cryptosporidium* testing
60	• Faecal wet preparation • Faecal flotation • *Cryptosporidium* testing

24.17 Suggested routine quarantine protocol for parasites.

Control of parasitic infections

As most of the parasites identified in captive reptiles have direct life cycles, strict hygiene is very important. There are a number of common factors that allow parasites to develop to large burdens in captivity.

Faecal material left in the tank of reptiles can be spread easily around the tank and contaminate food sources. Housing the reptile on particulate substrate makes it very difficult to remove all the faecal material and it is advised to house reptiles on sheets of newspaper in a spartan environment if they are undergoing screening or treatment for parasites. This enables thorough cleaning until effective treatment has been administered. Once the reptile is parasite free, then new cage furnishings and substrate can be provided.

Live invertebrate prey fed to insectivores can act as a source of reinfection by becoming contaminated with infective faecal material left in the vivarium. It is therefore important to ensure live food is eaten promptly or subsequently removed from the vivarium to avoid injury to the reptile. Live insect prey removed from the vivarium should not be returned to the tub as they could contaminate all the remaining live food. The insect prey can also contaminate other food and water sources.

Timing of treatment is also important. In the case of animals going into naturalistic vivaria or outside on to soil, treatment, with subsequent confirmation of the success of treatment, is required prior to release into an environment where parasite control is difficult to impossible. Animals that hibernate or brumate should be treated sufficiently early in the year to ensure effective treatment prior to entering hibernation/brumation.

Treatment options

It is important to ensure treatment has been effective, and, generally, direct administration parenterally, topically or orally is required to ensure the correct dosage has been provided for each animal. If recognized doses have been applied and environmental control has been rigorous, treatment failure may indicate resistance. In these cases, rotating different classes of drug may be indicated alongside monitoring of the parasite burdens of the reptiles being considered. Only commonly used agents, for a wide variety of parasitological problems, are discussed here.

Benzimidazoles

These are commonly used for gastrointestinal parasites, such as ascarids and oxyurids. It is important to accurately weigh and dose individual reptiles, as toxicity has been reported with these agents (Alvarado et al., 2001; Neiffer et al., 2005). Historically, treatment was commonly performed using oxfendazole but fenbendazole is routinely available as a companion-animal preparation in a liquid suspension and is generally preferred. However, it has been reported that fenbendazole-treated animals have positive faecal egg counts for longer (Giannetto et al., 2007). Common dosing regimens use a single high dose (100 mg/kg) orally, which may be repeated after 14 days, or a lower dose (25 mg/kg) repeated daily for 3–5 days, which is anecdotally reported to be more effective. Some reports do not support a repeat treatment at the 2-week interval (Giannetto et al., 2007), and repeat testing of an individual prior to readministering treatment is advised. High doses of fenbendazole have resulted in toxicity, with radiomimetic signs consistent with microtubule inhibition (Alvarado et al., 2001). Using lower doses over a few days is preferable.

Ivermectin

Ivermectin is commonly used in reptiles. It is important to note that toxicity – causing paresis and paralysis due to its gamma-aminobutyric acid (GABA) agonism – has been known in chelonians since 1983 (Teare and Bush, 1983) and similar signs can be seen in other species. However, milbemycin at a dose of 0.25–0.5 mg/kg by parenteral injection has been used with apparent effectiveness and no toxicity reported (Bodri and Hruba, 1992). Ivermectin is most commonly used as the treatment of choice for ectoparasites, both mites and ticks, in snakes and lizards. Deaths in chameleons have been reported when it has been used parenterally for treatment of filarial infections (Széll et al., 2001). Caution is also advised regarding indigo snakes, skinks and small lizards (Schneller and Pantchev, 2008a).

Levamisole

Levamisole is widely available in pet shops and commonly used to treat nematodes. Direct oral administration is advised as this is safer than parenteral administration owing to the narrow margin of safety. Care is needed as neurological signs have been reported (Rees Davis and Klingenberg, 2004). Typically, doses of 5–10 mg/kg have been used by injection and 10 mg/kg orally as a one-off dose. Higher doses of up to 50 mg/kg have been reported.

Fipronil

This is a GABA agonist widely used to control ectoparasites. The spray formulation (2.5 mg/ml) is sprayed on to a gauze swab and wiped across the surface of the reptile. This kills mites, and the wiping action may also dislodge them. The dose used in licensed species is 7.5 mg/kg and this should not be exceeded.

Toxic effects have been reported in chameleons and young boas, and risk is increased when the skin is more permeable during shedding (Schneller and Pantchev, 2008a).

Nitroimidazoles (e.g. metronidazole)

These are widely used for protozoal infections. The doses used are considerably higher than that used for its antibacterial action. Toxicity has been reported in indigo snakes, rattlesnakes and kingsnakes. Nitroimidazoles have action against ciliates and flagellates, but also amoeba trophozoites. Doses recommended are hugely variable, 40–100 mg/kg given as a single oral dose repeated after 14 days, or lower oral doses of 20–40 mg/kg q24h for 3–5 days.

Toltrazuril

Toltrazuril is commonly used to treat coccidiosis in reptiles. It is alkaline and is often diluted or mixed with food prior to oral dosing. The active metabolite ponazuril is also available and is less alkaline. Toltrazuril (15 mg/kg) or ponazuril (30 mg/kg) can be given orally every 48 hours, typically for two or three doses (Gibbons, 2014).

Trimethoprim/sulphonamides

These are used to treat coccidiosis. They are generally administered orally at a dose of 25 mg/kg for 3–5 days.

Permethrins

These have been recommended for control of ticks in many different species of reptile. Owing to the importance of reptile ticks as reservoirs for economically important diseases, a series of papers has been published. Permethrins have been shown to be superior in controlling ticks when compared with other agents such as fipronil (Burridge et al., 2002). Permethrin 5 mg/ml is sprayed directly on to tortoises (in the soft-tissue areas, generally for 10 seconds), but is not recommended for snakes and lizards. It has a wide safety margin in tortoises (Burridge et al., 2003).

Paromomycin

For amoeba cysts, 35–100 mg/kg is given daily by mouth. For the treatment of Cryptosporidium, 100 mg/kg is given daily for 7 days, then twice a week for 6 weeks (Grosset et al., 2011). Higher doses up to 800 mg/kg have been used in some species (Coke and Tristan, 1998).

Iodoquinol

This is given orally and is effective against amoeba cysts. A dose of 50 mg/kg q24h for 3 weeks is recommended.

Treatment of the environment

There are no specific therapeutic agents effective against nematode eggs, and eggs are resistant to disinfectants. Many protozoal oocysts are susceptible to disinfectants and these are detailed under the Protozoa section above. However, specific environmental treatments are used to control ticks and mites.

Ivermectin

Ivermectin has been used as an environmental spray to control mites. A topical pour-on solution (5 mg/ml) is mixed with propylene glycol and tap water to create an overall concentration of 5–10 mg/l. This can be easily achieved by mixing 1 ml of the pour-on solution with 1 ml of propylene glycol and 500 ml water in a hand-held sprayer. The mixture is then shaken and used immediately. Weekly application is advised.

Fipronil

This is used as an environmental spray (2.5 mg/ml) for mite control. The enclosure should be well ventilated prior to the animal being placed back inside to reduce the risk of toxicity. It is used once weekly for up to 6 weeks.

Permethrins

These have been used to successfully control ticks in naturalistic environments without the need for direct treatment of the reptiles, with the environment being treated every 2 weeks using a 5 mg/ml spray formulation. The animal and water sources are removed prior to treatment and returned the following morning once the enclosure is completely dry, to minimize the risk of toxicity (Burridge et al., 2003, 2004).

References and further reading

Alvarado TP, Garner MM, Gamble K et al. (2001) Fenbendazole overdose in four Fea's vipers (Azemiops feas). Proceedings of the Meeting of the American Association of Zoo Veterinarians, Association of Reptile and Amphibian Veterinarians, American Association of Wildlife Veterinarians, and National Association of Zoo and Wildlife Veterinarians, Orlando, Florida, pp. 28–29

Barnard SM and Upton SJ (1994) A Veterinary Guide to the Parasites of Reptiles, Volume I: Protozoa. Krieger, Malabar, FL, USA

Bielli M (2007) Preliminary notes on ivermectin to control Foleyella microfilaraemia in panther chameleon, Fucifer pardalis. Journal of Herpetological Medicine and Surgery 17(3), 104–106

Bodri MS and Hruba SJ (1992) Safety of milbemycin (A3–A4 oxime) in chelonians. Proceedings of the Joint Meeting of the American Association of Zoo Veterinarians and the American Association of Wildlife Veterinarians, pp. 156–157

Brownstein DG, Strandberg JD, Montali RJ, Bush M and Fortner J (1977) Cryptosporidium in snakes with hypertrophic gastritis. Veterinary Pathology 14, 606–617

Burridge MJ, Peter TF, Allan SA and Mahan SM (2002) Evaluation of safety and efficacy of acaricides for control of the African tortoise tick (Amblyomma marmoreum) on leopard tortoises (Geochelone pardalis). Journal of Zoo and Wildlife Medicine 33, 52–57

Burridge MJ, Simmons LA and Condie T (2004) Control of an exotic tick (Aponomma komodoense) infestation in a Komodo dragon (Varanus komodoensis) exhibit at a zoo in Florida. Journal of Zoo and Wildlife Medicine 35(2), 248–249

Burridge MJ, Simmons LA and Hofer CC (2003) Clinical study of a permethrin formulation for direct or indirect use in control of ticks on tortoises, snakes and lizards. Journal of Herpetological Medicine and Surgery 13, 16–19

Burridge MJ, Simmons LA, Simbi BH, Peter TF and Mahan SM (2000) Evidence of Cowdria ruminantium infection (heartwater) in Amblyomma sparsum ticks found on tortoises imported into Florida. Journal of Parasitology 86(5), 1135–1136

Campbell I and Tzipori S (1982) Effect of disinfectants on survival of Cryptosporidium oocysts. Veterinary Record 111, 414–415

Casemore DP, Armstrong M and Sands RL (1985) Laboratory diagnosis of cryptosporidiosis. Journal of Clinical Pathology 38, 1337–1341

Coke RL and Tristan TE (1998) Cryptosporidium infection in a colony of leopard geckos (Eublepharis macularius). Proceedings of the Association of Reptile and Amphibian Veterinarians Annual Conference, pp. 157–163

Cranfield MR and Graczyk TK (1996) Cryptosporidiosis. In: Reptile Medicine and Surgery, ed. DR Mader, pp. 359–363. WB Saunders, Philadelphia

Cutler SL (2004) Nematode-associated aural abscess in a Mediterranean tortoise, Testudo graeca. Journal of Herpetological Medicine and Surgery 14(3), 4–5

Deming C, Greiner E and Uhl EW (2008) Prevalence of Cryptosporidium infection and characteristics of oocyst shedding in a breeding colony of leopard geckos (Eublepharis macularius). Journal of Zoo and Wildlife Medicine 39(4), 600–607

Fayer R (2010) Taxonomy and species delimitation in Cryptosporidium. Experimental Parasitology 124, 90–97

Fitzgerald SD, Moisan PG and Bennett R (1998) Aural polyp associated with cryptosporidiosis in an iguana (Iguana iguana). Journal of Veterinary Diagnostic Investigation 10, 179–180

Foreyt WJ (2001a) Diagnostic parasitology. In: Veterinary Parasitology, 5th edition, ed. WJ Foreyt, pp. 3–9. Blackwell, Ames, IA

Foreyt WJ (2001b) Parasites of reptiles. In: Veterinary Parasitology, 5th edition, ed. WJ Foreyt, pp. 207–218. Blackwell, Ames, IA

Frye FL (1991) Applied clinical non-hemic parasitology of reptiles. In: Biomedical and Surgical Aspects of Captive Reptile Husbandry, Volume I, 2nd edition, ed. FL Frye, pp. 281–325. Krieger, Malabar, FL, USA

Giannetto S, Brianti E, Poglayen G et al. (2007) Efficacy of oxfendazole and fenbendazole against tortoise (Testudo hermanni) oxyurids. Parasitology Research 100(5), 1069–1073

Gibbons PM (2014) Advances in reptile clinical therapeutics. Journal of Exotic Pet Medicine 23(1), 21–38

Graczyk TK, Cranfield MR and Bostwick EF (1999) Hyperimmune bovine colostrum treatment of moribund leopard geckos (Eublepharis macularius) infected with Cryptosporidium sp.. Veterinary Research 30(4), 377–382

Graczyk TK, Cranfield MR and Bostwick EF (2000) Successful hyperimmune bovine colostrum treatment of savannah monitors (Varanus exanthematicus) infected with Cryptosporidium sp.. Journal of Parasitology 86(3), 631–632

Graczyk TK, Cranfield MR and Fayer R (1995) A comparative assessment of direct immunofluorescence antibody, modified acid fast stain and sucrose flotation techniques for the detection of Cryptosporidium serpentis oocysts in snake faecal specimens. Journal of Zoo and Wildlife Medicine 26(3), 396

Graczyk TK, Cranfield MR and Fayer R (1996a) Evaluation of commercial enzyme immunoassay (IFA) test kits for detection of Cryptosporidium oocysts other than Cryptosporidium parvum. American Journal of Tropical Medicine and Hygiene 54(3), 274–279

Graczyk TK, Cranfield MR, Helmer P, Fayer R and Bostwick EF (1998) Therapeutic efficacy of hyperimmune bovine colostrum treatment against clinical and subclinical Cryptosporidium serpentis infections in captive snakes. Veterinary Parasitology 74, 123–132

Graczyk TK, Cranfield MR and Hill SL (1996b) Therapeutical efficacy of spiramycin and halfuginone treatment against Cryptosporidium serpentis (Apicomplexa: Cryptosporiidiiae) infections in captive snakes. Parasitology Research 82(2), 143–148

Graczyk TK, Owens R and Cranfield MR (1996c) Diagnosis of subclinical cryptosporidiosis in captive snakes based on stomach lavage and cloacal sampling. Veterinary Parasitology 67, 143–151

Greenblatt RJ, Work TM, Balazs GH et al. (2004) The Ozobranchus leech is a candidate mechanical vector for the fibropapilloma-associated turtle herpesvirus found latently infecting skin tumors on Hawaiian green turtles (Chelonia mydas). Virology 321, 101–110

Greiner EC and Mader DR (2006) Parasitology. In: Reptile Medicine and Surgery, 2nd edition, ed. DR Mader, pp. 343–364. WB Saunders, St Louis

Grosset C, Villeneuve A, Brieger A et al. (2011). Cryptosporidiosis in juvenile bearded dragons (Pogona vitticeps): effects of treatment with paromomycin. Journal of Herpetological Medicine and Surgery 21, 10–15

Hedley J, Eatwell K and Shaw DJ (2013) Gastrointestinal parasitic burdens in UK tortoises: a UK survey of tortoise owners and potential risk factors. Veterinary Record 173, 525–526

Hollamby S, Murphy D and Schiller C (2000) An epizootic of amoebiasis in a mixed species collection of juvenile tortoises. Journal of Herpetological Medicine and Surgery 10, 9–15

Innis CJ, Garner MM, Johnson AJ et al. (2007) Ante-mortem diagnosis and characterization of nasal intranuclear coccidiosis in Sulawesi tortoises (Indotestudo forsteni). Journal of Veterinary Diagnostic Investigations 19, 660–667

Jacobson E (2007) Parasites and parasitic diseases of reptiles. In: Infectious Diseases and Pathology of Reptiles: Color Atlas and Text, pp. 571–665. CRC Press, Boca Raton, FL

Jacobson ER, Green DE, Undeen AH, Cranfield M and Vaughn KL (1998) Systemic microsporidiosis in inland bearded dragons (Pogona vitticeps). Journal of Zoo and Wildlife Medicine 29, 315–323

Jacobson ER, Schumacher J, Telford SR Jr et al. (1994) Intranuclear coccidiosis in radiated tortoises (Geochelone radiata). Journal of Zoo and Wildlife Medicine 25, 95–102

Johnson CA, Griffith JW, Tenorio P, Hytrek S and Lang CM (1998) Fatal trematodiasis in research turtles. Laboratory Animal Science 48(4), 340–343

Kik MJ, Van Asten A, Lenstra JA and Kirpensteijn J (2011) Cloaca prolapse and cystitis in green iguana (Iguana iguana) caused by a novel Cryptosporidium species. Veterinary Parasitology 175, 165–167

Klaphake E, Cross CA, Patton S and Head J (2005) Gastric impaction in a milk snake, Lampropeltis triangulum, caused by Kalicephalus sp. Journal of Herpetological Medicine and Surgery 15(1), 21–23

McArthur SM, McLellan L and Brown S (2004) Gastrointestinal system. In: BSAVA Manual of Reptiles, 2nd edition. BSAVA Publications, Gloucester, UK

McConnahie EW (1955) Studies of Entamoeba invadens Rodhain, 1934 in vitro, and its relationship to some other species of Entamoeba. Parasitology 45, 452–481

Mancianti F, Magi M, Bicchi F, Salvadori M and Verni F (2001) Filariasis in wild-caught chameleons. Veterinary Record 149(19), 596

Martinez-Silvestre A (2011) Massive Tachygonetria (Oxyuridae) infection in a Herman's tortoise (Testudo hermanni). Consult Journal (Special Edition) 409–412

Neiffer DL, Lydick D, Burks K and Doherty D (2005) Haematologic and plasma biochemical changes associated with fenbendazole administration in Hermann's tortoise (Testudo hermanni). Journal of Zoo and Wildlife Medicine 36(4), 661–672

Ozaki K, Matsuo K, Tanaka O and Narama I (2000) Amoebosis in the flat-shelled spider tortoise (Acinixys planicauda). Journal of Comparative Pathology 123(4), 299–301

Paré JA (1997) Treatment of cryptosporidiosis in Gila monsters (Heloderma suspectum) with paromomycin. Proceedings of the Association of Reptilian and Amphibian Veterinarians Annual Conference, p. 23.

Pedraza-Díaz S, Ortega-Mora LM, Carrión BA, Navarro V and Gómez-Bautista M (2009) Molecular characterization of Cryptosporidium isolates from pet reptiles. Veterinary Parasitology 23(160), 3–4

Philbey W (2006) Amoebic enterocolitis and acute myonecrosis in leopard tortoises (Geochelone pardalis). Veterinary Record 158, 567–569

Rees Davies R and Klingenberg RJ (2004) Therapeutics and medication In: BSAVA Manual of Reptiles, 2nd edition, ed. SJ Girling and P Raiti, pp. 115–130. BSAVA Publications, Gloucester

Riley J and Self JT (1980) On the systematics and life-cycle of the pentastomid Kiricephalus Sambon, 1922 with descriptions of three new species. Systematic Parasitology 1(2), 127–140

Sales MJ, Ferrer D, Castellà J, Borràs D and Hall MJ (2003) Myiasis in two Hermann's tortoises (Testudo hermanni). Veterinary Record 153(19), 600–601

Schmidt V, Dyachenko V, Aupperle H et al. (2008) Case report of systemic coccidiosis in a radiated tortoise (Geochelone radiata). Parasitology Research 102(3), 431–436

Schneller P and Pantchev N (2008a) General parasitology in snakes, lizards and chelonians. In: Parasitology in Snakes, Lizards and Chelonians: A Husbandry Guide, pp. 32–35. Edition Chimaira, Frankfurt am Main

Schneller P and Pantchev N (2008b) Parasitology in Snakes, Lizards and Chelonians: A Husbandry Guide, pp. 105–172. Edition Chimaira, Frankfurt am Main

Schneller P and Pantchev N (2008c) Parasitology in Snakes, Lizards and Chelonians. A Husbandry Guide. Edition Chimaira, Frankfurt am Main

Schultz H (1975) Human infestation by Ophionyssus natricis snake mite. British Journal of Dermatology 93(6), 695–697

Stidworthy M, Storm J, Hale G, Everett KG and Rodriguez Barbon A (2008) Microsporidial conjunctivitis in bearded dragons (Pogona vitticeps). Proceedings of the British Veterinary Zoological Society, p. 48

Széll Z, Sréter T and Varga I (2001) Ivermectin toxicosis in a chameleon (Chamaeleo senegalensis) infected with Foleyella furcata. Journal of Zoo and Wildlife Medicine 32(1), 115–117

Teare JA and Bush M (1983) Toxicity and efficacy of ivermectin in chelonians. Journal of the American Veterinary Medical Association 183(11), 1195–1197

Terrell SP, Uhl EW and Funk RS (2003) Proliferative enteritis in leopard geckos (Eublepharis macularius) associated with Cryptosporidium sp. infection. Journal of Zoo and Wildlife Medicine 34(1), 69–75

Thapar GS (1925) Studies on the oxyurid parasites of reptiles. Journal of Helminthology 3(3–4), 83–150

Upton SJ, McAllister CT, Freed PS and Barnard SM (1989) Cryptosporidium spp. in wild and captive reptiles. Journal of Wildlife Disease 25(1), 20–30

Wiechert JM (2007) Infection of Hermann's tortoises, Testudo hermanni boettgeri, with the common snake mite, Ophionyssus natricis. Journal of Herpetological Medicine and Surgery 17(2), 53–54

Wilkinson R (2004) Clinical pathology. In: Medicine and Surgery of Tortoises and Turtles, ed. S McArthur, R Wilkinson and J Meyer, pp. 141–186. Blackwell, Oxford, UK

Wozniak EJ and DeNardo DF (2000) The biology, clinical significance, and control of the common snake mite, Ophionyssus natricis, in captive reptiles. Journal of Herpetological Medicine and Surgery 10(3), 4–10

Wozniak EJ and Telford SR Jr (1991) The fate of Hepatozoon species naturally infecting Florida black racers and watersnakes in potential mosquito and soft tick vectors, and histological evidence of pathogenicity in unnatural host species. International Journal for Parasitology 21(5), 511–516

Xiao L, Ryan UM, Graczyk TK et al. (2004) Genetic diversity of Cryptosporidium spp. in captive reptiles. Applied and Environmental Microbiology 70(2), 891–899

Zajac AM and Conboy GA (2012) Faecal examination for the diagnosis of parasitism. In: Veterinary Clinical Parasitology, ed. AM Zajac and GA Conboy, pp. 3–170. Wiley-Blackwell, Chichester

Zwart P and Truyens EHA (1975) Hexamitiasis in tortoises. Veterinary Parasitology 1, 175–183

Chapter 25

Infectious diseases

Rachel Marschang and John Chitty

This chapter covers infectious diseases caused by viruses, bacteria and fungi. Infections of protozoa and other parasites are covered in Chapter 24. The conditions described are those caused by agents normally considered to be infectious, although in many cases the agents are secondary factors in disease situations. Exposure to infected animals often will not result in disease unless underlying factors are present and carrier status is common, with 'pathogens' routinely isolated from healthy animals. While Koch's postulates have been fulfilled in experimental situations for some agents (e.g. the *Chrysosporium* anamorph of *Nannizziopsis vriesii* (CANV); Paré *et al.*, 2006a), in the clinical situation these agents may be part of a multifactorial disease. The clinical approach reflects this (Figure 25.1) and requires a full appreciation of the animal's husbandry in addition to identification of infectious agents. If nothing else, the reptile's immune response appears to be related to environmental factors, particularly temperature (Stacy and Pessier, 2007).

Accordingly, apparent disease outbreaks within a collection may not be solely due to transmission of one infectious agent but may also reflect a shared husbandry defect (Figure 25.2) as well as multiple potential pathogens. The presence of opportunistic invaders further complicates diagnosis. Agents entering a naïve population, especially if

Disease	Primary factors	Secondary agents	Tertiary invaders
Scale rot in a vivarium of garter snakes	Poor hygiene, excess water in substrate, low temperature	e.g. *Pseudomonas aeruginosa*	Environmental bacteria
Upper respiratory tract infection in a colony of spur-thighed tortoises	Low temperature, poor body condition, unnatural climate	*Mycoplasma*, chelonid herpesvirus	Bacteria, yeasts

25.2 Examples of infectious diseases and associated stressors.

those individuals are stressed or have concurrent underlying disease, may be more pathogenic, e.g. a novel chelonid herpesvirus entering a naïve population of newly imported tortoises.

Viral infections

Reptile virology is an evolving field. Over the years, an increasing number of viruses have been detected in reptiles. New sequencing techniques have recently led to the detection of multiple probable viral pathogens in reptiles, e.g. arenaviruses associated with inclusion body disease (IBD) in boas and pythons (Stenglein *et al.*, 2012) and nidoviruses associated with respiratory disease in pythons (Stenglein *et al.*, 2014). Koch's postulates have only been fulfilled for a small number of these; for others, association with disease is based on pathological and histological findings or, in some cases, pure speculation. In some cases, viruses may be involved in disease processes when found in conjunction with other factors (environmental) or with other infectious agents, including other viruses. Viruses that have been described in reptiles are listed in Figures 25.3 to 25.7. Some of the common and important viral diseases found in reptiles most frequently kept as pets (tortoises, snakes and lizards) are discussed below in more detail.

When diagnosing viral infection in reptiles, it is important to remember that diagnostic tests have not been standardized and that the tests available will depend on the laboratory. A short overview of techniques that can be used for the detection of viruses in reptiles is provided.

Primary underlying factors = stressors
e.g. poor husbandry
These MUST be corrected

↓

Secondary infectious agents
e.g. viruses, bacteria, fungi
These require treatment

↓

Tertiary invaders
e.g. bacteria, fungi
These sometimes require treatment

25.1 A clinical approach to infectious diseases in reptiles.

Virus	Species	Clinical importance	Clinical and pathological signs	Common diagnostic methods	Samples for diagnostics
Adenoviridae: Siadenovirus	Sulawesi tortoises, impressed tortoises, Burmese star tortoises, leopard tortoise	+ to +++	Anorexia, lethargy, mucosal ulcerations, nasal and ocular discharge, diarrhoea	PCR, EM	Nasal flush, oral and cloacal swabs, plasma, liver
Adenoviridae: 'Testadenovirus'	Multiple tortoise species	+ to ++	Unknown. Found in clinically healthy turtles as well as in animals with mixed viral infections	PCR	Oral and cloacal swabs, liver, intestine
Herpesviridae	Wide range of tortoise spp., all chelonians should be considered susceptible	+++	Rhinitis, conjunctivitis, stomatitis and glossitis	PCR Serology: VNT	Oral swabs, tongue, trachea and oesophagus, liver, intestine, kidney and brain
Iridoviridae: Ranavirus	Wide range of tortoise species, viruses not species specific	+++	Upper respiratory tract disease, pneumonia, tracheitis, oesophagitis, pharyngitis, hepatitis, enteritis	PCR	Oral swabs, blood, liver, tongue
Papillomaviridae	Russian tortoise	(?)	Stomatitis	EM	Lung wash
Paramyxoviridae: Ferlavirus	Spur-thighed, Hermann's and leopard tortoises	(+++)	Pneumonia, dermatitis described in one case	RT-PCR	Oral and cloacal swabs, tracheal wash, lung, intestine, liver, kidney, trachea
Picornaviridae ('Topivirus', virus 'x')	Many tortoise species, including spur-thighed, marginated, Egyptian, and leopard tortoises	++	Softening of the carapace in young tortoises, diphtheroid necrotizing stomatitis and pharyngitis, conjunctivitis, rhinitis, pneumonia, enteritis, ascites	Virus isolation, RT-PCR Serology: VNT	Oral swabs, tongue, intestine, liver, kidney
Poxviridae	Hermann's tortoise	(+)	Skin lesions around the eye	Histology, EM	Material from lesions
Reoviridae	Hermann's and spur-thighed tortoises	(++)	Cachexia, stomatitis, glossitis, increased mortality, splenomegaly	Virus isolation, RT-PCR	Oral swabs, tongue, intestine, lung, liver
Togaviridae: WEE virus	Texas tortoises	–	None described have been shown to be infected	RT-PCR	Blood

25.3 Select viruses of land tortoises. Clinical importance in parentheses = only individual report or reports available, virus appears to be uncommon in these animals; +++ = highly pathogenic; – = no pathology associated with infection in available reports; ? = pathology unknown; EM = electron microscopy; PCR = polymerase chain reaction; RT-PCR = reverse transcriptase polymerase chain reaction; VNT = virus neutralization test. (Adapted from Jacobson (2007), Marschang (2011) and information presented in this chapter)

Virus	Species	Clinical importance	Clinical and pathological signs	Common diagnostic methods	Samples for diagnostics
Adenoviridae: 'Testadenovirus'	Box turtles, sliders	? to +++	Hepatitis, sudden death, also found in clinically healthy animals	PCR	Oral and cloacal swabs, liver, intestine
Bunyaviridae	Texas soft-shelled turtle	–	None described	Virus isolation	Blood
Circoviridae	Painted turtle	(+++)	Necrosis in spleen and liver	EM	
Herpesviridae	Water turtles, various species	? to +++	Stomatitis, lethargy, anorexia, subcutaneous oedema, pulmonary oedema, hepatic necrosis	PCR	Liver, oral and cloacal swabs
	Green sea turtles	++	Grey patch disease, necrotizing dermatitis	PCR	Skin, possibly liver
	Green, Pacific Ridley, olive Ridley, hawksbill, and loggerhead turtles	+++	Associated with fibropapillomatosis, fibropapillomas on the skin, in some cases the cornea, internal tumours also possible	PCR	Papillomas
	Green turtles	+++	Lung, eye and trachea disease (LETD): dyspnoea, buoyancy abnormalities, periglottal necrosis, necrotizing tracheitis, bronchopneumonia	PCR	Ocular and oral swabs, trachea, lung
	Loggerhead turtles	(++)	Loggerhead genital-respiratory HV (LGRV)	PCR	Oral and cloacal swabs, trachea, cloaca
	Loggerhead turtles	(++)	Loggerhead orocutaneous HV (LOCV)	PCR	Oral swabs, material from plaques, lung

25.4 Select viruses of box turtles, turtles and sea turtles. Clinical importance in parentheses = only individual report or reports available, virus appears to be uncommon in these animals; +++ = highly pathogenic; – = no pathology associated with infection in available reports; ? = pathology unknown; EM = electron microscopy; HV = herpesvirus; PCR = polymerase chain reaction; RT-PCR = reverse transcriptase polymerase chain reaction. (continues) (Adapted from Jacobson (2007), Marschang (2011) and information presented in this chapter)

▶

Virus	Species	Clinical importance	Clinical and pathological signs	Common diagnostic methods	Samples for diagnostics
Iridoviridae: Ranavirus	Wide range of species, particularly box turtles, but also sliders and other turtle species	+++	Upper respiratory tract disease, pneumonia, tracheitis, oesophagitis, pharyngitis, 'red neck disease', hepatitis, enteritis	PCR	Oral swabs, blood, liver
Papillomaviridae	Bolivian side-necked turtle	(+)	Skin lesions	Histology, EM	Skin lesions
	Loggerhead turtle	(+)	Small white papules on skin	EM, PCR	Skin lesions
	Green turtle	(+)	Small white papules on skin	EM, PCR	Skin lesions
Retroviridae	Green turtles	?	Found in tissues of turtles with fibropapillomatosis, not believed to be the causative agent of this disease	EM	
Togaviridae and *Flaviviridae*	Various turtle species	–	Various species have been found to be susceptible to infection with arboviruses from the togaviruses (e.g. eastern equine encephalitis (EEE) virus) and flaviviruses (e.g. Japanese encephalitis virus, West Nile virus). No pathology associated with infection	RT-PCR	Blood
'Tornovirus'	Green turtles	?	Animals also had severe fibropapillomatosis (HV infection)	Metagenomics	

25.4 (continued) Select viruses of box turtles, turtles and sea turtles. Clinical importance in parentheses = only individual report or reports available, virus appears to be uncommon in these animals; +++ = highly pathogenic; – = no pathology associated with infection in available reports; ? = pathology unknown; EM = electron microscopy; HV = herpesvirus; PCR = polymerase chain reaction; RT-PCR = reverse transcriptase polymerase chain reaction.
(Adapted from Jacobson (2007), Marschang (2011) and information presented in this chapter)

Virus	Species	Clinical importance	Clinical and pathological signs	Common diagnostic methods	Samples for diagnostics
Adenoviridae: Atadenovirus	Various snake species including boas, pythons, colubrids and viperids	++	Hepatitis, pneumonia, regurgitation, head tilt	PCR	Cloacal swabs, liver, intestine
Arenaviridae	Boas and pythons	+++	IBD-associated virus	RT-PCR	Oesophageal swabs, whole blood, brain, liver, pancreas
Bornaviridae	Vipers, pythons, colubrids	– to ++	Associated with neurological disease in some cases	RT-PCR	Oral and cloacal swabs, brain
Caliciviridae	Rattlesnakes	(++)	Enteritis, hepatitis	EM, virus isolation	Intestine, liver
Herpesviridae	Boa constrictor, monocled cobra, horned vipers	(++ to +++)	Lethargy, anorexia, dyspnoea, liver necrosis, poor venom quality	PCR	Altered tissues
Iridoviridae: erythrocytic virus	A number of different snake species, including free-ranging and captive-bred snakes	?	From no clinical signs to anaemia and systemic disease	Histology, EM	Blood
Iridoviridae: Ranavirus	Green tree pythons, other snake species also susceptible	(+++)	Ulceration of nasal mucosa, hepatic necrosis, severe necrotizing inflammation of the pharyngeal submucosa	Virus isolation, PCR	Oral swabs, oral mucosa, liver
Nidovirales: Torovirinae	Pythons, rarely found in boas	+++	Stomatitis, proliferative pneumonia	RT-PCR	Oral swabs, tracheal washes, lung, intestine
Paramyxoviridae (PMV): Ferlavirus	Viperid, colubrid, elapid and boid snakes	+++	Respiratory disease and CNS disorders	RT-PCR	Oral and cloacal swabs, tracheal washes, lung, liver, kidney, pancreas
Parvoviridae	Kingsnakes	(+++)	Gastroenteritis	Histology, EM	Intestine

25.5 Select viruses of snakes. Clinical importance in parentheses = only individual report or reports available, virus appears to be uncommon in these animals; +++ = highly pathogenic; – = no pathology associated with infection in available reports; ? = pathology unknown; CNS = central nervous system; EM = electron microscopy; IBD = inclusion body disease; PCR = polymerase chain reaction; RT-PCR = reverse transcriptase polymerase chain reaction. (continues)
(Adapted from Jacobson (2007), Marschang (2011) and information presented in this chapter)

Virus	Species	Clinical importance	Clinical and pathological signs	Common diagnostic methods	Samples for diagnostics
Picornaviridae	Aesculapian snake		Gastrointestinal disease	Histology, EM	Intestine
Retroviridae	Boas, pythons, vipers, colubrids	– to ++	From none to neoplasia; endogenous retroviruses detected in various species. Retroviruses also detected in a number of snakes with IBD but not considered the cause of disease	Histology, EM, virus isolation, PCR	Liver, kidney, affected tissues
Reoviridae	Multiple snake species	+ to +++	Pneumonia, stomatitis, wasting, CNS signs	Virus isolation, RT-PCR	Oral swabs, lung, liver, brain
Sunviridae	Pythons	+ to +++	Respiratory and CNS disease	RT-PCR	Oral and cloacal swabs, lung, brain
Togaviridae and *Flaviviridae* (e.g. western equine encephalitis, eastern equine encephalitis, Japanese encephalitis and West Nile viruses)	Various colubrid species	–	None (arboviruses capable of infecting mammals)	RT-PCR	Blood

25.5 (continued) Select viruses of snakes. Clinical importance in parentheses = only individual report or reports available, virus appears to be uncommon in these animals; +++ = highly pathogenic; – = no pathology associated with infection in available reports; ? = pathology unknown; CNS = central nervous system; EM = electron microscopy; IBD = inclusion body disease; PCR = polymerase chain reaction; RT-PCR = reverse transcriptase polymerase chain reaction.
(Adapted from Jacobson (2007), Marschang (2011) and information presented in this chapter)

Virus	Species	Clinical importance	Clinical and pathological signs	Common diagnostic methods	Samples for diagnostics
Adenoviridae: Atadenovirus	Many different species of lizards, particularly common in bearded dragons	+ to +++	None seen in some cases; anorexia, opisthotonus, hepatitis, enteritis, nephritis	PCR	Cloacal swabs, liver, intestine
Bunyaviridae	Australian skink	–	None (arboviruses also capable of infecting mammals)	Virus isolation	Blood
Herpesviridae	Iguanas, agamas, plated lizards, monitors	+ to +++	Cutaneous papillomas, hepatic necrosis, stomatitis, pneumonia	PCR	Oral and cloacal swabs, liver, material from lesions
Iridoviridae: erythrocytic virus	Several different species including wild-caught animals	– to ++	No pathology observed in some cases, anaemia possible, systemic disease possible	Histology, EM, PCR	Blood
Iridoviridae: invertebrate iridovirus (IIV)	Multiple lizard species, particularly bearded dragons and chameleons	?	Cachexia, pneumonia, skin lesions	PCR	Skin, liver
Iridoviridae: Ranavirus	Numerous lizard species	+++	Granulomatous lesions on the tongue and tail, hepatitis, skin lesions	PCR, virus isolation	Oral and cloacal swabs, skin, liver
Papillomaviridae	European green lizards	+	Skin lesions	Histology, EM	Skin
Paramyxoviridae: Ferlavirus	Several lizard species including Caiman lizards	– to +++	Proliferative pneumonia	RT-PCR	Oral and cloacal swabs, lung
Parvoviridae	Bearded dragons	(?)	Found together with adenovirus infections in individual animals	EM	Liver
Poxviridae	Flap-necked chameleon, tegu	(+)	Skin lesions	Histology, EM	Skin, spleen, liver
Reoviridae	Multiple lizard species	++	Often associated with respiratory and neurological disease	Virus isolation, RT-PCR	Oral and cloacal swabs, lung
Rhabdoviridae	Australian house gecko, teiid lizards	(–)	None (arboviruses also capable of infecting mammals)	Virus isolation	Blood
Togaviridae and *Flaviviridae* (e.g. western equine encephalitis, eastern equine encephalitis, Japanese encephalitis, and West Nile viruses)	Various species including iguanas and skinks have been shown to be susceptible to infection	–	None (arboviruses also capable of infecting mammals)	Virus isolation, EM	Blood

25.6 Select viruses of lizards. Clinical importance in parentheses = only individual report or reports available, virus appears to be uncommon in these animals; +++ = highly pathogenic; – = no pathology associated with infection in available reports; ? = pathology unknown; EM = electron microscopy; PCR = polymerase chain reaction; RT-PCR = reverse transcriptase polymerase chain reaction.
(Adapted from Jacobson (2007), Marschang (2011) and information presented in this chapter)

Virus	Species	Clinical importance	Clinical and pathological signs	Common diagnostic methods	Samples for diagnostics
Adenoviridae	Nile crocodiles	(+++)	Underweight, delayed development, hepatic necrosis	Histology, EM	Liver
Flaviviridae: West Nile virus	American alligators; other crocodilians can also be infected	++ to +++	CNS signs, star gazing, stomatitis, hepatitis, myocardial degeneration, pneumonia, skin lesions (arboviruses also capable of infecting mammals)	Virus isolation, RT-PCR	Blood
Herpesviridae	Various crocodile species and American alligators	(+–++)	Skin lesions, lesions around the cloaca, lymphoid proliferation, encephalitis, pharyngitis	Virus isolation, PCR	Material from lesions
Poxviridae	Caimans and crocodiles	+ to ++	Wart-like skin lesions	Histology, EM, PCR in crocodiles	Skin
Retroviridae	Crocodilians	–	Endogenous retroviruses found in multiple species	PCR	

25.7 Select viruses of crocodilians. Clinical importance in parentheses = only individual report or reports available, virus appears to be uncommon in these animals; +++ = highly pathogenic; – = no pathology associated with infection in available reports; CNS = central nervous system; EM = electron microscopy; PCR = polymerase chain reaction; RT-PCR = reverse transcriptase polymerase chain reaction.
(Adapted from Jacobson (2007), Marschang (2011) and information presented in this chapter)

Herpesviridae

Herpesviruses are large enveloped viruses with a double-stranded DNA genome and an icosahedral capsid (Figure 25.8). Studies on tortoise herpesviruses have shown that they probably belong in the *Alphaherpesvirinae* subfamily (Bicknese *et al.*, 2010), in the newly accepted genus *Scutavirus* (Davison and McGeoch, 2010), which currently contains a fibropapilloma-associated virus of sea turtles. Herpesviruses can cause latent infections in animals, and any animal that has undergone infection must be considered a lifelong carrier. Among reptiles, herpesviruses are most commonly reported as important pathogens in tortoises, although they have also been described in other chelonians as well as in snakes, lizards and crocodilians. There are at least four genetically distinct tortoise herpesviruses. Two of these have been isolated in cell culture from tortoises in Europe and are also serologically distinct.

Tortoise herpesviruses

Species affected: Herpesviruses have been found in a wide range of tortoise species. They are most commonly described in the spur-thighed, Hermann's and Horsfield's tortoises, but all tortoise species should be considered susceptible. Different species may have different susceptibility to disease and different virus strains may differ in their pathogenicity. Hermann's and Horsfield's tortoises are highly susceptible to common herpesvirus infections, while spur-thighed tortoises appear to be relatively resistant, although they also sometimes develop disease. This difference in reaction to infection makes it particularly important not to mix species when keeping or treating tortoises.

Clinical signs and pathology: Herpesvirus infections in tortoises are commonly associated with rhinitis, conjunctivitis, stomatitis and glossitis. This frequently develops into a diphtheroid necrotizing stomatitis and glossitis, with diphtheroid membranes covering parts of the oral cavity and extending down into the trachea and oesophagus (Figure 25.9). Oedema of the neck is a common sign. Animals are generally anorexic and lethargic. Herpesvirus infection appears to be an important cause of upper respiratory tract disease (URTD) and is, therefore, an important differential diagnosis for mycoplasmosis in tortoises. Animals that survive acute herpesvirus infection may develop central nervous system (CNS) disorders including paralysis or incoordination. Infected animals may become latently infected and either shed virus inapparently or develop disease at a later date.

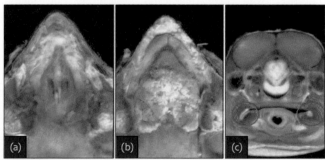

25.9 Post-mortem sections of a herpesvirus-infected Horsfield's tortoise with (a) stomatitis, (b) glossitis and (c) oesophagitis.
(Courtesy of Udo Hetzel)

Histology: Herpesviruses cause eosinophilic intranuclear inclusions in infected tissues, most frequently in epithelial cells of the tongue, oral mucosa and upper respiratory tract, as well as in the gastrointestinal tract, typically from the oesophagus to the duodenum (Figure 25.10). Inclusions can also be found in epithelial cells of the urinary tract and in the brain, liver and spleen. Inclusions may not be visible if there is extensive necrosis, or may only be visible in focal areas on the edges of necrotic areas (McArthur *et al.*, 2002).

25.8 Electron micrograph of herpesvirus nucleocapsids. This herpesvirus was isolated from the tongue and oesophagus of a Horsfield's tortoise. (Negative staining of cell culture supernatant with phosphotungstic acid)

`100 nm`

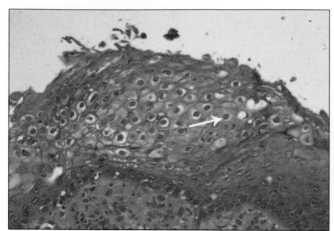

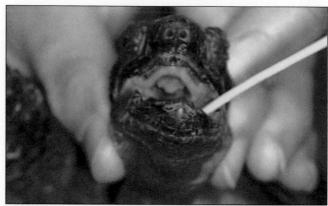

25.11 Oral swabs can be used to diagnose herpesvirus infections in tortoises.

25.10 Histopathology of the tongue of a leopard tortoise infected with herpesvirus, showing ballooning degeneration of epithelial cells. Eosinophilic intranuclear inclusions and margination of chromatin are visible in numerous epithelial cells. (Haematoxylin and eosin; original magnification X20)
(Courtesy of Horst Posthaus)

Diagnosis: There are a number of tests available for the diagnosis of herpesviruses in tortoises. These include serological tests and methods for direct virus detection.

For serological testing, a virus neutralization test and an enzyme-linked immunosorbent assay (ELISA) have been described (Origgi *et al.*, 2001); the virus neutralization test is more widely available. Both tests are influenced by the tortoise species being tested and the virus serotype used in the test. Not all tortoise species will seroconvert equally; for example, spur-thighed tortoises tend to seroconvert readily and have measurable antibody titres, while Hermann's and Horsfield's tortoises tend to have lower to non-existing titres. The virus serotype is also important, since the two serotypes that have been described do not cross-react and exposure to one serotype cannot be measured using a test against the other serotype. Seroconversion against herpesviruses in tortoises may take 4–9 weeks, so that the time point at which serology is carried out after infection is also important. It is advisable to retest negative animals after at least 2 months. Latently infected animals may not always have measurable antibody titres.

Both immunohistochemistry and *in situ* hybridization methods have been described to identify herpesvirus infection in histological samples (Teifke *et al.*, 2000; Origgi *et al.*, 2003). In live animals the use of impression smears of the tongue for herpesvirus diagnosis in tortoises has been described (Müller *et al.*, 1990). In some cases, intranuclear inclusions can be observed in the epithelial cells. This method can be difficult to interpret and is relatively non-specific.

Detection of viral DNA by polymerase chain reaction is the method of choice for the detection of tortoise herpesviruses. Several different polymerase chain reaction tests (PCRs) have been used to detect herpesviruses in samples from tortoises (Origgi *et al.*, 2000; Teifke *et al.*, 2000; Une *et al.*, 2000). In general, a pan-herpesvirus PCR is used to screen samples (van Devanter *et al.*, 1996; Marschang *et al.*, 2006), which can be followed by a second PCR or sequencing for further confirmation and typing. Virus isolation has also been used as a diagnostic tool. It is much slower than PCR but can be helpful in some cases. For virus detection (both PCR and virus isolation) in dead animals, tongue is the best tissue, followed by trachea and oesophagus, liver, intestine, kidney and brain. For live animals, oral swabs can be used (Figure 25.11). Nasal flushes have also been successfully used for herpesvirus diagnosis in tortoises.

Treatment and prevention: Herpesvirus-infected animals should be separated from other tortoises. It is important to divide groups of tortoises according to species, especially during a disease outbreak. Supportive care, including tube feeding, fluid substitution and treatment of oral lesions, along with antibiotic therapy, has been reported to be successful in some cases. Aciclovir has been suggested for the treatment of herpesvirus infections in tortoises. Suggested treatments include topical use of a 5% ointment orally once daily (Cooper *et al.*, 1988) and oral dosage of 80 mg/kg q24h (Schumacher, 1996). However, the efficacy of this treatment and the pharmacokinetics of aciclovir in tortoises need further investigation. Immunomodulators, for example Zylexis (inactivated *Parapoxvirus ovis*) (Zoetis, New Jersey, USA), have also been suggested for use in herpesvirus-infected tortoises. Any animal that survives a herpesvirus infection should be considered a lifelong carrier.

Quarantine of incoming tortoises should be practised as a matter of course. The quarantine period should be at least 6 months and should include various environmental conditions, including hibernation, if possible. Incoming animals can be tested for exposure to herpesviruses serologically and by PCR, or by virus isolation using oral swabs. Tests should be repeated at least once during quarantine.

Iridoviridae

Iridoviruses are important pathogens of invertebrates and ectothermic vertebrates. They have been described as possible pathogens of reptiles since the 1960s. Iridoviruses are large (125–300 nm) double-stranded DNA viruses with icosahedral symmetry and containing a lipid membrane. The family *Iridoviridae* is currently divided into five genera: *Iridovirus*, *Chloriridovirus*, *Lymphocystivirus*, *Megalocytivirus* and *Ranavirus*. Viruses belonging to the genera *Iridovirus* and *Chloriridovirus* generally infect invertebrates, while lymphocystiviruses and megalocytiviruses infect bony fish. Ranaviruses have been shown to cause systemic infection and death in a wide range of ectothermic vertebrate species. They include important pathogens of fish and have been considered responsible for large die-offs in wild and captive amphibian populations (Chinchar, 2002). A sixth genus, *Hemocytivirus*, has been proposed to contain erythrocytic viruses found in various ectothermic vertebrates.

Three genetically distinct types of iridoviruses have been described in reptiles:

* Erythrocytic viruses in lizards, snakes and turtles
* Ranaviruses in chelonians, lizards and snakes
* Invertebrate iridovirus-like viruses in lizards.

Viral erythrocytic infections associated with iridovirus-like viruses have been described in fish and amphibians as well as lizards, snakes and turtles (Wolf, 1988). These viruses have been preliminarily classified as iridoviruses. They are associated with inclusions in erythrocytes of infected animals, and these inclusions were originally believed to be parasites, e.g. *Toddia* and *Pirhemocyton* (Stehbens and Johnston, 1966; Wolf, 1988). Pathology associated with viral erythrocytic infections in reptiles is unclear, but morphological changes in infected erythrocytes have been documented and they have been associated with progressive anaemia in geckos (Clark and Lunger, 1981; Smith *et al.*, 1994). A transmission study conducted with Iberian mountain and emerald lizards showed that infection with these agents can, in some cases, become systemic and may lead to death (Alves de Matos *et al.*, 2002). Recent studies on the partial characterization of erythrocytic viruses in snakes from Florida and lizards from Portugal (Wellehan *et al.*, 2008; Alves de Matos *et al.*, 2011) have shown that these probably represent a new genus in the family *Iridoviridae*, and the addition of a new genus, 'Hemocytivirus', to the family has been proposed.

Ranaviruses have been increasingly shown to be important pathogens of ectothermic animals. They have been regularly isolated from reptiles since the late 1990s. They have been mostly described in chelonian species worldwide, including eastern box turtles, Florida box turtles, red-eared sliders, Chinese soft-shelled turtles, Horsfield's tortoises, Hermann's tortoises, Egyptian tortoises, marginated tortoises, spur-thighed tortoises, Burmese star tortoises, gopher tortoises and a leopard tortoise (Mao *et al.*, 1997; Chen *et al.*, 1999; Marschang *et al.*, 1999; De Voe *et al.*, 2004; Benetka *et al.*, 2007; Johnson *et al.*, 2007; Blahak and Uhlenbrok, 2010; Uhlenbrok 2010; Allender *et al.*, 2011; Duffus *et al.*, 2015). In these species, viral infection has been associated with hepatitis, enteritis, pneumonia, ulcerative stomatitis and 'red-neck disease' (Figure 25.12). Histologically, ranaviruses have been associated with basophilic intracytoplasmic inclusions in epithelial cells of the gastrointestinal tract and hepatocytes in a few cases. Recently, ranavirus infections have been increasingly described in lizard species, including a flat-tailed gecko, brown and green anoles, green iguanas, bearded dragons, Asian glass lizards, an Iberian mountain lizard and green striped tree dragons (Marschang *et al.*, 2005; Alves de Matos *et al.*, 2011; Behncke *et al.*, 2013; Stöhr *et al.*, 2013; Duffus *et al.*, 2015). Infected lizards have been reported to show granulomatous lesions and hepatic necrosis. In many of the recently reported cases, skin lesions consisting of

purulent to ulcerative necrotizing dermatitis and hyperkeratosis were detected (Figure 25.13). In snakes, ranavirus infection has been described in green pythons in Australia, showing ulceration of the nasal mucosa, hepatic necrosis and severe necrotizing inflammation of the pharyngeal submucosa (Hyatt *et al.*, 2002).

Invertebrate iridoviruses (IIVs) belonging to the genus *Iridovirus* have been discussed as possible pathogens of insectivorous lizards. These viruses are widespread in the pet trade as pathogens of feeder insects. Viruses that have been shown to be similar to cricket viruses have been isolated from several different lizard species, including bearded dragons, four-horned and high-casqued chameleons, frilled lizards and a green iguana (Just *et al.*, 2001;

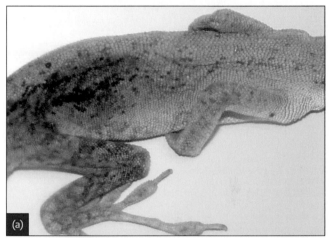
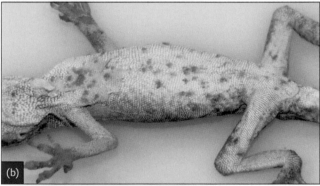
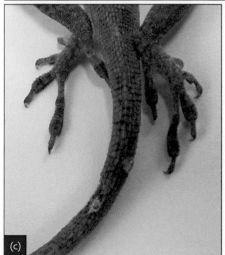

25.13 Skin alterations observed in green anoles infected with a ranavirus. (a) Beige–grey discoloration of the skin on the lateral abdomen. (b) Multiple ulcers on the ventral abdominal surface. (c) Grey lesions on the skin of the tail.
(Reproduced from Stöhr *et al.*, 2013)

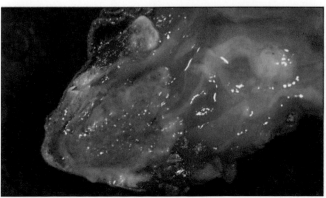

25.12 The tongue of a Hermann's tortoise with stomatitis and pharyngitis. This animal was infected with a ranavirus.
(Courtesy of Lucca Bacciarini)

Marschang *et al.*, 2002; Weinmann *et al.*, 2007). In most cases the animals died suddenly and in some cases many animals in the collection died. The most commonly observed pathology in infected animals has been skin lesions of various types, ranging from loss of scales to widespread pox-like lesions (Figure 25.14). The pathology of IIVs for lizards is not certain and they may only be involved in disease processes under specific circumstances, e.g. inadequate husbandry and presence of other infectious agents.

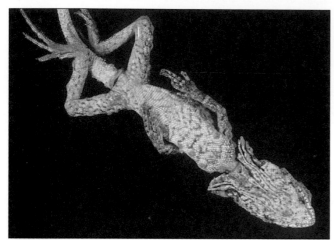

25.14 Skin lesions on an Australian frilled lizard. A virus that was similar to invertebrate iridoviruses was isolated from this animal.
(Courtesy of Silvia Blahak)

Diagnosis

Viral erythrocytic infections are diagnosed by detection of intracytoplasmic inclusions in erythrocytes, followed by electron microscopic evaluation of the inclusions. PCRs have been described for the detection of these viruses and may become more widely available as more information on the genomes of related viruses is published.

Both ranaviruses and IIVs have been diagnosed in reptiles by isolation in cell culture (Figure 25.15). These viruses grow well in a wide range of cell lines at 28°C. Exact identification of the viruses involves further studies, including sequencing a portion of the genome. A number of PCRs have been described for the detection of ranaviruses in swabs or blood as well as in tissues (especially liver) from reptiles. ELISAs have been developed for the detection of antibodies to ranaviruses in various reptile species (Ariel, 1997; Johnson *et al.*, 2010), but these are not widely available. A nested PCR and a real-time PCR have been used for the detection of IIVs in reptiles. When these viruses are detected in reptiles it is important to remember that feeder insects may contain large virus loads, so that virus detection in oral or cloacal swabs or in the intestine may only reflect the presence of virus in the insects rather than infection of the lizard.

Paramyxoviridae

The family *Paramyxoviridae* contains pleomorphic enveloped viruses with a helical capsid and a negative-sense single-stranded RNA genome (Figure 25.16). The majority of paramyxoviruses (PMVs) found in reptiles have been grouped together in the genus *Ferlavirus* (Kurath *et al.*, 2004; Marschang *et al.*, 2009). These viruses have also been called ophidian PMV (oPMV) and were originally detected in fer-de-lance vipers in Switzerland (Fölsch and

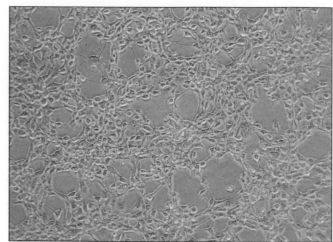

25.15 Typical ranavirus cytopathic effect in cells of the TH-1 cell line. Cell lysis and round cell formation are visible. (Original magnification X100)

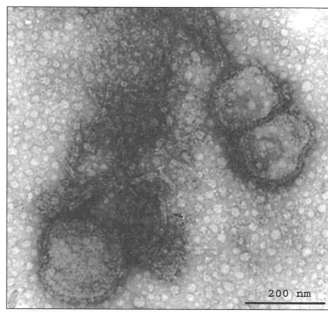

200 nm

25.16 Electron micrograph of paramyxovirus particles and filamentous nucleocapsid material with a herringbone structure. This virus was isolated from an oral swab from a timber rattlesnake. (Negative staining of cell culture supernatant with phosphotungstic acid)

Leloup, 1976). While they are most commonly found in viperid and colubrid snakes, they can also infect various other snake species as well as lizards and tortoises (Marschang *et al.*, 2009). Koch's postulates have been fulfilled for PMV-associated respiratory disease in rattlesnakes (Jacobson *et al.*, 1997) and in corn snakes (Pees *et al.*, 2016).

Ferlavirus infections

Ferlaviruses have been found in a wide range of snake species. They are most common in viperids but have also been found in colubrids, elapids and boids. They have also been detected in lizards in a number of cases, as well as in tortoises.

Clinical signs: These most commonly involve the respiratory system and CNS. They can include gaping of the mouth, mucus or blood in the oral cavity, gagging, regurgitation, convulsions, abnormal behaviour, loss of equilibrium, and opisthotonus (Hyndman *et al.*, 2013). In lizards, ferlavirus infection has been associated with pneumonia in individual cases (Jacobson *et al.*, 2001), while no clinical signs have been observed in some cases (Marschang *et al.*, 2009; Abbas *et al.*, 2012). Respiratory disease has been reported in tortoises with ferlavirus infection (Marschang *et al.*, 2009; Papp *et al.*, 2011).

Pathology: Pathological findings include congested lungs, serous exudate to caseous necrotic cellular debris within the lumen of the lungs and air sacs, and thickened and oedematous lungs. Less frequently, changes can involve the liver, with hepatomegaly and white nodules in the hepatic parenchyma and enlargement of the pancreas (Hyndman *et al.*, 2013). The pulmonary lesions are considered highly suggestive but not pathognomonic of PMV.

Histology: Histologically, ferlavirus infections are frequently characterized by proliferative interstitial pulmonary disease. Mononuclear inflammatory cells and heterophils may infiltrate the interstitium. Hyperplasia and hypertrophy of septal and faveolar epithelial cells are a common finding (Oros *et al.*, 2001). These cells may contain eosinophilic intracytoplasmic inclusions (Jacobson *et al.*, 1992). In cases with CNS disease, demyelination and degeneration of axon fibres, with moderate ballooning of axon sheaths, and meningoencephalitis with eosinophilic intracytoplasmic inclusions in glial cells have been described (West *et al.*, 2001).

Diagnosis: A number of methods are available for the diagnosis of PMV infections in snakes. Serological tests are available to detect antibodies against ferlaviruses; haemagglutination inhibition tests are most commonly used for this purpose. Time to seroconversion can take several weeks and may depend on the host species and virus strain involved, so that acutely ill animals may or may not have detectable antibodies (Gaskin *et al.*, 1989; Neul *et al.*, 2016). Ferlaviruses can be isolated in cell culture, but the most common detection method used is a reverse transcription-PCR targeting the L gene of ferlaviruses (Ahne *et al.*, 1999). The method is very sensitive and capable of detecting all of the ferlaviruses described so far. However, it is not very specific and confirmation of results by other means (e.g. sequencing of PCR products) is recommended. Virus is most commonly detected in lung, followed by kidney, intestine, pancreas and brain (Blahak, 1995; Pees *et al.*, 2016). In live animals, virus can be detected in oral and cloacal swabs as well as tracheal washes.

Treatment and prevention: There is no specific treatment available for PMV infections. Antibiotic therapy may be helpful in reducing secondary bacterial infections. During an outbreak, it is important to reduce the amount of contact between snakes as much as possible. This can be done by dividing larger collections into several groups at different locations with no contact between the groups. New snakes coming into a healthy collection should be quarantined for at least 90 days in a separate quarantine room. No snakes showing abnormal behaviour, poor feeding, regurgitation or anorexia should be introduced into the collection. The virus can likely be transmitted via aerosol, so air circulation should also be considered. Cleaning and disinfection of cages of dead snakes with PMV can be carried out with 0.15% sodium hypochlorite or any viricidal disinfectant. Cages should remain vacant for 2 weeks following disinfection. Allow at least 2 months following the last death before adding new snakes to the affected collection (Jacobson *et al.*, 1992).

A study using an inactivated ferlavirus as a vaccine in a group of western diamondback rattlesnakes led to seroconversion in several of the snakes (Jacobson *et al.*, 1991). However, the seroconversion was variable and transient, so that no vaccine for this disease in snakes is currently in sight.

Inclusion body disease – Arenaviridae

Inclusion body disease (IBD) is a chronic progressive disease in boas and pythons. It is believed to be due to a viral infection and arenaviruses have been shown to be the most likely cause of this disease (Stenglein *et al.*, 2012).

Species affected and distribution

All boid and pythonid snakes should be considered susceptible to IBD. Common boas currently appear to be most commonly affected (Jacobson *et al.*, 1999). IBD appears to affect captive snake collections worldwide, although it has not been reported in wild populations. The mode of transmission of this disease is unknown. It has been theorized that droplets in the air or contaminated bowls might play a role; that it might be transmitted as a venereal disease, and that snake mites (*Ophionyssus natricis*) may serve as a vector (Jacobson *et al.*, 1999). Young snakes born to infected parents are frequently infected and develop disease relatively quickly, suggesting that vertical transmission is possible.

Clinical signs

IBD appears to cause immune suppression and has been associated with many different clinical signs. CNS signs, including ataxia, opisthotonus and anisocoria (Figure 25.17) are most commonly observed. Other typical signs are regurgitation, anorexia, stomatitis and pneumonia. IBD may present as refractory infections of varying organ systems and has also been associated with neoplasia (cutaneous, leukaemias) (Jacobson *et al.*, 1999). IBD is a slowly progressing debilitating disease that frequently leads to the death of affected snakes. This can take months or even years, and inclusions have been detected in clinically healthy animals. The disease is more acute in pythons, with neurological signs being seen in the early stages of the condition. In boas, chronic regurgitation is seen initially, with CNS signs appearing later on in the course of the disease (see Chapter 21).

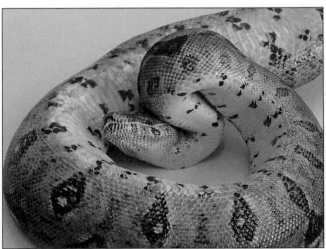

25.17 Inclusion body disease in a common boa, showing typical CNS signs.

Histology

IBD is defined by the typical histological changes observed in tissues of infected snakes. These are non-membrane-bound eosinophilic intracytoplasmic inclusions, made up of electron-dense material that has been shown to be composed of a unique protein called inclusion body disease protein. The inclusions can be found in the liver and the pancreas; in epithelial cells of the respiratory, gastrointestinal and urogenital tracts; in cells of the central and peripheral nervous systems; and in haemopoietic and lymphatic tissues (Figure 25.18). In pythons, inclusions are mostly found within neurons in the CNS, while they are often more widely distributed in boa constrictors (Chang and Jacobson, 2010).

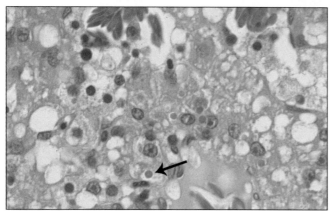

25.18 Inclusion body disease in a common boa. Eosinophilic intracytoplasmic inclusions (arrowed) of variable size are visible in several cells in this liver section. (Haematoxylin and eosin; original magnification X40)
(Courtesy of Udo Hetzel)

Diagnosis

IBD is diagnosed by detection of typical inclusions in tissues of infected snakes. For diagnosis in living snakes, biopsies of oesophageal tonsils, gastric mucosa, liver and kidneys have been suggested (Jacobson et al., 1999). Biopsy material should be fixed in neutral buffered 10% formalin and processed for light microscopy. Inclusions can sometimes also be found in peripheral blood cells. Since the identification of reptarenaviruses as the probable aetiological agent of IBD, it has also become possible to detect these by PCR using the same samples as for inclusion body detection. In live animals, blood and oesophageal swabs can also be used for virus detection. There are no serological tests available. In necropsied animals, inclusions are most commonly found in liver, pancreas, oesophageal tonsils and kidney (Jacobson et al., 1999). In pythons it is important to test brain tissues and detection in live pythons is unreliable.

Treatment and prevention

There is no treatment available for IBD. Euthanasia has been recommended for animals with inclusions. If this is not done, such animals should be permanently removed from breeding populations and excluded from further contact with healthy animals. A quarantine of new animals before introduction into collections of at least 3–6 months has been recommended in order to prevent the introduction of infected animals. No recommendations have yet been developed for clinically healthy animals that are tested arenavirus positive, but these should also be considered potential sources of infection.

Adenoviridae

Adenoviruses are non-enveloped double-stranded DNA viruses with icosahedral capsids. They have been detected in all reptile subgroups, but they are most commonly found in squamates. Squamate adenoviruses characterized so far have been placed into the genus *Atadenovirus*. Several authors have reported co-infection of reptiles with adenoviruses and other pathogens, suggesting that immunosuppression may be a cofactor in the development of adenoviral disease. Koch's postulates have been fulfilled in one case for an adenoviral hepatitis in a common boa (Jacobson et al., 1985).

Species affected

Adenovirus infections have been detected in a wide range of reptile species including chelonians, crocodilians, snakes and lizards. They are most commonly described in squamates, particularly in bearded dragons. They appear to occur worldwide in captive populations, and antibodies to adenoviruses have been detected in wild snakes from Costa Rica and the USA. In more recent years, adenoviruses have also repeatedly been described in chelonians in Europe and the USA, including tortoises, turtles and terrapenes (Rivera et al., 2009; Doszpoly et al., 2013).

Clinical signs

A range of clinical signs has been described. Some animals may show no clinical signs and simply be found dead. Anorexia is relatively common in infected animals and can be associated with lethargy. CNS signs, including head tilt, opisthotonus and circling, may occur (Jacobson et al., 1985; Kim et al., 2002). In individual cases, stomatitis (Heldstab and Bestetti, 1984) and dermatitis (Perkins et al., 2001) have been described. In chelonians, adenovirus infection has been associated with anorexia, lethargy, mucosal ulcerations, nasal and ocular discharge, and diarrhoea (Rivera et al., 2009). In other cases, clinically healthy chelonians have been found to be shedding viral DNA (Doszpoly et al., 2013).

Pathology and histology

Pathology of adenovirus-infected animals is generally non-specific and is frequently restricted to the liver, which may be enlarged and with petechiae or pale areas scattered throughout. Histology most commonly shows hepatic necrosis. The intestine may also be affected and the duodenum may be dilated with hyperaemia of the mucosa. Basophilic intranuclear inclusions are a typical finding. They are mostly present in hepatocytes, generally associated with areas of necrosis. They have also been described in enterocytes (Heldstab and Bestetti, 1984; Jacobson et al., 1996; Kim et al., 2002), myocardial endothelial cells (Jacobson and Kollias, 1986), renal epithelial cells (Julian and Durham, 1982), endocardium and epithelial cells of the lung (Schumacher et al., 1994).

Diagnosis

Diagnosis is generally accomplished by PCR detection of viral DNA in affected tissues (Wellehan et al., 2004); the liver and intestine should be included in such studies. In live animals, cloacal swabs can be used for diagnostic testing. In several cases, virus has been isolated from infected snakes and, in a few cases, from lizards in cell culture. Neutralization tests for the detection of antibodies against squamate adenoviruses isolated from various snake and lizard species have been described (Marschang *et al.*, 2003; Ball *et al.*, 2013), but are not generally available for diagnostic purposes.

Diagnostic tests
Samples

It is always important to contact the laboratory to which samples will be sent as soon as possible to discuss diagnostic methods and procedures. The success of viral detection methods will depend a great deal on the samples that are collected and sent to the laboratory. Important factors include the choice of tissues, timing, and method of collection and handling of samples.

- The choice of samples will depend on the type of animal, whether the animal is still alive and the phase of the infection. Different tissues may contain virus in acute and chronic phases of disease; sampling should always include all tissues that appear morphologically changed.
- In live animals, oral and cloacal swabs and nasal flushes as well as whole blood have been useful for virus detection in reptiles. Biopsy samples can be used for microscopic evaluation and virus detection.
- In necropsied animals, samples should be collected from all major organs. In the case of animals with CNS signs, this should also include the brain. It can be helpful to freeze samples from necropsied animals for later virus detection efforts.
- Virological samples for virus isolation should be collected as aseptically as possible. Samples should be collected dry or placed in a buffered solution at neutral pH. The solution should contain antibiotics to inhibit bacterial growth.
- Samples that will be sent to the laboratory within 1 week should be cooled but not frozen. Samples that must be stored for longer than 1 week should be frozen at –70°C if possible. Repeated freezing and thawing must be avoided.
- Formalin-fixed tissues can be used for PCR detection of viral RNA or DNA. However, formalin will lead to degradation of nucleic acids, so that virus detection from fixed tissues is less sensitive and fixation for longer than 2 days should be avoided.

Virus detection methods

Virus isolation: Viruses can be isolated on cell culture from a wide range of specimens. There are a number of cell lines available for reptile virology. The most commonly used include: terrapene heart cells (TH-1, ATCC, Manassas, VA; CCL 50), which are used for the isolation of herpesviruses from tortoises; viper heart cells (VH2, ATCC, CCL 140), which have been used for the isolation of PMVs and adenoviruses in snakes among others; and iguana heart cells (IgH2, ATCC, CCL 108). Growth of virus in cell culture is usually determined by the development of a cytopathic effect (CPE) followed by methods for virus identification.

Virus isolation requires live virus in the samples. It also requires some expensive equipment and expertise. It is a relatively slow method, and final identification of the isolated viruses can be time-consuming and expensive. Isolation of a virus allows further study of the agent, the development of additional tests (e.g. serological tests) and transmission studies. In reptile medicine, virus isolation is also a method that can lead to the description of new agents capable of infecting reptiles.

Light microscopy: This can be used to detect virus-specific changes in infected cells, generally inclusions. These may have typical staining properties, morphology and location. Examples are herpesvirus infections, IBD and adenovirus infections. This method is often a first step in identifying a viral infection but should be complemented by more specific methods. Not all viruses cause typical microscopic changes, and changes will not be detectable in all virus-infected animals.

Electron microscopy: This can be used to detect virus particles in tissues and other samples (e.g. faeces). It requires expensive equipment and experience, well preserved samples and a large number of viruses in the samples in order to have a chance of finding anything. Electron microscopy is most often used to complement other methods; it can be used to identify the cause of changes observed by light microscopy or to identify viruses that have been isolated in cell culture.

Antigen detection: There are only few cases in which antibodies have been produced against reptile viruses and can be used for virus detection assays. These can include immunohistochemistry (immunofluorescence and immunoperoxidase staining) and antigen ELISAs. The success of immunohistochemistry depends on the quality of the specimens, how the slides are prepared and the specificity of the antigen used. In reptile virology, these methods have been described for a few viruses including herpesviruses of tortoises and ferlaviruses of snakes. The techniques are generally limited to individual laboratories where they have been developed and might not be commercially available.

Nucleic acid detection

Polymerase chain reaction: PCR is an extremely sensitive method for the detection of viral DNA or RNA. It is the most common method used for the detection of specific viruses in reptiles. It has a number of important advantages including the relative speed and ease with which it can be carried out. It also carries several inherent drawbacks. These include possible contamination of diagnostic material, leading to false positive results, as well as the possible presence of inhibitory factors in samples leading to false negative results. In reptile virology, PCRs have been developed for the detection of many different viruses, including ranaviruses, herpesviruses, adenoviruses, reoviruses, paramyxoviruses and arenaviruses (see Figures 25.3–25.7). The high specificity of this test can be a disadvantage in some cases in reptile medicine, since only closely related viruses, with correct sequences at the primer binding sites, will be positive. This has been shown to be a problem in the case of herpesvirus infections of tortoises.

Hybridization: Where sequences are available from reptile viruses or from related viruses, *in situ* hybridization can be used to detect virus-specific nucleic acids in tissues of infected animals. The success of this method depends on a number of factors, as does immunohistochemistry, including the actual sequence of the viral genome and the sequence used for hybridization. It can be used to detect virus in tissues that may otherwise appear negative. In reptile virology, this method has been used to detect herpesviruses in tissue samples of tortoises and adenoviruses in tissue samples of snakes. It is currently not commercially available for reptile viruses.

Next generation sequencing: This is a term used for various modern sequencing technologies allowing high-throughput sequencing of many different types of sample. In reptile medicine, these techniques have been used for the detection of possible viral pathogens in tissues from diseased animals, leading to the detection of, for example, reptarenaviruses associated with IBD and nidoviruses of pythons. The methods are still expensive and require extensive analysis, but they have been used increasingly in reptile virology and have led to important discoveries and diagnostic advances.

Serology

Serological detection methods have been described for a number of viral infections in reptiles. The most commonly used method is a virus neutralization test, which measures the ability of antibodies in the serum to prevent a given amount of virus from infecting cells and causing a cytopathic effect (CPE). This type of test has been used for the detection of antibodies against herpesviruses in tortoises. A haemagglutination inhibition test is similar and measures the ability of antibodies in the serum to prevent virus from haemagglutinating chicken red blood cells. This type of test is used for the detection of antibodies against ferlaviruses.

ELISAs have also been developed for use in reptile virology. These require secondary antibodies against specific reptilian antibodies, but may be more sensitive than the tests mentioned above. They have been developed for the detection of antibodies against herpesviruses in tortoises, among others, but are not widely available at this time. When carrying out serological tests on reptiles, it is important to remember that reptiles may be slow in developing antibodies to infectious agents, and that antibody production will depend on a number of environmental factors such as temperature and time of year.

Bacterial infections

It is important to note that few, if any, bacterial agents can be considered primary pathogens. The role of underlying disease and poor husbandry in the aetiology of bacterial disease in reptiles cannot be overstated. Even seemingly straightforward bacterial abscesses may be linked to underlying factors – for example, aural abscesses in eastern box turtles have been linked to both hypovitaminosis A and environmental organochlorine compounds (Chinnadurai and DeVoe, 2009).

A typical bacterial 'syndrome' would be necrotic dermatitis, where a range of potential underlying factors (physical, husbandry, metabolic) may predispose to various viral, fungal, bacterial or parasitic infections. The degree of pathogenicity of the infective agent is important in determining how much of an underlying factor is required to facilitate infection. In these cases, an holistic approach to the case must be taken in terms of the whole animal and its environment/husbandry (Maas, 2013).

However, certain bacterial species may be considered more pathogenic than others. The more pathogenic species are those that are most capable of causing infection in otherwise healthy animals, and hence are those most likely to be isolated from lesions (Figure 25.19). In general, Gram-negative rods appear to be more commonly isolated from lesions in reptiles than Gram-positive rods or cocci. However, these species are still likely to originate from normal commensal populations (especially in the gut) or from the environment; therefore, 'screening' procedures and prophylactic antibiosis cannot be recommended as a means of eradicating pathogenic species. Diagnosis of a bacteria-related disease should prompt further investigation of underlying disease and/or husbandry problems, especially where bacteria of low pathogenicity are isolated. Pathogenicity may be increased by the presence of other bacteria, e.g. combined *Pseudomonas aeruginosa* and *Aeromonas hydrophila* infection in snakes.

Species	Pathogenicity	Comments
Acinetobacter	+++	One study reports this bacterium as being a common isolate in the oral cavity of normal snakes – 28% in this study (Jho *et al.*, 2011)
Actinobacillus	+++	May be zoonotic (Johnson-Delaney, 2009)
Aeromonas	++++	Waterborne bacterium – generally *A. hydrophila*. More of a problem in aquatic species though may be seen in terrestrial species from contaminated water or environments (Ebani *et al.*, 2008)
Bacteroides	+++	Anaerobes usually are found associated with lesions in reptiles (Stewart, 1990) and are less common in studies of healthy animals. However, one study (Cooper *et al.*, 1985) did isolate *Bacteroides* from healthy animals
Chlamydia	+++	Mixed species isolated, including *C. psittaci* and *C. pneumoniae*, and all may be associated with respiratory disease (see Chapter 18)
Citrobacter freundii	++++	Most commonly found in lesions of aquatic chelonians
Clostridium	+++	See comments re. *Bacteroides* above
Corynebacterium	++++	Often associated with abscesses but may also be found in the faeces of healthy animals (Pessoa, 2009)
Escherichia coli	++	Less commonly isolated from reptiles than from mammals or birds. Many strains show multiple drug resistances (Gopee *et al.*, 2000)
Edwardsiella	+++	*E. tarda* has been found as a common isolate in reptile faeces, especially tortoises and snakes (Roggendorf and Müller, 1976)
Enterobacter	+++	Also found as a common isolate in lizard faeces (Roggendorf and Müller, 1976)
Klebsiella	++++	A common faecal isolate in reptiles (Graves *et al.*, 1988)
Micrococcus	–	Non-pathogenic
Morganella	++++	*M. morganii* has been isolated from skin lesions
Mycobacteria	++++	Many species – see text
Mycoplasma	+++	Pathogenicity varies with species – see text and also Chapter 18

25.19 Bacteria in reptiles. Note that, unless stated, these bacteria are capable of causing disease in any species of reptile. – = not pathogenic; ++++ = highly pathogenic. (continues)

Species	Pathogenicity	Comments
Pasteurella	+++	*P. haemolytica* and *P. testudinis* appear more common isolates than *P. multocida* (Snipes, 1984), cf. mammals
Proteus	++++	Various species isolated – *P. mirabilis*, *P. rettgeri*, *P. vulgaris* (Roggendorf and Müller, 1976)
Providencia	+++	*P. rettgeri* (Kycko *et al.*, 2013) has been isolated from a granulomatous pneumonia in a crocodile monitor lizard, although it is often seen as a commensal
Pseudomonas	++++	Waterborne bacterium. More of a problem in aquatic species, though may be seen in terrestrial species from contaminated water or environments. A wide range of species have been isolated from lesions, especially *P. aeruginosa* (Ebani *et al.*, 2008)
Salmonella	Variable	Very wide variation in pathogenicity between different strains and in different species – see text
Serratia	++++	*S. marcescens* has also been reported as a cause of cellulitis in people bitten by iguanas. It would therefore be presumed that this is a part of that species' normal oral flora (Hsieh and Babl, 1999; Grim *et al.*, 2010). Both *S. marcescens* and *S. fonticola* have been associated with lesions (particularly abscesses) in reptiles (Garcia *et al.*, 2008)
Coagulase-positive staphylococci	+++	There do not appear to be reports of methicillin-resistant *Staphylococcus aureus* (MRSA)-type infections in reptiles
Coagulase-negative staphylococci	–	Non-pathogenic
Beta-haemolytic *Streptococcus*	+++	May originate from mammalian food source (Hetzel *et al.*, 2003)

25.19 (continued) Bacteria in reptiles. Note that, unless stated, these bacteria are capable of causing disease in any species of reptile. – = not pathogenic; ++++ = highly pathogenic.

Clinical signs

Clinical signs relate to the organ(s) affected. In many cases infection is localized; the reader should consult individual chapters for clinical syndromes relating to each organ system. Infections may range from acute to (more commonly) chronic with granuloma or abscess formation. However, infection may disseminate to other organ systems, especially by haematogenous spread. This means that even small localized lesions have the potential to cause systemic illness if left untreated.

Septicaemia and bacteraemia

- Septicaemia is a systemic disease associated with the presence and persistence of bacteria in the blood. Bacterial organisms may be identified within circulating white blood cells.
- Bacteraemia is the temporary presence of bacteria in the blood. These bacteria are not associated with clinical signs but may cause embolic infections; this may be normal in healthy reptiles (Hanel *et al.*, 1999).

Septicaemia may occur as an acute condition following inoculation of bacteria into the animal via the skin or gut, or as a more chronic situation where localized infection has not been noticed or has not been adequately treated. Clinical signs may be non-specific (lethargy, anorexia, weakness progressing to collapse and death) but may include signs of embolic infection, e.g. polyarthritis, endocarditis, tail embolism and skin petechiae (Figure 25.20). Where any bacterial disease is suspected, especially where petechiae are present or where there are multiple sites of infection or abscesses, the heart should be auscultated using a 8-MHz Doppler probe. The finding of a harsh murmur typical of endocarditis indicates a poor or grave prognosis. This can be confirmed via echocardiography.

Diagnosis of septicaemia is difficult. Blood culture is of little use as any bacteria cultured may represent a 'normal' bacteraemia and there is difficulty in obtaining samples without skin contamination (Hanel *et al.*, 1999). Haematology may show raised, normal or low total white cell counts. However, heterophils and/or macrophages will normally show toxicity and phagocytosed bacteria may be

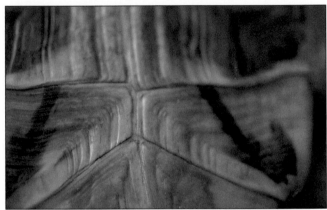

25.20 Cutaneous signs of septicaemia in a tortoise. Note the reddening of the shell.

visible. This latter change should be differentiated from the finding of 'free' bacteria within the blood smear with no evidence of phagocytosis or toxic changes in the white cells; this may represent bacterial contamination of the sample or bacteraemia.

Clinical approach

In general, where bacterial disease is suspected lesions should be sampled and specimens tested in the following manner.

Cytology

Aspirates smeared on slides or direct impression smears from open lesions can be examined. Ideally, both a Gram stain and a trichrome stain (e.g. Diff-Quik®) should be used. The finding of inflammatory cells is always suggestive of infection and bacteria may be seen. A sparse mixed population of bacteria suggests contamination or commensal organisms, whereas many monomorphic forms suggests greater significance, especially where Gram-negative rods are seen. The presence of phagocytosed bacteria in inflammatory cells is especially significant. This enables a rapid provisional diagnosis and prompt 'first-guess' antibiosis based on bacterial morphology.

Bacteriology

A swab should be submitted from any bacterial lesions for bacteriology and sensitivity testing (Figure 25.21). Culture should be performed at 37°C and 22°C; this is because many of these organisms (of environmental origin) have adapted to grow at lower temperatures than those normally used. Both aerobic and anaerobic/microaerophilic culture conditions should be used, as many of these organisms are adapted to lower oxygen concentrations (Macdonald J and Frye F (2002) personal communications). Rather than these culture requirements reflecting conditions found in the normal reptile, they reflect why the 'cold' or 'hypoxic' reptile is more vulnerable to bacterial infection. Sensitivity tests are essential, as antibiotic resistance is commonly encountered. Contamination by environmental or faecal bacteria makes interpretation very difficult. Swabs should always be taken from deeper parts of the lesion in order to avoid confusion with environmental contaminants. Blood culture may produce false positive results due to the presence of bacteraemia; however, the heavy pure growth of a bacterium from the bloodstream in a diseased animal may indicate the presence of septicaemia. Also, biopsy samples may be submitted for culture (Figure 25.22).

Histopathology

This will reveal infectious organisms and any cellular response to them, which may help distinguish infection from contamination.

Importantly, when chronic granulomata are present, the numbers of infective organisms within lesions may be quite low, which will affect their identification by culture or histopathology. In these cases, *in situ* hybridization techniques may assist owing to their greater sensitivity.

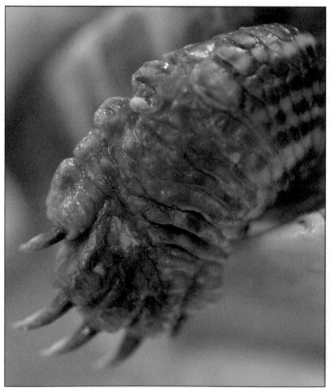

25.21 Ulcerative necrotic dermatitis in a turtle. The turtle was also septicaemic. Treatment involved antibiosis (based on culture and sensitivity test results from deep-tissue samples), supportive care (fluid therapy) and environmental correction (temperature, water quality).

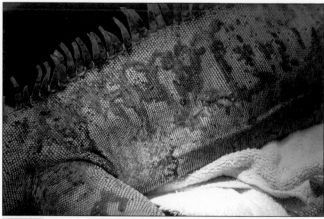

25.22 Granulomatous dermatitis in a green iguana. Bacterial infection was confirmed by biopsy. Culture revealed the presence of *Escherichia coli*. Environmental evaluation revealed a low temperature and some vivarium materials that may have traumatized the skin. Treatment involved antibiosis, topical cleaning (with povidone iodine solution and silver sulfadiazine cream) and correction of environmental temperature.

Treatment

Although systemic antibiosis is generally important to avoid embolic spread or septicaemia, surgery is often required to remove bacterial lesions.

Salmonella

These organisms have a variable degree of pathogenicity for reptiles. They are normal inhabitants of the reptile gastrointestinal tract; hence their frequent appearance as invading agents in lesions or in a gut dysbiosis/overgrowth. A number of *Salmonella enterica* serovars have been implicated as pathogens causing septicaemia, pneumonia, coelomitis, abscesses, granulomas, hypovolaemic shock and death: Agioboo; Anatum; Carrau; Chameleon; Durham; Infantis; Krefeld; Marinum; Montevideo; Muenchen; Oslo; Pomona; Thompson; Typhimurium; Saintpaul; subgenus II and subgenus IV. However, the vast majority of these have also been isolated from healthy reptiles (Johnson-Delaney, 1996). Scheelings *et al.* (2011) suggest that wild Australian reptiles are not natural carriers of *Salmonella* spp. and that higher prevalence in captive reptiles may reflect effects of diet and/or captivity.

Although not a significant hazard to the reptile, these species may constitute a significant zoonotic risk. Accordingly, a lot of research has been undertaken to establish screening methods and/or methods of producing *Salmonella*-free reptiles. To date these have generally been unsuccessful (Mitchell and Shane, 2001; Mitchell *et al.*, 2001a and b, 2003), and most use of disinfectants and antibiotics in the reptile or in the environment of aquatic species cannot be recommended. However, more recently 'Baquacil', hydrogen peroxide and 'Sanocil' (surfactant, hydrogen peroxide, silver) have shown some capability in suppressing or eliminating *Salmonella* spp. in red-eared slider eggs and hatchlings (Mitchell *et al.*, 2009). Care should also be taken with use of antibiotics for other bacterial infections, as these drugs will also affect the normal gut bacteria, including *Salmonella* spp., and may result in the development of antibiotic resistance (Mitchell and Shane, 2001).

The standard means of diagnosis is culture, although this is fairly insensitive and so should not be used as a screening test. All reptiles should be considered carriers.

PCRs are more sensitive in both clinical and environmental samples. However, if specific serotyping is required, culture is essential (Mitchell, 2006). Means of preventing human reptile-associated salmonellosis are discussed in Chapter 2.

Mycobacteria

Mycobacteriosis is a potential zoonosis as 'mycobacteria other than tuberculosis' (MOTT) are found in lesions in reptiles. Typically these lesions resemble human disease, with tubercles found in many different organs (Hoop, 1997; Paré *et al.*, 2006b; Mitchell, 2012). Clinical signs relate to the location of the lesions but often include lethargy and wasting. The species typically found include: *Mycobacterium avium* complex (MAC); *M. marinum*; *M. chelonae*; *M. fortuitum*; *M. ulcerans*; *M. haemophilum*; *M. terrae*; *M. smegmatis*; *M. phamnopheos* and *M. phlei* (Hoop, 1997; Paré *et al.*, 2006b; Mitchell, 2012).

Suspicion should be aroused on finding typical granulomatous lesions, either topical or systemic, especially those that do not respond to antibiotic therapy. Unfortunately, many reptile abscesses fit this description. Samples (aspirates, biopsy samples or excised lesions) should be submitted for acid-fast staining and/or PCR (Figure 25.23). If positive, culture may be attempted.

There is no recommended therapy and in view of the zoonotic potential of these organisms, euthanasia of the affected animal is generally an appropriate course of action, unless there is a single localized lesion that may be completely excised. In-contact animals should be screened and vivaria used by the affected animal disposed of. When a suspected case is being hospitalized in the clinic the patient should be barrier nursed and great care used when handling it to avoid human infection.

Chlamydia

Chlamydia (formerly *Chlamydophila*) has been reported as causing pneumonia with hepatitis; a granulomatous pericarditis/myocarditis has been reported in a group of puff adders (Jacobson *et al.*, 1989). It has also been described as causing disease (regurgitation and death) in emerald tree boas, with lesions in small intestine, heart and oesophageal tonsils (Jacobson *et al.*, 2002), and a fatal

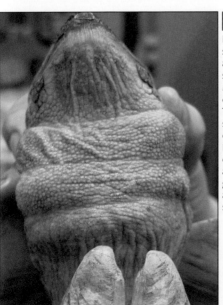

25.23

Hard subcutaneous swelling in the neck of a male sulcata (African spurred tortoise). Mycobacteriosis was confirmed by biopsy. The animal was subsequently euthanased. Post-mortem examination revealed a typical granulomatous appearance on the cut surfaces of the lesion.

pneumonia in spur-thighed tortoises (Vanrompay *et al.*, 1994). In both cases diagnosis was based on post-mortem histopathology and immunohistochemical staining of antigens. Organisms were not cultured.

Chlamydiosis should be suspected as a differential in cases of granulomatous disease and appropriate stains requested on histopathology. However, low numbers of organisms in such lesions can make identification challenging and PCR may be a more sensitive testing method.

In chelonian species showing respiratory signs, PCR of nasal lavage specimens or pharyngeal swabs should be undertaken (Jacobson, 2007; Pericard and Blahak, 2013).

A variety of *Chlamydia* species may be identified (Pericard and Blahak, 2013), so generic *Chlamydia* PCR should be used rather than specific *C. psittaci* probes. In some cases in these studies, *C. pneumoniae* has been identified so a zoonotic threat may be present.

Treatment of chlamydial granulomatous disease has rarely been attempted. However, fluoroquinolones (Ruegg *et al.*, 2015) or tetracyclines may be used in chelonian chlamydiosis. Where disease is occurring in a group, prophylactic treatment of in-contact animals would be advisable, as well as ensuring husbandry is optimal.

Mycoplasma

Mycoplasmosis has emerged as a major factor in respiratory disease of chelonians and crocodilians. In tortoises it may be a significant component of the upper respiratory tract disease (URTD) complex and has been reported as a cause of pneumonia.

The major species involved, *Mycoplasma agassizii*, has been isolated from a range of species including gopher tortoises, desert tortoises and many Mediterranean tortoises. Clinical signs are typical of URTD, with a serous, mucoid or purulent nasal and/or ocular discharge. Pneumonia may also be a consequence of infection (see Chapter 18). While transmission studies in desert and gopher tortoises have shown that this agent does fulfil Koch's postulates and may be considered a potential primary pathogen, it should be noted that this agent may also be detected in clinically normal tortoises. Pathogenicity may, therefore, also depend on host species, strain of agent, and health/immune status of the host. *M. testudinis* has also been isolated from gopher tortoises but does not appear to be pathogenic. However, *M. testudineum* does appear to cause URTD in gopher tortoises (Jacobson, 2007).

Diagnosis

Culture: Specific culture and transport media should be used and the laboratory contacted prior to sending the sample. Ideally, a specialized laboratory should be used.

Serology: An ELISA test has been developed for antibodies against *Mycoplasma agassizii* (Schumacher *et al.*, 1993). Although specific monoclonal antibodies are used, there may be cross-reactions with other tortoise antibodies and levels of antibody appear to fluctuate with season (Jacobson and Origgi, 2002). As with all serological tests, a positive reaction merely indicates exposure, not presence of the organism.

PCR: PCR is available for mycoplasmal DNA in swabs taken from the mouth and should be more sensitive than culture, indicating the presence of the organism in lesions. It has also shown carriage of the organism in clinically normal tortoise mouths. In one study (Soares *et al.*, 2003), presence of mycoplasmal antigen could not be correlated with presence of lesions, which may indicate that this organism is a part of the normal tortoise oral flora or, more likely, that latent infection is common and that even 'healthy' tortoises may be regarded as carriers. Interestingly, this study also suggested that Horsfield's tortoises may be more likely to be associated with this organism, although a different study showed that carriage was higher in spur-thighed than in Hermann's tortoises (Mathes, 2003).

Treatment and control

Details of control and therapy may be found in Chapter 18. Fluoroquinolones, clarithromycin and doxycycline appear useful in treatment. Given the presence of a carrier state, control is essential, with quarantine of new animals entering a colony, no mixing of tortoise species and attention paid to the animals' overall health status. Mycoplasmas may be transmitted by direct contact, so the quarantine control should be strict to avoid transmission via fomites. Similarly, sick tortoises in the veterinary clinic may also be capable of transmitting or being infected by this agent. Barrier nursing of ALL hospitalized tortoises is essential (Jacobson *et al.*, 2000; Jacobson and Origgi, 2002; Soares *et al.*, 2003).

Devriesea agamarum

This Gram-positive rod has been described as a pathogen in spiny-tailed lizards. In these animals it may cause a hyperkeratotic dermatitis, cheilitis (Figure 25.24) and potentially septicaemia. It has also been found as a commensal organism in the mouths of bearded dragons (though it can cause hyperkeratotic lesions when inoculated into the skin of this species). This, therefore, is the likely source of infection in spiny-tailed lizards in mixed collections. *Devriesea* has also been found to survive for up to 5 months in humid sand and/or water, so environmental contamination is also a potential source of infection.

Diagnosis is via histopathology and culture/sensitivity of biopsy samples from lesions.

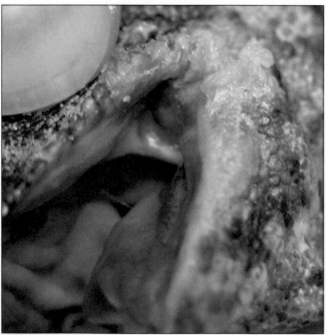

25.24 Cheilitis caused by *Devriesea agamarum* infection in a spiny-tailed lizard.

Treatment involves surgical debridement of lesions, and systemic ceftiofur (5 mg/kg q24h for 12–18 days (spiny-tailed lizards and *Pogona* spp.)). This should be combined with thorough environmental cleaning and disinfection. Fluoroquinolones are not effective (Pasmans *et al.*, 2010; Latney and Wellehan, 2013)

Fungal infections

Systemic mycoses are much less common than bacterial infections. Nevertheless, they are considerably more common in reptiles than in endothermic species. It is therefore important for the clinician to take samples for mycological as well as bacteriological tests, especially when there has been an apparent 'antibiotic failure'.

Fungi rarely act as primary pathogens, with infection representing opportunistic infection of the compromised reptile from the environment, with entry via gut, skin or respiratory system. However, *Fusarium incarnatum* infections of the skin/carapace of gopher tortoises have appeared to be primary infections with no underlying causes readily apparent (Rose *et al.*, 2001). *Ophidiomyces ophiodiicola* has also been associated with disease after experimental challenge in cottonmouths (Allender *et al.*, 2015; Lorch *et al.*, 2015). This has recently been described as the cause of snake fungal disease (SFD) in the United States (https://www.usgs.gov/science-explorer-results?es=Ophidiomyces+ophiodiicola), a disease of wild snakes. The full impact of this disease is not yet understood, nor the impact of primary factors allowing entry of the fungal pathogen (Guthrie *et al.*, 2015; Bohuski *et al.*, 2015).

The genera isolated most frequently include *Aspergillus*, *Mucor*, *Candida*, *Penicillium*, *Paecilomyces*, *Fusarium*, *Acremonium* and *Geotrichum*, although a wide variety of species have been isolated from lesions. Mixed fungal infections may also be found.

Clinical signs

Dermatomycoses and subcutaneous mycoses (see Chapter 15) are the most common form of fungal disease in reptiles (Paré, 2003; Schumacher, 2003). Generally, they present as localized abscesses or granulomas and may be a common cause of 'shell rot' in chelonians.

Signs of systemic mycoses relate to whether disease is caused by invasion of tissue or release of toxins from more localized lesions, or by ingestion of contaminated foodstuffs (mycotoxicosis). For this reason, even small localized lesions should be viewed seriously. Rarely, hypersensitivity to the fungus may be an issue although this has not been described in reptiles (Quinn *et al.*, 1994).

Systemic mycoses generally originate from the respiratory or gastrointestinal systems (Schumacher, 2003) Clinical signs relate to the organ system principally affected, e.g. mycotic pneumonia grossly resembles bacterial pneumonia or may present as a non-specific weakness or lethargy. Signs may only be seen when disease is already advanced.

Abscesses or granulomas are the most common lesions seen. Thick caseous or creamy exudates may also be found.

Chrysosporium anamorph of *Nannizziopsis vriesii* (CANV) complex

Recent DNA work suggests this is not a single fungal species, but rather a complex of different species causing similar disease in different reptile species (Sigler *et al.*, 2013). Specific fungal species will be mentioned in this section, but all can be considered a part of the CANV complex. The importance of this is that the relationship of specific isolates to disease in specific species implies different susceptibilities and concerns when controlling outbreaks in mixed-species collections. There has previously been evidence that CANV may be zoonotic to immunocompromised individuals. However, Sigler *et al.* (2010) did not isolate human-associated CANV species from reptiles. Nonetheless, it is generally recommended that potentially susceptible handlers always wear gloves to handle or, preferably, avoid handling the reptile and avoid cleaning out the vivarium until infection is cleared.

This fungal pathogen has been shown to fulfil Koch's postulates (Pare *et al.*, 2006a) and has been seen as primary disease in a wide range of reptiles, especially inland bearded dragons and chameleons.

An excellent overview of this condition is found in Mitchell and Walden (2013) and the disease is also discussed in Chapter 15.

Clinical signs consist mainly of cutaneous crusting and ulceration (Figure 25.25). Systemic spread is seen in debilitated/immunosuppressed individuals. Lesions in bearded dragons (due to *Nannizziopsis guarroi*; this can also infect iguanas) are particularly aggressive, starting with yellow cutaneous crusts (hence the name 'yellow fungus disease') and progressing into subcutaneous tissues, muscle and bone.

In snakes a necrotizing dermatitis is seen with lesions found mainly on the head and ventrum – lesions in snakes tend to be associated with *Ophidiomyces ophiodiicola* (part of the CANV complex). This has been a problem with wild colubrids and viperids in the United States (see https://www.usgs.gov/science-explorer-results?es=Ophidiomyces+ophiodiicola).

Diagnosis of CANV is partly based on clinical signs in some species (e.g. bearded dragons), although signs are fairly non-specific in others (e.g. snakes). Otherwise, deep-tissue samples should be taken for histopathology, fungal (and bacterial) culture and/or PCR. CANV is rarely cultured from skin samples of healthy reptiles (Paré *et al.*, 2003), so positive culture/PCR results are always of significance. An holistic approach should be taken to these cases, with radiography to assess invasion into deeper structures and haematology/biochemistry to assess immune response and underlying health issues.

Itraconazole and voriconazole have both been found to be effective treatments in cutaneous disease, although there is growing evidence of itraconazole resistance in these species. In addition, van Waeyenberghe *et al.* (2010) report apparent high mortality levels in bearded dragons being treated for CANV infection using itraconazole. Their findings were that voriconazole (10 mg/kg orally q24h) appeared much safer and more effective for this infection in this species. The deeper the infection, the poorer the prognosis. An excellent review of therapy is found in Mitchell and Walden (2013).

The source of infection is unknown, although (given typical lesion distribution) substrate is implicated. Alternatively, invertebrate food sources have also been implicated, especially given the keratophilic nature of CANV, suggesting it is adapted to invertebrates.

Where CANV is diagnosed, it is very important to maintain good hygiene and optimal conditions within the vivarium. There is a report of CANV infection in an HIV sero-positive person although the source of infection was not confirmed. However, it is wise to suggest taking hygiene precautions if potentially immunocompromised individuals are working with CANV positive animals (Mitchell and Walden (2013).

Dermatophytosis

While ringworm has generally been considered rare in reptiles, there are increasing numbers of case reports of these infections in reptiles. *Trichophyton* species appear most implicated and have been described in a Tenerife lizard and a group of iguanas (Khosravi *et al.*, 2012; Oros *et al.*, 2013). Reports suggest disease occurs in immunocompromised animals.

Diagnosis is complicated by the similar culture characteristics and morphology to CANV. However, species can be distinguished by use of specific PCR techniques. Underlying husbandry factors are important in the pathogenesis of these infections.

Diagnostics

Ideally, samples from lesions (aspirates, scrapes, swabs or biopsy samples) should be submitted to a specialist laboratory for fungal culture. However, it may be difficult to isolate fungi owing to their sensitive nature or culture needs, or because of overgrowth of environmental bacterial or fungal contaminants. Samples should therefore be taken from deep within lesions. This is particularly important for cutaneous lesions, especially of chelonian shells.

Culture may take a long time and this may hamper diagnosis, especially as many fungal diseases are well advanced by the time of presentation. More rapid diagnosis may be facilitated by submission of biopsy samples for histopathology or of aspirates, smears or fluid exudates/washes for cytological examination for fungal organisms.

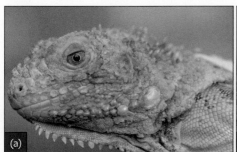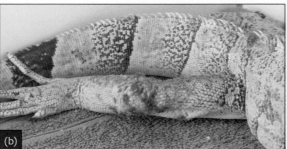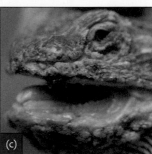

25.25 CANV infection in (a–b) two iguanas and (c) a bearded dragon. The diagnosis was confirmed via culture and histopathology. (b) Note the deep ulceration extending into the subcutaneous tissues on the limb of the iguana. (c) Note the typical yellow crusts on the head of the bearded dragon. The iguana recovered following 3 months' treatment with itraconazole (at 10 mg/kg orally q24h) and cleaning with topical povidone iodine solution. The bearded dragon was euthanased after showing no response to treatment.

Special staining (e.g. periodic acid–Schiff or silver stain) may be required to identify fungal hyphae, so the pathologist should always be advised when fungal disease is suspected. Haematoxylin and eosin will not always stain fungal hyphae.

Treatment

Antifungal agents (especially itraconazole or voriconazole) are the mainstays of therapy (see Chapter 11). It is vital to correct any underlying factors and to treat concurrent or primary disease. It should also be noted that, with the nature of the typical fungal lesion, surgical removal or debridement of lesions is usually necessary. In the case of systemic mycoses the prognosis is usually poor. In many cases the diagnosis will have been made following necropsy, so therapy is aimed at preventing disease in other animals in the group.

Acknowledgements

The authors are grateful to: Udo Hetzel, Institute für Veterinärpathologie of the Justus Liebig University Giessen, Germany (current address: University of Zurich, Switzerland); Horst Posthaus and Lucca Bacciarini, Institut für Veterinärpathologie, Bern University, Switzerland; and Silvia Blahak, Staatliches Veterinäruntersuchungsamt Detmold, Germany, for the contribution of photographs.

References and further reading

Abbas MD, Ball I, Ruckova Z et al. (2012) Virological screening of bearded dragons (Pogona vitticeps) and the first detection of paramyxoviruses in this species. Journal of Herpetological Medicine and Surgery 22(3–4), 86–90

Ahne W, Batts WN, Kurath G and Winton JR (1999) Comparative sequence analysis of sixteen reptilian paramyxoviruses. Virus Research 63, 65–74

Allender MC, Abd-Eldaim M, Schumacher J et al. (2011) Ranavirus in free-ranging eastern box turtles (Terrapene carolina carolina) at rehabilitation centers in three southeastern US states. Journal of Wildlife Diseases 47, 759–764

Allender MC, Baker S, Wylie D et al. (2015) Development of snake fungal disease after experimental challenge with Ophidiomyces ophiodiicola in cottonmouths (Agkistrodon piscivorous) PLoS One 10(10), e0140193

Alves de Matos AP, Caeiro MF, Papp T et al. (2011) New viruses from Lacerta monticola (Serra da Estrela, Portugal): further evidence for a new group of nucleo-cytoplasmic large deoxyriboviruses (NCLDVs). Microscopy and Microanalysis 17, 101–108

Alves de Matos AP, Paperna I and Crespo E (2002) Experimental infection of lacertids with lizard erythrocytic viruses. Intervirology 45, 150–159

Ariel E (1997) Pathology and serological aspects of Bohle iridovirus infections in six selected water-associated reptiles in North Queensland. PhD thesis, James Cook University, Townsville, QLD

Ball I, Öffner S, Funk RS et al. (2013) Detection of antibodies against adenoviruses in lizards and snakes. Proceedings of the Association of Reptilian and Amphibian Veterinarians Annual Conference, Indianapolis, IN, p. 12

Behncke H, Stöhr AC, Heckers K, Ball I and Marschang RE (2013) Mass-mortality in green striped tree dragons (Japalura splendida) associated with multiple viral infections. Veterinary Record 173, 248

Benetka V, Grabensteiner E, Gumpenberger M et al. (2007) First report of an iridovirus (genus Ranavirus) infection in a leopard tortoise (Geochelone pardalis pardalis). Veterinary Medicine Austria/Wiener Tierärztliche Monatsschrift 94, 243–248

Bicknese EJ, Childress AL and Wellehan JFX (2010) A novel herpesvirus of the proposed genus Chelonivirus from an asymptomatic bowsprit tortoise (Chersina angulata). Journal of Zoo and Wildlife Medicine 41, 353–358

Blahak S (1995) Isolation and characterization of paramyxoviruses from snakes and their relationship to avian paramyxoviruses. Journal of Veterinary Medicine B 42, 216–224

Blahak S and Uhlenbrok C (2010) Ranavirus infections in European terrestrial tortoises in Germany. Proceedings of the 1st International Conference on Reptile and Amphibian Medicine, Munich, Germany, pp. 17–23

Bohuski E, Lorch JM, Griffin KM, and Blehert DS (2015) TaqMan real-time polymerase chain reaction for detection of Ophidiomyces ophiodiicola, the fungus associated with snake fungal disease. BMC Veterinary Research 11(1), 1

Chang L-W and Jacobson ER (2010) Inclusion body disease, a worldwide infectious disease of boid snakes: a review. Journal of Exotic Pet Medicine 19, 216–225

Chen Z, Zheng J and Jiang Y (1999) A new iridovirus isolated from soft-shelled turtle. Virus Research 63, 147–151

Chinchar VG (2002) Ranaviruses (family Iridoviridae): emerging cold-blooded killers. Archives of Virology 147, 447–470

Chinnadurai SK and DeVoe RS (2009) Selected infectious diseases of reptiles. Veterinary Clinics of North America: Exotic Animal Practice 12, 583–596

Clark HF and Lunger PD (1981) Viruses. In: Diseases of the Reptilia, Volume 1, ed. JE Cooper and OF Jackson, pp. 135–164. Academic Press, London

Cooper JE (2000) Reptilian microbiology. In: Laboratory Medicine: Avian and Exotic Pets, ed. A Fudge, pp. 223–228. WB Saunders, Philadelphia

Cooper JE, Gschmeissner S and Bone RD (1988) Herpes-like virus particles in necrotic stomatitis of tortoises. Veterinary Record 123, 544

Cooper JE, Needham JR and Lawrence K (1985) Studies on the cloacal flora of three species of free-living British reptile. Journal of Zoology 207(4), 521–525

Davison A and McGeoch D (2010) Create genus Scutavirus (type species: the currently unassigned species Chelonid herpesvirus 5) in subfamily Alphaherpesvirinae, family Herpesviridae. Code 2010.016a-eV. 2010.016a-eV.A.v2.Scutavirus.pdf, International Committee on Taxonomy of Viruses (ICTV): http://talk.ictvonline.org/files/ictv_official_taxonomy_updates_since_the_8th_report/m/vertebrate-official/4176

De Voe R, Geissler K, Elmore S et al. (2004) Ranavirus-associated mortality in a group of eastern box turtles (Terrapene carolina carolina). Journal of Zoo and Wildlife Medicine 35, 534–543

Doszpoly A, Wellehan JF Jr, Childress AL et al. (2013) Partial characterization of a new adenovirus lineage discovered in testudinoid turtles. Infection Genetics and Evolution 17, 106–112

Duffus ALJ, Waltzek TB, Stöhr et al. (2015) Distribution and Host Range of Ranaviruses. In: Ranaviruses: Lethal Pathogens of Ectothermic Vertebrates, ed. MJ Gray and VG Chinchar, pp. 9–58. SpringerOpen. DOI 10.1007/978-3-319-13755-1

Ebani VV, Fratini F, Ampola M et al. (2008) Pseudomonas and Aeromonas isolates from domestic reptiles and study of their antimicrobial in vitro sensitivity. Veterinary Research Communications 32, 195–198

Fölsch DW and Leloup P (1976) Fatale endemische Infektion in einem Serpentarium. Tierärztliche Praxis 4, 527–536

Garcia ME, Lanzarot P, Costas E et al. (2008) Isolation of Serratia fonticola from skin lesions in a Nile crocodile (Crocodylus niloticus) with an associated septicaemia. Veterinary Journal 176(2), 254–256

Gaskin JM, Haskell M, Keller N and Jacobson ER (1989) Serodiagnosis of ophidian paramyxovirus infections. Proceedings of the Third International Colloquium on the Pathology of Reptiles and Amphibians, pp. 21–23

Gopee NV, Adesiyun AA and Caesar K (2000) A longitudinal study of Escherichia coli strains isolated from captive mammals, birds, and reptiles in Trinidad. Journal of Zoo and Wildlife Medicine 31(3), 353–360

Graves SR, Rawlinson PA, Kennelly-Merrit SA et al. (1988). Enteric bacteria of reptiles on Java and the Krakatau Islands. Philosophical Transactions of the Royal Society of London B 322(1211), 355–361

Grim KD, Doherty C and Rosen T (2010) Serratia marcescens bullous cellulitis after iguana bites. Journal of the American Academy of Dermatology 62(6), 1075–1076

Guthrie AL, Knowles S, Ballmann AE, and Lorch JM (2015) Detection of snake fungal disease due to Ophidiomyces ophiodiicola in Virginia, USA. Journal of Wildlife Diseases 52(1), 143–149

Hanel R, Heard DJ, Ellis GA and Nguyen A (1999) Isolation of Clostridium spp. from the blood of captive lizards. Bulletin of the Association of Reptilian and Amphibian Veterinarians 9(2), 4–8

Heldstab A and Bestetti G (1984) Virus associated gastrointestinal disease in snakes. Journal of Zoo Animal Medicine 15, 118–128

Hetzel U, König A, Yildirim AÖ, Lämmler C and Kipar A (2003) Septicaemia in emerald monitors (Varanus prasinus Schlegel 1839) caused by Streptococcus agalactiae acquired from mice. Veterinary Microbiology 95(4), 283–293

Hoop RK (1997) Public health implications of exotic pet mycobacteriosis. Seminars in Avian and Exotic Medicine 6, 3–8

Hsieh S and Babl FE (1999) Serratia marcescens cellulitis following an iguana bite. Clinical Infectious Diseases 28(5), 1181–1182

Hyatt AD, Williamson M, Coupar BEH et al. (2002) First identification of a ranavirus from green pythons (Chondropython viridis). Journal of Wildlife Diseases 38, 239–252

Hyndman TH, Marschang RE, Wellehan JF Jr and Nicholls PK (2012) Isolation and molecular identification of Sunshine virus, a novel paramyxovirus found in Australian snakes. Infection, Genetics and Evolution 12, 1436–1446

Hyndman TH, Shilton CM and Marschang RE (2013) Paramyxoviruses in reptiles: a review. Veterinary Microbiology 165, 200–213

Jacobson ER (2007) Bacterial diseases of reptiles. In: Infectious Diseases and Pathology of Reptiles, ed. ER Jacobson, pp. 461–526. CRC Press, Boca Raton, FL, USA

Jacobson ER, Adams HP, Geisbert TW et al. (1997) Pulmonary lesions in experimental ophidian paramyxovirus pneumonia of Aruba island rattlesnakes, Crotalus unicolor. Veterinary Pathology 34, 450–459

Jacobson ER, Brown DR, Schumacher IM et al. (2000) An update on mycoplasmal respiratory disease of tortoises. Proceedings of the Association of Reptilian and Amphibian Veterinarians Annual Conference, pp. 131–132

Jacobson ER, Gaskin JM, Flanagan JP and Odum A (1991) Antibody responses of western diamondback rattlesnakes (*Crotalus atrox*) to inactivated ophidian paramyxovirus vaccines. *Journal of Zoo and Wildlife Medicine* **22**, 184–190

Jacobson ER, Gaskin JM and Gardiner CH (1985) Adenovirus-like infection in a boa constrictor. *Journal of the American Veterinary Medical Association* **187**, 1226–1227

Jacobson ER, Gaskin JM and Mansell J (1989) Chlamydial infection in puff adders (*Bitis arietans*). *Journal of Zoo and Wildlife Medicine* **20**, 364

Jacobson ER, Gaskin JM, Wells S, Bowler K and Schumacher J (1992) Epizootic of ophidian paramyxovirus in a zoological collection: pathological, microbiological, and serological findings. *Journal of Zoo and Wildlife Medicine* **23**, 318–327

Jacobson ER, Klingenberg RJ, Homer BL and Mader DR (1999) Roundtable: inclusion body disease. *Bulletin of the Association of Reptilian and Amphibian Veterinarians* **9**, 18–25

Jacobson ER and Kollias GV (1986) Adenovirus-like infection in a savannah monitor. *Journal of Zoo Animal Medicine* **17**, 149–151

Jacobson ER, Kopit W, Kennedy FA and Funk RS (1996) Coinfection of a bearded dragon, *Pogona vitticeps*, with adenovirus- and dependovirus-like viruses. *Veterinary Pathology* **33**, 343–346

Jacobson ER and Origgi F (2002) Use of serology in reptile medicine. *Seminars in Avian and Exotic Pet Medicine* **11(1)**, 33–45

Jacobson ER, Origgi F, Heard D and Detrisac C (2002) Immunohistochemical staining of chlamydial antigen in emerald tree boas (*Corallus caninus*). *Journal of Veterinary Diagnostic Investigation* **14**, 487–494

Jacobson ER, Origgi F, Pessier AP et al. (2001) Paramyxovirus infection in Caiman lizards (*Draecena guianensis*). *Journal of Veterinary Diagnostic Investigation* **13**, 143–151

Jho YS, Park DH, Lee JH, Cha SY and Han JS (2011) Identification of bacteria from the oral cavity and cloaca of snakes imported from Vietnam. *Laboratory Animal Research* **27(3)**, 213–217

Johnson AJ, Pessier AP and Jacobson ER (2007) Experimental transmission and induction of ranaviral disease in western ornate box turtles (*Terrapene ornata ornata*) and red-eared sliders (*Trachemys scripta elegans*). *Veterinary Pathology* **44**, 285–297

Johnson AJ, Wendland L, Norton TM, Belzer B and Jacobson ER (2010) Development and use of an indirect enzyme-linked immunosorbent assay for detection of iridovirus exposure in gopher tortoises (*Gopherus polyphemus*) and eastern box turtles (*Terrapene carolina carolina*). *Veterinary Microbiology* **142**, 160–167

Johnson-Delaney CA (1996) Reptile zoonoses and threats to public health. In: *Reptile Medicine and Surgery*, ed. DR Mader, pp. 20–33. WB Saunders, Philadelphia

Johnson-Delaney CA (2009) Precautions against zoonotic disease transmission from companion birds, reptiles and exotic pets. Available at: www.veterinariosenweb.com/campus/cdvl/memorias/material/136_Zoonosesexoticos.pdf

Julian AF and Durham JK (1982) Adenoviral hepatitis in a female bearded dragon (*Amphobolurus barbatus*). *New Zealand Veterinary Journal* **30**, 59–60

Just F, Essbauer S, Ahne W and Blahak S (2001) Occurrence of an invertebrate iridescent-like virus (Iridoviridae) in reptiles. *Journal of Veterinary Medicine B* **48**, 685–694

Khosravi AR, Shokri H, Rostami A et al. (2012) Severe dermatophytosis due to *Trichophyton mentagrophytes* var. *interdigitale* in flocks of green iguanas (*Iguana iguana*). *Journal of Small Animal Practice* **53**, 286–291

Kim DY, Mitchell MA, Bauer RW, Poston R and Cho D-Y (2002) An outbreak of adenoviral infection in inland bearded dragons (*Pogona vitticeps*) coinfected with dependovirus and coccidial protozoa (*Isospora* sp.). *Journal of Veterinary Diagnostic Investigation* **14**, 332–334

Kurath G, Batts WN, Ahne W and Winton JR (2004) Complete genome sequence of fer-de-lance virus reveals a novel gene in reptilian paramyxoviruses. *Journal of Virology* **78**, 2045–2056

Kycko A, Kozaczyński W, Jasik A et al. (2013) Granulomatous pneumonia and hepatitis associated with *Providencia rettgeri* infection in a crocodile monitor lizard (*Varanus salvadorii*). *Acta Veterinaria Hungarica* **61(1)**, 51–58

Latney LV and Wellehan J (2013) Selected emerging diseases of Squamata. *Veterinary Clinics of North America: Exotic Animal Practice* **16**, 319–338

Lorch JM, Lankton J, Werner K et al. (2015) Experimental infection of snakes with *Ophidiomyces ophiodiicola* causes pathological changes that typify snake fungal disease. *mBio* **6(6)**, e01534-15

Maas AK (2013) Vesicular ulcerative and necrotic dermatitis of reptiles. *Veterinary Clinics of North America: Exotic Animal Practice* **16**, 737–755

McArthur S, Blahak S, Kölle P et al. (2002) Roundtable: chelonian herpesviruses. *Journal of Herpetological Medicine and Surgery* **12**, 14–31

Mao J, Hedrick RP and Chinchar VG (1997) Molecular characterization, sequence analysis, and taxonomic position of newly isolated fish iridoviruses. *Virology* **229**, 212–220

Marschang RE (2011) Viruses infecting reptiles. *Viruses* **3**, 2087–2126, doi:10.3390/v311208

Marschang RE, Becher P and Braun S (2002) Isolation of iridoviruses from three different lizard species. *Proceedings of the Association of Reptilian and Amphibian Veterinarians Annual Conference*, pp. 99–100

Marschang RE, Becher P, Posthaus H et al. (1999) Isolation and characterization of an iridovirus from Hermann's tortoises (*Testudo hermanni*). *Archives of Virology* **144**, 1909–1922

Marschang RE, Braun S and Becher P (2005) Isolation of a ranavirus from a gecko (*Uroplatus fimbriatus*). *Journal of Zoo and Wildlife Medicine* **36**, 295–300

Marschang RE, Gleiser CB, Papp T et al. (2006) Comparison of eleven herpesvirus isolates from tortoises using partial sequences from three conserved genes. *Veterinary Microbiology* **117**, 258–266

Marschang RE, Michling R, Benkö M et al. (2003) Evidence for widespread *Atadenovirus* infection among snakes. *Proceedings of the 6th International Congress of Veterinary Virology*, p. 152

Marschang RE, Papp T and Frost JW (2009) Comparison of paramyxovirus isolates from snakes, lizards and a tortoise. *Virus Research* **144**, 272–279

Mathes K (2003) Untersuchungen zum Vorkommen von Mykoplasmen und Herpesviren bei freilebenden und in Gefangenschaft gehaltenen Mediterranen Landschildkröten (*Testudo hermanni*, *Testudo graeca graeca* und *Testudo graeca ibera*) in Frankreich und Marokko. *Veterinary Medical Dissertation*, Justus Leibig University, Giessen, Germany

Mitchell MA (2006) *Salmonella*: diagnostic methods for reptiles. In: *Reptile Medicine and Surgery, 2nd edition*, ed. DR Mader, pp. 900–905. Elsevier, St Louis

Mitchell MA (2012) Mycobacterial infections in reptiles. *Veterinary Clinics of North America: Exotic Animal Practice* **15**, 101–111

Mitchell MA, Barron B, Singh R et al. (2009) Evaluating the efficacy of four different antimicrobials against *Salmonella* in red-eared slider turtles. *Proceedings of the Association of Reptilian and Amphibian Veterinarians 16th Annual Conference*, p. 80

Mitchell MA, Nehlig R, Holley M-C, Diaz-Figueroa O and Riggs SR (2003) Evaluating the efficacy of Baquacil against *Salmonella* spp. in the aquatic environment of the red-eared slider (*Trachemys scripta elegans*). *Proceedings of the Association of Reptilian and Amphibian Veterinarians Annual Conference*, p. 109

Mitchell MA and Shane SM (2001) *Salmonella* in reptiles. *Seminars in Avian and Exotic Pet Medicine* **10(1)**, 25–35

Mitchell MA, Shane SM, Nevarez J et al. (2001a) Establishing a *Salmonella*-free iguana, *Iguana iguana*, model using enrofloxacin. *Proceedings of the Association of Reptilian and Amphibian Veterinarians Annual Conference*, pp. 189–190

Mitchell MA, Shane SM, Pesti D et al. (2001b) Effect of avirulent *Salmonella* vaccine on *Salmonella* colonisation of hatchling green iguanas, *Iguana iguana*. *Proceedings of the Association of Reptilian and Amphibian Veterinarians Annual Conference*, pp. 187–188

Mitchell MA and Walden MR (2013) *Chrysosporium* anamorph of *Nannizziopsis vriesii*: an emerging fungal pathogen of captive and wild reptiles. *Veterinary Clinics of North America: Exotic Animal Practice* **16**, 659–668

Müller M, Sachsse W and Zangger N (1990) Herpesvirus-Epidemie bei der griechischen (*Testudo hermanni*) und der maurischen Landschildkröte (*Testudo graeca*) in der Schweiz. *Schweizer Archiv für Tierheilkunde* **132**, 199–203

Neul A, Schrödl W, Marschang RE et al. (2017) Immunologic responses in corn snakes (*Pantherophis guttatus*) after experimentally induced infection with ferlaviruses. *American Journal of Veterinary Research* **78**, 482–494

Origgi FC, Klein PA, Mathes K et al. (2001) Enzyme-linked immunosorbent assay for detecting herpesvirus exposure in Mediterranean tortoises. *Journal of Clinical Microbiology* **39**, 3156–3163

Origgi FC, Klein PA, Tucker SJ and Jacobson ER (2000) Serological and molecular diagnostic techniques for chelonian herpesviruses. *Proceedings of the 5th International Congress of the European Society for Veterinary Virology*, pp. 113–114

Origgi FC, Klein PA, Tucker SJ and Jacobson ER (2003) Application of immunoperoxidase-based techniques to detect herpesvirus infection in tortoises. *Journal of Veterinary Diagnostic Investigation* **15**, 133–140

Oros J, Hernandez JD, Gallardo J, Lupiola P and Jensen HE (2013) Dermatophytosis caused by *Trichophyton* spp. in a Tenerife lizard (*Gallotia galloti*): an immunohistochemical study. *Journal of Comparative Pathology* **149**, 372–375

Oros J, Sicilia J, Torrent A et al. (2001) Immunohistochemical detection of ophidian paramyxovirus in snakes in the Canary Islands. *Veterinary Record* **149**, 21–23

Papp T, Seybold J and Marschang RE (2011) Paramyxovirus infection in a leopard tortoise (*Geochelone pardalis babcocki*) with respiratory disease. *Journal of Herpetological Medicine and Surgery* **20**, 64–68

Paré JA (2003) Fungi and fungal diseases of reptiles. *Proceedings of the Association of Reptilian and Amphibian Veterinarians Annual Conference*, pp. 128–131

Paré JA, Coyle KA, Sigler I et al. (2006a) Pathogenicity of the *Chrysosporium* anamorph of *Nannizziopsis vriesii* for veiled chameleons (*Chamaeleo calyptratus*). *Medical Mycology* **44**, 25–31

Paré JA, Sigler L, Rosenthal KL and Mader DR (2006b) Microbiology: fungal and bacterial diseases of reptiles. In: *Reptile Medicine and Surgery, 2nd edition*, ed. DR Mader, pp. 217–238. Elsevier, St Louis

Paré JA, Sigler L, Rypien KL et al. (2003) Cutaneous mycobiota of captive squamate reptiles with notes on the scarcity of *Chrysosporium* anamorph of *Nannizziopsis vriesii*. *Journal of Herpetological Medicine and Surgery* **13**, 10–15

Pasmans F, Hellebuck T, Haesebrouck F and Martel A (2010) Dermatitis and septicaemia caused by *Devriesea agamarum*: an overview including recent developments in disease management. *Proceedings of the 1st International Conference on Reptile and Amphibian Medicine*, Munich, Germany, pp. 105–106

Pees M, Neul A, Müller K et al. (2016) Virus distribution and detection in corn snakes (*Pantherophis guttatus*) after experimental infection with three different ferlavirus strains. *Veterinary Microbiology* **182**, 213–222

Pericard JM and Blahak S (2013) Occurrence of Mycoplasma, Chlamydia and herpesvirus in land tortoises with respiratory or ocular diseases in the south of France. *Proceedings of the 1st International Conference on Avian, Herpetological and Exotic Mammal Medicine*, Wiesbaden, Germany, p. 140

Perkins LEL, Campagnoli RP, Harmon BG *et al.* (2001) Detection and confirmation of reptilian adenovirus infection by *in situ* hybridization. *Journal of Veterinary Diagnostic Investigation* **13**, 365–368

Pessoa CA (2009) Bacterial and fungal microbiota evaluation in the companion tortoise (*Geochelone carbonaria*) and the analysis of the potential risk to human health. Doctoral dissertation, Faculdade de Medicina Veterinária e Zootecnia, Universidade de São Paulo

Quinn PJ, Markey BK, Carter ME and Carter GR (1994) Introduction to the pathogenic fungi. In: *Veterinary Clinical Microbiology*, pp. 367–380. Mosby Wolfe, London

Rivera S, Wellehan JF Jr, McManamon R *et al.* (2009) Systemic adenovirus infection in Sulawesi tortoises (*Indotestudo forsteni*) caused by a novel siadenovirus. *Journal of Veterinary Diagnostic Investigation* **21**, 415–426

Roggendorf M and Müller HE (1976) (Enterobacteria of reptiles (author's transl.)). Zentralblatt für Bakteriologie, Parasitenkunde, Infektionskrankheiten und Hygiene. Erste Abteilung Originale. *Reihe A: Medizinische Mikrobiologie und Parasitologie* **236(1)**, 22–35

Rose FL, Koke J, Koehn R *et al.* (2001) Identification of the etiological agent for necrotizing scute disease in the Texas tortoise. *Journal of Wildlife Diseases* **37**, 223–228

Ruegg S, Regenscheit N, Origgi F, Kaiser C and Borel N, (2015) Detection of *Chlamydia pneumoniae* in a collection of captive snakes and response to treatment with marbofloxacin. *Veterinary Journal* **205(30)**, 424–426

Scheelings TF, Lightfoot D and Holz P (2011) Prevalence of *Salmonella* in Australian reptiles. *Journal of Wildlife Diseases* **47(1)**, 1–11

Schumacher IM, Brown MB, Jacobson ER, Collins BR and Klein PA (1993) Detection of antibodies to a pathogenic mycoplasma in desert tortoises (*Gopherus agassizii*) with upper respiratory tract disease. *Journal of Clinical Microbiology* **31**, 1454–1460

Schumacher J (1996) Viral diseases. In: *Reptile Medicine and Surgery*, ed. DR Mader, pp. 224–234. WB Saunders, Philadelphia

Schumacher J (2003) Fungal disease of reptiles. *Veterinary Clinics of North America: Exotic Animal Practice* **6**, 327–335

Schumacher J, Jacobson ER, Burns R and Tramontin RR (1994) Adenovirus-like infection in two rosy boas (*Lichanura trivirgata*). *Journal of Zoo and Wildlife Medicine* **25**, 461–465

Sigler L, Hambleton S and Páre JA (2013) Molecular characterization of reptile pathogens currently known as members of the *Chrysosporium anamorph* of *Nannizziopsis vriesii* complex and relationship with some human-associated isolates. *Journal of Clinical Microbiology* **51(10)**, 3338–3357

Smith TG, Desser SS and Hong H (1994) Morphology, ultrastructure and taxonomic status of *Toddia* sp. in northern water snakes (*Nerodia sipedon sipedon*) from Ontario. *Canadian Journal of Wildlife Diseases* **30**, 169–175

Snipes KP (1984) *Pasteurella* in reptiles. In: *Diseases of Amphibians and Reptiles*, eds GL Hoff, FL Frye and ER Jacobsen, pp. 25–35. Springer, New York

Soares JF, Chalker VJ, Erles K *et al.* (2003) Prevalence of *Mycoplasma agassizii* and Chelonian Herpesvirus in captive tortoises (*Testudo* spp.) in the United Kingdom. *Proceedings of the Association of Reptilian and Amphibian Veterinarians Annual Conference*, p. 91

Stacy BA and Pessier AP (2007) Host response to infectious agents and identification of pathogens in tissue section. In: *Infectious Diseases and Pathology of Reptiles*, ed. ER Jacobson, pp. 257–298. CRC Press, Boca Raton, FL, USA

Stehbens WE and Johnston MRL (1966) The viral nature of *Pirhemocyton tarentolae*. *Journal of Ultrastructural Research* **15**, 543–554

Stenglein MD, Jacobson ER, Wozniak EJ *et al.* (2014) Ball python nidovirus: a candidate etiologic agent for severe respiratory disease in *Python regius*. *mBio* **5(5)**, e01484-14

Stenglein MD, Sanders C, Kistler AL *et al.* (2012) Identification, characterization, and *in vitro* culture of highly divergent arenaviruses from boa constrictors and annulated tree boas: candidate etiological agents for snake inclusion body disease. *mBio* **3(4)**, e00180-12

Stewart JS (1990) Anaerobic bacterial infections in reptiles. *Journal of Zoo and Wildlife Medicine* **(21)**, 180–184

Stöhr AC, Blahak S, Heckers KO *et al.* (2013) Ranavirus infections associated with skin lesions in lizards. *Veterinary Research* **44**, 84, doi:10.1186/1297-9716-44-84

Teifke JP, Löhr CV, Marschang RE, Osterrieder N and Posthaus H (2000) Detection of chelonid herpesvirus DNA by nonradioactive *in situ* hybridization in tissues from tortoises suffering from stomatitis–rhinitis complex in Europe and North America. *Veterinary Pathology* **37**, 377–385

Uhlenbrok C (2010) Nachweis von Ranavirusinfektionen bei Landschildkröten und Charakterisierung von Virusisolaten (Detection of ranavirus infections in tortoises and characterization of virus isolates). Inaugural thesis for the degree of Dr. med. vet. with specialist area veterinary medicine, Justus-Liebig-Universität Giessen, Germany

Une Y, Murakami M, Uemura K *et al.* (2000) Polymerase chain reaction (PCR) for the detection of herpesvirus in tortoises. *Journal of Veterinary Medical Science* **62**, 905–907

van Devanter DR, Warrender P, Bennett L *et al.* (1996) Detection and analysis of diverse herpesviral species by consensus primer PCR. *Journal of Clinical Microbiology* **34**, 1666–1671

Vanrompay D, De Meurichy W, Ducatelle R and Haesebruck F (1994) Pneumonia in Moorish tortoises (*Testudo graeca*) associated with avian serovar A *Chlamydia psittaci*. *Veterinary Record* **135**, 284–285

van Waeyenberghe L, Baert K, Pasmans F *et al.* (2010) Voriconazole, a safe alternative for treating infections caused by the *Chrysosporium* anamorph of *Nannizziopsis vriesii* in bearded dragons (*Pogona vitticeps*). *Medical Mycology* **48(6)**, 880–885

Weinmann NT, Papp T, Alves de Matos AP, Teifke JP and Marschang RE (2007) Experimental infection of crickets (*Gryllus bimaculatus*) with an invertebrate iridovirus isolated from a high-casqued chameleon (*Chamaeleo hoehnelii*). *Journal of Veterinary Diagnostic Investigation* **19**, 674–679

Wellehan JF, Johnson AJ, Harrach B *et al.* (2004) Detection and analysis of six lizard adenoviruses by consensus primer PCR provides further evidence of a reptilian origin for the atadenoviruses. *Journal of Virology* **78**, 13366–13369

Wellehan JF Jr, Strik NI, Stacy BA *et al.* (2008) Characterization of an erythrocytic virus in the family Iridoviridae from a peninsula ribbon snake (*Thamnophis sauritus sackenii*). *Veterinary Microbiology* **131**, 115–122

West G, Garner M, Raymond J, Latimer KS and Nordhausen R (2001) Meningoencephalitis in a Boelen's python (*Morelia boeleni*) associated with paramyxovirus infection. *Journal of Zoo and Wildlife Medicine* **32**, 360–365

Wolf K (1988) Viral erythrocytic necrosis. In: *Fish Viruses and Fish Viral Disease*, ed. K Wolf, pp. 389–398. Comstock Publishing, Ithaca, NY

Chapter 26

Crocodilians

Darryl Heard

Crocodilians should not be kept as pets. All are dangerous and have the potential to maim or kill. Many species are critically endangered. All require large terrestrial and aquatic habitats, as well as warm temperatures for optimum health. Veterinary surgeons (veterinarians) are most likely to be consulted for animals housed in zoological or research facilities, or crocodilian farms. This chapter is an introduction to the medical management of these fascinating reptiles. For further reading this author recommends Richardson *et al.* (2000), Huchzermeyer (2003) and Jacobson (2007).

All living crocodilians belong to the family Crocodylidae, subdivided into crocodiles, false gavials, alligators, caimans and gharials. Figure 26.1 illustrates some commonly kept species.

Biology

Anatomy

All living crocodilians are similar in structure. The main differences between species are in adult size, skull structure and skin. The skin is covered with scales or scutes arranged in different patterns for each species. The skin of the skull is closely adhered to the underlying bone. Bony plates (osteoderms) are present in the dorsal as well as ventral scales of some species. These calcified structures may obscure radiographic visualization of internal structures and interfere with needle placement for blood collection (Figure 26.2). Although tough and heavily protected, the skin is well innervated with pain and thermal receptors and mechanoreceptors. Paired holocrine glands are present lateral to the cloacal opening (cloacal or paracloacal) and in the posterior intermandibular skin (mandibular or gular). Each large paracloacal gland empties through a single duct. These glands may be mistaken for abscesses during necropsy. The mandibular glands may be everted during physical restraint in alligators and other species.

The external nares are located at the dorsorostral end of the skull, and are closed tightly except during inhalation and exhalation (Figure 26.3). The opening to the ear is located caudal to the eye and is covered by a flap (Figure 26.4). During diving, sphincters close the nares and a depressor muscle closes the auricular flap. Manipulation of the nares or the earflaps in an awake animal will usually elicit a violent reaction. The eyes can be retracted and closed tightly, making ophthalmic examination difficult. An opaque third eyelid covers the cornea during submersion (Figure 26.5). As in birds, the iris is composed of striated rather than smooth muscle. Prominent supratemporal fossae, located dorsal and posterior to the eyes, can be indicative of muscle wasting in some species (Figure 26.6). The cranial cavity lies between the orbits and the supratemporal fossae.

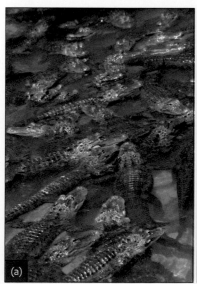

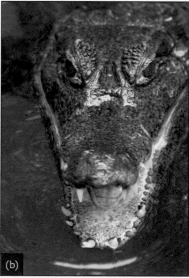

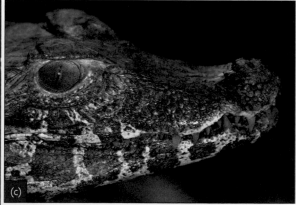

26.1 Crocodilians are not recommended as pets. Some species that may, however, be encountered by veterinary surgeons (veterinarians) include (a) the American alligator, (b) spectacled caiman and (c) the dwarf caiman. Some crocodilians can tolerate high densities as juveniles (e.g. alligators), but not as adults.

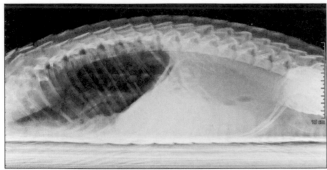

26.2 Lateral radiograph of a dwarf caiman. Note the presence of the osteoderms (bony plates) within the scales.

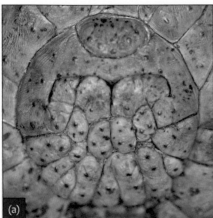

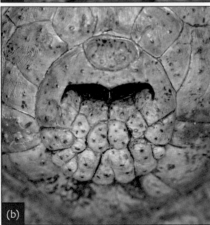

26.3 Crocodilian nares are located at the dorsorostral end of the maxilla. (a) The nares are usually tightly closed, except (b) during inhalation and exhalation. Crocodilians strenuously resist sampling from within the nares.

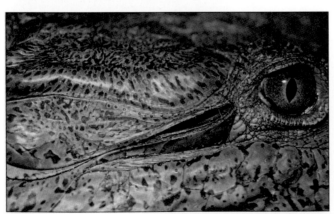

26.4 The openings to the ears are located immediately behind the eyes and covered by the auricular flap. The tympanic membrane can be visualized when this flap is raised, but awake animals will violently resist this movement. Leeches can occasionally be found under the flap.

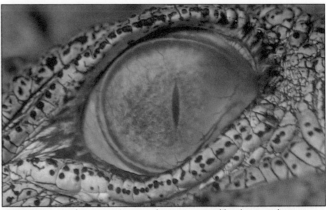

26.5 As in this estuarine or saltwater crocodile, the translucent third eyelid covers the eye during diving. It is well vascularized and contains inflammatory cells that may react to irritants and infectious agents.

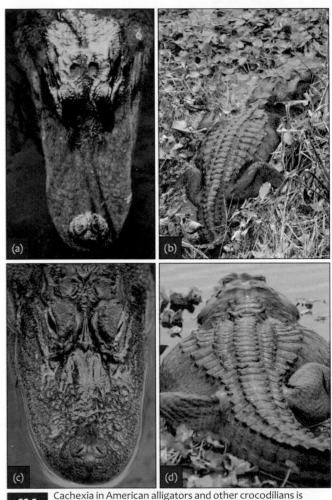

26.6 Cachexia in American alligators and other crocodilians is indicated by (a) prominent supratemporal fossae and (b) obvious pelvic bones and narrow neck, compared with (c–d) healthy animals. In severe cachexia the tail will turn laterally owing to loss of muscle mass.

The homomorphic (same shape) teeth are replaced constantly throughout life, although this process slows as the animal ages. The teeth should be pointed and sharp and are usually white (Figure 26.7). In crocodiles the first mandibular canine is the longest and often extends above the snout. In some animals mandibular incisors penetrate the maxilla to produce 'false nares'. The teeth are surrounded by mechanoreceptors and pain receptors, as well as taste buds.

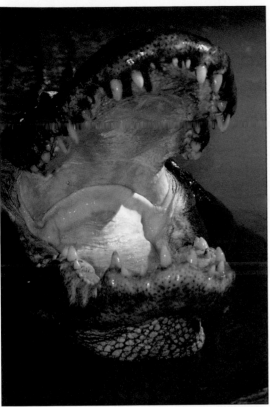

26.7 The oral cavity of an adult American alligator. Note the large sharp white teeth, the gular flap at the back of the throat, the large relatively immobile tongue and the wide powerful gape.

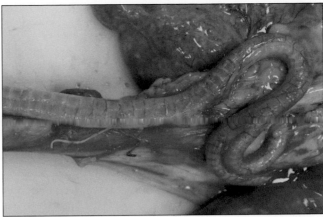

26.8 The trachea of a Philippine crocodile, showing a normal lateral deviation of the trachea.

The large tongue covers the floor of the mouth, but is attached laterally and is relatively immobile (see Figure 26.7). Its dorsal surface contains mucus glands associated with lymphoid tissue. Crocodiles also have salt glands on the dorsal surface of the tongue. In hypovitaminosis A the lingual glands may be altered by squamous metaplasia, leading to caseous abscesses. The powerful jaw muscles attach to the medial mandibular surfaces. The jaw articulation is behind the atlanto-occipital joint, allowing a very wide mouth opening (see Figure 26.7). The closing force of the jaws of an adult American alligator is sufficient to crush the shell of a large freshwater turtle.

The oral cavity is separated from the pharynx by the gular flap (see Figure 26.7). This flap allows crocodilians to open their mouths underwater. The simple glottis lies immediately behind this flap, is linked to the internal nares and closes during swallowing. Both Eustachian tubes enter the pharynx through a common opening slightly posterior to the internal nares. Close to this opening are two lateral mucosal folds containing tonsillar tissue. This tissue is important to sample during a necropsy for evidence of infectious disease. As would be expected, the thoracic inlet is big to allow large portions of unmasticated food to be swallowed. In crocodiles, but not alligators, the trachea bends to the left inside the thorax before its bifurcation (Figure 26.8).

All the vertebrae have dorsal spinous processes and both the cervical and thoracic vertebrae have ribs. The ribs connected to the sternum are partially cartilaginous, allowing them to collapse during diving. The caudal vertebrae have ventral spinous processes (haemal arches) protecting the coccygeal vessels. The pubic bones are connected to the sternum by a fibrous membrane containing abdominal ribs (gastralia). This membrane supports the abdominal viscera.

The humerus, radius and ulna are short; the hindlimbs are twice as long as the forelimbs. The fore- and hindlimbs have five and four toes, respectively. Claws are present on the first three toes of each limb. The pelvic girdle consists of an ilium and ischium and a cranioventrally directed pubis.

The lungs are highly vascularized, thick walled and multisaccular. They lie in pleural chambers separated by a complete mediastinum. Although there is no diaphragm, two transverse membranes divide the thorax from the abdomen. These fibrous and muscular membranes attach the caudal lung to the liver and the liver to the os pubis. During inspiration the liver is pulled caudally, increasing the volume of the lungs and generating a negative pressure. Expiration is both passive and active. In alligators, and probably all crocodilians, airflow through the lungs is unidirectional. Crocodilians make a range of sounds by forcing air through the compressed glottal opening. They are able to remain submerged for 30 minutes or more. Owing to their low metabolic rate they also have a large respiratory reserve; crocodilians rarely show clinical signs of respiratory distress even when much of the lungs has been compromised.

The oesophagus has many longitudinal folds to accommodate large chunks of food. The stomach lies to the left, immediately behind the left lobe of the liver. There is a well-defined sphincter between the cardia and the oesophagus. The small bulbous pyloric antrum lies slightly to the right of the cardia and opens into the duodenum. The pyloric opening is very small, preventing the escape of foreign bodies. The gastric wall is strongly muscularized, giving the stomach a gizzard-like appearance. Stones (gastroliths) are commonly found in the stomach, but their function is unknown. The intestine, as in other vertebrates, is composed of duodenum, jejunum, ileum and colorectum emptying into the cloaca. The duodenum is looped, sometimes doubly in crocodiles. The intestinal mucosa is formed into a system of complex zigzagging ridge-like folds.

The proximal pancreas lies within the duodenal loop, while the distal part surrounds the cranial spleen. The liver is bilobed, the right being slightly larger than the left, and separated by the heart. The gall bladder lies between the two lobes and receives bile from both. The pear-shaped spleen lies in the mesentery close to the base of the duodenal loop. The four chambers of the heart are completely separated and crocodilians have two aortic arches.

The mesenteries, especially those of the small intestine, are areas of fat deposition. In addition, crocodilians have a creamy rhomboid to triangular solid fat body.

During periods of anorexia the fat is slowly resorbed causing the structure to become smaller and reddish to orange in colour. Inexperienced clinicians may misidentify the fat body as either a neoplasm or an inflammatory structure.

The two kidneys are firmly attached to the dorsal abdominal wall in the caudal coelom. They lack a capsule and are not embedded in fat. The renal tissue is folded over: in a single fold in the dwarf crocodile and in multiple folds in other species. Crocodilians do not have a urinary bladder; the two ureters open into the cloaca.

Sexing

Most crocodilians are not sexually dimorphic, although adult males are usually larger than females. The male gharial develops a protuberance on the end of its nose, the ghar, when sexually mature. The sex of all crocodilians can be determined by palpation of the anterior cloaca for a phallus in the male (Figure 26.9). Females possess a similar, but much smaller, structure. This phallus can occasionally be extruded in juveniles by gently palpating the cloacal area. Males have paired internal testes close to the kidneys. Females have paired ovaries and all species are oviparous.

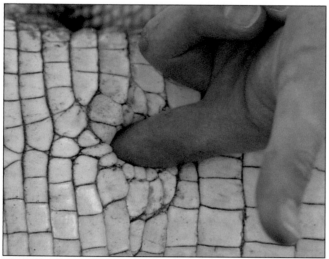

26.9 All crocodilians can be sexed by palpating the phallus on the ventral floor of the male cloaca.

Husbandry

Inappropriate husbandry and malnutrition are the main causes of disease in captivity.

Housing

Detailed online information for housing is provided by Britton (2012). Adult crocodilians should not be housed in mixed-species exhibits. Cannibalism is common when small individuals are housed with large (Figure 26.10). Compatibility will change depending on sexual status, housing density, body size and for unknown reasons. Even animals housed together for many years may become aggressive to each other. Providing adequate hiding areas in an appropriately sized enclosure can reduce aggression. Alligators and dwarf crocodiles can make extensive tunnels into the banks of natural aquatic enclosures. For a pair of crocodiles, it is recommended the minimum land area be three times the largest animal's snout–vent length

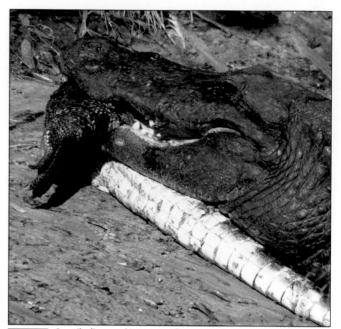

26.10 Cannibalism and intraspecific aggression is common in crocodilians. This is a major reason why usually animals of different sizes should not be housed together.

(SVL) wide and four times SVL long. The minimum water area should be at least four times the largest animal's SVL wide and five times SVL long, and minimum depth must be 0.3 times SVL.

Crocodilians are adapted to environments with moderate to high humidity and warm temperatures. Most have a preferred body temperature of approximately 30°C (29–34°C). Air temperatures in enclosures can range from 36°C during the day to 20°C at night, but water temperatures are maintained around 27–31°C. It is important that animals do not overheat; temperatures above 40°C should be avoided. Conversely, long periods of hypothermia will depress appetite, slow digestion and growth, and impair immune function. In small- to medium-sized enclosures the water can be heated with submersible aquarium heaters capable of using 1 watt of power to heat 1 litre of water. All heaters must have a thermostat to prevent overheating, be pretested before adding an animal to the enclosure and be connected to a ground-fault circuit interrupter. At least one basking area over land is required in the enclosure for each crocodilian. A thermostat is used to accurately control the temperature. When environmental temperatures are measured they are taken at the level where the animal's head or back is likely to be. The temperatures to aim for are the higher ends of the preferred body temperatures. The surface temperature of the substrate must also be measured because a cold surface, even in a warm environment, will make an animal hypothermic.

Incandescent bulbs are commonly used as heating elements. Other heat sources suitable for larger enclosures include ceramic heat emitters. Higher wattages require a ceramic lamp holder because the lamps become very hot. To prevent thermal injury ensure the animals cannot reach the heater. An advantage of a ceramic heat emitter is that it can be used at night without emitting light to disrupt the circadian cycle. Many crocodilians are active at night, but do not require a night light.

The land area should be large enough for every animal to emerge from the water into an area either within or outside the basking spot. Most crocodilians require a day (12–13 hours)/night period. Daylight can be provided using incandescent bulbs or fluorescent tubes, or simply natural light if the day length is sufficient. Dim light at night can be provided with coloured incandescent bulbs, or natural moonlight when it is available. Although controversial, it is recommended that a fluorescent light emitting both UVA and UVB wavelengths be used for animals not exposed to sunlight. Some species of crocodilians, such as the dwarf caimans and the dwarf crocodile, often spend considerable amounts of their daytime hidden in burrows or under dense vegetation in the wild.

Contaminated water and unclean enclosures will predispose to disease, and reflect ignorance or poor husbandry. Any uneaten food should be removed from the enclosure as soon as possible, and faeces should be cleaned up immediately. A filtration system should be used to keep the water clean. Unless the water is replaced frequently, it is recommended that a bacterial system be used to break down ammonia and other toxic contaminants. Protein films that form on the water surface should be removed with skimmers. No matter the type of filtration system, frequent water changes are recommended. The enclosure must also be cleaned periodically (every week or two).

Diet

All crocodilians are carnivores. Although the ideal diet should mimic that eaten in the wild, the diet and nutritional requirements of many crocodilian species have not been defined. All crocodilians should have access to water for drinking and bathing. Some species, e.g. the estuarine or saltwater crocodile, can drink salt water. Dietary supplementation should be unnecessary if the animals are fed a complete balanced diet. Crocodilians can be fed whole prey items (e.g. rodents, rabbits, etc.), a commercial pelleted diet or, in the case of fish eaters, whole fish or a fish gel. This author recommends the use of commercial pellets because they are balanced and inexpensive, and it is easy to monitor the food intake of an animal. Similarly, the fish gels are balanced and less expensive than feeding fresh fish. Contrary to popular opinion, crocodilians do not like eating rotten food. The best guide to whether you feed something to a crocodilian is whether you would eat it yourself. Several nutritional deficiency syndromes have been identified, including metabolic bone disease, hypovitaminosis A and E, and thiamine deficiency. Steatitis may be associated with hypovitaminosis E. Obesity is also a major nutritional problem of captive crocodilians (Figure 26.11). Lead toxicosis is a possible complication of feeding prey that has been shot, or urban wildlife (e.g. pigeons) contaminated with lead.

Handling and restraint

Physical restraint or chemical immobilization is required for examination and collection of diagnostic samples. Techniques for restraint of juvenile and adult crocodilians are well described by Vliet (2014). If you have no experience restraining a crocodilian, especially medium to large animals, you must seek help from people who have.

All crocodilians are dangerous. Although the teeth are the most obvious potential cause of injury, the tail can also inflict severe injury. Although some crocodilians will show behavioural indications of impending aggression (e.g. hissing), most do not. Aggressive responses are explosive and crocodilians may not immediately respond to touch or a close approach. When restrained they will roll to escape.

Small crocodilians are caught using either protective gloves or a heavy towel. All are approached from behind and the immediate target of capture is to grasp the animal behind the head and press it down to the ground. The opening force of the jaws is weak and they can be taped shut with electrical tape. The tape must avoid the nares. If the jaws are taped for long periods of time the animal will become dehydrated, even if immersed in water. When the mouth is taped shut, exposed teeth can still injure or lacerate when the head is swung. The legs must not be tied above the back because of the potential for muscle injury. Struggling crocodilians will develop lactic acidaemia. Large crocodilians can be restrained using flat boards and strapping (Figure 26.12). Captive crocodilians may also be trained to enter restraint crates for blood collection, reproductive ultrasonography and other minor diagnostic procedures.

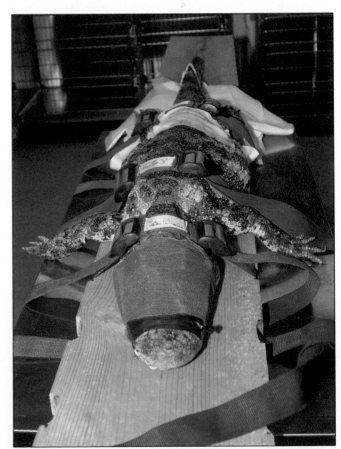

26.12 Medium to large crocodilians may be restrained on purpose-built boards with straps, to allow transport and minor diagnostic procedures. This caiman has its jaws taped shut with plumber's tape, its eyes covered with bandage wrap and seat-belt straps for body restraint. This set-up is suitable for performing a computerized axial tomography (CAT) scan in small- to medium-sized awake animals.

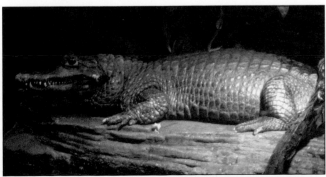

26.11 As in this yacare caiman, obesity is a common nutritional problem in captive crocodilians. Note the large jowls, abdominal distension and swollen limbs. Oedema from vasculitis, as in septicaemia, may resemble these clinical signs, but animals would also be depressed and weak.

Diagnostic approach

The history, especially of husbandry, is very important in evaluating crocodilian patients (Figure 26.13).

Physical examination

Physical examination first begins at a distance, observing the enclosure and the animal. The animal is assessed for body position, abnormal swellings or discharges, respiration rate, body condition (see Figures 26.6 and 26.11), relationship to its physical surroundings, interaction with other animals in the enclosure, and response to feeding and other stimuli (e.g. noise, approach of a human and touch). Figure 26.14 gives details for systematic examination.

General

Date .... Client identification .... Animal identification ....

Species (common and scientific names) .... Sex and age ..

Presenting problem(s) ....

Where did you obtain this animal and when? ....

Do you have the appropriate permits? .... Was this animal captive bred or caught wild? ....

If owned previously, do you know by whom and for how long? ....

What medical problems, if any, has this animal had previously? ....

If group housed, have there been any health problems in the other animals? ....

Housing

Is this animal housed indoors, outdoors or both? ....

Please describe or draw the enclosure with approximate dimensions ....

Is the aquatic environment fresh water or salt water? ....

How is the water cleaned and what filtration, if any, is used? ....

Environment

How is heat provided on land and in the water? ....

Maximum, minimum and average day/night temperatures ....

How do you monitor environmental temperatures? ....

Is humidity varied and monitored? ....

What lighting is provided? ....

What is the photoperiod and how is it managed? ....

Nutrition

What and how much food is fed? How often and when? ....

Does the animal eat all of its food? .... Does food vary with season? ....

Any mineral or vitamin supplements? ....

How is food prepared? ....

Observations

Activity and appetite ....

How often are faeces passed? ....

Reproductive data

Age at sexual maturity ....

Has this animal laid eggs and if so when? .... Does this animal build a nest and defend it? ....

Kept in isolation or as part of group? .... Last contact with opposite sex? ....

Disease control

Do you have a quarantine programme? .... How long is the quarantine period? ....

What disinfectants are used, how and when? ....

When did this animal last meet a new crocodilian? ....

26.13 Sample history form and questions.

26.14   A physical examination checklist.

Sample collection

Blood

Approximately 10% of the blood volume can be collected safely, assuming the animal is not severely anaemic. In reptiles this is approximately 0.6–1.0% of bodyweight (1 ml = 1 g). For example, 30–60 ml could be collected from a 5 kg animal. Blood for a complete blood count (CBC) and plasma biochemical panel can be collected into a heparinized syringe, and then placed into serum tubes. Alternatively, blood for the CBC can be collected into a non-heparinized syringe and placed in an edetate calcium disodium tube. This anticoagulant does not appear to haemolyse crocodilian blood as it does in other reptiles. Prepare several air-dried smears. One heparinized blood sample should be centrifuged immediately, and the plasma separated, decanted and frozen until analysis.

There are several blood collection sites in crocodilians. These include the spinal vein (supravertebral sinus) (Zippel *et al.*, 2003; Myburgh *et al.*, 2014), and ventral and dorsal coccygeal vessels. The skin at all blood collection sites should be cleaned and disinfected before needle insertion.

The spinal vein arises from an enlarged occipital sinus over the medulla and extends the whole length of the vertebral column. It lies immediately above the spinal cord. The indentation immediately behind the back of the skull is palpated and the needle inserted in the midline at the point of greatest depression (Figure 26.15a) located between the atlas and axis (C1 and C2). In Nile crocodiles this depression is just cranial to the first cervical osteoderms. Once the needle is inserted through the skin, the plunger of the syringe is pulled back to generate a small amount of negative pressure. The needle, oriented 90 degrees to perpendicular, is then slowly advanced until blood enters the syringe (Figure 26.15b). The hub of the needle is steadied with one hand resting on the animal. If the animal twitches or clear liquid enters the needle, it has gone too far. If the needle contacts bone, withdraw and redirect the needle. Needle sizes depend on the animal. The largest needle required for an adult would be 60–80 mm long, while 30 mm should be adequate for most small- to medium-sized crocodilians. The dorsal coccygeal vessels described below are an extension of the spinal vein. This author has used a 7.5 MHz ultrasound probe to identify the vessel in medium to large crocodilians.

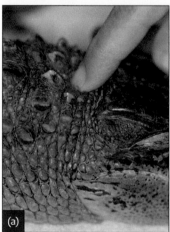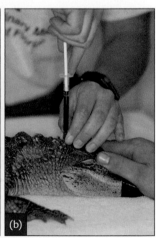

26.15   Blood collection from the supravertebral sinus. After disinfecting the skin, (a) the deepest depression (C1–C2) behind the skull is palpated, (b) the needle is inserted perpendicularly in the midline and, with a slight suction on the syringe, advanced until blood is aspirated.

The ventral coccygeal vessels are located in the midline immediately below the vertebral bodies (Figure 26.16a). They include both an artery and vein(s) and are protected by ventral spinous processes formed into haemal arches. These arches angle caudoventrally. The coccygeal vessels can be accessed using either a ventral or a lateral approach. For the ventral approach, the animal is placed either in dorsal recumbency or left in sternal recumbency, and the tail lifted and gently flexed to expose the ventral surface. Hyperflexion of the distal tail of a dwarf caiman may cause it to break off. The needle is inserted in the midline and advanced cranially at a 45–40 degree angle until either the vertebral body or vessels are contacted. If bone is touched, withdraw gently with a slight negative pressure and redirect.

The lateral approach allows the animal to remain in ventral recumbency (Figure 26.16ab). The transverse process is palpated, and the needle inserted between the process and the ventral midline. The needle is perpendicular to the long axis, but angled upwards at 45 degrees. The needle is then advanced until it contacts the bone of the vertebral body, then 'walked' ventrally until it enters the coccygeal vessels. The ventral coccygeal vessels can be catheterized for fluid administration (Wellehan *et al.*, 2004) (Figure 26.16c).

The dorsal coccygeal vessel(s) can be accessed in the midline, similarly to the supravertebral sinus discussed

Blood culture: Blood culture is useful for identifying circulating bacteria, both aerobic and anaerobic, associated with pathological processes. More importantly, once identified, sensitivity testing can be performed to direct antimicrobial therapy. Samples of 2–5 ml of blood are placed in the appropriate media bottles. If the animal is undergoing antibiotic therapy, special bottles are used to bind the antibiotic. It is very important that the blood sample is collected in as sterile a manner as possible to avoid environmental contamination. The skin must be disinfected, sterile surgical gloves should ideally be worn by the collector and the needle used for collection must be changed for a sterile new needle before insertion into the blood culture bottle.

Faecal examination

Faeces are usually eliminated into the water. Fresh samples collected from water with a dip net may be examined, as for any other mammal. Since the sample is from water, care must be taken in interpreting the significance of motile protozoa. As crocodilians are carnivores, parasites and their ova from prey items will also pass through in the digesta.

Urinalysis

The primary nitrogenous excretory product is ammonia (Pidcock *et al.*, 1997). Crocodilians do not have a bladder. Their urine is excreted into water and is usually not recoverable. A technique for the collection of a clear urine sample directly from the urodeum in Nile crocodiles has been described by Myburgh *et al.* (2012). Some crocodilians will void faeces and urine when handled. Crocodiles, unlike alligators, are able to tolerate salt water without increases in plasma sodium and chloride.

Cerebrospinal fluid analysis

The subdural space lies immediately below the spinal vein. To obtain a sample uncontaminated by blood it is necessary to use a spinal needle directed through the sinus into the space. This author has used ultrasonography to identify this space and direct a needle into the subarachnoid space. Normal reference ranges have not been defined for cerebrospinal fluid in either crocodilians or other reptiles.

Nasal swab

Nasal swabs are indicated when upper respiratory disease is suspected. Unfortunately, it is very difficult to pass a swab into an awake animal. It may be possible to wait for inhalation and rapidly insert. Alternatively, in anaesthetized crocodilians a nasal flush is preferable for sample collection.

Imaging

Radiography, as in domestic animals, is an important diagnostic tool (see Figure 26.2). Unfortunately, the large size of many crocodilians may exceed the capability of many small veterinary radiology units. The osteoderms also make interpretation difficult. Computerized axial tomography (CAT scan) imaging is very useful for evaluating lung disease (Figure 26.17) (Hall *et al.*, 2011). Magnetic resonance imaging (MRI) is valuable for assessing soft-tissue structures (e.g. the central nervous system). On plain radiographs the gastrointestinal tract should contain little to no air (see Figure 26.2). Lead fragments ingested in prey items are readily identified on radiographs.

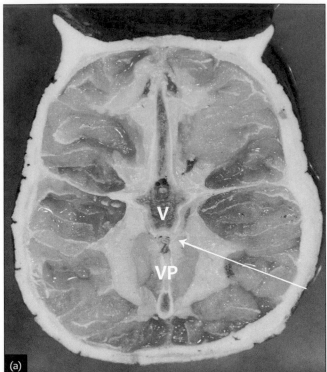

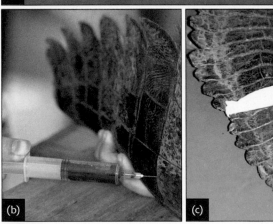

26.16 (a) The ventral coccygeal vessels (artery and veins) are located immediately below the vertebral body (V) as shown in this cross-section of the tail of an American alligator. They can be accessed from the ventral midline between the ventral spinous processes (VP) or (a–b) from the ventrolateral surface of the tail (arrowed). (c) The ventral coccygeal vessels can be catheterized for fluid administration.

above. The space between the spinous processes on the tail is palpated and the needle inserted in the midline until blood is aspirated. Unfortunately, although this technique works well for juveniles, in adults the insertion site is protected by osteoderms.

Although there are several publications of reference ranges for blood values in crocodilians (e.g. Huchzermeyer, 2003), they are not included in this chapter. The CBC and plasma biochemical values of crocodilians are very similar to those of other reptiles; white blood cell counts are usually below 10,000. Electrolyte values are the same as in mammals and birds. Mature females are seasonally hyperalbuminaemic, hyperglobulinaemic and hypercalcaemic. Calcium will be elevated in females undergoing folliculogenesis, but the phosphorus levels should not be higher than calcium levels: this would suggest renal dysfunction. Normal and abnormal values given by laboratories must be treated with caution. For many species there are no reference data. Massive seasonal changes in normal haematology and biochemistry values are possible.

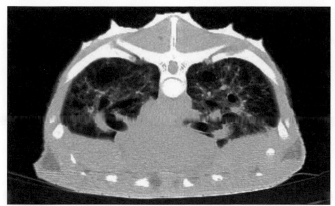

26.17 A computerized axial tomography (CAT scan) cross-sectional image of the lung of an American alligator. This is the recommended diagnostic modality for identifying respiratory disease (including fungal pneumonia) in crocodilians.

Endoscopy

Endoscopy has been evaluated for the assessment of lung disease (LaFortune *et al.*, 2005). It can be performed in small crocodilians awake. Unfortunately, this author has found it to be of limited value in identifying and characterizing respiratory disease and prefers CAT scans (see Figure 26.17). This is because lung lesions are usually walled off and material is rarely expelled into the respiratory system. The CAT scan can guide transcutaneous aspirates of the lung lesions for cytological examination and culture. Endoscopy is also used for evaluating the upper gastrointestinal tract for disease and foreign bodies.

Common conditions

Figure 26.18 summarizes common disease processes based on the body system involved, and can be used as a beginning guide to formulating a differential diagnosis list. The most common health problems in captive crocodilians are related to husbandry and trauma. Parasites are not usually a major concern, except when animals are exposed to parasites from a different geographical area. This may occur by housing animals from different regions together, or feeding local wildlife (e.g. fish) containing parasite intermediate stages. The most important pathogenic parasites are pentastomids. There are several species; all have intermediate stages in fish, and most reside in the lungs as adults. The main infectious causes of disease are Gram-negative bacteria producing bacteraemia and septicaemia. Although other infectious diseases have been described (e.g. mycoplasmosis, West Nile virus, chlamydiosis), they are usually a problem of large collections or crocodilian farms.

Zoonoses

Salmonellosis is the most important reptilian zoonosis. West Nile virus has recently been described in several disease outbreaks in alligator farms in North America and represents a potential for human transmission. *Trichinella* has also been identified in the skeletal muscle of several crocodile species, but would only be of significance if the animal were eaten, and even then its zoonotic potential is unknown.

Disease	Cause(s)	Clinical signs	Diagnosis	Therapy
Skin				
Pox	Pox virus	White to dark brown multifocal crusty lesions	Biopsy – histopathology with typical intracytoplasmic inclusions; PCR; EM	No treatment. Antimicrobial therapy for secondary bacterial infection
Bacterial dermatitis	Usually Gram negative, occasionally Gram positive. *Dermatophilus* sp.	Skin discoloration, swollen scales, ulceration, haemorrhage into scales, skin sloughing	Biopsy, culture, PCR	Antimicrobial therapy, removal from water, increase in environmental temperature, removal of obvious sources of stress
Leeches	Variety of species	Leeches present in oral cavity, eyelids, under ear flaps or axillae	Visual	Physically remove, bathe in salt water
Mycotic dermatitis	Many species	Similar to bacterial	Histopathology, culture, PCR	Systemic and/or topical therapy. Mixed mycotic/bacterial infection common. Predisposed to by low environmental temperatures
Nutritional	Hypovitaminosis A	Skin infection	Histopathology, blood retinoic acid levels, dietary review	Vitamin A injection, dietary correction
Trauma	Intraspecific aggression	Lacerations	History, visual	Supportive care, antimicrobial therapy, topical cleansing
Eyes				
Trauma	Intraspecific aggression	Corneal laceration, ruptured globe	History, visual examination	Symptomatic wound management
Conjunctivitis	Trauma, bacteria (including *Chlamydia* spp.), fungi	Swollen lids, discharge, discoloration	Cytology, culture, PCR	Systemic antimicrobial therapy, subconjunctival antibiotic injection
Glaucoma	Congenital, infectious, trauma	Globe distension	Ophthalmic examination, intraocular pressures	Treat underlying infection, symptomatic therapy, enucleation?

26.18 Common disease problems. AST = aspartate aminotransferase; CAT = computerized axial tomography; CSF = cerebrospinal fluid; EM = electron microscopy; ERG = electroretinogram; MRI = magnetic resonance imaging; PCR = polymerase chain reaction; UV = ultraviolet. (continues) ▶
(Huchzermeyer, 2003; Jacobson, 2007)

Disease	Cause(s)	Clinical signs	Diagnosis	Therapy
Eyes continued				
Third eyelid prolapse	Periocular inflammation	Swollen prolapsed eyelid	Cytology, culture, PCR	Symptomatic treatment
Blindness	Trauma, congenital, albinism	Panophthalmitis, collapsed globe, corneal or lens opacity	Ophthalmic examination, ocular ultrasonography, ERG, cytology, culture, PCR	Treat underlying infections, enucleation. Blind crocodilians are very dangerous because they will strike at any nearby movement, vibration or sound
Teeth				
Tooth loss	Normal, trauma, vitamin A deficiency, metabolic bone disease, osteomyelitis	Small broken teeth, no tooth replacement	Histopathology, dietary assessment, culture, radiography	Correct nutritional deficiencies
Abnormal mineralization	Dietary calcium deficiency, calcium/phosphorus imbalance, inadequate UV exposure?	Translucent teeth, easily damaged or lost	Histopathology, dietary assessment, culture, radiography	Correct nutritional deficiencies
Protruding incisors	Dietary calcium deficiency, calcium/phosphorus imbalance, inadequate UV exposure?	Horizontal incisors, swollen jaws	Histopathology, dietary assessment, culture, radiography	Correct nutritional deficiencies
Abnormal position	Dietary calcium deficiency, calcium/phosphorus imbalance, inadequate UV exposure?	Malleable jaws (rubber jaws)	Histopathology, dietary assessment, culture, radiography	Correct nutritional deficiencies
Gums (Gingivitis)				
Traumatic	Intraspecific aggression	Lacerations, fractures	Visual	Symptomatic wound management
Pox	Pox virus	White to dark brown multifocal crusty lesions	Biopsy – histopathology with typical intracytoplasmic inclusions; PCR; EM	No treatment. Antimicrobial therapy for secondary bacterial infection
Bacterial	Gram-negative bacteria	Ulceration, swelling	Cytology, biopsy, culture	Antimicrobial therapy
Hyperkeratosis	Hypovitaminosis A	Tooth loss, gingival swelling, tongue abscesses	Biopsy, dietary history, blood retinoic acid levels	Vitamin A injection, correct diet
Stomach				
Ulcers	Stress, bacteria, foreign bodies, malnutrition, endoparasitism	Anorexia, weight loss, regurgitation, bloating	History, endoscopy and biopsy with histopathology/culture/PCR	Antimicrobial therapy, correct husbandry and diet, remove foreign bodies
Gastritis	Bacteria, endoparasitism, heavy metals, viruses, mycosis	Anorexia, weight loss, regurgitation, bloating	History, endoscopy and biopsy with histopathology/culture/PCR	Antimicrobial therapy, chelation therapy, parasiticides
Intestines				
Enteritis	Bacteria, endoparasites, heavy metals, viruses (e.g. adenovirus), mycosis	Anorexia, regurgitation, weight loss, septicaemia/ bacteraemia, diarrhoea, abnormal flotation	Blood electrolytes, acid–base, endoscopy and biopsy/culture/ PCR, radiography, ultrasonography	Although common, endoparasites rarely cause clinical disease. Most enteritis is associated with Gram-negative bacteria. Depressed immune function due to poor husbandry and malnutrition predispose to secondary infection. Heavy metals ingested either in gun-shot prey (lead) or as coins (zinc) tossed by the public
Occlusion	Foreign body, severe enteritis, ileus	Anorexia, regurgitation, bloating, weight loss, abnormal flotation	Blood electrolytes, acid–base, endoscopy and biopsy/culture/ PCR, radiography, ultrasonography	Antimicrobial therapy, parenteral fluids, surgery
Liver				
Adenoviral hepatitis	Adenovirus	Non-specific debilitation, elevated AST	Liver biopsy and histopathology, PCR	Supportive care, antimicrobial therapy for secondary bacterial infection
Bacterial hepatitis	Gram-negative bacteria	Non-specific debilitation	Liver aspirate or biopsy for histopathology	Antimicrobial therapy
Chlamydial hepatitis	Chlamydia	Non-specific debilitation	Liver aspirate or biopsy for histopathology, PCR, culture	Antimicrobial therapy – oxytetracycline, doxycycline, enrofloxacin

26.18 (continued) Common disease problems. AST = aspartate aminotransferase; CAT = computerized axial tomography; CSF = cerebrospinal fluid; EM = electron microscopy; ERG = electroretinogram; MRI = magnetic resonance imaging; PCR = polymerase chain reaction; UV = ultraviolet. (continues)

(Huchzermeyer, 2003; Jacobson, 2007)

Disease	Cause(s)	Clinical signs	Diagnosis	Therapy
Kidneys				
Pyelonephritis	Ascending bacterial infection	Non-specific debilitation	Difficult – clinicopathological indicators of diminished renal function; urine sample; ultrasonography	Antimicrobial therapy
Gout	Renal injury – drugs, bacteria	Non-specific debilitation (visceral form). Swollen joints. Decreased activity, reluctance to leave water, difficulty in walking	Uricaemia – may not be present depending on stage of disease. Periarticular and articular swelling. Joint aspirate – characteristic crystals	Treat renal disease. Symptomatic therapy
Reproductive system				
Uterine prolapse	Egg laying	Tissue protruding from cloaca	Cloacoscopy, ultrasonography	Surgical replacement or removal. Antimicrobial therapy to cover secondary infection
Oophoritis and preovulatory stasis	Immunosuppression, inappropriate environment for egg-laying	Non-specific, cessation of egg-laying, debilitation	Radiography, CAT scan, MRI, coelomic aspirate to detect free egg yolk and inflammation	Surgery. Antimicrobial therapy for secondary bacterial infection
Ectopic eggs and egg yolk coelomitis	Repetitive breeding, metritis, older animal	Non-specific, cessation of egg-laying, debilitation	Radiography, CAT scan, MRI, coelomic aspirate to detect free egg yolk and inflammation	Surgical removal. Antimicrobial therapy for secondary bacterial infection
Nervous system				
Encephalitis/meningitis	Bacteria (Including chlamydia), mycosis, mycoplasma, West Nile virus	Depression, debilitation, ataxia, paresis, paralysis, torticollis	CSF tap, culture, cytology, MRI, serology	Antimicrobial therapy. Mycoplasmosis, chlamydiosis and West Nile virus infections have been described in large collections
Encephalomalacia	Thiamine deficiency – feeding fish deficient in thiamine and/or endogenous thiaminases	Opisthotonus, depression, debilitation, ataxia, paresis, paralysis	History, clinical signs, CSF tap, culture, cytology, MRI, response to therapy, thiamine blood levels	Thiamine injections, correct diet
Respiratory system				
Rhinitis	Trauma, bacteria, fungi, mycoplasma, chlamydia	Nasal discharge, perinasal ulceration	Cytology, culture, radiography, CAT scan, MRI	Antimicrobial therapy, increase environmental temperature, remove other stressors, assess and correct diet
Pneumonia	Parasites, bacteria, fungi, mycoplasma, chlamydia	No clinical signs usually. Abnormal floatation	Tracheal wash, cytology, culture, radiography, CAT scan, MRI, endoscopy	Antimicrobial therapy, increase environmental temperature, remove other stressors, assess and correct diet
Pentastomiasis	Pentastomids, several species	Debilitation, secondary respiratory disease	Faecal and tracheal wash examination for ova, endoscopy of lungs	No drug therapy. Physical removal impractical if large numbers present. Intermediate stages go through fish – do not feed wild-caught fish
Musculoskeletal system				
Metabolic bone disease	Dietary calcium deficiency, calcium/phosphorus imbalance, inadequate UV exposure?	Pathological fractures, hindlimb paresis, muscle fasciculations	Radiography, blood calcium usually normal	Correct diet, UV exposure?
Trauma	Intraspecific aggression	Fractures, limb swelling, haemorrhage, purulent discharge	Radiography	Fracture repair and wound management. Even severe wounds may heal if kept clean. Antimicrobial therapy for secondary infection
Arthritis	Trauma, bacteria, mycoplasma, fungi, articular gout	Swollen joints, difficulty or reluctance to move	Radiography, joint aspirate with cytology and culture	Antimicrobial therapy. Joint lavage
Swollen leg(s)	Bacterial cellulitis secondary to bite wounds, ulcerative pododermatitis	Swollen leg	Radiography, aspirate and cytological examination	Antimicrobial therapy

26.18 (continued) Common disease problems. AST = aspartate aminotransferase; CAT = computerized axial tomography; CSF = cerebrospinal fluid; EM = electron microscopy; ERG = electroretinogram; MRI = magnetic resonance imaging; PCR = polymerase chain reaction; UV = ultraviolet. (Huchzermeyer, 2003; Jacobson, 2007)

Supportive care

Hospitalization

Crocodilians should be hospitalized in a heated enclosure, especially for long-term management. Medium to large crocodilians require specialized housing, and most will be treated at the facility in which they are housed. The enclosure should be waterproof and easily cleaned. Cat and dog cages are unsuitable for even small crocodilians. For most, a plastic tank with a haul-out area is suitable. Where animals are kept out of water, regular misting is advisable. In humid environments, plastic mats limit ground contact where excreta may predispose to ventral scale infections. Some crocodilians can be trained to enter chutes or restraint cages, facilitating drug administration and diagnostic sampling.

Drug administration

Intravenous drugs should **not** be administered into the spinal vein because of the possibility of accidental injection into the subdural space. As described above, the ventral coccygeal vessels can be catheterized for intravenous drug administration (Wellehan *et al.*, 2004) (see Figure 26.16c). Intramuscular injections are preferably given in the forelimbs because of the renal portal system. This author will, however, inject medium to large crocodilians in the hindlimbs or tail for handler safety, and because pharmacokinetic studies suggest the clinical effect of the renal portal system is minor. This author has injected edetate calcium disodium intracoelomically for chelation of lead without evidence of pain or tissue injury. The injection is made off midline in the caudal coelomic cavity.

Fluid therapy and nutritional support

Oral methods

Nutritional support or oral fluid therapy can be given by stomach tubing. This assumes gastrointestinal motility and gastric emptying is normal. The animal must also be at an appropriate body temperature for normal digestion to occur. Animals that have been anorexic for prolonged periods of time should be fed conservatively, beginning with electrolyte solutions first, and then gradually adding in liquefied solids. For chronic administration of enteral fluids and food it is recommended an oesophageal tube be placed (Figure 26.19). If the tube is sufficiently long, it allows food administration from behind the animal.

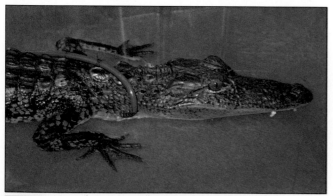

26.19 A juvenile American alligator with a surgically placed oesophageal tube for repetitive enteral feeding and drug administration. This route is useful in animals that are anorexic, but otherwise have normal gastrointestinal function. The tube can be extended down the back to facilitate safe administration.

Non-enteral fluid therapy

Intravenous fluids can be administered through a catheter placed in the ventral coccygeal vessels (Wellehan *et al.*, 2004) (see Figure 26.16c). Although 'reptile-specific' fluids have been described, this author routinely uses commercially available fluids such as lactated Ringer's solution, etc., without adverse effects. Intraosseous fluid administration is impossible because of the dense bone structure of the appendicular skeleton, even in juvenile animals.

Anaesthesia and analgesia

Anaesthesia has been reviewed by Fleming (2014) (Figure 26.20) and always involves some form of physical restraint. Mask induction of small crocodilians with an inhalant anaesthetic is possible, but may be prolonged because of breath holding and involuntary excitement. Alternatively, small crocodilians can be physically restrained; have a mouth block placed, the gular flap displaced and local anaesthetic applied to the glottis; and then be intubated and ventilated with an inhalant anaesthetic. Isoflurane and sevoflurane both provide rapid induction and recovery. This author also uses nitrous oxide with these inhalants when there is no evidence of either hypoxaemia or closed gas-filled spaces in the body.

Drug	Dosage	Comments
Parenteral anaesthetics		
Propofol	2–6 mg/kg i.v.	Large alligators start with 2 mg/kg
Alfaxalone	2–6 mg/kg i.v., i.m.	Large injection volume precludes intramuscular route in large animals
Tiletamine/ zolazepam	4–8 mg/kg i.m., i.v.	Prolonged induction and recovery
Medetomidine	100–150 µg/kg i.m.	Used in large saltwater crocodiles
Medetomidine: Ketamine	100 µg/kg: 5–10 mg/kg i.m., i.v.	
Muscle relaxants	**Not recommended**	No analgesia, animal aware, succinylcholine causes pain during muscle fasciculations, low therapeutic index
Inhalant anaesthetics		
Isoflurane	3–5% induction, 1.5–2.5% maintenance	
Sevoflurane	5–8% induction, 2.5–4% maintenance	
Nitrous oxide	2:1 to 1:1 nitrous oxide: oxygen	Do not use in hypoxaemia or in animals with closed air spaces
Analgesics		
Morphine	0.5–3 mg/kg i.m., i.v., q24h	
Buprenorphine	0.01–0.03 mg/kg i.m., i.v., q24–12h	
Butorphanol	0.2–0.5 mg/kg i.m., i.v., q24–12h	
Meloxicam	0.1–0.3 mg/kg i.m., i.v., q24h	

26.20 Analgesics and anaesthetics. Lower dosages should be used in larger animals and for intravenous administration.
(Fleming, 2014)

When safety is of primary concern, this author recommends intramuscular administration of a zolazepam/tiletamine combination. Induction to safe immobilization is approximately 45 minutes. This drug combination is also recommended for darting of animals that cannot be approached closely. Anaesthesia should not occur in water because of the possibility of drowning. Medetomidine alone or combined with ketamine has been described for use in alligators and crocodiles, but high dosages are required. Alternatively, if intravenous access is obtained, propofol or alfaxalone can be used for induction. Although muscle relaxants have been used in the past to immobilize crocodilians, this author does not recommend their use in captive animals because of the availability of alternatives. Muscle relaxants are not analgesic – the animals are conscious unless other drugs are used; succinylcholine causes pain during muscle depolarization and may produce hyperkalaemia.

Endotracheal intubation

Once an animal is sufficiently relaxed a mouth block is placed, the gular flap (see Figure 26.7) is displaced and the glottis is visualized. The endotracheal tube can then be readily placed through the glottis. Since the glottis will usually be closed, the end of the tube is gently placed between the lips of the glottis and then opened.

Monitoring and supportive care

The metabolic rate of crocodilians is very low, and recommended ventilation rate under anaesthesia is approximately 1–2 breaths/minute. Pulse oximetry has not been calibrated for reptiles, including crocodilians. A capnograph is useful for monitoring adequacy of ventilation. A Doppler flow probe can be placed directly over the heart or the eye or into the cloaca to detect blood flow. Occasionally, blood flow can be detected on the ventral tail and in the femoral and axillary triangles.

Analgesia

It appears crocodilians are similar to mammals in being mu-opioid-receptor predominant. Since pharmacokinetics has not been described for these drugs, it is recommended the same dosage be given as for mammals, but less often. Similarly, for non-steroidal anti-inflammatory drugs use a mammalian dosage, but less frequently (see Figure 26.20). Local anaesthetic blocks are also recommended for limb amputations, dentistry and biopsies (Wellehan et al., 2006).

Common surgical procedures

Surgery is not commonly performed on crocodilians. The most common indication is for trauma and amputation of injured limbs. Retained infected egg yolks are a cause of poor growth in juvenile crocodilians and can be surgically removed through a midline laparotomy. Exploratory coeliotomy in adult crocodilians is not common. Adult crocodilians have a lot of fibrous adhesions/tissue within the coelomic cavity and abdominal wall dehiscence is common postoperatively. A paralumbar surgical approach is recommended when possible. Metal and nylon haemoclips and monofilament suture materials are appropriate to reptilian surgery. Skin sutures may be removed after

4–6 weeks. Laparoscopic surgery requires further evaluation, but will allow more rapid return to normal function, including immersion.

Microchipping

The microchip is best placed at the base of the neck. A reader on the end of a pole can then be used to read the microchip.

Euthanasia

Euthanasia involves first anaesthetizing the animal, and then injecting euthanasia solution intravenously. Pithing can be performed only when an animal is unconscious. The use of muscle relaxants to immobilize an animal prior to pithing is inappropriate since the animal is conscious. Although destruction of the brain with a bullet or captive bolt is appropriate, it is usually impractical in a captive setting. The brain of a large crocodile is small and protected by thick bone.

Drug formulary

Care must be taken in selecting drug dosages because of the wide range of body size between juvenile and adult animals (see Appendix 2; Figure A2.2). In general, the larger the crocodilian, the lower the dosage and frequency of administration. There may also be differences between species. Alligators appear to require lower drug dosages than crocodiles of a similar size. **Ivermectin must not be used**; there are several anecdotal, but unpublished, reports of paralysis and death at recommended therapeutic dosages. Care should also be taken when using benzimidazoles; low doses every day for 5 days are preferred to a single large bolus.

References and further reading

Britton A (2012) Crocodilians: Natural History and Conservation. Available at: http://crocodilian.com/

Brown DR, Nogueira MF, Schoeb TR et al. (2001) Pathology of experimental Mycoplasma alligatoris infection in American alligators. Journal of Wildlife Diseases 37, 671–679

Brown DR, Schumacher IM, Nogueira MF et al. (2001) Detection of antibodies to a pathogenic mycoplasma in American alligators (Alligator mississippiensis), broad-nosed caimans (Caiman latirostris), and Siamese crocodiles (Crocodylus siamensis). Journal of Clinical Microbiology 39, 285–292

Buenviaje G, Ladds P and Martin Y (1998) Pathology of skin diseases in crocodiles. Australian Veterinary Journal 76, 357–363

Clippinger TL, Bennett RA, Johnson CM et al. (2000) Morbidity and mortality associated with a new mycoplasma species from captive American alligators (Alligator mississippiensis). Journal of Zoo and Wildlife Medicine 31, 303–314

Fleming G (2014) Crocodilians (crocodiles, alligators, caimans, gharials). In: Zoo Animal and Wildlife Immobilization and Anesthesia, 2nd edition, ed. G West, DJ Heard and N Caulkett. Blackwell Publications, Ames, IA

Hall NH, Conley K, Berry C et al. (2011) Computed tomography of granulomatous pneumonia with oxalosis in an American alligator (Alligator mississippiensis) associated with Metarhizium anisopliae var anisopliae. Journal of Zoo and Wildlife Medicine 42, 700–708

Huchzermeyer FW (2003) Crocodiles: Biology, Husbandry and Diseases. CABI Publishing, Cambridge, Massachusetts

Huchzermeyer FW, Gerdes GH, Foggin CN, Huchzermeyer KDA and Limper LC (1994) Hepatitis in farmed hatchling Nile crocodiles (Crocodylus niloticus) due to chlamydial infection. Journal of the South African Veterinary Association 65, 20–22

Huchzermeyer FW, Langelet E and Putterill JF (2008) An outbreak of chlamydiosis in farmed crocodiles (Crocodylus porosus): clinical communication. Journal of the South African Veterinary Association 79, 99–100

Jacobson E (2007) Infectious Diseases and Pathology of Reptiles: Color Atlas and Text. CRC Press, Boca Raton, FL, USA

Jacobson ER, Ginn PE, Troutman JM *et al.* (2005) West Nile virus infection in farmed American alligators (*Alligator mississippiensis*) in Florida. *Journal of Wildlife Diseases* **41**, 96–106

LaFortune M, Gobel T, Jacobson ER *et al.* (2005) Respiratory bronchoscopy of subadult American alligators (*Alligator mississippiensis*) and tracheal wash evaluation. *Journal of Zoo and Wildlife Medicine* **36(1)**, 12–20

Martelli P, Lai OR, Krishnasamy K *et al.* (2009) Pharmacokinetic behavior of enrofloxacin in estuarine crocodile (*Crocodylus porosus*) after single intravenous, intramuscular, and oral doses. *Journal of Zoo and Wildlife Medicine* **40**, 696–704

Myburgh JG, Huchzermeyer FW, Soley JT *et al.* (2012). Technique for the collection of clear urine from the Nile crocodile (*Crocodylus niloticus*). *Journal of the South African Veterinary Association* **83(1)**, 6 pages, dx.doi. org/10.4102/jsava.v83i1.8

Myburgh JG, Kirberger RM, Steyl JC *et al.* (2014) The post-occipital spinal venous sinus of the Nile crocodile *Crocodylus niloticus*: its anatomy and use for blood sample collection and intravenous infusions. *Journal of the South African Veterinary Association* **85**, 965–975

Pidcock S, Taplin LE and Grigg GC (1997) Differences in renal-cloacal function between *Crocodylus porosus* and *Alligator mississippiensis* have implications for crocodilian evolution. *Journal of Comparative Physiology B* **167**, 153–158

Pye GW, Brown DR, Nogueira MF *et al.* (2001) Experimental inoculation of broad-nosed caimans (*Caiman latirostris*) and Siamese crocodiles (*Crocodylus siamensis*) with *Mycoplasma alligatoris*. *Journal of Zoo and Wildlife Medicine* **32**, 196–201

Richardson KC, Webb GJW and Manolis SC (2000) *Crocodiles: Inside Out. A Guide to Crocodilians and their Functional Morphology.* Surrey Beatty and Sons, Sydney

Vliet K (2014) Crocodilian capture and restraint. In: *Zoo Animal and Wildlife Immobilization and Anesthesia, 2nd edition*, ed. G West, DJ Heard and N Caulkett. Blackwell Publications, Ames, IA

Wellehan JFX, Gunkel CI, Kledzik D, Robertson S and Heard DJ (2006) Use of a nerve locator to facilitate administration of mandibular nerve blocks in crocodilians. *Journal of Zoo and Wildlife Medicine* **37**, 405–408

Wellehan JFX, LaFortune M, Gunkel C *et al.* (2004) Coccygeal vascular catheterization in lizards and crocodilians. *Journal of Herpetological Medicine and Surgery* **14**, 26–28

Zippel KC, Lillywhite HB and Mladinich CRJ (2003) Anatomy of the crocodilian spinal vein. *Journal of Morphology* **258**, 327–335

Chapter 27

Sea turtles

Estelle Rousselet and Terry Norton

Natural history and conservation

There are seven species of sea turtles; the flatback, green, hawksbill, Kemp's ridley, leatherback, loggerhead and olive ridley. The leatherback is the only representative of the Dermochelyidae family, and has a soft shell composed of blubber overlying the ribs and vertebrae that is covered dorsally with waxy skin and embedded dermal ossicles. Longitudinal ridges along the carapace allow the shell to collapse during deep dives. Members of the Cheloniidae family have a shell composed of bone covered by keratinous scutes. Species from this family can be distinguished using key characteristics such as the number of prefrontal scales on top of the nares, the form of the jaw, and the number and pattern of the carapacial scutes (Wyneken, 2001).

Sea turtles can be found in all oceans except for the Arctic (Figure 27.1). Sea turtles navigate by sensing the declination and inclination of the earth's magnetic field.

The flatback turtle is found solely on the northern coast of Australia. All species of sea turtles are listed as threatened or endangered.

Sea turtles are long-lived, with some species taking decades to reach sexual maturity. They have adapted to high egg and juvenile mortality rates, but not to high levels of adult mortality. Significant threats to sea turtle populations include loss of habitat, light pollution, contaminants and marine debris, poaching and illegal use of their meat and eggs for consumption and body parts for a variety of purposes, mortality in various fisheries, boat-strike injuries, harmful algal blooms, and infectious diseases.

The knowledge base for sea turtle medicine and surgery has expanded significantly in the last decade and has become quite sophisticated. Rehabilitation alone is primarily a humanitarian effort; however, when combined with education and health-related research the conservation impacts are enhanced dramatically (Feck and Hamann, 2013).

Sea turtle species	Ecosystem occupation	Nestings	Distribution
Loggerhead (most abundant species)	Oceanic	Atlantic; Masirah Island (Oman); South Florida (USA)	Circumglobal: temperate and tropical regions – Atlantic, Pacific and Indian Oceans; Mediterranean Sea
	Neritic (nearshore coastal areas)	Australia Cape Verde Islands; Brazil and Caribbean; Mediterranean Sea (eastern); North Pacific: Japan	
Green	Open ocean Coastal areas: benthic feeding	Central America: Tortuguero (Costa Rica) Great Barrier Reef in Australia: Raine Island USA: Florida (south-east)	Globally distributed: tropical and subtropical Atlantic, Pacific and Indian Oceans
Kemp's ridley	Neritic	95% of worldwide nesting in arribada (synchronized large-scale nesting) in Tamaulipas, Mexico: • Rancho Nuevo • Tepehuajes • Barra del Tordo + Veracruz (Mexico) and Texas	Gulf of Mexico; western Atlantic – Florida to New England; occasionally near the Azores, the waters off Morocco and within the Mediterranean Sea
Olive ridley	Pelagic Inhabit coastal areas	Solitary (40 countries) Arribadas in the eastern Pacific (Mexico, Nicaragua, Costa Rica, Panama) and India	Globally distributed in the tropical regions of the South Atlantic, eastern Pacific and Indian Oceans
Hawksbill	Associated with healthy coral reefs Post-hatchlings: pelagic Juveniles: oceanic	Solitary nesters: Puerto Rico and the USA. Throughout the Caribbean, Virgin Islands, south-east coast of Florida and the Florida Keys, Hawaii, American Samoa, and Guam Largest nesting population in Australia	Tropical Atlantic, Pacific and Indian Oceans: Caribbean Sea, southern Florida and Gulf of Mexico, Republic of Seychelles, Indonesia and Australia
Leatherback	Pelagic Forage in coastal waters	Around the world Largest nesting population on the coasts of northern South America and West Africa Within the USA: US Virgin Islands and south-east Florida	Critical habitats: coastal waters adjacent to Sand Point, St Croix, US Virgin Islands, USA west coast Sighted along the entire continental east coast of the USA

27.1 Natural history and distribution of six sea turtle species.

Unique anatomical characteristics

A detailed description of sea turtle anatomy can be downloaded from https://repository.library.noaa.gov/view/noaa/8502. Some sea turtle anatomical peculiarities useful for the clinician are described below.

The sea turtle oesophagus is lined with a series of sharp keratinized papillae, which point inward towards the stomach. Their role is to avoid damage from abrasive prey items (e.g. crabs, jellyfish, whelks) and to trap prey while salt water is expelled (Wyneken, 2001). It can be a challenge to place a stomach tube and perform oesophageal and gastric endoscopy on sea turtles, in part because of the prominent oesophageal papillae. In the green sea turtle, the ileum ends in a muscular sphincter and the proximal end of the colon is enlarged and functions as a caecum (Wyneken, 2001). This caecal-like structure harbours a rich microflora that degrades plant material with a high degree of efficiency. Both captive and wild green sea turtles tend to have more gastrointestinal disorders than the more carnivorous sea turtle species (Erlacher-Reid et al., 2013).

Sea turtles cannot concentrate urine hyperosmotic to blood. They possess large lobular salt glands located adjacent to the eye orbits, which serve as the major electrolyte excretion route to maintain homeostasis (Williard, 2013). Salt glands are modified lacrimal glands, capable of secreting tears with osmotic concentration as high as twice the concentration of seawater. They are activated in response to hypernatraemia. Freshwater baths, often used to kill or loosen epibionts and for rehydration during the initial stage of rehabilitation, should be maintained for a maximum of 24 hours. Salinity should then be increased slowly over several days to allow the salt gland to adjust.

The sea turtle heart has four chambers: a sinus venosus, two large atria and a ventricle. The ventricle is thick-walled and internally subdivided into three compartments, the cavum venosum, cavum arteriosum, and cavum pulmonale, which are separated only partially from one another (Wyneken, 2001). This configuration results in some mixing of oxygenated and non-oxygenated blood. The blood route through the heart differs depending upon whether blood is shunted towards the lungs and the body or primarily towards the body. Separation of the intracardiac flow (pulmonary and systemic outflows) is not distinct. Right-to-left shunts, bypassing the lungs, limit the amount of inhalant anaesthetic uptake during the induction period and slow anaesthetic elimination. Therefore, these shunts can delay the induction to, and recovery from, inhaled anaesthesia. Sea turtles have a short trachea with complete cartilaginous rings; thus, they should be intubated with an uncuffed endotracheal tube and care should be taken not to insert the endotracheal tube into a bronchus. The left lung is attached to the stomach via the gastropulmonary ligament and the right lung is attached to the right lobe of the liver by the hepatopulmonary ligament (Wyneken, 2001). Blunt-force trauma may cause tears where these ligaments attach to the lungs, leading to a pneumocoelom.

The skull is divided into the neurocranium, which is the inner braincase containing the brain, and an outer bony superstructure, the splanchnocranium (Wyneken, 2001). Fractures of the neurocranium typically cause brain injury and may require euthanasia, whereas splanchnocranial fractures can be repaired.

Diagnostic work-up

General examination

Debilitated or weak sea turtles may require being dry-docked on a padded surface, or placed on a waterbed or in shallow water. With dry-docking, sea turtles should be kept moist by regular misting and, if prolonged, application of vitamin A and D ointment on the skin. Upon arrival, carefully observe the turtle prior to handling. Observations should be made on the turtle's activity level, respiratory rate and sounds, external wounds, body condition and epibiotic load. The visual examination will be helpful in preparing for the physical examination, diagnostic work-up and initial therapeutic plan. If the turtle is stable enough it can be placed in water, where its activity level and attitude usually improve dramatically. An in-water visual examination should be performed with subsequent evaluations.

A systematic physical examination should be performed. Body temperature correlates with the turtle's recent environmental temperature. A laser thermal monitoring device (Raytek Corporation, Santa Cruz, CA) directed at the inguinal area correlates well with core body temperature and is less stressful than using a deep cloacal temperature probe (Norton and Walsh, 2012). Heart rate and rhythm can be assessed with a Doppler or ultrasound probe placed on the skin between the distal cervical region and a proximal front flipper. Bradycardia is common in sea turtles with hypothermia, certain neurological diseases (Jacobson et al., 2006), or potentially other illnesses and when using some anaesthetics. Bodyweight, a subjective body-condition score, and standardized digital images of the turtle and any wounds or lesions should be taken upon arrival and regularly throughout the rehabilitation process. Perform a brief neurological examination on every patient and a more detailed neurological evaluation on patients exhibiting neurological signs. Chrisman et al. (1997) adapted a dog and cat neurological examination for sea turtles. It includes three parts: an in-water assessment and an out-of-water assessment in ventral and dorsal recumbency, which will ultimately assist in localizing the lesion (Figures 27.2 and 27.3). For example, a spinal-cord lesion may be localized using general observations and withdrawal reflexes of the front and rear flippers and tail. An upper motor-neuron lesion is characterized by a decrease of flipper strength, increased tone and reflexes, and minimal to no muscle atrophy, whereas decreased tone, reflexes

Examination steps
Step 1: General observations in water and out of water
• Mentation • Head posture/movement • Gait = swimming • Body posture • Compulsive circling • General activity
Step 2: Postural reaction in water
• Movement/strength of limbs, tail movement • Visual avoidance • Righting response • Tonic neck reaction and nociception

27.2 Neurological examination of sea turtles. The steps include examinations in the water and out of the water in dorsal and ventral recumbency. These steps will help to localize the neurological lesion. (continues)

(Adapted from Chrisman et al. (1997))

Examination steps

Step 3: Thoracic limb reflexes out of water

- Tone
- Withdrawal (flexor) reflex
- Nociception: periosteal and dermal

Step 4: Pelvic limb and tail reflexes out of water

- Tone
- Withdrawal (flexor) reflex
- Nociception: periosteal and dermal
- Tail nociception
- Clasp response
- Cloacal reflex

Step 5: Released reflexes, dorsal recumbency out of water

- Crossed extensor reflex of pelvic limbs

Step 6: Cranial nerves (CN), ventral recumbency out of water

- CN I olfaction
- CN II, VII menace
- CN II, III pupillary light
- CN III, IV, VI strabismus
- CN V jaw tone and strength
- CN V, VII palpebral reflex
- CN VIII vestibular nystagmus
- CN IX, X swallow
- CN XII tongue

27.2 (continued) Neurological examination of sea turtles. The steps include examinations in the water and out of the water in dorsal and ventral recumbency. These steps will help to localize the neurological lesion.
(Adapted from Chrisman et al. (1997))

Central nervous system – brain

- Cerebrum
- Diencephalon:
  - Hypothalamus
  - Thalamus, pituitary
  - Pineal
  - Optic chiasma
- Cerebellum
- Medulla
- Vestibular system

Central nervous system – spinal cord

- Cranial cervical
  - UMN thoracic and pelvic
- Cervico-thoracic enlargement
  - LMN thoracic and UMN pelvic
- Thoracolumbar
  - UMN pelvic
- Lumbosacral enlargement and sacral region
  - LMN pelvic

Peripheral nervous system

- Cranial nerves
- Brachial plexus
- Lumbosacral plexus
- Peripheral vestibular system

27.3 Localizing the neurological lesion following the neurological examination outlined in Figure 27.2. LMN = lower motor-neuron lesion; UMN = upper motor-neuron lesion.
(Adapted from Chrisman et al. (1997))

and muscle atrophy are typical of lower motor-neuron lesions. Lesion localization will assist in prioritizing the next steps for diagnostic testing such as advanced imaging. Serial neurological examination will assist in prognostication and evaluation of response to treatment.

Clinical pathology

The preferred blood-collection site in most sea turtle species is the external jugular vein (dorsal cervical sinus).

For greens, positioning the turtle with the head directed in a ventral position is often helpful (Figure 27.4). The lateral jugular vein has been described for blood drawing and intravenous catheterization (Wyneken et al., 2006; Di Bello et al., 2010), and the ventral caudal tail vein and femoral and interdigital vessels are alternative blood-collection sites for leatherbacks (Norton and Walsh, 2012; Innis et al., 2014b). Lymph contamination can occur and will cause erroneous results. Lithium or sodium heparin is the preferred anticoagulant because ethylenediamine tetra-acetic acid (EDTA) causes red-blood-cell lysis in sea turtles.

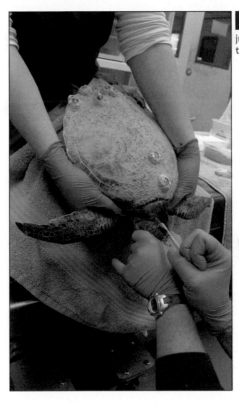

27.4 Blood draw in a juvenile green sea turtle.

A minimum database should consist of a haematocrit (normal 25–35%), total solids (normal 30–40 g/l) and glucose. Glucose can be measured using a human glucometer, but will be approximately 1.11 mmol/l; 20 g/dl lower than if performed on a chemistry machine. A complete blood count and plasma biochemical panel should be performed on the initial evaluation. Ideally, a blood sample for bacterial culture should be collected using sterile technique before initiating antimicrobial therapy; however, this may be cost-prohibitive to do on every case. Blood cultures should be performed at room temperature because most of the microbial pathogens in reptiles do not grow at the higher temperatures typically used for blood cultures in mammals. A blood gas analysis is very useful in critical patients. Blood gases need to be corrected for the patient's body temperature (Innis et al., 2007). Plasma and other biomaterials should be banked for future studies.

Morphological classification of blood cells (Figure 27.5) has been reported (Stacy et al., 2011), and further information can be found at http://www.seaturtleguardian.org/clinical-pathology-of-sea-turtles (Mettee, 2014). Reference ranges for complete blood count, clinical chemistry and plasma electrophoresis for various sea turtle species from different geographical regions have been reported (Figures 27.6 and 27.7). See http://accstr.ufl.edu/resources/blood-chemistry-data, for an ongoing database of clinical pathology reference values.

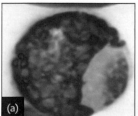 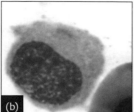 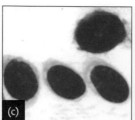 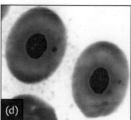 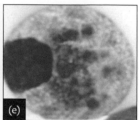

27.5 Photomicrographs of peripheral blood cells in a Kemp's ridley sea turtle representative of white blood cells. (a) A heterophil; (b) a monocyte; (c) a lymphocyte next to three thrombocytes; (d) erythrocytes with basophilic inclusions (degenerate organelles; no clinical significance); (e) an eosinophil. (Original magnification X100 oil)
(Courtesy of Dr Nicole Stacy)

Study	Green turtle				Loggerhead turtle			
	Work *et al.* (1998)	Flint *et al.* (2010)	Casal *et al.* (2009)	Keller *et al.* (2004)	Stamper *et al.* (2005)	Kakizoe *et al.* (2007)	Bradley *et al.* (1998)	Rousselet *et al.* (2013)
	Unopette Wild immature, range	WBC estimate Wild male immature, reference interval	NH Wild juveniles, range	NH Wild juveniles, range	NH Wild residential, median	Unopette Captive 1–36 months of age, range of means	Unopette Captive 2–12 months of age, range of means	Unopette Captive 8–56 months of age, range
Length SCL (cm)	41–59	38.9–107.2	16.5–49.3	45.7–77.3	64.55	4.5–58.2	8.46–20.6	8.8–56.5
Weight (kg)	>10	5.5–149	1.4–26	14.4–56.6	41	0.02–26.7	0.11–14.4	0.11–23.4
PCV (%)	17–35	13.4–53.2	17–45	23–38	32	16–26.2	16.4–20.3	17–32
Total WBC (10³/µl)	5.9–23.6	0.8–30.1	2–18.9	5.8–20.7	15.8	4.7–10.2	0.38–6.19	2.1–27.3
Lymphocytes (%)	72.5				65	24.6–58.6	8.6–32.8	41–100
Lymphocytes (x 10³/µl)	3.6–18.6	0.6–22.3	0.1–1.8	4.6–15	9.92	1.3–5.2		2–25.3
Heterophils (%)	10.1				27	35.8–73.3	55.4–85.9	0–41
Heterophils (× 10³/µl)	0.3–3.2	0.04–6.8	1.8–7.3	1.3–8.2	3.48	2.5–5.1		0–2.4
Monocytes (%)	5.8				3	0–2.2	23–24	0–10
Monocytes (x 10³/µl)	0.1–1.9	0.07–3.4	0–0.3	0.17–1.5	0.75			0–2.1
Eosinophils (%)	12.3				6		1.9–7	0–9
Eosinophils (x 10³/µl)	0.7–3.2	0.01–1.7	0–1.2	0.14–2.7	0.88			0–0.6
Basophils (%)	0				0		0.17–0.8	0–7
Basophils (x 10³/µl)	0–1	0	0–10⁻⁶	0–0.38	0			0–0.9

27.6 Summary of morphometric and haematological parameters of loggerhead and green sea turtles reported in various studies. NH = Natt and Herrick; PCV = packed cell volume; SCL = straight carapace length; WBC = white blood cell count.
(Adapted from Rousselet *et al.*, 2013)

Study	Green turtle				Loggerhead turtle			
	Jacobson *et al.* (2007)	Flint *et al.* (2010)	Kakizoe *et al.* (2007)	Jacobson *et al.* (2007)	Deem *et al.* (2009)	Keller *et al.* (2004)	Casal *et al.* (2009)	Rousselet *et al.* (2013)
	Juveniles, range	Large immature, reference interval	1–36 months of age, range of means	SCL >60 cm, range	Foraging juveniles, range	Wild juveniles, range	Juveniles after rehabilitation, range	8–56 months of age, range
Total protein (g/l)	30–50	20.8–62	15–33	29–41	16–56	24–59	20–110	13–27
Albumin (g/l)	10–29	6.9–17.5	5.6–13.7	7–31	8–16	0–15	10–14	5–12
Uric acid (mmol/l)	41.6–83.3	22.0–131.4	8.3–57.1	35.7–83.3	11.9–71.4	17.8–202.2	<50.1–99.9	17.8–65.4
BUN (mmol/l)	1.4–12.5	0–25.5	14.8–50.8	10.0–26.4	0.36–38.2	8.9–70.3	1.8–67.3	5.9–18.3
Glucose (mmol/l)	4.0–7.1	3.7–9.9	6.8–9.2	9.6–6.2	3.9–7.6	4.2–7.9	1–16.2	3.6–10.5
Cholesterol (mmol/l)	2.4–5.4		2.7–5.0	1.4–5.9	1.2–5.2		1.3–10.3	0.76–3.9
CK (IU/l)	181–3145	326–2728.5	400–2810.6	319–1742	3–1899	281–5667		83.0–2829.0
AST (IU/l)	99–343	74.1–244.6		149–318	2–255	128–355	<10–844	57.0–298.0
Phorphorus (mmol/l)	2.0–3.4	1.6–3.6	2.0–5.4	1.9–3.1	1.3–2.6	1.7–2.9		1.5–2.85
Calcium (mmol/l)	1.3–2.8	0.2–2.2	1.5–2.1	1.1–1.9	1.4–2.1	1.4–2.85	0.7–3.1	1.17–1.85
Sodium (mmol/l)	147–174	139.2–157.8	143.2–154.4	150–168	135–175	154–164		84.0–155.0
Potassium (mmol/l)	4.0–5.1	3.0–7.1	3.2–4.48	3.5–7.9	3.3–13.9	3.1–5.6		2.1–4.7
Chloride (mmol/l)	94–119	100.7–121.1	103.0–120.6	103–128	107–158	110–125		63.0–212.0

27.7 Summary of blood chemistry parameters of loggerhead and green sea turtles reported in various studies. AST = aspartate aminotransferase; BUN = blood urea nitrogen; CK = creatine kinase; SCL = straight carapace length.
(Adapted from Rousselet *et al.*, 2013)

Endoscopy and imaging

Rigid endoscopy has been used for gender determination, evaluation of reproductive activity, exploring the coelomic cavity and organ biopsy for histopathology. Both rigid and flexible systems can be used to visualize the location of fish hooks in the oesophagus. Flexible endoscopes can be used to evaluate the upper and lower gastrointestinal tract (GIT), and to visualize the trachea, bronchi and the anterior lung. Saline can be instilled through the scope to distend the cloaca giving a better view of the bladder, rectum, distal ureteral openings and reproductive tract. A more detailed radiographic evaluation of the lower GIT can be performed by instilling contrast media directly into the lower colon (see Chapter 9). Similar techniques can be used to perform an enema with saline or other solutions.

A dorsoventral (DV) radiograph should be performed as part of the initial diagnostic database. Even with a heavy barnacle load, foreign bodies such as fish hooks, gas in the GIT and long-bone fractures may be detected. Once the patient is stable, barnacles should be removed from the shell so they do not interfere with radiographic interpretation. Three views should be performed: anteroposterior, lateral and DV views (Figure 27.8). For larger sea turtles, four radiographs may be required to assess the entire coelom from a DV view. To evaluate gastrointestinal motility, barium-impregnated polyethylene spheres (BIPS) may be placed in a food item, with subsequent serial radiography (Figure 27.9). Contrast media such as barium sulfate and non-ionic iodinate can be used to diagnose intestinal obstruction, motility disorder and foreign bodies (Erlacher-Reid et al., 2013). Normal transit times have been established for loggerheads (Di Bello et al., 2006b). The skull and limbs may need to be radiographed separately in larger turtles.

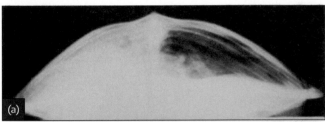

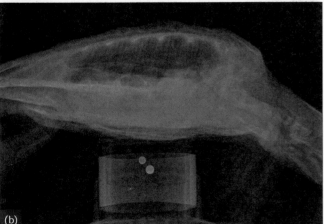

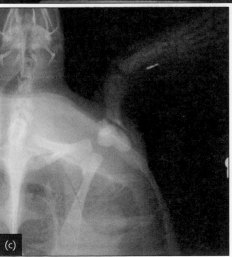

27.8 Radiographs of sea turtles.
(a) Anteroposterior view demonstrates severe opacity of right pulmonary lobe. (b) Lateral view.
(c) Dorsoventral view demonstrating a right proximal humeral fracture in a juvenile green sea turtle.

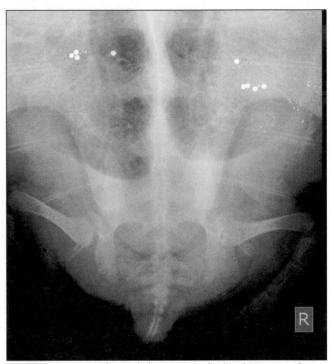

27.9 Contrast radiograph demonstrates barium-impregnated polyethylene spheres used to assess gastrointestinal motility in a green sea turtle.

Ultrasonography has been used to evaluate reproductive status, internal fibropapillomas, intestinal plication and integrity of ocular structures. Several acoustic windows are used to perform a systematic ultrasound evaluation, including inguinal (evaluation of kidneys, distal intestines, coelomic fluid), between the head and pectoral limb (liver, gall bladder and heart), the ventral neck (oesophagus), and the lateral neck vessels for catheter placement.

Computed tomography (CT) is useful for assessing spinal and head injuries, especially to differentiate between neurocranial and splanchnocranial fractures (Figure 27.10), and to visualize free air pockets in the coelom, pneumonia, bronchiolar blockage (Valente et al., 2007) and internal fibropapillomatosis (Page-Karjian et al., 2014). Normal CT skull anatomy has been established in loggerheads (Arencibia et al., 2005). Compared with CT, magnetic resonance imaging (MRI) provides better resolution for soft tissue, spinal cord and brain. Normal MRI of internal anatomical structures has been established in loggerheads (Valente et al., 2006), and this technology has been used to detect internal fibropapillomas. Open MRI imaging is useful for larger sea turtles that do not fit into the CT or MRI chambers. Anaesthesia is usually required when performing an MRI, because of the length of the procedure. The turtle should be measured to make sure it fits into the advanced imaging chamber prior to transport.

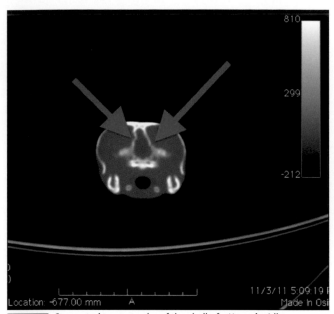

27.10 Computed tomography of the skull of a Kemp's ridley sea turtle. Fracture involves the neurocranium (arrowed).

Husbandry

Husbandry is the key to success and is part of the veterinary management of rehabilitated animals. Good water quality and nutrition are critical for maintaining the health of sea turtles in captivity. Important basic principles and recommendations for water quality are summarized in Figure 27.11, and additional information can be obtained from Bluvias and Eckert (2010).

Tank	• Avoid aggression: add divider if necessary • Fibropapillomatosis: keep affected and healthy animals in different areas • Quarantine new arrivals • Tanks should be circular with non-abrasive fibreglass inside surfaces, and free of anything small enough for turtles to bite, swallow or ingest
Water parameters	• Salinity: 32 ppt unless freshwater soak is indicated • pH: between 7.5 and 8.5 • Temperature: 24°C ideal, a bit higher for new arrivals (exception: cold-stunned turtle). Monitor daily to multiple times/day • Disinfection protocols should be in place with options being ozone, ultraviolet (UV) sterilization and chlorine (<1.0 parts per million (ppm)). Chlorine can cause ocular irritation and other health issues (skin and respiratory tract) • Coliform bacteria: <1000 most probable number per 100 ml of water • Monthly testing is recommended • Water clear enough to allow viewing of sea turtles in any part of the tank
Lighting	• Artificial lighting: full-spectrum bulbs (UVA/UVB 280–320 nm) are recommended for small tanks. Animal needs to be in close proximity to the light to be effective • Access to natural sunlight for a few hours a week (warmer months) is beneficial • Photoperiod: similar to a natural photoperiod (summer- and winter-season daylight hours). No more than 14 hours of light per 24-hour period • Provide dark/shaded areas, especially if outside, to protect from the sun and to provide hiding/resting areas

27.11 Major husbandry parameters include adequate tanks, water quality (salinity, pH, temperature and coliform bacteria) and lighting. ppt = parts per thousand

A diagnostic table for sea turtles is provided in Figure 27.12.

Common clinical presentations
• Debilitation • Fibropapillomatosis • Cold-stunned • Fish hook and line ingestion • Trauma, including predator bites and boat entanglement • Harmful algae bloom
Step 1: General examination
• History • Morphometrics • Weight • Visual examination • Physical examination • Neurological examination
Step 2: Clinical pathology
• Haematology • Biochemistry • Blood gas • Blood work
Step 3: Imaging diagnostic

• Ultrasonography:
  • Internal fibropapillomatosis
  • Intestinal plication
  • Coelomic cavity
  • Eye, vessels, joints
• Radiography with or without contrast:
  • Three views:
    – AP, lateral, DV
  • Foreign bodies
  • Lungs
  • Bone
  • GI motility
• Computed tomography (CT):
  • Neurological examination:
    – Spinal cord lesion, skull lesions
  • Lung:
    – Pneumonia
  • Internal fibropapillomatosis
• Magnetic resonance imaging (better resolution than CT for soft tissue):
  • Spinal cord lesion
  • Brain lesions
  • Tendon-ligaments

Step 4: Endoscopy

• Rigid:
  • Inguinal:
    – Lung, kidneys, liver, gonads
    – Fibropapillomatosis biopsies
• Flexible:
  • Trachea, bronchi, anterior lung
  • Oesophagus, stomach, small intestine
• Rigid and flexible:
  • Respiratory
  • Upper gastrointestinal and distal gastrointestinal/cloaca
    – Enema and contrast media

Step 5: Additional diagnostics
• Blood culture • Cytology • Histology • Polymerase chain reaction for fibropapillomatosis • Parasitology • Harmful algae toxins, chemical analysis • Lung lavage/tracheal wash

27.12 Steps of a diagnostic work-up in sea turtles in the context of different clinical presentations. Including general examination, clinical pathology, imaging diagnostics, endoscopy and additional diagnostics. Refer to Stacy and Boylan (2014) for further information.

Veterinary support

Adapted medical treatments for specific ailments are described below. The following recommendations will help the veterinary surgeon (veterinarian) focus on what has been commonly used with success.

- Fluid therapy (Figure 27.13)
- Anaesthesia and analgesia (Figure 27.14)
- Antibiotics and antifungals (Figure 27.15)
- Miscellaneous drugs (Figure 27.16).

Fluids or drugs	Dosage and frequency	Comments
Crystalloid fluids: • Lactated Ringer's solution (LRS) • 0.9% sodium chloride	Maintenance dose: 10–20 ml/kg i.v., s.c. (inguinal fossa, medially in the forelimb fossa)/orally q24h	Base choice of fluids on plasma electrolytes and glucose level
Dextrose 2.5%, 5% or 10% diluted in lactated Ringer's or saline	5% dextrose + LRS 10–20 ml/kg preferentially i.v, as a last option i.c.; 10% dextrose 5 ml/kg i.v.	Oral route can be used if venous access difficult; honey given orally works well for hypoglycaemia in small sea turtles
Colloid fluids: Hetastarch, diluted 1:2 with 0.9% saline	Author uses 5 ml/kg i.v. bolus for hypoproteinaemic and hypovolaemic patients	
Blood transfusion: blood in acid citrate dextrose or heparin	May be indicated if the packed cell volume (PCV) <5%. The donor and recipient should be the same species and cross-matching is recommended. Technique is similar to that for dogs and cats	
Calcium gluconate 100 mg/kg	100 mg/kg s.c. q24h	Hypocalcaemia
Potassium chloride	20 mEq/l of fluid: 1 mEq/kg given over 1 hour i.v., oral administration if eating or tube feeding	Hypokalaemia
Sodium bicarbonate 8.4% solution with 1 mEq/ml	1 mEq/kg diluted in 0.9% saline, given over 1 hour, i.v., or s.c. for slower absorption	If plasma pH <7.20

27.13 Fluid therapy. LRS = lactated Ringer's solution.
(Adapted from Norton (2005))

Drugs	Dosage and frequency	Comments
Dexmedetomidine (DM)	Author's preferences include one dose 25–100 µg/kg i.v. or i.m. alone or two doses <25 µg/kg for debridement or compromised patient	Dosage as low as 5 µg/kg i.v. used in some patients for analgesia during debridement Combined with ketamine and/or butorphanol in sea turtles and intubate for general anaesthesia
Atipamezole	Same volume as DM	Antagonist/reversal DM
Ketamine (K)	2.5–5 mg/kg + DM ± butorphanol i.v. for general anaesthesia induction	
Opioids	0.2–0.4 mg/kg i.v.	Added for additional analgesia and sedation (use with DM or DM/K)
Propofol	5–7 mg/kg i.v. initial dose and then half-dose increments for supplementation	
Midazolam	0.1–1 mg/kg i.m., i.v. (0.3 mg/kg is a good starting point)	Seizure control, muscle relaxation
Lidocaine	5 mg/kg maximum dose	Local anaesthetic (FP removal and other procedures) Buffer 1:1 with sodium bicarbonate
Tramadol	5–10 mg/kg s.c., orally q48–72h	Pharmacokinetic study in sea turtles
Alfaxalone	5 mg/kg i.m., i.v.	

27.14 Pain management and anaesthetics. DM = dexmedetomidine; FP = fibropapillomatosis; K = ketamine.
(Data from Norton et al. (2015); Norton TM et al. (2012))

Drug	Family	Dosage and frequency	Comments
Amikacin (A)	Aminoglycoside	Loading dose 5 mg/kg s.c. then maintenance dose 3 mg/kg s.c. q72h	Gram-negative Potentially nephrotoxic
Ceftazidime (C)	Beta-lactam Third-generation cephalosporin	20 mg/kg s.c., i.m., i.v. q72h	Broad spectrum More Gram-negative (PK1)
Ampicillin	Beta-lactam aminopenicillin	Loading dose 20 mg/kg s.c. then 10 mg/kg q24h	20–30 mg/kg s.c., i.m. q24h in association with A for Enterococcus spp. in Kemp's Ridley (Innis et al., 2014a)
Ticarcillin	Beta-lactam	50 mg/kg q24h or 100 mg/kg q48h i.m.	Gram-negative, Pseudomonas aeruginosa in association with clavulanic acid to get a synergetic effect between a beta-lactam and clavulanic acid and prevent resistance (PK2)
Chloramphenicol	Phenicol Bacteriostatic	30–50 mg/kg q24h or 100 mg/kg q48h i.m., s.c., orally	Aerobic and anaerobic, causes aplastic anaemia in humans

27.15 Table of antibiotics and antifungals. PK = pharmacokinetic studies in sea turtles. PK1 = Stamper et al. (1999); PK2 = Manire et al. (2005); PK3 = Jacobson et al. (2005); PK4 = Lai et al. (2009); PK5 = Marin et al. (2008); PK6 = Manire et al. (2003). (continues)

Drug	Family	Dosage and frequency	Comments
Enrofloxacin (E)	Fluoroquinolone	5 mg/kg s.c. q24–48h 10–20 mg/kg orally q5d (PK3)	Irritating to tissue, dilute 1:10 with saline (PK3)
Marbofloxacin	Fluoroquinolone	2 mg/kg orally/i.m., i.v., s.c. q24h	PK4
Danofloxacin	Fluoroquinolone	6 mg/kg i.m./s.c. q48h	PK5
Oxytetracycline	Tetracycline Bacteriostatic	Loading dose 41 mg/kg i.m. then 21 mg/kg i.m. q72h	Gram-positive and Gram-negative
Metronidazole	Nitroimidazole	20 mg/kg orally q24–48h	Anaerobic, can be used with A, C, E to broaden antibacterial spectrum
Itraconazole	Triazole antifungal	5 mg/kg orally q24h 15 mg/kg orally q72h	PK6

27.15 (continued) Table of antibiotics and antifungals. PK = pharmacokinetic studies in sea turtles. PK1 = Stamper *et al.* (1999); PK2 = Manire *et al.* (2005); PK3 = Jacobson *et al.* (2005); PK4 = Lai *et al.* (2009); PK5 = Marin *et al.* (2008); PK6 = Manire *et al.* (2003).

Drugs	Dosage and frequency	Comments
Cisapride	0.5–2 mg/kg orally q24h	Generalized GIT motility enhancer
Metoclopramide	0.5 mg/kg orally/s.c./i.m./i.v.	Upper GIT motility enhancer
Sucralfate	0.5–1 g/animal orally q12–24h	Coats gastric ulcers
Iron dextran	5–10 mg/kg i.m.	Anaemia, iron deficiency. Use with caution: iron accumulation in liver
Vitamin K1 (phytomenadione)	0.5–1 mg/kg i.m./s.c. q14d	Suspected clotting issues
Methylprednisolone Sodium succinate	20 mg/kg i.v.	Central nervous system trauma
Mannitol	0.5–1.5 g/kg i.v. slow bolus	Severe head trauma, do not use in hypovolaemic patients
Glycopyrronium (glycopyrrolate)	0.01 mg/kg or 0.05 ml/kg i.v./i.m./s.c.	Bradycardia
Atropine sulphate	0.01–0.02 mg/kg i.v./i.m./s.c.	Bradycardia
Praziquantel	25 mg/kg three times in 1 day, repeat 2 weeks	Pharmacokinetic study in sea turtles (Jacobson *et al.*, 2003), spirorchiid trematodes
Fenbendazole	25 mg/kg orally q24h for 3 days, repeat 2 weeks	Do not give if severely anaemic. May cause bone marrow suppression

27.16 Table of miscellaneous drugs. GIT = gastrointestinal tract.

Common medical ailments

Traumatic injuries

Traumatic injuries are a common reason for sea turtles to present for rehabilitation. Head trauma, lacerations and fractures of various body parts are frequently caused by boat strikes, predator bites, fishing gear entanglement and entrapment in dredging equipment (Upite *et al.*, 2012). If head trauma is suspected, a neurological examination, skull radiographs and advanced imaging should be performed to establish a prognosis and appropriate treatment plan early in the course of rehabilitation. Fractures of the neurocranium carry a poor prognosis. Samples collected for cytology, histopathology and culture of various microorganisms can be helpful in directing therapy, especially in chronic wounds that are slow to heal.

Sea turtles with severe traumatic injuries often require intensive emergency and critical care. Therapeutic strategies are very similar to human and domestic-animal medicine. For traumatic head injuries, treatment may include fluid therapy (see Figure 27.13) to maintain adequate perfusion, oxygen, and mannitol or hypertonic saline administered by intravenous bolus. Analgesics (see Figure 27.14), broad-spectrum antibiotics (see Figure 27.15) and supportive care are usually indicated.

Stable long-bone and shell fractures typically do well without orthopaedic intervention; however, unstable fractures will require stabilization. Modified external fixators have been used to repair skull fractures involving the splanchnocranium and bone plates have been used to repair displaced unstable long-bone fractures. The authors have used zip ties reinforced with marine epoxy to temporarily repair an unstable carapace fracture followed by placement of orthopaedic plates (Figure 27.17). Although the aquatic environment presents many challenges, wound management techniques used for sea turtles are similar to those for humans and domestic animals. Initially, the wound is cleaned and large debris is pulled out of the wound. Copious lavage with saline or lactated Ringer's, dilute chlorhexidine or povidone iodine is important. The turtle should be positioned so the flushed solution drains ventrally, especially if the coelomic cavity integrity is compromised. Regular debridement of dead and infected tissue is critical, especially in the early stages of wound management. In stable patients that require regular heavy debridement, dexmedetomidine (5–100 µg/kg) administered intravenously and subsequently reversed with atipamezole provides mild to heavy sedation and excellent analgesia. The dosage used is tailored to the specific patient. The goal is to keep the dose as low as possible while still providing analgesia and sedation if needed.

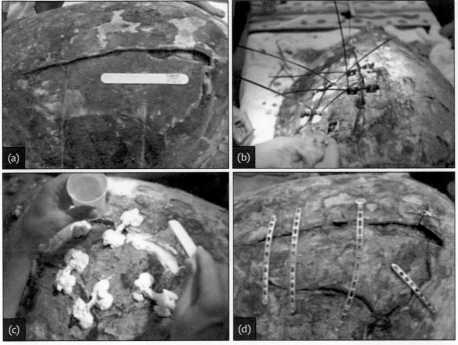

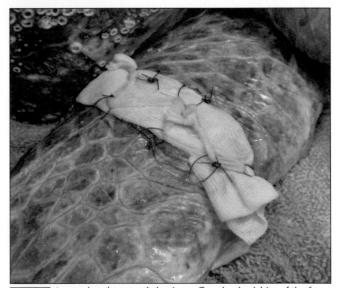

27.17 Carapace fracture in a subadult loggerhead sea turtle (*Caretta caretta*) illustrating zip ties and plates for shell repair. (a) An unstable carapace fracture. (b) Zip tie bases and zip ties are secured with epoxy and used to temporarily stabilize the fracture. (c) Marine epoxy is used to reinforce the zip ties and RediHeal® and bone cement are placed in the open portions of the fracture. (d) Five bone plates were used for long-term stabilization of the fracture. The fracture healed in approximately 8 weeks. RediHeal® and bone cement were changed weekly with flushing and debridement of the wound prior to reapplication.

A variety of topical products for open-wound management have been used successfully by the authors. The choice of a particular product depends on the wound, stage of healing and frequency of treatment. For relatively minor wounds on the shell, silver-containing products such as Silver Collasate® Postoperative Dressing (PRN Pharmacal, Pensacola, FL, USA) and silver sulfadiazine cream mixed with Ilex paste (Medcon Biolab Technologies, Grafton, MA, USA) for waterproofing can be applied after cleaning and debridement (Norton and Walsh, 2012). Commercially available medicinal honey products come in a variety of forms (gel, liquid, sticky bandages, etc.) that may be used on a variety of wounds, but may not be cost-effective, especially for larger wounds (Figure 27.18). Fresh honey is an alternative. Honeycomb has been used to pack deep wounds. Frequent wound management is usually necessary and a waterproof bandage is often needed to keep the honey in place. A waterproof bandage consists of placement of petroleum jelly-impregnated gauze over the topical product, Tegaderm® (3M, Maplewood, MN, USA) or similar sticky bandaging material with superglue placed around the edges, and finally waterproof tape placed over the entire area with another application of superglue. RediHeal® (borate-based biological glass containing factors that promote angiogenesis, Avalon Medical, Stillwater, MN) applied to deep wounds with exposed bone is often very effective. It can be placed within the wound and then covered with bone cement, which may be impregnated with an antibiotic. Doxycycline gel has been useful for treating exposed bone and stays on well in the aquatic environment. Superglue is placed on the outer edges of the products once dry, to provide further waterproofing. Weekly wound management is usually adequate when using these products. Large skin defects are often difficult to bandage. The wound is packed with the preferred topical product and petroleum jelly-impregnated gauze and then suture loops are placed around the wound and umbilical tape or suture material is placed through the loops to hold the dressing in place (Figure 27.18). A modified vacuum-assisted wound-care protocol (Figure 27.19) has been very effective in treating a variety of wounds in sea turtles, especially if the coelomic

27.18 Loggerhead sea turtle having suffered a shark bite of the front flipper. The wound was dressed using suture loops, Medihoney-, honeycomb- and Vaseline-impregnated gauze bandage.

cavity has been compromised (Marin *et al.*, 2014). Therapeutic laser therapy has been useful at the Georgia Sea Turtle Center for accelerating wound healing.

Hook and marine-debris ingestion

Medical issues related to the GIT are a common cause of morbidity and mortality in sea turtles. Sea turtles often ingest plastics, oil and tar, and fishing line with or without attached fishhooks. Some of the ingested material, especially smaller items, may pass through the GIT without any issues. Alternatively, the foreign material may cause mucosal irritation; lacerate or perforate the GIT (e.g. fishhooks); or may lead to obstruction, plication, intussusception (fishing line) and death (Wyneken *et al.*, 2006). A DV radiograph including the neck and head should be performed on every sea turtle at admission to rule out

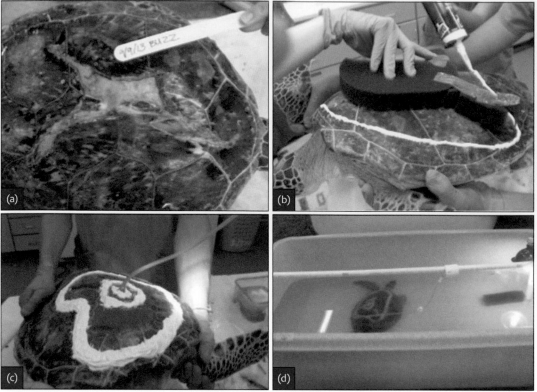

27.19 Waterproof vacuum-assisted wound-care therapy for a juvenile green sea turtle. (a) Boat strike injury with lung exposed in a juvenile green sea turtle. Marsh mud and debris were packed between the lung and the carapace. (b) Vacuum- assisted wound care (VAC) application: appropriate size pore sponge is cut to fit the wound with one layer of silicone applied around the wound where the sticky bandage will be applied. (c) Sticky bandage placed with additional layers of silicone placed, a quarter size hole is cut in the dorsal aspect of the sticky bandage to allow placement of the suction apparatus. Silicone is applied for an airtight seal. (d) Green turtle in the water with waterproof VAC in place. The turtle can move freely in the tank.

fishhook and/or line ingestion. If the hook is in the mouth, it may be relatively easy to cut and remove it. Mid-oesophageal hooks may be removed under heavy sedation using a relatively non-invasive technique, taking advantage of the highly mobile oesophagus, which may be slightly prolapsed, for better access and visualization (Parga, 2012). Endoscopy can be used to visualize the hook and line. Hooks found in the mid to lower oesophagus, stomach or intestinal tract may require anaesthesia and surgery for removal. An oesophageal incision may be required to remove some hooks in the midoesophagus. If the shaft of the hook can be visualized and grasped with forceps, then the point of the hook may be rotated to the ventral oesophagus. A small skin incision can be made over the point and the barb pushed out of the incision where the hook is cut below the barb. The remainder of the hook can then be removed from the mouth. A larger oesophageal incision or a supraplastron incision may be necessary for some hooks in the mid to lower oesophagus. To access the entire stomach, a left axillary-region approach (along the cranial margin of the plastron) has been used successfully, while the left and right inguinal approaches can access the remainder of the GIT (Di Bello et al., 2006a). Dehooking devices are available but should only be used if the hook can be visualized from the oral cavity, owing to the risk of tearing the oesophagus, trachea and surrounding vessels. The hook may need to be left in place depending on the anatomical location, type of hook (e.g. biodegradable) and circumstances (e.g. remote area). Enemas, fluids, petroleum laxatives and other supportive care may aid in passage of the hook and/or line. If plication or intussusception is present then surgery must be performed immediately. If fishing line is coming out of the mouth or cloaca, it should not be pulled upon. The line can be secured to the carapace during transport so tension is not placed upon it.

Fibropapillomatosis

Fibropapillomatosis (FP) is most likely caused by an alpha herpesvirus or chelonid fibropapilloma-associated herpesvirus (CFPHV). The use of polymerase chain reaction has demonstrated the association of this virus with FP tumours (Page-Karjian et al., 2014). Since the mid-1980s, the disease has been documented in most sea turtle species, with a higher frequency and severity in greens. The prevalence of the disease is associated with human activities (pollution, agricultural run-off, coastline with high human density), warm water and/or biotoxin-producing algae. A strong association exists between FP-affected turtles and immunosuppression (Work et al., 2001).

Common sites for FP tumours include the eyes (especially eyelids, conjunctiva and cornea) and skin (head, neck, axillary and inguinal regions, around the cloaca and flippers). Fibropapillomas may be solitary to highly invasive with a diversity of presentations, often starting as mild ulcerations and plaques, which may progress to sessile-like lesions, papillomatous, or polypoid smooth masses. These masses may impair vision (Figure 27.20), hydrodynamics and mobility of the turtle, leading to inability to find food and swim, with subsequent starvation. A tumour-scoring system is used for prognostication (Page-Karjian et al., 2014). Internal FP and severe ocular and bone involvement are associated with a poor prognosis (Page-Karjian et al., 2014), and humane euthanasia is often indicated.

Initial treatment consists of fluid therapy, nutritional support and antimicrobial therapy. Turtles with FP should be quarantined from unaffected turtles. Excellent water quality is critical, especially postoperatively. CO_2 laser surgery is currently the preferred surgical modality because the tumours can be removed quickly with minimal bleeding. The surgical sites are left open to heal by second intention while the turtle is maintained on systemic and possibly topical antimicrobials. Once the wounds have

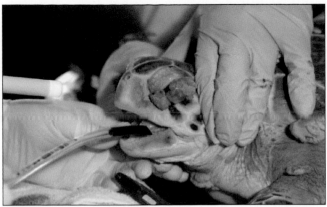

27.20 Juvenile green sea turtle with fibropapillomas on the sclera and nictitating membrane.

healed and there is no return of tumours, then it is appropriate to release the turtle in the same area that it was originally found. The clinician may elect to leave small tumours that are not affecting the turtle's health, mobility or vision. Regression of tumours has been documented (Page-Karjian et al., 2014).

Cold stunning or severe hypothermia

Hypothermia in sea turtles occurs when the water temperature suddenly drops below 10°C. Affected animals are unable to swim and dive, and often float on the surface. Secondary complications such as pneumonia and osteomyelitis (Norton, 2005; Innis et al., 2007, 2014a) are common and may not be clinically apparent for weeks. Acutely cold-stunned sea turtles are lethargic with poor response to external stimuli, have bradycardia (heart rate as low as four beats per minute), and low body temperature (<10°C). Dehydration, corneal ulcerations and lesions on the skin and shell are frequent findings. Abnormal laboratory findings may include heterophilic leucocytosis or leucopenia, electrolyte alterations, and metabolic and respiratory acidosis (Innis et al., 2007). It is important to monitor packed cell volume (PCV), total solids (TS) and glucose. In addition, pH, pCO_2 and pO_2 should be regularly assessed as they provide clinical and prognostic information (Keller et al., 2012; Stacy et al., 2013). Body temperature should be slowly increased, because an accelerated temperature increase may lead to acidaemia, hypercapnia and secondarily hyperkalaemia. See Figure 27.21 for median values of selected clinicopathological variables with significant differences between survivor and non-survivor cold-stunned Kemp's ridley turtles (Keller et al., 2012; Stacy et al., 2013). The causes of hyperkalaemia include renal function impairment, dehydration, compensatory response, hypoglycaemia and insulin resistance. Hyperkalaemia >5.5 mmol/l carries a poor prognosis (Stacy et al., 2013). Both hypoglycaemia (<2.2 mmol/l; 40 mg/dl)

Parameter	Survival	Non-survival
Acidosis pH (median)	pH = 7.57	pH = 7.35
Hypercarbia pCO_2 mmHg (median)	pCO_2 = 22.4	pCO_2 = 35.4
Hypoxia pO_2 mmHg (median)	pO_2 = 50.4	pO_2 = 33.4
Hyperkalaemia K^+ mmol/l (median)	K^+ = 3.0	K^+ = 5.03

27.21 Blood gas parameters in survival and non-survival cold-stunned Kemp's ridley turtles. Values were corrected using the temperature of the patient. Bicarbonate concentration (mmol/l) (median): 31.3 for survival and 25.7 for non-survival. (Keller et al., 2012)

and hyperglycaemia (>11.1 mmol/l; 200 mg/l) have been observed in cold-stunned sea turtles (Norton, 2005; Innis et al., 2007; Keller et al., 2012; Stacy et al., 2013). The causes of hypoglycaemia in cold-stunned turtles include anorexia, exhaustion, altered metabolism and sepsis. Hyperglycaemia may be due to stress, metabolic disease and iatrogenic injection of dextrose (Keller et al., 2012).

The treatment plan for hypothermic sea turtles should include a slow increase in body temperature (3°C/day) until reaching 24°C, prophylactic antibiotics, fluid therapy and nutritional support (Norton, 2005). Ideally, antimicrobial therapy should not be started until the body temperature reaches approximately 20°C (Norton and Walsh, 2012). Corneal ulceration can be difficult to manage medically if severe. Conjunctival flaps have been used occasionally by the authors with severe corneal ulceration. The therapeutic plan should be based on serial blood-gas and electrolyte evaluations. Fluid therapy for rehydration, including crystalloids and colloids as well as specific drugs to correct acid–base and electrolyte status, is described in Figure 27.13. Hyperkalaemia therapy includes calcium administration to alter the threshold potential of cells, sodium bicarbonate to alter the flux of potassium into cells and correct metabolic acidosis, and glucose, which facilitates cellular uptake of potassium (Pascoe, 2012). Respiratory acidosis due to an excess of CO_2 can be corrected by delivering oxygen via mechanical ventilation. In case of metabolic acidosis, including lactic acidosis, small doses of sodium bicarbonate should be administered slowly to increase the pH. Sodium bicarbonate increases the production of CO_2, thus, care should be taken when administered to patients with respiratory depression (Pascoe, 2012). It is essential that ventilation increases to allow removal of CO_2 from the body. Assessment of body temperature and heart rate is used for monitoring treatment progress.

Starvation/debilitated sea turtle syndrome

Debilitation in sea turtles (Figure 27.22) is a common presenting problem and can occur in any species. In 2003, a large number of debilitated loggerhead sea turtles were stranded along the south-eastern United States (Norton, 2005). Standardized diagnostic and necropsy protocols were established and utilized. The final results indicated

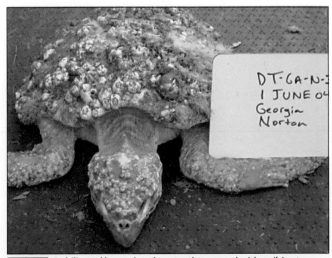

27.22 Debilitated loggerhead sea turtle covered with epibionts. Barnacles are not uncommonly found on the shell, but finding a heavy load on the skin is usually a sign of a severely ill animal. Cases of pericardial and cardiac tears have been documented in debilitated sea turtles.

that this condition was probably end-stage disease with the causes being multifactorial and the primary aetiology being masked by secondary problems.

When a loggerhead sea turtle presents in a debilitated state, initial diagnostics include a physical examination, complete blood count and plasma chemistry profile and radiographs. Physical examination often reveals heavy epibiosis, ulcers and other deep wounds on the skin and shell, severe emaciation, and fluid in the coelomic cavity. Blood work typically reveals a non-regenerative anaemia, hypoproteinaemia, hypoalbuminaemia, hypoglycaemia or hyperglycaemia, and low blood urea nitrogen. Radiographic findings often reveal colonic impactions from chitinous exoskeleton and shell parts (Figure 27.23) secondary to ileus. An ulcerative colitis has been documented in many cases.

Successful treatments include crystalline and colloidal fluid therapy intravenously (see Figure 27.13); total parenteral nutrition (Manire *et al.*, 2014); blood transfusions (see Figure 27.13); motility-modifying drugs (see Figure 27.16); and oral nutritional support with a highly absorbable elemental diet (Norton, 2005), deboned and debeaked prey items, careful iron supplementation (see Figure 27.16), specific vitamin and mineral supplementation, antimicrobial therapy, endoscopy-guided saline enemas and cortisone suppositories, and treatment of spirorchiid trematodes and other parasites. Additional treatments including blood transfusion are listed in Figures 27.13, 27.14, 27.15 and 27.16.

Harmful algae blooms

Harmful algal blooms occur worldwide and are caused by a variety of different algal species. Several episodes of morbidity and mortality in sea turtles associated with brevetoxicosis on the west coast of Florida and saxitoxins in Central America have been documented. Brevetoxicosis is caused by *Karenia brevis*, a dinoflagellate (Norton and Walsh, 2012). Fish, birds, marine mammals and several sea turtle species can be affected. Neurological signs are usually observed, with severity varying significantly among the different species of sea turtles. Clinical signs in Kemp's ridley and green turtles are relatively mild and include head bobbing, muscle twitching and jerky body movements. Loggerheads typically have more severe clinical signs, which may include generalized lethargy to coma, oedema, chemosis, and prolapsed cloaca and penis (Manire *et al.*, 2013).

Kemp's ridleys and greens affected by brevetoxicosis typically respond to removing them from the contaminated environment and providing supportive care. Loggerheads, on the other hand, require fairly intensive therapy (Manire *et al.*, 2013) including:

- Furosemide: 5 mg/kg i.m. or s.c. q24h for 3 days
- Withholding of all parenteral fluids for the first 2 days
- Diphenhydramine to reduce chemosis: 2 mg/kg i.m. q24h
- Penile and/or cloacal prolapse should be manually reduced, lubricated and potentially bandaged.

References and further reading

Arencibia A, Rivero MA, Casal AB *et al.* (2005) CT and cross-sectional anatomy of the normal head of the loggerhead sea turtle (*Carreta caretta*). *Anatomia Histologia Embryologia* **34(S1)**, 3–31

Bluvias JE and Eckert KL (2010) *Marine Turtle Trauma Response Procedures: A Husbandry Manual*. Wider Caribbean Sea Turtle Conservation Network (WIDECAST) Technical Report No. 10. Ballwin, MO. Available at: www.widecast.org/Resources/Docs/Bluvias_and_Eckert_Sea_Turtle_Husbandry_Manual_2010.pdf

Chrisman CL, Walsh MT, Meeks JC *et al.* (1997) Neurologic examination of sea turtles. *Journal of the American Veterinary Medical Association* **211**, 1043–1047

Di Bello A, Valastro C, Freggi D *et al.* (2010) Ultrasound-guided vascular catheterization in loggerhead sea turtles (*Caretta caretta*). *Journal of Zoo and Wildlife Medicine* **41**, 516–518

Di Bello A, Valastro C and Staffieri F (2006a) Surgical approach to the coelomic cavity through the axillary and inguinal regions in sea turtles. *Journal of the American Veterinary Medical Association* **228**, 922–925

Di Bello A, Valastro C, Staffieri F *et al.* (2006b) Contrast radiography of the gastrointestinal tract in sea turtles. *Veterinary Radiology and Ultrasound* **47**, 351–354

Erlacher-Reid C, Norton T, Harms C *et al.* (2013) Intestinal and cloacal strictures in free ranging and aquarium-maintained green sea turtles (*Chelonia mydas*). *Journal of Zoo and Wildlife Medicine* **44(2)**, 408–429

Feck AD and Hamann M (2013) Effect of sea turtle rehabilitation centres in Queensland, Australia, on people's perceptions of conservation. *Endangered Species Research* **20**, 153–165

Harms CA, Papich MG, Stamper MA *et al.* (2004) Pharmacokinetics of oxytetracycline in loggerhead sea turtles (*Caretta caretta*) after single intravenous and intramuscular injections. *Journal of Zoo and Wildlife Medicine* **35(4)**, 477–488

Innis CJ, Braverman H, Cavin JM *et al.* (2014a) Diagnosis and management of *Enterococcus* spp. infections during rehabilitation of cold-stunned Kemp's Ridley turtles (*Lepidochelys kempii*): 50 cases (2006–2012). *Journal of the American Veterinary Medical Association* **245(3)**, 315–323

Innis CJ, Merigo C, Cavin JM *et al.* (2014b) Serial assessment of the physiological status of leatherback turtles (*Dermochelys coriacea*) during direct capture events in the northwestern Atlantic Ocean: comparison of post-capture and pre-release data. *Conservation Physiology* **2(1)**, cou048; doi.org/10.1093/conphys/cou048

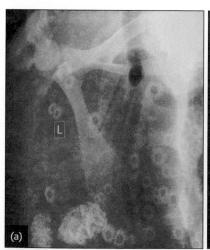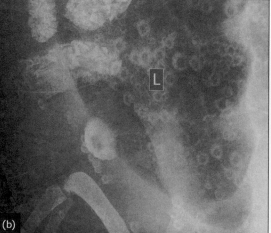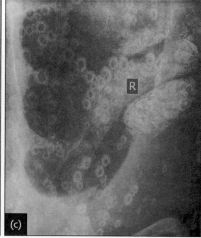

27.23 Radiographs of a subadult loggerhead sea turtle with intestinal impaction from shells and chitinous exoskeleton parts from prey items ingested (left (L) and right (R) sides of coelomic cavity, increased radiopacity). Numerous epibionts were also present on top of the carapace. (a) Cranial left quadrant of the coelomic cavity. (b) Caudal left quadrant of the coelomic cavity. (c) Caudal right quadrant of the coelomic cavity.

Innis CJ, Tlusty M, Merigo C *et al.* (2007) Metabolic and respiratory status of cold-stunned Kemp's ridley sea turtles (*Lepidochelys kempii*). *Journal of Comparative Physiology B* **177(6)**, 623–630

Jacobson ER, Gronwall R, Maxwell LK *et al.* (2005) Plasma concentrations of enrofloxacin after single-dose oral administration in loggerhead sea turtles (*Caretta caretta*). *Journal of Zoo and Wildlife Medicine* **36(4)**, 628–634

Jacobson ER, Harman GR, Maxwell LK *et al.* (2003) Plasma concentrations of praziquantel after oral administration of single and multiple doses in loggerhead sea turtles (*Caretta caretta*). *American Journal of Veterinary Research* **64(3)**, 304–309

Jacobson ER, Homer BL, Stacy BA *et al.* (2006) Neurological disease in wild loggerhead sea turtles *Caretta caretta*. *Diseases of Aquatic Organisms* **12(70)**, 139–154

Keller KA, Innis CJ, Tlusty MF *et al.* (2012) Metabolic and respiratory derangements associated with death in cold-stunned Kemp's ridley turtles (*Lepidochelys kempii*): 32 cases (2005–2009). *Journal of the American Veterinary Medical Association* **240(3)**, 317–323

Lai OR, Marin P, Laricchiuta P *et al.* (2009) Pharmacokinetics of marbofloxacin in loggerhead sea turtles (*Caretta caretta*) after single intravenous and intramuscular doses. *Journal of Zoo and Wildlife Medicine* **40(3)**, 501–507

Manire CA, Anderson ET, Byrd L *et al.* (2013). Dehydration as an effective treatment for brevetoxicosis in loggerhead sea turtles (*Caretta caretta*). *Journal of Zoo and Wildlife Medicine* **44(2)**, 447–452

Manire CA, Hunter RP, Koch DE *et al.* (2005) Pharmacokinetics of ticarcillin in the loggerhead sea turtle (*Caretta caretta*) after single intravenous and intramuscular injections. *Journal of Zoo and Wildlife Medicine* **36(1)**, 44–53

Manire CA, Montgomery NB, Cassle SE *et al.* (2014) Slow bolus administration of parenteral nutrition to chronic debilitated sea turtles. In: *Proceedings from the Annual International Association for Aquatic Animal Medicine Conference*

Manire CA, Rhinehart HL, Pennick GJ *et al.* (2003) Steady-state plasma concentrations of itraconazole after oral administration in Kemp's ridley sea turtles, *Lepidochelys kempi*. *Journal of Zoo and Wildlife Medicine* **34(2)**, 171–178

Marin ML, Norton TM and Mettee NS (2014) Vacuum-assisted wound closure in Chelonians. In: *Current Therapy in Reptile Medicine and Surgery*, ed. DR Mader and SJ Divers, pp. 197–204. Elsevier, St Louis

Marin P, Bayón A, Fernández-Varón E *et al.* (2008) Pharmacokinetics of danofloxacin after single dose intravenous, intramuscular and subcutaneous administration to loggerhead turtles *Caretta caretta*. *Diseases of Aquatic Organisms* **82(3)**, 231–236

Mettee N (2014) *Marine Turtle Trauma Response Procedures: A Veterinary Guide*. WIDECAST Technical Report No. 16. Available at: www.seaturtleguardian.org

Norton TM (2005) Chelonian emergency and critical care. *Seminars in Avian and Exotic Pet Medicine* **14(2)**, 106–130

Norton TM and Walsh MT (2012) Sea turtle rehabilitation. In: *Fowler's Zoo and Wild Animal Medicine Current Therapy, 7th edition*, ed. RE Miller and ME Fowler, pp. 239–246. Elsevier Saunders, St Louis

Norton TM, Cox S, Nelson SE Jr *et al.* (2015) Pharmacokinetics of tramadol and o-desmethyltramadol in loggerhead sea turtles (*Caretta caretta*). *Journal of Zoo and Wildlife Medicine* **46(2)**, 262–265

Page-Karjian A, Norton TM, Krimer P *et al.* (2014) Factors influencing survivorship of rehabilitating green sea turtles (*Chelonia mydas*) with fibropapillomatosis. *Journal of Zoo and Wildlife Medicine* **45(3)**, 507–519

Parga ML (2012) Hooks and sea turtles: a veterinarian's perspective. *Bulletin of Marine Science* **88(3)**, 731–741

Pascoe PJ (2012) Perioperative management of fluid therapy. In: *Fluid, Electrolyte, and Acid–Base Disorders in Small Animal Practice, 4th edition*, ed. SP DiBartola and WB Saunders, pp. 405–435. Elsevier Saunders, St Louis

Rousselet E, Stacy NI, LaVictoire K *et al.* (2013) Hematology and plasma biochemistry in five age classes of immature captive-reared loggerhead sea turtles (*Caretta caretta*). *Journal of Zoo and Wildlife Medicine* **44(4)**, 859–874

Stacy BA, Foley AM, Greiner E *et al.* (2010) Spirorchiidiasis in stranded loggerhead *Caretta caretta* and green turtles *Chelonia mydas* in Florida (USA): host pathology and significance. *Diseases of Aquatic Organisms* **89**, 237–259

Stacy NI, Alleman AR and Sayler KA (2011) Diagnostic hematology of reptiles. *Clinics in Laboratory Medicine* **31(1)**, 87–108

Stacy NI and Boylan S (2014) Clinical pathology of sea turtles. In: *Clinical Pathology. Marine Turtle Trauma Response Procedures: A Veterinary Guide*, ed. N Mettee. WIDECAST Technical Report No. 16. Available at www.seaturtleguardian.org/clinical-pathology-of-sea-turtles

Stacy NI, Innis CJ and Hernandez JA (2013) Development and evaluation of three mortality prediction indices for cold-stunned Kemp's ridley sea turtles (*Lepidochelys kempii*). *Conservation Physiology* **1(1)**, cot003; doi.org/10.1093/conphys/cot003

Stamper MA, Papich MG, Lewbart GA *et al.* (1999) Pharmacokinetics of ceftazidime in loggerhead sea turtles (*Caretta caretta*) after single intravenous and intramuscular injections. *Journal of Zoo and Wildlife Medicine* **30(1)**, 32–35

Upite C, Murray KT, Stacy BA *et al.* (2012) *Serious Injury and Mortality Determinations for Sea Turtles in US Northeast and Mid-Atlantic Fishing Gear, 2006–2010*. Northeast Fisheries Science Center Technical Memorandum NMFS-NE-222

Valente ALS, Cuenca R, Zamora M *et al.* (2007) Computed tomography of the vertebral column and coelomic structures in the normal loggerhead sea turtle (*Caretta caretta*). *Veterinary Journal* **174(2)**, 362–370

Valente ALS, Cuenca R, Zamora MA *et al.* (2006) Sectional anatomic and magnetic resonance imaging features of coelomic structures of loggerhead sea turtles. *American Journal of Veterinary Research* **67**, 1347–1353

Williard AS (2013) Physiology as integrated systems. In: *The Biology of Sea Turtles, Volume 3*, ed. J Wyneken, KJ Lohmann and JA Musick, pp. 1–30. CRC Press, Boca Raton, FL, USA

Work TM, Raymeyer RA, Balazs GH *et al.* (2001) Immune status of free ranging green turtles with fibropapillomatosis from Hawaii. *Journal of Wildlife Diseases* **37**, 574–581

Wyneken J (2001) *The Anatomy of Sea Turtles*. US Department of Commerce National Oceanic and Atmospheric Administration Technical Memorandum NMFS-SEFSC-470. Available at: www.noaa.gov and search for turtles/TM_470_Wyneken.pdf

Wyneken J, Mader DR, Weber ES *et al.* (2006) Medical care of sea turtles. *In: Reptile Medicine and Surgery, 2nd edition*, ed. DR Mader, pp. 972–1007. Elsevier, St Louis

Differential diagnosis for clinical signs in reptiles

This table summarizes the differential diagnoses that should be considered for clinical signs in reptiles and the diagnostic procedures that will be useful in determining a diagnosis. The columns are organized alphabetically; there is no indication of incidence of the various diseases, nor order or relative importance of the tests. Page numbers in italics indicate Figures.

Abbreviations: CBC = cellular blood count; CNS = central nervous system; CSF = cerebrospinal fluid; ECG = electrocardiography; FNA = fine–needle aspiration; GI = gastrointestinal; IBD = inclusion body disease; LRT = lower respiratory tract; MBD = metabolic bone disease; PCV = packed cell volume; RTA = road traffic accident; TP = total protein; TSH = thyroid stimulating hormone; T4 = thyroxine; URT = upper respiratory tract.

Clinical sign	Differential diagnoses	Diagnostic procedures (relevant chapter or page numbers in parentheses)
Anaemia/pale mucous membranes	Cardiovascular failure Endoparasites Haemolytic anaemia: haemoparasites; nutritional; viral Haemorrhage Neoplasia: bone marrow or blood–borne leukaemia Renal failure Respiratory disease Toxaemia/septicaemia	History and physical examination (see Chapter 6) Blood: CBC, PCV, TP (119–23, 124, 343–4); parasites (121, 336–7) Bone marrow cytology (128) Faeces: parasites (129, 284, 302–4, 411–15) Radiography: lungs (135–7, 313)
Anorexia	GI obstruction or parasites Inappropriate diet Intra/interspecies fighting (e.g. aggressive breeding male iguanas; inappropriate species mix in chelonians) Liver disease (e.g. hepatic lipidosis) Nutritional disease (e.g. hypocalcaemia, hypovitaminosis A) Gravidity and physiologically 'NORMAL' anorexia: females in later stages of folliculogenesis; males in search of females during breeding season; hibernation; aestivation (e.g. Horsfield's tortoise) Poor husbandry (temperature, light, humidity) Post-hibernation anorexia in chelonians Psychological (e.g. excessive noise, disruptive light patterns) Respiratory disease (e.g. pneumonia, URT infection, rhinitis) Sensual deprivation: loss of sight (e.g. cataracts, frost damage, corneal lipidosis); loss of smell (e.g. severe URT infection) 'Stress': postoperative, post–traumatic Urogenital disease (e.g. follicular stasis/egg retention, renal failure, cystic calculi)	History and physical examination (see Chapter 6) Assess husbandry (see Chapter 3) Assess nutrition (see Chapters 4 and 22) Blood: renal/liver disease (124, 296–8, 343–7) Coelioscopy (167–72) Faeces (129, 284, 411–15) Radiography and ultrasonography: reproductive tract (140–1, 150, 152–3, 155, 348); liver (149–52, 154, 157); GI tract (149–52, 154, 285–6) Respiratory tract sampling (127–8, 314, 320) Urinalysis (129, 344–5) Virology (129–31, 433–4)
Articular swelling (*see* Swollen joints)		
Ataxia and circling	CNS infection: viral (e.g. boid IBD); bacterial; fungal; parasitic (e.g. visceral larval migrans, protozoal) Frost damage Hepatoencephalopathy Iatrogenic (e.g. ivermectin toxicity) Metabolic disease (e.g. hypocalcaemia, ketoacidosis, hypovitaminosis B1, biotin deficiency, hypoglycaemia) Toxicity (e.g. insecticide) Trauma (e.g. dropped, RTA) Vestibular disease (e.g. otitis media/interna)	History and physical examination (see Chapter 6) Blood: CBC (119–124, 124–5); liver disease (119–124, 124–5, 296–8) CSF analysis (128, 356) Neurological examination (353–5) Radiography: spine and head (see Chapter 9) Virology (129–31, 359, 423–434)
Beak overgrowth (*see* Nail and beak overgrowth)		*continues* ▶

Clinical sign	Differential diagnoses	Diagnostic procedures (relevant chapter or page numbers in parentheses)
Blepharoedema/blepharospasm	Corneal damage (keratitis, conjunctivitis): viral (e.g. papillomas in Lacerta); bacterial (e.g. *Mycoplasma*, *Chlamydia*); fungal Foreign body Hypovitaminosis A Oedema Restraint (e.g. engorgement of periocular venous sinuses in iguanas and chelonians)	History and physical examination (see Chapter 6) Assess husbandry (see Chapter 3) Blood: protein (124, 125); renal function (124–5, 125–126, 344) Cardiovascular assessment (327–334) Direct sampling (127); fluid analysis/cytology (127, 279–80) Ophthalmic examination (96, 274–5)
Blindness (apparent)	Cataracts CNS disease (e.g. amoebic meningoencephalitis, IBD in snakes) Corneal damage: keratitis; conjunctivitis; spectacle removal Frost damage in chelonians Hypovitaminosis A Trauma	History and physical examination (see Chapter 6) Assess husbandry (see Chapter 3) Assess nutrition (see Chapter 4 and 22) Ophthalmic examination (96, 274–5) CSF (128, 356) Radiography: head (see Chapter 9)
Burns	Bonfires (garden tortoises) Bush/forest fires (wild species) Debilitated individual restricted to area under heat lamps/on heat mats Unsuitable heat source	History and physical examination (see Chapter 6); position of burns on body/shell may indicate source
Circling behaviour (*see* Ataxia and circling)		
Cloacal prolapse (may be prolapsed cloaca, bowel, or reproductive organs)	Cloacitis Constipation Cystic calculi Dystocia Enteritis Obstructive bowel disease (e.g. neoplasia, foreign body, intussusception) Salpingitis Trauma (e.g. post–mating)	History and physical examination (see Chapter 6); identify prolapsed organ (292–3) Cloacal swab/wash culture (128, 433) Coelioscopy (167–72) Faeces: parasites (129, 284, 302–4 411–15) Radiography and ultrasonography: urogenital, GI and respiratory tracts (see Chapter 9) Urinalysis (129, 344–5)
Cloacitis (with straining and/or haemorrhage)	Cloacolith/faecolith Cystic calculi Dystocia/egg binding Endoparasitism Infection: viral; bacterial; fungal (e.g. yeasts) Myiasis Trauma (e.g. post–mating)	History and physical examination (see Chapter 6) Cloacal swabs/wash for culture (128, 412, 433) Endoscopy: cloaca (164–5) Faeces: parasites (129, 284, 302–4, 411–15) Radiography (see Chapter 9) Urinalysis (129, 344–5)
Constipation/reduced faecal output	Cloacolith/faecolith Cystic calculi Dystocia Foreign body/gastroliths Intussusception Lethargy Poor husbandry (e.g. too cold)	History and physical examination (see Chapter 6) Assess husbandry (see Chapter 3) Cloacal swabs/wash for culture (128, 412, 433) Coelioscopy (167–72) Faeces: parasites (129, 284, 302–4 411–15) Radiography and ultrasonography: urogenital and GI tracts (see Chapter 9)
Corneal opacity	Arcus lipoides (chelonians and monitor lizards): age–related change Infection (keratitis): viral; bacterial (e.g. *Mycoplasma*; *Chlamydia*); fungal Corneal lipidosis in chelonians/monitors Normal appearance prior to ecdysis Scar tissue (e.g. post–keratitis, post–frost damage) Subspectacular abscess Tearduct blockage (leading to bullous spectaculopathy)	History and physical examination (see Chapter 6) Corneal sampling, culture andand cytology (127, 279, 433) Ophthalmic examination (96, 274–5)
Dermatitis/skin infection	Burns Ectoparasites High room humidity (RH) Iatrogenic (e.g. trauma, hypervitaminosis A) Infection: viral (e.g. papillomavirus, poxvirus, herpesvirus, iridovirus); bacterial; fungal (e.g. dermatophytosis, aspergillosis, CANV) Nutritional disease (e.g. hypovitaminosis A and E) Poor husbandry (e.g. poor hygiene, abrasive substrate, heater burns) Trauma (e.g. dog bites, chemical burns)	History and physical examination (see Chapter 6); slough/skin (98, 126–7, 258–61) Assess nutrition (see Chapters 4 and 22) Exudate culture (127, 260, 433) Skin biopsy (260) Virology (129–31, 433–4) Mycology (438)
Diarrhoea	Endoparasites (e.g. *Entamoeba* in snakes) Inappropriate diet (e.g. fermented fruit/vegetables) Infection: viral; bacterial; fungal (esp. post–antibiotic yeasts) 'Normal' if mixed large volume of urine and faeces excreted Obstructive bowel disease (e.g. intussusception, foreign body, neoplasia) Poor husbandry: too cold (e.g. lack of basking area) Septicaemia Toxaemia	History and physical examination (see Chapter 6) Assess husbandry (see Chapter 3) Assess nutrition (see Chapter 4 and 22) Blood culture (132, 435–6) Coelioscopy (167–173) Faeces: culture (129, 284, 436); parasites (129, 284, 302–4 411–15) Radiography and ultrasonography: GI tract (see Chapter 9 and 285–6)

continues ▶

Clinical sign	Differential diagnoses	Diagnostic procedures (relevant chapter or page numbers in parentheses)
Distension of coelomic cavity	Cardiovascular disease Coelomitis (e.g. egg yolk coelomitis) Cystic calculi Endoparasites (e.g. helminths) GI distension (e.g. intussusception, ileus, obstruction) Gravidity Hepatomegaly (e.g. hepatitis, hepatic lipidosis) Neoplasia/granuloma Obesity Oedema/ascites Pre–ovulatory/post–ovulatory stasis Renomegaly	History and physical examination (see Chapter 6); palpation/transillumination (99, 343, 347) Blood: renal/hepatic damage (119–126, 296–8, 344) Coelomic fluid cytology (127) Faeces (129, 284, 411–15) Radiography and ultrasonography: GI and urogenital tracts (see Chapter 9) Urinalysis (129, 344–5) Virology (129–31, 433–4)
Dysecdysis: excessive skin sloughing	Burns Dirty environment; secondary infection Ectoparasites (mites, ticks) Hypo/hyperthyroidism Ischaemic necrosis (e.g. frost damage, thromboemboli) Nutritional causes (e.g. hypo/hypervitaminosis A)	History and physical examination (see Chapter 6); slough/skin (98, 126–7, 258–61) Assess husbandry (see Chapter 3) Assess nutrition (see Chapters 4 and 22) Blood: T4 (267) Culture 'weeping' areas (127, 434–8)
Dysecdysis: excessive sloughing of scutes (chelonians)	High–protein/low Ca:P diets Hypo/hypervitaminosis A Infection: local; renal; septicaemia Rapid growth	History and physical examination (see Chapter 6); slough/skin (98, 126–7, 258–61) Assess husbandry (see Chapter 3) Assess nutrition (see Chapters 4 and 22) Blood: biochemistry (124–5); haematology (119–123, 124–5) Culture affected areas (127, 434–8)
Dysecdysis: retained slough. NB: retained scutes can be seen in aquatic chelonians that are not provided with basking areas.	Dehydration Dermatitis Ectoparasites Poor husbandry (e.g. low RH, too hot, lack of abrasive surfaces) Malnutrition Scarring (old)	History and physical examination (see Chapter 6); slough/skin (98, 126–7, 258–61) Assess husbandry (see chapter 3); examine water dish for mites Assess nutrition (see Chapters 4 and 22) Blood: PCV, TP (119–23, 124–5) Culture 'weeping' areas (127, 434–8) Virology (129–31, 261–2, 433–4)
Dyspnoea	Neoplasia Nutritional disease (e.g. hypovitaminosis A) Pneumonia: viral (e.g. paramyxovirus); bacterial (e.g. *Mycoplasma*, *Chlamydia*, *Pasteurella*); fungal; parasitic (e.g. Entomelas in lizards); aspirational (if tube feeding) Poor husbandry (e.g. too hot) Topical irritants (e.g. disinfectant fumes) Cardiac disease causing pulmonary oedema	History and physical examination (see Chapter 6) Assess husbandry (see Chapter 3) Assess nutrition (see Chapters 4 and 22) Endoscopy: URT and lungs (165–7, 310, 313–14, 318) Lung wash cytology and microbiology (127–8, 314, 318, 424) Radiography: lungs (144, 313) Virology (129–131, 433–4) Diagnostic techniques (438)
Dystocia ± straining	Cystic calculi Trauma caused by intra/interspecies aggression Narrowing of pelvic canal (e.g. fractures, neoplasia) Poor husbandry: humidity; temperature Salpingitis Systemic illness (e.g. hypocalcaemia, dehydration)	History and physical examination (see Chapter 6) Assess husbandry (see Chapters 3 and 5) Blood: (e.g. hypocalcaemia, dehydration (119–124, 124–5) Endoscopy: reproductive tract (165–7) Radiography: pelvis/reproductive tract (see Chapter 9 and 347, 348, 350)
Erythema (*see* Skin petechiae and erythema)		
Flotation problems (aquatic species)	Bloat: nutritional; obstructive; incorrect temperature Gastrolith/foreign body Gravidity Pneumonia	History and physical examination (see Chapter 6) Assess husbandry (see Chapter 3) Assess nutrition (see Chapters 4 and 22) Blood: CBC (119–24, 127) Endoscopy: LRT and lungs (165–7, 310, 313, 318) Lung sample/wash: parasites and microbiology (127–8, 314, 318, 424) Radiography: GI, reproductive and respiratory tracts (see Chapter 9) Virology (129–131, 433–4)
Hemipenile prolapse (*see* Penile/hemipenile prolapse)		
Inguinal/prefemoral distension (chelonians)	Cardiovascular disease Coelomitis (e.g. egg yolk coelomitis) Cystic calculi Endoparasites (e.g. *Hexamita*, amoebiasis) Gravidity Hepatomegaly (e.g. hepatitis, hepatic lipidosis) Obesity Oedema/ascites Neoplasia/granulomas Pre/postovulatory stasis	History and physical examination (see Chapter 6) Blood: renal/hepatic damage (119–126, 296–8, 344) Coelioscopy (167–72) Faeces (129, 284, 411–415) Radiography and ultrasonography (see Chapter 9) Sampling coelomic fluid (127) Urinalysis (129, 344–5)

continues ▶

Clinical sign	Differential diagnoses	Diagnostic procedures (relevant chapter or page numbers in parentheses)
Jaundice	Haemolytic disease Hepatic disease: intrahepatic; post–hepatic obstruction	History and physical examination (see Chapter 6) Blood: liver function (124–5, 296–8); renal function (119–126, 344); CBC, PCV (119–24, 127); parasites (119–24, 335–7) Bone marrow cytology (128) Endoscopy ± biopsy: liver (167–72) Faecal parasites (129, 284, 302–4 411–15) Radiography and ultrasonography (see Chapter 9 and 285–6) Virology (129–131, 433–4)
Lameness	Dislocation Fracture (traumatic/pathological) Gout Infection (local and septicaemia) Metabolic bone disease Pseudogout Tendon/ligament damage	History and physical examination (see Chapter 6) Assess nutrition (see Chapter 4 and 22) Blood: uric acid (124–5, 344–5) Radiography: spine and limbs (see Chapter 9)
Lethargy	GI obstruction or parasites Liver disease (e.g. lipidosis) Loss of sight (e.g. cataracts, intraocular disease) Musculoskeletal disease (e.g. poor mineralization) Neurological disease (e.g. frost damage, meningoencephalitis) Nutritional disease (e.g. hypocalcaemia, hypovitaminosis A) Poor husbandry: temperature; light; humidity; lack of UV light Post–hibernation anorexia in chelonians Psychological (e.g. excessive noise, disruptive light patterns) Respiratory disease (e.g. pneumonia, URT infection) Sensual deprivation: loss of sight (e.g. cataract, frost damage, corneal lipidosis) Starvation/cachexia 'Stress': postoperative, post-traumatic Urogenital disease (e.g. follicular stasis/egg retention, renal failure, cystic calculi)	History and physical examination (see Chapter 6) Assess husbandry (see Chapter 3) Assess nutrition (see Chapter 4 and 22) Blood: renal/liver disease (119–126, 296–8, 344) Coelioscopy (167–72) Faeces (129, 284, 411–15) Neurological examination (353–5) Ophthalmic examination (96, 274–5) Radiography and ultrasonography: reproductive, GI and respiratory tracts (see Chapter 9) Respiratory tract sampling (127–8, 314, 320) Virology (129–131, 433–4) Urogenital system (see Chapter 20)
Mouth rot see Stomatitis		
Nail and beak overgrowth	Husbandry: lack of abrasive substrate 'Normal' features: e.g. forelimbs of male terrapins; hindlimbs of female leopard tortoises Nutritional: excess protein (e.g. cat/dog food); low Ca:P diet Rapid growth in juveniles	History and physical examination (see Chapter 6) Assess growth (see Chapter 4) Assess husbandry (see Chapter 3) Assess nutrition (see Chapters 4 and 22)
Nasal exudate	Foreign body in URT or pharynx Infection: viral; bacterial (e.g. Mycoplasma, Chlamydia) Neoplasia Normal salt gland excretion (e.g. iguanas) Nutritional disease (e.g. hypovitaminosis A) Poor husbandry: humidity; temperature Stomatitis Topical irritants (e.g. disinfectant fumes)	History and physical examination (see Chapter 6) Assess husbandry (see Chapter 3) Assess nutrition (see Chapters 4 and 22) Biopsy/cytology for neoplasia (129, 397) Culture lesions (131–2, 289, 313–15, 319, 434–8) Endoscopy: URT and LRT (165–7) Radiography: respiratory tract (144, 313–14) Virology (129–131, 433–4)
Oedema	Cardiovascular failure Coelomitis (e.g. intestinal perforation, egg yolk coelomitis) Hypoproteinaemia: enteropathy (e.g. severe parasitism); hepatopathy; nephropathy (e.g. Hexamita) Hypothyroidism (especially giant chelonians) Lymphatic disease/obstruction Poison/toxin (e.g. bacterial endotoxins, insect bites/stings)	History and physical examination (see Chapter 6) Assess nutrition (see Chapter 4 and 22) Blood: TP, liver/kidney disease (119–126, 296–8, 344); thyroid (267) Blood culture (132, 435–6) ECG/echocardiography (329–333) Radiography and ultrasonography: reproductive tract (see Chapter 9 and 348)
Oviductal prolapse	Constipation Cystic calculi Egg binding Salpingitis	History and physical examination (see Chapter 6) Radiography of urogenital and GI tracts (see Chapter 9)
Pale mucous membranes (see Anaemia/pale mucous membranes)		
Paresis, weakness and flaccidity	Carapacial trauma CNS infection: viral (boid IBD); bacterial; fungal; parasitic (e.g. visceral larva migrans, protozoal) Cystic calculi Hypocalcaemia Peripheral neuropathies (e.g. in hypothyroidism) Renomegaly Spinal trauma (often sequel to MBD with collapse of vertebral bodies) Toxicity (e.g. pesticides, ivermectin)	History and physical examination (see Chapter 6) Assess nutrition (see Chapters 4 and 22) Blood: CBC (119–124, 124–5); liver disease (119–124, 124–5, 296–8); hypocalcaemia (124–5); hypothyroidism (267, 296) CSF (128, 356) Radiography: spine/head and urinary system (see Chapter 9) Virology (129–131, 433–4)

continues ▶

Clinical sign	Differential diagnoses	Diagnostic procedures (relevant chapter or page numbers in parentheses)
Penile/hemipenile prolapse	Cachexia and debility Cloacitis Constipation Cystic calculi in chelonians Endoparasites Poor husbandry: gender mix; poor substrate Spinal damage Trauma (e.g. post–mating, post–probing)	History and physical examination (see Chapter 6); Jackson's ratio (94) Assess husbandry (see Chapters 3 and 5) Faeces: parasites (129, 284, 302–4 411–15) Neurological examination (353–5) Radiography and ultrasonography: GI and urogenital tracts (see Chapter 9, 347–8, 350–1) Urinalysis (129, 344–5)
Regurgitation (see Vomiting/regurgitation)		
Shell deformity ('pyramid/ cornish pasty' effect)	Congenital/birth defect Metabolic bone disease Nutritional secondary hyperparathyroidism (NSHP) Rapid early growth (high–protein diets)	History and physical examination (see Chapter 6) Assess nutrition (see Chapter 4 and 22) Radiography (see Chapter 9)
Shell discoloration/ fracture	Burns Petechiae/ecchymoses Septicaemia 'Shell rot' ± osteomyelitis Trauma: animal attack; being dropped; road traffic accident; lawnmowers	History and physical examination (see Chapter 6); skin/shell (98, 126–7, 258–61) Blood: parasites (119–24, 335–7) Blood culture (132, 435–6) Culture affected areas (127, 434–8)
Shell softening	Local infection/abscess Metabolic bone disease Nutritional secondary hyperparathyroidism Rapid early growth (high–protein diets) Septicaemia	History and physical examination (see Chapter 6); skin/shell (98, 126–7, 258–61) Assess nutrition (see Chapters 4 and 22) Blood culture (132, 435–6) Culture affected areas (127, 434–8) Radiography (see Chapter 9)
Skin discoloration	Burns Ectoparasites (e.g. mites) Natural/behavioural changes (e.g. anoles, chameleons) Petechiae/ecchymoses Septicaemia Trauma (e.g. animal attacks)	History and physical examination (see Chapter 6); skin/shell (98, 126–7, 258–61) Blood: parasites (119–24, 335–7) Blood culture (132, 435–6) Culture affected areas (127, 434–8)
Skin petechiae and erythema	Abscess (if discrete lesion on shell) Burns Iatrogenic (e.g. hypervitaminosis A) Intravascular haemolysis (e.g. nutritional, haemoparasitic) Septicaemia (if generalized in skin or on shell)	History and physical examination (see Chapter 6) Blood: parasites (119–24, 335–7) Blood culture (132, 435–6)
Skin swelling (discrete)	Foreign body Iatrogenic: injection site reaction Infection: abscess/granuloma/fibriscess; cellulitis; mycobacteria; viral (e.g. papillomas) Joint inflammation: articular gout; pseudogout Neoplasia (incl. viral papillomas) Parasites: cutaneous (e.g. ticks); subcutaneous (e.g. filarial worms, esp. chameleon; botfly) Sebaceous cysts (esp. tail of green iguana)	History and physical examination (see Chapter 6) Assess husbandry/housing (see Chapter 3) Biopsy/FNA/impression smear (126–7, 261, 398) Blood: renal damage (119–126, 344) Radiography (see Chapter 9)
Skin tenting	Age–related wasting Dehydration	History and physical examination (see Chapter 6) Blood: dehydration/renal disease, etc. (119–126, 344) Urinalysis (129, 344–5)
Skin/shell wounds	Burns Iatrogenic (e.g. dropped) Interspecific fighting (inappropriate mixing) Intraspecific fighting (e.g. mating trauma in green iguana) Metabolic bone disease (pathological fractures) Substrate abrasion Trauma (e.g. animal wounds, lawnmowers, motor boats)	History and physical examination (see Chapter 6); skin/shell (98, 126–7, 258–61) Assess husbandry (see Chapter 3) Culture affected areas (127, 434–8)
Skin ulcers	Burns Infection Myiasis Trauma (esp. rostrum in Asian water dragon)	History and physical examination (see Chapter 6); slough/skin (98, 126–7, 258–61) Culture affected areas (127, 434–8) Look for ecto/endoparasites (see chapter 24 and 261, 265–6)
Stomatitis and excessive salivation	Foreign body reactions Infectious periodontal disease: (inappropriate diet in agamids, potentiated by immunosuppression as in/after hibernation); viral (e.g. chelonian herpesvirus); bacterial; fungal Nutritional disease (e.g. hypovitaminosis A or C) Renal disease Topical irritants (e.g. disinfectants for cleaning bowls) Toxicosis Oral neoplasia	History and physical examination (see Chapter 6) Assess husbandry (see Chapter 3) Assess nutrition (see Chapter 4 and 22) Culture lesions (131–2, 289, 313–15, 319, 434–8) Virology (129–131, 433–4) Cutaneous tumours (402)

continues ▶

Clinical sign	Differential diagnoses	Diagnostic procedures (relevant chapter or page numbers in parentheses)
Swollen head	Abscess of middle ear Oedema Trauma	History and physical examination (see Chapter 6) Culture affected areas (127, 434–8) Radiography: musculoskeletal system (see Chapter 9)
Swollen joints	Gout/pseudogout Infection Metabolic bone disease Neoplasia Trauma	History and physical examination (see Chapter 6) Assess nutrition (see Chapter 4 and 22) Biopsy/FNA (127, 398) Blood: renal disease (119–126, 344); calcium (124–5) Radiography: musculoskeletal system (see Chapter 9) Urinalysis (129, 344–5)
Swollen limbs	Articular gout Callus formation ± MBD Infection: cellulitis or osteomyelitis (mainly bacterial, e.g. mycobacteria) Metabolic bone disease Neoplasia Oedema	History and physical examination (see Chapter 6) Assess nutrition (see Chapter 4 and 22) Blood: renal disease (119–126, 344) FNA (127) Radiography: musculoskeletal system (see Chapter 9) Urinalysis (129, 344–5)
Urine discoloration	Biliverdinuria: haemolysis; *Hexamita*; liver disease/cholestasis Porphyrinuria Uroliths Haematuria secondary to trauma or cystic calculi	History and physical examination (see Chapter 6) Assess nutrition (see Chapter 4 and 22)Blood: liver enzymes (119–124, 124–5, 296–8); CBC (119–124, 124–5); parasites (119–24, 335–7) Endoscopy ± biopsy: liver (167–72) Foodstuffs may cause colour directly, e.g. pink from beetroot) Urinalysis (e.g. Hexamita) (129, 344–7)
Vomiting/regurgitation	Endoparasites (e.g. ascarids/strongyles, protozoans) Gastritis In snakes when handled shortly after consuming prey Iatrogenic: drug toxicity; excessive fluid volumes when stomach tubing; stress after force feeding Inappropriate ambient temperature Infection (e.g. IBD in snakes) Obstructive disease: foreign body; intussusception; GI neoplasia Septicaemia	History and physical examination (see Chapter 6) Assess husbandry (see Chapter 3) Blood culture (132, 435–6) Endoscopy ± biopsy: stomach (164) Faeces: parasites (129, 284, 302–4 411–15) Radiography and ultrasonography: GI tract (see Chapter 9 and 285–6) Stomach wash (127, 299) Virology (129–131, 433–4)
Weight gain	Cystic calculi Excessive fluid therapy Gravidity/follicular stasis/ egg binding Hypothyroidism/goitre Inappropriate diet (hepatic lipidosis) Oedema (e.g. cardiovascular disease, renal failure, hypoproteinaemia) Overfeeding	History and physical examination (see Chapter 6); weigh –Jackson's ratio (94) Assess nutrition (see Chapters 4 and 22) Blood: thyroid (267) ECG/echocardiography (329–333) Radiography and ultrasonography: reproductive tract (see Chapter 9)
Weight loss	Endoparasites Inappropriate diet Poor husbandry: temperature; humidity Progressive dehydration (e.g. renal failure, lack of fresh vegetables/fruit/free water, diarrhoea) Starvation	History and physical examination (see Chapter 6) Assess husbandry (see Chapter 3) Assess nutrition (see Chapters 4 and 22) Blood: TP, liver/kidney disease (119–126, 296–8, 344) Faeces: parasites (129, 284, 302–4 411–15) Virology (129–131, 433–4)

Acknowledgement

The Editors would like to thank Stuart McArthur for his help with this table.

A formulary of drugs for reptiles

This formulary is intended to provide a guide to commonly used drug dosages in reptiles. The class Reptilia contains between 8000 and 9000 different species; therefore, while the following dosages are taken from peer-reviewed trials and texts, there is always an inherent danger in extrapolating from one species to another, as there are simply not enough data on all species seen in captivity. Antibacterial and antifungal doses are based on pharmacokinetic studies at preferred optimum temperature zones whenever individual species are cited.

The reader is strongly urged by the Editors that when dealing with a species not specifically listed below, or with any unfamiliar species, they should contact veterinary surgeons (veterinarians) who are known to specialize in reptile medicine for advice on drugs to be used, their dosages, frequencies and routes of administration. Figure A2.1 is a formulary of drugs for chelonians, lizards and snakes and Figure A2.2 is a formulary of drugs for crocodilians.

Drug	Dosages	Indications and comments
Antiviral agents		
Aciclovir	80 mg/kg orally q8–24h Topical ointment (5%) also available	Tortoises with chelonian herpesvirus
Antibacterial agents		
Amikacin	5 mg/kg i.m. once, then 2.5 mg/kg q72h, based on gopher snakes 3.48 mg/kg i.m. once only in the royal ball python	Ensure adequate hydration and renal function prior to use of aminoglycosides. Generally considered less nephrotoxic than gentamicin. Low environmental temperatures reduce clearance and increase risks of toxicity
Amoxicillin	10–22 mg/kg orally q24h	Reported in chameleons. Useful for *Staphylococcus*, *Streptococcus* and some anaerobic bacteria
Ampicillin	3–6 mg/kg orally, s.c., i.m. q12–24h 20 mg/kg i.m. q24h 50 mg/kg i.m. q12h	Most species Chelonians Tortoises
Azithromycin	10 mg/kg orally q2–7d	Ball pythons. Useful against *Mycoplasma* spp.
Carbenicillin	400 mg/kg s.c. or i.m. q48h in tortoises; q24h in lizards and snakes	Increased efficacy against Gram-negative bacteria, e.g. *Pseudomonas*
Cefoperazone	125 mg/kg i.m. q24h, based on tegus 100 mg/kg i.m. q96h, based on false water cobras	Similar spectrum of activity to ceftazidime, but excreted by the liver and not the kidneys
Cefotaxime	20–40 mg/kg i.m. q24h	Can be used with an aminoglycoside to enhance activity against Gram-negative bacteria
Ceftazidime	20–40 mg/kg s.c., i.m. or i.v. q48–72h, based on various snakes	Very useful against Gram-negative bacteria, particularly *Vibrio*, *Pseudomonas* and *Aeromonas*. Acts synergistically with aminoglycosides and possibly with fluoroquinolones
Ceftiofur	5 mg/kg s.c., i.m. q24h 4 mg/kg i.m. q24h 2.2 mg/kg i.m. q48h	Lizards Tortoises: Particularly useful with bacterial respiratory tract infections (e.g. *Pasteurella*, Gram-negative bacteria) Snakes
Cefuroxime	100 mg/kg i.m. q24h	Can be used with an aminoglycoside to enhance activity against Gram-negative bacteria
Chloramphenicol	50 mg/kg orally, s.c. or i.m. q24h in boids; q12h in rat/king/indigo snakes; q72h in water snakes Topical eyedrops also available	Concerns re. public health and bone marrow suppression; has caused anaemia in juvenile water snakes. Useful against rickettsias, *Chlamydia*, anaerobes in the upper respiratory tract and eye infections in chelonians

A2.1 Formulary of drugs for chelonians, lizards and snakes. (continues) ▶

BSAVA Manual of Reptiles, third edition. Edited by Simon J. Girling and Paul Raiti. ©BSAVA 2019

Drug	Dosages	Indications and comments
Antibacterial agents continued		
Chlortetracycline	200 mg/kg orally q24h	Most species
Ciprofloxacin	10 mg/kg orally q48h	Most species. Use with care in juveniles due to damaging effects of fluoroquinolones on growing cartilage. Useful for *Pseudomonas, Mycoplasma, Chlamydia*
Clarithromycin	15 mg/kg orally q48–72h	Useful in pasteurellosis and *Mycoplasma*-associated upper respiratory tract infection in chelonians
Clindamycin	5 mg/kg orally q12h	Most species. Useful for anaerobes and osteomyelitis
Danofloxacin	6 mg/kg s.c. q48h x 30 days	Tortoises (mycoplasmosis)
Doxycycline	5–10 mg/kg orally q24h x 10–45 days 50 mg/kg i.m. once, then 25 mg/kg q72h	Most species (mycoplasmosis) Used in Hermann's tortoise against *Staphylococcus* and *Klebsiella*. Also likely to be effective against *Chlamydia* and rickettsias
Enrofloxacin	5–10 mg/kg orally or i.m. q24h (large chelonians suggested 5 mg/kg i.m. q12–24h)	Useful for *Pseudomonas, Mycoplasma, Chlamydia* and Gram-negative bacteria. Drug causes discomfort and tissue necrosis at site of injection, particularly subcutaneously. Oral solution achieves good systemic bioavailability. Has been associated with occasional regurgitation and excessive salivation in chelonians. Use with care in juveniles due to damaging effects of fluoroquinolones on growing cartilage
Gentamicin	2.5–5 mg/kg i.m. q72h For Gram-negative respiratory infections: 10–20 mg/15 ml saline and then nebulized for 15–30 min q8–12h	May be combined with third-generation cephalosporin (e.g. ceftazidime) to enhance activity against *Pseudomonas* and other Gram-negative bacteria Ensure adequate hydration and healthy renal function; risks of nephrotoxicity relatively high in snakes
Marbofloxacin	10 mg/kg orally q48h 10 mg/kg i.m., s.c. q24h	Ball pythons Most species (author's experience) See notes on ciprofloxacin and enrofloxacin. Good activity against Gram-negative bacteria
Metronidazole	20 mg/kg orally q24h; q48h in yellow ratsnakes and green iguanas May be used at 12.5 mg/kg orally once in snakes as an appetite stimulant	Useful for anaerobes. May combine with amikacin to broaden spectrum of activity. Duration of treatment usually >10 days, but beware of hepatotoxicity if using q24h
Piperacillin	50–100 mg/kg i.m. q24h for 1–2 wk For respiratory infections: 100 mg/10 ml saline and then nebulized for 15–30 min q8–12h	Broad spectrum of activity; useful for respiratory infections. May be used with an aminoglycoside to increase activity against Gram-negative bacteria
Silver sulfadiazine cream	Apply topically q24h	Broad-spectrum antibacterial (particularly effective against Gram-negatives, e.g. *Pseudomonas*). Some fungicidal activity
Antifungal agents		
Amphotericin B	0.5–1 mg/kg i.v. or intracoelomically q24–72h for 2–4 wk For respiratory infections: 5 mg/150 ml saline and then nebulized for 30–60 min q12h	Useful for aspergillosis and candidiasis. Potentially nephrotoxic; ensure adequate hydration and renal function Useful for fungal and some bacterial respiratory infections
Clotrimazole	Apply topically q12–24h	Fungal dermatitis or stomatitis
Enilconazole	1:50 dilution with water applied topically q2–3d	Fungal dermatitis
Fluconazole	21 mg/kg s.c. loading dose; then 10 mg/kg s.c. q5d, based on loggerhead turtles 5 mg/kg orally q24h	Fungal infection Lizards
Itraconazole	5 mg/kg orally q24h	Most species. May be effective against CANV infections but hepatotoxicity side-effects may be noted
Ketoconazole	15–30 mg/kg orally q24h for 2–4 weeks	Studies in gopher tortoises. Beware hepatotoxicity
Malachite green	0.15 mg/l water as a 1 hour bath q24h for 2 weeks for soft-shelled turtles	Fungal and algal dermatitis
Nystatin	100,000 IU/kg orally q24h for 10 days	Fungal gut infections, e.g. enteric candidiasis
Voriconazole	10 mg/kg orally q24h x 5–8 weeks	Long-term treatment is necessary for *Chrysosporium* spp. infection. No hepatotoxicity noted in bearded dragons
Antiparasitic agents		
Albendazole	50 mg/kg orally	Most species (ascaridosis)
Chloroquine	125 mg/kg orally q48h on 3 occasions	Blood parasites in tortoises
Fenbendazole	25–100 mg/kg orally once; repeat after 2 and 4 weeks 20–50 mg/kg orally q24h for 3 days	Nematodes, some cestodes

A2.1 (continued) Formulary of drugs for chelonians, lizards and snakes. (continues) ▶

Drug	Dosages	Indications and comments
Antiparasitic agents continued		
Fipronil	Spray on cloth first and wipe over reptile surface q7–14d until negative tests for parasites. Advised to wash off after 5 minutes to minimize toxicity	Ectoparasites, particularly mites and ticks. Beware as toxicity issues have been seen – possibly due to alcohol carrier base
Imidacloprid + moxidectin	0.2 mg/kg topically q14d x 3 treatments	Lizards (hookworms, pinworms)
Ivermectin	0.2 mg/kg orally or s.c. once; repeat q10–14d until negative tests for parasites 1 mg/kg orally q14d for pentastomiasis in tokay and day geckos Topical spray: 5 mg/l water every 7–10 days as for snakes and vivaria (add 1 part propylene glycol to 2 parts ivermectin to aid mixing with water)	Mites, ticks and nematodes. Do not use in chelonians or indigo snakes. Some suggestion of toxicity in crocodilians, chameleons and skinks
Levamisole	10 mg/kg i.m. once; repeat q2wk until negative tests for parasites	Nematodes, particularly lungworms in snakes. Use with care in chelonians
Metronidazole	125–250 mg/kg orally once Kingsnakes and indigo snakes: 40 mg/kg orally once; repeat after 2 and 4 weeks	Protozoans (flagellates, amoebae). Beware toxicity at higher doses Kingsnakes and indigo snakes sensitive to toxic side effects
Oxfendazole	66 mg/kg orally once; repeat q2wk until negative tests for parasites	Nematodes
Paromomycin	Entamoebiasis: 35–60 mg/kg orally q7d for 2 weeks Cryptosporidiosis: 300–350 mg/kg orally q48h for 3 weeks; then q5d for 3 months	Long-term cure not proven for cryptosporidiosis
Permethrin (10%)	Dilute to 1% solution and apply topically; repeat after 10 days	Treatment for mites. Less toxic than pyrethrins, but beware toxicity and ensure adequate ventilation after treatment
Ponazuril	30 mg/kg orally q48h x 2	Bearded dragons (coccidiosis)
Praziquantel	5–8 mg/kg orally once; repeat after 2 and 4 weeks	Cestodes and trematodes
Pyrantel pamoate	5 mg/kg orally q14d 25 mg/kg orally q24h x 3d, repeat in 3 weeks	Most species (nematodes) Most species (nematodes)
Quinacrine	19–100 mg/kg orally q48h for 14–21 days	Haemo-protozoans
Spiramycin	160 mg/kg orally q24h for 10 days	Cryptosporidiosis in snakes; not proven to cure but reduces numbers of parasites and may prolong survival
Sulfadiazine	25 mg/kg orally q24h for 21 days	Coccidiosis. Ensure adequate hydration/renal function as potentially nephrotoxic
Sulfadimethoxine	90 mg/kg orally once; then 45 mg/kg orally q24h	Coccidiosis. Ensure adequate hydration/renal function as potentially nephrotoxic
Sulfadimidine	0.3–0.6 mg/kg orally q24h for 10 days (33% solution)	Coccidiosis. Ensure adequate hydration/renal function as potentially nephrotoxic
Sulfamethazine	50 mg/kg q24h for 3 days; then no treatment for 3 days; then repeat for 3 days	Coccidiosis. Ensure adequate hydration/renal function as potentially nephrotoxic
Toltrazuril	5–15 mg/kg orally q24h x 3 days 15 mg/kg orally q48h x 10 days discontinue for 2 weeks, repeat q24h x 10 days	Lizards (coccidiosis) Tortoises (intranuclear coccidiosis)
Trimethoprim/sulfadiazine	30 mg/kg orally q24h x 2 days once, then q48h x 21 days 30 mg/kg i.m. q24h x 2 days once then 15 mg/kg i.m. q48h x 10–28 days	Most species (coccidiosis) Most species (coccidiosis) Ensure adequate hydration/renal function as potentially nephrotoxic
Trimethoprim/ sulfamethoxazole	15–20mg/kg orally q24–48h for 7–14 days	Bearded dragons (coccidiosis). Ensure adequate hydration/renal function as potentially nephrotoxic
Anaesthetic and analgesic agents		
Acepromazine	0.1–0.5 mg/kg i.m. 1 hour prior to anaesthesia	Pre-anaesthetic sedation
Alfaxalone	3–10 mg/kg i.v. or 20–40 mg/kg i.m.	Induction of anaesthesia and short period of surgical anaesthesia
Atipamezole	Dose at 5 times the dose (mg/kg) of medetomidine used, i.m. once	Reversal agent for medetomidine
Atropine	0.01–0.04 mg/kg s.c., i.v., i.m. or intracoelomically once	Pre-anaesthetic. Reduces respiratory tract secretions and inhibits bradycardia in some reptiles but may make secretions very tenacious and actually enhance blockage of endotracheal tubes
Bupivacaine	1–2 mg/kg local injection	Local anaesthetic. Do not exceed 4 mg/kg as a maximum dose or cardiotoxicity reported
Buprenorphine	0.01–1 mg/kg i.m.	Analgesic. Sedation at doses above 0.05 mg/kg

A2.1 (continued) Formulary of drugs for chelonians, lizards and snakes. (continues) ▶

Drug	Dosages	Indications and comments
Anaesthetic and analgesic agents continued		
Butorphanol	Analgesia: 0.5–1 mg/kg i.m. Pre-anaesthetic sedation: 0.4 mg/kg + 2 mg/kg midazolam i.m. Sedation (green tree monitor): 0.4 mg/kg + 0.08 mg/kg medetomidine i.m.	
Carprofen	2–4 mg/kg s.c., i.m. or orally q24h	Analgesia. Beware use with renal insufficiency/dehydration
Dexmedetomidine	0.03–0.08 mg/kg i.m.	Sedative. Can be combined with ketamine for short periods of anaesthesia at 5 mg/kg ketamine
Diazepam	Sedative in chelonians: 0.2–1 mg/kg i.m. Sedative in snakes: 0.2–0.8 mg/kg + 20–60 mg/kg ketamine i.m. Seizures: 2.5 mg/kg i.m. or i.v.	Chelonians: used with ketamine to help with muscle relaxation Snakes: used as a sedative (low dose ketamine) or anaesthetic (high dose) to help with muscle relaxation
Fentanyl	2.5 µg/hour as a transdermal patch	Analgesic. Difficulty titrating dosage with patch size. Thickness of reptile skin may also make this route ineffective in some species
Fumazenil	0.1–0.2 mg/kg i.m.	Benzodiazepine reversal agent
Gallamine	0.3–1.5 mg/kg i.m.	Reversible neuromuscular blocking agent (with neostigmine); provides no analgesia. Crocodilians: immobilization 15–30 mins; recovery 1.5–15 hours. Generally used only in crocodiles currently Unsafe in alligators at dosages above 1 mg/kg with deaths reported in American alligators and false gharials
Glycopyrronium (glycopyrrolate)	0.01 mg/kg i.m., i.v. or s.c. once	Pre-anaesthetic. Prevents bradycardia
Haloperidol	0.5–10 mg/kg i.m. q7–14d	Used to manage aggression in boids
Halothane	3–5% induction; 1–3% maintenance	Isoflurane is the preferred gaseous anaesthetic
Hydromorphone	0.5 mg/kg s.c.	Analgesia. Beware use with liver disease
Isoflurane	3–5% induction; 2–4% (av. 2.5%) maintenance	Licensed anaesthetic for reptiles in UK; preferred gaseous anaesthetic
Ketamine	Chelonians: 3–60 mg/kg i.m or i.v. Lizards: 25–60 mg/kg i.m. or i.v. Snakes: 20–80 mg/kg i.m. or i.v. Crocodilians: 10–50 mg/kg i.m. or i.v.	Sedative on its own. See also butorphanol, diazepam, medetomidine and midazolam for combinations
Lidocaine (lignocaine)	Local infiltration s.c. to effect	Local anaesthetic. Total doses >5 mg/kg may be cardiotoxic. Consider diluting 1:1 with sterile saline prior to injection
Medetomidine	100–200 µg/kg i.m. + 5–10 mg/kg ketamine i.m.	Anaesthetic. Dose per kg varies with size of patient (see Chapter 12)
Meloxicam	0.1–1 mg/kg orally or i.m. q24h	Analgesia. Beware use with renal insufficiency/dehydration
Methadone	3–5 mg/kg i.m. s.c.	Analgesia. Beware use with liver disease
Midazolam	Premedication: 1–2 mg/kg i.m. Chelonian sedation/anaesthesia: ≤2 mg/kg + 20–60 mg/kg ketamine i.m.	Premedication 20 min prior to induction of anaesthesia. Chelonians: sedation (low dose ketamine) to anaesthesia (high dose ketamine) with improved muscle relaxation over ketamine alone
Morphine	1–5 mg/kg s.c.	Analgesia. Beware use with liver disease. May cause sedation
Neostigmine	0.25 mg/kg i.m.	Reversal agent for gallamine muscular blocking agent. Adding 75 mg hyaluronidase may enhance reversal. May cause vomiting and laccrimation
Pethidine	20 mg/kg i.m. q24h	Analgesia
Prednisolone (or prednisone)	2–5 mg/kg orally	Analgesic for chronic pain or soft tissue inflammation
Propofol	3–20 mg/kg i.v. or intraosseously (i.o.) 0.3–0.5 mg/kg/min i.v. or i.o. as constant rate infusion	Induction agent; short-acting anaesthetic
Sevoflurane	Induction: 6–8% Maintenance: 3–5%	Similar properties to isoflurane. Less irritating to mucous membranes and therefore less breath-holding observed
Succinycholine	0.25–1 mg/kg i.m.	Has been used in chelonians, lizards and alligators. No analgesia and low margin of safety. No antidote. Recovery occurs due to metabolism. Intermittent positive-pressure ventilation (IPPV) often required due to respiratory muscle paralysis
Tiletamine/zolazepam	Lizards: 4–10 mg/kg i.m. Snakes: 3–20 mg/kg i.m.	Sedative Snakes: premedicant to allow intubation

A2.1 (continued) Formulary of drugs for chelonians, lizards and snakes. (continues) ▶

Drug	Dosages	Indications and comments
Anaesthetic and analgesic agents continued		
Tramadol	5–25 mg/kg orally, s.c.	Analgesia. Start low dosage and increase to effect. High dosages may produce sedation
Xylazine	0.1–1 mg/kg i.m.	Used infrequently; may be used as pre-anaesthetic to ketamine, particularly in crocodilians
Yohimbine	0.1 mg/kg i.m.	Reversal agent for xylazine
Miscellaneous		
Allopurinol	10–20 mg/kg orally q24h Green iguanas: 25 mg/kg orally q24h Chelonians: 50 mg/kg orally q24h has recently been suggested as more effective	Prevents uric acid synthesis; useful in treating gout
Aluminium hydroxide	100 mg/kg orally q24h	Used as a phosphate binder in chronic renal disease associated with hyperphosphataemia
Aminophylline	2–4 mg/kg i.m. once	Bronchodilator
Arginine vasotocin	0.01–1 µg/kg i.v. or intracoelomically once	Uterine muscle stimulant; more potent than oxytocin
Atenolol	7 mg/kg orally Combined with 100 mg/kg calcium gluconate s.c. and followed the next day with 1–3 IU/kg oxytocin	Tortoises to promote oviposition by relaxing vaginal sphincter
Atropine	0.1–0.2 mg/kg q24h	Organophosphate toxicity
Bromhexine	Scatter powder on food at 'a pinch' per kilogram of food 0.1–0.2 mg/kg i.m. q24h	Bronchial mucolytic
Calcitonin	50 IU/kg i.m. once; repeat after 2 weeks	Secondary hyperparathyroidism in juvenile iguanas. Must ensure blood calcium levels are within normal range prior to use otherwise may cause fatal hypocalcaemic fits
Calcium glubionate	10 mg/kg orally q12–24h	Dietary calcium supplementation for hypocalcaemia
Calcium gluconate	100 mg/kg i.m., s.c. or intracoelomically q6h until normal blood calcium levels attained 1 ml/kg q24h of oral solution	Treatment of acute hypocalcaemic tetany in iguanas
Calcium EDTA	10–40 mg/kg i.m. q12h	Heavy metal chelation agent. Ensure hydration as may be nephrotoxic
Calcium lactate	10 mg/kg i.m. q24h	Treatment of acute hypocalcaemia
Cimetidine	4 mg/kg orally, i.m. q8h	Antacid
Cisapride	0.5–2 mg/kg orally q24h	Gastric and intestinal motility enhancer
Dexamethasone	0.03–0.15 mg/kg i.m.	Treatment of septic shock. Soft tissue anti-inflammatory
Doxapram	4–12 mg/kg i.m. or i.v.	Central respiratory stimulant
Furosemide	2–5 mg/kg i.m. q12–24h	Diuretic
Haemoglobin glutamer-200 (bovine)	1–2 ml/kg i.v. or intraosseous, once; slow bolus injection	Severe blood loss where transfusion not feasible
Itopride	2 mg/kg orally q24h	Most species; intestine motility modifier
Lactulose	0.5 ml/kg orally q24h	Lizards and chelonians. May act as a laxative and help with liver disease management
Levothyroxine	0.02 mg/kg orally q24h	Hypothyroidism in giant tortoises. Part of supportive therapy for fatty liver syndrome and anorexia in Mediterranean tortoises
Methimazole	1–2 mg/kg orally q24h for 30 days	Hyperthyroidism. Recheck blood values after 30 days. Treatment may be repeated
Methylprednisolone	5–10 mg/kg i.m. or i.v. once	Shock. Spinal or head trauma
Metoclopramide	0.05 mg/kg orally q24h x 7 days 1–10 mg/kg orally q24h	Most species, gastric motility stimulant Tortoises (≥1 mg/kg)
Milk thistle	4–15 mg/kg orally q8–12h	Lizards and chelonians, hepatoprotectant
Nandrolone	0.5–5 mg/kg i.m. q7–28d 1 mg/kg i.m. q7–28d	Most species (hepatic lipidosis) Lizards (anabolic, reduces protein catabolism) May increase appetite and promote erythropoiesis
Oxytocin	Chelonians: 10 IU/kg i.m. Lizards: 5–20 IU/kg i.m. Snakes: 20–40 IU/kg i.m.	Uterine muscle stimulant. May be repeated q24h on a maximum of four occasions. Useful to prime oviducts with calcium gluconate injection first
Pimobendan	0.2 mg/kg orally q24h	Therapy of cardiac failure; vasodilatation
Sucralfate	0.5–1 g/kg orally q12h	Gastric protectant

A2.1 (continued) Formulary of drugs for chelonians, lizards and snakes. (continues) ▶

Drug	Dosages	Indications and comments
Miscellaneous		
Vitamin A	1000–2000 IU/kg orally or s.c. q7d	Hypovitaminosis A. Parenteral doses of 7000–10,000 IU/kg have been associated with skin sloughing in chelonians, even on a one-dose basis
Vitamin B1 (thiamine)	Thiamine deficiency: 25–35 mg/kg orally, i.m. or s.c. q24h Diet high in thiaminases: 30 g/kg in food q24h	
Vitamin B12 (cyanocobalamin)	0.05 mg/kg i.m. or s.c.	May act as appetite stimulant in lizards
Vitamin C	10–20 mg/kg i.m. q7d	Hypovitaminosis C. Useful in stomatitis
Vitamin D3	100 IU/kg i.m. once; repeat after 2 weeks	Fibrous osteodystrophy
Vitamin E	1 IU/kg i.m.	Hypovitaminosis E. Steatitis
Vitamin K1	0.5 mg/kg i.m. q24h	Liver disease. Warfarin/coumarin toxicity

A2.1 (continued) Formulary of drugs for chelonians, lizards and snakes.

Drug	Dosages	Indications and comments
Amikacin	2.25 mg/kg i.m. q3–5d	Antibiotic Gram-negative bacteria, no efficacy against anaerobes. Combine with either penicillin or metronidazole for broad-spectrum coverage
Calcium gluconate	10–50 mg/kg i.m., i.v.	Emergency treatment of hypocalcaemic tetany
Ceftazidime	20 mg/kg i.m. q3d	Gram-negative bacteria
Ciprofloxacin	5–10 mg/kg, orally q2–3d	Antibiotic Gram-negative bacteria, mycoplasmosis, no efficacy against anaerobes
Edetate calcium disodium	73 mg/kg i.c. q24h for 5 days	Chelation therapy for lead, zinc, cadmium
Enrofloxacin	5 mg/kg i.m., orally q2–3d	Antibiotic Gram-negative bacteria, mycoplasmosis, no efficacy against anaerobes. Avoid intramuscular injection if possible because of tissue injury
Fenbendazole	10–20 mg/kg orally q24h for 5 days	Nematode parasites
Fluconazole	5–10 mg/kg orally q2–3d	Systemic mycotic infections
Itraconazole	5–10 mg/kg orally q2–3d	Systemic mycotic infections
Metronidazole	20 mg/kg orally q2d for five treatments	Anaerobic bacterial and protozoal infections
Oxytocin	10 IU/kg i.m., i.v.	Non-obstructive egg binding – used with calcium gluconate, warmth
Oxytetracycline	10–20 mg/kg i.m. q5–7d	*Mycoplasma*, *Chlamydia*, Gram-negative bacteria
Procaine penicillin	20,000–30,000 IU/kg q5–7d	Gram-positive and anaerobic bacteria
Praziquantel	5–10 mg/kg i.m., orally once, repeat in 2 weeks	Cestodes
Sulfadimethoxine	50 mg/kg q2d for five treatments	Coccidiosis
Trimethoprim/sulphonamide	10–20 mg/kg orally q24h for 2 days, then every other day	Antibiotic Gram-negative bacteria, no efficacy against anaerobes
Vitamin A (retinyl palmitate)	3–6 ml 200,000 IU/ml i.m.	For treatment of vitamin A deficiency. The palmitate must be metabolized to the active form and, therefore, is safer
Vitamin B1 (Thiamine)	10 mg/kg i.m. q24h for 5 days	For treatment of thiamine deficiency
Vitamin E	3–6 ml 300 IU/ml i.m.	For treatment of vitamin E deficiency

A2.2 Formulary of drugs for crocodilians; in general, use the lower dose (mg/kg) for larger animals.

References and further reading

Carpenter JW, Klaphake E and Gibbons PM (2014) Reptile formulary and laboratory normal. In: *Current therapy in reptile medicine and surgery*, ed. DR Mader and SJ Divers, pp. 382–410. Saunders Elsevier, St. Louis

Carpenter JW, Mashima TY and Rupiper DJ (1996) *Exotic Animal Formulary*. Greystone Publications, Manhattan, KS

Funk RS (2000) A formulary for lizards, snakes, and crocodilians. *Veterinary Clinics of North America: Exotic Animal Practice* **3**, 333–358

Funk RS, Diethelm G (2006) Reptile formulary. In: *Reptile Medicine and Surgery*, 2nd edn, ed. DR Mader, pp. 1119–1139. Saunders Elsevier, St. Louis

Kauffman GE (1997) Pharmacology, pharmacodynamics and drug dosing. In: *The Biology, Husbandry and Health Care of Reptiles, Vol III, The Health Care of Reptiles*, ed. L Ackerman, pp. 803–821. TFH Publications, Inc, Neptune, NJ

Mader DR (1991) Antibiotic therapy. In: *Biomedical and Surgical Aspects of Captive Reptile Husbandry*, ed. FL Frye, pp. 621–633. Krieger, Malabar, FL

Stein G (1996) Reptile and amphibian formulary. In: *Reptile Medicine and Surgery*, ed. DR Mader, pp. 465–472. WB Saunders, Philadelphia

Special considerations for venomous reptiles

Donal M. Boyer

Venomous reptiles (Figure A3.1) have long aroused fascination, reverence and/or fear in humans. The role these reptiles play in various ecosystems is only slowly being revealed and through modern molecular techniques evolutionary relationships are being refined. Toxicological research into venom is contributing important benefits to human medicine; for example, a chemical compound has been isolated from Gila monster venom to serve as a model for an experimental diabetes drug. Global climate change and habitat destruction are impacting on a number of species which may require conservation intervention if extinction is to be prevented (Figures A3.1c–d)

Exotic venomous reptiles are held legally by zoos, researchers and licensed private collectors but are also maintained illegally by private collectors. In the UK it is estimated that thousands of exotic snakes comprising 75 different species are held legally and illegally. Illegal ownership of exotic venomous snakes is often revealed when bitten owners seek medical attention. Whether one is a research scientist or hobbyist, captive animals can develop health problems that require the specialized expertise of the veterinary surgeon (veterinarian). There is an inherent risk of working with these creatures but it can be ameliorated to some degree by following wise management practices and sound safety protocols.

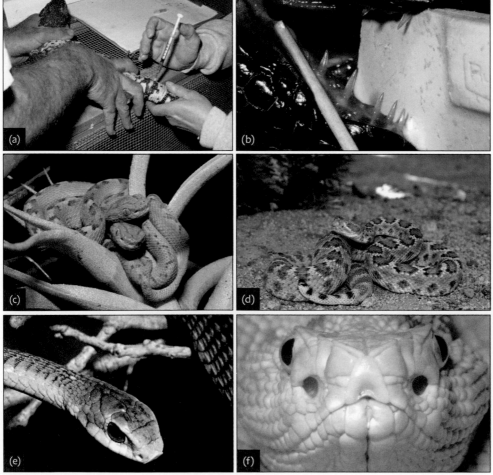

A3.1 Some venomous reptiles. (a) During a procedure with a venomous reptile a trained assistant restrains the animal, allowing the veterinary surgeon (veterinarian) to concentrate on the procedure. In this case blood is being collected from the tail of a Gila monster restrained in dorsal recumbency. (b) Beaded lizards and Gila monsters have large grooved teeth on the lower jaw towards the rear of the mouth. These lizards deliver venom through a chewing motion. The venom is drawn up the groove and into the wound. (c) Rowley's palm pit viper has a very small range, occurring only in several remote mountain ranges of the Mexican states of Oaxaca and Chiapas maybe negatively impacted by climate change. (d) The Santa Catalina rattlesnake is an insular endemic restricted to one very small island in the Gulf of California. It is listed by the International Union for Conservation of Nature (IUCN) as critically endangered. (e) The boomslang is a rear-fanged colubrid. This alert agile species can be difficult to handle and its bite has caused human fatalities. (f) Pit vipers have forward-facing heat-sensing loreal fossae or 'pits'. These are evident in this rattlesnake and enable it to direct a strike accurately, even in total darkness. (c, Courtesy of Alan Kardon; d, Courtesy of Ian Recchio; e, Courtesy of JH Tashjian)

Prior to obtaining a venomous reptile, one should have a protocol that includes established emergency procedures and handling guidelines. Some species of venomous reptiles are capable of inflicting life-threatening or seriously debilitating bites. The outcome of envenomation is hard to predict, due to a large number of variables such as species involved, amount of venom delivered, victim's health, location of bite, time until medical care is rendered, etc.. While it seems intuitive, the best measure of safety in working with venomous reptiles is to avoid being bitten; however, even with the best planning, accidents may occur. At such times, a well-planned emergency protocol is invaluable and may save lives.

Housing

While venomous reptiles can be kept in a wide variety of enclosures, from small glass aquaria to large walk-in enclosures, the most practical for the clinic setting are probably commercially available modular plastic enclosures. This type of caging is available through specialized reptile dry goods dealers. Units can be stacked on top of each other and are thereby space-efficient. These are easy to disinfect because the seams are sealed and all corners rounded. Whether caging is purchased or custom-made, the following points should be borne in mind:

- Enclosures should be easy to clean and disinfect and close securely with some sort of locking mechanism. Environmental requirements for proper husbandry are addressed in Chapter 3
- Enclosures should be placed in an uncluttered room with sufficient space to allow a safe work distance and room to retreat if needed
- The room should have smooth flooring and good quality ambient lighting. A smooth floor provides less traction for snake locomotion, although it certainly does not prevent it
- The room should have emergency lighting. In the event of a power failure, emergency lights are activated automatically
- Room doors should have sealed thresholds, screened windows and vents that will prevent escape from the room if a snake escapes from its enclosure
- Escape routes under enclosures and behind furnishing should be minimized
- Snakes are very good at escaping if given the opportunity. A plastic or metal rubbish bin acts as a holding enclosure (with a series of small holes drilled in the lid for ventilation) when the enclosure is being cleaned. The lid should lock securely or be secured to prevent escape. A handle in the middle of the lid will help prevent bites to fingers while lifting it.

These features will give staff a safe workspace to handle and manipulate venomous reptiles.

Labelling

- Any container housing a venomous reptile for more than a few moments (e.g. while cleaning a cage) should be labelled (Figure A3.2).
- All venomous reptile enclosures should be clearly labelled with two duplicate tags indicating:

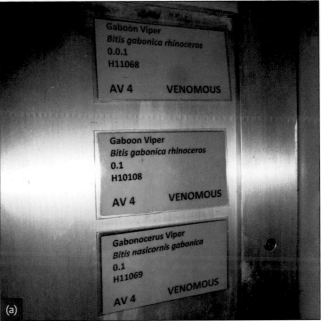

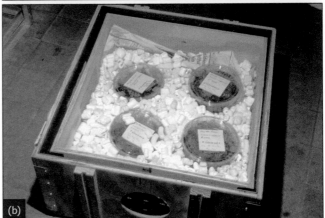

A3.2 Venomous reptile enclosures should always be clearly labeled as venomous providing common name, scientific name, and number of specimens present. (a) Examples of removable venomous labels attached with velcro to enclosure door. (b) Transportation of venomous reptiles also requires special packing guidelines. The proper authorities must be consulted prior to shipping.

- The species is venomous (bright red or orange coloured labels often indicate a venomous reptile in the USA zoo setting)
- Common and scientific names
- First-aid procedures
- Recommended antivenom product.
- An additional tag should indicate the number of specimens in the enclosure.

Handling

It is strongly advised that in order to work with venomous reptiles someone on the staff should possess expertise in handling techniques. Competent handling is a skill learned through experience and practice. A wide variety of handling techniques are used and some techniques expose the handler to unnecessary risk. The guidelines described here are designed to reduce risk but do not eliminate it altogether.

Risk factors

- Temperament, behaviour and risk factors vary among venomous species:
  - A small pit viper may be relatively quiet and not difficult to manipulate; however, a large adult mamba may present a serious challenge which requires a higher skill and confidence level (Aitimari, 1998)
  - This is not to imply that small species cannot be dangerous or that their bites are inconsequential; far from it
  - Venomous reptiles are venomous from birth or the moment they hatch; therefore, hatchlings should be treated with the same caution as when handling adults (Figure A3.3)
  - Know the species you are working with and do not get in over your head!

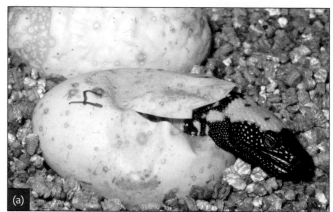

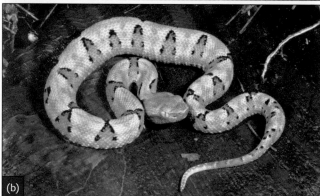

A3.3 Venomous reptiles are venomous from birth. (a) Hatchling Gila monster. Egg incubation containers should be clearly labelled as containing venomous species. (b) Venom composition may vary between young and adult snakes but young venomous species, such as this Brazilian lancehead pit viper, can inflict a serious bite.

Risks from dead reptiles

- Dead venomous reptiles can cause envenomation by accidental injury through contact with the fangs.
- Use caution while examining the head portion of a snake. Some pathologists insist on decapitation of the specimens before necropsy on the rest of the body is performed.
- Venom can remain stable for a period of time and for much longer if frozen.
- Dead venomous reptiles should be clearly labelled (see above) and should be placed in containers that prevent accidental mechanical injury to staff. Bodies should be stored this way until incinerated or returned to the owner.

Training

- A training programme for staff should include:
  - A literature review
  - Demonstration of competency in venomous snakebite emergency protocols
  - Demonstration of competency in venomous reptile handling techniques.
- In zoos, reptile keepers are typically trained in venomous snake handling methods through supervised hands-on sessions with senior members of staff.

Handling equipment

- There is a wide variety of equipment on the market. Basic tools needed for handling are snake hooks, tongs, bag sticks, clear plastic restraint tubes and long forceps (Figure A3.4; see also Chapter 6).
- Snake hooks should be provided in a variety of sizes to accommodate a variety of species and to keep the handler out of striking range.
- It is important to maintain an assortment of snake hooks and tongs in a variety of sizes and styles. Although the tongs may not generally be used to restrain snakes, they should be kept to hand when performing procedures with very aggressive, fast-moving agile species.
- A snake bag stick is useful when bagging snakes for capture or transport. The bag is attached to a long handle and held wide open. There is a sleeve located on the bottom of the bag to enable tube immobilization directly from the bag.
- Clear acrylic tubes in a graduated series of diameters are utilized for immobilization, a method widely employed by zoos in venomous snake restraint (Murphy, 1971).
- If spitting cobras are maintained, several clear full-face shields should be kept by the enclosures and a sign should alert of the hazard. Spitting cobras can very accurately spit venom at your eyes and face.
- An alarm system, first-aid and eyewash stations should be present in every area where venomous reptiles are maintained.

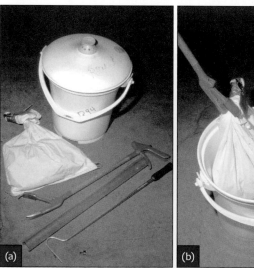

A3.4 (a) Basic venomous-reptile handling tools include a snake hook, plastic restraint tube, tongs, snake bag and locking bucket. (b) Even when the snake has been secured in a bag, care should be taken to avoid close contact with the bagged snake to avoid bites. Tongs should be used to manipulate the bag thus eliminating bite risk.

Handling techniques

While there are a wide variety of techniques used to manipulate venomous reptiles certain established techniques are widely used in the zoo community. Many of these techniques are discussed by Boyer (1995).

- Be clear about, and consistent in, your handling practices.
- While working with venomous reptiles, two staff members should be present who have completed venomous reptile training. The second person can assist if something goes awry.
- Be sure that all staff are aware that a procedure is being conducted on potentially dangerous reptiles.
- All staff must know emergency snakebite protocols, which should be periodically reviewed.
- Maintain communication with snakebite physicians, and meet periodically to review protocols and new species additions, tour the facilities, and speak with veterinary staff. Everyone should have a clear understanding of the emergency steps that must be carried out in the event of a venomous bite.

Physical observation

In order to carry out preliminary observations on specimens, clear plastic jars or larger plastic boxes are useful.

Anaesthesia

Clear containers may be used for the induction of anaesthesia using inhalant agents for incapacitating particularly dangerous or agile species. However, a widely used and fairly safe method of venomous snake restraint in zoos involves clear plastic tubes (see above). This method of restraint can be practiced to reduce risk and is harmless to snakes. Once a specimen is restrained in the tube one has access to the lower two thirds of the snake's body or, by sliding the snake further forward, to the head.

To induce general anaesthesia with an inhalant agent:

1. Immobilize the snake in a tube.
2. Place a gas induction mask over the tube at the end closest to the snake's head. This should fit the tube tightly through the use of the appropriate sized bell or mask with rubber gasket.
3. Once the righting reflex is lost and the snake is unresponsive to caudal pinching, move the snake forward.
4. Administer gas anaesthesia through tracheal intubation. Take great care when intubating venomous species. A solid mouth gag secured in place is essential, e.g. a block of wood or plastic to keep the jaws open or a plastic pipe through which intubation is attempted.
5. Assign a trained staff member to monitor the snake and to restrain it manually if necessary.
6. Once the procedure is complete and the snake begins to regain consciousness, remove the tracheal tube and slide the snake back into the restraint tube or straight back into a transport container or its enclosure for recovery.

Many zoos also use, and indeed may prefer, injectable anaesthetics. Once the reptile is restrained safely, ketamine or propofol may be administered (see Chapter 12 for doses).

Developing an emergency protocol

- Contact the local hospital or zoo to find medical doctors and toxicologists experienced in treating envenomations:
  - They should be familiar with the medical management of venomous snake bite
  - With a serious bite, time is an important factor and it behoves one to have a physician that is knowledgeable, will act decisively and is familiar with the use of antivenom products
  - Zoo professionals can be a very good source of information and advice, not only on protocol issues but also management and husbandry practices.
- Ask the physician to develop a list of emergency consultants with snakebite expertise
- Put together a list of emergency contact numbers that include:
  - Ambulance service
  - Doctor's 24-hour contact information
  - Antivenom source contact numbers
  - Hospital and Poison Control Centre information.

Print the list and give copies to your staff, and also post a list by the telephone.

In the United Kingdom, risk assessments must be completed at places of work. These must be read and signed by all staff working with the venomous reptile(s).

Antivenom

In the event of an envenomation emergency, access to antivenom is required. For a private practice it may be impractical to maintain antivenom due to cost. If this is the case, research product availability and set up a contact at the institution. It is vital to have 24-hour contact information.

In the UK, venomous reptiles are only legally kept by private owners with a Dangerous Wild Animals Act licence. This would normally specify that the owners have a supply of antivenom, where appropriate. This information should be obtained from the owner before they bring the animal to the surgery. Not all venomous species have an antivenom developed; in some species antivenom provides cross neutralization of other taxonomically related species. Antivenom choice in these situations is best left to the medical expertise of the doctors. Antivenom is not always necessary and the overall medical management of the case is reliant on the physician's expertise. Some species which may be popular with private collectors but have no antivenom are the Gila monsters and beaded lizards, African bush viper species and shield nosed cobra. Snake species such as boomslang or Asian keelback may have limited or no antivenom available outside of the range countries in which they occur.

Sources

External sources of antivenom should not be relied upon in the event of an emergency. The personnel dealing with venomous species have a responsibility to themselves and their staff to ensure the appropriate emergency treatment is available.

- Most zoos maintain antivenom stock for the species in their collection.

- Universities that are conducting research on venomous reptiles usually maintain a supply of antivenom.
- If you only work with your regional endemic venomous herpetofauna, the local hospital probably stocks the appropriate antivenom. In the UK, the only native venomous snake is the adder *Vipera berus*.
- The American Zoo and Aquarium Association (AZA) in collaboration with the American Association of Poison Control Centers (AAPCC) has an online antivenom index which is administered by the University of Arizona College of Pharmacy. The AZA and AAPCC have limited access to its members only. Another online resource is the WCH Clinical Toxinology Resources (www.toxinology.com). This site is designed for health professionals seeking information on diagnosis and treatment of envenoming and poisoning animals and plants.
- A list of commercially available antivenom has been published (Theakston and Warrell, 1991). Prior to ordering, check the legality of foreign antivenom importation. Importing antivenom can at times be a difficult task due to the lack of response from foreign companies or lack of current product supply. In the USA, most foreign antivenom is considered an experimental drug due to the lack of Federal Drug Administration approval; importation of such antivenom requires special permits. Zoos are the main source for antivenom products on an emergency basis.

Types

- If you have the resources to stock your own antivenom and wish to do so, you will need to determine which types to stock. It would be impractical to stock all available types.
- There are two basic types of antivenom (Figure A3.5):
    - Monovalent antivenom is made for a single species
    - Polyvalent antivenom is made to offer coverage for multiple species, generally within a similar geographical region.

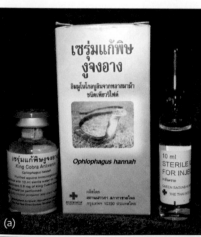
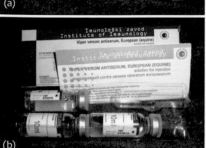

A3.5 Antivenom products are either lyophilized or liquid serum in a preservative suspension. (a) Monovalent king cobra antivenom from the Thai Red Cross is a lyophized product. (b) Polyvalent European viper antivenom from the Institute of Immunology, is a liquid serum.

- Do some research to determine which to stock based on the venomous species you work with most commonly.

Storage

- Purchase enough antivenom to offer coverage for two serious bites. Should an envenomation occur you will then only have used half your stock. Bear in mind replacing product can be a lengthy process, at times taking 6 months or more.
- Antivenom should be stored according to the manufacturer's recommendations.
- Antivenom is produced either in a lyophilized state or in a liquid form in a phenol suspension. Both product forms will have the manufacturer's expiry date listed. The lyophilized type generally has a longer shelf-life. Stored properly, antivenom has a longer efficacy than listed; however, this is an issue for your snakebite consultants.
- Antivenom products should be refrigerated.
- Keep an inventory of your supply, noting expiration date. Ideally, new antivenom should be ordered prior to the expiration of existing stock.

Alarm systems

- In most zoos venomous snakebite alarms, first-aid stations and an emergency telephone are present in all venomous reptile areas.
- At least two staff members trained in your emergency procedures should be present or in range of the alarm system.
- Should a bite occur and the victim becomes incapacitated the second person is invaluable. In the event of a bite the victim activates the alarm. This alarm should have an audible tone which can be heard anywhere in the building.

Emergency procedures

1. The first person on the scene should ensure that the venomous reptile is secured (the point being to avoid multiple envenomations), and then make telephone contact with the ambulance service. Do not delay in calling.
2. This person then performs the designated first-aid procedures. Your snakebite consultant can advise on what these procedures should be. Several basic first aid methods are available:
    - For all viperid (pit viper and true viper) rings, watches and any jewellery which may constrict blood flow as oedema occurs should be removed.
    - In most elapid bites a Sutherland wrap is applied and the involved limb is splinted to reduce movement. This technique utilizes a flexible crepe bandage that is wrapped to about the same thickness you would use for a sprain injury, in a distal to proximal fashion (Sutherland *et al.*,1979). This technique provides broad restriction of lymphatic flow but does allow for arterial circulation. This method has been shown to slow down greatly the onset of the life-threatening symptoms of elapid envenomation.
3. Keep victim calm and immobilize the bitten limb with a sling.

4. If antivenom is stocked, half of the existing stock of the appropriate antivenom is placed in a small cooler with an ice pack that will accompany the victim to hospital.
5. If possible, a knowledgeable staff member should accompany the victim to hospital.
6. Once the victim has left in the ambulance, make phone contact with the primary care physicians, informing them of the details and that a bite victim is on the way to the designated hospital.

Legal considerations

- In most cases the veterinary surgeon is not the owner of the venomous reptile and it is not his/her responsibility to hold the necessary permits and documentation.
- Veterinary surgeons in the UK should consult their Health and Safety advisor on the legal obligations of an employer when staff are treating venomous animals.
- Other legal requirements may have an impact. For example, you could have a practice in a township in the USA that forbids ownership or possession of venomous reptiles. In the USA, maintaining foreign antivenom requires permits from several federal agencies and there is also an annual reporting obligation whether or not any antivenom product has been used.

- Legal requirements vary from country to country, within the country, state or province, or even at municipal level. Check with your local city, county and state wildlife authorities ahead of time. Federal permits and/or foreign permits may be required for any specimens listed in the Convention on International Trade in Endangered Species of Wild Fauna and Flora (CITES) categories I, II and III. These permits also apply to dead specimens, or any derived parts such as blood and tissues.
- Shipment guidelines for crating requirements may apply at the local or country level. The International Air Transportation guidelines apply to international shipments.

References and further reading

Altimari W (1998) Venomous snakes: a safety guide for keepers. *SSAR Herpetological Circular* No. 26

Boyer DM (1995) Venomous reptiles: an overview of families, handling, restraint techniques and emergency protocol. *Proceedings of the Association of Reptilian and Amphibian Veterinarians*, pp. 83–95

Murphy JB (1971) A method for immobilizing snakes at the Dallas Zoo. *International Zoo Yearbook* **11**, 233

Sutherland SK, Coulter AR and Harris RD (1979) Rationalisation of the first-aid measures for elapid snakebite. *The Lancet* 1183–1186

Theakston RDG and Warrell DA (1991) Antivenoms: a list of hyperimmune sera currently available for the treatment of envenoming by bites and stings. *Toxicon* **29**, 1419–1470

Warrell DA (2005) Treatment of bites by adders and exotic venomous snakes. *British Medical Journal* **331**, 1244–1247

Common and scientific names

Common names have been used throughout this book for readability. This table gives the equivalent taxonomic names. Reptile nomenlature is continually in a state of flux, but every effort has been made to list the most current scientific names. The following references have been used:

- Ernst CH and Barbour RW (1989) *Turtles of the World*. Smithsonian Institution Press, Washington DC
- Henkel F and Schmidt W (1995) *Geckoes*. Krieger Publishing, Malabar, FL
- The IUCN Red List of Threatened Species. Version 2018–1. www.iucnredlist.org.
- Mehrtens JM (1987) *Living Snakes of the World*. Sterling Publishing, New York

- Obst FJ *et al.* (1988) *The Completely Illustrated Atlas of Reptiles and Amphibians for the Terrarium*. TFH Publications, Neptune, NJ
- Rogner M (1997) *Lizards. Volumes 1 and 2*. Krieger Publishing, Malabar, FL
- Roskov Y, Abucay L, Orrell T *et al.* (2018) Species 2000 and ITIS Catalogue of Life, 2018 Annual Checklist. Digital resource at www.catalogueoflife.org/annual-checklist/2018. Species 2000: Naturalis, Leiden, the Netherlands. ISSN 2405-884X

The Editors would like to acknowledge the assistance of William Cermak in the preparation of this Appendix.

Chelonians: tortoises and turtles

Common name	Scientific name
Afghan tortoise *see* Horsfield's tortoise	
African spurred tortoise	*Centrochelys sulcata*
African tent tortoise	*Psammobates tentorius*
Aldabran tortoise	*Aldabrachelys gigantea*
Alligator snapping turtle	*Macrochelys temminckii*
Argentine side-necked turtle	*Phrynops hilarii*
Argentine tortoise *see* Chaco tortoise	
Asian box turtle *see* Malayan box turtle	
Asian temple turtle	*Hieremys annandalei*
Barbour's map turtle	*Graptemys barbouri*
Bell's hingeback tortoise	*Kinixys belliana*
Big-headed turtle	*Platysternon megacephalum*
Black marsh turtle	*Siebenrockiella crassicollis*
Black side-necked turtle	*Pelusios subniger*
Black terrapin	*Pelusios niger*
Blanding's turtle	*Emydoidea blandingii*
Bolivian side-necked turtle *see* Chaco side-necked turtle	
Bolson tortoise	*Gopherus flavomarginatus*
Brazilian freshwater turtle	*Phrynops geoffroanus*
Burmese brown tortoise	*Manouria emys*
Burmese star tortoise	*Geochelone platynota*
California desert tortoise *see* Desert tortoise	
Celebes tortoise	*Indotestudo forstenii*
Central American wood turtle *see* Mexican spotted wood turtle	
Central American river turtle	*Dermatemys mawii*

Common name	Scientific name
Ceylon terrapin *see* Indian black turtle	
Chaco side-necked turtle	*Acanthochelys pallidipectoris*
Chaco tortoise	*Chelonoidis chilensis*
Chilean tortoise *see* Chaco tortoise	
Chinese box turtle	*Cuora flavomarginata*
Chinese soft-shelled turtle	*Pelodiscus sinensis*
Cogwheel turtle	*Heosemys spinosa*
Common long-necked turtle	*Chelodina longicollis*
Common snake-necked turtle *see* Common long-necked turtle	
Common snapping turtle	*Chelydra serpentina*
Cooter	*Pseudemys floridana*
Desert tortoise	*Gopherus agassizii*
Diamondback terrapin	*Malaclemys terrapin*
Eastern box turtle	*Terrapene carolina carolina*
Egyptian tortoise	*Testudo kleinmanni*
European pond turtle	*Emys orbicularis*
Flap-shelled turtle *see* Indian flap-shelled turtle	
Flatback turtle	*Natator depressus*
Fly River turtle	*Carettochelys insculpta*
Galapagos tortoise	*Chelonoidis nigra*
Giant Aldabra tortoise *see* Aldabran tortoise	
Gopher tortoise	*Gopherus polyphemus*
Greek tortoise *see* Spur-thighed tortoise	
Green sea turtle	*Chelonia mydas*
Hawksbill turtle	*Eretmochelys imbricata*
Helmeted turtle	*Pelomedusa subrufa*
Hermann's tortoise	*Testudo hermanni*
Hingeback tortoises	*Kinixys* spp.
Horsfield's tortoise	*Agrionemys horsfieldi*

Common name	Scientific name
Impressed tortoise	*Manouria impressa*
Indian black turtle	*Melanochelys trijuga*
Indian flap-shelled turtle	*Lissemys punctata*
Indian roofed terrapin	*Pangshura tectum*
Indian star tortoise	*Geochelone elegans*
Kemp's ridley sea turtle	*Lepidochelys kempii*
Leatherback turtle	*Dermochelys coriacea*
Leopard tortoise	*Stigmochelys pardalis*
Loggerhead turtle	*Caretta caretta*
Macquarie River turtle	*Emydura macquarii*
Malayan box turtle	*Cuora amboinensis*
Map turtles	*Graptemys* spp.
Marginated tortoise	*Testudo weissingeri*
Mata mata	*Chelus fimbriata*
Mediterranean spur-thighed tortoise see Spur-thighed tortoise	
Mexican spotted wood turtle	*Rhinoclemmys rubida*
Mobile terrapin see Red-eared terrapin	
Mud turtles	*Kinosternon* spp.
Musk turtle	*Kinosternon odoratum*
Narrow-breasted snake-necked turtle	*Chelodina oblonga*
Olive ridley sea turtle	*Lepidochelys olivacea*
Ornate box turtle	*Terrepene ornata*
Painted turtle	*Chrysemys picta*
Pancake tortoise	*Malacochersus tornieri*
Piedmont terrapin see River cooter	
Radiated tortoise	*Geochelone radiata*
Red-eared slider see Red-eared terrapin	
Red-eared terrapin	*Trachemys scripta elegans*
Red-footed tortoise	*Chelonoidis carbonarius*
River cooter	*Pseudemys concinna*
Russian tortoise see Horsfield's tortoise	
Soft-shelled turtle	*Trionyx* spp.
Speke's hingeback tortoise	*Kinixys speckii*
Spider tortoise	*Pyxis arachnoides oblonga*
Spiny softshell turtle	*Apalone spinifera*
Spotted turtle	*Clemmys guttata*
Spur-thighed tortoise	*Testudo graeca*
Star tortoise see Indian star tortoise	
Stinkpot see Musk turtle	
Sulawesi tortoise see Celebes tortoise	
Sulcata tortoise	*Centrochelys sulcata*
Texas tortoise	*Gopherus berlandieri*
Tunisian tortoise	*Testudo graeca nabeulensis*
Turkish tortoise	*Testudo graeca ibera*
Twist-necked turtle	*Platemys platycephala*
Western pond turtle	*Emys marmorata*
Wood turtle	*Glyptemys insculpta*
Yellow-footed tortoise	*Chelonoidis denticulata*
Yellow-headed temple turtle see Asian temple turtle	
Yellow-spotted Amazon river turtle	*Podocnemis cayennensis*

Lizards

Common name	Scientific name
Amazon streak lizard	*Gonatodes humeralis*
Ameivas	*Ameiva* spp.
Andros island iguana	*Cyclura cychlura cychlura*
Anole lizards	*Anolis* spp.
Asian water dragon	*Physignathus cocincinus*
Asian water monitor	*Varanus salvator*
Australian frilled lizard	*Chlamydosaurus kingii*
Australian water dragon	*Intellagama lesueurii*
Basilisk lizard see Common basilisk	
Beaded lizard	*Heloderma horridum*

Common name	Scientific name
Bearded dragon see Inland bearded dragon	
Bell's dab lizard	*Uromastyx acanthinura*
Bengal monitor	*Varanus bengalensis*
Berber skinks	*Eumeces* spp.
Black iguana	*Ctenosaura similis*
Black tegu	*Tupinambis teguixin*
Black-throated monitor	*Varanus albigularis ionidesi*
Black-lined plated lizard	*Gerrhosaurus nigrolineatus*
Blue-tailed day gecko	*Phelsuma cepediana*
Blue-tongue lizards see Blue-tongued skinks	
Blue-tongued skinks	*Tiliqua* spp.
Bosc monitor see Savannah monitor	
Caiman lizard	*Dracaena guianensis*
Central bearded dragon see Inland bearded dragon	
Chinese crocodile lizard	*Shinisaurus crocodilurus*
Chinese water dragon	*Physignathus cocincinus*
Chuckwallas	*Sauromalus* spp.
Coastal bearded dragon	*Pogona barbata*
Collared lizard	*Crotophytus collaris*
Common agama see Rainbow lizard	
Common basilisk	*Basiliscus basiliscus*
Common blue-tongued skink	*Tiliqua scincoides*
Common chameleon	*Chamaeleo chamaeleon*
Common lizard	*Lacerta vivipara*
Common wall lizard	*Zootoca vivipara*
Crested gecko	*Correlophus ciliatus*
Crocodile lizard see Chinese crocodile lizard	
Crocodile Monitor	*Varanus salvadorii*
Cuban knight anole	*Anolis equestris*
Day geckos	*Phelsuma* spp.
Desert iguana	*Dipsosaurus dorsalis*
Desert monitor	*Varanus griseus*
Desert spiny lizard	*Sceloporus magister*
Drakensberg crag lizard	*Pseudocordylus melanotus*
East Indian water lizard	*Hydrosaurus amboinensis*
Eastern blue-tongued skink	*Tiliqua scincoides*
Eastern fence lizard	*Sceloporus undulatus*
Eastern water dragon see Australian water dragon	
Egyptian spiny-tailed lizard	*Uromastyx aegyptia*
Egyptian uromastyx see Egyptian spiny-tailed lizard	
Emerald tree monitor	*Varanus prasinus*
European green lizard	*Lacerta viridis*
European wall lizard	*Podarcis muralis*
Eyed lizard	*Timon lepidus*
Fijian iguanas	*Brachylophus* spp.
Fischer's chameleon	*Kinyongia fischeri*
Flap-necked chameleon	*Chamaeleo dilepis*
Flat-tailed gecko	*Uroplatus fimbriatus*
Florida worm lizard	*Rhineura floridana*
Four-horned chameleon	*Trioceros quadricornis*
Frilled lizard see Australian frilled lizard	
Galapagos land iguana	*Conolophus subcristatus*
Gargoyle gecko	*Rhacodactylus* spp.
Giant day gecko	*Phelsuma grandis*
Gila monster	*Heloderma suspectum*
Gould's monitor	*Varanus gouldii*
Grand Cayman iguana	*Cyclura lewisi*
Gray's monitor	*Varanus olivaceus*
Great plated lizard	*Gerrhosaurus major*
Green anole	*Anolis carolinensis*
Green crested basilisk see Plumed basilisk	
Green iguana	*Iguana iguana*
Green tree monitor	*Varanus prasinus*
Guatemalan beaded lizard	*Heloderma horridum charlesbogerti*

Common name	Scientific name
Hardwick's spiny-tailed lizard	*Saara hardwickii*
Henkel's leaf-tailed gecko	*Uroplatus henkeli*
High-casqued chameleon	*Chamaeleo hoehnelii*
Horned lizard	*Phrynosoma spp.*
Iberian emerald lizard	*Lacerta schreiberi*
Iberian mountain lizard	*Iberolacerta monticola*
Indian monitor	*Varanus bengalensis*
Inland bearded dragon	*Pogona vitticeps*
Italian wall lizard	*Podarcis siculus*
Jackson's chameleon	*Trioceros jacksonii*
Jamaican iguana	*Cyclura collei*
Knob-scaled lizards	*Xenosaurus spp.*
Knob-tailed geckos	*Nephrurus spp.*
Komodo dragon	*Varanus komodoensis*
Lace monitor	*Varanus varius*
Leopard gecko	*Eublepharis macularius*
Madagascar day gecko	*Phelsuma madagascariensis*
Malaysian monitor lizard *see* Asian water monitor	
Mali uromastyx	*Uromastyx dispar maliensis*
Mangrove monitor	*Varanus indicus*
Marbled velvet gecko	*Oedura marmorata*
Mediterranean house gecko	*Hemidactylus turcicus*
Meller's chameleon	*Trioceros melleri*
Mexican beaded lizard *see* Beaded lizard	
Monitor lizards	*Varanus spp.*
Montane chameleons	*Trioceros spp.*
Moorish gecko	*Tarentola mauritanica*
Mountain-horned dragons	*Acanthosaura spp.*
Mountain chameleon	*Trioceros montium*
Namib sanddiver	*Meroles anchietae*
New Caledonian giant geckos	*Rhacodactylus spp.*
Nile monitor	*Varanus niloticus*
Ornate uromastyx	*Uromastyx ornata*
Oustalet's chameleon	*Furcifer oustaleti*
Panther chameleon	*Furcifer pardalis*
Parson's chameleon	*Calumma parsonii parsonii*
Pink-tongued skink	*Cyclodomorphus gerrardii*
Plated lizard	*Gerrhosaurus spp.*
Plumed basilisk	*Basiliscus plumifrons*
Prehensile-tailed skink	*Corucia zebrata*
Rainbow lizard	*Agama agama*
Rankin's dragon lizards	*Pogona henrylawsoni*
Rhinoceros iguana	*Cyclura cornuta*
Ricord's iguana	*Cyclura ricordii*
Rough knob-tailed gecko	*Nephrurus asper*
Roughneck monitor lizard	*Varanus rudicollis*
Round Island skink	*Leiolopisma telfairii*
Saharan spiny-tailed lizard	*Uromastyx geyri*
Sailfin lizard	*Hydrosaurus spp.*
Sand lizard	*Lacerta agilis*
Sandfish	*Scincus spp.*
Savannah monitor	*Varanus exanthematicus*
Shingleback lizards	*Tiliqua spp.*
Shingleback skink	*Tiliqua rugosa*
Six-lined racerunner	*Aspidoscetis sexlineata*
Slow worm	*Anguis fragilis*
Smooth knob-tailed gecko	*Nephrurus levis*
Solomon island monkey-tailed skink *see* Prehensile-tailed skink	
Spiny-tailed goanna	*Varanus acanthurus acanthurus*
Spiny-tailed iguana	*Ctenosaura similis*
Standing's day gecko	*Phelsuma standingi*
Stump-tail skink *see* Shingleback skink	
Sudan plated lizard	*Broadleysaurus major*
Tegu lizards	*Tupinambis spp.*
Texas spiny lizard	*Sceloporus olivaceous*
Thai water dragon *see* Asian water dragon	

Common name	Scientific name
Three-horned chameleon *see* Jackson's chameleon	
Tokay gecko	*Gekko gecko*
Trinidad gecko	*Gonatodes humeralis*
Two-legged worm lizards	*Bipes spp.*
Variegated gecko	*Gehyra variegata*
Veiled chameleon	*Chamaeleo calyptratus*
Water dragon *see* Asian water dragon	
Western fence lizard	*Scleroporus occidentalis*
Whiptail lizards	*Cnemidophorus spp.*
White-throated monitor	*Varanus albigularis*
Worm lizards	*Amphisbaena spp.*
Yellow monitor	*Varanus flavescens*
Yellow-spotted monitor	*Varanus panoptes*
Yellow tree monitor	*Varanus reisingeri*
Yemen chameleon *see* Veiled chameleon	
Zonures	*Smaug spp.*

Snakes

Common name	Scientific name
Adder	*Vipera berus*
Aesculapian snake	*Zamenis longissimus*
African house snakes	*Lamprophis spp.*
African rock python	*Python sebae*
Amazon tree boa	*Corallus hortulanus*
American water snakes	*Nerodia spp.*
Amethystine python	*Simalia amethistina*
Anaconda	*Eunectes murinus*
Arabian sand boa	*Eryx jaculus*
Aruba island rattlesnake	*Crotalus durissus unicolor*
Assam trinket snake	*Coelognathus spp.*
Asian water snake	*Natrix piscator*
Ball python *see* Royal python	
Black kingsnake	*Lampropeltis nigra*
Black mamba	*Dendroaspis polylepis*
Black-headed python	*Aspidites melanocephalus*
Blind snakes	*Typhlops spp.,* *Rhamphotyphlops spp.*
Blind worm snake *see* Brahminy blind snake	
Blood python	*Python curtus*
Boa constrictor *see* Common boa	
Boa constrictor imperator	*Boa constrictor imperator*
Boelen's python	*Simalia boeleni*
Boomslang	*Dispholidus typus*
Brahminy blind snake	*Indotyphlops braminus*
Brazilian lancehead	*Bothrops moojeni*
Broad-banded copperhead *laticinctus*	*Agkistrodon contortrix*
Brown python	*Liasis fuscus*
Brown tree snake	*Boiga irregularis*
Bullsnake	*Pituophis melanoleucas sayi*
Burmese python	*Python bivittatus*
Bushmaster	*Lachesis spp.*
California mountain kingsnake	*Lampropeltis zonata*
Cape coral snake	*Aspidelaps lubricus*
Carpet python	*Morelia spilota variegata*
Children's python	*Antaresia childreni*
Chinese 100 flower snake *see* Moellendorff's trinket snake	
Coastal carpet python	*Morelia spilota mcdowelli*
Common boa	*Boa constrictor imperator*
Common kingsnake	*Lampropeltis getula*
Copperhead	*Agkistrodon contortrix*
Copperhead viper *see* Copperhead	
Corn snake	*Pantherophis guttatus*
Cribo	*Drymarchon corais*
Death adder	*Acanthophis antarcticus*
Deckert's ratsnake	*Pantherophis obsoletus*

Common name	Scientific name
Dekay's snake	*Storeria dekayi*
Diamond python	*Morelia spilota spilota*
Dice snakes *see* Eurasian water snakes	
Dumeril's boa	*Acrantophis dumerili*
Eastern diamondback rattlesnake	*Crotalus adamanteus*
Eastern kingsnake	*Lampropeltis getula getula*
Eastern milk snake	*Lampropeltis t. triangulum*
Eastern ribbon snake	*Thamnophis sauritus*
Eastern tiger snake	*Notechis scutatus*
Egg-eating snakes	*Dasypeltis* spp.
Elephant trunk snake	*Acrochordus javanicus*
Emerald tree boa	*Corallus caninus*
Eurasian water snakes	*Natrix* spp.
European adder	*Vipera berus*
European viper *see* European adder	
Everglades ratsnake	*Pantherophis alleghaniensis*
Eyelash viper	*Bothriechis schlegelii*
False water cobra	*Hydrodynastes gigas*
Fea's viper	*Azemiops feae*
Four-lined snake	*Elaphe quatuorlineata*
Gaboon viper	*Bitis gabonica gabonica*
Garter snake	*Thamnophis sirtalis*
Gopher snakes	*Pituophis catenifer*
Grass snake	*Natrix natrix*
Green anaconda *see* Anaconda	
Green tree python	*Morelia viridis*
Grey-banded kingsnake	*Lampropeltis mexicana*
Hognose snakes	*Heterodon* spp.
Honduran milk snake	*Lampropeltis abmorma*
Horned vipers	*Cerastes* spp.
Hungarian meadow viper	*Vipera ursinii rakosiensis*
Indian python	*Python molurus*
Indigo snake *see also* Cribo	*Drymarchon couperi*
Jamaican boa	Chilabothrus subflavus
Jungle corn snake	*Pantherophis guttatus* X *Lampropeltis getula*
King cobra	*Ophiophagus hannah*
Kingsnakes	*Lampropeltis* spp.
Leopard snake	*Zamenis situla*
Long-nosed snake	*Rhinocheilus lecontei*
Madagascar boa / Malagasy ground boa	*Acrantophis madagascariensis*
Madagascar ground boa *see* Dumeril's boa	
Massasauga rattlesnake	*Sistrurus catenatus*
Mexican burrowing python	*Loxocemus bicolor*
Milk snake	*Lampropeltis triangulum* subspp.
Moellendorff's trinket snake	*Orthriophis moellendorfi*
Mole kingsnake	*Lampropeltis calligaster rhombomaculata*
Mole vipers	*Atractaspis* spp.
Monocled cobra	*Naja kaouthia*
Namibian house snake *see* African house snakes	
Neotropical rattlesnake	*Crotalus durissus* ssp.
North American whipsnakes	*Coluber* spp.
Olive python	*Liasis olivaceus*
Oriental green snake	*Cyclophiops major*
Palm viper	*Bothriechis marchi*
Peninsula ribbon snake	*Thamnophis sauritus sackenii*
Pine snake	*Pituophis melanoleucas* ssp.
Pipe snakes	*Cylindrophis* spp.

Common name	Scientific name
Prairie rattlesnake	*Crotalus viridis*
Puff adder	*Bitis arietans*
Racers	*Coluber* spp.
Rainbow boa	*Epicrates cenchria*
Rattlesnakes	*Crotalus* spp.
Red-tailed boa *see* Common boa	
Red coachwhip snake	*Masticophis flagellum piceus*
Red diamond rattlesnake	*Crotalus ruber*
Red spitting cobra	*Naja Quesodilio*
Reticulated python	*Malayopython reticulatus*
Rhino ratsnake	*Gonyosoma boulengeri*
Rhinoceros viper	*Bitis nasicornis*
Ridge-nosed rattlesnake	*Crotalus willardi*
Rock python see African rock python and Indian python	
Rosy boa	*Lichanura trivirgata*
Rough green snake	*Opheodrys aestivus*
Round Island boa	*Casarea dussumieri*
Royal python	*Python regius*
Russell's viper	*Daboia russelii*
Russian viper	*Vipera raddei*
Saharan horned viper	*Cerastes cerastes*
Sand boa	*Eryx colubrinus*
Schweitzer's viper	*Macrovipera schweitzeri*
Smooth green snake	*Opheodrys vernalis*
Snail-eating snake	*Dipsas indica*
Solomon Island boa	*Candoia paulsoni*
South American tree boa	*Corallus hortulanus enydris*
Speckled rattlesnake	*Crotalus pyrrhus*
Spitting cobra	*Naja nigricollis*
Stimson's python	*Antaresia stimsoni*
Sunbeam snakes	*Xenopeltis* spp.
Texas ratsnake	*Pantherophis obsoletus lindheimeri*
Thread snakes	*Leptotyphlids*
Timber rattlesnake	*Crotalus horridus*
Timor Island python	*Malayopython timoriensis*
Tortuga Island rattlesnake	*Crotalus atrox tortugensis*
Tree python see Green tree python	
Uracoan rattlesnake	*Crotalus durissus vegrandis*
Urutu	*Bothrops alternatus*
Warty water snakes	*Acrochordus* spp.
Water moccasin	*Agkistrodon piscivorus*
Western diamondback rattlesnake	*Crotalus atrox*
Western fence lizard	*Scleroporus occidentalis*
Western hognose snake	*Heterodon nasicus*
Whipsnakes	*Coluber* spp.
Yellow ratsnake	*Pantherophis obsoletus quadrivittatus*
Yellow-bellied racer	*Coluber constrictor*
Yellow-bellied watersnake	*Nerodia erythrogaster flavigaster*

Others

Common name	Scientific name
American alligator	*Alligator mississippiensis*
Broad-snouted caiman	*Caiman latirostris*
Caiman	*Caiman* spp.
Gavials	*Gavialis gangeticus*
Nile crocodile	*Crocodylus niloticus*
Siamese crocodile	*Crocodylus siamensis*
Spectacled caiman	*Caiman crocodilus*
Tuatara	*Sphenodon punctatus*
West African dwarf crocodile	*Osteolaemus osborni*
Yacare caiman	*Caiman yacare*

CITES and UK legislation

CITES

The 'Washington' Convention on International Trade in Endangered Species (CITES) legislation has been implemented by many countries around the world. In Europe the EU has directly imposed these regulations on its member states under the following pieces of legislation:

- Council Regulation EC No. 338/97 and associated legislation
- Commission Regulation EC No. 1808/2001 and associated legislation
- Control of Trade in Endangered Species (Enforcement) Regulations (COTES) 1997

Broadly, the majority of CITES category I species are protected and included in Annex A of the COTES Regulations, as are many CITES II species such as the Mediterranean spur-thighed, Hermann's and marginated tortoises. Trade, capture and breeding of these species is strictly controlled, a licence being required from the appropriate government authority (in the UK the Department for Environment, Food and Rural Affairs, DEFRA) to allow the sale, barter or breeding of these and similarly classified species, and ensures that the EU COTES Regulations are more restrictive than the similar CITES regulations. More information regarding UK legislation associated with the CITES and COTES Regulations can be found currently at www.ukcites.gov.uk

Dangerous Wild Animals Act 1976; Dangerous Wild Animals Act 1976 (Modification Order) 2007; The Legislative Reform (Dangerous Wild Animals) (Licensing) Order 2010

This applies to the private keeping of species, outwith the provisions for pet shops, zoos, circuses or areas designated under the Animals (Scientific Procedures) Act 1986, considered dangerous to public health and welfare as laid down by the 1984 Order. This includes many reptile species, including most of the species of venomous snakes, such as rattlesnakes, cobras and pit vipers, as well as the two venomous lizards, the beaded lizard and the Gila monster, and crocodile, caiman, alligator and gharial families.

Basic standards of husbandry are demanded of the owner, and secure accommodation is required for the licensed pet as well as an annual veterinary inspection and annual renewal of the licence, for which a fee is payable to the local authority.

Although this Act does not affect veterinary surgeons in their legal ability to treat animals listed by the Act, they should be aware that clients should be in receipt of a valid DWA licence for their pet, and failure to gain a licence prior to obtaining a pet so listed is a criminal offence. The British Veterinary Zoological Society has produced guidance for its members on how to carry out a DWA inspection on behalf of a Local Authority.

Health and Safety at Work etc. Act 1974

Following on from the DWA Act it is logical that any veterinary practice seeing animals listed by the DWA Act 1976 (as amended by the DWA (Modification) Order 1984) has an obligation to its staff to minimize risks wherever possible and to have in place a Risk Assessment plan should they choose to treat such species. This includes provision for training of staff, relevant equipment (e.g. snake hooks, protective visors in the case of spitting cobras), antivenom and suitable local medical support. The Health and Safety Executive has produced guidance for zoo reptiles covering many of the venomous and other dangerous species, which is recommended to be read in conjunction with the Secretary of State's Standards of Modern Zoo Practice (see References and further reading).

Animal Welfare Act (2006) as amended; Animal Health and Welfare Act (Scotland) (2006) as amended

The Animal Welfare Act (2006) (applies to England and Wales) and the Animal Health and Welfare Act (Scotland) (2006) in Scotland cover the welfare of all captive vertebrates (and cephalopods) and as such, therefore, include reptiles. The Act not only makes it an offence to cause suffering deliberately but also by omission, e.g. failing to provide the correct food and water.

The Welfare of Animals (Transport) Order 1997 (as amended 2006)

This covers all forms of animals and governs their safe transport to prevent unnecessary suffering, or injury. These guidelines ensure that the IATA (see below) and CITES guidelines are also adhered to.

This is further reinforced by the International Air Transport Association's (IATA) Live Animals Regulations, which dictate cage sizes and composition for the transport of all forms of animals, as well as temperatures at which they should be kept, lighting regimes, and food and water requirements while in flight.

Veterinary Surgeons Act 1966 and supplementary legislation

This ensures that, in the UK, only veterinary surgeons and veterinary practitioners registered with the Royal College of Veterinary Surgeons have the right to practise veterinary surgery in respect to mammals, birds and reptiles, and to prescribe prescription only medications.

Medicines Act 1968; Veterinary Medicines Regulations 2013 SI 2033 (VMR) and Veterinary Medicines Guidance Notes (VMGN) and RCVS Code of Conduct

These pieces of legislation/guides ensure the compliance with medicines legislation, e.g. prescribing, supplying and labelling of prescription-only medicines, which includes prescribing for reptile species. It ensures that veterinary surgeons in the UK can only prescribe for reptiles 'under their care' (cf. Guide to Professional Conduct, RCVS, 2012), and that the 'cascade' is followed when prescribing a drug outwith its marketing authorization (cf. British Veterinary Association 2007; Veterinary Medicines Directorate 2015).

Wildlife and Countryside Act 1981 as amended; Wildlife and Natural Environment (Scotland) Act 2011 and EU Invasive Alien Species Regulations (1143/2014)

These pieces of legislation protect many of the native species of reptile in the UK, including the common lizard, glass snake and smooth snake. It prevents their deliberate capture, injury or killing and their possession. It does not apply to veterinary surgeons attempting to heal injured native species if the aim is to return the fully fit reptile back to the wild.

The UK-based legislation also prohibits the release of non-native species of reptile into the wild (e.g. red-eared terrapins, which have been regularly abandoned into the UK's waterways by owners unable to cope with their needs as they outgrow their hatchling purchase size). The EU Invasive Alien Species (IAS) Regulations (1143/2014) has further enforced the ban on releasing non-native species and also specifically covers the red-eared terrapin.

References and further reading

British Veterinary Zoological Society (2014) *Dangerous Wild Animals Act 1976: Templates, Species Guide and Advice*, www.bvzs.org

British Veterinary Association (2007) *Veterinary Medicines Good Practice Guide*. BVA Publications, London

DEFRA: Guidance notes on aspects of the CITES Regulations. DEFRA, Bristol https://www.gov.uk/guidance/cites-controls-import-and-export-of-protected-species

DEFRA: Secretary of State's Standards of Modern Zoo Practice, 2012. DEFRA, Bristol. https://www.gov.uk/government/publications/secretary-of-state-s-standards-of-modern-zoo-practice

Health and Safety Executive (2012) *Managing Health and Safety in Zoos*. HMSO, London ISBN 978 0 7176 2058 6

IATA: *Live Animal Regulations*. International Air Transport Association, Montreal and Geneva (annual publication)

Royal College of Veterinary Surgeons (2012) *Guide to Professional Conduct*. RCVS, London

Veterinary Medicines Directorate (2015) *The Cascade: Prescribing Unauthorised Medicines*, Addlestone, Surrey https://www.gov.uk/guidance/the-cascade-prescribing-unauthorised-medicines

> The CITES and UK legislation set out in Appendix 5 was accurate at the time of going to press. In light on ongoing Brexit negotiations, the editors advise referring to the Department for Environment, Food and Rural Affairs (DEFRA) and other appropriate government authorities for any updates to existing legislation.

Conversion tables for units

Temperature

SI unit	Conversion factor	Conventional unit
°C	(x 9/5) + 32	°F

Haematology

Parameter	SI unit	Conversion factor	Conventional unit
Red blood cell count	10^{12}/l	1	10^6/μl
Haemoglobin	g/l	0.1	g/dl
MCH	pg/cell	1	pg/cell
MCHC	g/l	0.1	g/dl
MCV	fl	1	μm³
Platelet count	10^9/l	1	10^3/μl
White blood cell count	10^9/l	1	10^3/μl

Biochemistry

Parameter	SI unit	Conversion factor	Conventional unit
Alanine aminotransferase	IU/l	1	IU/l
Albumin	g/l	0.1	g/dl
Alkaline phosphatase	IU/l	1	IU/l
Aspartate aminotransferase	IU/l	1	IU/l
Bilirubin	μmol/l	0.0584	mg/dl
Blood urea nitrogen (BUN)	mmol/l	2.8	mg/dl
Calcium	mmol/l	4	mg/dl
Carbon dioxide (total)	mmol/l	1	mEq/l
Cholesterol	mmol/l	38.61	mg/dl
Chloride	mmol/l	1	mEq/l
Cortisol	nmol/l	0.362	ng/ml
Creatine kinase	IU/l	1	IU/l
Creatinine	μmol/l	0.0113	mg/dl
Glucose	mmol/l	18.02	mg/dl
Insulin	pmol/l	0.1394	μIU/ml
Iron	μmol/l	5.587	μg/dl
Magnesium	mmol/l	2	mEq/l
Phosphorus	mmol/l	3.1	mg/dl
Potassium	mmol/l	1	mEq/l
Sodium	mmol/l	1	mEq/l
Total protein	g/l	0.1	g/dl
Thyroxine (T4) (free)	pmol/l	0.0775	ng/dl
Thyroxine (T4) (total)	nmol/l	0.0775	μg/dl
Tri-iodothyronine (T3)	nmol/l	65.1	ng/dl
Triglycerides	mmol/l	88.5	mg/dl

BSAVA Manual of Reptiles, third edition. Edited by Simon J. Girling and Paul Raiti. ©BSAVA 2019

Hypodermic needles

Parameter	Metric	Non-metric
Needle gauge	0.8 mm	21 G
	0.6 mm	23 G
	0.5 mm	25 G
	0.4 mm	27 G
Needle length	12 mm	½ inch
	16 mm	⅝ inch
	25 mm	1 inch
	30 mm	1.25 inch
	40 mm	1.5 inch

Suture material sizes

Metric (Ph. Eur.)	USP
0.4	8/0
0.5	7/0
0.7	6/0
1	5/0
1.5	4/0
2	3/0
3	2/0
3.5	0
4	1
5	2
6	3

Reference values for haematology and biochemistry in common species

Parameter	Corn snake (ZIMS, 2018)	Boa constrictor (Machado et al., 2006; ZIMS, 2018)	Burmese python (ZIMS, 2018)	Garter snake (Wack et al., 2012; ZIMS, 2018)
Red blood cell count (x 10¹²/l)	0.35–1.77 (mean 0.93)	0.404–0.520	0.31–1.89 (mean 0.83)	0.5–1.3
Haemoglobin (mg/dl)	0.6–14.1 (mean 9.1)	7.2–7.4	3.7–11.4 (mean 8.6)	5.2–13.2
Packed cell volume (l/l)	0.16–0.44 (mean 0.31)	0.217–0.232	0.150–0.391 (mean 0.271)	0.189–0.420
Mean cell volume (fl)	16.8–584.8 (mean 322.2)	382–412	302.3 (mean)	NR
Mean cell haemoglobin (pg)	86.4 (mean)	122.6 (mean)	101.2 (mean)	NR
Mean cell haemoglobin concentration (g/dl)	16.7–42.2 (mean 30.4)	30.9–33.7	32.7 (mean)	NR
White blood cell count (x 10⁹/l)	0.7–15 (mean 6.6)	5.90–10.13	2–19.5 (mean 8.5)	3.1–13.7
Heterophil count (x 10⁹/l)	0.26–5.339 (mean 1.788)	1.21–1.24	0.374–6.013 (mean 2.181)	0.23–0.37
Lymphocyte count (x 10⁹/l)	0.206–12.507 (mean 4.134)	2.14–5.82	0.409–16.883 (mean 4.583)	1.66–15.1
Monocyte count (x 10⁹/l)	0.012–2.493 (mean 0.677)	0.094–2.07	0–2.958 (mean 0.515)	0.695 (mean)
Azurophils (x 10⁹/l)	0.097–4.674 (mean 1.250)	1.98–2.02	0.066–6.097 (mean 1.884)	0.19–1.94
Eosinophil count (x 10⁹/l)	0–0.465 (mean 0.117)	0–1.043 (mean 0.23)	0.253 (mean)	NR
Basophil count (x 10⁹/l)	0.014–0.9 (mean 0.259)	0–1.111 (mean 0.301)	0–0.643 (mean 0.161)	0.65–0.86
Thrombocyte count (x 10⁹/l)	NR	6.76–12.37	NR	NR
AST (IU/l)	0–117 (mean 28)	0–67 (mean 19)	4–54 (mean 19)	8–48
Creatinine kinase (IU/l)	25–969 (mean 281)	70–2500 (mean 721)	47–2554 (mean 600)	17–1428
Glucose (mmol/l)	0.6–5.1 (mean 2.9)	0.4–4.6 (mean 1.7)	0.1–2.8 (mean 1.3)	2.94–9.27
Calcium (total) (mmol/l)	2.4–5.3 (mean 4.0)	2.2–5.4 (mean 3.8)	2.6–7.3 (mean	2.93–4.15
Phosphorus (mmol/l)	0.58–2.31 (mean 1.26)	0.76–3.02 (mean 1.54)	0.76–3.78 (mean 1.59)	0.58–2.45
Sodium (mmol/l)	148–178 (mean 162)	144–175 (mean 159)	146–172 (mean 157)	136–166
Potassium (mmol/l)	1.5–9.8 (mean 5.1)	0–6.9 (mean 4.4)	1.8–10.3 (mean 5.2)	1.8–7
Total protein (g/l)	33–99 (mean 68)	34–100 (mean 69)	47–95 (mean 69)	41–79
Albumin (g/l)	12–32 (mean 22)	16–44 (mean 29)	12–31 (mean 20)	10–21
Globulins (g/l)	23–73 (mean 46)	20–70 (mean 40)	22–72 (mean 46)	0–70
Uric acid (µmol/l)	16–894 (mean 342)	37–1022 (mean 319)	22–809 (mean 298)	101–952

A7.1 Blood parameters of some commonly kept snakes; NR = none reported.

Parameter	Bearded dragon (Ellman, 1997; ZIMS 2018)	Basilisk lizards (Dallwig et al., 2011; ZIMS, 2018)	Green iguana (Harr et al., 2001)	Panther chameleon (Laube et al., 2016; ZIMS, 2018)
Red blood cell count (x 10¹²/l)	0.68–1.21 (mean 0.97)	NR	1–1.8	0.45–1.67
Haemoglobin (g/dl)	6.7–12 (mean 9.5)	8.6–9.1 (mean 8.9)	6.7–12.2	NR
Packed cell volume (l/l)	0.19–0.40 (mean 0.30)	0.20–0.52 (mean 0.314)	0.29–0.47	0.11–0.56
Mean cell volume (fl)	236–397 (mean 311)	NR	228–331	200–418 (mean 330)
Mean cell haemoglobin (pg)	8.1–14.0 (mean 10.8)	NR	NR	NR

A7.2 Blood parameters of some commonly kept lizards; NR = none reported. (continues) ▶

BSAVA Manual of Reptiles, third edition. Edited by Simon J. Girling and Paul Raiti. ©BSAVA 2019

Parameter	Bearded dragon (Ellman, 1997; ZIMS 2018)	Basilisk lizards (Dallwig et al., 2011; ZIMS, 2018)	Green iguana (Harr et al., 2001)	Panther chameleon (Laube et al., 2016; ZIMS, 2018)
Mean cell haemoglobin concentration (g/dl)	24–45 (mean 34)	22–29 (mean 26)	23–31	NR
White blood cell count (x 10⁹/l)	1.99–23 (mean 8.14)	3.9–35.5 (mean 18.7)	8–25	1.3–28.1 (mean 10.2)
Heterophil count (x 10⁹/l)	0.35–4.99 (mean 2.17)	3.1–24.1 (mean 13.2)	0.6–6.4	0.115–7.766 (mean 2.629)
Lymphocyte count (x 10⁹/l)	0.57–17 (mean 4.68)	0.77–7.4 (mean 3.6)	5–17.2	0.231–21.678 (mean 5.973)
Monocyte count (x 10⁹/l)	0.03–2.72 (mean 0.7)	0.08–4.2 (mean 1.4)	0.2–2.7	1.101 (mean)
Eosinophil count (x 10⁹/l)	0.06–0.27 (mean 0.15)	0	0–0.4	0.171 (mean)
Basophil count (x 10⁹/l)	0.05–1.01 (mean 0.39)	0.19–0.39 (mean 0.28)	0.1–1.2	0.195 (mean)
AST (IU/l)	0–77 (mean 27)	19.5–115 (mean 48.3)	7–102	5–49.3
Creatinine kinase (IU/l)	59–7000 (mean 1211)	2497–8893 (mean 6323)	174–8768 (mean 1876)	95–836
Glucose (mmol/l)	7.72–16.15 (mean 11.66)	6–15.49 (mean 10.71)	3.89–18.60	3.25–21.95
Calcium (total) (mmol/l)	2.15–6.75 (mean 2.95)	2.08–2.33 (mean 2.65)	2.15–3.5	Mean (summer) 2.4 male; 3.5 female
Phosphorus (mmol/l)	0.87–4.88 (mean 1.84)	1.32–3 (mean 1.8)	0.90–3.00	0.9–7.9
Sodium (mmol/l)	137–190 (mean 153)	142–167 (mean 153.5)	152–172	143 (mean)
Potassium (mmol/l)	1–6.5 (mean 3.6)	2.3–7.9 (mean 5.4)	2–6.1	4.9 (mean)
Total protein (g/l)	36–64 (mean 50)	31–66 (mean 44)	44–76	37–70
Albumin (g/l)	13–36 (mean 26)	13–26 (mean 18)	13–30	13–33
Globulins (g/l)	10–44 (mean 23)	16–47 (mean 26)	25–52	29–46
Uric acid (μmol/l)	95.17–678.07 (mean 309.30)	35.69–172.49 (mean 101.12)	53.53–398.52	17.8–1261

A7.2 (continued) Blood parameters of some commonly kept lizards; NR = none reported.

Parameter	Hermann's tortoise (Andreani et al., 2014; Bielli et al., 2015).	Hermann's tortoise (Andreani et al. 2014; Bielli et al., 2015)	Leopard tortoise (ZIMS, 2018)	Red eared terrapin (Jacobson, 1988; ZIMS, 2018)
Red blood cell count (x 10¹²/l)	0.42–1.02 (median 0.8)	0.43–1.05	0.16–1.06 (mean 0.52)	0.33–2.21 (mean 0.84)
Haemoglobin (g/dl)	2.6–11.5 (median 6.8)	4.1–13.5	7.3 (mean)	10–12.2 (mean 11.1)
Packed cell volume (l/l)	0.11–0.32 (median 0.24)	0.11–0.40	0.063–0.4 (mean 0.234)	0.1–0.411 (mean 0.255)
Mean cell volume (fl)	193–350 (median 310)	193–350	534 (mean)	179–697 (mean 409)
Mean cell haemoglobin (pg)	54.8–125.8 (median 100)	54.8–125.8	114.6 (mean)	108 (mean)
Mean cell haemoglobin concentration (g/dl)	21.6–43.3 (median 32.5)	21.6–43.3	33.7 (mean)	30 (mean)
White blood cell count (x 10⁹/l)	4.1–14 (median 9.4)	4.1–14	1.1–14.9 (mean 4.8)	1.23–15.5 (mean 5.97)
Heterophil count (x 10⁹/l)	0.79–4.74 (median 2.31)	0.79–4.74	0.181–6.563 (mean 2.216)	0.251–8.365 (mean 2.461)
Lymphocyte count (x 10⁹/l)	1.44–8.49 (median 4.44)	1.44–8.49	0.176–6.576 (mean 1.886)	0.246–6.598 (mean 2.192)
Monocyte count (x 10⁹/l)	0.18–1.34 (median 0.48)	0.18–1.34	0–1.007 (mean 0.238)	0.023–1.234 (mean 0.284)
Eosinophil count (x 10⁹/l)	0.36–2.4 (median 0.97)	0.36–2.4	0.008–0.541 (mean 0.174)	0.014–2.296 (mean 0.635)
Basophil count (x 10⁹/l)	0–0.19 (median 0.085)	0–0.19	0.013–0.615 (mean 0.144)	0.011–5.029 (mean 1.237)
AST (IU/l)	18–628	0–359	6–142 (mean 58)	41–608 (mean 171)
Creatinine kinase (IU/l)	19–1346	0–732	17–1660 (mean 408)	109–5275 (mean 1136)
Glucose (mmol/l)	2.05–9.82	0.83–6.66	0.2–10.9 (mean 4.1)	1.2–5.5 (mean 2.8)
Calcium (total) (mmol/l)	2.68–7.05	1.2–5.13	1.9–5.6 (mean 3.2)	1.9–6.5 (mean 3.3)
Phosphorus (mmol/l)	0.58–2.81	0.19–1.78	0.3–2.46 (mean 0.96)	0.43–3.5 (mean 1.28)
Sodium (mmol/l)	119–150	116–143	111–154 (mean 132)	116–160 (mean 135)
Potassium (mmol/l)	3.5–8.7	3.5–7.7	2.9–11 (mean 5.9)	0.2–7.7 (mean 3.9)
Total protein (g/l)	19–55	24–61	10–67 (mean 44)	15–76 (mean 44)
Albumin (g/l)	5–22	8–26	2–31 (mean 17)	4–28 (mean 14)
Globulins (g/l)	NR	11.2–40.1	8–49 (mean 28)	2–50 (mean 28)
Uric acid (μmol/l)	41–468	0–309	24–321 (mean 124)	6–164 (mean 52)

A7.3 Blood parameters of some commonly kept chelonian; NR = none reported.

References and further reading

Andreani G, Carpene E, Cannavacciuolo A *et al.* (2014) Reference values for hematology and plasma biochemistry variables, and protein electrophoresis of healthy Hermann's tortoises (*Testudo hermanni* ssp.) *Veterinary Clinical Pathology* **47(4)**, 573–583

Bielli M, Nardini G, Di Girolamo N and Savarino, P (2015) Hematological values for adult eastern Hermann's tortoise (*Testudo hermanni boettgeri*) in semi-natural conditions. *Journal of Veterinary Diagnostic Investigation* **27(1)**, 68–73

Dallwig RK, Paul-Murphy J, Thomas C *et al.* (2011) Hematology and clinical chemistry values of free-ranging Basilisk lizards (*Basiliscus plumifrons*) in Costa Rica. *Journal of Zoo and Wildlife Medicine* **42(2)**, 205–231

Ellmann MM (1997) Hematology and plasma chemistry of the Inland bearded dragon *Pogona vitticeps*. *Bulletin of the Association of Reptile and Amphibian Veterinarians* **7**, 10–12

Harr KE, Alleman AR, Dennis PM *et al.* (2001) Morphologic and cytochemical characteristics of blood cells and hematologic and plasma biochemical reference ranges in green iguanas. *Journal of the American Veterinary Medical Association* **218**, 915–921

Jacobson ER (1988) Evaluation of the reptile patient In: *Exotic Animals*, ed ER Jacobson and GV Kollias Jnr, pp. 35–48. Churchill Livingstone, New York

Laube A, Pendl H, Claus M, Altherr B and Hatt J–M (2016) Plasma biochemistry and hematology reference values of captive panther chameleons (*Furcifer pardalis*) with special emphasis on seasonality and gender differences. *Journal of Zoo and Wildlife Medicine* **47(3)**, 743–753

Machado CC, Silva LFN, Ramos PRR and Takahira RK (2006) Seasonal influence on hematologic values and haemoglobin electrophoresis in Brazilian *Boa constrictor amarali*. *Journal of Zoo and Wildlife Medicine* **37(4)**, 487–491

Wack RF, Hansen E, Small M *et al.* (2012) Hematology and plasma biochemistry values for the giant garter snake (*Thamnophis gigas*) and valley garter snake (*Thamnophis sirtalis fitchi*) in the central valley of California. *Journal of Wildlife Diseases* **48(2)**, 307–313

ZIMS (Zoological Information Management System) (2018) Species expected test results. Apple Valley, MN. Accessed 17.09.18

Index